T0309576

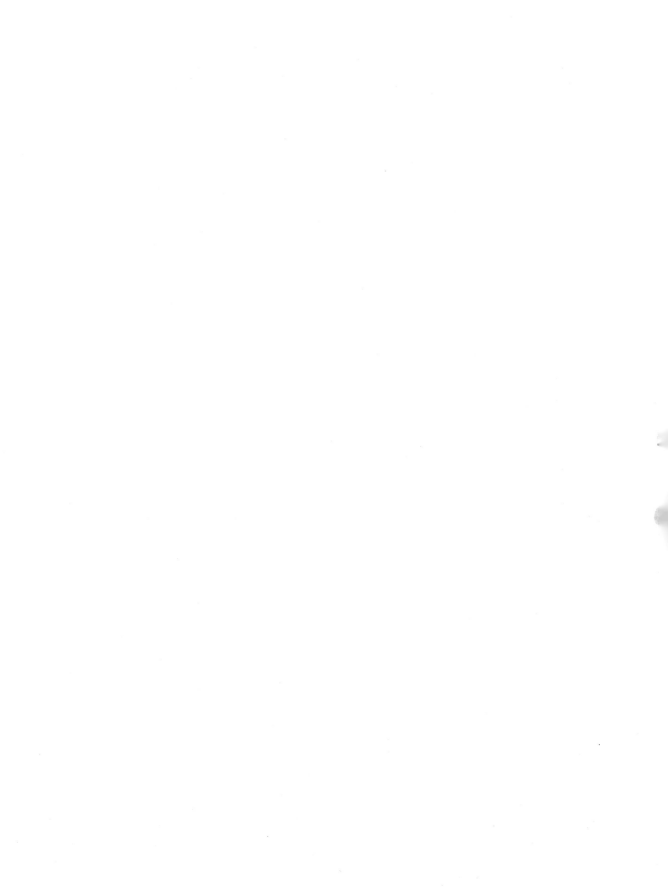

CLINICAL TRIALS

SECOND EDITION

CLINICAL TRIALS

Study Design, Endpoints and Biomarkers, Drug Safety, and FDA and ICH Guidelines

SECOND EDITION

Tom Brody, Ph.D.

AMSTERDAM • BOSTON • HEIDELBERG • LONDON
NEW YORK • OXFORD • PARIS • SAN DIEGO
SAN FRANCISCO • SINGAPORE • SYDNEY • TOKYO

Academic Press is an imprint of Elsevier

Academic Press is an imprint of Elsevier
125, London Wall, EC2Y 5AS.
525 B Street, Suite 1800, San Diego, CA 92101-4495, USA
50 Hampshire Street, 5th Floor, Cambridge, MA 02139, USA
The Boulevard, Langford Lane, Kidlington, Oxford OX5 1GB, UK

Second Edition 2016

ISBN: 978-0-12-804217-5

British Library Cataloguing-in-Publication Data
A catalogue record for this book is available from the British Library.

Library of Congress Cataloging-in-Publication Data
A catalog record for this book is available from the Library of Congress.

For Information on all Academic Press publications
visit our website at http://store.elsevier.com/

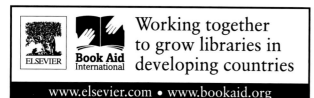

www.elsevier.com • www.bookaid.org

Publisher: Mica Haley
Acquisition Editor: Kristine Jones
Editorial Project Manager: Molly McLaughlin
Production Project Manager: Julia Haynes
Designer: Greg Harris

Typeset by MPS Limited, Chennai, India
www.adi-mps.com

Dedication

To Shideh and Dawnia

Contents

13. Oncology Endpoints: Overall Survival and Progression-Free Survival

14. Oncology Endpoints: Time to Progression

15. Oncology Endpoint: Disease-Free Survival

16. Oncology Endpoint: Time to Distant Metastasis

34. Patents

Acknowledgments

I thank Julia Haynes, Molly McLaughlin, Kristine Jones, and April Graham of Elsevier, Inc., for their devotion and expertise in the editing and production phases of this book.

I am indebted to Dr Waihei A. Chu, PharmD, for his guidance in the field of regulatory writing. In his own words: I thank the following people for answering specific questions during the course of this project. Nearly all of these persons are physicians and principal investigators in clinical trials in oncology, multiple sclerosis, and infectious diseases. Many of these persons are thought-leaders in the field of study design or are tenured professors in medical schools. I thank Masha Hareli, Amit Bar-Or, and Olaf Steve, for authoritative guidance on multiple sclerosis. I thank Christina Slover for guidance on drug–drug interactions. I am grateful to Patrick Archdeacon, Patricia Harley, Michelle Eby, and Joette M. Meyer, all of the FDA, for information on various aspects of the FDA approval process. I am grateful to Peter C. Raich for granting permission to reproduce his consent forms, and I thank David Cella for sending me these forms. I thank Marc Buyse, Tomasz Burzykowski, Daniel J. Sargent, Gerold Bepler, Sally Stenning, John Hainsworth, Sanjiv S. Agarwala, Clifford A. Hudis, Axel Grothey, Wen-Jen Hwu, Keith Wheatley, Joseph A. Sparano, Elizabeth A. Eisenhauer, Miguel Martin, and Linda Colangelo, for their expert guidance on endpoints. I am deeply grateful to Frank Worden and Bruce E. Johnson for guidance on run-in periods. I am most grateful to David Cella, Barbara Vickrey, Andrea (Andy) Trotti, and Jinny Tavee, for help on health-related quality-of-life (HRQoL) instruments. I thank Jeffrey A. Cohen for his detailed responses to my questions on multiple sclerosis. Also, I am grateful to Ching-Hon Pui, James B. Nachman, Eric E. Hedrick, Stacey L. Berg, and Tanja Hartmann for their insights regarding the leukemias. I acknowledge Margaret von Mehren for information on gastrointestinal stromal tumors. I thank Bruce A. Roe for modifying my diagram of the Philadelphia chromosome, and I thank Adele K. Fielding for further guidance on this chromosome. I am also grateful to Jake Liang and Robert E. Lanford for explaining relations between IFN-alpha and IFN-gamma, as they apply to hepatitis C virus.

I thank Martin E. Stryjewski, Jonathan S. Berek, James Cassidy, Olivier Leroy, and Michael E. Pichichero, for help on per protocol analysis and intent-to-treat analysis. I thank Lawrence Rubinstein, Thomas G. Roberts Jr, Thomas J. Lynch, Murray D. Norris, Bradley R. Prestidge, and Igor Sherman, for information on subgroups or on inclusion/exclusion criteria.

I am grateful to Peter J. Barrett-Lee for information on drug safety. I thank Anthony Viera for information on randomization. I thank Syed Y. Zafar and Richard L. Schilsky for their expertise on best supportive care and palliative care. I acknowledge Karen Mosher for her expertise on decision aids, as it relates to consent forms. I am grateful to Elizabeth B. Andrews, Balall Naeem, Michael Klepper, and Barry D.C. Arnold, for their knowledge regarding the CIOMS I form. I thank Patricia Mozzicato for her time answering questions about the MedDRA terminology. Moreover, I thank Tiiamari Pennanen for information on the history of the European Medicines Agency, and Dominic Stevenson and Sarah Heffer for advice on the Yellow Card. For the first edition of this book, I thank Jenna Elder and Harvey Motulsky for reviewing the draft chapter on biostatistics.

Preface

This book is a pharmacology textbook. It can serve a handbook for all personnel involved in regulated clinical trials, including employees at the US Food and Drug Administration (FDA) and the European Medicines Agency (EMA). The book quotes extensively from comments by FDA reviewers, which are published on the FDA's website at the time that the FDA grants approval to a drug. In other words, along with the FDA's approval letter, the FDA also publishes its *Medical Reviews*, *Clinical Reviews*, *Pharmacology Reviews*, and other documents, each of which includes comments from various FDA personnel.

The content of these reviews closely tracks the Sponsor's *Integrated Summary of Safety* (ISS), submitted as part of an NDA or BLA. It is therefore the case that this book provides an accurate representation of what the FDA looks for (and complains against), during its review of submissions from a Sponsor's phase II and phase III clinical trials. In all, the author made use of the *Medical Reviews* and *Clinical Reviews* that accompanied about 75 of the FDA's approval letters.

In this book, the words "Sponsor" and "investigator" are sometimes used interchangeably, though it should be noted that the Sponsor is the party that initiates a clinical trial, while an investigator is the party that actually does the work, such as the work of writing the Clinical Study Protocol and other FDA-submissions, enrolling study subjects,

administering the study drug, and collecting data on efficacy and safety (1).

Also, to ensure that the book is a lively and compelling textbook and handbook, the text provides the history of consent forms using the example of Walter Reed's yellow fever study, the history of the FDA and the EMA, background information on assay methods in biochemistry and immunology, and quotations from published courtroom opinions relating to clinical trials.

This book fulfills various unmet needs, as detailed below.

THE STUDY SCHEMA AND STUDY DESIGN

The best way to communicate trial design is with a flow chart or table called the *schema*.

The author observed that the schema is rarely detailed in any explicit way by books or journal articles. Unfortunately, books on clinical trials generally refrain from disclosing much on trial design, for example, regarding the various goals of the run-in period, or regarding decision trees that may modify drug dosing during the course of an ongoing trial. This book provides a thorough introduction to study design, includes many representative diagrams of the study schema, and details several distinct reasons for including a run-in period.

---

[1]American Academy or Pediatrics Policy Statement. Off-label use of drugs in children. Pediatrics 2014;133:563−7.

INTENT-TO-TREAT ANALYSIS AND PLACEBOS

Second, the authors observed that other aspects of clinical trials are inadequately described in textbooks, for example, they were covered only by a short paragraph. These aspects include intent-to-treat (ITT) analysis, modified ITT (mITT) analysis, and per protocol (PP) analysis. ITT analysis is a term that is almost universally used in clinical trials, but the available textbooks on clinical trial design typically fail to describe ITT analysis, mITT analysis, or PP analysis, and how to choose between these three types of data analysis. This book contains an entire chapter on ITT, mITT, and PP analyses. It is also the case that most or all books on clinical trials fail to include any organized account of placebos. This book has an entire chapter on placebos.

HOW TO CHOOSE ENDPOINTS

Third, definitions of endpoints used in oncology clinical trials are frequently disclosed in the available textbooks, but unfortunately, textbooks generally fail to state the advantages of any given endpoint over another, and fail to state situations where a particular endpoint gives ambiguous information or where an endpoint cannot be used. These oncology endpoints include objective response rate (ORR), overall survival (OS), progression-free survival (PFS), time to progression (TTP), time to distant metastasis (TDM), disease-free survival (DFS), 6-month PFS, and health-related quality of life (HRQoL). The FDA's Guidance for Industry (2) provides a fine introduction to these endpoints, but refrains from detailing, for example, situations where any given endpoint is likely to be unreliable or unusable.

This book fulfills an unmet need by providing a more detailed account on how to choose the most appropriate oncology endpoint, and on when to refrain from using a given endpoint.

DIAGNOSTIC TESTS

Fourth, this book takes care to integrate diagnostic tests with each disease. What are described are disability status questionnaires, HRQoL questionnaires, blood counts, flow cytometry, immunoassays, polymerase chain reaction (PCR), microarrays, and magnetic resonance imaging (MRI). Moreover, this book provides an introduction to the process of FDA approval for diagnostics tests.

MECHANISM OF ACTION

Fifth, the book describes the mechanisms of various diseases and the mechanisms of action of various drugs. These mechanisms are integrated into the context of clinical trials, in commentary demonstrating how the mechanism of action can influence the inclusion/exclusion criteria, warnings on consent forms, and information on package inserts. This book also describes how the mechanism of action can influence study design, that is, the particular combination and timing of administered drugs. The book reveals that a knowledge of the mechanism of action can encourage regulatory agencies to allow a clinical trial to be initiated.

STANDARDS

Sixth, the text emphasizes the role of various standards that apply to clinical trials. These standards include criteria for measuring

---

[2] U.S. Department of Health and Human Services. Food and Drug Administration. Guidance for industry. Clinical trial endpoints for the approval of cancer drugs and biologicals; 2007 (19 pp.).

physical fitness, such as the Eastern Cooperative Oncology Group (ECOG) score, Karnofsky score, and the Kurtzke Expanded Disability Status Scale (EDSS) score, criteria for measuring tumor size and number (Response Evaluation Criteria in Solid Tumors, RECIST criteria), and criteria for staging tumors [Tumor Node Metastasis (TNM) staging; Dukes' staging]. The text provides a warning about potential confusion that can arise, when two different sets of standards are applied to one disease. This warning takes the form of a narrative on the Will Rogers Phenomenon.

The administrative law, and guidance documents from regulatory agencies, constitute another type of standard. These standards are also revised from time to time. The ICH Guidelines and the FDA's Guidance for Industry documents constitute a recurring theme in this textbook.

FDA'S WARNING LETTERS

This textbook uses the FDA's Warning Letters as a source material. The FDA issues Warning Letters to manufacturers of drugs, medical devices, foods, and dietary supplements. Generally, these letters include complaints about a company's failure to comply with one or more sections of Title 21 of the Code of Federal regulations. The FDA uses two different instruments for complaining about failures to follow various sections of Title 21 of the Code of Federal Regulations, for the situation where the failures are detected during an FDA inspection of the Sponsor's clinical facilities or manufacturing facilities.

These two instruments are the FDA's Form 483 notices and the FDA's Warning Letters. Quotations from the FDA's Warning Letters are included at various points in this book. A sustained account of the FDA's Warning Letters, as well as a description of their relation to the FDA's Form 483, appears in one of the last chapters in this book.

CLINICALTRIALS.GOV AND OTHER REGISTRIES FOR CLINICAL TRIALS

ClinicalTrials.gov is a registry of clinical trials, developed by the FDA and NIH, and first operational in 2000 (3). In 2007, the Food and Drug Administration Amendments Act (FDAAA) imposed the requirement that sponsors of clinical trials register and report summary results at www.ClinicalTrials.gov (4). As of Jan. 2009, ClinicalTrials.gov had more than 67,000 registered trials (5). About one-quarter of these trials are sponsored by pharmaceutical companies. Zarin et al. (6) describe the content of this website.

The European Union provides the EU Clinical Trials Registry, which contains information on clinical trials that were conducted in the European Union, starting after May 1, 2004. This Registry contains information that was entered by Sponsors of clinical trials. The information, which appears in the EudraCT database, can be searched by the public, and the information includes the trial design, Sponsor, medicine, therapeutic area, summary of results, and whether the trial is merely authorized, or is ongoing or complete. EudraCT is provided

[3]Steinbrook R. Public registration of clinical trials. New Engl. J. Med. 2004;351:315−7.

[4]Anderson ML, et al. Compliance with results reporting at ClinicalTrials.gov. New Engl. J. Med. 2015;372:1031−9.

[5]Wood AJ. Progress and deficiencies in the registration of clinical trials. New Engl. J. Med. 2009;360:824−30.

[6]Zarin DA, Tse T, Williams RJ, Califf RM, Ide NC. The ClinicalTrials.gov results database—update and key issues. New Engl. J. Med. 2011;364:852−60.

in 24 different languages. The step at which the user can select the language, is provided on the world wide web at: www.eudrapharm.eu/eudrapharm/. Any member of the public can input query terms such as the trade name or the chemical name of the drug.

Registries that are not affiliated with any governmental agency include, for example, the TYSABRI Pregnancy Exposure Registry. This registry is identified on the package insert for Tysabri, which states that, "[i]f a woman becomes pregnant while taking TYSABRI, consider enrolling her in the TYSABRI Pregnancy Exposure Registry by calling 1-800-456-2255" (7).

Each study has a unique registration number. Another registry used for clinical trials is the International Standard Randomised Controlled Trial Number (ISRCTN) (8). Where a clinical trial is conducted in only one country, study information should be entered only in one register, to avoid duplication and confusion. However, companies that perform international clinical studies may be required to register their trial in a national clinical study register, as well as in an international clinical study register (9). The WHO International Clinical Trials Registry Platform (ICTRP) provides a search portal to locate trials from many primary registries worldwide (http://www.who.int/ictrp/en/). This registry began operating in 2005 (10).

A similar service for ongoing and completed studies is available from the International Federation of Pharmaceutical Manufacturers & Associations (IFPMA) (http://www.ifpma.org/clinicaltrials) (11).

The FDA Amendments Act, enacted in Sep. 2007. Congress expanded the requirements for sponsors and investigators to post information about clinical trials, including selected aspects of trial results, on ClinicalTrials.gov (12). Requirements relevant to registration are set forth in Section 801 of this Act. Section 801 mandates registration on ClinicalTrials.gov of all new controlled clinical investigations (other than phase I) of drugs, biologics, and devices subject to regulations by the FDA. This applies to research for any condition, regardless of sponsor type, for example, industry, government, or academic (13). New clinical studies must be registered within 21 days after the first patient is enrolled, where updates of the registry information must occur at least every 12 months. Recruitment status should be updated within 30 days of any change. Dec. 2007 was the due date to start registering new studies or updating all required information fields for ongoing studies (14,15). One of the FDA's Guidance for Industry documents, *Providing Regulatory Submissions in Electronic Format*, provides guidance for registering your clinical trial (16).

[7]TYSABRI (natalizumab) Injection Full Prescribing Information. Biogen IDEC, Inc.; January 1, 2012 (32 pp.).

[8]Thomas KB, Tesch C. Clinical trial disclosure-focusing on results. The Write Stuff. 2008;17:70−3.

[9]Thomas KB, Tesch C. Clinical trial disclosure-focusing on results. The Write Stuff. 2008;17:70−3.

[10]Sim I. Trial registration for public trust: making the case for medical devices. J. Gen. Intern. Med. 2008;23 (Suppl. 1):64−8.

[11]Thomas KB, Tesch C. Clinical trial disclosure-focusing on results. The Write Stuff. 2008;17:70−3.

[12]Wood AJ. Progress and deficiencies in the registration of clinical trials. New Engl. J. Med. 2009;360:824−30.

[13]Thomas KB, Tesch C. Clinical trial disclosure-focusing on results. The Write Stuff. 2008;17:70−3.

[14]Thomas KB, Tesch C. Clinical trial disclosure-focusing on results. The Write Stuff. 2008;17:70−3.

[15]Wood AJJ. Progress and deficiencies in the registration of clinical trials. New Engl. J. Med. 2009;360:824−30.

[16]U.S. Department of Health and Human Services. Food and Drug Administration. Providing regulatory submissions in electronic format—drug establishment registration and drug listing; May 2009 (13 pp.).

Although Public Law No. 110-85 contains a section named, Section 801, the law only has 88 sections. Section 801 is reproduced, in part, below (17):

> (i) SEARCHABLE CATEGORIES.—The Director of NIH shall ensure that the public may, in addition to keyword searching, search the entries in the registry data bank by 1 or more of the following criteria:
>
> (I) The disease or condition being studied in the clinical trial, using Medical Subject Headers (MeSH) descriptors.
>
> (II) The name of the intervention, including any drug or device being studied in the clinical trial.
>
> (III) The location of the clinical trial.
>
> (IV) The age group studied in the clinical trial, including pediatric subpopulations.
>
> (V) The study phase of the clinical trial.
>
> (VI) The sponsor of the clinical trial, which may be the National Institutes of Health or another Federal agency, a private industry source, or a university or other organization.
>
> (VII) The recruitment status of the clinical trial.
>
> (VIII) The National Clinical Trial number or other study identification for the clinical trial.

The International Committee of Medical Journal Editors (ICMJE) adopted the policy that clinical trials be registered at the onset of patient enrollment, as a condition for publication (18). In observing that trial registration is largely voluntary, and that registries contain only a small proportion of trials, the ICMJE proposed that trial registration be a solution to the problem of selective awareness, and set forth the goal that ICMJE member journals require (as a condition of consideration for publication) registration in a public trials registry (19,20). Trials must register at or before the onset of patient enrollment. Hirsch (21) and others (22,23) provide comments on this policy. In a survey of editorial policies of 165 medical journals, Hopewell et al. (24), found that 44 specially require that the clinical trial be registered before submitting the manuscript to the journal.

According to the FDA's Guidance for Industry document on good pharmacovigilance practices, a sponsor may establish or create a new registry, for example, for the goals of evaluating safety signals identified from spontaneous case reports or from literature reports, and for evaluating factors that affect the risk of adverse outcomes, such as dose, timing of exposure, or patient characteristics (25).

[17] Public Law 110-85. 110th Congress. September 27, 2007. Food and Drug Administration Amendments of 2007.

[18] Foote M. Clinical trial registries and publication of results—a primer. In: Foote M, editor. Clinical trial registries a practical guide for sponsors and researchers of medicinal products. Basel, Switzerland: Birkhäuser Verlag; 2006. pp. 1–12.

[19] De Angelis CD, Drazen JM, Frizelle FA, et al. Is this clinical trial fully registered?—A statement from the International Committee of Medical Journal Editors. New Engl. J. Med. 2005;352:2436–8.

[20] De Angelis CD, Drazen JM, Frizelle FA, et al. Clinical trial registration: a statement from the International Committee of Medical Journal Editors. J. Am. Med. Assoc. 2004;292:1363–4.

[21] Hirsch L. Trial registration and results disclosure:impact of US legislation on sponsors, investigators, and medical journal editors. Curr. Med. Res. Opin. 2008;24:1683–9.

[22] Bonati M, Pandolfini C. Trial registration, the ICMJE statement, and paediatric journals. Arch. Dis. Child 2006;91:93.

[23] Sekeres M, Gold JL, Chan AW, et al. Poor reporting of scientific leadership information in clinical trial registers. PLoS One 2008;3:e1610.

[24] Hopewell S, Altman DG, Moher D, Schulz KF. Endorsement of the CONSORT Statement by high impact factor medical journals: a survey of journal editors and journal 'Instructions to Authors'. Trials 2008;9:20.

[25] U.S. Department of Health and Human Services. Food and Drug Administration. Guidance for industry. Good pharmacovigilance practices and pharmacoepidemiologic assessment; March 2005 (20 pp.).

This book emphasizes cancer for a number of reasons. Therapy for cancer involves more variables, more drug candidates, and more drug combinations, than therapy for other diseases. Hence, there is a greater need to provide a harmonious description of trial design and endpoints, as it applies to cancer. Also, the number of cancer clinical trials is greater than for other diseases. In Jan. 2011, about 27,000 cancer trials, 4190 trials on immunological diseases (sum of arthritis, multiple sclerosis, lupus, psoriasis, Crohn's disease, and ulcerative colitis), 5180 trials on diabetes, and 690 trials on atherosclerosis, were identified on www.ClinicalTrials.gov.

Introduction

Where a drug or medical device is tested on human subjects, the test may be called a clinical trial. Clinical trials may be conducted in an academic setting, where the goals are to obtain knowledge on the mechanism of action, efficacy, and pharmacokinetics of the drug. Clinical trials are also conducted by the pharmaceutical industry, where the goals are to obtain knowledge on safety, efficacy, pharmacokinetics, and mechanism of action, and to obtain regulatory approval.

The structure of clinical trials is set forth in a document called the Clinical Study Protocol. Clinical Study Protocols contain a number of common elements, or concepts, despite the variety of drugs being tested, and the variety of diseases. These common elements include inclusion and exclusion criteria for the study subjects, subgroups of the study population, methods for stratifying the study subjects, techniques for recruitment, obtaining consent, randomization, and allocation, and statistical methods for data presentation and analysis. The Clinical Study Protocol includes a summary called the synopsis and a flow chart called the study schema. The schema provides the study design, the identity of the study drug and control, and an identification of some of the endpoints.

Endpoints in any given clinical trial may relate, for example, to tumor size, the number of lesions in an organ or tissue, the concentration of bacteria or viruses in the bloodstream, or to a metabolite or hormone in the bloodstream. Endpoints can take the form of relatively subjective data from questionnaires filled out by study subjects, or of relatively objective data, such as laboratory values in chemistry and hematology, or images from computed tomography and magnetic resonance imaging (MRI).

In clinical trials, the main goals are capturing and analyzing data on safety and efficacy. It is usually not the goal to ensure that study subjects recover from their disorder.

Trials intended for regulatory approval by the US Food and Drug Administration (FDA), as well as monitoring activities in the post-approval context, are regulated by the United States Code (USC) and by the administrative law, that is, the Code of Federal Regulations (CFR). The term "administrative law" refers to the rules in the CFR. The USC contains statutes, whilst the CFR contains rules. The relevant statutes are found in Title 21 of the USC (21 USC §355).

The relevant administrative law (or rules) is found in Title 21 and Title 45 of the CFR, as indicated below:

- Investigational New Drug (IND) (21 CFR §312)
- New Drug Application (NDA) (21 CFR §314)
- Investigator's Brochures (IB) (21 CFR §312)
- Integrated Summary of Safety (ISS) (21 CFR §314.50 (d)(5))
- Integrated Summary of Efficacy (ISE) (21 CFR §314.50 (d)(5))
- Consent form (21 CFR §50 and 45 §CFR 46)
- Package insert (21 CFR §201.10 and 21 CFR §201.56)
- Data Monitoring Committee Charter (DMC Charter) (21 CFR §312.50 and 45 CFR §46).

I. GOOD CLINICAL PRACTICE

Clinical trials intended for regulatory approval should conform to a set of guidelines known as, Good Clinical Practice (GCP). According to the ICH Guidelines:

> Good Clinical Practice is an international ethical and scientific quality standard for designing, conducting, recording and reporting trials that involve the participation of human subjects. Compliance with this standard provides public assurance that the rights, safety and well-being of trial subjects are protected, consistent with the principles that have their origin in the Declaration of Helsinki, and that the clinical trial data are credible [1].

GCP encompasses the requirement that the clinical study be approved by an independent ethics board, such as an Institutional Review Board (IRB), prior to initiating the clinical study. GCP also encompasses the requirements that study subjects give informed consent prior to entering the study, that records of study subjects be kept confidential, that investigators be properly qualified by education and training, that adequate medical care be given to any study subjects who suffer from study-related adverse events, that serious adverse events be immediately reported to the sponsor, and that study drugs and placebo (if any) be manufactured according to Good Manufacturing Practices (GMP).

The ICH Guideline for Good Clinical Practice also provides the organization and content of the Clinical Study Protocol. The Clinical Study Protocol is, in essence, the instruction manual used by persons involved in conducting the trial. Additionally, the ICH Guideline for Good Clinical Practice details the organization and content of the Investigator's Brochure (IB), a document that compiles relevant clinical data and non-clinical data. These data include those arising apart from the study, for example, from reports from animal studies and from clinical trials conducted by other investigators, as well as data from human subjects arising from the study itself. Most of the information set forth in this textbook can be viewed in the context of Good Clinical Practice.

The ICH Good Clinical Practice Guidelines sets forth international standards for the quality, safety, and efficacy of developmental-stage pharmaceutical products. The ICH Good Clinical Practice Guidelines were made binding by the EU Clinical Trials Directive in 2004.[2] They require the sponsor to verify the qualifications of the investigators, obtain informed consent before each subject's participation in the trial, ensure the trials are adequately monitored, and that the institutional review board (IRB) reviews and approves the Clinical Study Protocol, and oversee the trial.

This textbook frequently refers to the ICH Guidelines and the FDA's Guidance for Industry documents, and uses these documents as anchor points for the various narratives.

II. FDA'S DECISION-MAKING PROCESS IN GRANTING APPROVAL TO A DRUG

This textbook is unique in its extensive use of documents published by the FDA at the time the FDA grants approval to a drug. These document are published by the FDA, in its response to an NDA or BLA submitted by a Sponsor. The decision-making processes leading to regulatory approval of various drugs are available, in part, on the website of the FDA. The available documents, which are published

---

[1]ICH Harmonised Tripartite Guidelines. Guideline for Good Clinical Practice E6 (R1). Step 4 version, June 1996.

[2]Hathaway CR, Manthei JR, Haas JB, Scherer CA. Looking abroad: clinical drug trials. Food and Drug Law Journal. 2008; 63:673–681.

at the time that the FDA grants approval to a drug, include:

- Approval Letter
- Package Insert
- Medical Review or Clinical Review
- Pharmacology Review
- Statistical Review
- Package Insert
- Administrative Documents and Correspondence.

For the Reviews, it is the case that FDA reviewers reproduce some of the data that had been submitted by the Sponsor, re-analyze the results, and come to their own conclusions. The Reviews include clearly labeled comments from the reviewers. These comments provide invaluable guidance from the ultimate authority on the types of study design and data that are needed to influence the FDA to grant approval. These comments sometimes take the form of complaints, however, since the Reviews are published at the time of FDA approval, it is generally not the case that the complaints are harsh enough to bring a halt to the drug-approval process. On occasion, parts of the FDA's Reviews that correspond to an earlier phase of the drug-approval process will reveal

harsh complaints, such as those involving a *Clinical Hold* or a *Refuse to File* notice, and where these complaints were eventually overcome by the Sponsor. Moreover, because the Reviews are published at the time of FDA approval, it is the case that these Reviews often emphasize postmarketing requirements that were imposed by the FDA, for example, the requirement to conduct confirmatory clinical trials, in the case of a trial that had received an accelerated approval, or the requirement to include an REMS in the postmarketing situation.

III. DISCLAIMER

The following is a disclaimer. The present writing does not constitute legal advice, and it does not establish any relationship between the reader and the authors. A goal of the present writing is to facilitate communication between investigators in pharmaceutical companies and their attorneys, in matters limited to consent forms, package inserts, and patents. The opinions set forth herein do not necessarily reflect the opinions of the authors' past, present, or future employers.

Abbreviations and Definitions

ADCC antibody-dependent cell cytotoxicity

ADME absorption, distribution, metabolism, and excretion

ADR adverse drug reaction

AE adverse event

ALL acute lymphocytic leukemia; acute lymphoblastic leukemia

AML acute myeloid leukemia; acute myelogenous leukemia

APC antigen presenting cell. APCs include cells of the immune system, for example, dendritic cells and macrophages. Antigens, which take the form of peptides and oligopeptides, are noncovalently bound to MHC, and are presented to T cells by way of the MHC, where presentation occurs in an immune synapse that involves the APC and a T cell

ASCO American Society of Clinical Oncology

AUC area under the curve of concentration, in serum or plasma, over time. The AUC represents the overall impact of a drug, over the course of time, to organs, tissues, and cells, in the physiological milieu

bid "bid in die," which is Latin for twice a day

C_{max} maximum concentration in plasma or serum. Plasma refers to blood containing an anticoagulant, with blood cells removed. Serum prepared by allowing blood naturally to clot, followed by discarding the clot and the blood cells

C_{min} minimum concentration in plasma or serum

CBER Center for Biologics Evaluation and Research

CD cluster of differentiation. The CD nomenclature refers to cell-surface proteins of immune cells, and is used to identify immune cells

CDER Center for Drug Evaluation and Research

CFR; C.F.R. Code of Federal Regulations

CI confidence interval

CIOMS Council for International Organizations of Medical Sciences

CLL chronic lymphocytic leukemia; chronic lymphoblastic leukemia

CMI Consumer Medication Information

CML chronic myeloid leukemia; chronic myelogenous leukemia

CONSORT Consolidated Statement of Reporting Trials

COPD chronic obstructive pulmonary disease

CR complete response. Complete response is a type of objective response. "Objective response" means assessing tumor size and number, as described by the RECIST criteria. CR is also used to refer to a totally different parameter, complete remission

CRF Case Report Form

CRP C-reactive protein

CTCAE Common Terminology Criteria for Adverse Events

DC dendritic cell

DFS disease-free survival

DMC Data Monitoring Committee

DNA deoxyribonucleic acid

DSMC Data and Safety Monitoring Committee

ECG electrocardiogram

ECOG Eastern Cooperative Oncology Group

ECRIN European Clinical Infrastructure Network

EGF epidermal growth factor

EMA; EMEA European Medicines Agency. EMEA was the formerly used abbreviation, but in Dec. 2009 the abbreviation was changed to EMA

FDA US Food and Drug Administration

FDA Form 356h the form used to submit an NDA or BLA

FDA Form 483 Form 483 is sometimes issued during the time of an FDA inspection of a clinical or manufacturing facility. If the problems are not corrected in due course, FDA may follow-up by issuing a Warning Letter

FDA Form 1571 the form used to submit an IND

FOLFIRI anticancer therapy using folinic acid, fluorouracil, and irinotecan. Folinic acid, also known as leucovorin, is a trivial name for 5-formyl-tetrahydrofolic acid

FPI Full Prescribing Information. FPI is the US Food and Drug Administration's name for part of the package insert

5-FU 5-fluorouracil

GCP Good Clinical Practices

GLP Good Laboratory Practices

Gy Gray (1 gray = 1 J/kg and also equals 100 rad). The gray is a unit of absorbed energy per mass of tissue

HCV hepatitis C virus

HERG gene human ether-related a-go-go gene

HIPAA Health Insurance Portability and Accountability Act

HR hazard ratio

HRQoL health-related quality of life, or simply, QoL.

IB Investigator's Brochure

ICH International Conference Harmonization

ICMJE International Committee of Medical Journal Editors

ICSR Individual Case Safety Reports

IM intramuscular

IND Investigational New Drug application

IP intraperitoneal or intraperitoneally

ITT intent to treat, as in, "intent-to-treat analysis"

IV intravenous or intravenously

IVRS interactive voice response systems

LDH lactic dehydrogenase

LLOQ lower limit of quantification

M molarity; moles per liter

MABEL minimum anticipated biological effect level

MDS myelodysplastic syndromes (MDS is a genus of related diseases)

MedDRA Medical Dictionary for Regulatory Activities Terminology

MHC major histocompatibility complex. The MHC is a complex of membrane-bound proteins, expressed by a dendritic cell, that is used to hold antigenic peptides. The MCH presents the antigenic peptides to a T cell, that is, to the T cell receptor of a T cell. In response, the T cell is activated. The complex of MHC (residing on a dendritic cell) and the T cell receptor (residing on a T cell) is called the immune synapse

MHRA Medicines and Healthcare products Regulatory Agency

miRNA micro-RNA; micro-ribonucleic acid

mL milliliter

MOG myelin oligodendrocyte glycoprotein

MRD minimal residual disease. MRD refers to the amount of leukemic blood cells following therapy against leukemia. For MRD analysis, the blood cells can be acquired from the bone marrow or from peripheral blood, and then identified. Identification employs the polymerase chain reaction, a technique that can detect mRNA specific to leukemic cells

MTX methotrexate. Methotrexate, a drug used for treating cancer and arthritis. MTX is a chemical analog of folic acid

NK cell natural killer cell. NK cells can kill target cells by way of ADCC. In ADCC, an antibody binds to the NK cell by way of the constant region of the antibody and an Fc receptor. Also, the same antibody binds to a target cell by way of its variable region, and a specific antibody on the target cell. In ADCC, various ligand and receptors, expressed on the surface of the NK cell and the target cell must be compatible with each other. When the above conditions are met, the NK cell kills the target cell

NOAEL no-observed adverse effect level. This term is used in toxicology, in the context of using animal studies to arrive at a human dose

NS2 nonstructural protein 2 of hepatitis C virus

NS5A nonstructural protein 5A of hepatitis C virus

OR objective response

OS overall survival

P **value** assuming that there is no actual difference in the means between two groups of data, the *P* value is the probability of finding a difference (a difference arising by chance alone) between the means of the two groups that is as large, or larger, than the experimentally observed difference

PBMCs peripheral blood mononuclear cells. The term PBMCs refers to a preparation of bulk leukocytes. PBMCs include T cells, B cells, NK cells, and monocytes, and they may include circulating tumor cells. PBMCs do not include red blood cells and polymorphonuclear leukocytes (neutrophils)

PCR polymerase chain reaction. PCR is a technique for reproducing, in a reiterative and exponential manner, a region of double-stranded DNA

PD progressive disease

PDR Physician's Desk Reference. The PDR contains reproductions of package inserts, including the black box warnings of the inserts

PFS progression-free survival

pH negative log of hydrogen ion concentration

PK pharmacokinetics. PK refers to drug concentrations, over the course of time, during absorption, distribution, metabolism, and excretion, of any administered drug. Pharmacodynamics, in contrast, refers to the physiological responses of organs, tissues, cells, and genes, to an administered drug

PP per protocol, as in "per protocol analysis"

PPI Patient Package Insert

PR partial response

PSUR Periodic Safety Update Reports

QT interval Time (ms) between Q wave and T wave

QTc interval corrected QT interval

RCT randomized controlled trial; randomised controlled trial (British spelling)

RECIST Response Evaluation Criteria In Solid Tumors

REMS Risk Evaluation and Mitigation Strategy

RTF Refuse to File

RFS relapse-free survival

RNA ribonucleic acid

RTOG Radiation Therapy Oncology Group

SAE serious adverse event

SC subcutaneous

SNP single nucleotide polymorphism

SPA request for Special Protocol Assessment

SVR sustained virological response

SWOG Southwest Oncology Group

T cells thymus-derived cells

TDM time to distant metastasis

TdP Torsade de pointes

Th1 Th1 refers to Th1-type helper T cells. Th1 also refers to any Th1-type cytokine, for example, IFN-gamma, without regard to the cell origin

Th2 Th2 refers to Th2-type helper T cells. Th2 also refers to any Th2-type cytokine, for example, IL-4, IL-5, IL-10, and IL-13, without regard to the cell origin

tid "ter in die," which is Latin for three times a day

q3w every three weeks

USC; U.S.C. United States Code

USPTO United States Patent and Trademark Office

WHO World Health Organization

Biographies

The author received his PhD from the University of California at Berkeley in 1980, and conducted postdoctoral research at University of Wisconsin-Madison and also at U.C. Berkeley. Most of his 20 research publications concern the enzymology, metabolism, and pharmacokinetics of folates and related amino acids (1,2,3,4). Also, he cloned, sequenced, and expressed an oncogene (*XPE* gene) (5,6,7). Later, he performed research on the structure of an antibody (natalizumab) used for treating multiple sclerosis (8). The author has 15 years of pharmaceutical industry experience, acquired at Schering-Plough, Cerus Corporation, and Athena Neurosciences (Elan Pharmaceuticals), and has contributed to FDA-submissions for the indications of multiple sclerosis, melanoma, head and neck cancer, liver cancer, pancreatic cancer, and hepatitis C. At an earlier time, he wrote two editions of *Nutritional Biochemistry*, published by Elsevier, Inc. (9). *Nutritional Biochemistry* describes the clinical features, diagnosis, treatment, and mechanisms of action of 40 drugs, relating to the metabolic diseases. More recently, the author acquired 3 years of experience in FDA regulations, as applied to package inserts, as well as further experience in medical writing in oncology, immune disorders, and infections, at Baker Hostetler, LLP, Costa Mesa, CA. The author has 16 years of training and experience in the Code of Federal regulations, as it applies to pharmaceuticals and clinical trial design.

[1]Brody T, Stokstad ELR. Folate oligoglutamate:amino acid transpeptidase. J. Biol. Chem. 1982;257:14271−9.

[2]Brody T, Watson JE, Stokstad ELR. Folate pentaglutamate and folate hexaglutamate mediated one-carbon metabolism. Biochemistry 1982;21:276−82.

[3]Brody T, Stokstad ELR. Nitrous oxide provokes changes in folylpenta- and hexaglutamates. J. Nutr. 1990;120:71−80.

[4]Brody T, Stokstad ELR. Incorporation of the 2-ring carbon of histidine into folylpolyglutamate coenzymes. J. Nutr. Biochem. 1991;2:492−8.

[5]Brody T, Keeney S, Linn S. Human damage-specific DNA binding protein p48 subunit mRNA, GenBank, Accession # U18299; 1995.

[6]Keeney S, Eker AP, Brody T, et al. Correction of the DNA repair defect in xeroderma pigmentosum group E by injection of a DNA damage-binding protein. Proc. Natl Acad. Sci. 1994;91:4053−6.

[7]Dualan R, Brody T, Keeney S, et al. Chromosomal localization and cDNA cloning of the genes (DDB1 and DDB2) for the p127 and p48 subunits of a human damage-specific DNA binding protein. Genomics 1995;29:62−9.

[8]Brody T. Multistep denaturation and hierarchy of disulfide bond cleavage of a monoclonal antibody. Analytical Biochem. 1997;247:247−56.

[9]Brody T. Nutritional biochemistry. 2nd ed. San Diego, CA: Academic Press; 1999.

Dr Jennifer A. Elder, PhD, author of Chapter 10, *Biostatistics: Part II*, is Chief Scientific Officer at PharPoint Research, Inc., in Durham, NC. Dr Elder has performed statistical analyses for clinical trials for 15 years, with 11 of those years being in the CRO industry. Dr Elder served as the lead statistician on pivotal studies for various compounds, and has participated in the completion of several NDA, MAA, sNDA, and IND applications, and provided strategic consulting, and statistical analysis oversight for over 75 projects.

1

Origins of Drugs

I. INTRODUCTION

Drugs have a number of origins, as outlined:

- Natural products, for example, chemicals from plants and microorganisms.
- Analogs of naturally occurring chemicals that reside in various biosynthetic pathways of mammals.
- Antibodies that bind to naturally occurring targets in the body.
- Discovery that an existing drug, established as effective for a first disease, is also effective for treating an unrelated second disease.
- Drugs identified by screening libraries of chemicals.

Some drugs are based on natural products, where the natural products were known to have pharmacological effects. The term "natural products" is a term of the art that generally refers to chemicals derived from plants, fungi, or microorganisms. Drugs that are derived from natural products, or that actually are natural products, include warfarin (1), penicillin (2,3), cyclosporine (4), aspirin (5,6), paclitaxel (7), fingolimod (8), and reserpine (9). Many other drugs have structures based on chemicals that occur naturally in the human body, that

[1]Wardrop D, Keeling D. The story of the discovery of heparin and warfarin. Br. J. Haematol. 2008;141:757—63.

[2]Diggins FW. The true history of the discovery of penicillin, with refutation of the misinformation in the literature. Br. J. Biomed. Sci. 1999;56:83—93.

[3]Fleming A. On the antibacterial action of cultures of a penicillium, with special reference to their use in the isolation of B. influenzae. 1929. Bull. World Health Organ. 2001;79:780—90.

[4]Heusler K, Pletscher A. The controversial early history of cyclosporin. Swiss Med. Wkly 2001;131:299—302.

[5]Lafont O. From the willow to aspirin. Rev. Hist. Pharm. (Paris) 2007;55:209—16.

[6]Mahdi JG, Mahdi AJ, Mahdi AJ, Bowen ID. The historical analysis of aspirin discovery, its relation to the willow tree and antiproliferative and anticancer potential. Cell Prolif. 2006;39:147—55.

[7]Socinski MA. Single-agent paclitaxel in the treatment of advanced non-small cell lung cancer. Oncologist 1999;4:408—16.

[8]Adachi K, Chiba K. FTY720 story. Its discovery and the following accelerated development of sphingosine 1-phosphate receptor agonists as immunomodulators based on reverse pharmacology. Perspect. Medicin. Chem. 2007;1:11—23.

[9]Rao EV. Drug discovery from plants. Curr. Sci. 2007;93:1060.

Clinical Trials.
DOI: http://dx.doi.org/10.1016/B978-0-12-804217-5.00001-1

is, where the drugs are analogs of these chemicals. These include analogs of intermediates or final products of biosynthetic pathways. Drugs that are analogs of chemicals in biosynthetic pathways include methotrexate, cladribine, and ribavirin.

Still other drugs originated by first identifying a target cell, or target protein, and then by preparing antibodies that bind to that target. Vaccines have a similar origin. Once a target protein is identified, this target protein (or a derivative of it) can be formulated as a vaccine. Typically, vaccines take the form of the target protein derivative, called an "antigen," in combination with a second compound that is an immune adjuvant.

Drugs are also derived using a screening assay and by testing hundreds or thousands of purified candidate compounds using that assay. Where the screening method is automated, the method is called high-throughput screening. The screening assay may consist of tumor cells that are cultured in vitro, where a robot determines if the candidate drug inhibits a particular enzyme in the tumor cell or if the candidate drug kills the tumor cell.

II. STRUCTURES OF DRUGS

A knowledge of the structure of a drug to be used in a clinical trial is needed for the following reasons. First, the issue of whether a drug is hydrophobic or hydrophilic will dictate the nature of the excipient. If a drug is not water-soluble, then the excipient might need to include a solubilizing agent, such as a solvent. Second, the structure can also provide an idea of stability during long-term storage and thus in need of protection from light or in need of cold storage. Third, the structure can dictate the route of administration, and enable a prediction of pharmacokinetics of the drug and pathways of metabolism, transport, and excretion. Fourth, the structure of the drug can help the investigator predict adverse events that might be expected from the drug. For example, if the drug belongs to a class of compounds that activates cytochrome P450, some of the adverse events can be predicted. Fifth, regulatory submissions to the US Food and Drug Administration (FDA), such as the Investigational New Drug (IND), Investigator's Brochure, and the package insert, typically contain a drawing of the drug structure.

a. Origin of Warfarin

Warfarin is a drug that is widely used to prevent blood clotting, for example, in people at risk of heart attacks or strokes [10]. A natural product produced during the spoiling of sweet clover inspired warfarin's design. The drug was not named after any kind of warfare, even though it is used in warfare against mice and rats; it was named after the *Wisconsin Alumni Research Foundation*.

Spoiled sweet clover contains coumarin, a compound that inhibits an enzyme in the liver, where the end-result is impaired blood clotting. Blood clotting factors are biosynthesized in the liver, and then released into the bloodstream. Farmers in the mid-West found that cattle bled to death during the process of de-horning, where the cattle had eaten spoiled sweet clover. Eventually, one particular farmer in Wisconsin took a bucket of unclotted blood to researchers at the University of Wisconsin. The researchers examined the blood, as well as samples of spoiled sweet clover, and discovered that the culprit was dicoumarol, a degradative product of coumarin. Researchers synthesized and tested about 50 analogs of this compound. The analogs were

[10] Yeh CH, et al. Evolving use of new oral anticoagulants for treatment of venous thromboembolism. Blood 124:1020−8.

tested in rabbits. It was discovered that the best analog was warfarin (11). Warfarin is also the active ingredient in rodent poison.

Warfarin

b. Origins of Methotrexate and 5-Fluorouracil

The natural substrate of one particular enzyme, dihydrofolate reductase, inspired the design of methotrexate. This natural substrate is *dihydrofolic acid* (12). Dihydrofolic acid is the end-product of the biosynthetic pathway of folates (13). Anticancer drugs that inhibit dihydrofolate reductase were designed by synthesizing and screening chemicals that resembled dihydrofolate (14,15,16). Methotrexate, which is an analog of dihydrofolic acid, and also an analog of folic acid, inhibits dihydrofolic acid reductase. Another antifolate drug used in oncology is 5-fluorouracil. Fluorouracil was invented by Charles Heidelberger (17,18). The drug was developed on the basis of findings in the 1950s that cancer cells incorporated a larger amount of the uracil base into the DNA than normal cells. In testing a number of halogen-substituted uracil compounds, 5-fluorouracil appeared to be the most active and promising drug. Fluorouracil is a *suicide inhibitor* of thymidylate synthase. This means that the enzyme's own catalytic activity results in the activation of the drug, where this activation causes the drug to react covalently with the enzyme, thereby destroying the enzyme's catalytic activity.

Methotrexate

[11]Link KP. The discovery of dicumarol and its sequels. Circulation 1959;19:97−107.

[12]Folic acid is used as a vitamin supplement and for enzymatic studies of dihydrofolic acid reductase. But folic acid is not a naturally occurring chemical. Folic acid is formed during the breakdown of dihydrofolic acid, upon exposure to oxygen. Dihydrofolic acid is a natural product made by microorganisms and plants.

[13]Brown GM, Williamson JM. Biosynthesis of riboflavin, folic acid, thiamine, and pantothenic acid. Adv. Enzymol. Relat. Areas Mol. Biol. 1982;53:345−81.

[14]Friedkin M. Enzymatic aspects of folic acid. Annu. Rev. Biochem. 1963;32:185−214.

[15]Bertino JR. The mechanism of action of folate antagonists in man. Cancer Res. 1963;23:1286−306.

[16]Brody T. Folic acid. In: Machlin LJ, editor. Handbook of vitamins. New York: Marcel Dekker, Inc.; 1990. p. 453−89.

[17]Muggia FM, Peters GJ, Landolph Jr JR. XIII International Charles Heidelberger Symposium and 50 years of fluoropyrimidines in cancer therapy held on September 6 to 8, 2007 at New York University Cancer Institute, Smilow Conference Center. Mol. Cancer Ther. 2009;8:992−9.

[18]Heidelberger C. On the rational development of a new drug: the example of the fluorinated pyrimidines. Cancer Treat. Rep. 1981;65(Suppl. 3):3−9.

c. Origin of Ribavirin

Ribavirin was discovered by synthesizing analogs of a compound participating in the pathways of nucleotide biosynthesis. In designing, synthesizing, and testing a variety of analogs of intermediates in nucleotide biosynthetic pathways, the result was the discovery of ribavirin, also known as virazole (19,20).

Ribavirin, in combination with one or more drugs, is used to treat HCV infections (21,22,23,24,25,26,27,28,29). The other drugs in this combination include sofosbuvir, dasabuvir, and pegylated interferon-alfa. Ribavirin alone has been used to treat hepatitis E virus (30).

Ribavirin

[19]Witkowski JT, Robins RK, Sidwell RW, Simon LN. Design, synthesis, and broad spectrum antiviral activity of 1-beta-D-ribofuranosyl-1,2,4-triazole-3-carboxamide and related nucleosides. J. Med. Chem. 1972;15:1150−4.

[20]Te HS, Randall G, Jensen DM. Mechanism of action of ribavirin in the treatment of chronic hepatitis C. Gastroenterol. Hepatol. 2007;3:218−25.

[21]Feld JJ, Kowdley KV, Coakley E, et al. Treatment of HCV with ABT-450/r-ombitasvir and dasabuvir with ribavirin. New Engl. J. Med. 2014;370:1594−603.

[22]Kwo PY, Mantry PS, Coakley E, et al. An interferon-free antiviral regimen for HCV after liver transplantation. New Engl. J. Med. 2014;371:2375−82.

[23]Zeuzem S, Dusheiko GM, Salupere R, et al. Sofosbuvir and ribavirin in HCV genotypes 2 and 3. New Engl. J. Med. 2014;370:1993−2001.

[24]Afdhal N, Zeuzem S, Kwo P, et al. Ledipasvir and sofosbuvir for untreated HCV genotype 1 infection. New Engl. J. Med. 2014;370:1889−98.

[25]Ferenci P, Bernstein D, Lalezari J, et al. ABT-450/r-ombitasvir and dasabuvir with or without ribavirin for HCV. New Engl. J. Med. 2014;370:1983−92.

[26]Gane EJ, Stedman CA, Hyland RH, et al. Nucleotide polymerase inhibitor sofosbuvir plus ribavirin for hepatitis C. New Engl. J. Med. 2013;368:34−44.

[27]Kamar N, Izopet J, Tripon S, et al. Ribavirin for chronic hepatitis E virus infection in transplant recipients. New Engl. J. Med. 2014;370:1111−20.

[28]Lawitz E, Mangia A, Wyles D, et al. Sofosbuvir for previously untreated chronic hepatitis C infection. New Engl. J. Med. 2013;368:1878−87.

[29]Rodriguez-Torres M, Jeffers LJ, Sheikh MY, et al. Peginterferon alfa-2a and ribavirin in Latino and non-Latino whites with hepatitis C. New Engl. J. Med. 2009;360:257−67.

[30]Zeuzem S, Soriano V, Asselah T, et al. Faldaprevir and deleobuvir for HCV genotype 1 infection. New Engl. J. Med. 2013;369:630−9.

d. Origin of Paclitaxel

Paclitaxel (Taxol®), an anticancer drug, was discovered in extracts of the Pacific yew tree, *Taxus brevifolia*. In 1963, a crude extract from Pacific yew bark was found to have activity against tumors in experimental animals (31). In 1991, the active component, paclitaxel, was approved by the FDA as an anticancer drug. Paclitaxel, which is a class of drugs called taxanes, acts on the cytoskeleton of the cell. Specifically, the drug acts on tubulin, disrupts the normal behavior of the cytoskeleton in mediating cell division, and causes cell death (32). Docetaxel (Taxotere®) is a semisynthetic analog of paclitaxel (33) having a mechanism and anticancer properties similar to those of paclitaxel. Docetaxel can be synthesized using a precursor extracted from needles of the European yew, *Taxus baccata* (34). Paclitaxel finds use in treating various cancers, in a formulation where paclitaxel is bound to albumin (35,36,37). The albumin confers water-solubility to paclitaxel, which is not soluble in water.

Paclitaxel

e. Origin of Cladribine

Cladribine (2-chloro-2'-deoxyadenosine) is a small molecule that is a nucleotide analog. Cladribine is an analog of deoxyadenosine. After administration, cladribine enters various cells and once inside the cell, the enzyme deoxycytidine kinase catalyzes the attachment of three phosphate groups. The result is the conversion of cladribine to cladribine triphosphate. Cladribine triphosphate, in turn, inhibits DNA synthesis, inhibits DNA repair, and results in apoptosis (death of the cell). The drug is most

[31]Socinski MA. Single-agent paclitaxel in the treatment of advanced non-small cell lung cancer. Oncologist 1999;4:408−16.

[32]Pusztai L. Markers predicting clinical benefit in breast cancer from microtubule-targeting agents. Ann. Oncol. 2007;18(Suppl. 12):xii15−20.

[33]Bissery MC, Guénard D, Guéritte-Voegelein F, Lavelle F. Experimental antitumor activity of taxotere (RP 56976, NSC 628503), a taxol analogue. Cancer Res. 1991;51:4845−52.

[34]Verweij J. Docetaxel (Taxotere): a new anti-cancer drug with promising potential? Br. J. Cancer 1994;70:183−4.

[35]Socinski MA. Update on taxanes in the first-line treatment of advanced non-small-cell lung cancer. Curr. Oncol. 2014;21:e691−703.

[36]Socinski MA, et al. Weekly *nab*-paclitaxel in combination with carboplatin versus solvent-based paclitaxel plus carboplatin as first-line therapy in patients with advanced non-small-cell lung cancer: final results of a phase III trial. J. Clin. Oncol. 2012;30:2055−62.

[37]Viudez A, et al. Nab-paclitaxel: a flattering facelift. Crit. Rev. Oncol. Hematol. 2014;92:166-80.

active in cells with high levels of deoxycytidine kinase, such as lymphocytes (38,39). Cladribine is used to treat multiple sclerosis and a type of leukemia (hairy cell leukemia) (40).

The connection between deoxynucleotides and killing lymphocytes, as it applies to cladribine, is as follows. Inherited deficiencies of the enzyme adenosine deaminase interfere with lymphocyte development while sparing most other organ systems (41). The accumulation of deoxyadenosine nucleotides in the lymphocytes, that is, in lymphocytes of people suffering from adenosine deaminase deficiency, reduces the number of lymphocytes. As a consequence, the patients suffer from severe immunodeficiency.

Carson et al. (42) realized that the elimination of adenosine deamidase activity can halt lymphocytes that are pathological, such as the lymphocytes in leukemia (leukemia is a cancer of lymphocytes). This elimination was accomplished by cladribine. Cladribine, in effect, mimics the inherited disease (adenosine deaminase deficiency) because cladribine resists the effects of adenosine deaminase. Cladribine naturally resists deamination catalyzed by adenosine deaminase. (For cladribine to be effective in destroying lymphocytes, it is not necessary that patients be suffering from adenosine deaminase deficiency.) Just as the normally occurring deoxyadenosine kills lymphocytes in people with the genetic disease adenosine deaminase deficiency, cladribine kills lymphocytes when administered to normal humans (43). It was about 10 years after the use of cladribine to treat leukemia that cladribine was first used to treat multiple sclerosis (44,45).

This summarizes the pathway of the discovery of cladribine for multiple sclerosis. First, it was known that an inherited genetic disease involved the accumulation of deoxyadenosine nucleotides in the cell, and resulted in death of lymphocytes. Second, researchers developed a drug that, when administered to a human subject, mimicked the effects of this disease (due to the inability of adenosine deaminase to act on the drug). Third, the drug was used to treat leukemia. Fourth, the drug was used to treat multiple sclerosis (46).

[38]Klanova M, Lorkova L, Vit O, et al. Downregulation of deoxycytidine kinase in cytarabine-resistant mantle cell lymphoma cells confers cross-resistance to nucleoside analogs gemcitabine, fludarabine and cladribine, but not to other classes of anti-lymphoma agents. Mol. Cancer 2014;13:159 (14 pp.).

[39]Piro LD, Carrera CJ, Beutler E, Carson DA. 2-Chlorodeoxyadenosine: an effective new agent for the treatment of chronic lymphocytic leukemia. Blood 1988;72:1069−73.

[40]Rosenburg JD. Clinical characteristics and long-term outcome of young hairy cell leukemia patients treated with cladribine: a single-institution series. Blood 2014;123:177−83.

[41]Carson DA, Kaye J, Seegmiller JE. Lymphospecific toxicity in adenosine deaminase deficiency and purine nucleoside phosphorylase deficiency: possible role of nucleoside kinase(s). Proc. Natl Acad. Sci. USA 1977;74:5677−81.

[42]Carson DA, Wasson DB, Taetle R, Yu A. Specific toxicity of 2-chlorodeoxyadenosine toward resting and proliferating human lymphocytes. Blood 1983;62:737−43.

[43]Piro LD, Carrera CJ, Beutler E, Carson DA. 2-Chlorodeoxyadenosine: an effective new agent for the treatment of chronic lymphocytic leukemia. Blood 1988;72:1069−73.

[44]Sipe JC, Romine JS, Koziol JA, McMillan R, Zyroff J, Beutler E. Cladribine in treatment of chronic progressive multiple sclerosis. Lancet 1994;344:9−13.

[45]Beutler E, Koziol JA, McMillan R, Sipe JC, Romine JS, Carrera CJ. Marrow suppression produced by repeated doses of cladribine. Acta Haematol. 1994;91:10−15.

[46]Giovannoni G, Comi G, Cook S, et al. A placebo-controlled trial of oral cladribine for relapsing multiple sclerosis. New Engl. J. Med. 2010;362:416−26.

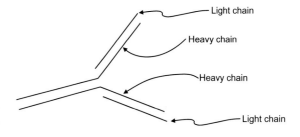

f. Origins of Therapeutic Antibodies

Antibodies designed with the aid of animal models are used to treat various cancers and immune diseases. For example, antibody drugs include trastuzumab (Herceptin®) (47), which binds to epidermal growth factor, and which is used to treat breast cancer. Antibody drugs also include bevacizumab (Avastin®) (48), which binds to vascular endothelial growth factor receptor (VEGFR), and is used to treat a variety of cancers. Moreover, an antibody drug used to treat various immune diseases is natalizumab (Tysabri®) (49). This antibody binds to a protein called integrin, which occurs on the surface of white blood cells. Natalizumab is used to treat two autoimmune diseases, multiple sclerosis and Crohn's disease.

Developing antibody drugs includes the step of refining the polypeptide sequence of the antibody into a drug suitable for administering to humans (50,51,52). This refinement step is called humanization (53). Humanization refers to the process of using genetic engineering to convert any protein of animal origin to a protein that can be injected into people, where the injected protein fails to elicit an immune reaction against itself.

Antibodies take the form of four polypeptides, two light chains and two heavy chains, as indicated in the diagram below. The first light chain and first heavy chain are covalently attached to each other by disulfide bonds, to form a first complex. The second light chain and second heavy chain are covalently attached to each by disulfide bonds to form a second complex. The first complex and second complex are also covalently attached to each other by way of disulfide bonds.

[47]Verma S, Lavasani S, Mackey J, et al. Optimizing the management of her2-positive early breast cancer: the clinical reality. Curr. Oncol. 2010;17:20−33.

[48]Eskens FA, Sleijfer S. The use of bevacizumab in colorectal, lung, breast, renal and ovarian cancer: where does it fit? Eur. J. Cancer 2008;44:2350−6.

[49]Coyle PK. The role of natalizumab in the treatment of multiple sclerosis. Am. J. Manag. Care 2010;16(6 Suppl.): S164−70.

[50]Kent SJ, Karlik SJ, Cannon C, et al. A monoclonal antibody to alpha 4 integrin suppresses and reverses active experimental allergic encephalomyelitis. J. Neuroimmunol. 1995;58:1−10.

[51]Yednock TA, Cannon C, Fritz LC, et al. Prevention of experimental autoimmune encephalomyelitis by antibodies against alpha 4 beta 1 integrin. Nature 1992;356:63−6.

[52]Brody T. Multistep denaturation and hierarchy of disulfide bond cleavage of a monoclonal antibody. Analyt. Biochem. 1997;247:247−56.

[53]Presta LG. Molecular engineering and design of therapeutic antibodies. Curr. Opin. Immunol. 2008;20:460−70.

As an example of an antibody drug, the amino acid sequence of the light chain and the amino acid sequence of the heavy chain of trastuzumab are shown below (54).

The amino acid sequence of the light chain of trastuzumab, as found at the cited accession numbers (55,56), is shown below. The light chain, shown below, has 214 amino acids.

```
DIQMTQSPSSLSASVGDRVTITCRASQDVNT
AVAWYQQKPGKAPKLLIYSASFLYSGVPSRFSGS
RSGTDFTLTISSLQPEDFATYYCQQHYTTPPTFG
QGTKVEIKRTVAAPSFIFPPSDEQLKSGTASVVC
LLNNFYPREAKVQWKVDNALQSGNSQESVTEQDS
KDSTYSLSSTLTLSKADYEKHKVYACEVTHQGLS
SPVTKSFNRGEC
```

The amino acid sequence of the heavy chain of this antibody, which has 451 amino acids and can be found at the cited accession number (57), is shown below.

```
EVQLVESGGGLVQPGGSLRLSCAASGFNIKD
TYIHWVRQAPGKGLEWVARIYPTNGYTRYADSVK
GRFTISADTSKNTAYLQMNSLRAEDTAVYYCSRW
GGDGFYAMDYWGQGTLVTVSSASTKGPSVFPLA
PSSKSTSGGTAALGCLVKDYFPEPVTVSWNSGAL
TSGVHTFPAVLQSSGLYSLSSVVTVPSSSLGTQT
YICNVNHKPSNTKVDKKVEPPKSCDKTHTCPPCP
APELLGGPSVFLFPPKPKDTLMISRTPEVTCVVV
DVSHEDPEVKFNWYVDGVEVHNAKTKPREEQYNS
TYRVVSVLTVLHQDWLNGKEYKCKVSNKALPAPI
EKTISKAKGQPREPQVYTLPPSRDELTKNQVSLT
CLVKGFYPSDIAVEWESNGQPENNYKTTPPVLDS
DGSFFLYSKLTVDKSRWQQGNVFSCSVMHEALHN
HYTQKSLSLSPGK
```

The three-dimensional structure of this antibody drug can be found at: www.drugbank. ca/drugs/DB00072

Let us dwell on the structure of the light chain and heavy chain for a moment. In testing and marketing any polypeptide drug, pharmaceutical companies are concerned with the following drug stability issues. First, it is the case that long-term storage of polypeptides results in the spontaneous deamination of residues of glutamine (Q) and asparagine (N). Deamination can occur at various steps in the manufacturing process, during shipment, and during storage. Also, oxidation of cysteine (C) residues can occur during manufacturing, shipping, and storage. These types of damage may lower the potency of polypeptide drugs. The reader will be able to find the locations of Q, N, and C, in the polypeptide chains of trastuzumab.

III. THE 20 CLASSICAL AMINO ACIDS

This reviews the 20 classical amino acids (Table 1.1). Twenty *classical* amino acids exist, and these are listed, along with their abbreviations in Table 1.1. The *nonclassical* amino acids include homocysteine, selenocysteine (58), methionine sulfoxide, ornithine, gamma-carboxyglutamate (GLA) (59), phosphotyrosine, hydroxyproline (60), sarcosine, and betaine. A *protein* is a long polypeptide that is a linear

[54]Fong S, Hu Z. Therapeutic anti-HER2 antibody fusion polypeptides. U.S. Pat. Appl. Publ. 2009/0226466; 2009. September 10.

[55]Cho HS, Mason K, Ramyar KX, et al. GenBank Accession No. PDB:1N8Z_A (submitted November 21, 2002).

[56]http://www.drugbank.ca/drugs/DB00072

[57]Trastuzumab (DB00072) DrugBank Accession No. DB0072. Creation date June 13, 2005, updated June 2, 2009.

[58]Brody T. Nutritional biochemistry. 2nd ed. San Diego, CA: Academic Press; 1999. p. 21 and 825−7.

[59]Brody T, Suttie JW. Evidence for the glycoprotein nature of vitamin K-dependent carboxylase from rat liver. Biochim. Biophys. Acta 1987;923:1−7.

[60]Brody T. Nutritional biochemistry. 2nd ed. San Diego, CA: Academic Press; 1999. p. 21 and 619−23.

TABLE 1.1 The 20 Classical Amino Acids

Amino Acid	One-Letter Abbreviation	Three-Letter Abbreviation
AMINO ACIDS WITH CHARGED SIDE GROUP		
Glutamic acid	E	Glu
Aspartic acid	D	Asp
Lysine	K	Lys
Histidine	H	His
Arginine	R	Arg
Asparagine	N	Asn
Glutamine	Q	Gln
AMINO ACIDS WITH LIPOPHILIC (HYDROPHOBIC) SIDE CHAIN		
Phenylalanine	F	Phe
Tyrosine	Y	Tyr
Leucine	L	Leu
Isoleucine	I	Ileu
Valine	V	Val
Tryptophan	W	Trp
AMINO ACID WITH HYDROXYL GROUP		
Serine	S	Ser
Threonine	T	Thr
AMINO ACIDS WITH SULFUR ATOM		
Cysteine	C	Cys
Methionine	M	Met
OTHER AMINO ACIDS		
Glycine	G	Gly
Alanine	A	Ala
Proline	P	Pro

polymer of amino acids, typically about 100–500 amino acids in length. The term *oligopeptide* refers to shorter polymers of amino acids in the range of about 10–50 amino acids. Some nonclassical amino acids, such as homocysteine, exist only in the free state, and do not become incorporated into any polypeptide. But other nonclassical amino acids, such as GLA and phosphotyrosine, occur in naturally occurring proteins because of a process called *post-translational modification*.

Table 1.1 identifies which amino acids have a side chain that is charged, and thus interact well with water, and amino acids with an uncharged side chain, and thus do not much interact with water. The terms hydrophilic and hydrophobic are used to refer to chemicals, or to regions of chemicals, that are charged and that are uncharged, respectively. Hydrophilic groups include carboxyl groups, amino groups, and hydroxyl groups. Hydrophobic groups include alkane chains and aromatic rings. Although the term "hydrophobic" is in common use, it has been pointed out that there does not exist any force or interaction in nature that is a hydrophobic force or interaction (61).

A knowledge of the amino acids is needed to understand:

- drug stability during manufacturing and storage,
- point of attachment of polyethylene glycol (PEG) to the drug, where relevant,
- unwanted immunogenicity,
- immunogenicity that is desired and essential for drug efficacy.

This concerns in vitro stability. For drugs that are oligopeptides or proteins, stability

---

[61]Hildebrand JH. Is there a "hydrophobic effect"? Proc. Natl Acad. Sci. 1979;76:194.

during manufacturing and storage is an issue because of spontaneous deamidation. Aswad and coworkers have detailed the deamidation of biologicals (62,63). The stability of proteins can also be compromised by degradation catalyzed by contaminating proteases and by the related issue of aggregation (64,65,66). Proteases can occur as contaminants during the drug-manufacturing process, and proteases also occur in the human body. Polyethylene glycol can be connected to recombinant enzymes and cytokines to enhance the stability and lifetime of the drug in the bloodstream. Polypeptide drugs that are modified in this way are called, pegylated polypeptides (67,68,69), where the polyethylene glycol can be attached to residues of lysine or arginine (70,71,72).

For drugs that are antibodies, enzymes, cytokines, and hormones, what is desired is that the drug not be immunogenic. In striking contrast, for drugs that are vaccines, what is desired and essential, is that the drug stimulate a vigorous immunogenic response. A knowledge of the amino acids is needed for understanding all of the above issues. Undesired immunogenicity arises where the drug takes the form of extract from a tissue or organ from an animal, or where the drug takes the form of a recombinant version of an animal protein. Undesired immunogenicity can be reduced or eliminated by the process of "humanization," where the genetic engineer alters the primary sequence of the animal protein so that it matches the primary sequence of the corresponding human protein (73).

[62]Paranandi MV, Guzzetta AW, Hancock WS, Aswad DW. Deamidation and isoaspartate formation during in vitro aging of recombinant tissue plasminogen activator. J. Biol. Chem. 1994;269:243–53.

[63]Aswad DW, Paranandi MV, Schurter BT. Isoaspartate in peptides and proteins: formation, significance, and analysis. J. Pharm. Biomed. Anal. 2000;21:1129–36.

[64]Simpson RJ. Stabilization of proteins for storage. Cold Spring Harb. Protocol. 2010;2010(5).

[65]O'Fágáin C. Storage and lyophilisation of pure proteins. Methods Mol. Biol. 2011;681:179–202.

[66]Chi EY, Krishnan S, Randolph TW, Carpenter JF. Physical stability of proteins in aqueous solution: mechanism and driving forces in nonnative protein aggregation. Pharm. Res. 2003;20:1325–36.

[67]Ramos EL. Preclinical and clinical development of pegylated interferon-lambda 1 in chronic hepatitis C. J. Interferon Cytokine Res. 2010;30:591–5.

[68]Hershfield MS, Roberts LJ II, Ganson NJ, et al. Treating gout with pegloticase, a PEGylated urate oxidase, provides insight into the importance of uric acid as an antioxidant in vivo. Proc. Natl Acad. Sci. USA 2010;107:14351–6.

[69]Fishburn CS. The pharmacology of PEGylation: balancing PD with PK to generate novel therapeutics. J. Pharm. Sci. 2008;97:4167–83.

[70]Lee H, Park TG. Preparation and characterization of mono-PEGylated epidermal growth factor: evaluation of in vitro biologic activity. Pharm. Res. 2002;19:845–51.

[71]Veronese F, Sartore L, Orsolini P, Deghenghi R. U.S. Pat. No. 5,286,637.

[72]Gauthier MA, Klok HA. Arginine-specific modification of proteins with polyethylene glycol. Biomacromolecules 2011;12:482–93.

[73]Kuramochi T, et al. Humanization and simultaneous optimization of monoclonal antibody. Methods Mol. Biol. 2014;1060:123–37.

IV. ANIMAL MODELS

a. Introduction to Animal Models of Human Diseases

Animals are used for studying the biochemistry, molecular biology, and genetics of various diseases, that is, the disease mechanism. Once a suitable animal has been found where the mechanism is similar to that of a corresponding disease in humans, that particular animal may be used as an animal model for testing efficacy of candidate drugs. For oncology, animal models are typically injected with tumor cells. For immune disorders, animals are administered an agent that provokes inflammation. And for infections, animals are exposed to the relevant microorganism or virus.

For these reasons, animal models are described in this chapter. For the sake of continuity, what is also included are specialized topics on animals, such as validation, the Animal Rule, and use of animal data to arrive at doses for humans.

Regulatory approval for drugs requires data on safety and efficacy in animals. While data on safety can be acquired from studies on mice, rats, rabbits, dogs, and primates, with little or no need for correspondence of mechanisms of an animal disease with mechanisms of a human disease, data on efficacy can only be acquired where there is an available animal model of the disorder in question. Where the goal of the drug is to enhance wound healing, it is easy to find a suitable animal model (all that is needed is to surgically remove a circle of skin from the animal). However, where the goal of the drug is to treat diseases such as cancer, immune diseases, or infections, there is a need to find an appropriate animal model. Brody (74) describes animal models for various diseases, and reveals the criteria needed for an animal model to predict the efficacy of a drug for the disease in humans.

While rodents spontaneously develop various cancers, it is not practical to acquire a group of rodents with the same type of cancer, and at the same stage of the cancer, at the same time. The variety of tumors that occurs spontaneously in rats has been exhaustively documented (75,76).

Separate animal models are available for various types of cancer. Marks (77) identified sources of various animal cancer models. Nandan and Yang (78), Kuperwasser et al. (79), Soda et al. (80), and Noonan et al. (81), discuss animal models for colorectal cancer, breast cancer, nonsmall-cell lung cancer, and melanoma, respectively.

[74]Brody T. Enabling claims under 35 USC §112 to methods of medical treatment or diagnosis, based on *in vitro* cell culture models and animal models. J. Patent Trademark Office Soc. 2015;97:328−411.

[75]Son WC, Bell D, Taylor I, Mowat V. Profile of early occurring spontaneous tumors in Han Wistar rats. Toxicol. Pathol. 2010;38:292−6.

[76]Bomhard E. Frequency of spontaneous tumors in Wistar rats in 30-months studies. Exp. Toxicol. Pathol. 1992;44:381−92.

[77]Marks C. Mouse Models of Human Cancers Consortium (MMHCC) from the NCI. Dis. Model Mech. 2009;2:111.

[78]Nandan MO, Yang VW. Genetic and chemical models of colorectal cancer in mice. Curr. Colorectal Cancer Rep. 2010;6:51−9.

[79]Kuperwasser C, Dessain S, Bierbaum BE, et al. A mouse model of human breast cancer metastasis to human bone. Cancer Res. 2005;65:6130−8.

[80]Soda M, Takada S, Takeuchi K, et al. A mouse model for EML4-ALK-positive lung cancer. Proc. Natl Acad. Sci. USA 2008;105:19893−7.

[81]Noonan FP, Dudek J, Merlino G, De Fabo EC. Animal models of melanoma: an HGF/SF transgenic mouse model may facilitate experimental access to UV initiating events. Pigment Cell Res. 2003;16:16−25.

Similarly, animal models for certain infections are available. Animal models for infectious diseases include the woodchuck (82), which is the animal model of choice for hepatitis B virus, the chimpanzee (83), which is an appropriate large-animal model for HCV, and the armadillo (84), which is the animal model for *Mycobacterium leprae*, the cause of leprosy (Hansen's disease). A suitable small-animal model for hepatitis C infections has not yet been found.

In proposing and using animal models for disorders that have an immune component, it is useful to be aware of the similarities (and differences) between the mouse immune system and the human immune system. Mestas and Hughes (85) outline some of these similarities and differences. Researchers conducting animal models on diseases with an immune component, that is, cancer, autoimmune diseases, and inflammatory disorders, need to be aware of similarities and differences in the immune systems between their animal and humans. For example, comparisons between mouse and human dendritic cells (86), T cells (87), B cells (88), NK cells (89), macrophages (90), eosinophils (91), and toll-like receptors (TLRs) (92), are available.

Animal models for immune disorders include the following. A rodent model for multiple sclerosis, called EAE (93), involves injecting animals with myelin basic protein (94). A mouse model for rheumatoid arthritis involves injecting

[82]Menne S, Cote PJ. The woodchuck as an animal model for pathogenesis and therapy of chronic hepatitis B virus infection. World J. Gastroenterol. 2007;13:104−24.

[83]Bukh J, Thimme R, Meunier JC, et al. Previously infected chimpanzees are not consistently protected against reinfection or persistent infection after reexposure to the identical hepatitis C virus strain. J. Virol. 2008;82:8183−95.

[84]Hamilton HK, Levis WR, Martiniuk F, Cabrera A, Wolf J. The role of the armadillo and sooty mangabey monkey in human leprosy. Int. J. Dermatol. 2008;47:545−50.

[85]Mestas J, Hughes CC. Of mice and not men: differences between mouse and human immunology. J. Immunol. 2004;172:2731−8.

[86]Boonstra A, Asselin-Paturel C, Gilliet M, et al. Flexibility of mouse classical and plasmacytoid-derived dendritic cells in directing T helper type 1 and 2 cell development: dependency on antigen dose and differential toll-like receptor ligation. J. Exp. Med. 2003;197:101−9.

[87]Walzer T, Arpin C, Beloeil L, Marvel J. Differential in vivo persistence of two subsets of memory phenotype CD8 T cells defined by CD44 and CD122 expression levels. J. Immunol. 2002;168:2704−11.

[88]Frasca D, Landin AM, Riley RL, Blomberg BB. Mechanisms for decreased function of B cells in aged mice and humans. J. Immunol. 2008;180:2741−6.

[89]Ehrlich LI, Ogasawara K, Hamerman JA, et al. Engagement of NKG2D by cognate ligand or antibody alone is insufficient to mediate costimulation of human and mouse CD8 + T cells. J. Immunol. 2005;174:1922−31.

[90]Sunderkötter C, Nikolic T, Dillon MJ, et al. Subpopulations of mouse blood monocytes differ in maturation stage and inflammatory response. J. Immunol. 2004;172:4410−7.

[91]Dyer KD, Percopo CM, Xie Z, Yang Z, et al. Mouse and human eosinophils degranulate in response to platelet-activating factor (PAF) and lysoPAF via a PAF-receptor-independent mechanism: evidence for a novel receptor. J. Immunol. 2010;184:6327−34.

[92]Janssens S, Beyaert R. Role of Toll-like receptors in pathogen recognition. Clin. Microbiol. Rev. 2003;16:637−46.

[93]Mix E, Meyer-Rienecker H, Zettl UK. Animal models of multiple sclerosis for the development and validation of novel therapies—potential and limitations. J. Neurol. 2008;255(Suppl. 6):7−14.

[94]Zaller DM, Osman G, Kanagawa O, Hood L. Prevention and treatment of murine experimental allergic encephalomyelitis with T cell receptor V beta-specific antibodies. J. Exp. Med. 1990;171:1943−55.

collagen (95). A mouse model for inflammatory bowel disease employs a strain of mice that naturally develops inflammation of the intestinal tract (96). Psoriasis (97), lupus (98), asthma (99), and other immune disorders also have well-characterized animal models.

b. FDA Regulations and Animal Models

Animal models are used to provide data on safety and efficacy, where the data are included in various FDA submissions. Relevant issues include:

- disease mechanisms,
- validation,
- good laboratory practice (GLP),
- animal rule.

Animals are used in the following situations. The first is for discovering the mechanisms of a disease. Second, animals are used for discovering the mechanisms of drug action (with or without regard to any disease). In other words, the ability of the anticancer drug *ibrutinib* to inhibit Bruton's tyrosine kinase can be studied in noncancerous cells, as well as in cancer cells (100). Third, the issue of animals arises when there is a need to develop a suitable animal model for a disease. Fourth, the issue of animals occurs in the validation of an existing animal model for a disease. And fifth, the issue of animals occurs when

conducting animal studies in compliance with GLP. GLP governs many laboratory practices in addition to those involving animals. The following comments also disclose adverse consequences to a Sponsor, where the Sponsor's use of animals fails to comply with various FDA regulations, as set forth by 21 CFR §58 and by GLP.

c. Disease Mechanisms

An animal model may be ideally suited for determining the mechanism of a disease, and for the screening of candidate drugs, but may be inappropriate and ill-suited for determining efficacy or safety of a particular type of therapy for that disease. The fruitfly is one type of an animal model that is not likely to be accepted by the FDA, for convincing the FDA of a drug's efficacy and safety. The proven utility of the fruitfly model is as follows. According to Poidevin et al. (101), the fruitfly *Drosophila melanogaster* is:

> a premiere model system for the study of human neurodegenerative diseases, due to the realization that flies and humans share many structurally and functionally related gene families. Development of such disease models in the fly allows ... the existing fruit fly models of human neurological disorders to identify small-molecule leads that could potentially be further developed for therapeutic use.

[95]Cho YG, Cho ML, Min SY, Kim HY. Type II collagen autoimmunity in a mouse model of human rheumatoid arthritis. Autoimmun. Rev. 2007;7:65−70.

[96]Wilk JN, Bilsborough J, Viney JL. The mdr1a-/- mouse model of spontaneous colitis: a relevant and appropriate animal model to study inflammatory bowel disease. Immunol. Res. 2005;31:151−9.

[97]Schön MP. Animal models of psoriasis: a critical appraisal. Exp. Dermatol. 2008;17:703−912.

[98]Cohen PL, Maldonado MA. Animal models for SLE. Curr. Protoc. Immunol. 2003;Chapter 15:Unit 15.20.

[99]Takeda K, Gelfand EW. Mouse models of allergic diseases. Curr. Opin. Immunol. 2009;21:660−5.

[100]Woyach J, Furman RR, Liu TM, et al. Resistance mechanisms for Bruton's tyrosine kinase inhibitor ibrutinib. New Engl. J. Med. 2014;370:2286−94.

[101]Poidevin M, et al. Small-molecule screening using *Drosophila* models of human neurological disorders. Methods Mol. Biol. 2015;1263:127−38.

Moreover, Pandey and Nichols (102) state that the fruitfly is useful for determining the mechanisms and for drug screening for a variety of human disorders. According to these authors, the fruitfly:

> can effectively be used for ... high-throughput drug screens as well as in target discovery ... [and for] models of human diseases and opportunities for therapeutic discovery for central nervous system disorders, inflammatory disorders, cardiovascular disease, cancer, and diabetes.

Guidance on why certain animal models are not appropriate for establishing efficacy of any given drug comes from an agency of the US government other than FDA, namely, the US Patent and Trademark Office (USPTO). From the USPTO, superlative and consistent guidance on certain issues is provided by the Patent Trial and Appeal Board (PTAB). This guidance takes the form of many thousands of published opinions from the Board, for example, *Ex parte Steffan* (103).

Ex parte Steffan concerned a proposal to treat a human disease (Huntington's disease) with a drug, where this proposal was based on data from an animal model. The animal model was a genetically altered fruitfly. In the fruitfly study, the investigators discovered that the neurological disease in the fruitfly could be cured by mutating one of the fruitfly's genes. The gene was the *smt3* gene. The mutation in the *smt3* gene suppressed neurodegeneration in the fruitfly, just as the eventual goal of

the investigators was to suppress neurodegeneration in human patients. The Patent Office refused to accept the fruitfly model as a suitable model for treating Huntington's disease in humans. The reasons for refusing to accept the fruitfly model include the following:

• Invertebrates models are unpredictable.
• Drugs cannot be administered to flies. Please note that invertebrates have an open circulatory system, and do not have any arteries or veins (104).
• The method that successfully prevented the disease in the fruitflies (mutating the *smt* gene in the chromosome) cannot be performed on human patients.
• Mammalian animal models are closer to humans than invertebrates. The Patent Office stated that, "non-human mammals ... more closely replicate the essential features of the pathophysiology of the disease in humans, as compared to invertebrate models" (105).

In a similar published opinion from the Board, the Board considered the ability of a genetically modified mouse to be a model for treatment of human degenerative diseases. As described in *Ex parte Franzoso* (106) the genetically modified mouse was engineered to have a mutation in the *Gadd45beta* gene. The eventual goal of the investigators was to develop an administrable drug that inhibits the *Gadd45beta* gene in humans. However, the Board refused to accept the mouse model.

---

[102]Pandey UB, Nichols CD. Human disease models in *Drosophila melanogaster* and the role of the fly in therapeutic drug discovery. Pharmacol. Rev. 2011;63:411–36.

[103]*Ex parte* Steffan, No. 2009-005999 (B.P.A.I. Mar. 2, 2010).

[104]Brody T, Mathews TD. The release of zinc from leukocytes provoked by A23187 and EDTA is associated with the release of enzymes. Comp. Biochem. Physiol. Part A 1989;94:693–7.

[105]Examiner's Answer of Aug. 5, 2008, at 7, in file history of U.S. Patent Application No. 10/789,518.

[106]*Ex parte* Franzoso, No. 2007–2724 (B.P.A.I. Mar. 12, 2008).

To summarize, fruitflies and other animals such as zebrafish (107) (model for cardiovascular diseases), as well as treatment of mice by mutating a particular gene, are commonly used as animal models for human diseases. However, it is not likely that animals such as these will be accepted by the FDA to establish safety and efficacy for a given drug in humans, to the extent that the FDA will be persuaded to approve the initiation of a clinical trial. The present commentary helps to provide a definition of an acceptable animal model for treating a disease, by an example of what is *not an acceptable model*.

d. Developing an Accepted Animal Model for a Disease

The first step in arriving at an animal model for a disease is to develop an animal model that resembles the human condition, in view of the physiology of the disease, symptoms of the disease, and response to therapeutic interventions, such as to an administered drug. Varga et al. (108) used the term "valid animal model" to refer to an animal model that resembles the human condition, but this use of the word "valid" is not the same as the defined process of "validation."

Regarding the history of the development of animal models, one of the first steps in adopting the rat as a standard animal took place at the University of Wisconsin-Madison, where E.V. McCollum advocated using rats instead of cows. Initially, the idea was met with adversity, as documented by McCollum's statement that, "Professor Hart was astonished and offended at my pronouncement on the cow project. He was contemptuous of my suggestion that we turn to the rat as an experimental animal" (109). Over the course of decades, rats as well as other animals, became standard models for testing various pharmaceuticals, as demonstrated by a guidance document issued by the FDA (110).

A conventional animal model for arthritis involves the generation of arthritis-like symptoms by injecting antibodies raised against type II collagen into the animal (111,112). A conventional animal model for multiple sclerosis, called EAE, involves injecting myelin-derived proteins into the animal (113,114). Recombinant animals that are animal models for diseases include the PDAPP transgenic mouse model for Alzheimer's disease, which is engineered to express a mutant human amyloid precursor protein (115). An animal model

[107]Asnani A, Peterson RT. The zebrafish as a tool to identify novel therapies for human cardiovascular disease. Dis. Model Mech. 2014;7:763−7.

[108]Varga OE, et al. Validating animal models for preclinical research: a scientific and ethical discussion. Alternat. Lab Anim. 2010;38:245−8.

[109]McCollum EV. The paths to the discovery of vitamins A and D. J. Nutr. 1967;91(Suppl. 1):11−6.

[110]U.S. Department of Health and Human Services. Food and Drug Administration. Guidance for industry. Estimating the safe starting dose in clinical trials for therapeutics in adult healthy volunteers; 2002.

[111]Nandakumar KS, et al. Collagen type II-specific monoclonal antibody-induced arthritis in mice: description of the disease and the influence of age, sex, and genes. Am. J. Pathol. 2002;163:1827−37.

[112]Stuart JM, et al. Collagen autoimmune arthritis. Annu. Rev. Immunol. 1984;2:199−218.

[113]Yednock TA, et al. Prevention of experimental autoimmune encephalomyelitis by antibodies against alpha 4 beta 1 integrin. Nature 1991;356:63−6.

[114]MacKay IR, et al. Immunopathological comparisons between experimental autoimmune encephalomyelitis and multiple sclerosis. Clin. Exp. Immunol. 1973;15:471−82.

[115]Schenk D, et al. Immunization with amyloid-beta attenuates Alzheimer-disease-like pathology, the PDAPP mouse. Nature 1999;400:173−7.

that was created with recombinant technology is the "Harvard Mouse," which is a mouse engineered to express an oncogene, such as the *c-myc* gene (116).

The European Medicines Agency (EMA) has provided guidance for assessing the validity of a given animal model for use in testing the efficacy of a drug for a particular disease. According to the EMA (117):

> Qualitative and quantitative differences may exist in biological responses in animals compared to humans. For example, there might be differences in affinity for molecular targets, tissue distribution of the molecular target, cellular consequences of target binding, cellular regulatory mechanisms, metabolic pathways, or compensatory responses to an initial physiological perturbation.

e. Validation of Animal Models

After an animal model has been identified or developed, one can establish the validity of that model by way of the process of "validation." According to Varga et al. (118), validating an animal model includes development of a particular procedure or test that uses a specific type of animal, followed by employing the laboratory procedure, independently conducted in a blind trial, by at least three different laboratories. This interlaboratory trial is followed by data analysis and an evaluation of the outcome of the study in comparison with predefined performance criteria. The final step in validation may take the form of acceptance by a regulatory

agency, such as a national or international organization.

f. GLP, as It Applies to Animal Studies

GLP is a set of standards set forth by the FDA.

Before the FDA grants approval to a Sponsor to initiate recruiting of human subjects and to conduct a clinical trial, the Sponsor is required to submit nonclinical safety and toxicology studies to demonstrate that the proposed drug entity is likely to be safe with testing in a clinical trial on human subjects. The term "nonclinical studies" encompasses studies with animals, in vitro cell culture, and the Ames bacterial mutagenicity test. These nonclinical studies are governed by GLP regulations (119). GLP is regulated by Title 21 CFR §58. Title 21 CFR §58 is entitled, "Good Laboratory Practice for Nonclinical Laboratory Studies." If there are deficiencies in GLP, for example, in the maintenance of the animal facility, the FDA may issue a *Refuse to File* (RTF) notice. The consequence of the RTF notice is that the FDA halts any further review of the Sponsor's application, until the Sponsor takes appropriate remedial action. Title 21 CFR §58 provides concrete guidance on what is required for animal studies. For example, 21 CFR §58.90 sets forth requirements for animal care:

> Animal cages, racks and accessory equipment shall be cleaned and sanitized at appropriate

[116]Pattengale PK, et al. Animal models of human disease. Pathology and molecular biology of spontaneous neoplasms occurring in transgenic mice carrying and expressing activated cellular oncogenes. Am. J. Pathol. 1989;135:39−61.

[117]European Medicines Agency. Committee for Medicinal Products for Human Use (July 2007) Guideline on Strategies to Identify and Mitigate Risks for First-in-Human Clinical Trials with Investigational Medicine Products (12 pp.).

[118]Varga OE, et al. Validating animal models for preclinical research: a scientific and ethical discussion. Alternat. Lab Anim. 2010;38:245−8.

[119]Adamo JE, Bauer G, Berro, M, et al. A roadmap for academic health centers to establish good laboratory practice-compliant infrastructure. Acad. Med. 2012;87:279−84.

intervals ... [f]eed and water used for the animals shall be analyzed periodically to ensure that contaminants known to be capable of interfering with the study and reasonably expected to be present in such feed or water are not present at levels above those specified in the protocol. Documentation of such analyses shall be maintained as raw data.

To give another example about animal care, 21 CFR §58.120 sets forth requirements about written protocols, records of test articles (drugs), animal weight, and diet:

Each study shall have an approved written protocol that clearly indicates the objectives and all methods for the conduct of the study. The protocol shall contain ... [i]dentification of the test and control articles by name, chemical abstract number, or code number ... [t]he number, body weight range, sex, source of supply, species, strain, substrain, and age of the test system ... [a] description and/or identification of the diet ... [e]ach dosage level, expressed in milligrams per kilogram of body weight or other appropriate units, of the test or control article to be administered and the method and frequency of administration.

Thus, it is self-evident that GLP encompasses a number of topics relating to the Sponsor's laboratories. These topics overlap those used in basic research, but with the following exception. In basic research, laboratory procedures are likely to change every month, in response to experimental results. However, GLP allows for little flexibility and hence is not compatible with most types of basic research.

If a sponsor is found not to comply with GLP, then the FDA may respond by disqualifying a testing facility (21 CFR §58.202). Grounds for disqualification include a situation where noncompliance adversely affects the validity of the animal studies or any other nonclinical laboratory studies, or where the Sponsor ignores warnings from the FDA.

The term "483" is known throughout the pharmaceutical industry (120). Following an inspection of a testing facility by FDA officials, the FDA may issue a warning on a document called, Form FDA-483. The nature of Form FDA-483 is as follows (121):

The FDA-483 is the written notice of objectionable practices or deviations from the regulations that is prepared by the FDA investigator at the end of the inspection. The items listed on the form serve as the basis for the exit discussion with laboratory management at which time management can either agree or disagree with the items and can offer possible corrective actions to be taken.

Regarding validation of each written protocol, it is the case that the FDA acknowledged the need for flexibility in how the Sponsor establishes validity. To this end, the FDA's Guidance for Industry states that (122):

Who assesses protocol validity (Number of animals, test article dosage, test system, etc.)? This is done by the study scientists using the scientific literature, published guidelines, advice from regulatory agencies, and prior experimental work.

If a Sponsor submits data from animal studies, as part of an FDA submission, the FDA may respond by sending a RTF notice to the Sponsor. According to the FDA's *Manual of Policies and Procedures*, the FDA issues a RTF if, "[t]he application does not contain a statement for each nonclinical laboratory study that it was

---

[120]Pritchett T. A 483 Primer. Learning from the mistakes of others. BioProcess Int.; March 2011 (4 pp.).

[121]U.S. Department of Health and Human Services. Food and Drug Administration. Guidance for industry. Good laboratory practices questions and answers; July 2007 (25 pp.).

[122]U.S. Department of Health and Human Services. Food and Drug Administration. Guidance for industry. Good laboratory practices questions and answers; July 2007 (25 pp.).

conducted in compliance with the requirements set forth in 21 CFR Part 58" (123). The FDA has commented on the frequency of RTF decisions, where these decisions are based on a number of problems, not merely on issues in test animals that occur in nonclinical studies (124).

GLP is applied, for example, to in vivo mutagenicity studies, acute toxicity studies, chronic toxicity studies, and carcinogenicity studies. However, GLP does not apply to clinical studies, or to studies on veterinary drugs in animals (125). A quality assurance manager, quality control analysts, and standard operating procedures (SOPs), are used in laboratories operating under GLP (126).

g. Examples of FDA Form 483 Warning Letters, as Applied to Animal Studies

FDA Form 483 warning letters are available on the FDA's website. Problems relating to animals are only one of the many problems that can provoke the FDA to issue a Form 483. Please note the following. Although Form 483 letters are available on the FDA's website

device that is called, "Warning Letters," it is not the case that Form 483 is exactly the same thing as a Warning Letter. Form 483 letters are issued with a minimal amount of review while, in contrast, Warning Letters are issued by the FDA only after high-level review by attorneys employed by the FDA (127). It is common for Form 483 to be referred to as a "warning letter" (128). For convenience, the present commentary refers to Form 483 as a "warning letter."

The following Warning Letter complained about the Sponsor's *failure to clean animal cages*. The Warning Letter refers to a SOP, and to the failure of the Sponsor to comply with this particular SOP (129):

> Dear Dr. [REDACTED]:
> The FDA investigators met with you and other members of your staff to review [your] Corporation's conduct of nonclinical laboratory studies ... performed under the Good Laboratory Practice (GLP) for Nonclinical Laboratory Studies regulations [21 CFR Part 58] ... [a]t the end of the inspection a Form FDA 483, Inspectional Observations, was issued and discussed with you ... we conclude that [your company] has violated GLP regulations governing the

[123]U.S. Department of Health and Human Services. Food and Drug Administration. Manual of policies and procedures. Good review practice: refuse to file; October 11, 2013 (21 pp.).

[124]According to Janet Rehnquist, "[a]lthough FDA can refuse to file applications, it rarely does so. The CDER refused to file 4 percent of submitted applications in FY 2000, down from 17 percent in 1993. In part, this decrease may be attributable to the advice FDA provides sponsors that helps them prepare higher quality applications." See, Rehnquist, J. FDA's review process for new drug applications. A management review. Department of Health and Human Services; March 2003 (47 pp.).

[125]Adamo JE, Bauer G, Berro M, et al. A roadmap for academic health centers to establish good laboratory practice-compliant infrastructure. Acad. Med. 2012;87:279—84.

[126]Adamo JE, Bauer G, Berro M, et al. A roadmap for academic health centers to establish good laboratory practice-compliant infrastructure. Acad. Med. 2012;87:279—84.

[127]According to Cooper and Fleder, "[a] #483 is issued by one or more FDA investigators at the conclusion of a site inspection, and usually is not reviewed by a compliance officer, district director, or an official in FDA's headquarters before it is issued. An FDA warning letter, on the other hand, is issued by a district director or headquarters official of similar seniority, and only after review by FDA's Office of Chief Counsel." See, Cooper RM, Fleder JR. Responding to a Form 483 Warning Letter: a practical guide. Food Drug Law J. 2005;60:479.

[128]Senger JM. Emerging issues in FDA regulation: warning Letters, internet promotion, and tobacco. J. Health Care Policy 2010;13:211—25.

[129]Warning Letter, CBER-09-01, January 5, 2009.

proper conduct of nonclinical studies as published under 21 CFR Part 58 … [y]our firm did not check every animal cage for feed and water each day, or clean the animal cages for study (b)(4) for twelve days … [a]s a result, the animals were not checked (b)(4) as required in the *Animal Care Schedule* SOP.

To provide another example, the following Warning Letter complained about the Sponsor's *failure to analyze a specimen* from a test animal (130):

Dear Mr. [REDACTED]:
FDA investigator … met with … members of your staff to review your firm's conduct of study [REDACTED] performed under the Good Laboratory Practices (GLP) regulations [21 CFR Part 58] … [a]t the end of the inspection, a Form FDA 483 … was issued and discussed with … your staff … [t]hese specimens represent eight of the … animals in one of the … dose cohorts required for … studies at the … week time point. The box packed on 12/8/05 was not found until almost one year later during the FDA inspection. The final report for study … was signed by the study director on 04/06/06 with no indication that these samples were missing, as evidenced by the lack of protocol deviation report in the study file. Your letter acknowledges that these samples were not analyzed. You explain that these animals were administered an [REDACTED] test article dose and were not included in the final study report. We disagree with your claim that these samples had no bearing or impact on the study data.

h. Animal Rule

Where a Sponsor seeks FDA approval of a drug, but where use of human subjects would be unethical, the FDA permits use of animal model data as the basis for approval for administration in humans. For example, FDA approval for treatments for plague due to *Yersinia pestis* was granted using the African green monkey model, approval for a treatment for cyanide poisoning was granted using a dog model, and approval for a treatment for smallpox (variola virus) was granted using monkeypox virus in primates and rabbitpox in rabbits (131). To provide another example, the FDA has also described the hypothetical treatment of a drug to treat gastrointestinal disorders resulting from acute radiation exposure in the case of a nuclear detonation (132).

This avenue for drug approval is called the Animal Rule. The Animal Rule finds a basis in Sections 314.600 (small molecule drugs) and 601.90 (biologicals) of the Code of Federal Regulations. According to the FDA's Guidance for Industry (133):

The Animal Rule states that for drugs developed to ameliorate or prevent serious or life threatening conditions caused by exposure to lethal or permanently disabling toxic substances, when human challenge studies would not be ethical to perform and field trials to study effectiveness after accidental or intentional human exposure have not been feasible, FDA may grant marketing approval based on adequate and well-controlled animal efficacy studies when the results of those studies establish that the drug is reasonably likely to produce clinical benefit in humans.

In addition to the requirement that use of human subjects not be ethical, the FDA requires that the mechanism of action of the disorder in the animal model correspond to the mechanism of action of the disorder in humans, and that the mechanism of action of the proposed treatment in the animal model

---

[130]Warning Letter, CBER-07-007, March 23, 2007.

[131]U.S. Department of Health and Human Services. Food and Drug Administration. Guidance for industry. Product development under the animal rule; May 2014 (53 pp.).

[132]U.S. Department of Health and Human Services. Food and Drug Administration. Guidance for industry. Product development under the animal rule; May 2014 (53 pp.).

[133]U.S. Department of Health and Human Services. Food and Drug Administration. Guidance for industry. Product development under the animal rule; May 2014 (53 pp.).

also correspond to the mechanism of action of the treatment in humans. Regarding the need for mechanisms in the animal model to track mechanisms in humans, the FDA refers to the example of treatment of pneumonic plague caused by *Y. pestis*. The FDA states that infection by this bacterium can occur by way of flea bites, which causes bubonic plague, while infection by inhalation of the bacterium causes pneumonic plague. Thus, for obtaining regulatory approval for a drug against pneumonic plague, the animal model must use an inhalation route (not a flea bite route) for the bacterium (134). To provide one more example of the need for the mechanisms in the animal model to track those in the human, the FDA states that, "[i]f the thresholds in humans and in the animal model differ greatly, the suitability of the animal model may be called into question and the model should be discussed with FDA" (135).

Use of the Animal Rule for gaining FDA approval for drugs for human patients has been detailed for the indications of smallpox (136,137), pneumonic plague (138), ebola virus (139), anthrax (140), and radiation (141).

i. FDA's Decision-Making Process in Evaluating Raxibacumab, for Treating *Bacillus anthracis* Infections

At the time of drug approval, the FDA publishes its *Approval Letter* along with its *Medical Review* or *Clinical Review*, *Pharmacological Review*, *Statistical Review*, and other reviews. The following is from the FDA's approval of *raxibacumab*, for treating *B. anthracis* infections. The drug is an antibody for treating anthrax.

Thus, it can be readily understood that it is rarely or never the case that any human subjects will be available for this type of clinical trial. This example is from BLA 125349, which is available from December 2012 of the FDA's website. Please note that efficacy data were collected from studies on rabbits and monkeys, while safety data were collected from studies on human volunteers. The human volunteers where healthy, and were only treated with the study drug (and not exposed to any anthrax bacteria).

The FDA reviewer stated that the animal studies indicate that the study drug shows

---

[134]U.S. Department of Health and Human Services. Food and Drug Administration. Guidance for industry. Product development under the animal rule; May 2014 (53 pp.).

[135]U.S. Department of Health and Human Services. Food and Drug Administration. Guidance for industry. Product development under the animal rule; May 2014 (53 pp.).

[136]Trost LC, et al. The efficacy and pharmacokinetics of brincidofovir for the treatment of lethal rabbitpox virus infection: a model of smallpox disease. Antiviral Res. 2014;117:115−21.

[137]Olson VA, Smith SK, Foster S. In vitro efficacy of brincidofovir against variola virus. Antimicrob. Agents Chemother. 2014;58:5570−1.

[138]Graham VA, et al. Efficacy of primate humoral passive transfer in a murine model of pneumonic plague is mouse strain-dependent. J. Immunol. Res. 2014;2014:807564.

[139]Sullivan NJ, et al. Correlates of protective immunity for Ebola vaccines: implications for regulatory approval by the animal rule. Nat. Rev. Microbiol. 2009;7:393−400.

[140]Williamson D. Approaches to modeling the human immune response in transition of candidates from research to development. J. Immunol. Res. 2014;2014:395302 (6 pp.).

[141]Gluzman-Poltoruk Z, et al. Randomized comparison of single dose of recombinant human IL-12 versus placebo for restoration of hematopoiesis and improved survival in rhesus monkeys exposed to lethal radiation. J. Hematol. Oncol. 2014;7:31 (12 pp.).

"potential survival benefit" to humans suffering from anthrax. Also, the reviewer described the animal models as, "two representative animal models of inhalation anthrax in NZW rabbits (35–44% survival) and cynomolgus macaques (69% survival) when treatment was initiated postexposure at the time when all animals were toxemic/febrile."

Please note that the study design was a stringent one, in that the study drug was administered after infection, rather than prior to infection. The study with human subjects was only for assessing safety and in referring to these studies, the FDA reviewer pointed out that, "[s]afety of raxibacumab ... single intravenous infusion was established in ... 326 healthy human volunteers."

V. ESTIMATING HUMAN DOSE FROM ANIMAL STUDIES

a. Introduction

The most appropriate dose of a drug for humans can be derived from animal studies. The FDA provides guidance on converting effective doses from animal studies, to corresponding doses that are likely to be effective in human subjects (142). Two approaches with animals are in common use. The first is to arrive at the highest drug dose that is not toxic. This approach is commonly used for small-molecule drugs for cancer. The second is to arrive at the dose of a drug that is optimally effective, as determined by tests sensitive to efficacy. With the information of the dose in hand, investigators then scale up the dose derived from animal studies, and then calculate a dose for first use in humans. Lowe et al. (143), Reigner and Blesch (144), Contrera et al. (145), and Sharma and McNeill (146) review methods for using animal studies to arrive at doses for humans. These methods include methods based on body surface area, and methods based on pharmacokinetic (PK) data. Sawyer and Ratain (147) and Kouno et al. (148) discuss the common formulas used to calculate body surface area.

b. NOAEL Approach

The No Adverse Effect Dose Level (NOAEL) is determined in animal safety

---

[142] U.S. Department of Health and Human Services. Food and Drug Administration. Guidance for Industry. Estimating the Safe Starting Dose in Clinical Trials for Therapeutics in Adult Healthy Volunteers. U.S. Department of Health and Human Services, Food and Drug Administration. 2002; 24 pp.

[143] Lowe PJ, Hijazi Y, Luttringer O, Yin H, Sarangapani R, Howard D. On the anticipation of the human dose in first-in-man trials from preclinical and prior clinical information in early drug development. Xenobiotica 2007;37:1331–54.

[144] Reigner BG, Blesch KS. Estimating the starting dose for entry into humans: principles and practice. Eur. J. Clin. Pharmacol. 2002;57:835–45.

[145] Contrera JF, Matthews EJ, Kruhlak NL, Benz RD. Estimating the safe starting dose in phase I clinical trials and no observed effect level based on QSAR modeling of the human maximum recommended daily dose. Regul. Toxicol. Pharmacol. 2004;40:185–206.

[146] Sharma V, McNeill JH. To scale or not to scale: the principles of dose extrapolation. Br. J. Pharmacol. 2009;157:907–21.

[147] Sawyer M, Ratain MJ. Body surface area as a determinant of pharmacokinetics and drug dosing. Invest. New Drugs 2001;19:171–7.

[148] Kouno T, Katsumata N, Mukai H, Ando M, Watanabe T. Standardization of the body surface area (BSA) formula to calculate the dose of anticancer agents in Japan. Jpn J. Clin. Oncol. 2003;33:309–13.

studies performed in the most sensitive and relevant animal species. The NOAEL method is commonly used to arrive at a first-in-humans dose. The relevant dose is then reduced by an appropriate safety factor, for example, by reducing the dose by a factor of 10. According to the FDA's *Guidance for Industry* (149), NOAEL is determined as follows. For selecting a starting dose, the following is used, namely, the highest dose level that does not produce a significant increase in adverse effects in comparison to the control group.

c. MABEL Approach

Another approach for arriving at a suitable dose for humans, is use of the Minimal Anticipated Biological Effect Level (MABEL) approach (150). The MABEL approach provides the dose level leading to a biological effect of interest. The biological effect of interest can be saturation of a drug transport mechanism, stimulation of a cell signaling pathway, or activation of a cell. Calculating MABEL makes use of in vitro and in vivo information available from PK data and pharmacodynamics (PD) data.

The concentrations of drug which need to be achieved in the bloodstream of a patient during actual treatment, can be estimated by studies with cultured human and animal cells. According to guidance from the EMEA (151),

in vitro data with cultured cells can be used to determine, "target binding and receptor occupancy studies *in vitro* in target cells from human and the relevant animal species ... concentration—response curves *in vitro* in target cells from human and the relevant animal species and dose/exposure—response *in vivo* in the relevant animal species."

d. Scaling-Up the Drug Dose, Acquired From Animal Studies, for Use in Humans

When an appropriate dose is found from animal studies, that is, by using the NOAEL approach or the MABEL approach, an appropriate first dose for use in humans can be calculated using body surface area measurements and by incorporating a safety factor. For any given patient, for example, in a clinical study or during ordinary everyday clinical practice, the recommended drug dose may be expressed in terms of body surface area. Hence, where toxicology studies or efficacy studies with animals result in an appropriate dose, and where researchers have expressed this dose in terms of body surface area, the same dose may be appropriate for humans. The FDA provides a conversion table for changing a dose found appropriate for animals to a corresponding dose for humans, where this conversion is based on body surface area (152). The FDA's

[149]U.S. Department of Health and Human Services. Food and Drug Administration. Guidance for industry. Estimating the maximum safe starting dose in initial clinical trials for therapeutics in adult healthy volunteers; July 2005 (27 pp.).

[150]Milton MN, Horvath CJ. The EMEA guideline on first-in-human clinical trials and its impact on pharmaceutical development. Toxicol. Pathol. 2009;37:363—71.

[151]European Medicines Agency (EMEA). Guideline on strategies to identify and mitigate risks for first-in-human clinical trials with investigational medicinal products; July 2007.

[152]U.S. Department of Health and Human Services. Food and Drug Administration. Guidance for industry. Estimating the maximum safe starting dose in initial clinical trials for therapeutics in adult healthy volunteers; July 2005 (27 pp.).

conversion table also includes a factor of 0.1, where the dose arrived at by the calculation is multiplied by 0.1, in order to ensure that the dose in humans will not be toxic (153). The resulting dose, as found with the FDA's table, is expected to be the dose that results in no observed adverse effect, where higher doses or concentrations would result in an adverse effect. The table provides separate conversion factors, for converting animal doses to human doses, for the mouse, rat, rabbit, dog, monkey, and pig. After the investigator applies the scaling factor, the resulting number is called the human equivalent dose (HED) (154). The species that generates the lowest HED is called the most sensitive species. After arriving at the HED, the HED is further modified by applying a safety factor. Thus, according to the FDA's Guidance for Industry (155), "[a] safety factor should then be applied to the HED to increase assurance that the first dose in humans will not cause adverse effects."

e. Examples From Clinical Study Protocols of Using Animal Studies to Arrive at Appropriate Human Dose

1. *Drug for Non-small Cell Lung Cancer*

A Clinical Study Protocol for a cancer clinical trial detailed how animal studies were used to arrive at an appropriate dose for humans. The drug, LDK378, also known as ceritinib, was subsequently FDA-approved for the indication of non-small cell lung cancer (NSCLC) (156). The term "GLP" means "Good Laboratory Practice," which is a set of standards relating to the care and handling of laboratory animals. The concepts in the quoted excerpt include:

- *STD$_{10}$*. The term "STD$_{10}$" means "severely toxic dose 10 (the dose causing severe toxicity in approximately 10% of all animals)."
- *AUC*. Area under the curve. This refers to a value, determined by integration, of blood plasma concentration of the drug over a given period of time. Plasma AUC$_{0-24}$ refers to integration from time zero to 24 h.
- *Safe starting dose*. The safe starting dose for humans was calculated using data from rat studies.
- *Efficacious dose*. The efficacious dose in humans was calculated using PK data from animals. This textbook refrains from providing background information on these calculations.
- *HNSTD*. HNSTD means, "highest nonseverely toxic dose" (157).
- *BSA*. BSA is body surface area.

[153]Ochoa R, Rousseaux C. The role of the toxicologic pathologist in risk management. Toxicol. Pathol. 2009;37:705–7.

[154]U.S. Department of Health and Human Services. Food and Drug Administration. Guidance for industry. Estimating the maximum safe starting dose in initial clinical trials for therapeutics in adult healthy volunteers; July 2005 (27 pp.).

[155]U.S. Department of Health and Human Services. Food and Drug Administration. Guidance for industry. Estimating the maximum safe starting dose in initial clinical trials for therapeutics in adult healthy volunteers; July 2005 (27 pp.).

[156]Khozin S, Blumenthal GM, Zhang L, et al. FDA approval: ceritinib for the treatment of metastatic anaplastic lymphoma kinase-positive non-small cell lung cancer. Clin. Cancer Res. 2015;21:2436–9.

[157]Saber H, Leighton JK. An FDA oncology analysis of antibody-drug conjugates. Regul. Toxicol. Pharmacol. 2015;71:444–52.

The Clinical Study Protocol stated that (158):

Dose selection. The selection of starting dose was based on the rat STD_{10} from the 4-week GLP study (50 mg/kg/day). Expressing 50 mg/kg in the rat based on body surface area is equivalent to 300 mg/m^2. Applying a safety factor of 10, the starting dose in humans would be 1/10th of the STD_{10} in rats or 1/10th of 300 mg/m^2 = 30.0 mg/m^2. Since 1/10th of the STD_{10} in rat is below the HNSTD in the monkey (30 mg/kg or 360 mg/m^2), this dose is expected to be well tolerated by the monkey. Therefore, the rat is considered an appropriate species. Thus, based on an average BSA of 1.73 m^2, the recommended safe flat starting dose of LDK378 [study drug] is 51.9 mg/patient (50 mg/patient).

The human efficacious dose was estimated by tumor kinetic PK/PD modeling. By fitting plasma LDK378 [study drug] PK and tumor regression dynamics in two xenograft models, key tumor regression parameters (tumor doubling time) and drug effect (IC50 and Hill coefficient) can be estimated. Target exposure of tumor inhibition ranging from ... stable disease ... to 90% regression ... can be calculated and considered potentially therapeutic in patients. Derived from tumor kinetic PK/PD modeling, plasma AUC_{0-24} values ranging from 3000 to 12408 ng*hr/mL are considered potentially therapeutic target exposures in patients and were used to estimate the potentially therapeutic dose range humans. The following equation was employed: Dose (human) = (CL/F)* (AUC_{tau}), where AUC_{tau} corresponds to the exposure at steady-state leading to the desired pharmacologic effects, CL represent the predicted human clearance, and F is the human absolute bioavailability and estimated to be 0.7. Therefore, the human efficacious dose range is estimated to be 120 to 480 mg/day, based on exposures associated with *in vivo* tumor growth inhibition, i.e., tumor stasis to 90% tumor regression in the ... rat models.

2. *Drug for a Disease of the Intestinal Mucosa (Crohn's Disease)*

An interesting nuance for the technique for extrapolating from mouse dose to human dose, comes from a clinical trial on a drug used to treat an autoimmune disease (colitis) of the gut. The Clinical Study Protocol explained (159):

After careful consideration of the appropriate basis for extrapolating efficacious doses in mice to humans, a judgment was made that this should be based on the intestinal mucosal surface area. The primary rationale for this is that the product, when delivered orally, is only minimally absorbed systemically and is essentially delivered topically to the intestinal epithelium. Therefore, the human-equivalent efficacious dosage was calculated as described ... [t]he surface area of the colon and terminal ileum of the mice used in the above experiments is 947.5 mm^2 ... so, it is 265 fold smaller than the corresponding human surface area, which is approximately 251,000 mm^2. Since the therapeutic dose in mice with colitis was 0.125 mg/mouse, we established the dose to use in humans by multiplying this value for 265. The calculated dose (33 mg).

VI. ORIGIN OF DRUGS THAT ARE BIOSIMILARS

"Biosimilars" refers to a class of drug called biologicals. Biologicals include antibodies, viruses, vaccines, serums, blood products, and polypeptides (160). Polypeptides that are biosimilars are those made by expression in living cells, and do not include polypeptides made by organic synthesis. The term biosimilars is

[158]Oncology Clinical Trial Protocol CLDK378X2101. A phase I, multicenter, open-label dose escalation study of LDK378, administered orally in adult patients with tumors characterized by genetic abnormalities in anaplastic lymphoma kinase (ALK); August 19, 2010.

[159]A phase II multicenter, randomized, double-blind, controlled vs placebo, dosefinding study on the efficacy and safety of GED-0301, in patients with active Crohn's disease (Ileo-Colitis). Protocol: GED-301-01-11. EUDRACT NUMBER 2011-002640-27.

[160]Abraham J. Developing oncology biosimilars: an essential approach for the future. Semin. Oncol. 2013;40 (Suppl. 1):S5−24.

used in the context of regulatory approval. According to comments from FDA officials, the US Congress authorized the FDA to grant approval to drugs that are biosimilars, where the source of motivation was to improve access of the public to drugs that are biologicals (161).

A "biosimilar" is a biological that is similar to, or nearly identical to, an existing FDA-approved reference biological. A corresponding term exists for small-molecule drugs, where this term is "generic drug." Generic drugs are usually small molecules that are absolutely identical to an existing, reference drug. It is difficult for two different manufacturers to produce biologicals that are identical to each other, because of variability in post-translational modification, such as, glycosylation, phosphorylation (162), and carboxylation (163), because of differences in degradation, aggregation, or deamination (164), in view of differences in conformational changes (165), as well as in immunogenicity. Processes for synthesizing biologicals, such as the production of recombinant antibodies by cell culture, and conditions of storage (time; temperature) have a much greater influence on biologicals than on small molecules.

The FDA defines a biosimilar as, "the biological product is highly similar to the reference product notwithstanding minor differences in clinically meaningful differences between the biological product in terms of safety, purity, and potency of the product," adding that, for a biosimilar, "there are no clinically meaningful differences between the biological product and the reference product in terms of safety, purity, and potency of the product" (166).

Where a Sponsor wishes to gain FDA-approval of a biosimilar, the FDA recommends conducting side-by-side tests of the biosimilar and the reference compound. In this recommendation, the FDA stated that, "analytical studies and at least one clinical pharmacokinetic … study … must include an adequate comparison of the proposed biosimilar product directly with the U.S.-licensed reference product" (167).

VII. ORIGIN OF DRUGS THAT ARE ORPHAN DRUGS

a. Rare Diseases

The Orphan Drug Act classifies a rare disease as one that afflicts under 200,000 people in the United States. About 5000—8000 rare conditions exist in the United States and Europe. In the United States, about 25 million people (8%) are afflicted with rare diseases (168). Rare diseases include Fabry's

[161]Kozlowski S, et al. Developing the nation's biosimilars program. New Engl. J. Med. 2011;365:385—8.

[162]Weise M, Bielsky M-C, De Smet K, et al. Biosimilars: what clinicians should know. Blood 2012;120:5111—7.

[163]Brody T, Suttie JW. Evidence for the glycoprotein nature of vitamin K-dependent carboxylase from rat liver. Biochim. Biophys. Acta 1987;923:1—7.

[164]Bui LA, Taylor C. Developing clinical trials for biosimilars. Semin. Oncol. 2014;41:S15—25.

[165]Brody T. Multistep denaturation and hierarchy of disulfide bond cleavage of a monoclonal antibody. Analyt. Biochem. 1997;247:247—56.

[166]U.S. Department of Health and Human Services. Food and Drug Administration. Guidance for industry. Clinical pharmacology data to support a demonstration of biosimilarity to a reference product; May 2014 (15 pp.).

[167]U.S. Department of Health and Human Services. Food and Drug Administration. Guidance for industry. Clinical pharmacology data to support a demonstration of biosimilarity to a reference product; May 2014 (15 pp.).

[168]Arnon SS. Creation and development of the public service orphan drug human botulism immune globin. Pediatrics 2002;19:785—9.

disease (5000), Gaucher's disease (2500), tyrosinemia type I (2500), and mucopolysaccharidosis (200), where the numbers indicate the number of afflicted persons in the United States (169). Another rare disease, Morquio A syndrome, occurs at a prevalence of about one case per 76,000 to 640,000 people in the populations of Ireland and Australia, respectively (170).

Impediments to conducting clinical trials on rare diseases include low numbers of volunteers available for clinical trials, lack of blood and tissue samples for use in research, and insufficient basic research on the mechanisms of the diseases. FDA-regulated clinical trials on drugs require from about 350 to 4000 subjects (171). A drug can receive status as an orphan drug, at the request of a Sponsor, if it is used to treat a rare disease or condition.

b. Orphan Drug Act

For a drug to qualify for orphan status, both the drug and the disease or condition must meet certain criteria specified in the Orphan Drug Act and 21 CFR §316.

The granting of orphan status does not alter the standard regulatory requirements and process for obtaining marketing approval. In other words, the nature of the Sponsor's submitted data on efficacy, safety, PK, and statistics, is substantially the same for conventional drugs and for drugs intended for orphan drug status. Clinical trials are still required for demonstrating efficacy and safety for orphan drugs. The Code of Federal Regulations reveals some differences between FDA submissions for regular drugs and FDA submissions for orphan drugs, in its writing about the requirement for animal toxicology experiments (172).

Orphan status, also called, orphan designation, qualifies the Sponsor of the drug for various development incentives, including tax credits for clinical testing. The Orphan Drug Act provides Sponsors with three incentives (173):

- Federal funding to perform clinical trials of orphan products
- A tax credit of 50 percent of clinical testing costs
- An exclusive right to market the orphan drug for 7 years from the date of marketing approval. This protects orphan drug manufacturers from competition for 7 years.

The Orphan Drug Act of 1983 encourages the research and development of drugs for treating rare diseases, for which a very limited patient market could otherwise dampen a Sponsor's interest in the product. According to

---

[169]Zitter M. Managing drugs for rare genetic diseases: trends and insights. Managed Care 2005;14:52−67.

[170]Leadley RM, et al. A systematic review of the prevalence of Morquio A syndrome: challenges for study reporting in rare diseases. Orphanet J. Rare Diseases 2014;9:173 (17 pp.).

[171]Gites B, et al. Benefits of the orphan drug act for rare diseases treatments. TuftScope Express Online. Spring 2010 (3 pp.).

[172]Please see commentary in 21 CFR 316.20(b)(4) regarding the need to submit, "data from in vitro laboratory studies, preclinical efficacy studies conducted in an animal model for the human disease or condition, and clinical experience with the drug in the rare disease or condition that are available to the sponsor, whether positive, negative, or inconclusive. *Animal toxicology studies are generally not relevant* to a request for orphan-drug designation" (emphasis added).

[173]Kesselheim AS. B. Innovation and the Orphan Drug Act, 1983−2009: regulator and clinical characteristics of approved orphan drugs. Washington, DC: National Academies Press; 2010. 28 pp.

one commentator (174), the opportunity to seek and acquire approval of orphan status of a drug may provide the following benefits. The opportunity encourages manufacturers to seek out orphan indications for drugs that could otherwise be tested in more general populations (this benefits patients). It provides public subsidies for the development of products (this benefits companies). Also, it may lead to the approval of drugs then widely used off-label without supporting data (this benefits patients, because of the supporting data).

Please note that the Code of Federal Regulations allows Sponsors to submit a request for orphan drug status, even if the disease is not a rare disease. Requests for diseases that are not rare will be accepted by the FDA if the Sponsor has information that it is not likely that any company will be developing drugs for that nonrare disease. The relevant law is in 21 CFR §316.20(b)(8)(ii), and is reproduced in footnote (175).

c. Examples of Drugs That Have Been Granted Orphan Drug Status

FDA has granted orphan drug status to various drugs to be used for the indications described in the following list. Documents written by FDA reviewers in the approval of all drugs, including orphan drugs, can be found on the FDA's website using the procedure in footnote (176). The following list identifies the indication, as well as the location (on FDA's website) of the FDA's Approval Letter and other documents that supported the FDA's decision to approve the drug:

- *Ibrutinib* for mantle cell lymphoma (MCL). Documents available on the FDA's website at November 2013.
- *Imatinib* for chronic myeloid leukemia, a disease characterized by a chromosomal location called, Philadelphia chromosome. Documents available on the FDA's website at January 2013.
- *Obinutuzumab* for chronic lymphocytic leukemia (CLL). Documents available on the FDA's website at November 2013.
- *Afatinib* for nonsmall-cell lung cancer where tumors have a deletion in exon 19 of the gene encoding epidermal growth factor receptor or a mutation in exon 21 that involves change of a leucine residue to an arginine residue (L858R). Documents available on the FDA's website at July 2013.
- *Velaglucerase alpha* for type 1 Gaucher disease. Documents available on the FDA's website at November 2013.
- *Glycerol phenylbutyrate* for urea cycle disorders. Documents available on the FDA's website at January 2013.
- *Cysteamine bitartrate* for nephropathic cystinosis. Documents available on the FDA's website at April 2013.
- *Riociguat* for pulmonary arterial hypertension. Documents available on the FDA's website at October 2013.

---

[174]Kesselheim AS. Using market exclusivity incentives to promote pharmaceutical innovation. New Engl. J. Med. 2010;363:1855–62.

[175]For a drug intended for diseases or conditions affecting 200,000 or more people, or for a vaccine, diagnostic drug, or preventive drug to be administered to 200,000 or more persons per year in the United States, there is no reasonable expectation that costs of research and development of the drug for the indication can be recovered by sales of the drug in the United States as specified in §316.21(c).

[176]On the FDA website, click on DRUG tab, click on Search Drug Approvals by Month Using Drugs@FDA, then choose the month and year, then choose the drug, and finally click on Approval History, Letters, Reviews, and related documents. As a result of this process, you will gain access to the Approval Letter, Medical Review, Pharmacological Review, Statistical Review, and other documents that were prepared by FDA employees.

- *Sapropterin* for hyperphenylalaninemia in patients with phenylketonuria. Documents available on the FDA's website at December 2013.
- *Elosuflase alpha* for Morquio A syndrome, also known as mucopolysaccharidosis IVA. The drug, which takes the form of the enzyme *N*-acetylgalactosamine sulfatase, replaces an enzyme that is missing in the patient's body. Documents available on the FDA's website at February 2014.

d. Orphan Status for Ibrutinib for the Indication of MCL

This section introduces a number of topics that are detailed in later chapters. As such, this is a preview of what is to come, and defines some of the main goals of this textbook. The topics are:

- The hematological cancers
- Biomarkers that define subgroups in patient populations
- Biomarkers that can be used to predict outcome of a disease, if left untreated
- Biomarkers that can predict efficacy or safety of a given drug
- Drug safety
- FDA's Approval Letter and documents from FDA reviewers, made available on the FDA website at the time of drug approval.

According to Dr Richard Pazdur, an FDA official, "FDA also granted ibrutinib ... orphan-product designation because the drug is intended to treat a rare disease" (177). This is background information on the genetics and prevalence of the rare disease, MCL. Non-Hodgkin lymphoma has over 30 subtypes. Each of these subtypes has different clinical and genetic features. MCL is a rare subtype of non-Hodgkin lymphoma.

MCL is characterized by the chromosomal translocation, t(11:14)(q13;q32). In addition to this chromosomal translocation, genetic mutations that also commonly occur in MCL include mutations in the genes encoding ATM (ATM senses DNA damage), *NOTCH1/2*, *WHSK1*, and *MLL2* (178). This author points out that all of these mutations are likely of interest as biomarkers, for example, for predicting survival of a nontreated patient (prognosis), and for predicting efficacy and safety in response to any given drug.

The symptoms of MCL include loss of appetite, fatigue, night sweats, and fevers. There were about 15,000 MCL patients in the United States in 2014 (179). MCL has one of the worst outcomes of all the lymphomas, and it remains incurable. As of 2015, four drugs were licensed by the FDA for use in treating MCL, namely, ibrutinib (Imbruvica), bortezomib (Velcade), temsirolimus (Torisel), and lenalidomide (Revlimid) (180).

Ibrutinib inhibits the enzyme, Bruton's tyrosine kinase. As stated above, ibrutinib is effective for treating MCL. Older forms of chemotherapy for MCL include use of the combination of etoposide, methylprednisolone, cytarabine, and cisplatin, but this

---

[177]Pazdur R. FDA approves ibrutinib for mantle cell lymphoma. The ASCO Post 2013;4(issue 19).

[178]Campo E, Rule S. Mantle cell lymphoma: evolving management strategies. Blood 2015;125:48–55.

[179]Wang Y, Shuangge M. Racial differences in mantle cell lymphoma in the United States. BMC Cancer 2014;14:764 (8 pp.).

[180]Campo E, Rule S. Mantle cell lymphoma: evolving management strategies. Blood 2015;125:48–55.

drug combination has a poor safety profile. In contrast, therapy with ibrutib is relatively nontoxic (181).

Ibrutinib is also effective for treating another type of cancer, CLL. CLL is the most common leukemia in adults (182). A subgroup of CLL patients is characterized by the chromosomal deletion, 17p13.1. This subgroup of CLL patients fails to respond to older forms of chemotherapy, such as the combination of fludarabine and anti-CD20 antibody, or the combination of fludarabine, cyclophosphamide, and anti-CD20. In other words, this subgroup responds poorly to chemoimmunotherapy. In contrast, response to ibrutinib appears to be independent of whether the patient has, or does not have, the 17p13.1 deletion (183). To summarize, the above commentary illustrates the value of subgroup analysis that involves biomarkers, such as chromosomal abnormalities and genetic mutations.

VIII. SUMMARY

Drugs are generally classified as small molecules and biologicals. Because a chemistry background is needed in order to write FDA-submissions, this chapter includes a brief account of the concepts of hydrophilic and hydrophobic, a generic diagram of an antibody, a picture of a polypeptide chain with all of its amino acids, and a table of the 20 classical amino acids.

Further regarding animal models, data on efficacy and safety, as acquired from animal models, are used by a Sponsor for submitting to the FDA by way of the IND application. The goal of the IND is to acquire permission to initiate clinical trials in human subjects. Data from animal models are also used to support the warnings statement appearing on package labels of drugs. The FDA states that the warning can, in part, be based on animal data, in its writing that, "[a]nimal data raise substantial concern about the potential occurrence of the adverse reaction in humans (eg, animal data demonstrating that a drug has teratogenic effects" (184).

Hence, animal data are used prior to engaging any communications with the FDA, as well as in the final stages of the drug-approval process when the package label is being perfected.

During the course of drug development, animals are used to establish the mechanisms of action of the disease and of the drug. As the degree of engagement with the FDA increases, there is an increase in the need to comply with regulations regarding the use of animals. These regulations include those set forth by Good Laboratory Practices (GLP), as well as the need to follow validated Standard Operating Procedures (SOPs).

[181]Wang ML, Rule S, Martin M, et al. Targeting BTK with ibrutinib relapsed or refractory mantle-cell lymphoma. New Engl. J. Med. 2003;369:507−16.

[182]Byrd JC, Furman RR, Coutre SE, et al. Targeting BTK with ibrutinib in relapsed chronic lymphocytic leukemia. New Engl. J. Med. 2013;369:32−42.

[183]Byrd JC, Furman RR, Coutre SE, et al. Targeting BTK with ibrutinib in relapsed chronic lymphocytic leukemia. New Engl. J. Med. 2013;369:32−42.

[184]U.S. Department of Health and Human Services. Food and Drug Administration. Guidance for industry. Warnings and precautions, contraindications, and warning sections of labeling for human prescription drug and biological products—content and format; October 2011 (13 pp.).

The bulletpoints appearing below outline the big picture of adverse consequences (to the Sponsor) for failures in various aspects of drug development. These adverse consequences can result by deficiencies in the Sponsor's use of animals, as well as by issues unrelated to animals. RTF and *Clinical Hold* are defined in the footnotes and are detailed in the account of the timeline for FDA-approval, as set forth in Chapter 23. This chapter concluded with an account of origins of drugs that are defined by FDA-regulations, that is, by the FDA-defined categories that are "biosimilars" and "orphan drugs."

- RTF (185,186),
- *Clinical Hold* (187,188),
- FDA Form 483.

---

[185] According to FDA's Guidance for Industry, a Refuse to File notice is issued by FDA, "if the paper or electronic portions are illegible, uninterpretable, or otherwise clearly inadequate, including incompatible formats and inadequate organization." See, U.S. Department of Health and Human Services. Food and Drug Administration. Guidance for industry. Providing regulatory submissions to the Center for Biologics Evaluation and Research (CBER) in electronic format—biologics marketing application; November 1999 (63 pp.).

[186] According to FDA's website, "New Drug Applications that are incomplete become the subject of a formal "refuse-to-file" action. In such cases, the applicant receives a letter detailing the decision and the deficiencies that form its basis." See, FDA website. Drug development and review definitions; December 17, 2014.

[187] According to the FDA's Guidance for Industry, a Clinical Hold is, "[a]n order issued by FDA to the sponsor of an IND to delay or to suspend a clinical investigation for reasons described in 21 CFR 312.42." See, U.S. Department of Health and Human Services. Food and Drug Administration. Guidance for industry. Submitting and reviewing complete responses to clinical holds; October 2000 (5 pp.).

[188] According to the FDA's website, "[a] clinical hold is the mechanism that CDER uses when it does not believe, or cannot confirm, that the study can be conducted without unreasonable risk to the subjects/patients." See, the FDA website's disclosure of drug development and review definitions; December 17, 2014.

2

Clinical Trial Design

I. INTRODUCTION TO REGULATED CLINICAL TRIALS

Clinical trials are classified as phase I, phase II, and phase III clinical trials. The goals of these trials are to acquire data on safety and efficacy, to receive regulatory approval for the relevant drug or medical device, and to provide safe and effective treatments for the relevant disease or condition. Regulatory approval is granted by agencies such as the US Food and Drug Administration (FDA), the European Medicines Agency (EMA), and the Pharmaceuticals and Medical Devices Agency (PMDA) in Japan (1,2,3,4,5,6).

Phase I clinical trials are distinguished as being the initial trials conducted on human subjects. Phase I trials are sometimes called "first in human studies" (7) or "first in man studies" (8).

Before any drug is used in humans, the drug must be created, tested in animals, and characterized in terms of its structure, stability, and purity. Animal testing involves tests on toxicity, efficacy, pharmacokinetics (PK), and pharmacodynamics (PD). In the United States, an Investigational New Drug (IND) application must be submitted to the FDA in order to gain approval for initiating clinical trials (9). The IND summarizes data on the chemistry and stability of the active drug substance,

[1]Sihna G. Japan works to shorten "drug lag," boost trials of new drugs. J. Natl. Cancer Inst. 2010;102:148−51.

[2]Dal Pan GJ, Arlett PR. The US Food and Drug Administration-European Medicines Agency collaboration in pharmacovigilance: common objectives and common challenges. 2015;38:13−5.

[3]Ehmann F, et al. Pharmacogenomic information in drug labels: European Medicines Agency perspective. Pharmacogenomics 2015; http://dx.doi.org/10.1038/tpj.2014.86.

[4]Asano K, et al. Regulatory challenges in the review of data from global clinical trials: the PMDA perspective. Clin. Pharmacol. Ther. 2013;195−8.

[5]Kuribayashi R, et al. Regulation of generic drugs in Japan: the current situation and future prospects. AAPS J. May 6, 2015; Epub ahead of print.

[6]Ishiguro A. Current PMDA activities for use of biomarkers in drug evaluation. Yakugaku Zasshi 2015;135:681−4.

[7]European Medicines Agency (EMEA). Guideline on strategies to identify and mitigate risks for first-in-human clinical trials with investigational medicinal products; July 2007.

[8]Mehta S, et al. Phase I (first-in-man) prophylactic vaccine's clinical trials: selecting a clinical trial site. Perspect. Clin. Res. 2015;6:77−81.

[9]Tamimi NA, Ellis P. Drug development: from concept to marketing! Nephron Clin. Pract. 2009;113:c125−1231.

studies using in vitro methods, such as studies with cultured cells, data on toxicity, and efficacy acquired from animal studies, and any available data on humans. The term "clinical data" only refers to data from studies on human subjects (not to data from animal studies).

The main goals of a phase I clinical trial are to assess safety and to determine an effective dose suitable for subsequent phase II trials. In clinical trials on anticancer drugs, phase I trials are often configured to determine the minimal dose that can cause significant toxicity. From this particular dose, it is often assumed that the dose is that which will be most effective against the cancer. In other words, the most appropriate dose is that which is just below a dose that produces unacceptable toxicity. But this method is not used to arrive at the dose used in clinical trials for diseases that are not cancers.

Phase I clinical trials begin by administering a small dose of the study drug to a group of three or more patients. Subsequently, cohorts of patients receive increasing doses, first by 100%, then 66%, 50%, 40%, and 33%, a progression that is loosely based on the Fibonacci sequence (10,11). Regarding another progression, Mussai et al. (12) describe the 3 + 3 design and the rolling-6 design for increasing drug doses in phase I clinical trials. The trial ends when severe or dose-limiting toxicities (DLTs) are experienced by a large fraction of subjects at a given dosage level. The dose just below that which was associated with excessive DLT is defined as the maximum tolerated dose (MTD). In the case of oncology clinical trials, the dose that is the MTD may be recommended for phase II and phase III clinical trials. In view of the fact that it may be impossible to predict the toxicity of a newly synthesized chemical, it necessarily follows that many phase I clinical trials include doses that are too low to be effective against cancers. It has been estimated that about half of the subjects treated with the lowest doses receive doses that are "subtherapeutic" (13).

Where subjects are titrated with a drug, it is not that case that any given subject initially receives a lower drug dose, and then receives a higher dose, and then receives an even higher dose. ICH Guidelines (14) warn against conducting a titration scheme with any one, particular subject:

> A critical disadvantage is that by itself, this study design cannot distinguish response to increased dose from response to increased time on drug therapy or a cumulative drug dosage effect. It is therefore an unsatisfactory design where response is delayed, unless treatment at each dose is prolonged. Even where the time-until-development of effect is known to be short (from other data), this design gives poor information on adverse effects, many of which have time-dependent characteristics.

In other words, conducting the entire titration scheme with a single human subject cannot distinguish between the drug's effects that

[10]Saber H, Leighton JK (2015) An FDA oncology analysis of antibody-drug conjugates. Regul. Toxicol. Pharmacol. 71:444–52.

[11]Koyfman SA, Agrawal M, Garrett-Mayer E, et al. Risks and benefits associated with novel phase 1 oncology trial designs. Cancer 2007;110:1115–24.

[12]Mussai FJ, et al. Challenges of clinical trial design for targeted agents against pediatric leukemias. Front. Oncol. 2015;4:Article 374 (7 pp.).

[13]Koyfman SA, Agrawal M, Garrett-Mayer E, et al. Risks and benefits associated with novel phase 1 oncology trial designs. Cancer 2007;110:1115–24.

[14]ICH Harmonised Tripartite Guideline. Dose-response information to support drug registration E4; March 1994. 12 pp.

are a consequence of only the highest dose (the highest dose in the titration scheme), or if they are a consequence of the cumulative effects of the lowest, intermediate, and highest doses. This source of concern applies to efficacy data and to safety data.

Additional information on arriving at an optimal dose, from the ICH Guidelines, emphasizes the fact that an effective dose and an unacceptably toxic dose may be in a similar or overlapping range, or may reside in well-separated ranges, for any given drug. Facts on whether these ranges are well separated, or are not separate, can guide the clinician in choosing the starting dose in a phase I trial (15):

> For example, a relatively high starting dose (on or near the plateau of the effectiveness dose-response curve) might be recommended for a drug with a large demonstrated separation between its useful and undesirable dose ranges or where a rapidly evolving disease process demands rapid effective intervention. A high starting dose, however, might be a poor choice for a drug with a small demonstrated separation between its useful and undesirable dose ranges. In these cases, the recommended starting dose might best be a low dose exhibiting a clinically important effect in even a fraction of the patient population, with the intent to titrate the dose upwards as long as the drug is well-tolerated.

Phase II trials are sometimes divided into phase IIa trials and phase IIb trials. In the phase IIa trial, the drug is tested in a small group of subjects (12–100). In this context, the drug may be used only at a single high dose, that is, at the maximum tolerated dose. In the subsequent phase IIb trial, several dose levels may be tested (dose-ranging studies) in order to define the minimally effective dose and also to decide the optimal dose, based on efficacy and safety (16,17).

The final stage of drug development is the phase III clinical trial. Phase III clinical trials confirm the dose level, frequency, and timing, of doses. Phase III trials can involve up to several thousands subjects. This large number of subjects is needed to ensure detection of less-frequently arising drug-related toxicities, to acquire a confident assessment of efficacy, and to serve as a basis for the package insert or the drug label (18,19). In addition to being used for clinical trials on drugs, phase I, phase IIa, phase IIb, and phase III clinical trials are also used for gaining FDA approval of diagnostics (20).

a. Logistics of Increasing Dose of Study Drug During the Course of a Phase I Clinical Trial

A Clinical Study Protocol for a phase I trial on an anticancer drug provides guidance on the logistics of deciding on dosing, during a

[15]ICH Harmonised Tripartite Guideline. Dose-response information to support drug registration E4; March 1994. 12 pp.

[16]Bonderman D, et al. Riociguat for patients with pulmonary hypertension caused by systolic left ventricular dysfunction: a phase IIb double-blind, randomized, placebo-controlled, dose-ranging hemodynamic study. Circulation 2013;128:502–11.

[17]Tamimi NA, Ellis P. Drug development: from concept to marketing! Nephron Clin. Pract. 2009;113:c125–1231.

[18]U.S. Dept. of Health and Human Services. Food and Drug Administration. Guidance for Industry. Labeling for human prescription drug and biological products—implementing the PLR content and format requirements; February 2013 (30 pp.).

[19]Tamimi NA, Ellis P. Drug development: from concept to marketing! Nephron Clin. Pract. 2009;113:c125–1231.

[20]Colli A, et al. The architecture of diagnostic research: from bench to bedside – research guidelines using liver stiffness as an example. Hepatology 2014;60:408–18.

dose-escalating trial. By "logistics," what is meant is the process by which company employees agree upon an appropriate dose. The term "DLT" means dose-limiting toxicity, and MTD means maximum tolerated dose (21). CTCAE, which is used in oncology clinical trials, is a standard dictionary of adverse events, that is, it grades toxicity to various organs in the body (22). PK refers to pharmacokinetics. Reference to "cohort" and to "next cohort" means a group of study subjects administered a lower dose, and a subsequent group of study subjects receiving a higher dose.

Regarding the logistics, the Clinical Study Protocol included the instructions (23):

> **Dose-selection process:** At the end of each treatment cohort, [the Sponsor] will convene a teleconference with the investigators of the escalation phase. At the dose escalation teleconference the clinical course (safety information including both DLTs and all ≥ CTCAE Grade 2 toxicity data during Cycle 1, and PK data) for each patient in the current dose cohort will be described in detail. Updated safety data on other ongoing patients, including data in later cycles, will be discussed as well.
>
> To determine the dose regimen for the next cohort, the available toxicity information (including adverse events that are not DLTs), PK, PD, and efficacy information, as well as the recommendations from the BLRM will be evaluated by the Investigators and [the Sponsor's] study personnel … at the dose decision meeting. The parties must reach a consensus on whether to declare MTD, escalate the dose any further, or whether to de-escalate and/or expand recruitment into particular cohorts. [The Sponsor] will prepare minutes from these meetings

and circulate them to each investigator for comment prior to finalization. Drug administration at the next dose level may not proceed until the investigator receives written confirmation from [the Sponsor] that the results of the previous dose level were evaluated and the higher dose level is estimated not to have exceeded the MTD. Dose escalation will continue until identification of the MTD or PK futility (defined as no substantive increase in exposure despite administration of increasing doses) is encountered.

b. FDA's Decision-Making Process in Arriving at the Best Dose, From Phase I Trial Data

At the time the FDA grants approval to a drug, the FDA publishes its *Approval Letter*, *Medical Review*, *Pharmacological Review*, and other reviews. The FDA's comments in these reviews reveals the FDA's decision-making process, its interpretation of the Sponsor's data, as well as its comments on specific features of trial design.

This example discloses the arrival at the proper drug dose, which was part of the approval process for a drug used for treating colorectal cancer. The information is from BLA 125084, located on February 2014 of the FDA website. The drug was cetuximab, an antibody (24). The phase I trial contained a pharmacodynamics study, where the influence of drug on its target was measured. The target of the drug was a protein expressed by tumor cells. This protein was epidermal growth factor receptor (EGFR). In addition, the study

---

[21]Braun TM. The current design of oncology phase I clinical trials: progressing from algorithms to statistical models. Chin. Clin. Oncol. 2014;3:2. http://dx.doi.org/10.3978/j.issn.2304-3865.2014.02.01.

[22]National Cancer Institute (NCI)/National Institutes of Health (NIH) Common Terminology Criteria for Adverse Events, version 4 (CTCAE v4.0).

[23]Oncology Clinical Trial Protocol CLDK378X2101. A phase I, multicenter, open-label dose escalation study of LDK378, administered orally in adult patients with tumors characterized by genetic abnormalities in anaplastic lymphoma kinase (ALK); August 19, 2010.

[24]Martinelli E, De Palma R, Orditura M, De Vita F, Cirdiello F. Anti-epidermal growth factor receptor monoclonal antibodies in cancer therapy. Clin. Exp. Immunol. 2009;158:1−9.

also assessed safety. Study subjects received increasing amounts of drug, where the influence of drug dose on EGFR expression and on toxicity was measured.

In the phase I clinical trial, study subjects received 50, 100, 250, 400, or 500 mg antibody/m^2. (Each subject received only one level of dose. It was not the case that any given subject received more than one dose level.) The term "meter-squared" refers to body surface area of the patient. In other words, drug dose was based on the body surface area, rather than the patient's weight. The dose escalation study showed that an acceptable safety profile was found at up to and including 400 mg/m^2. But at the higher level of 500 mg/m^2, the result was an unacceptable *high incidence of toxicity to the skin* (25). Regarding the influence of escalating doses on expression of EGFR by tumors, *maximal inhibition of EGFR expression* occurred at 250–500 mg/m^2. But at doses below 250 mg/m^2, the researchers found that increases in EGFR expression occurred. The FDA reviewer concluded that therapeutic activity would best be maintained at a drug dose of 250 mg/m^2 or above. Hence, the data from this FDA *Medical Review* implicated the best dose as one that is at or above 250 mg/m^2, but lower than 500 mg/m^2 (26). The recommended dose on the *package insert was 400 mg/m^2*. Thus, the *Medical Review* reveals how data from a phase I study were used to arrive at the most appropriate dose for the package insert.

II. STUDY DESIGN

Clinical studies take various forms. At its simplest, one person takes a drug, and the person's response to the drug is measured. The response can takes the form of various parameters, such as blood pressure, data from an electrocardiogram (27,28), and titer of a given bacterium or virus, where these parameters are measured shortly before, as well as after, taking the drug.

Phase I clinical trials, which typically involve only a small number of subjects, focus on drug safety, pharmacokinetics, the influence of food on the PK of the drug, the dose providing the greatest efficacy, and the most appropriate route of dosing. Regarding the dosing route, drugs may be administered orally (per os), intramuscularly (IM), intravenously (IV), subcutaneously (SC), rectally, or by inhalation.

Large clinical trials include one or more study arms. For example, a two-arm clinical trial can take the form of a study drug group and a placebo group. Also, a two-arm clinical trial can take the form of a study drug group and an active control group. The term "active control" usually refers to an older drug that has been the standard of care for the disease of interest. Moreover, a three-arm clinical trial can include a study drug group, placebo group, and active control group. The terms placebo and active control are further defined below. Other features of clinical trial design include a run-in period and a follow-up period.

[25]Pai-Scherf LH, Thornton M, Andrich M, Mills G, Keegan P. STN/BLA 125084. Medical Review. Erbitux (cetuximab). February 12, 2004.

[26]Pai-Scherf LH, Thornton M, Andrich M, Mills G, Keegan P. STN/BLA 125084. Medical Review. Erbitux (cetuximab). February 12, 2004.

[27]U.S. Dept. of Health and Human Services. Food and Drug Administration. E14 clinical evaluation of QT/QTc interval prolongation and proarrhythmic potential for non-antiarrhythmic drugs; October 2012 (9 pp.).

[28]Giorgi MA, Bolaños R, Gonzalez CD, Di Girolamo G. QT interval prolongation: preclinical and clinical testing arrhythmogenesis in drugs and regulatory implications. Curr. Drug Saf. 2010;5:54–7.

Large clinical trials focus on safety and efficacy, but other types of information may additionally be collected, for example, data on pharmacokinetics, correlations between a drug's efficacy and the subject's genetic makeup, and correlations between the drug's adverse effects and the subject's genetic makeup.

The instructions for conducting a clinical trial are contained in a document called a Clinical Study Protocol. The Clinical Study Protocol may include a flow chart in the form of a stick-diagram, or a table called a schema. The schema is the best way to communicate the structure and timeline of any clinical trial. Shown below are various hypothetical study schema, followed by a collection of representative schema from actual clinical trials.

III. THE STUDY SCHEMA

a. Introduction

The treatment schedule or timeline used in clinical trials is represented by the study schema. When included in a Clinical Study Protocol, or in a research publication, the schema aids in understanding the dosing schedule. Moreover, when designing a clinical trial,

the principal investigator may draw several versions of the schema, before arriving at the final version to be used in the study.

Where only writing is used to describe the study design, and where the study design includes multiple branching points (or multiple segments), and where the entire study is described in a single lengthy sentence, the narrative risks ambiguity.

Additionally, where only writing is used to describe study design, and where the sentences include multiple periods, and where the exact meaning depends on the placement of each comma, ambiguity is the predictable result. Moreover, the term "biweekly," which is often used to describe trial design, is distinguished in that it has two different meanings. "Biweekly" means twice per week. "Biweekly" also means once every 2 weeks. For the above reasons, a schema should be considered for even the simplest trial designs.

At its simplest, the study schema might take the form shown in Fig. 2.1. This particular study schema can be used for clinical trials in oncology, infectious diseases, immune disorders, metabolic diseases, and so on. The schema shown below has two arms, where one arm receives the study drug and the other arm receives a placebo. The schema has six boxes and four arrows (Fig. 2.1).

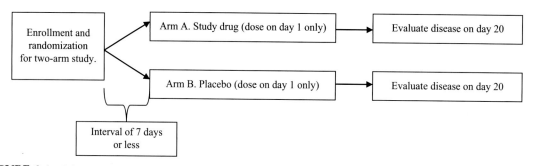

FIGURE 2.1   Schema with two study arms. This schema shows the step of enrollment, the interval of time between enrollment and treatment, and the steps of treatment and evaluation of efficacy.

The study design may also be one that contains only one arm, that is, a single-arm study, as shown in Fig. 2.2. The schema contains four blocks and two arrows. In a single-arm study, the patient may serve as his own control. In this situation, the patient's health immediately prior to enrolling in the study (baseline) is used for comparison purposes. In another type of single-arm study, the outcome for each patient may be compared to the outcome of a historical control. The historical control group can be from the same institution or the same investigators as in the present single-arm study, or it can be from a totally unrelated group of investigators.

Figure 2.3 discloses a schema that includes a run-in period. Run-in periods are used for a variety of reasons, as detailed in Chapter 3. The common feature of all of these run-in periods is that they occur immediately prior to randomization of the subjects, and immediately prior to allocation of the subjects to the various study arms.

The schema (Fig. 2.3) contains seven boxes and six arrows. This run-in period is used to

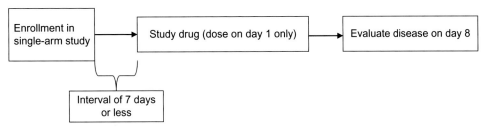

FIGURE 2.2 Schema with one study arm. The schema shows the step of enrollment, the interval of time from enrollment to beginning treatment, and the step of evaluating efficacy of treatment.

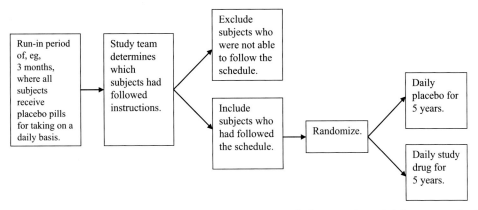

FIGURE 2.3 Schema including a run-in period. The study design includes a run-in period that screens for the ability of potential subjects to follow the treatment schedule.

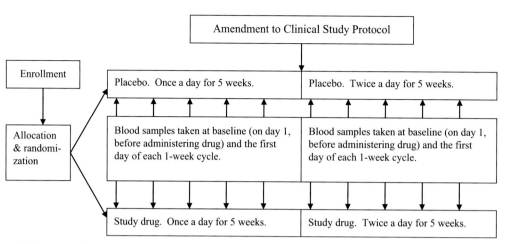

FIGURE 2.4 Schema of a two-arm study where the study design was changed during the study. The schema shows the date when the study design was changed. Also shown are dates when blood samples were withdrawn.

test the ability of potential study subjects to adhere to a timely and orderly schedule of pill-taking. Information on patient adherence is especially critical for clinical studies on drugs that are intended for *chronic administration*. Drugs intended for chronic administration include atorvastatin (marketed as Lipitor®), which is used to prevent heart attacks, and finasteride (Proscar®) (29,30) which is used to prevent prostate cancer. Several drugs for *chronic administration* are also used to prevent breast cancer (31).

Figure 2.4 provides a hypothetical schema revealing various procedural issues, such as the existence of an amendment to the Clinical Study Protocol. The procedural issues in this schema also include the step of enrollment, the steps of allocation and randomization, and the taking of

blood samples. The goal of the amendment was to get permission to increase the drug dose.

The following provides a selection of representative schema from real clinical trials. Oncology clinical trials are usually more complex than clinical trials for other diseases, because of the use of multiple drugs, often with staggered dosing schedules, and sometimes used in combination with radiation therapy. For this reason, the following schema are from oncology clinical trials.

Study designs sometimes include a decision tree. Typically, decision trees in clinical trials require assessment of the response at a particular date, and deciding whether to increase or decrease the dose given to each individual subject, or deciding to remove the subject from the trial.

[29]Moinpour CM, Lovato LC, Thompson IM. Profile of men randomized to the prostate cancer prevention trial: baseline health-related quality of life, urinary and sexual functioning, and health behaviors. J. Clin. Oncol. 2000;18:1942−53.

[30]Moinpour CM, Darke AK, Donaldson GW, et al. Longitudinal analysis of sexual function reported by men in the prostate cancer prevention trial. J. Natl. Cancer Inst. 2007;99:1025−35.

[31]Sestak I. Preventative therapies for healthy women at high risk of breast cancer. Cancer Manag. Res. 2014;6:423−30.

As is evident, various schema emphasize different aspects of the trial, for example, details on the run-in period, schedules of drug dosing, decision trees that take into account drug toxicity, and schedules for blood sample collection.

The concepts illustrated by the following study schema are summarized by the bulletpoints.

- Staging (32,33,34). Staging refers to identifying the stage (severity) of a particular disease
- Staging followed by restaging (35)

- Schemas showing a decision tree (36,37)
- Schema for a dose-escalation clinical trial (38,39,40)
- Run-in period that determines expression of a biomarker (41)
- Schema indicating days for evaluating pharmacokinetics (42)
- Schema with a run-in period where risk for an adverse event is assessed (43)
- What to do about placebo dosing, where two arms of the clinical trial receive two different volumes of a study drug (44)

[32]Reeves HL, Aisen AM. Hepatocellular carcinoma: optimal staging impacts survival. Gastroenterology 2015; pii: S0016-5085(15)00582-X. http://dx.doi.org/10.1053/j.gastro.2015.04.026.

[33]Prat J, et al. FIGO's staging classification for cancer of the ovary, fallopian tube, and peritoneum: abridged republication. J. Gynecol. Oncol. 2015;26:87−9.

[34]Blumenschein GR, Khuri FR, von Pawel J, et al. Phase III trial comparing carboplatin, paclitaxel, and bexarotene with carboplatin and paclitaxel in chemotherapy-naive patients with advanced or metastatic non-small-cell lung cancer: SPIRIT II. J. Clin. Oncol. 2008;26:1879−85.

[35]Czito BG, Willett CG, Bendell JC, et al. Increased toxicity with gefitinib, capecitabine, and radiation therapy in pancreatic and rectal cancer: phase I trial results. J. Clin. Oncol. 2006;24:656−62.

[36]Baselga J, Zambetti M, Llombart-Cussac A, et al. Phase II genomics study of ixabepilone as neoadjuvant treatment for breast cancer. J. Clin. Oncol. 2009;27:526−34.

[37]Katsumata N, Watanabe T, Minami H, et al. Phase III trial of doxorubicin plus cyclophosphamide (AC), docetaxel, and alternating AC and docetaxel as front-line chemotherapy for metastatic breast cancer: Japan Clinical Oncology Group trial (JCOG9802). Ann. Oncol. 2009;20:1210−5.

[38]Marshall J, Chen H, Yang D, et al. A phase I trial of a Bcl-2 antisense (G3139) and weekly docetaxel in patients with advanced breast cancer and other solid tumors. Ann. Oncol. 2004;15:1274−83.

[39]Moore M, Hirte HW, Siu L, et al. Phase I study to determine the safety and pharmacokinetics of the novel Raf kinase and VEGFR inhibitor BAY 43-9006, administered for 28 days on/7 days off in patients with advanced, refractory solid tumors. Ann. Oncol. 2005;16:1688−94.

[40]Van Cutsem E, Verslype C, Beale P, et al. A phase Ib dose-escalation study of erlotinib, capecitabine and oxaliplatin in metastatic colorectal cancer patients. Ann. Oncol. 2008;19:332−9.

[41]Dy GK, Miller AA, Mandrekar SJ, et al. A phase II trial of imatinib (ST1571) in patients with c-kit expressing relapsed small-cell lung cancer: a CALGB and NCCTG study. Ann. Oncol. 2005;16:1811−6.

[42]Marshall J, Chen H, Yang D, et al. A phase I trial of a Bcl-2 antisense (G3139) and weekly docetaxel in patients with advanced breast cancer and other solid tumors. Ann. Oncol. 2004;15:1274−83.

[43]Ganz PA, Hussey MA, Moinpour CM, et al. Late cardiac effects of adjuvant chemotherapy in breast cancer survivors treated on Southwest Oncology Group protocol s8897. J. Clin. Oncol. 2008;26:1223−30.

[44]Reck M, von Pawel J, Zatloukal P, et al. Phase III trial of cisplatin plus gemcitabine with either placebo or bevacizumab as first-line therapy for nonsquamous non-small-cell lung cancer: AVAil. J. Clin. Oncol. 2009;27:1227−34.

- Run-in period, that determines response to chemotherapy, where chemotherapy is provided before initiation of the clinical trial (45)
- Two study arms, where one arm uses sequential dosing with two drugs, while the other arm uses concurrent administration of the same two drugs (46)
- Comparing neoadjuvant therapy with adjuvant therapy (47)
- Schema where each study arm uses both neoadjuvant therapy, followed by surgery, followed by adjuvant therapy (48)
- Two study arms, where the first arm uses a specific order of administration of two different drugs, while the second arm uses the reverse order of administration of the two drugs (49)

- Patients receiving three different drugs, each drug having its own different schedule (50).

Burstein et al. (51) provide an interesting thumbnail diagram depicting a dozen different schema for various oncology clinical trials. Chittick et al. (52) provide a particularly interesting schema from a clinical trial on infections.

b. Sequential Treatment Versus Concurrent Treatment—The Perez Schema

In a clinical trial with three arms, Perez et al. (53) disclosed the first arm as the control arm, the second arm as a sequential arm, and

[45]Hanna NH, Sandier AB, Loehrer Sr PJ, et al. Maintenance daily oral etoposide versus no further therapy following induction chemotherapy with etoposide plus ifosfamide plus cisplatin in extensive small-cell lung cancer: a Hoosier Oncology Group randomized study. Ann. Oncol. 2002;13:95—102.

[46]Perez EA, Suman VJ, Davidson NE, et al. Cardiac safety analysis of doxorubicin and cyclophosphamide followed by paclitaxel with or without trastuzumab in the North Central Cancer Treatment Group N9831 adjuvant breast cancer trial. J. Clin. Oncol. 2008;26:1231—8.

[47]Gianni L, Baselga J, Eiermann W, et al. Phase III trial evaluating the addition of paclitaxel to doxorubicin followed by cyclophosphamide, methotrexate, and fluorouracil, as adjuvant or primary systemic therapy: European Cooperative Trial in Operable Breast Cancer. J. Clin. Oncol. 2009;27:2474—81.

[48]Untch M, Möbus V, Kuhn W, et al. Intensive dose-dense compared with conventionally scheduled preoperative chemotherapy for high-risk primary breast cancer. J. Clin. Oncol. 2009;27:2938—45.

[49]Puhalla S, Mrozek E, Young D, et al. Randomized phase II adjuvant trial of dose-dense docetaxel before or after doxorubicin plus cyclophosphamide in axillary node-positive breast cancer. J. Clin. Oncol. 2008;26:1691—7.

[50]Sekine I, Nishiwaki Y, Noda K, et al. Randomized phase II study of cisplatin, irinotecan and etoposide combinations administered weekly or every 4 weeks for extensive small-cell lung cancer (JCOG9902-DI). Ann. Oncol. 2003;14:709—14.

[51]Burstein HJ, Prestrud AA, Seidenfeld J, et al. American Society of Clinical Oncology clinical practice guideline: update on adjuvant endocrine therapy for women with hormone receptor-positive breast cancer. J. Clin. Oncol. 2010;28:3784—96.

[52]Chittick GE, Zong J, Blum MR, et al. Pharmacokinetics of tenofovir disoproxil fumarate and ritonavir-boosted saquinavir mesylate administered alone or in combination at steady state. Antimicrob. Agents Chemother. 2006;50:1304—10.

[53]Perez EA, Suman VJ, Davidson NE, et al. Cardiac safety analysis of doxorubicin and cyclophosphamide followed by paclitaxel with or without trastuzumab in the North Central Cancer Treatment Group N9831 adjuvant breast cancer trial. J. Clin. Oncol. 2008;26:1231—8.

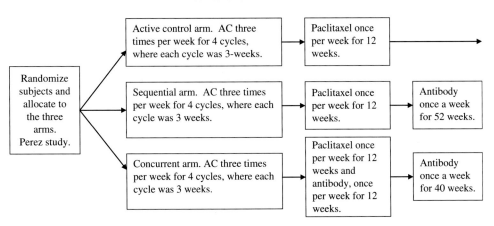

FIGURE 2.5 Schema of a three-arm study. The first arm received an active control treatment. The second arm received small-molecule drug plus antibody on different, nonoverlapping weeks (sequential treatment), while the third arm received small-molecule drug and antibody at the same time, that is, during the same week (concurrent treatment).

the third arm as a concurrent arm (Fig. 2.5). In the control arm, patients received an active control (AC) followed by paclitaxel. The abbreviation "AC" refers to doxorubicin, which is an anthracycline (AC) drug. In the sequential arm, patients received the same drugs as in the active control arm, but followed by an antibody (trastuzumab). In the concurrent arm, patients received the same drugs as in the active control arm, but with the antibody given at the same time (concurrently) as paclitaxel. Trastuzumab (Herceptin®) is an antibody that binds to HER2.

The goal of the study was to determine which treatment was least toxic to the heart. Arm A, which did not include the antibody, was the least cardiotoxic (cardiac damage in 0.3% of subjects). Arm B was more toxic (2.8% cardiotoxic). Arm C was the most toxic (3.3%

cardiac damage), but only slightly more toxic than Arm B.

As a general proposition, sequential chemotherapy is preferred over combination chemotherapy, where reducing toxicity is especially needed, for example, with patients who are elderly (54). In other words, toxicity is expected to be a bigger problem where two drugs are administered on the same day, and a lesser problem where two different drugs are administered on separate days. Raetz et al. (55) provide a dramatic example of sequential chemotherapy, but for a different reason. In this study, three different blocks of chemotherapy were administered. Each of these three blocks delivered a different collection of drugs. The goal of using these three blocks of time (nonoverlapping blocks) of chemotherapy was to ensure a lengthy period of remission.

[54]Miles D, von Minckwitz G, Seidman AD. Combination versus sequential single-agent therapy in metastatic breast cancer. Oncologist 2002;7(Suppl. 6):13−9.

[55]Raetz EA, Borowitz MJ, Devidas M, et al. Reinduction platform for children with first marrow relapse of acute lymphoblastic leukemia: A Children's Oncology Group Study. J. Clin. Oncol. 2008;26:3971−8.

c. Neoadjuvant Chemotherapy Versus Adjuvant Chemotherapy—The Gianni Schema

Gianni et al. (56) provide a schema for a three-arm clinical trial, where two arms use adjuvant chemotherapy and one arm uses neoadjuvant chemotherapy (Fig. 2.6).

The term "adjuvant chemotherapy" refers to chemotherapy that follows surgery. In contrast, the term "neoadjuvant chemotherapy," sometimes called "induction chemotherapy," refers to chemotherapy that precedes surgery.

In one adjuvant arm, patients received surgery followed by A, which was followed by CMF. In another adjuvant arm, patients received surgery followed by AT, which was followed by CMF. But in the neoadjuvant arm, patients received AT, and then CMF, and finally surgery.

"A" refers to doxorubicin, a drug that is an anthracycline group (A). "T" refers to paclitaxel, a drug that is a taxane (T). "CMF" refers to the combination of cyclophosphamide, methotrexate, and 5-fluorouracil. The take-home lesson from this schema is as follows. In designing the clinical trial, the investigator is free to test surgery followed by drugs (adjuvant), as well as drugs followed by surgery (neoadjuvant).

d. Neoadjuvant Chemotherapy Plus Adjuvant Chemotherapy—The Untch Schema

The clinical study of Untch et al. (57) uses a schema where, for every patient, chemotherapy was given before surgery and also after surgery (Fig. 2.7). Hence, the schema involved neoadjuvant therapy as well as adjuvant therapy, for every patient.

It is interesting to point out that one study arm involved concurrent chemotherapy (both drugs at once) while the other study arm involved sequential chemotherapy (drugs administered, not on the same day, but on different days).

CMF refers to the combination of three drugs, cyclophosphamide, methotrexate, and 5-fluorouracil. Although randomization was part of the trial design, the schema shown below does not contain a box representing the event of randomization.

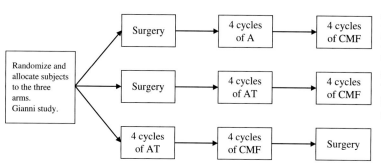

FIGURE 2.6 Schema showing three-arm study where subjects received adjuvant therapy or neoadjuvant therapy. The first two arms received adjuvant therapy, that is, surgery prior to drugs. The third arm received neoadjuvant therapy, that is, drugs for down-sizing the tumors prior to surgery.

[56]Gianni L, Baselga J, Eiermann W, et al. Phase III trial evaluating the addition of paclitaxel to doxorubicin followed by cyclophosphamide, methotrexate, and fluorouracil, as adjuvant or primary systemic therapy: European Cooperative Trial in Operable Breast Cancer. J. Clin. Oncol. 2009;27:2474—81.

[57]Untch M, Möbus V, Kuhn W, et al. Intensive dose-dense compared with conventionally scheduled preoperative chemotherapy for high-risk primary breast cancer. J. Clin. Oncol. 2009;27:2938—45.

e. Forwards Sequence and Reverse Sequence—The Puhalla Schema

The clinical trial of Puhalla et al. (58) contains two arms (Fig. 2.8). Subjects in the first arm received drugs in this order: D followed by AC.

In detail, subjects received docetaxel on the first day of each cycle, for four cycles, where each cycle was 14 days long. This was followed by doxorubicin (an anthracycline drug) plus cyclophosphamide, on the first day of each cycle, for four cycles. Each cycle was 2 weeks long.

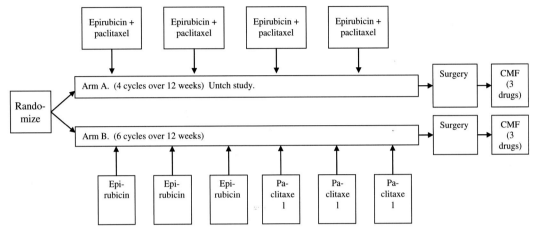

FIGURE 2.7 Schema showing two-arm study. Subjects in the first arm received chemotherapy before as well as after surgery. Subjects in the second arm also received chemotherapy prior to and after surgery. The neoadjuvant chemotherapy in arm A was concurrent, what that in arm B was sequential.

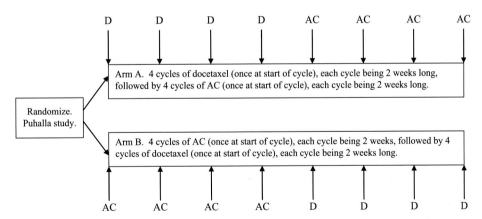

FIGURE 2.8 Schema showing a two-arm study. In this two-arm study drugs were administered in a "forward" sequence for arm A, and in a "reverse" sequence for arm B.

[58]Puhalla S, Mrozek E, Young D, et al. Randomized phase II adjuvant trial of dose-dense docetaxel before or after doxorubicin plus cyclophosphamide in axillary node-positive breast cancer. J. Clin. Oncol. 2008;26:1691−7.

Now, this is about the second arm. Subjects in the second arm received drugs in the reverse order, that is, AC followed by D. The investigators chose a two-arm study design, where each arm was the reverse of the other, because it was not possible to predict which order would provide the best outcome.

Utility in trial design, where one arm uses a "forward sequence" of two drugs, and another arm uses the "reverse sequence" of the two drugs, sometimes finds a basis in the mechanism of action of certain drugs. The following specifically concerns chemotherapy involving paclitaxel and gemcitabine. As explained by Paccagnella et al. (59), for a clinical trial on lung cancer, "[s]everal reports have shown that the sequence of administration of gemcitabine and paclitaxel may also affect the efficacy of this combination chemotherapy, since paclitaxel increases the concentration of active metabolite of gemcitabine (dFdCTP) when administered first."

f. Both Arms Received Three Drugs, Each Arm at a Different Schedule—The Sekine Schema

In a clinical trial of lung cancer, Sekine et al. (60) administered three drugs to all subjects in arm A and the same three drugs to all subjects in arm B (Fig. 2.9). Different schedules were used for each of the three drugs. The two arms

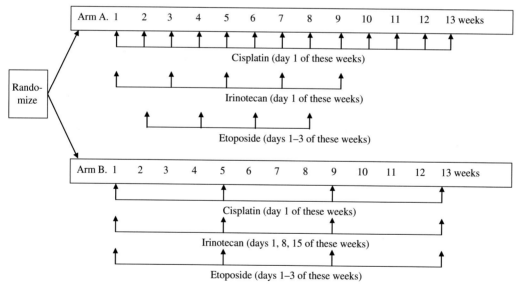

FIGURE 2.9   Schema showing a two-arm study. Each arm received the same three drugs, but with different timing for each of the three drugs.

[59]Paccagnella A, Oniga F, Bearz A, et al. Adding gemcitabine to paclitaxel/carboplatin combination increases survival in advanced non-small-cell lung cancer: results of a phase II-III study. J. Clin. Oncol. 2006;24:681−7.

[60]Sekine I, Nishiwaki Y, Noda K, et al. Randomized phase II study of cisplatin, irinotecan and etoposide combinations administered weekly or every 4 weeks for extensive small-cell lung cancer (JCOG9902-DI). Ann. Oncol. 2003;14:709−14.

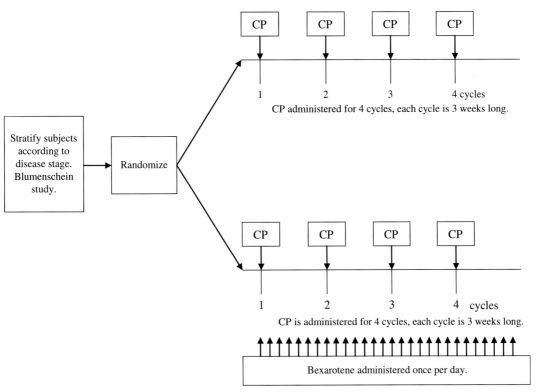

FIGURE 2.10   Schema showing a two-arm study. The schema shows the steps of stratification and randomization. The daily administration of bexarotene is unambiguous, as the schema shows a separate arrow for each of the 28 days of administration of this drug.

were different from each other in that different schedules were used for administering the drugs.

The three drugs shown on the schema, cisplatin, irinotecan, and etoposide, are small-molecule drugs. Subjects also received a fourth drug, granulocyte colony stimulating factor (G-CSF). G-CSF is a polypeptide, not a small molecule. For clarity in presentation, G-CSF is not shown on the schema. Blood samples and chest X-rays were taken at various intervals

(not shown). Blood counts were run twice a week, and chest X-rays were conducted once a week. Chest X-rays are used during the diagnosis and treatment of lung cancer (61).

g. Staging—The Blumenschein Schema

The schema of Blumenschein et al. (62) reveals three different steps in the trial design (Fig. 2.10). These are the steps to stratifying patients according to disease stage, the step of

[61]Gohagan JK, Marcus PM, Fagerstrom RM, et al. Final results of the Lung Screening Study, a randomized feasibility study of spiral CT versus chest X-ray screening for lung cancer. Lung Cancer 2005;47:9−15.

[62]Blumenschein Jr GR, Khuri FR, von Pawel J, et al. Phase III trial comparing carboplatin, paclitaxel, and bexarotene with carboplatin and paclitaxel in chemotherapy-naive patients with advanced or metastatic non-small-cell lung cancer: SPIRIT II. J. Clin. Oncol. 2008;26:1879−85.

randomization, and the step of drug administration. Although most clinical trials in oncology stratify patients before randomization, this particular schema is unique in that the published flow chart actually includes a box showing the step of stratification. Subjects in the two arms received the same drugs, except that arm B received an additional drug, bexarotene. CP refers to carboplatin plus paclitaxel. Carboplatin is in a class of drugs called platinum drugs. Paclitaxel is in a class of drugs called taxanes.

h. Staging and Restaging—The Czito Schema

In a clinical study involving chemotherapy and radiation, Czito et al. (63) provided a schema that indicates steps where staging occurred (Fig. 2.11). Although staging is used in clinical trials in oncology, infections, immune diseases, and other disorders, it is only on occasion that the step of staging is actually depicted in the schema. Staging was specifically included in this schema to emphasize the fact that staging was done at two different points during the course of the clinical trial.

The trial was a single-arm trial. Because the trial had only one arm, the subjects were not randomized. In other words, subjects were not randomized to be treated with arm A drugs or arm B drugs, because there was only one arm. As this was a phase I trial, the main purpose was to determine the DLT, that is, to determine a dose suitable for using in a subsequent phase II trial.

Chemotherapy was given every day for 38 days. Radiation was given on the same days as the drugs, except not on Saturdays or Sundays. The days for radiation treatment are made unambiguous by the schema, as it shows arrows only on week days (not on weekends).

i. Methodology Tip—Staging

The term *staging* refers to measuring the parameters of a cancer, with respect to a set of criteria accepted by the medical profession. For most cancers, there are established, published criteria for determining whether the cancer is at, for example, stage I, stage II, stage III, or stage IV. By staging, what is meant is the determination of the size, number, and location of tumors, and the comparison of these values

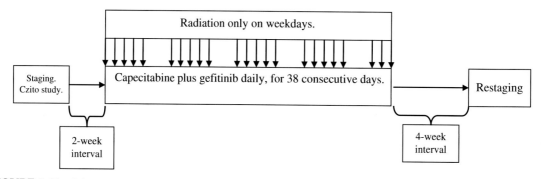

FIGURE 2.11 Schema of a single-arm clinical trial. Staging of the tumors occurred at two time points, as indicated.

[63]Czito BG, Willett CG, Bendell JC, et al. Increased toxicity with gefitinib, capecitabine, and radiation therapy in pancreatic and rectal cancer: phase I trial results. J. Clin. Oncol. 2006;24:656–62.

with established standards for different stages for the cancer. By *restaging*, what is meant is repeating the determination of the size, number, and location of the tumors, and comparing these values with the standard for staging of the cancer in question. Staging encompasses the acts of determining whether the tumors are resectable, locally advanced, or metastatic. Staging can be accomplished using computed tomography, endoscopic ultrasound, and surgical evaluation.

j. Decision Tree—The Baselga Schema

The schema of Baselga et al. (64) depicts two points where a decision needed to be made (Fig. 2.12). These two points are indicated by the forked arrows. The decision involved assessing the tumor's response to therapy (at that time point) for every individual patient. Based on the tumor's response, the patient was assigned to one of two different therapies.

The Baselga clinical trial could be characterized as a single-arm trial, because there was no control group and no placebo group. The goal of the trial was to detect correlations between gene expression, as determined by measuring gene expression in tumor biopsies, and positive response to drug treatment. The expression of 200 genes was measured, where these genes were chosen before the study. This clinical trial involved neoadjuvant chemotherapy. Neoadjuvant refers to the fact that chemotherapy was administered before surgery (not after surgery). Where the schema reads, "tumors shrink or remain stable" or "tumors progress," this indicates that the physician had examined the patient, determined the status of the tumors, and made the decision to use the treatment that is

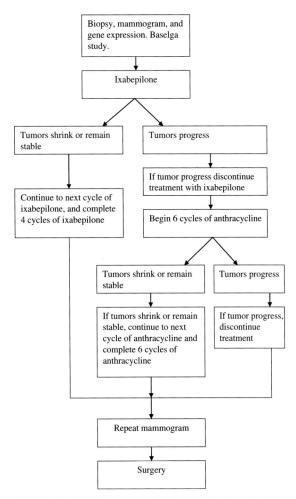

FIGURE 2.12 Schema with boxes showing decision points. Forked arrows indicate time points when tumors were assessed, and when a decision was made to proceed with the indicated course of action.

disclosed in the subsequent (lower) arrows on the flow chart.

Where the trial design includes a decision point or decision tree, the medical writer should use forked arrows in the schema to indicate the decision.

[64]Baselga J, Zambetti M, Llombart-Cussac A, et al. Phase II genomics study of ixabepilone as neoadjuvant treatment for breast cancer. J. Clin. Oncol. 2009;27:526−34.

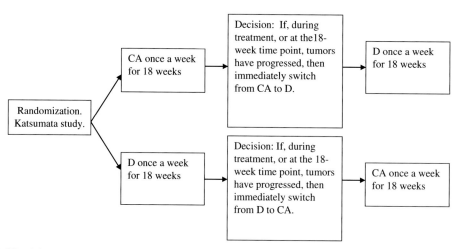

FIGURE 2.13   Schema showing a two-arm study. Each of the two arms incorporated a cross-over design.

k. Decision Tree—The Katsumata Schema

Decision trees occur in the schema of Katsumata et al. (65), where the decision is triggered by an increase (if any) in tumor size (Fig. 2.13). At each decision point, the decision takes the form of crossing over to the alternate therapy, or of continuing with the same type of drug. The letter "A" represents doxorubicin, an anthracycline compound (66). C represents cyclophosphamide. Thus, AC means the combination of doxorubicin plus cyclophosphamide. D represents docetaxel.

The decision to switch drugs was triggered by detection of tumor progression either during the first 18 weeks of treatment or after completion of the first 18 weeks of treatment. In the words of the investigators, "[o]n treatment failure or disease progression during or after treatment, patients were crossed over from AC to D, or from D to AC" (67).

The Katsumata schema shows a cross-over design (Fig. 2.13). Cross-over means that subjects receiving CA therapy, upon encountering the decision tree, were crossed over to D therapy. And subjects receiving D therapy, upon encountering the decision tree, were crossed over to CA therapy. If no tumor progression was detected, then patients were not switched to a different drug. (The clinical trial actually included a third arm, but for clarity in presentation, this arm was omitted from the schema shown below.)

[65]Katsumata N, Watanabe T, Minami H, et al. Phase III trial of doxorubicin plus cyclophosphamide (AC), docetaxel, and alternating AC and docetaxel as front-line chemotherapy for metastatic breast cancer: Japan Clinical Oncology Group trial (JCOG9802). Ann. Oncol. 2009;20:1210–5.

[66]O'Shaughnessy J, Twelves C, Aapro M. Treatment for anthracycline-pretreated metastatic breast cancer. Oncologist 2002;7(Suppl. 6):4–12.

[67]Katsumata N, Watanabe T, Minami H, et al. Phase III trial of doxorubicin plus cyclophosphamide (AC), docetaxel, and alternating AC and docetaxel as front-line chemotherapy for metastatic breast cancer: Japan Clinical Oncology Group trial (JCOG9802). Ann. Oncol. 2009;20:1210–5.

The following defines the cross-over design. According to Donner (68), the cross-over design involved a single group of subjects, where each subject served as his own control for comparing two treatments. Subjects were randomized to one of two treatment sequences, where half the subjects received the treatments in the order EC, the other half in the order CE. The advantage of this design is that it allows the effects of the treatments to be compared within the same subjects.

The cross-over design may be used for various different goals. One goal is to gain regulatory approval for only one of the drugs, that is, for a treatment scheme that uses only one of the two drugs. Another goal is to gain regulatory approval for the combination of the two drugs, for a treatment scheme where drug A is given for a period of time followed by drug B for a separate period of time.

In comments about the desirability of a cross-over scheme used in clinical practice, Katsumata et al. (69) stated that, "[a]lternating chemotherapy is an approach designed to produce maximal antitumor activity by alternating noncross-resistant regimens of chemotherapy. Alternating chemotherapy has been suggested to be effective in Hodgkin's disease and small-cell lung cancer." In this type of cross-over design, it is desirable that there are "carry-over effects." In other words, it is hoped that the carry-over effects produced by the cross-over design improve the efficacy of the treatment.

ICH Guidelines (70) provide a general comment and warning on the cross-over study design. These comments refer to a cross-over design where the goal is to evaluate the efficacy of just one of the two drugs used in the study (not where it is the goal to evaluate the efficacy of the combination of the two drugs, when the two drugs are administered sequentially):

> A randomized multiple cross-over study of different doses can be successful if drug effect develops rapidly and patients return to baseline conditions quickly after cessation of therapy, if responses are not irreversible (cure, death), and if patients have reasonably stable disease. This design suffers, however, from the potential problems of all cross-over studies: it can have analytic problems if there are many treatment withdrawals; it can be quite long in duration for an individual patient; and there is often uncertainty about carry-over effects (longer treatment periods may minimize this problem), baseline comparability after the first period, and period-by-treatment interactions.

The cross-over design is sometimes used in clinical trials where there is a placebo arm (71,72). Where one group of subjects is initially assigned to the placebo arm, those subjects are assigned to receive the placebo until the endpoint of interest arrives. Typically, the endpoint of interest, at least in oncology

[68]Donner A. Approaches to sample size estimation in the design of clinical trials—a review. Stat. Med. 1984;3:199−214.

[69]Katsumata N, Watanabe T, Minami H, et al. Phase III trial of doxorubicin plus cyclophosphamide (AC), docetaxel, and alternating AC and docetaxel as front-line chemotherapy for metastatic breast cancer: Japan Clinical Oncology Group trial (JCOG9802). Ann. Oncol. 2009;20:1210−5.

[70]ICH Harmonised Tripartite Guideline. Dose-response information to support drug registration E4; March 1994, 12 pp.

[71]Ratain MJ, Sargent DJ. Optimising the design of phase II oncology trials: the importance of randomisation. Eur. J. Cancer 2009;45:275−80.

[72]Seymour L, Ivy SP, Sargent D, et al. The design of phase II clinical trials testing cancer therapeutics: consensus recommendations from the clinical trial design task force of the national cancer institute investigational drug steering committee. Clin. Cancer Res. 2010;16:1764−9.

clinical trials, is growth of the tumors beyond a predetermined point. The event where a tumor grows beyond a predetermined point is known as "progression." For any given subject in the placebo arm, at the time that this end-point is reached, that subject is then crossed-over to the drug (the active treatment) that was used in the study drug arm. Where a cross-over design is used in clinical trials involving a placebo, this design can improve recruitment of subjects in the trial who are not particularly eager to be assigned to the placebo treatment (73,74).

l. Methodology Tip—What Is "Tumor Progression"?

In the clinical trial of Katsumata et al. (75), increases in tumor size were compared to an accepted standard. The accepted standard was as follows: an increase in tumor dimensions of 20% or greater, in the interval between starting chemotherapy and a subsequent tumor assessment.

The term *progression*, in the context of oncology, refers to an increase in tumor size and number, where the increase progresses beyond a certain minimal limit set by these criteria. Progression can be with reference to the RECIST criteria (76,77,78). Some investigators prefer to use an older set of criteria, the WHO response criteria (79,80). The Katsumata study assessed tumors with respect to the WHO criteria.

m. Methodology Tip—Unit of Drug Dose Expressed in Terms of Body Surface Area

The following explains the unit used in the drug dose, "doxorubicin 40 mg/m^2," used above in the study of Katsumata et al. (81). In the words of the investigators, arm A of the clinical trial received, "doxorubicin 40 mg/m^2

[73]Ma BB, Britten CD, Siu LL. Clinical trial designs for targeted agents. Hematol. Oncol. Clin. North Am. 2002;16:1287–305.

[74]Gray R, Manola J, Saxman S, et al. Phase II clinical trial design: methods in translational research from the Genitourinary Committee at the Eastern Cooperative Oncology Group. Clin. Cancer Res. 2006;12:1966–9.

[75]Katsumata N, Watanabe T, Minami H, et al. Phase III trial of doxorubicin plus cyclophosphamide (AC), docetaxel, and alternating AC and docetaxel as front-line chemotherapy for metastatic breast cancer: Japan Clinical Oncology Group trial (JCOG9802). Ann. Oncol. 2009;20:1210–5.

[76]Eisenhauer EA, Therasse P, Bogaerts J, et al. New response evaluation criteria in solid tumours: revised RECIST guideline (version 1.1). Eur. J. Cancer 2009;45:228–47.

[77]Therasse P, Arbuck SG, Eisenhauer EA, et al. New guidelines to evaluate the response to treatment in solid tumors. European Organization for Research and Treatment of Cancer, National Cancer Institute of the United States, National Cancer Institute of Canada. J. Natl. Cancer Inst. 2000;92:205–16.

[78]Schwartz LH, Bogaerts J, Ford R, et al. Evaluation of lymph nodes with RECIST 1.1. Eur. J. Cancer 2009;45:261–7.

[79]World Health Organization. Handbook for reporting results of cancer treatment. Geneva, Switzerland: World Health Organization; 1979, publication 48.

[80]Park JO, Lee SI, Song SY, et al. Measuring response in solid tumors: comparison of RECIST and WHO response criteria. Jpn. J. Clin. Oncol. 2003;33:533–7.

[81]Katsumata N, Watanabe T, Minami H, et al. Phase III trial of doxorubicin plus cyclophosphamide (AC), docetaxel, and alternating AC and docetaxel as front-line chemotherapy for metastatic breast cancer: Japan Clinical Oncology Group trial (JCOG9802). Ann. Oncol. 2009;20:1210–5.

plus cyclophosphamide 500 mg/m^2 (AC) every 3 weeks for six cycles." The investigators also wrote that patients in arm B of the trial received, "docetaxel 60 mg/m^2 (D), administered by IV infusion over the course of 1 h every 3 weeks for six cycles."

A question that arises is, "What is the meaning of the unit: mg/m^2?"

Drug doses are sometimes expressed in terms of body surface area (meters-squared). According to Felici et al. (82) and others (83,84), many anticancer drugs have a narrow therapeutic window. This means that a small change in dose can lead to poor antitumor effects or unacceptable toxicity. The rationale for using body surface area is to normalize the drug dose among patients. Using body surface area in the unit of drug dosing seems to work best for drugs where there is a relationship between body surface area and a pharmacokinetic parameter, such as the parameter of half-life in the bloodstream.

n. Run-In Period—The Schema of Dy

The schema of Dy et al. (85) discloses a run-in period (Fig. 2.14). Where a clinical trial includes a run-in period, it occurs before randomization of subjects and before allocating subjects to the various arms of the trial.

Run-in periods are used for a variety of purposes, for example, for determining whether patients are willing or capable of taking medications on time, or if patients find the study drug to be intolerably toxic.

As shown in the following schema, the run-in period was used to screen patients for expression of a biomarker, c-kit. Where tumors were negative for c-kit, the subject was not included in the trial. Where tumors were positive for c-kit, patients were included in the trial, and were then treated with imatinib.

While all clinical trials have inclusion criteria and exclusion criteria, whether they be in oncology, infectious diseases, or immune disorders, the clinical trial of Dy et al. (86) is

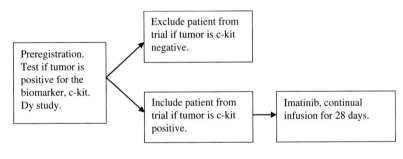

FIGURE 2.14 Study schema of a single-arm trial. The schema includes a run-in period that is used to determine eligibility of each potential subject.

[82]Felici A, Verweij J, Sparreboom A. Dosing strategies for anticancer drugs: the good, the bad and body-surface area. Eur. J. Cancer 2002;38:1677—84.

[83]Sawyer M, Ratain MJ. Body surface area as a determinant of pharmacokinetics and drug dosing. Invest. New Drugs. 2001;19:171—7.

[84]Kouno T, Katsumata N, Mukai H, Ando M, Watanabe T. Standardization of the body surface area (BSA) formula to calculate the dose of anticancer agents in Japan. Jpn. J. Clin. Oncol. 2003;33:309—13.

[85]Dy GK, Miller AA, Mandrekar SJ, et al. A phase II trial of imatinib (ST1571) in patients with c-kit expressing relapsed small-cell lung cancer: a CALGB and NCCTG study. Ann. Oncol. 2005;16:1811—6.

[86]Dy GK, Miller AA, Mandrekar SJ, et al. A phase II trial of imatinib (ST1571) in patients with c-kit expressing relapsed small-cell lung cancer: a CALGB and NCCTG study. Ann. Oncol. 2005;16:1811—6.

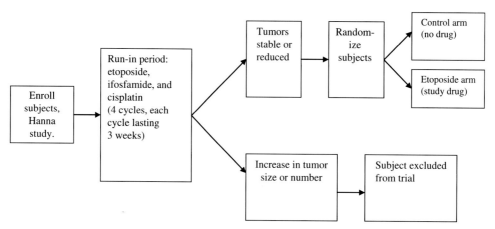

FIGURE 2.15 Study schema of a two-arm study that included a run-in period. The run-in period was used to determine eligibility of the potential study subjects.

unique in that the schema clearly identifies one of the inclusion criteria. The criterion shown in the flow chart is positive expression of c-kit.

Once enrolled in the trial, patients received repeated cycles of imatinib, each cycle lasting 28 days, for a total time of 16 weeks. Imaging was obtained after every other 28-day cycle, where imaging provided data on tumor size and number.

o. Run-In Period—The Hanna Schema

The run-in period of Hanna et al. (87) took the form of a miniature clinical trial where the goal was to determine whether patients would respond favorably to a combination of three drugs (Fig. 2.15).

The three drugs were etoposide, ifosfamide, and cisplatin. After treatment with these three drugs during the run-in period, the patient's

tumors were measured to determine tumor size and number. Where tumor size and number remained constant, or where tumors shrank, patients were then enrolled in the clinical trial, randomized, and assigned to arm A or arm B. But where the combination of the three drugs failed to control tumors, the patient was excluded from further study.

As shown in the schema (Fig. 2.15), patients with tumors controlled by the three drugs were randomized and assigned to arm A (control arm), where patients received no other drug, or to arm B, where patients received etoposide (study drug arm).

Belani et al. (88) also provide a schema with a run-in period, where the run-in period takes the form of a miniature clinical trial occurring before randomization. In the words of these authors, "[a]fter the completion of two cycles of chemotherapy, patients were reassessed with chest CT to ensure the absence of

[87]Hanna NH, Sandier AB, Loehrer Sr PJ, et al. Maintenance daily oral etoposide versus no further therapy following induction chemotherapy with etoposide plus ifosfamide plus cisplatin in extensive small-cell lung cancer: a Hoosier Oncology Group randomized study. Ann. Oncol. 2002;13:95–102.

[88]Belani CP, Wang W, Johnson DH, et al. Phase III study of the Eastern Cooperative Oncology Group (ECOG 2597): induction chemotherapy followed by either standard thoracic radiotherapy or hyperfractionated accelerated radiotherapy for patients with unresectable stage IIIA and B non-small-cell lung cancer. J. Clin. Oncol. 2005;23:3760–7.

metastatic progression. In the absence of meta-static progression, patients were randomly assigned to one of two different ... regimens." The particular type of trial design used by Hanna et al. (89) and by Belani et al. (90) is called, "randomized discontinuation" (91). A run-in period in a clinical trial that has a randomized discontinuation feature serves to enrich the study population for patients likely to respond positively to the study drug.

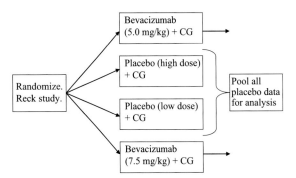

FIGURE 2.16   Study schema with four arms.

p. How to Maintain Blinding of the Treatment When the Study Drug and the Control Treatment Are Provided by Different-Sized Pills (or by Different Volumes of Solutions)—The Reck Schema

The following concerns studies requiring a "double dummy" design, such as the study of Reck et al. (92) (Fig. 2.16). This concerns trials with two different study arms. Subjects in each study arm are assigned to receive a different number of pills (or a different injected volume). For example, subjects in arm A may receive 1 pill/day and subjects in arm B receive 4 pills/day. To provide another example, subjects in arm A receive an injection of 5 mL/day, and subjects in arm B receive an injection of 20 mL/day. This poses the vexing problem of designing the placebo arm.

The problem can be articulated as follows. What approach should be used for arm C (placebo arm) of the study?

The FDA has specifically recognized this situation, writing, "[s]ome trials may study more than one dose of the test treatment ... [i]n these cases, it may be easier for the investigator to use more than one placebo (double-dummy) than to try to make all treatments look the same." Thus, the best solution might be for arm C (placebo) to receive an injection of 5 mL/day of placebo and arm D (also placebo) to receive an injection of 10 mL/day of placebo (93). Thus, for maintaining blinding in this situation, a common approach is to use a double dummy.

[89]Hanna NH, Sandier AB, Loehrer Sr PJ, et al. Maintenance daily oral etoposide versus no further therapy following induction chemotherapy with etoposide plus ifosfamide plus cisplatin in extensive small-cell lung cancer: a Hoosier Oncology Group randomized study. Ann. Oncol. 2002;13:95−102.

[90]Belani CP, Wang W, Johnson DH, et al. Phase III study of the Eastern Cooperative Oncology Group (ECOG 2597): induction chemotherapy followed by either standard thoracic radiotherapy or hyperfractionated accelerated radiotherapy for patients with unresectable stage IIIA and B non-small-cell lung cancer. J. Clin. Oncol. 2005;23:3760−7.

[91]Fu P, Dowlati A, Schluchter M. Comparison of power between randomized discontinuation design and upfront randomization design on progression-free survival. J. Clin. Oncol. 2009;27:4135−41.

[92]Reck M, von Pawel J, Zatloukal P, et al. Phase III trial of cisplatin plus gemcitabine with either placebo or bevacizumab as first-line therapy for nonsquamous non-small-cell lung cancer: AVAil. J. Clin. Oncol. 2009;27:1227−34.

[93]Dept. of Health and Human Services. Food and Drug Administration. Guidance for Industry. E10. Choice of control group and related issues in clinical trials; May 2001.

In the clinical trial of Reck et al. (94), the formulation of the study drug, bevacizumab, was in liquid form, and was injected in patients in two different study arms, one arm receiving a smaller dose and the other arm receiving a larger dose. The two different doses were 7.5 mg/kg body weight and 15 mg/kg body weight.

The problem facing the investigators was how to configure the placebo. The study drug was available in a vial of only one size, and was available at only one concentration. Thus, some of the study drug patients needed to receive the contents of one vial, and the other study drug patients needed to receive the contents of two vials. To avoid bias in the trial, two different placebos were used, one with a small volume and the other with a larger volume, where the volumes corresponded to those of the study drug.

The end-result was that any physician administering a large volume would not likely be capable of guessing whether the large volume dose contained placebo or study drug. Bevacizumab or placebo was administered intravenously and concurrently with chemotherapy every 3 weeks on day 1.

Patients in all four arms of the trial received cisplatin and gemcitabine (CG). Cisplatin was administered on day 1, and gemcitabine was administered on days 1 and 8, of each 21-day cycle. Drug administration was continued for six cycles. Regarding the two placebo groups, Reck et al. (95), stated that, "[p]atients assigned to high- and low-dose placebo were pooled into one placebo group for all analyses."

Another example of using two different placebos, each corresponding to a lower dose and higher dose of study drug, comes from the example of cladribine for treating multiple sclerosis (96).

The following provides two situations where a double-dummy design can be used. In all cases, the double-dummy design is a technique for retaining the blind when administering supplies in a clinical trial, when the two treatments cannot be made identical (97).

The first design, which is from an example from the ICH Guidelines (98), involves a two-arm study where the first arm receives a study drug and the second arm receives another drug, that is, an active control drug. (This study design does not involve any placebo group.)

- *Arm A.* All subjects in arm A receive a round pill that is the active control drug plus a flat pill that is the placebo.
- *Arm B.* All subjects in arm B receive a flat pill that is the study drug plus a round pill that is the placebo.

The second design, also shown below, is a four-arm study, where two arms receive only drugs, and where the remaining two arms receive only placebo.

- *Arm A.* Round pill study drug.
- *Arm B.* Round pill placebo.
- *Arm C.* Flat pill active control drug.
- *Arm D.* Flat pill placebo.

---

[94]Reck M, von Pawel J, Zatloukal P, et al. Phase III trial of cisplatin plus gemcitabine with either placebo or bevacizumab as first-line therapy for nonsquamous non-small-cell lung cancer: AVAil. J. Clin. Oncol. 2009;27:1227−34.

[95]Reck M, von Pawel J, Zatloukal P, et al. Phase III trial of cisplatin plus gemcitabine with either placebo or bevacizumab as first-line therapy for nonsquamous non-small-cell lung cancer: AVAil. J. Clin. Oncol. 2009;27:1227−34.

[96]Giovannoni G, Comi G, Cook S, et al. A placebo-controlled trial of oral cladribine for relapsing multiple sclerosis. New Engl. J. Med. 2010;362:416−26.

[97]ICH Harmonised Tripartite Guideline Statistical Principles for Clinical Trials E9; February 1998 (46 pp).

[98]ICH Harmonised Tripartite Guideline Statistical Principles for Clinical Trials E9; February 1998 (46 pp).

q. Dose Escalation—The Moore Schema

For many small-molecule drugs used in chemotherapy, it is assumed that the higher the dose, the more effective will be the antitumor treatment (99). Hence, the goal of phase I dose-escalation clinical trials is to determine the highest tolerable dose. The adverse events that are measured are used to define the *DLT*. The DLT informs the investigator which dose is the *maximally tolerable dose* (MTD).

In a clinical trial of solid tumors, Moore et al. (100) administered increasing levels of drug (sorafenib) to different groups of patients (Fig. 2.17). Totally different groups of patients received each particular dose. It was never the

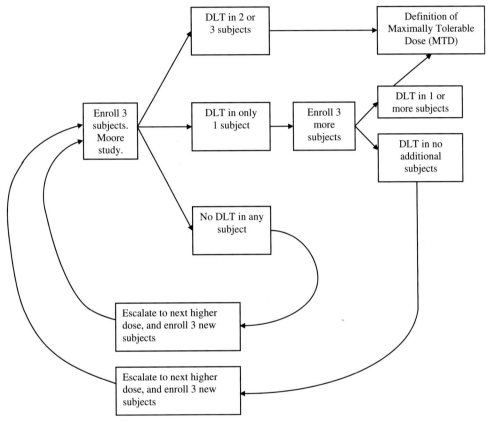

FIGURE 2.17 Schema used in dose-escalation study. The schema involves a number of decision trees where the decisions are in response to toxicities that are present in the study subjects, and where the decisions are to increase the dose for subsequently enrolled subjects.

[99]Postel-Vinay S, Arkenau HT, Olmos D, et al. Clinical benefit in Phase-I trials of novel molecularly targeted agents: does dose matter? Br. J. Cancer 2009;100:1373–8.

[100]Moore M, Hirte HW, Siu L, et al. Phase I study to determine the safety and pharmacokinetics of the novel Raf kinase and VEGFR inhibitor BAY 43-9006, administered for 28 days on/7 days off in patients with advanced, refractory solid tumors. Ann. Oncol. 2005;16:1688–94.

case that one patient received one particular dose and, at a later point in the trial, was tested with a higher dose of the same drug. This dose-escalating trial followed a typical and conventional design of dose-finding trials.

According to Lin and Shih (101), the goal of dose-escalating phase I clinical trials is to find the highest tolerable dose, as it is believed that maximal benefit to the patient can be achieved at this dose. This generalization applies to small molecules used in oncology. Once the phase I trial is completed, the investigator then uses the maximally tolerable dose (MTD), or one dose below the MTD, as the recommended dose for a subsequent phase II trial. This approach to finding the optimal dose is not used for biologicals, such as antibodies and cytokines, or to drugs for infections, immune disorders, or metabolic diseases. (It should be noted that it is common medical practice, when treating infections, immune disorders, and metabolic diseases, for the physician to increase dosing when a lower dose is not effective.)

In the Moore study, increasing sorafenib doses were:

- 50 mg every 4 days
- 50 mg every other day
- 50 mg per day
- 100 mg per day
- 200 mg per day
- 400 mg per day
- 800 mg per day and
- 1200 mg per day.

The schema reveals that three subjects were enrolled at first (Fig. 2.17). They were given the lowest dose. Then, according to a decision tree, if DLT occurred in two out of three subjects, this defined the MTD. But if DLT occurred in only one subject, then three new subjects were enrolled in the trial, and provided with the next highest dose. Also, if no DLT occurred in any of the three subjects, then here also, three new subjects were enrolled and provided with the next highest dose. This process was reiterated until the arrival of a value for the MTD.

Treatment was continued until *tumor progression*, at which point treatment was halted, or until *toxicity to the patient*, at which point treatment was halted. The dose that resulted in toxicity represented the DLT and was used to define the maximum tolerated dose (MTD). All patients in the trial were victims of incurable cancer, and had already been treated for incurable cancer. What is described above is standard procedure in the pharmaceutical industry.

The result of the Moore et al. (102) study was that the MTD was 800 mg sorafenib per day. The authors recommended that this dose be used for subsequent phase II and phase III trials. Van Cutsem et al. (103) provide a similar schema used for another dose-escalating trial.

r. Pharmacokinetics—The Marshall Schema

The schema provided by Marshall et al. (104) is distinguished in that it indicates the time points relating to analytical methods

[101]Lin Y, Shih WJ. Statistical properties of the traditional algorithm-based designs for phase I cancer clinical trials. Biostatistics 2001;2:203–15.

[102]Moore M, Hirte HW, Siu L, et al. Phase I study to determine the safety and pharmacokinetics of the novel Raf kinase and VEGFR inhibitor BAY 43-9006, administered for 28 days on/7 days off in patients with advanced, refractory solid tumors. Ann. Oncol. 2005;16:1688–94.

[103]Van Cutsem E, Verslype C, Beale P, et al. A phase Ib dose-escalation study of erlotinib, capecitabine and oxaliplatin in metastatic colorectal cancer patients. Ann. Oncol. 2008;19:332–9.

[104]Marshall J, Chen H, Yang D, et al. A phase I trial of a Bcl-2 antisense (G3139) and weekly docetaxel in patients with advanced breast cancer and other solid tumors. Ann. Oncol. 2004;15:1274–83.

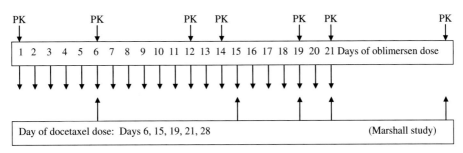

FIGURE 2.18 Study schema showing time points for withdrawing blood. Blood was withdrawn from study subjects at the time points indicated by arrows, to characterize the pharmacokinetic and pharmacodynamic properties of the drug.

(Fig. 2.18). The indicated time points are dates when blood was withdrawn. Blood samples were taken for use in the analysis of plasma drugs and drug metabolites, and for the characterization of the pharmacokinetic and pharmacodynamic properties of the drug. The term *pharmacodynamics* refers to the drug's influence on physiology, biochemistry, and molecular biology over the course of time.

Although most clinical trials include an analysis of pharmacokinetics, the Marshall et al. (105) schema is one of the few that indicate dates of blood collection.

The clinical trial of Marshall et al. (106) is a dose-escalation study (Fig. 2.18). Dose-escalation studies are used in phase I clinical trials, where the goal is to arrive at the dose that is likely to be most effective, without resulting in intolerable toxicity. In the words of the investigators, "[e]nrollment to successive dose cohorts could not occur until all patients at the previous dose had received the 4-week treatment without dose limiting toxicity (DLT)" (107). This was a single-arm, dose-escalation study.

The study drugs were docetaxel and oblimersen. Oblimersen is in a class of compounds called reverse sense RNA. When administered in vitro to cultured cells, or when administered to an animal or human subject, oblimersen inhibits expression of the Bcl-2 gene. Oblimersen is used in cancers where the tumor overexpresses the Bcl gene.

The dose of docetaxel was fixed throughout the entire study. But the dose of oblimersen was increased, in the indicated steps, in successive groups (cohorts) of subjects. For each individual subject, the subject was only exposed to one particular dosage, and that particular subject was never treated subsequently with a higher dosage. In detail, two subjects were used for a dose of 5 mg/kg/day, then four subjects were used for the 7 mg/kg/day regimen, and finally, four subjects were used for the 9 mg/kg/day regimen.

For each of the three escalating doses, the following schedule was used. In other words, the following schedule was repeated three times. The notation "PK" indicates the days that blood samples were taken for chemical

---

[105]Marshall J, Chen H, Yang D, et al. A phase I trial of a Bcl-2 antisense (G3139) and weekly docetaxel in patients with advanced breast cancer and other solid tumors. Ann. Oncol. 2004;15:1274–83.

[106]Marshall J, Chen H, Yang D, et al. A phase I trial of a Bcl-2 antisense (G3139) and weekly docetaxel in patients with advanced breast cancer and other solid tumors. Ann. Oncol. 2004;15:1274–83.

[107]Marshall J, Chen H, Yang D, et al. A phase I trial of a Bcl-2 antisense (G3139) and weekly docetaxel in patients with advanced breast cancer and other solid tumors. Ann. Oncol. 2004;15:1274–83.

analysis of plasma oblimersen. Also, blood samples taken on these days were used for measuring the in vivo influence of oblimersen on expression of the Bcl gene in white blood cells. Morris et al. (108) also provide a schema with extensive markings showing days of laboratory tests.

IV. FURTHER CONCEPTS IN CLINICAL TRIAL DESIGN

Additional concepts in study design include:

- *Active control*
- *Add-on design active control*
- *Three-arm study*
- *Dose modification and dose discontinuation.*

a. Active Control

Clinical trials typically use an active control treatment, including clinical trials that test new drugs, new surgical methods, and new medical devices. Where an established therapy exists, and where the efficacy and safety of the established therapy is reasonably predictable or uniform, an active control might be the preferred clinical trial design. Consider the hypothetical where a new drug is compared with a placebo. Assume the new drug works better than the placebo. However, even if the new drug works better than the placebo, the results do not provide any direct information on whether the drug works better than the established therapy. This comparison can only be established in a clinical trial where one arm contains the study drug, and where a control arm contains an active control that is an established therapy.

Examples of active controls are disclosed in the schema appearing above, that is, in the clinical trials of Perez et al. (109), Untch et al. (110), Puhalla et al. (111), and Sekine et al. (112). The FDA has specifically warned investigators, in choosing a drug for the active control, to avoid using an active drug that is outmoded or that has been replaced by another drug (113).

Sobrero and Guglielmi (114) noted the phenomenon where, over the course of decades, clinical trials in oncology using an active control design, have produced diminishing returns. In other words, with the passing of

[108]Morris MJ, Huang D, Kelly WK, et al. Phase 1 trial of high-dose exogenous testosterone in patients with castration-resistant metastatic prostate cancer. Eur. Urol. 2009;56:237—44.

[109]Perez EA, Suman VJ, Davidson NE, et al. Cardiac safety analysis of doxorubicin and cyclophosphamide followed by paclitaxel with or without trastuzumab in the North Central Cancer Treatment Group N9831 adjuvant breast cancer trial. J. Clin. Oncol. 2008;26:1231—8.

[110]Untch M, Möbus V, Kuhn W, et al. Intensive dose-dense compared with conventionally scheduled preoperative chemotherapy for high-risk primary breast cancer. J. Clin. Oncol. 2009;27:2938—45.

[111]Puhalla S, Mrozek E, Young D, et al. Randomized phase II adjuvant trial of dose-dense docetaxel before or after doxorubicin plus cyclophosphamide in axillary node-positive breast cancer. J. Clin. Oncol. 2008;26:1691—7.

[112]Sekine I, Nishiwaki Y, Noda K, et al. Randomized phase II study of cisplatin, irinotecan and etoposide combinations administered weekly or every 4 weeks for extensive small-cell lung cancer (JCOG9902-DI). Ann. Oncol. 2003;14:709—14.

[113]U.S. Dept. Health and Human Services. Food and Drug Administration. Guidance for Industry. Non-inferiority clinical trials; March 2010.

[114]Sobrero A, Guglielmi A. Current controversies in the adjuvant therapy of colon cancer. Ann. Oncol. 2004;15 (Suppl. 4):iv 39—41.

decades, it is easy to discover new anticancer drugs, but it becomes progressively more difficult to find a new anticancer drug that works significantly better than other recently available drugs.

Where a new drug is devised, but where it is not certain whether a significant difference will be found between the new drug and an active control, the trial design may shift its perspective. The shifted perspective takes the form of a noninferiority trial. The main goal of a noninferiority trial is to show that the study drug is not less effective than the active control.

A clinical trial on a study drug that shows noninferiority to the active control can provide marketing advantages to the study drug, for the following reasons. As summarized by Lesaffre (115), these advantages include:

- While the efficacy of the study drug may be merely noninferior to the active control drug, the study drug may have a far better safety profile
- The study drug may be easier to administer. An example of this is fingolimod (116,117), which is a pill for multiple sclerosis, in contrast to natalizumab, which is injected
- The study drug may be administered by a flexible schedule, while the active control may require a strict, disciplined schedule.

b. Add-On Design Active Control

With an add-on design, the study drug is administered in combination with a previously established drug, and the control group receives only the previously established drug (118). According to the ICH Guidelines, "[a]n add-on study is a placebo-controlled trial of a new agent conducted in people also receiving standard treatment. Such studies are particularly important when available treatment is known to decrease mortality or irreversible morbidity, and when a noninferiority trial with standard treatment as the active control cannot be carried out or would be difficult to interpret. It is common to study anticancer, antiepileptic, and heart failure drugs this way" (119). The FDA has recognized that add-on design clinical studies are common in clinical trials in oncology, heart failure, seizure disorders, and human immunodeficiency virus (120).

According to Roberts et al. (121), it may be easier to obtain regulatory approval for an anticancer drug when the trial uses an add-on design, writing that, "most agents with first-line indications are approved for use in combination (eg, irinotecan plus fluorouracil and leucovorin for first-line colon cancer)."

[115]Lesaffre E. Superiority, equivalence, and non-inferiority trials. Bull. N.Y.U. Hosp. Jt. Dis. 2008;66:150–4.

[116]Cohen JA, Barkhof F, Comi G, et al. Oral fingolimod or intramuscular interferon for relapsing multiple sclerosis. New Engl. J. Med. 2010;362:402–15.

[117]Kappos L, Radue EW, O'Connor P, et al. A placebo-controlled trial of oral fingolimod in relapsing multiple sclerosis. New Engl. J. Med. 2010;362:387–401.

[118]Daugherty CK, Ratain MJ, Emanuel EJ, Farrell AT, Schilsky RL. Ethical, scientific, and regulatory perspectives regarding the use of placebos in cancer clinical trials. J. Clin. Oncol. 2008;26:1371–8.

[119]ICH Harmonised Tripartite Guideline. Choice of control group and related issues in clinical trials E10. (Step 4 version, July 2000) 33 pp.

[120]U.S. Dept. Health and Human Services. Food and Drug Administration. Guidance for Industry. Non-inferiority clinical trials; March 2010.

[121]Roberts TG, Lynch TJ, Chabner BA. The phase III trial in the era of targeted therapy: unraveling the "go or no go" decision. J. Clin. Oncol. 2003;21:3683–95.

In a clinical trial on nonsmall-cell lung cancer, Rosell et al. (122), used an add-on design. The new drug was an antibody (cetuximab). The established therapy was the combination of two small molecules, namely, cisplatin and vinorelbine. In the words of the investigators, "[t]he main purpose of this study was to assess the add-on activity of cetuximab."

Add-on design clinical trials were also used to gain FDA approval of anakinra and abatacept. Unfortunately, as observed by Ottolenghi et al. (123), the report from the add-on design study did not provide a list of adverse events that were unambiguously caused by the study drug alone, but only provided adverse events that are caused by the combination of the study drug and the previously approved drug.

c. Three-Arm Study—Clinical Trial With Two Different Active Control Arms

Clinical trials can include more than one control arm. In addition to an arm that receives study drug, the trial design can also include two active control arms, each receiving a different active control. In a clinical trial for *Staphylococcus aureus* infections, Stryjewkski et al. (124), included a study drug arm (telavancin), plus a first active control arm (vancomycin) and a second active control arm (penicillin), as summarized below:

- Study drug arm (telavancin)
- First active control arm (vancomycin)
- Second active control arm (penicillin).

Two active control arms were used for the following reasons. First, vancomycin and penicillin are both standards of care, that is, they are both suitable for use as an active control. Secondly, the infecting agent, *S. aureus*, is heterogeneous. This heterogeneity took the following form. *Staphylococcus aureus*, occurs in methicillin-resistant (MRSA) and methicillin-susceptible (MSSA) forms. Vancomycin is effective against MRSA, but may not be effective against MSSA (125). Conversely, penicillin is effective against MSSA, but not MRSA. If only one active control had been used, the results of this clinical study could have led investigators to overstate the efficacy of the study drug, relative to the efficacy of the standard of care.

Clinical study design using two different active controls can be used in studies of infections, as well as for clinical studies in oncology, immune disorders, metabolic diseases, and neurological disorders.

d. Dose Modification and Dose Discontinuation

Dose modification is a component clinical trial design that encompasses dose reductions, dose increases, and interruptions or delays in dosing. Dose discontinuation refers to permanent cessation of dosing to a particular study subject.

Although a dose modification and discontinuation can be indicated in the study schema diagram, they are more often indicated only in the text of the Clinical Study Protocol. Dose

---

[122]Rosell R, Robinet G, Szczesna A, et al. Randomized phase II study of cetuximab plus cisplatin/vinorelbine compared with cisplatin/vinorelbine alone as first-line therapy in EGFR-expressing advanced non-small-cell lung cancer. Ann. Oncol. 2008;19:362−9.

[123]Ottolenghi L, et al. Limits of add-on trials: antirheumatic drugs. Eur. J. Clin. Pharmacol. 2009;65:33−41.

[124]Stryjewski ME, Chu VH, O'Riordan WD, et al. Telavancin versus standard therapy for treatment of complicated skin and skin structure infections caused by gram-positive bacteria: FAST 2 study. Antimicrob. Agents Chemother. 2006;50:862−7.

[125]Stryjewski ME. E-mail of October 10, 2010.

modification and discontinuation refer to a decision that is made for individual subjects, not for simultaneous changes in dose levels that are used for all subjects in one particular arm of the study. Generally, these are triggered by the materialization of an adverse event in a given subject. Also, dose modification is triggered where the investigator determines that the study drug is not effective, and where the investigator wishes to increase the dose for a given subject.

The following commentary on dose modification introduces the terms, "adverse event" and "CTCAE" (126). CTCAE is a dictionary of terms for various adverse events. This dictionary accounts for the fact that any given adverse event can occur at increasing levels of severity. CTCAE provides definitions of each adverse event when it occurs at these increasing levels of severity.

An adverse event, as set forth by CTCAE, as well as by other dictionaries used in clinical trials, includes abnormal laboratory values, such as high serum bilirubin, as well as clinical problems, such as skin rash, pain, or cardiac arrhythmias. When used in the clinical trial documents, the term "adverse event" is used *without regard* to whether there is any connection or causal influence by the study drug. Further information on adverse events and on CTCAE are found in Chapter 25.

1. Dose Modifications in Clinical Study Protocol for Nonsmall-Cell Lung Cancer

The Clinical Study Protocol (127) for an anticancer drug, ceritinib, provided for *dose reductions, dose delay, and dose escalations*. The study drug was used for nonsmall-cell lung cancer. The Protocol stated that dose reductions and delays were for use when drug toxicity was encountered, in its statement that, "[f]or patients who experience dose-limiting toxicity with LDK378, dose adjustments are permitted if it is considered in the best interest of the patient to continue therapy." Regarding the dose reductions that were to be used when toxicity was encountered, the Protocol provided the following instructions:

> For each patient, a maximum of 3 dose reductions will be allowed after which the patient should be discontinued from the study. For each patient, once a dose level reduction has occurred, the dose level may not be re-escalated during subsequent treatment cycles with LDK378. Dose reduction for LDK378 means treatment at a lower LDK378 dose level. Provisional dose levels for LDK378 are listed in Table 5-1.

After the clinical trial had been conducted, the investigator published comments about the dose reductions and delays that had actually occurred in the clinical trial, stating that, "[a] total of 66 of 130 patients (51%) required at least one dose reduction, and the median duration of treatment interruption was 7.3 days" (128).

The Protocol also provided for *dose delay*, in its instructions that, "[i]f a patient requires a dose delay of >21 days due to an LDK378-related toxicity, then the patient must be discontinued from the study unless the patient has experienced evidence of clinical benefit."

The Protocol also set forth instructions for dose increases, stating that *dose increases* were forbidden until after the study subject had

---

[126]CTCAE means Common Terminology Criteria for Adverse Events. CTCAE is published by National Cancer Institute of the National Institutes of Health (NIH), and is periodically revised by NIH.

[127]Shaw AT, Kim D-W, Mehra R, et al. Ceritinib in *ALK*-rearranged non-small-cell lung cancer. New Engl. J. Med. 2014;370:1189−97.

[128]Shaw AT, Kim D-W, Mehra R, et al. Ceritinib in *ALK*-rearranged non-small-cell lung cancer. New Engl. J. Med. 2014;370:1189−97.

completed a given series of treatments. The instructions for dose increase read:

> [D]ose escalation is not permitted during the first 4 cycles of treatment. After the 4th cycle is completed, individual patients may be considered for treatment at a dose of LDK378 higher than the dose to which they were initially assigned. In order for a patient to be treated at a higher dose of LDK378, he or she must have received the lower dose for at least 4 cycles of therapy without a drug-related toxicity of CTCAE grade 2:: 2.

2. Dose Modifications in Clinical Study Protocol for Anemia

This concerns a Clinical Study Protocol that provided instructions for *increasing* or *decreasing* doses based on the efficacy of the drug. The study drug was *darbepoetin* (129). These instructions were keyed to efficacy values, not to any adverse events associated with the drug. To emphasize this point, even though the Protocol provided instructions for decreasing the dose, these were keyed with efficacy values, not with any drug-induced toxicity.

The drug was darbepoetin for treating anemia, and the efficacy was determined by blood values for hemoglobin (Hb), as well as the rate of increase over the course of time of blood hemoglobin. Instructions were provided by a table (Table 2.1). These instructions referred to prefilled syringes. The syringes contained the study drug in the amounts of 10, 15, 20, 30, 40, 50, 60, 80, 100, 150, 200, and 300 μg.

3. Dose Modifications in Clinical Study Protocol for Cushing's Disease

A Clinical Study Protocol (130) regarding a drug for treating Cushing's disease provided instructions for dose reduction and dose escalation, where the instructions identified specific adverse events. These adverse events

TABLE 2.1 Dose Modification Instructions for Clinical Trial on Darbepoetin for Anemia[a]

Hemoglobin (g/dL)	Hb Rate of Rise (g/dL/2 weeks)	Instruction
Under 12.2	Under 0.5	Increase to next higher prefilled syringe
Under 12.2	0.5–1.0	Maintain dose
Under 12.2	Greater than or equal to 1.0	Decrease to next lower prefilled syringe
12.5–13.5	Under 0.5	Maintain dose
12.5–13.5	0.5–1.0	Maintain dose
12.5–13.5	Greater than or equal to 1.0	Decrease to next lower prefilled syringe

[a]*Instructions slightly modified from table in Clinical Study Protocol of Solomon SD, Uno H, Lewis EF, et al. Erythropoietic response and outcomes in kidney disease and type 2 diabetes. New Engl. J. Med. 2010;363:1146–55.*

included hypoadrenalism, as defined by serum cortisol levels. The instructions also stated the amount of the dose reduction, and how to monitor the adverse event after the physician had imposed the dose reduction:

> The dose may be reduced at any time in steps of 300 μg b.i.d. in case of intolerance (1200 μg b.i.d. to 900 μg b.i.d., 900 μg b.i.d. to 600 μg b.i.d., 600 μg b.i.d. to 300 μg b.i.d.). The lowest dose that should be administered is 300 μg b.i.d. However, a lower dose (such as 150 μg b.i.d.) may be allowed as long as efficacy is maintained; otherwise, the patient should be discontinued from the study. Dose reductions are required for the following criteria: Evidence of hypoadrenalism: defined as an early morning (between 8 and 10 AM) serum cortisol <3 μg/dL and a UFC measurement < LLN or symptoms suggestive of hypoadrenalism (e.g. postural hypotension, nausea, and abdominal pain) and a UFC measurement < LLN ... [d]ose reductions are to be performed as follows: The dose will be reduced by 300 μg b.i.d. for one week. If the AE improves to grade ≤2 within one week, increase dose by 300 μg b.i.d.

[129]Solomon SD, Uno H, Lewis EF, et al. Erythropoietic response and outcomes in kidney disease and type 2 diabetes. New Engl. J. Med. 2010;363:1146–55.

[130]Colao A, Petersenn S, Newell-Price J, et al. A 12-month phase 3 study of pasireotide in Cushing's disease. New Engl. J. Med. 2012;366:914–24.

The Clinical Study Protocol (131) for Cushing's disease also set forth instructions for *dose escalation*, for use when efficacy was not achieved. The Protocol stated that, "[t]he dose may be increased at any time ... if response is not achieved/maintained. Dose increase is done in steps of 300 μg b.i.d. (300 μg b.i.d. to 600 μg b.i.d., 600 μg b.i.d. to 900 μg b.i.d., 900 μg b.i.d. to 1200 μg b.i.d.). The highest dose that can be administered is 1200 μg b.i.d."

At a greater step of complexity, was the *dose reduction* scheme in a study of hepatocellular carcinoma (132). The list of adverse events, in the dose reduction instructions, included an increase in serum enzymes, grade 3 hyponatremia, grade 4 hyponatremia, and cutaneous adverse events. The more detailed feature of this dose-reduction scheme, was the instruction regarding how to reduce the dose after the first, second, and third occurrence of any given type of adverse event. For example, after the first adverse event relating to bilirubin levels, the instructions stated to hold study drugs until bilirubin fell to under 3× the upper limit of normal. But after the third adverse event relating to bilirubin, the instructions stated to stop study drugs.

4. Dose Modifications in Clinical Study Protocol for Leukemia

In another exemplary dose reduction scheme, a Clinical Study Protocol for treating leukemia provided separate dose reductions for each type of adverse event, and also separate dose reductions for each grade of severity of that particular adverse event (133). The adverse events were serum enzymes (ALT/AST), bilirubin, neutropenia, and thrombocytopenia. For each of these adverse events, the instructions provided a different dose reduction for an adverse event of grade 1, grade 2, grade 3, and grade 4. Grade 0 includes all values that do not meet criteria for an abnormality of at least Grade 1. In the Clinical Study Protocol, these dose modifications took the form shown in Table 2.2. Please note that the units for adverse event severity, and the terminology of the particular adverse event, were those of CTCAE. Please note that high levels of enzymes and of bilirubin take the form of a "laboratory value" adverse event, while the rash takes the form of a "clinical" adverse event.

5. Introduction to Dose Discontinuations

Discontinuing the administration of a drug to a given study subject may be for a variety of reasons. These include toxicity, lack of efficacy of the drug, or lack of compliance (poor adherence) with the Clinical Study Protocol. As revealed by one analysis of drug discontinuations, also called treatment discontinuations, the rate of discontinuation can be analyzed according to subgroup, such as gender, racial group, or cigarette smoking, as well as whether it was due to the physician's decision or to the study subject's decision (134,135).

[131]Colao A, Petersenn S, Newell-Price J, et al. A 12-month phase 3 study of pasireotide in Cushing's disease. New Engl. J. Med. 2012;366:914–24.

[132]Johnson PJ, Qin, S, Park J.-W., et al. Brivanib versus sorafenib as first-line therapy in patients with unresectable, advanced hepatocellular carcinoma: results from the randomized Phase III BRISK-FL Study. J. Clin. Oncol. 2013;31:3517–26.

[133]Furman RR, Sharman JP, Coutre SE, et al. Idelalisib and rituximab in relapsed chronic lymphocytic leukemia. New Engl. J. Med. 2014;370:997–1007.

[134]Cicconi P, Cozzi-Lepri A, Castagna A, et al. Insights into reasons for discontinuation according to year of starting first regimen of highly active antiretroviral therapy in a cohort of antiretroviral-naive patients. HIV Med. 2010;11:104–13.

[135]Yuan Y, et al. Determinants of discontinuation of initial highly active antiretroviral therapy regimens in a US HIV-infected patient cohort. HIV Med. 2010;7:156–62.

TABLE 2.2   Dose Modifications for Idelalisib in Clinical Trial on Chronic Lymphocytic Leukemia[a]

Adverse Event	CTCAE Grade 1	CTCAE Grade 2	CTCAE Grade 3	CTCAE Grade 4
Liver enzymes (transaminases)	Less than ULN to 3× ULN	Over 3 to 5× ULN	Over 5 to 20× ULN	Over 20× ULN
Bilirubin	Over ULN to 1.5× ULN	Over 1.5 to 3× ULN	Over 3 to 10× ULN	Over 10× ULN
Dose recommendations, in response to increased levels of liver enzymes, or of bilirubin, depending on increase in level	Maintain dose level	Maintain dose level. Monitor enzyme levels and bilirubin, for at least 1 week until all abnormalities are grade 1 or less	Withhold study drug, and confirm abnormalities within 3 days. Monitor enzyme levels and bilirubin for at least 1 week until all abnormalities are grade 1 or less. May resume study drug at next lower level	
Rash	Grade 1. Mild rash	Grade 2. Moderate rash	Grade 3. Severe rash	Grade 4. Life-threatening or disabling rash
Dose modifications in response to rash, depending on severity of rash	Withhold study drug until toxicity reduces to grade 0. Resume study drug at current level. If rechallenge at same dose level results in recurrent rash, may resume study drug at next lower level		Withhold study drug until toxicity is grade 0. May resume study drug at next lower dose level	

The term "ULN" refers to Upper Limit of Normal. Thus, this table does not express the concentrations of enzymes or of bilirubin in terms of conventional units, such as micrograms per liter, but instead expresses the concentrations in terms of Upper Limit of Normal.
[a]*Data from, Furman RR, Sharman JP, Coutre SE, et al. Idelalisib and rituximab in relapsed chronic lymphocytic leukemia. New Engl. J. Med. 370:997–1007.*

Dr Richard Pazdur of the FDA commented that, "[d]iscontinuation may be a result of toxicity, patient preference, or a physician's reluctance to continue therapy. These factors are not a direct assessment of the effectiveness of a drug" (136). Dr Pazdur further warned that, when a drug is discontinued, "[s]urvival analysis may be confounded because of subsequent therapies administered after a study drug is discontinued."

FDA's Guidance for Industry takes into account dose discontinuation, in its account of endpoints in cancer clinical trials. The following concerns one particular endpoint, namely, time to treatment failure (TTF). According to the FDA, "TTF is defined as a composite endpoint measuring time from randomization to **discontinuation of treatment** for any reason, including disease progression, treatment toxicity, and death. TTF is not recommended as a regulatory endpoint for drug approval. TTF does not adequately distinguish efficacy from these additional variables" (137). Moreover, FDA states that, "[f]rom a regulatory point of

[136]Pazdur R. Endpoints for assessing drug activity in clinical trials. Oncologist 2008;13(Suppl. 2):19–21.

[137]U.S. Dept. Health and Human Services. Food and Drug Administration. Guidance for Industry. Clinical Trial Endpoints for the Approval of Cancer Drugs and Biologics; May 2007 (19 pp).

view, TTF is generally not accepted as a valid endpoint. TTF is a composite endpoint influenced by factors unrelated to efficacy ... [t]hese factors are not a direct assessment of the effectiveness of a drug" (138).

Thus, it can reasonably be concluded that dose modification, where ethical, is preferred over dose discontinuation.

V. FDA's DECISION-MAKING PROCESSES REGARDING DOSE MODIFICATION AND DISCONTINUATION

a. Dose Discontinuation, Rather Than Mere Dose Modification, May Result From Physician Inexperience

This concerns dose modification and discontinuation for the reason of toxicity. This is from a clinical trial for *everolimus*, a drug for preventing rejection of kidney transplants. The information is from NDA 21560, which is available from January 2015 on FDA's website. In the Medical Review, which accompanies FDA's Approval Letter, the FDA reviewer speculated on the reason why the rate of dose discontinuations was much higher in the study drug arm, as compared with the active control arm. The study drug was everolimus, while the control drug was mycophenolic acid (Myfortic®).

The reviewer wrote that the adverse events "leading to study drug [everolimus] discontinuation are not the same as dose adjustments ... [t]he fact that the everolimus ... group had a higher rate of discontinuations compared to Myfortic may have reflected ... the fact that ... investigators may not have had much experience in adjusting everolimus ... concentrations. As a result, they may have preferred to discontinue patients rather than adjust the dose. In contrast, clinicians are well versed in reducing Myfortic doses based on toxicities."

The lesson to take is that, as a general proposition, it is the Sponsor's goal to ensure that a maximal number of study subjects remain enrolled in the clinical trial, and not discontinue the drug. To ensure this goal, the Sponsor should include instructions for dose modification that correlate toxicity severity with a recommended dose reduction.

b. Need for Dose Modifications Seen as a Positive Feature

This is from the clinical trial for *everolimus*, described immediately above. The FDA reviewer observed the frequency of dose modifications (adjustments; interruption) of the active control drug that was used in the control arm of the clinical trial. The active control was *Myfortic*. The reviewer's opinion was that the need for dose modification need not be seen as a negative aspect for any given drug, and that it could even be viewed as a positive feature of the drug. The reviewer wrote:

> Myfortic group has a higher rate of dose adjustments and interruptions due to adverse events. The reviewer sees the higher rate of dose adjustments and interruptions due to AEs [adverse events] as **strength of the Myfortic regimen not as a weakness**, it proves the manageability of the Myfortic immunosuppressive regimen. The reviewer, as a physician who has taken care of transplant patients knows that it is very common in clinical practice to adjust the dose or temporarily stop MPA derivatives because of decreases in leukocyte counts or gastrointestinal symptoms like diarrhea, nausea or vomiting.

c. Where Discontinuation of the Study Drug Is Followed by Switching to a Different Drug, the Results May Become Biased

This is also from the clinical trial for *everolimus*, described above. The FDA reviewer warned about the situation where dose discontinuation was followed by switching to a drug that was

---

[138]Pazdur R. Endpoints for assessing drug activity in clinical trials. Oncologist 2008;13(Suppl. 2):19−21.

different from the study drug. The FDA reviewer wrote:

> A disproportionate rate of premature treatment discontinuation, driven by higher rates of adverse events, must be taken into consideration in the interpretation of both safety and efficacy outcomes in this study. More patients in both of the everolimus groups prematurely discontinued study treatment and were subsequently switched to alternate therapy than in the Myfortic group [control group], which may **bias the interpretation** of the study results.

VI. AMENDMENTS TO THE CLINICAL STUDY PROTOCOL

After the Clinical Study Protocol is submitted to the FDA, the Protocol may be changed in response to new needs that arise during the course of the clinical study, such as a needed change in the study design. The desired changes are submitted to the FDA by way of amendments.

These changes may require approval by an ethics committee, as well as by the FDA. Amendments to the Clinical Study Protocol find a basis in the Code of Federal Regulations (CFR), as shown by the following excerpt from the CFR (139):

> (b) *Changes in a protocol.* (1) A sponsor shall submit a protocol amendment describing any change in a Phase 1 protocol that significantly

affects the safety of subjects or any change in a Phase 2 or 3 protocol that significantly affects the safety of subjects, the scope of the investigation, or the scientific quality of the study. Examples of changes requiring an amendment under this paragraph include:

> (i) Any increase in drug dosage or duration of exposure of individual subjects to the drug beyond that in the current protocol, or any significant increase in the number of subjects under study.

> (ii) Any significant change in the design of a protocol (such as the addition or dropping of a control group).

> (iii) The addition of a new test or procedure that is intended to improve monitoring for, or reduce the risk of, a side effect or adverse event; or the dropping of a test intended to monitor safety.

A selection of actual amendments is documented below. The amendments usually fall into the categories of changes in dose, changes in number of subjects, changes in inclusion criteria for subjects, and changes in tests. This list of amendments to the Clinical Study Protocol provides an idea of the purpose of these amendments, but also serves as a summary of various elements that are typically found in clinical trials:

- Increase the dose (140)
- Eliminate the lowest dose (141)
- Change in inclusion criteria (142,143)
- Double the frequency of dosing (144)

---

[139]21 CFR 312.30 (b) (version of April 1, 2010).

[140]Bander NH, Milowsky MI, Nanus DM, et al. Phase I trial of 177lutetium-labeled J591, a monoclonal antibody to prostate-specific membrane antigen, in patients with androgen-independent prostate cancer. J. Clin. Oncol. 2005;23:4591−601.

[141]Zimmerman TM, Harlin H, Odenike OM, et al. Dose-ranging pharmacodynamic study of tipifarnib (R115777) in patients with relapsed and refractory hematologic malignancies. J. Clin. Oncol. 2004;22:4816−22.

[142]Palumbo P, Lindsey JC, Hughes MD, et al. Antiretroviral treatment for children with peripartum nevirapine exposure. New Engl. J. Med. 2010;363:1510−20.

[143]Hohnloser SH, Crijns HJ, van Eickels M, et al. Effect of dronedarone on cardiovascular events in atrial fibrillation. New Engl. J. Med. 2009;360:668−78.

[144]Raetz EA, Cairo MS, Borowitz MJ, et al. Chemoimmunotherapy reinduction with epratuzumab in children with acute lymphoblastic leukemia in marrow relapse: a Children's Oncology Group Pilot Study. J. Clin. Oncol. 2008;26:3756−62.

- Change requirements for blinding (145)
- Increase the number of enrolled subjects (146,147,148)
- Changing the method of statistical analysis (149)
- Dictating times for conducting statistical analyses (150)
- Reducing or discontinuing doses to reduce drug toxicity (151,152)
- Regarding use of a biomarker in the set of inclusion criteria (153)
- Halting enrollment in a study arm because of toxicity of the study drug (154)
- Changing the ratio of subjects in the active drug arm versus the placebo arm (155)
- Change in tests, for example, electrocardiogram, tests for pulmonary function, or urine tests (156,157,158)

[145]Reck M, von Pawel J, Zatloukal P, et al. Phase III trial of cisplatin plus gemcitabine with either placebo or bevacizumab as first-line therapy for nonsquamous non-small-cell lung cancer: AVAil. J. Clin. Oncol. 2009;27:1227–34.

[146]Temel JS, Greer JA, Muzikansky A, et al. Early palliative care for patients with metastatic non-small-cell lung cancer. New Engl. J. Med. 2010;363:733–42.

[147]Massie BM, O'Connor CM, Metra M, et al. Rolofylline, an adenosine A1-receptor antagonist, in acute heart failure. New Engl. J. Med. 2010;363:1419–28.

[148]André T, Boni C, Navarro M, et al. Improved overall survival with oxaliplatin, fluorouracil, and leucovorin as adjuvant treatment in stage II or III colon cancer in the MOSAIC trial. J. Clin. Oncol. 2009;27:3109–16.

[149]Serra AL, Poster D, Kistler AD, et al. Sirolimus and kidney growth in autosomal dominant polycystic kidney disease. New Engl. J. Med. 2010;363:820–9.

[150]Kaufmann M, Jonat W, Hilfrich J, et al. Improved overall survival in postmenopausal women with early breast cancer after anastrozole initiated after treatment with tamoxifen compared with continued tamoxifen: the ARNO 95 Study. J. Clin. Oncol. 2007;25:2664–70.

[151]Pfeffer MA, Burdmann EA, Chen CY, et al. A trial of darbepoetin alfa in type 2 diabetes and chronic kidney disease. New Engl. J. Med. 2009;361:2019–32.

[152]Le Cesne A, Blay JY, Judson I, et al. Phase II study of ET-743 in advanced soft tissue sarcomas: a European Organisation for the Research and Treatment of Cancer (EORTC) soft tissue and bone sarcoma group trial. J. Clin. Oncol. 2005;23:576–84.

[153]Perez EA, Suman VJ, Davidson NE, et al. HER2 testing by local, central, and reference laboratories in specimens from the North Central Cancer Treatment Group N9831 intergroup adjuvant trial. J. Clin. Oncol. 2006;24:3032–8.

[154]Vansteenkiste J, Lara PN Jr, Le Chevalier T, et al. Phase II clinical trial of the epothilone B analog, ixabepilone, in patients with non small-cell lung cancer whose tumors have failed first-line platinum-based chemotherapy. J. Clin. Oncol. 2007;25:3448–55.

[155]Sparano JA, Bernardo P, Stephenson P, et al. Randomized phase III trial of marimastat versus placebo in patients with metastatic breast cancer who have responding or stable disease after first-line chemotherapy: Eastern Cooperative Oncology Group trial E2196. J. Clin. Oncol. 2004;22:4683–90.

[156]Jeha S, Razzouk B, Rytting M, et al. Phase II study of clofarabine in pediatric patients with refractory or relapsed acute myeloid leukemia. J. Clin. Oncol. 2009;27:4392–7.

[157]Kappos L, Antel J, Comi G, et al. Oral fingolimod (FTY720) for relapsing multiple sclerosis. New Engl. J. Med. 2006;355:1124–40.

[158]Belch A, Kouroukis CT, Crump M, et al. A phase II study of bortezomib in mantle cell lymphoma: the National Cancer Institute of Canada Clinical Trials Group trial IND.150. Ann. Oncol. 2007;18:116–21.

- Allowing or requirement for a prophylactic drug, such as an antibiotic, in an oncology trial (159,160)
- Implement a requirement that study subjects had already received some sort of therapy for the disease (first-line therapy) before enrolling in the clinical study (161,162)
- Increase the maximally allowed timeframe between presentation of the disease and enrollment/randomization in the clinical trial (163). The mean timeframe for this clinical trial, which involved acute coronary syndrome, was 5.6 h.

Once the proposed amendment is approved, subsequent versions of the Clinical Study Protocol list the dates of the amendments on the title page of the Clinical Study Protocol (164).

VII. CONCLUDING REMARKS

The study schema is a flow chart that provides a snapshot of the study design. The schema is generally included in the Clinical Study Protocol, as well as in any research publications stemming from the clinical study.

The Clinical Study Protocol is an instruction manual for physicians and healthcare workers who are employed in FDA-regulated clinical trials. The utility of this instruction manual can be enhanced by including an accurate schema.

The schema reveals the number of study arms, the identities of the study drugs, control drugs, and placebos (if any). The well-drafted schema also indicates the drug dose and the timing of the doses. Potentially confusing or unusual aspects of trial design, such as run-in periods and decision trees should be included in the schema.

The Clinical Study Protocol optionally includes instructions for dose reduction, dose delay, dose escalation, or dose discontinuation. These instructions can take the form of separate instructions that are keyed for different adverse events, separate instructions that are keyed to severity or grade for any given type of adverse event, and instructions for when to reduce, monitor response, and eventually resume dosing for a given study subject.

[159]Bontenbal M, Creemers GJ, Braun HJ, et al. Phase II to III study comparing doxorubicin and docetaxel with fluorouracil, doxorubicin, and cyclophosphamide as first-line chemotherapy in patients with metastatic breast cancer: results of a Dutch Community Setting Trial for the Clinical Trial Group of the Comprehensive Cancer Centre. J. Clin. Oncol. 2005;23:7081−8.

[160]Martín M, Lluch A, Seguí MA, et al. Toxicity and health-related quality of life in breast cancer patients receiving adjuvant docetaxel, doxorubicin, cyclophosphamide (TAC) or 5-fluorouracil, doxorubicin and cyclophosphamide (FAC): impact of adding primary prophylactic granulocyte-colony stimulating factor to the TAC regimen. Ann. Oncol. 2006;17:1205−12.

[161]Schiller JH, Larson T, Ou SH, et al. Efficacy and safety of axitinib in patients with advanced non-small-cell lung cancer: results from a phase II study. J. Clin. Oncol. 2009;27:3836−41.

[162]Blackwell KL, Pegram MD, Tan-Chiu E, et al. Single-agent lapatinib for HER2-overexpressing advanced or metastatic breast cancer that progressed on first- or second-line trastuzumab-containing regimens. Ann. Oncol. 2009;20:1026−31.

[163]Giugliano RP, White JA, Bode C, et al. Early versus delayed, provisional eptifibatide in acute coronary syndromes. New Engl. J. Med. 2009;360:2176−90.

[164]Wood LF, Foote MA. Targeted regulatory writing techniques. Clinical documents for drugs and biologics. Basel/Switzerland: Birkhäuser Verlag; 2009. p. 55, 73, 77.

3

Run-In Period

I. INTRODUCTION

Clinical trials sometimes include a *run-in period*, also called a *run-in phase* or *lead-in phase* (1), as part of the study design. The run-in period encompasses a period of time occurring immediately before randomization of the study subjects, and before allocating subjects to either the study drug or control treatment. Only a minority of clinical trials include a run-in period.

When a run-in period is included, it is advisable to include it in the schema, that is, as a box in the flow chart that constitutes the schema.

The run-in period is described in the ICH Guidelines and in the Food and Drug Administration's (FDA) Guidance for Industry documents. The utility of run-in periods is revealed in the cited documents relating to diabetes (2), emphysema (3), arthritis (4), pancreatic products (5), package inserts (6), and statistics (7).

---

[1]Di Bisceglie AM, Shiffman ML, Everson GT, et al. Prolonged therapy of advanced chronic hepatitis C with low-dose peginterferon. New Engl. J. Med. 2008;359:2429–41.

[2]U.S. Department of Health and Human Services. Food and Drug Administration, Center for Drug Evaluation and Research (CDER). Guidance for industry diabetes mellitus: developing drugs and therapeutic biologics for treatment and prevention; February 2008.

[3]U.S. Department of Health and Human Services. Food and Drug Administration, Center for Drug Evaluation and Research (CDER). Guidance for industry. Acute bacterial exacerbations of chronic bronchitis in patients with chronic obstructive pulmonary disease: developing antimicrobial drugs for treatment; August 2008.

[4]U.S. Department of Health and Human Services. Food and Drug Administration, Center for Drug Evaluation and Research (CDER), Center for Biologics Evaluation and Research (CBER), Center for Devices and Radiologic Health (CDRH). Guidance for industry clinical development programs for drugs, devices, and biological products for the treatment of rheumatoid arthritis (RA); February 1999.

[5]U.S. Department of Health and Human Services. Food and Drug Administration, Center for Drug Evaluation and Research (CDER). Guidance for industry. Exocrine pancreatic insufficiency drug products—submitting NDAs; April 2006.

[6]U.S. Department of Health and Human Services. Food and Drug Administration, Center for Drug Evaluation and Research (CDER), Center for Biologics Evaluation and Research (CBER). Guidance for industry clinical studies section of labeling for human prescription drug and biological products—content and format; January 2006.

[7]ICH Harmonised Tripartite Guideline. Statistical principles for clinical trials E9; February 1998 (46 pp.).

This lists the variety of purposes that can be served by a run-in period:

1. To allow a washout period.
2. Permitting time to detect baseline adverse events.
3. To screen for and exclude potential study subjects who are likely to experience excessive safety issues during the study.
4. To screen for and include only study subjects with controllable pain.
5. To determine a maximally tolerable dose.
6. To achieve and ensure steady-state in vivo concentrations of study drug, where the study drug is administered during the run-in period.
7. To allow a period of adjustment of lifestyle of the study subjects, for example, changes in dietary patterns.
8. To ensure that metabolic characteristics of all study subjects are similar, prior to administering drugs.
9. To ensure that potential study subjects can adhere to, or comply with, the study protocol.
10. To allow time to confirm that all study subjects meet the inclusion and exclusion criteria.
11. Detecting potential study subjects who show a desired, or homogeneous, response to the study drug, with the goal of including only these subjects.
12. Decision tree to determine whether a subject should receive treatment A or treatment B.
13. To create a self-control group.

Details of these categories of run-in periods are provided below.

a. Washout Period

Washout periods can minimize the lingering effects of a previously administered drug. These lingering effects may influence data that are later collected regarding safety and efficacy of the study drug in question. Schwartz et al. (8) used a 2-week washout period in a study of asthma. Prior to enrollment in the study, study subjects had received chronic treatment with an anti-asthma drug. After the 2-week washout period, during which subjects did not take any drug for asthma, subjects were randomized and allocated to study drug or placebo.

b. Detecting Baseline Adverse Events

Kramer (9) illustrates the rationale of detecting lingering adverse events resulting from a previously administered drug. This rationale is to detect adverse events arising from previous drug therapy, but also to detect possible adverse events related to withdrawal of the previous drug therapy.

c. Excluding Potential Study Subjects Who Have Safety Issues Correlating With the Study Drug

Greenspan et al. (10) used a run-in period (3 months) as a miniature clinical trial, in order to exclude subjects who had adverse events (at least, during the run-in period) to the study drug. This refers to the drug used in the clinical trial of interest, and not to any drugs administered prior to the clinical trial. The study drug was hormone replacement therapy for preventing bone loss. After the run-in period, subjects

---

[8]Schwartz HJ, Blumenthal M, Brady R, et al. A comparative study of the clinical efficacy of nedocromil sodium and placebo. How does cromolyn sodium compare as an active control treatment? Chest 1996;109:945–52.

[9]Kramer M. Placebo run-in for antidepressant trials. Neuropsychopharmacology 1996;15:105.

[10]Greenspan SL, Resnick NM, Parker RA. Combination therapy with hormone replacement and alendronate for prevention of bone loss in elderly women: a randomized controlled trial. J. Am. Med. Assoc. 2003;289:2525–33.

were randomized to receive either placebo or study drug. In the words of the researchers, "[t]he rationale behind the run-in phase was to ensure that the 4 groups would be roughly equal [in size] after 3 years, such that women taking hormone replacement could be compared with women taking…combination therapy, or placebo." During the run-in period, 112 potential subjects were discontinued from the trial, where 73 of these were discontinued because of adverse drug reactions resulting from the study drug.

The Greenspan clinical trial is unusual, in that a drug, rather than merely a placebo, was administered during the run-in period. Even subjects eventually randomized to receive placebo received the study drug during the run-in period. Most clinical trials using a run-in period, as part of the study design, use that period to administer only the placebo.

d. To Include Only Study Subjects With Controllable Pain

Run-in periods can screen for study subjects with adequate pain control. In a study of breast cancer by Blum et al. (11), subjects were first entered in a 1-week run-in period, during which subjects were assessed for adequate pain control. Subjects with no pain or with stable pain intensity were allowed to continue with the clinical study. Similarly, Burris et al. (12) included a

run-in period in a study of pancreatic cancer in order to exclude subjects who were not able to obtain stable pain. Cartwright et al. (13) included a run-in period, where subjects were assessed for pain control, and where subjects with inadequate pain control were excluded. The run-in period was also used as a convenient time for measuring vital signs, physical measurements, and clinical laboratory tests, all of which were performed within 7 days before start of study drug treatment. In a study by Filiu et al. (14), the run-in period was only used to assess pain, and not to exclude subjects with uncontrolled pain. In the above-cited studies, pain was assessed using the Memorial Pain Assessment scale (15).

e. To Determine the Maximal Tolerable Dose

A run-in period can take the form of a phase I clinical trial, with a first group of study subjects, where a subsequent phase II trial uses a totally different group of study subjects. The goal of this sort of study design is to determine the safety profile of the study drug. In a study of lung cancer, Heymach et al. (16) used a run-in period on a small group of subjects in order to determine the safety profile of two different doses of study drug, that is, 200 mg vandetanib in combination with paclitaxel and carboplatin

[11]Blum JL, Jones SE, Aman U, Buzda AU, et al. Multicenter phase II study of capecitabine in paclitaxel-refractory metastatic breast cancer. J. Clin. Oncol. 1999;17:485−93.

[12]Burris HA, Rivkin S, Reynolds R, et al. Phase II trial of oral rubitecan in previously treated pancreatic cancer patients. The Oncologist 2005;10:183−90.

[13]Cartwright TH, Cohn A, Varkey JA, et al. Phase II study of oral capecitabine in patients with advanced or metastatic pancreatic cancer. J. Clin. Oncol. 2001;20:160−4.

[14]Feliu J, Escudero P, Llosa F, et al. Capecitabine as first-line treatment for patients older than 70 years with metastatic colorectal cancer: an oncopaz cooperative group study. J. Clin. Oncol. 2005;23:3104−11.

[15]Fishman B, Pasternak S, Wallestein SL, et al. The memorial Pain Assessment card: a valid instrument for the evaluation of cancer pain. Cancer 1987;60:1151−8.

[16]Heymach JV, Paz-Ares L, Braud FD, et al. Randomized phase II study of vandetanib alone or with paclitaxel and carboplatin as first-line treatment for advanced non-small-cell lung cancer. J. Clin. Oncol. 2008;26:5407−15.

(PC), or 300 mg vandetanib in combination with PC. Only 25 subjects in all were used for this run-in period. The results from the run-in study demonstrated that the higher dose was well-tolerated. According to the researchers, "[t]he primary objective of the run-in phase was to establish the appropriate dose of vandetanib to be administered with PC" (17). PC means the combination of PC. These 25 subjects were not included in the subsequent, larger clinical trial of 181 subjects (18). Following the run-in study, 181 different subjects were enrolled in a randomized placebo-controlled clinical trial, where the higher dose of vandetanib was used. The results from the 25-subject run-in period were separately published (19).

f. To Achieve and Ensure Steady-State In Vivo Concentrations of Study Drug

A run-in period can establish that steady-state concentrations of the study drug are achieved, as well as to ensure that steady-state concentrations of metabolites of the study drug are achieved. In addition, the run-in period can be used as an opportunity for assessing pharmacokinetic (PK) properties of the study drug.

In a study of head and neck cancer, using the combination of erlotinib and cisplatin (20), a run-in period was used where erlotinib only was administered to all study subjects. Erlotinib

was administered on a continuous daily schedule. For cycle 1 only, erlotinib was taken alone for the first 7 days as a run-in period, to enable a steady-state concentration to be reached at the time of cisplatin dosing. After the run-in period, dosing of erlotinib was continued on a daily schedule, with cisplatin given intravenously on day 1 every 3 weeks. Blood samples were collected before administration of the erlotinib dose on days −6, 1, 15, 22, and 43. The steady-state concentrations of erlotinib and of one of its metabolites were determined. The goal of the run-in period was to ensure steady-state concentrations of the study drug had been reached.

One rationale for needing steady-state levels of erlotinib was to ensure that steady-state levels were reached, and to ensure greater consistency in values of concentrations of erlotinib and of its metabolite (OSI-420), when blood samples were taken in time periods after the run-in period.

The difference between erlotinib's effect on physiology after a relatively short period of exposure to this drug, and after a relatively long period of exposure this drug, has been documented. Boehrer et al. (21) demonstrated that 3 days of exposure to erlotinib produced relatively little induction of P39 cell differentiation, while 6 days of exposure to erlotinib produced a relatively large induction of P39 cell differentiation.

Another rationale for needing steady-state concentrations of erlotinib was as follows.

[17]Heymach JV, Paz-Ares L, Braud FD, et al. Randomized phase II study of vandetanib alone or with paclitaxel and carboplatin as first-line treatment for advanced non-small-cell lung cancer. J. Clin. Oncol. 2008;26:5407−15.

[18]Johnson BE, Sallaway DL. E-mail of August 16, 2010.

[19]Heymach JV, West H, Kerr R, et al. ZD6474 in combination with carboplatin and paclitaxel as first-line treatment in patients with NSCLC: results of the run-in phase of a two-part randomized phase II study (Abstract). Lung Cancer 2005;49(Suppl. 2):S247.

[20]Siu LL, Soulieres D, Chen EX, et al. Phase I/II trial of erlotinib and cisplatin in patients with recurrent or metastatic squamous cell carcinoma of the head and neck: a Princess Margaret Hospital Phase II Consortium and National Cancer Institute of Canada Clinical Trials Group Study. J. Clin. Oncol. 2007;25:2178−83.

[21]Boehrer S, Ades L, Braun T. Erlotinib exhibits antineoplastic off-target effects in AML and MDS: a preclinical study. Blood 2008;111:2170−80.

The goal was to ensure that erlotinib was present at a steady-state level, so that when cisplatin was administered after the run-in period, the two drugs would act in synergy. Erlotinib acts in synergy with some anticancer agents (22).

Moreover, the run-in period also provided the investigators with PK properties of erlotinib. The run-in period was used to determine the PK properties of erlotinib in the absence of cisplatin, and the PK properties of erlotinib in the presence of cisplatin (23).

g. To Allow a Period of Adjustment of Lifestyle of the Study Subjects, for Example, Changes in Dietary Patterns

A run-in period can be used to allow for changes in the dietary habits of study subjects, where the clinical trial has a nutritional component. Gardner et al. (24) provided a 7-day run-in period in a study of dietary soy protein on blood cholesterol. Changes in the intake of several nutrients not provided by the supplement were observed between baseline and randomization for the group as a whole. The changes included decreases in total fat, saturated fat, cholesterol, fiber, and iron intakes, and an increase

in vitamin C intake. The run-in phase was successful in allowing for dietary changes to accommodate to the daily dietary supplement.

h. To Ensure That Metabolic Characteristics of All Study Subjects Are Similar, Prior to Administering Drugs

A run-in period can ensure that the metabolic characteristics of all study subjects has become adequately uniform prior to initiating the actual trial. Where some of the study subjects had been taking oral contraceptives, a run-in period involving no contraceptives can be used to ensure that expression of cytochrome enzymes has been made uniform in all subjects. Certain components of the diet, such as grapefruit juice (25,26,27), can influence the expression of proteins that modulate the metabolism of drugs used in clinical trials. Moreover, drugs that were taken prior to enrollment in the clinical study, such as oral contraceptives (28) or drugs for asthma (29), can influence the expression of enzymes that modulate the metabolism of drugs used in clinical trials. In particular, drugs and diet can influence the expression of cytochrome enzymes and of drug transport systems.

[22]Ling YH, Aracil M, Jimeno J, Perez-Soler R, Yiyu Zou Y. Molecular pharmacodynamics of PM02734 (elisidepsin) as single agent and in combination with erlotinib; synergistic activity in human non-small cell lung cancer cell lines and xenograft models. Eur. J. Cancer 2009;45:1855−64.

[23]Siu LL. E-mail of August 3, 2010.

[24]Gardner CD, Newell KA, Cherin R, Haskell WL. The effect of soy protein with or without isoflavones relative to milk protein on plasma lipids in hypercholesterolemic postmenopausal women. Am. J. Clin. Nutr. 2001;73:728−35.

[25]Lown KS, Bailey DG, Fontana RJ, et al. Grapefruit juice increases felodipine oral availability in humans by decreasing intestinal CYP3A protein expression. J. Clin. Invest. 1997;99:2545−53.

[26]Li Z, Vachharajani NN, Krishna R. On the assessment of effects of food on the pharmacokinetics of drugs in early development. Biopharm. Drug Dispos. 2002;23:165−71.

[27]Fuhr U. Drug interactions with grapefruit juice. Extent, probable mechanism and clinical relevance. Drug Saf. 1998;18:251−72.

[28]Teichmann AT. Influence of oral contraceptives on drug therapy. Am. J. Obstet. Gynecol. 1990;163:2208−13.

[29]Boobis A, Watelet JB, Whomsley R, Benedetti MS, Demoly P, Tipton K. Drug interactions. Drug Metab. Rev. 2009;41:486−527.

i. To Ensure That Potential Study Subjects Can Adhere to, or Comply With, the Study Protocol

Heritier et al. (30) advocated that, "[a]n active run-in phase may be feasible to identify patients who are likely to drop out." Partridge et al. (31) provided the general warning that drugs that produce adverse reactions, such as anticancer drugs, can reduce patient compliance. These authors suggest that a run-in period with oral placebo-only be used to eliminate subjects who are likely not to adhere to the oral study d rug, once the randomized phase of the trial with the study drug actually begins. The following clinical trials contained run-in periods where potential study subjects took only placebo, where compliance was measured, and where only potential subjects showing a reasonable degree of compliance were actually randomized and used in the trial.

Moinpour et al. (32,33) used a 3-month run-in period (placebo only) immediately prior to randomization. The goal of the run-in period was to assess adherence to a home-dosing schedule. The study concerned finasteride for preventing prostate cancer. The study was a lengthy 1—7 years long. For this reason, adherence needed to be assessed by a run-in period, and this period needed to be relatively long (3 months). The schema from Moinpour et al. (34) clearly shows the run-in period as a block on the flow chart.

In a clinical trial on colorectal cancer, Alberts et al. (35) used a 4-week run-in period to determine whether potential study subjects could reliably return to the clinic for visits, or if potential study subjects reliably took at least 75% of their placebo doses. In another study by the same investigators, a 3-month run-in period was used before randomization, followed by a 9-month study period (36). Again the goal of the run-in period was to assess adherence.

Similarly, a 5-year clinical trial on diabetes, which compared study drugs with a placebo, had a 2-week run-in period to screen for subjects able to adhere to the schedule of taking pills (37). Likewise, Brandt et al. (38) conducted a

[30]Heritier SR, Gebski VJ, Keech AC. Inclusion of patients in clinical trial analysis: the intention-to-treat principle. Med. J. Aust. 2003;179:438—40.

[31]Partridge AH, Avorn J, Wang PS, Winer EP. Adherence to therapy with oral antineoplastic agents. J. Natl Cancer Inst. 2002;94:652—61.

[32]Moinpour CM, Lovato LC, Thompson IM. Profile of men randomized to the prostate cancer prevention trial: baseline health-related quality of life, urinary and sexual functioning, and health behaviors. J. Clin. Oncol. 2000;18:1942—53.

[33]Moinpour CM, Darke AK, Donaldson GW, et al. Longitudinal analysis of sexual function reported by men in the prostate cancer prevention trial. J. Natl Cancer Inst. 2007;99:1025—35.

[34]Moinpour CM, Lovato LC, Thompson IM. Profile of men randomized to the prostate cancer prevention trial: baseline health-related quality of life, urinary and sexual functioning, and health behaviors. J. Clin. Oncol. 2000;18:1942—53.

[35]Alberts DS, Martínez ME, Hess LM, et al. Phase III trial of ursodeoxycholic acid to prevent colorectal adenoma recurrence. J. Natl Cancer Inst. 2005;97:846—53.

[36]Alberts DS, Ritenbaugh C, Story JA, et al. Randomized, double-blinded, placebo-controlled study of effect of wheat bran fiber and calcium on fecal bile acids in patients with resected adenomatous colon polyps. J. Natl Cancer Inst. 1996;88:81—92.

[37]Mauer M, Zinman B, Gardiner R, et al. Renal and retinal effects of enalapril and losartan in type 1 diabetes. New Engl. J. Med. 2009;361:40—51.

[38]Brandt KD, Mazzuca SA, Katz BP, et al. Effects of doxycycline on progression of osteoarthritis: results of a randomized, placebo-controlled, double-blind trial. Arthritis Rheum. 2005;52:2015—25.

30-month clinical trial on arthritis, which had a 4-week run-in period that determined adherence.

j. To Confirm That All Study Subjects Meet the Inclusion and Exclusion Criteria

Run-in periods can be used to ensure that potential study subjects meet all of the inclusion and exclusion criteria. Typically, potential study subjects are screened before they are randomized and allocated to study drug or control, where the goal of the screening is to ensure that they meet specific criteria. In a trial of a potential cholesterol-lowering agent, Berthold et al. (39) included a 6-week run-in period where all subjects took placebo only. Of the 215 enrolled subjects, 75 were excluded during the run-in phase for various reasons. Potential subjects were excluded for a number of reasons, including failure to meet all of the inclusion criteria. Before incorporating this kind of run-in period into the study design, statisticians need to ensure that it will not introduce bias into the results of the clinical trial. As explained in Chapter 8 on ITT analysis, excluding subjects because they deviate from certain requirements in the Clinical Study Protocol can introduce bias into the results.

k. Detecting Potential Study Subjects Who Show a Predetermined Desired Response to the Study Drug, With the Goal of Including Only These Subjects

In a review, Stadler (40) describes a type of run-in period that screens for and retains potential subjects who exhibit a desired, predetermined response to a study drug. During this type of run-in period, all potential subjects receive the study drug. The duration of the run-in period must not be too short, otherwise influence of the study drug may not be detected. Moreover, the duration of the run-in period must not be too long, at least in the context of anticancer drugs, because the (usually) inevitable event of death may occur. In detail, the run-in period detects and then excludes subjects where the drug is ineffective, and where the tumors increase in size. The same run-in period detects and then excludes subjects where the tumors shrink. The only subjects who are kept in the study, after the run-in period, are those where the tumors are stable. This group of subjects is then randomized, and allocated to receive placebo, or to continue receiving the study drug. The clinical trials described by Stadler (41) involve a class of drugs that inhibit tumor growth, but do not kill tumors. This class of drugs is further described below in the Methodology Tip.

[39]Berthold HK, Unverdorben S, Degenhardt R, Bulitta M, Gouni-Berthold I. Effect of policosanol on lipid levels among patients with hypercholesterolemia or combined hyperlipidemia. J. Am. Med. Assoc. 2006;295:2262−9.

[40]Stadler WM. The randomized discontinuation trial: a phase II design to assess growth-inhibitory agents. Mol. Cancer Ther. 2007;6:1180−5.

[41]Stadler WM. The randomized discontinuation trial: a phase II design to assess growth-inhibitory agents. Mol. Cancer Ther. 2007;6:1180−5.

In an article on renal cancer, Rosner et al. (42) used the term *randomized discontinuation design*, to refer to a trial that contains a run-in period, where the run-in period selects a subset of enrolled patients who are relatively homogeneous with respect to important prognostic factors and where the trial randomizes only these patients. This kind of run-in period takes the form of a short clinical trial, where efficacy is measured, and where only subjects who respond with predetermined criteria are kept in the study, and subsequently randomized to the study drug and control. Chow and Chang (43) called the above described trial design a *drop-the-losers design*.

In a study of melanoma treatment with sorafenib, Eisen et al. (44) used a run-in period (12 weeks) as a miniature clinical trial, in order to assess the response to the study drug. What was assessed was the response of the tumors to the drug. Where the tumor grew at a rapid rate during the run-in period, subjects were not included in the trial. Where there was a dramatic reduction in tumor size, subjects were also not included. Only subjects with an in-between response were used for the trial where, after the run-in, subjects were divided into the study drug group and the placebo group. The subjects who actually entered the trial were, "[t]hose patients who had an unconfirmed change in tumour size of <25% were randomised in a double-blind fashion to receive either sorafenib…or matching placebo from week 12 onwards." Ratain et al. (45) described this 12-week run-in period, as well as other details of the same melanoma study.

l. Methodology Tip—Anticancer Drugs That Inhibit Tumor Growth and Merely Stabilize Tumors

A review by Stadler (46) focuses on a type of response where a drug stabilizes tumor size, that is, where the effect of the drug is maintenance of tumor size, and not tumor shrinkage. The endpoint of tumor stabilization is preferred where the mechanism of action of the drug is inhibiting tumor cell growth, not killing tumors. Sorafenib is one such drug. Anticancer drugs that halt angiogenesis tend not to kill tumors, but instead merely inhibit tumor growth. Ma and Waxman (47) provide a review of about a dozen antiangiogenic drugs, including sorafenib. These authors expressly state that, "anti-angiogenics are generally cytostatic rather than cytoreductive."

m. Decision Tree

A run-in period can be used to create a branching point, where investigators determine whether the subject should receive treatment A or treatment B. In a clinical trial of head and

[42]Rosner GL, Stadler W, Ratain MJ. Randomized discontinuation design: application to cytostatic antineoplastic agents. J. Clin. Oncol. 2002;20:4478–84.

[43]Chow SC, Chang M. Adaptive design methods in clinical trials—a review. Orphanet J. Rare Dis. 2008;3:11.

[44]Eisen T, Ahmad T, Flaherty KT, et al. Sorafenib in advanced melanoma: a phase II randomised discontinuation trial analysis. Br. J. Cancer 2006;95:581–6.

[45]Ratain MJ, Eisen T, Stadler WM, et al. Phase II placebo-controlled randomized discontinuation trial of sorafenib in patients with metastatic renal cell carcinoma. J. Clin. Oncol. 2006;24:2505–12.

[46]Stadler WM. The randomized discontinuation trial: a phase II design to assess growth-inhibitory agents. Mol. Cancer Ther. 2007;6:1180–5.

[47]Ma J, Waxman DJ. Combination of antiangiogenesis with chemotherapy for more effective cancer treatment. Mol. Cancer Ther. 2008;7:3670–84.

neck cancer by Worden et al. (48,49), subjects were first treated with one cycle of cisplatin plus 5-fluorouracil (run-in period), followed by diagnosing response to this short period of therapy. Depending on the subject's response, the physician then treated the patient with either (1) chemoradiotherapy (CRT), or (2) surgery followed by radiation. In detail, where a patient achieved a greater than 50% response to the drugs provided in the run-in period, the patient was then treated with CRT. The benefit of this approach was preservation of the patient's tissues. But where a patient achieved a response of 50% or lower, the patient was then treated with surgery followed by radiation (this approach resulted in loss of tissues).

Hutchins et al. (50) also conducted a clinical trial that used a run-in period that contained a decision tree. In a clinical trial on breast cancer, volunteers were screened for inclusion/exclusion criteria, which provided a pool of potential subjects for the trial. Potential subjects found to be at high risk, according to the criteria of tumor size and expression of a hormone receptor, were randomized and allocated to the various study drugs. But potential subjects found to be at uncertain risk, according to the same criteria (tumor size and hormone receptor), were then further screened, where tumor cells were characterized by flow cytometry. Where flow cytometry indicated high risk, these subjects were then randomized and allocated to the various study drugs. But where flow cytometry indicated low risk, the subjects were not randomized and were not treated. Hence, the run-in period served as a supplement to the inclusion/exclusion criteria, where the benefit of the run-in period was to ensure a greater number of subjects enrolled in the trial.

n. To Create a Self-Control Group

The run-in period can be used to provide information on baseline adverse events, so that each subject can serve as his own control. In a study of infant formulas, Nakamura et al. (51) used a 7-day run-in period to study the volume of formula intake, the frequency of constipation, the frequency of diarrhea, and the fussiness frequency, of the infants enrolled in the trial. Following the run-in period, all infants were divided into four groups, where each group received a different formula diet. The authors reported, for example, that, "[t]here were no significant differences among the feeding groups in the numbers of infants who experienced constipation or diarrhea during the run-in period or feeding trial." Thus, a purpose of the run-in period was to provide additional controls. In other words, one set of controls was the basal formula during the randomized feeding trial. But another set of controls resulted from comparing each infant's characteristics during the run-in period and during the subsequent randomized trial.

---

[48]Worden FP, Kumar B, Lee JS. Chemoselection as a strategy for organ preservation in advanced oropharynx cancer: response and survival positively associated with HPV16 copy number. J. Clin. Oncol. 2008;26:3138−46.

[49]Prof. Warden agreed with the author's perception that this approach can be classified as a run-in period. E-mail of August 2, 2010.

[50]Hutchins LF, Green SJ, Ravdin PM, et al. Randomized, controlled trial of cyclophosphamide, methotrexate, and fluorouracil versus cyclophosphamide, doxorubicin, and fluorouracil with and without tamoxifen for high-risk, node-negative breast cancer: treatment results of Intergroup Protocol INT-0102. J. Clin. Oncol. 2005;23:8313−21.

[51]Nakamura N, Gaskins HR, Collier CT. Molecular ecological analysis of fecal bacterial populations from term infants fed formula supplemented with selected blends of prebiotics. Appl. Environ. Microbiol. 2009;75:1121−8.

II. FDA'S DECISION-MAKING PROCESSES IN EVALUATING RUN-IN PERIOD

When the FDA grants approval for a drug, it published *Medical Reviews*, *Pharmacology Reviews*, and other reviews. FDA's comments in these reviews provide an intimate picture of FDA's decision-making process. This concerns the run-in period of the study design from the FDA's reviews of clinical trials on boceprevir, omalizumab, and cysteamine bitartrate. The comments in the FDA's reviews provide insights into the rationales for including a run-in period as part of the study design.

a. Boceprevir for Hepatitis C Virus

The study drug was boceprevir. In the clinical trial, boceprevir was administered in combination with ribavir and pegylated interferon-2A. The information is from the FDA's review of NDA 202258, which can be found on May 2011 of the FDA's website.

The study drug arm received all three drugs, while the control arm received ribavir and pegylated interferon-2A. Subjects in the control arm received an active control, that is, a drug (or drug combination) that was already established to have efficacy in treating the disease. DiNubile (52) discusses some aspects of using a study design that includes an active control arm. In using an active control, the Sponsor needs to take care in assigning subjects to each arm. Care must be taken so that the likelihood for safety issues is equal, a priori, for subjects receiving the study drug and for subjects receiving the active control (the comparator drug). An active control arm

is also used, as part of the study design, when use of a placebo arm would be unethical (53).

In the clinical trial on boceprevir, the run-in period lasted 4 weeks, and in this period all subjects in the study drug arm and the active control arm received the combination of ribavir and pegylated interferon-2A. (Boceprevir was not given.) Then, after the 4-week run-in period, boceprevir was added to the study drug arm. According to the FDA reviewer, this run-in period had the following advantages:

- *Reduced possibility of drug resistance.* The 4-week run-in period reduced the viral load in all subjects, thus decreasing the likelihood of the viruses developing resistance upon exposure to boceprevir. In other words, the fewer viruses that are exposed to boceprevir, at the time that administration of boceprevir begins, the lesser is the likelihood that resistance to this drug will develop.
- *Ensuring that all three drugs are simultaneously active.* The run-in period enables the immune system to adjust to the immune stimulant, pegylated interferon-2A. The immune system's response, which has various components, to this drug may take days or weeks to develop maximally. If no run-in period was used, and if all three drugs were simultaneous administered from the very beginning, only the boceprevir and ribavirin would be exerting their full influence against the virus.
- *Identify study subjects who do not respond to interferon.* An additional advantage of the run-in period, is that it enables the Sponsor to identify study subjects with immune systems that fail to respond to interferon. Identifying these particular study subjects

---

[52]DiNubile MH. Double-blind active-control trials: beware the comparator you keep. Clin. Infectious Dis. 2008;47:1064−7.

[53]Kaul S, Diamond CA. Good enough: a primer on the analysis and interpretation of noninferiority trials. Ann. Intern. Med. 2006;145:62−9.

enables the Sponsor to remove them from the trial, prior to initiating boceprevir.

- *Identify study subjects who cannot tolerate interferon.* Yet another advantage, is that the run-in period allows the Sponsor to identify subjects who cannot tolerate the interferon or ribavirin, that is, who respond with severe adverse drug reactions. Identifying these subjects enables the Sponsor to remove them from the trial.

It is interesting to note that features of this run-in period were eventually incorporated in the package insert. The package insert is the sheet of paper, included inside boxes that contain drugs, that provides instructions and warnings, regarding drug use. The package insert for *boceprevir* (Victrelis®), included the following instructions for administration (54). Although the package insert stated that, "VICTRELIS must be administered in combination with peginterferon alfa and ribavirin," it went on to state that dose recommendations are different for some subgroups. For patients with cirrhosis, the package insert recommended that "[p]atients with…cirrhosis should receive 4 weeks peginterferon alfa and ribavirin followed by 44 weeks of VICTRELIS." In short, the package insert included directions for drug administration that, in effect, included the run-in period.

b. Cysteamine Bitartrate for Nephropathic Cystinosis

The study drug is a timed-release formulation of *cysteamine bitartrate*, to be taken once every 12 h. The information is from the FDA's review of NDA 203389, which can be found on April 2013 of the FDA's website. The study drug and the active control drug were both cysteamine bitartrate, where the study drug (Procysbi®) was a timed-release formulation for taking once every 12 h, and the control drug (Cystagon®) was a formulation that needed to be taken once every 6 h.

The goal of the run-in period was to ensure that all study subjects comply with the inclusion criteria.

The inclusion criteria required that the subjects be taking Cystagon, that white blood cell levels of cystine have a level of under 2 nanomoles of half-cystine per milligram of protein, and that the subjects be able to swallow the capsule. As stated in the FDA's *Medical Review*, the inclusion criteria required:

1. Male and female nephropathic cystinosis patients on a stable Cystagon regimen (ie, able to maintain WBC cystine level <2 nmol $^1/_2$ cystine/mg protein).
2. Able to swallow intact Cystagon capsule.

Please note that Clinical Study Protocols for most or all FDA-regulated clinical trials have a list of inclusion and exclusion criteria, for determining which subjects can be admitted to the trial.

In detail, the inclusion criteria for the Procysbi clinical trial required that all subjects be taking the active comparator (Cystagon), for a 2-week run-in period prior to randomization. Immediately after the run-in period, the subjects were randomized to receive the study drug (Procybi), or to continue receiving the comparator drug (Cystagon). The importance of the run-in period was the very real possibility that the study subjects would not be able to swallow the Cystagon capsules. The FDA reviewer described the "formulation issues (inability of children to swallow over-encapsulated capsules) and the inability to mask the sulfurous smell of drug metabolites that are excreted via the lungs." Thus, as is the case with a number of other clinical trials, the run-in period for this clinical trial was to ensure that the subjects could comply with the study design, and actually consume the drugs.

---

[54]Package insert for, VICTRELIS™ (boceprevir) Capsules. Merck & Co., Inc.; May 2011 (26 pp.).

c. Omalizumab for Asthma

The study drug was *omalizumab*, a recombinant antibody. The information is from the FDA's review of BLA 103976, which can be found on December 2011 of the FDA's website. The study design required a run-in period, where all subjects were administered a dose of inhaled corticosteroid, a small molecule known as beclomethasone. The dose of the inhaled corticosteroid was kept the same during the run-in period "to achieve a level of symptoms and PEFR [peak expiratory flow rate] 'acceptable' to the subject and investigator."

Further information on the goal of the run-in period is evident from the FDA reviewer's comments on the consequences, where any given subject failed to comply with the drug dosing that must be taken during the run-in period. The consequence is confusion as to the efficacy of the study drug (omalizumab). In the words of the FDA reviewer:

> Violations of run-in periods were the most common protocol violation...[a] too brief run-in period could potentially have introduced uncertainty in the corticosteroid dosing at the start of the steroid stabilization period. The most problematic outcome of this would be to introduce variability in efficacy measures, but the effect would likely be equal since the violation was equally distributed between treatment arms and was in the same direction (too short a period for both arms).

To conclude, the goal of the run-in period was to ensure that all study subjects had the same ability to breathe, as determined by peak expiratory flow rate, prior to randomizing to the study drug or placebo control. The study drug and placebo control were both administered intravenously.

III. CONCLUDING REMARKS

The simplest type of run-in period is one where a placebo is taken during this period, and only persons found to comply are actually enrolled in the trial. In a review, Senn (55) provided additional remarks on placebo run-in periods:

> Many trials...are preceded by a *placebo run in*, in which all patients are given placebo. The practice is common within the pharmaceutical industry and recommended by standard texts as a means of weeding out noncompliers before randomisation, eliminating placebo responders, ensuring that patients are stable, washing out previous treatment, or simply to provide a period for baseline measurement.

The list of Senn (56) discloses an unusual reason for a placebo run-in period, namely, eliminating *placebo responders*. This particular rationale might be desired in clinical trials on antidepressants, but it would be irrelevant to clinical trials in oncology or infections.

Run-in periods that are a step greater in complexity are those that screen potential subjects who are relatively free from safety issues, and run-in periods that conduct a screen that confirms a diagnosis of the disease in question. Run-in periods can be used to exclude potential subjects who are found not to comply with the inclusion/exclusion criteria set forth by the Clinical Study Protocol. For example, the run-in period used by Boushey

[55]Senn S. Are placebo run ins justified? Br. Med. J. 1997;314:1191–3.

[56]Senn S. Are placebo run ins justified? Br. Med. J. 1997;314:1191–3.

et al. (57) excluded potential subjects showing excessive symptoms, too few symptoms, withdrawal of consent, loss to follow-up, failure to meet adherence criteria, use of excluded medications, and presence of an excluded medical condition. This type of run-in period might be viewed as inconsistent with the tenets of intent-to-treat analysis. Hence, investigators planning to use a run-in period to detect subjects who do not meet the requirements of the Clinical Study Protocol should first consult with their statistician.

[57]Boushey HA, Sorkness CA, King TS, et al. Daily versus as-needed corticosteroids for mild persistent asthma. New Engl. J. Med. 2005;352:1519–28.

4

Inclusion/Exclusion Criteria, Stratification, and Subgroups—Part I

I. THE CLINICAL STUDY PROTOCOL IS A MANUAL THAT PROVIDES THE STUDY DESIGN

The Clinical Study Protocol ("Protocol") is an instruction manual used for clinical trials on human subjects. The content of the Protocol is determined by the principal investigator of the study, and it is written and edited by the investigator and medical writers. The Protocol is then subjected to approval processes by an ethics board and by the FDA (U.S. Food and Drug Administration). The ethics board is typically an Institutional Review Board (IRB) (1, 2, 3). The IRB, which finds a basis in the administrative law (4), ensures that, "[r]isks to subjects are minimized … [b]y using procedures which are consistent with sound research design and which do not unnecessarily expose subjects to risk" (5).

The importance of the Protocol as a guide is evident from the fact that records must be kept of any deviations from the Protocol. The term "deviations" refers to deviations that were intentional, deviations that were the result of errors, and deviations that were the result of events beyond the control of the study employees, and so on. These deviations include failures to administer required doses, failures to adhere to the dosing schedule, and failures to acquire endpoint data on the required calendar dates. The need to anticipate deviations from the Protocol finds a basis in the Code of Federal Regulations (CFR), which suggests that:

"In Phases 2 and 3, detailed protocols describing all aspects of the study should be submitted. A protocol for a Phase 2 or 3 investigation should be designed in such a way that, if the sponsor anticipates that some deviation from the study design may become necessary as the investigation progresses, alternatives or contingencies to provide for such deviation are built into the protocols at the outset" (6).

[1]Barchi F, et al. Fostering IRB collaboration for review of international research. Am. J. Bioeth. 2014;14:3−8.

[2]Byerly WG. Working with the institutional review board. Am. J. Health Syst. Pharm. 2009;66:176−84.

[3]Neff MJ. Institutional review board consideration of chart reviews, case reports, and observational studies. Respir. Care 2008;53:1350−3.

[4]21 CFR 56.101-124 (version of April 1, 2010).

[5]21 CFR 56.111(a)(1) (version of April 1, 2010).

[6]21 CFR 312.23 (version of April 1, 2010).

Clinical Trials.
DOI: http://dx.doi.org/10.1016/B978-0-12-804217-5.00004-7

The importance of the Protocol as the gold standard for the clinical study is evident from the fact that a formal amendment process is required by the CFR when changes are to be made in a Protocol, once the actual clinical study has been started. Amendments to the Protocol find a basis in the CFR, as shown by the following excerpt (7):

> (b) *Changes in a protocol.* (1) A sponsor shall submit a protocol amendment describing any change in a Phase 1 protocol that significantly affects the safety of subjects or any change in a Phase 2 or 3 protocol that significantly affects the safety of subjects, the scope of the investigation, or the scientific quality of the study.

a. Clinical Study Protocol Provides the Inclusion/Exclusion Criteria and Stratification

The Protocol sets forth inclusion criteria, exclusion criteria, and the stratification of the study subjects. These three concepts may overlap each other. Typically, the title of the clinical study identifies some, but certainly not all, of the inclusion criteria. The full list of the inclusion/exclusion criteria occurs in the synopsis, as well as in the body of the Protocol. It is possible to disclose the same criterion in the list of inclusion criteria, and also in the list of exclusion criteria. For example, the Protocol can have the *inclusion criterion*: "all subjects must be treatment naive," and also the *exclusion criterion*: "subjects must not have received prior treatment." Regarding

the possibility of having the same criterion in both lists, it has been recommended that this sort of duplicity be avoided to prevent confusion during subsequent revisions or versions of the document (8).

Examples of titles are shown below, for a number of cancers and infectious diseases. The title of the following Clinical Study Protocol is one of the longest titles ever given to a Clinical Study Protocol. The title reveals an *exclusion criterion*, namely, that the patients must not have been treated for their multiple myeloma. The title also reveals an *inclusion criterion* that takes the form of an "or" statement, that is, they must be either 65 years of age or older, or they must not be candidates for stem cells. Consider the following title, which is from the cited clinical trial (9):

- *Title:* A Phase III, Randomized, Open-Label, 3-Arm Study to Determine the Efficacy and Safety of Lenalidomide (Revlimid®) Plus Low-Dose Dexamethsome When Given Until Progressive Disease or for 18 Four-Week Cycles Versus the Combination of Melphalan, Prednisone, and Thalidomide Given for 12 Six-Week Cycles in Patients with Previously Untreated Multiple Myeloma Who Are Either 65 Years of Age or Older or Not Candidates for Stem Cell Transplantation (10)

According to the above title, one of the inclusion criteria is that the subjects must be women, and the women must have breast cancer. Another inclusion criterion is that the cancer must be at either stages 0, I, or II.

---

[7]21 CFR 312.30 (b) (version of April 1, 2010).

[8]Wood LF, Foote MA. Targeted regulatory writing techniques. Clinical documents for drugs and biologics. Basel/Switzerland: Birkhäuser Verlag; 2009. p. 56.

[9]Benboubker L, Dimopoulos MA, Dispenzieri A, et al. Lenalidomide and dexamethasone in transplant-ineligible patients with myeloma. N. Engl. J. Med. 2014;371:906–17.

[10]Benboubker L, Dimopoulos MA, Dispenzieri A, et al. Lenalidomide and dexamethasone in transplant-ineligible patients with myeloma. N. Engl. J. Med. 2014;371:906–17.

The following title (11) discloses the inclusion criterion that the patients must never have received chemotherapy (they must be chemotherapy-naive). Another inclusion criterion is that the patients must have progressive metastatic prostate cancer. Yet another inclusion criterion is a requirement for failure, that is, that they must have already been treated for this cancer with androgen deprivation, and that this therapy failed.

- *Title:* A Multinational Phase 3, Randomized, Double-Blind, Placebo-Controlled Efficacy and Safety Study of Oral MDV3100 in Chemotherapy-Naïve Patients with Progressive Metastatic Prostate Cancer Who Have Failed Androgen Deprivation Therapy (12)

The following title reveals that study subjects entering the trial must have received anti-EGFR antibody (13).

- *Title:* An Open Label, Partially Randomised Phase II Study to Investigate the Efficacy and Safety of BIBW 2992 in Patients with Metastatic Colorectal Cancer Who Never Received Prior Anti-EGFR (Epidermal Growth Factor Receptor) Treatment (14)

According to the next title (15), one of the inclusion criteria is that the virus infecting the study subjects be one of five different genotypes. As a general proposition, subtypes of a disease, such as genotype of a virus, or stage of a disease, can be part of the title.

- *Title:* An Open-Label Trial in Genotype 2, 3, 4, 5 and 6 Hepatitis C-infected Subjects to Evaluate the Antiviral Activity, Safety, Tolerability and Pharmacokinetics of TMC435350 Following 7 Days Once Daily Dosing as Monotherapy (16)

Published reports of clinical trials also describe the inclusion and exclusion criteria. Roh et al. (17) provide one of the most comprehensive sets of inclusion and exclusion criteria ever published in a medical journal.

b. Stratification of Study Subjects

Subjects enrolled in clinical trials are typically classified into various strata, in a process called stratification. Stratification occurs at about the same time as randomization, and it occurs before subjects receive the experimental or control treatments. Stratification refers to a scheme where subgroups of a study population are classified according to stage of disease, gender, age, location of the clinic, prior therapy (if any), cytogenetics, or biomarker

[11]Beer TM, Armstrong AJ, Rathkopf DE, et al. Enzalutamide in metastatic prostate cancer before chemotherapy. N. Engl. J. Med. 2014;371:424–33.

[12]Beer TM, Armstrong AJ, Rathkopf DE, et al. Enzalutamide in metastatic prostate cancer before chemotherapy. N. Engl. J. Med. 2014;371:424–33.

[13]Boehringer Ingelheim Pharmaceuticals. http://www.clinicaltrials.gov/ct2/show/NCT01152437?term=%22never + received%22&rank=14.

[14]Boehringer Ingelheim Pharmaceuticals. http://www.clinicaltrials.gov/ct2/show/NCT01152437?term=%22never + received%22&rank=14.

[15]Tibotec Pharmaceuticals. http://www.clinicaltrials.gov/ct2/show/NCT00812331?cond=hepatitis + c&rank=1 [accessed from www.clinicaltrials.gov on 27.09.10].

[16]Tibotec Pharmaceuticals. http://www.clinicaltrials.gov/ct2/show/NCT00812331?cond=hepatitis + c&rank=1 [accessed from www.clinicaltrials.gov on 27.09.10].

[17]Roh MS, Colangelo LH, O'Connell MJ, et al. Preoperative multimodality therapy improves disease-free survival in patients with carcinoma of the rectum: NSABP R-03. J. Clin. Oncol. 2009;27:5124–30.

expression (18). The essence of stratification is that roughly equal numbers of subjects are assigned to the experimental treatment and to the control treatment.

Stratification factors used in clinical trials at the time of randomization, include:

- *Biomarker level* (PD-L1-positive versus PD-L1-negative, upon staining of tumor) (19)
- *ECOG status* (0 vs 1) (20)
- *Serum protein* (high beta2-macroglobulin vs low) (21)
- *Prior drug treatment* (lenalidomide vs thalidomide) (22); (tamoxifen vs no tamoxifen) (23)
- *Age group* (50−59, 60−69, 70 or older) (24)
- *Study site* (Asia or Australia, Europe, Latin America, North America) (25)

- *Baseline disease* (NIHSS stroke score, 6-16 vs 17 or more) (26)
- *Location of lesion* (blood clot at carotid artery vs at cerebral artery) (27).

Stratification according to location (city; nation) is useful, for example, in the event that data from one of the locations is unusual. After data are collected, all of the data from one particular location or clinic might be viewed as outliers, thus inspiring recalculation of the study data, but excluding the outliers. van Dongen et al. (28) noted that location-to-location differences can arise from variations in treatment techniques, in the skills of surgeons as well as of pathologists and radiation oncologists, in the selection of patients for the trial, or in the distribution of risk factors

[18]Biomarkers include genes or proteins that are detected in biological samples, such as tumor biopsies, white blood cells, blood plasma, or urine. The term expression, in the context of genes or proteins, refers to measuring increased copy number of a gene in the chromosome, or altered expression of messenger RNA (mRNA), microRNA (miRNA), or polypeptides. MicroRNA is described in Bartels CL, Tsongalis GJ. MicroRNAs: novel biomarkers for human cancer. Clin. Chem. 2009;55:623−31.

[19]Roberts C, Schachter J, Long GV, et al. Pembrolizumab versus ipilimumab in advanced melanoma. N. Engl. J. Med. 2015. doi:10.1056/NEJMoa1503093.

[20]Roberts C, Schachter J, Long GV, et al. Pembrolizumab versus ipilimumab in advanced melanoma. N. Engl. J. Med. 2015. doi:10.1056/NEJMoa1503093.

[21]McCarthy P, Owzar K, Hofmeister CC, et al. Lenalidomide after stem-cell transplantation for multiple myeloma. N. Engl. J. Med. 2012;366:1770−81.

[22]McCarthy P, Owzar K, Hofmeister CC, et al. Lenalidomide after stem-cell transplantation for multiple myeloma. N. Engl. J. Med. 2012;366:1770−81.

[23]Mehta RS, Barlow WE, Albain KS, et al. Combination anastrozole and fulvestrant in metastatic breast cancer. N. Engl. J. Med. 2012;367:435−44.

[24]Lal H, Cunningham AL, Godeaux O, et al. Efficacy of an adjuvanted herpes zoster subunit vaccine in older adults. N. Engl. J. Med. 2015. doi:10.1056/NEJMoa1501184.

[25]Lal H, Cunningham AL, Godeaux O, et al. Efficacy of an adjuvanted herpes zoster subunit vaccine in older adults. N. Engl. J. Med. 2015. doi:10.1056/NEJMoa1501184.

[26]Jovin TG, Chamorro A, Cobo E, et al. Thrombectomy within 8 hours after symptom onset in ischemic stroke. N. Engl. J. Med. 2015. doi:10.1056/NEJMoa1503780.

[27]Jovin TG, Chamorro A, Cobo E, et al. Thrombectomy within 8 hours after symptom onset in ischemic stroke. N. Engl. J. Med. 2015. doi:10.1056/NEJMoa1503780.

[28]van Dongen JA, Voogd AC, Fentiman IS, et al. Long-term results of a randomized trial comparing breast-conserving therapy with mastectomy: European Organization for Research and Treatment of Cancer 10801 trial. J. Natl. Cancer Inst. 2000;92:1143−50.

within the population from which the patients were selected.

The stratification of subjects serves a number of purposes, as outlined below:

- *Equal balancing between study drug and control group.* To ensure that subjects with potentially confounding characteristics, such as extensive metastasis, are identified before allocating subjects to study drug and control, and to ensure that the proportion of subjects with these confounding characteristics are equally distributed in the study drug group and control group (29). In other words, the goal is to ensure that baseline characteristics of the study drug group and control group are as similar as possible (30).
- *Comparing different clinical studies.* Stratification ensures that efficacy and safety of the study drug can reasonably be compared with other clinical trials that use the same drug (31).
- *Enabling firm conclusions on efficacy and safety.* With analysis of the entire study population, it may be difficult to draw any firm conclusion, as to the difference between study drug group and control, as to efficacy and safety. But imposing stratification on the study population, which allows subgroup analysis, increases the chances of arriving at a conclusion. Focusing on results of one particular subgroup removes background noise that is supplied by other subgroups.

- *Data and Safety Monitoring Committee.* The principal investigator of a clinical trial receives guidance and feedback from at least three bodies, namely, the Data and Safety Monitoring Committee, the Institutional Review Board, and the Food and Drug Administration. The Committee reviews data on efficacy and safety, at specific intervals, and provides recommendations to the principal investigator or sponsor. This Committee does not control the trial, but only provides recommendations. Where the Committee finds that the study drug is significantly effective, that the drug does not work, or that the drug is excessively toxic, the Committee can recommend that the trial be prematurely stopped. For these three fact-patterns, stopping is for efficacy, futility, and safety. In other words, a Committee can recommend stopping a clinical trial where early data show that the drug is dramatically effective (efficacy), where the early data show that the drug is a hopeless failure (futility), or where the early data show that the drug has very serious toxicity issues (safety). Stratification of the patients into various subgroups can help the Committee in its decisions (32). For example, if the drug is found to be excessively toxic, but where toxicity presents mainly in one subgroup, the

[29]Sorbye H, Köhne CH, Sargent DJ, Glimelius B. Patient characteristics and stratification in medical treatment studies for metastatic colorectal cancer: a proposal for standardization of patient characteristic reporting and stratification. Ann. Oncol. 2007;18:1666—72.

[30]Sorbye H, Köhne CH, Sargent DJ, Glimelius B. Patient characteristics and stratification in medical treatment studies for metastatic colorectal cancer: a proposal for standardization of patient characteristic reporting and stratification. Ann. Oncol. 2007;18:1666—72.

[31]Sorbye H, Köhne CH, Sargent DJ, Glimelius B. Patient characteristics and stratification in medical treatment studies for metastatic colorectal cancer: a proposal for standardization of patient characteristic reporting and stratification. Ann. Oncol. 2007;18:1666—72.

[32]DeMets DL, Furberg CD, Friedman LM. Data monitoring in clinical trials. New York, NY: Springer; 2006. p. 24—29, 85—92, 302.

Committee can recommend removing this subgroup from the trial and discontinuing recruiting new patients for this subgroup, rather than recommending halting the entire trial. Moreover, if the drug is found to be dramatically effective in only one subgroup, but not significantly effective in the patient population as a whole, the Committee can recommend halting the trial for efficacy.

c. Words of Warning

Hirji and Fagerland (33) cautioned against defining subgroups *after* the clinical trial is completed. Creation of subgroups after the trial is completed can result in bias when reporting the study. Regarding the creation of subgroups *after* the trial, the authors warned, "[a]nalysis of improper subgroups, though seductive, can be extremely misleading, because a particular treatment effect may influence classification to the subgroup. Thus, an apparent subgroup effect may not be a true effect of treatment but rather the result of inherent characteristics of patients that led to a particular response or to the development of side effects."

As cautioned by Proestel (34), the investigator's efforts in defining subgroups in a clinical trial usually are directed only to exploratory ends. In the situation where subjects in a particular subgroup occur in roughly equal numbers in the study drug group and in the control group, and where the number of subjects in this subgroup is sufficient to provide a statistically meaningful value, then subgroup analysis can provide firm guidance regarding the efficacy or safety of the study drug. But otherwise, information from the subgroup analysis is merely exploratory or suggestive. Sun et al. (35) provide a warning about dividing the study population into a disproportionately large number of subgroups, for example, into 23 subgroups.

Still another word of caution relates to the fact that phase II clinical trials are relatively small, while phase III clinical trials are relatively large. McDermott et al. (36) addressed the problem of the small number of subjects used in phase II trials, with regard to subgroups: "[a]nother limitation of randomized phase II trials is the increased likelihood of imbalances between the treatment arms because the study design does not usually allow for extensive stratification of even the most common prognostic factors."

d. Staging of the Disease

Subjects can be stratified according to the stage of their disease. Subjects (37) enrolling in clinical trials are often classified by the stage, in a process called *staging*. Information on staging can ensure that the proportion of subjects with more severe forms of the disease,

[33]Hirji KF, Fagerland MW. Outcome based subgroup analysis: a neglected concern. Trials 2009;10:33.

[34]Proestel S. Subgroup analysis in clinical trials. N. Engl. J. Med. 2008;358:1199.

[35]Sun X, Briel M, Busse JW, et al. Subgroup analysis of trials is rarely easy (SATIRE): a study protocol for a systematic review to characterize the analysis, reporting, and claim of subgroup effects in randomized trials. Trials 2009;10:101.

[36]McDermott DF, Sosman JA, Gonzalez R, et al. Double-blind randomized phase II study of the combination of sorafenib and dacarbazine in patients with advanced melanoma: a report from the 11715 Study Group. J. Clin. Oncol. 2008;26:2178−85.

[37]The term "subjects" is sometimes used instead of "patients," in the context of clinical trials, for the following reasons. First, where a person is enrolled in a clinical trial and is allocated to the placebo group, the term "patient" is not accurate. Second, in the context of a phase I clinical trial, where the trial is a dose-escalating trial, and where it is not likely that the lowest dose has any effect, the term "patient" is not accurate. Third, Title 21 of the CFR refers to people enrolled in clinical trials as "subjects." See, eg, 21 CFR 56.101 and 21 CFR 601.2.

and less extreme forms of the disease, reflects the proportions found in patients in the entire population of the country (38).

In the context of medical treatment outside of clinical trials, staging of a disease guides the physician as to the best route of treatment (39). The physician may explain the staging scheme as part of the patient-education process, to help the patient understand the expected outcome. According to Hammer et al. (40), "What stage am I?" is a question every patient asks upon receiving a new diagnosis of breast cancer. In the process of stratification, subjects may or may not be stratified according to stage.

e. The Study Schema

The study schema can provide some of the inclusion criteria, exclusion criteria, and information on stratification. For any clinical study, the schema can take the form of a flow chart or of a table, where the table contains a calendar of the most important events occurring during the course of the clinical trial.

This provides an example of stratification from the schema of a published Clinical Study Protocol (41). The schema, in a somewhat simplified form, is shown below. The first box in the schema contains some of the inclusion criteria. The inclusion criteria require that all study subjects be breast cancer patients, with stage 0, I, or II breast cancer (and not breast cancer at more advanced stages).

The second box in the flow chart reveals stratification. Stratification into subgroups was by disease stage, physiological status of the patient, and biochemical features of the tumor.

For the clinical trial shown below in the schema, it will be a goal to ensure that the proportion of patients at the disease stage called *DCIS*, in arm A, is the same proportion of patients with the *DCIS* disease stage in arm B. It will also be a goal to ensure that the proportion of premenopausal women in arm A is the same as the proportion of premenopausal women in arm B. In other words, it is the goal to ensure that the subgroups are balanced in arm A and arm B.

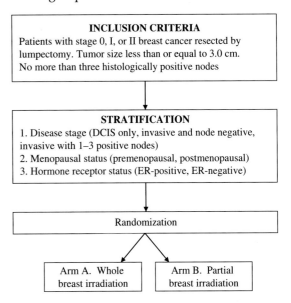

[38]Sorbye H, Köhne CH, Sargent DJ, Glimelius B. Patient characteristics and stratification in medical treatment studies for metastatic colorectal cancer: a proposal for standardization of patient characteristic reporting and stratification. Ann. Oncol. 2007;18:1666−72.

[39]Jeruss JS, Mittendorf EA, Tucker SL, et al. Staging of breast cancer in the neoadjuvant setting. Cancer Res. 2008;68:6477−81.

[40]Hammer C, Fanning A, Crowe J. Overview of breast cancer staging and surgical treatment options. Cleve. Clin. J. Med. 2008;75 (Suppl. 1):S10−6.

[41]NSABP Protocol B-39, RTOG Protocol 0413, A Randomized Phase III Study of Conventional Whole Breast Irradiation (WBI) Versus Partial Breast Irradiation (PBI) for Women with Stage 0, I, or II Breast Cancer (available from www.rtog.org).

The Clinical Study Protocol expressly states (see below) that one goal of the study scheme is to ensure that patients in the two study arms are *balanced*, as far as all of the stratification factors are concerned (42):

"Assignment of treatments to patients *will be balanced* with respect to disease stage (DCIS only, invasive disease with no positive nodes on pathological examination, invasive disease with 1−3 positive nodes on pathological examination), menopausal status, hormone receptor status (ER-positive and/or PgR-positive vs ER-negative and PgR-negative) …"

The following provides some of the inclusion/exclusion criteria from a Clinical Study Protocol used in a different clinical trial, namely a study of prostate cancer (43).

1. Inclusion Criteria for the RTOG 0232 Study of Prostate Cancer

1. Histologically confirmed adenocarcinoma of the prostate, clinical stage T1c−T2b, N0, M0. Lymph node evaluation by either CT, MRI, or node dissection is required.
2. Patient must be greater than or equal to 18 years of age.
3. Prostate-specific antigen (PSA) prior to study entry must be less or equal to 20 ng/ml.
4. Patients must sign a study-specific informed consent form prior to study entry.

2. Exclusion Criteria for the RTOG 0232 Study of Prostate Cancer

1. Stage of prostate cancer that is under stage T1c, T2c, T3, or T4

2. Lymph node involvement (*N1*)
3. Evidence of distant metastases (*M1*)
4. Previous hormonal therapy
5. Major medical or psychiatric illness, which in the investigator's opinion, would prevent completion of treatment.

f. Stratification of Subjects into Subgroups (Examples of Subgroups)

Where subjects are stratified, each stratum contains a specific subgroup. But even where subjects are not stratified, the investigator can classify each subject according to one or more subgroups. Subgroups may reflect characteristics expected for favorable prognosis (or unfavorable prognosis) in an untreated subject. Subgroups may also reflect data from a predictive marker, such as level of serum lactate dehydrogenase (LDH) or a tumor antigen, expected to be correlated with an expected response to the study drug. Subgroups may also be chosen to reflect characteristics that are purely exploratory, that is, where there is no particular expectation for outcome, for example, location of the clinic, or expression of a newly discovered gene.

This concerns a clinical trial for *olaparib* (Lynparaza®) for ovarian cancer. Information on the prognosis of a particular disease, or on predictability of drug efficacy or drug safety, can be acquired by subgroup analysis. A clinical trial on ovarian cancer involved the subgroups of genetic mutation (BRCA), age (under 50 years, 50−65 years, over 65 years), race, and the degree of response to drug therapy prior to enrolling in the clinical trial. Regarding the subgroup depending on prior

[42]NSABP Protocol B-39, RTOG Protocol 0413, A Randomized Phase III Study of Conventional Whole Breast Irradiation (WBI) Versus Partial Breast Irradiation (PBI) for Women with Stage 0, I, or II Breast Cancer (available from www.rtog.org).

[43]Radiation Therapy Oncology Group RTOG 0232. A phase III study comparing combined external beam radiation and transperineal interstitial permanent brachytherapy with brachytherapy alone for selected patients with intermediate-risk prostatic carcinoma (version March 29, 2010).

drug therapy, this subgroup involved a "[r]andomization [that] was stratified by the time to disease progression from the completion of the penultimate platinum therapy (6–12 months vs >12 months)" (44).

The Sponsor's goal of obtaining predictive information is revealed by the writing that, "[n]o predictive factors were identified … by subgroup" (45). Regarding the need for one or more subgroups that were defined by biomarkers, the researchers further added that, "[t]here is a need to identify biomarkers to select patients for this therapy."

g. FDA's Decision-Making Process in Evaluating Subgroups in the Olaparib Clinical Trial

This continues the narrative on *olaprib* (Lynparza®). At the time the FDA approves any drug, they publish the *Approval Letter*, *Medical Review*, *Pharmacological Review*, Statistical Review, and other reviews. The FDA's comments on these reviews provide an insider's account of how the FDA makes its decisions.

Data from the clinical trial on olaparib (Lynparza®) were also scrutinized by the FDA, during the FDA-review process of NDA 206162. In its *Medical Review*, the FDA referred to the study reported in the *New England Journal of Medicine* (46) as "Study 19" (47). The *Medical Review* is from December 2014, on FDA's website. The FDA reviewer stated that, "[f]urther subgroup analyses … were conducted by the FDA. These subgroups included patients with gBRCA1m, patients with gBRCA2m, and patients with tissue (somatic) BRCA mutations in the absence of germline mutations and patients with confirmed wtBRCA."

The FDA reviewer determined that the subgroups showing greatest efficacy were subjects with specific mutations in *BRCA* gene. These mutations were, *gBRCA1m* and *gBRCA2m*. The letter "g" indicates that the mutations were inherited, that is, a germline mutation. The reviewer stated that, "the treatment effect was consistent in the gBRCA1m and gBRCA2m populations." Regarding patients with wild-type *BRCA*, data in the *Medical Review* revealed that the study drug was effective in wild-type *BRCA* patients, but efficacy was less than in subjects with the *BRCA* mutations (48).

The *BRCA* mutation subgroup is reflected in the package insert for Lynparz, which states that, "Lynparza is indicated … in patients with … germline BRCA mutated … ovarian cancer" (49).

---

[44]Medical Review for olaparib (Lynparza®) for NDA 206162, from December 2014 on the FDA's website (page 88 of 131 page pdf file of Medical Review).

[45]Ledermann J, Harter P, Gourley C, et al. Olaparib maintenance therapy in platinum-sensitive relapsed ovarian cancer. N. Engl. J. Med. 2012;366:1382–92.

[46]Ledermann J, Harter P, Gourley C, et al. Olaparib maintenance therapy in platinum-sensitive relapsed ovarian cancer. New Engl. J. Med. 2012;366:1382-92.

[47]Medical Review for olaparib (Lynparza®) for NDA 206162, from December 2014 on the FDA's website.

[48]*Medical Review* for olaparib (Lynparza®) for NDA 206162, from December 2014 on the FDA's website (page 99 of 131 page pdf file having the *Medical Review*).

[49]Package insert for LYNPARZA™ (olaparib) capsules, for oral use (December 2014) (4 pages).

Typical subgroups are shown by the following bullet points:

- Location of study site (50, 51, 52, 53)
- Strain of virus infecting the patient (54)
- Titer of virus in patient's bloodstream (55)
- Biomarker expressed in a tumor biopsy (56, 57, 58)
- Size of tumor, eg, under 2 cm or 2 cm and above (59)

- Racial group of study subject, eg, white versus non-white (60)
- Age of study subject, eg, under 65 years or 65 years and over (61)
- Past history of medical treatment, prior to enrollment in the clinical study (62)
- Number of lymph nodes containing tumor cells, eg, three or fewer or greater than three (63)

[50]Treanor JJ, Campbell JD, Zangwill KM, Rowe T, Wolff M. Safety and immunogenicity of an inactivated subvirion influenza A (H5N1) vaccine. N. Engl. J. Med. 2006;354:1343–51.

[51]Hayden FG, Turner RB, Gwaltney JM, et al. Phase II, randomized, double-blind, placebo-controlled studies of ruprintrivir nasal spray 2-percent suspension for prevention and treatment of experimentally induced rhinovirus colds in healthy volunteers. Antimicrob. Agents Chemother. 2003;47:3907–16.

[52]Menezes AM, Hallal PC, Perez-Padilla R, et al. Tuberculosis and airflow obstruction: evidence from the PLATINO study in Latin America. Eur. Respir. J. 2007;30:1180–5.

[53]Roché H, Fumoleau P, Spielmann M, et al. Sequential adjuvant epirubicin-based and docetaxel chemotherapy for node-positive breast cancer patients: the FNCLCC PACS 01 Trial. J. Clin. Oncol. 2006;24:5664–71.

[54]Hayden FG, Turner RB, Gwaltney JM, et al. Phase II, randomized, double-blind, placebo-controlled studies of ruprintrivir nasal spray 2-percent suspension for prevention and treatment of experimentally induced rhinovirus colds in healthy volunteers. Antimicrob. Agents Chemother. 2003;47:3907–16.

[55]Study NV15942 described in Package Insert (May 2004) Ribavirin, Copegus™, Roche.

[56]Ma XJ, Hilsenbeck SG, Wang W, et al. The HOXB13:IL17BR expression index is a prognostic factor in early-stage breast cancer. J. Clin. Oncol. 2006;24:4611–9.

[57]Ejlertsen B, Mouridsen HT, Jensen MB, et al. Similar efficacy for ovarian ablation compared with cyclophosphamide, methotrexate, and fluorouracil: from a randomized comparison of premenopausal patients with node-positive, hormone receptor-positive breast cancer. J. Clin. Oncol. 2006;24:4956–62.

[58]de Azambuja E, Paesmans M, Beauduin M, et al. Long-term benefit of high-dose epirubicin in adjuvant chemotherapy for node-positive breast cancer: 15-year efficacy results of the Belgian multicentre study. J. Clin. Oncol. 2009;27:720–5

[59]Boccardo F, Rubagotti A, Puntoni M, et al. Switching to anastrozole versus continued tamoxifen treatment of early breast cancer: preliminary results of the Italian Tamoxifen Anastrozole Trial. J. Clin. Oncol. 2005;23:5138–47.

[60]Goldstein LJ, O'Neill A, Sparano JA, et al. Concurrent doxorubicin plus docetaxel is not more effective than concurrent doxorubicin plus cyclophosphamide in operable breast cancer with 0 to 3 positive axillary nodes: North American Breast Cancer Intergroup Trial E 2197. J. Clin. Oncol. 2008;26:4092–9.

[61]Chia S, Gradishar W, Mauriac L, et al. Double-blind, randomized placebo controlled trial of fulvestrant compared with exemestane after prior nonsteroidal aromatase inhibitor therapy in postmenopausal women with hormone receptor-positive, advanced breast cancer: results from EFECT. J. Clin. Oncol. 2008;26:1664–70.

[62]Treanor JJ, Campbell JD, Zangwill KM, Rowe T, Wolff M. Safety and immunogenicity of an inactivated subvirion influenza A (H5N1) vaccine. N. Engl. J. Med. 2006;354:1343–51.

[63]Boccardo F, Rubagotti A, Puntoni M, et al. Switching to anastrozole versus continued tamoxifen treatment of early breast cancer: preliminary results of the Italian Tamoxifen Anastrozole Trial. J. Clin. Oncol. 2005;23:5138–47.

- White blood cell count (64), eg, CD4$^+$ T cell count that is under 50 cells/mm^3, 50–100 cells/mm^3, or over 100 cells/mm^3.

These particular subgroups were chosen for reproduction in this chapter, because they were disclosed, by the cited reference, in the form of an organized format called a forest plot. A forest plot is a histogram. This plot acquired its name from the fact that the picture resembles a forest with many trees (65).

h. Prior Therapy

Prior therapy is often listed in the inclusion/exclusion criteria. The criteria may require the study subject to be treatment-naive or, in contrast, to have already been treated with the standard therapy. Subjects may be stratified according to whether he or she has received prior therapy.

The requirement that a patient be treatment-naive may reduce the pool of available participants, as documented by Bajetta et al. (66). However, there are a number of good reasons for requiring that subjects be treatment-naive. Poorer health status of patients already subjected to chemotherapy or radiotherapy may dictate use of treatment-naive subjects. Toxicity from prior therapy, that is cumulative or irreversible, may dictate use of treatment-naive subjects. Acquisition of resistance (by tumor cells) to the study drug, during earlier therapy, will mandate use of treatment-naive subjects. Another reason for using treatment-naive subjects is that prior hormone therapy can create artifacts in the expression of biomarkers. Moreover, prior therapy that establishes immune memory in a study subject, where this immune memory would interfere with the study, mandates exclusion of prior therapy.

But the trial design may also require that all of the study subjects have been treated with a given drug before enrolling in the clinical trial. One reason for this requirement is as follows. It may be easier to gain regulatory approval, where approval is for use of a given drug in *second-line therapy*. This means that the drug has been approved for use, only where another, more established drug, has failed for any given patient. In the words of Roberts et al. (67), "[i]t is generally true that most agents approved for second- and third-line indications are approved as single agents (eg, paclitaxel for second-line ovarian cancer and ifosfamide for third-line testicular cancer)." According to Dr T.G. Roberts (68) and Dr T.J. Lynch (69), oncology clinical trials that are called "second-line trials" require patients to have been exposed to a first-line regimen (before enrolling in the second-line trial). One reason for this requirement is to help ensure a homogeneous group of study subjects (70). Another reason, is to give study subjects a chance to have the best available treatment prior to enrolling in the second-line trial.

[64]Fätkenheuer G, Nelson M, Lazzarin A, et al. Subgroup analyses of maraviroc in previously treated R5 HIV-1 infection. N. Engl. J. Med. 2008;359:1442–55.

[65]Callcut RA, Branson RD. How to read a review paper. Respir. Care 2009;54:1379–85.

[66]Bajetta E, Catena L, Procopio G, et al. Is the new WHO classification of neuroendocrine tumours useful for selecting an appropriate treatment? Ann. Oncol. 2005;16:1374–80.

[67]Roberts TG, Lynch TJ, Chabner BA. The phase III trial in the era of targeted therapy: unraveling the "go or no go" decision. J. Clin. Oncol. 2003;21:3683–95.

[68]T.G. Roberts, Jr. e-mail of January 14, 2011.

[69]T.J. Lynch, e-mail of January 17, 2011.

[70]T.G. Roberts, Jr. e-mail of January 14, 2011.

Regarding this reason, FDA may mandate, for ethical reasons, that prior therapy be one of the inclusion criteria (71).

The inclusion/exclusion criteria for many thousands of clinical trials are available on www.clinicaltrials.gov. About 500 of these clinical trials concerns second-line therapy, that is, therapy for patients where a previous treatment has failed. The following is only one example of many. The example is from the trial, "Temsirolimus Versus Sorafenib as Second-Line Therapy in Patients with Advanced RCC Who Have Failed First-Line Sunitinib" (72). The list of inclusion criteria requires that, "subjects must have at least 1 cycle of sunitinib therapy." Another example, from a publication by the FDA, is a trial on multiple myeloma (73).

i. Poor Performance Status as a Basis for Exclusion

Potential subjects who have already been exposed to first-line therapy may have a declined performance status, due to drugs or radiation administered during the first-line therapy. Poor performance status has been defined as a score of 2 on the ECOG rating scale, as shown in Table 4.1. According to Wakelee and Belani (74), patients with poor performance status, as assessed by ECOG performance status, "are often excluded from clinical trials. They tend to have poorer responses to treatment and shorter survival than their counterparts with PS scores of 0—1. It is also

TABLE 4.1   ECOG Performance Status[a]

Grade	ECOG Performance Status
0	Fully active, able to carry on all predisease performance without restriction
1	Restricted in physically strenuous activity but ambulatory and able to carry out work of a light or sedentary nature, eg, light house work, office work
2	Ambulatory and capable of all selfcare but unable to carry out any work activities. Up and about more than 50% of waking hours
3	Capable of only limited selfcare, confined to bed or chair more than 50% of waking hours
4	Completely disabled. Cannot carry on any selfcare. Totally confined to bed or chair
5	Dead

[a]Oken MM, Creech RH, Tormey DC., et al. Toxicity and response criteria of the Eastern Cooperative Oncology Group. Am. J. Clin. Oncol. 1982;5:649—55.

generally believed that they are at greater risk for toxicity." Similarly, according to Hennessy et al. (75), "[e]lderly patients and patients with poorer performance statuses are often excluded from clinical trials ... where it was generally considered that these patients experienced higher toxicity rates ... [e]lderly patients often have comorbid conditions."

j. Irreversible and Cumulative Toxicity as a Basis for Exclusion

Although most chemotherapeutic agents have an associated toxicity, reversible side effects

[71]T.G. Roberts, Jr. e-mail of January 14, 2011.

[72]Clinicaltrials.gov identifier NCT00474786.

[73]Hazarika M, Rock E, Williams G, et al. Lenalidomide in combination with dexamethasone for the treatment of multiple myeloma after one prior therapy. Oncologist 2008;13:1120—7.

[74]Wakelee H, Belani CP. Optimizing first-line treatment options for patients with advanced NSCLC. Oncologist 2005;10 (Suppl. 3):1—10.

[75]Hennessy BT, Hanrahan EO, Breathnach OS. Chemotherapy options for the elderly patient with advanced non-small cell lung cancer. Oncologist. 2003;8:270—7.

impose fewer limitations on future treatment options (76). Topotecan's toxicity (neutropenia; leukopenia) is reversible and non-cumulative (77). Trastuzumab's toxicity (cardiotoxicity) tends to be reversible. According to Perez (78), "in contrast to anthracycline-induced cardiac toxicity, trastuzumab-related cardiac dysfunction does not appear to increase with cumulative dose or to be associated with ultrastructural changes in the myocardium and is generally reversible."

But, the toxicity of anthracyclines, such as doxorubicin, tends to be irreversible and cumulative. Doxorubicin's irreversible cardiac toxicity is well documented (79, 80). In the words of Montemurro et al. (81), "[a] steep increase in the risk for irreversible cardiotoxicity for cumulative doses of doxorubicin and epidoxorubicin ... represents the main limitation to rechallenge with these drugs."

Carboplatin can produce irreversible toxicity. Where carboplatin is used for treating a particular cancer, and where the cancer returns and where carboplatin is administered again, the result can be a hypersensitivity reaction in the form of tachycardia (82). Kandel et al. (83), suggest a strategy for overcoming cumulative carboplatin toxicity, where it is necessary to re-administer a platin drug. Re-administering platin drugs may be needed where there is a relapse of ovarian cancer, to give an example. The suggestion is to switch from one type of platinum drug to another type of platinum drug, that is, from carboplatin to cisplatin (84, 85).

[76]Dunton CJ. Management of treatment-related toxicity in advanced ovarian cancer. Oncologist 2002;7 (Suppl. 5):11−9.

[77]Dunton CJ. Management of treatment-related toxicity in advanced ovarian cancer. Oncologist 2002;7 (Suppl. 5):11−9.

[78]Perez EA. Cardiac toxicity of ErbB2-targeted therapies: what do we know? Clin. Breast Cancer 2008;8 (Suppl. 3): S114−20.

[79]Chan S, Friedrichs K, Noel D, et al. Prospective randomized trial of docetaxel versus doxorubicin in patients with metastatic breast cancer. J. Clin. Oncol. 1999;17:2341−54.

[80]Armenian SH, Sun CL, Francisco L, et al. Late congestive heart failure after hematopoietic cell transplantation. J. Clin. Oncol. 2008;26:5537−43.

[81]Montemurro F, Rossi V, Nolè F, et al. Underuse of anthracyclines in women with HER-2 + advanced breast cancer. Oncologist 2010;15:665−72.

[82]Markman M, Kennedy A, Webster K, et al. Clinical features of hypersensitivity reactions to carboplatin. J. Clin. Oncol. 1999;17:1141−5.

[83]Kandel MJ, Loehr A, Harter P, Traut A, Gnauert K, du Bois A. Cisplatinum rechallenge in relapsed ovarian cancer patients with platinum reinduction therapy and carboplatin hypersensitivity. Int. J. Gynecol. Cancer 2005;15:780−4.

[84]Ardizzoni A, Boni L, Tiseo M, Fossella FV, et al. Cisplatin- versus carboplatin-based chemotherapy in first-line treatment of advanced non-small-cell lung cancer: an individual patient data meta-analysis. J. Natl. Cancer Inst. 2007;99:847−57.

[85]Hartmann JT, Kollmannsberger C, Kanz L, Bokemeyer C. Platinum organ toxicity and possible prevention in patients with testicular cancer. Int. J. Cancer 1999;83:866−9.

In the non-small-cell lung cancer clinical trial of Ramlau et al. (86), the inclusion criteria required that all study subjects had received standard chemotherapy prior to enrolling in the Ramlau study. But this prior chemotherapy proved to be an issue during the analysis of adverse events that were captured during the Ramlau study. Ramlau's study drug was topotecan, a drug not known to cause neuropathy. But some of the topotecan-treated subjects had the adverse event of neuropathy. The authors attributed this neuropathy to chemotherapy received prior to entering the clinical trial, writing, "[b]ecause topotecan is not known to cause neuropathy, the neuropathy reported by patients in this group (8% topotecan vs 26% in the docetaxel group) is likely from first-line therapy or the malignant process itself."

Radiation can produce irreversible toxicity, for example, to the heart. Billingham et al. (87, 88) document the fact that radiation treatment can cause irreversible damage to the heart where, upon administering chemotherapy many years later, a cumulative effect is produced. These authors report that, "[t]his study indicates that radiation, even if remote, enhances adriamycin-induced cardiomyopathy. Therefore, adriamycin must be given cautiously in patients who have received previous mediastinal radiotherapy."

TABLE 4.2 Cumulative Toxicity[b]

Drug	Cumulative Toxicity
Cisplatin	Renal toxicity; neurotoxicity; high-tone hearing loss
Carboplatin	Thrombocytopenia
Paclitaxel	Peripheral neurotoxicity
Etoposide	Leukemia
Doxorubicin	Palmar-plantar erythrodysesthesia (PPE), cardiotoxicity
Gemcitabine	Cardiotoxicity, pulmonary toxicity, thrombotic microangiopathy
Topotecan	No cumulative toxicity

[b]Dunton CJ. Management of treatment-related toxicity in advanced ovarian cancer. The Oncologist. 2002;7 (Suppl. 5):11–9.

Cumulative toxicity refers to a situation where previous chemotherapy has been given, and more is contemplated at a later date, and where the toxicities of the earlier and later treatments are additive (89).

The above considerations provide a basis for inclusion criteria requiring that subjects be treatment-naive, and why some inclusion criteria stipulate the dose level of previous chemotherapy which must not have been exceeded (90).

The following table documents the cumulative and irreversible toxicities of some commonly used oncology drugs (Table 4.2).

[86]Ramlau R, Gervais R, Krzakowski M, et al. Phase III study comparing oral topotecan to intravenous docetaxel in patients with pretreated advanced non-small-cell lung cancer. J. Clin. Oncol. 2006;24:2800–7.

[87]Billingham ME, Bristow MR, Glatstein E, Mason JW, Masek MA, Daniels JR. Adriamycin cardiotoxicity: endomyocardial biopsy evidence of enhancement by irradiation. Am. J. Surg. Pathol. 197;1:17–23.

[88]Bird BR, Swain SM. Cardiac toxicity in breast cancer survivors: review of potential cardiac problems. Clin. Cancer Res. 2008;14:14–24.

[89]Barrett-Lee PJ. E-mail of October 12, 2010.

[90]Barrett-Lee PJ. E-mail of October 12, 2010.

k. Drug Resistance as a Basis for Exclusion

Prior treatment with a specific chemotherapeutic drug may be in the list of exclusion criteria, where the basis is drug resistance (resistance to both the earlier drug and the study drug). Resistance can arise from the fact that the earlier-administered drug induces genetic changes in the chromosomes of tumors, for example, changes in expression of drug transporters and changes that are mutations in oncogenes.

Resistance to a drug does not necessarily mean that the tumor had experienced a genetic change. Resistance can also present when a tumor is heterogeneous, for example, where it contains two types of cancer cells, where the first type is chemosensitive but the second type is chemoresistant. Koletsis et al. (91) observed that, at least in the context of lung cancer, non-responsiveness to chemotherapy can result where tumors are heterogeneous, that is, where lung tumors are a mixture of cells with the histology of small-cell lung cancer and non-small-cell lung cancer.

II. BIOCHEMISTRY OF DRUG RESISTANCE

a. Biochemistry of the ABC Drug Transporters

During chemotherapy against tumors, most drugs target proteins or nucleic acids that are located inside the tumor cell. Unfortunately, tumors have a number of transport systems that are able to pump drugs back out of the tumor cell. O'Brien et al. (92) and Burtness et al. (93) describe a number of drug transporters. One of these transport systems is a system called the ABC transporters. As reviewed by Elliott and Al-Hajj (94), the human genome encodes nearly 50 ABC transporters. Of these transporters, those used for multidrug transport are listed below.

In the following list of drug transporters, the alternate names are disclosed, for example, ABCC1 is the same protein as MRP1:

MRP1/ABCC1; MRP2/ABCC2; MRP3/ABCC3; MRP4/ABCC4; MRP5/ABCC5; MRP6/ABCC6; MRP7/ABCC10; MRP8/ABCC11; and MRP9/ABCC12 (95).

According to various publications (96, 97), the transporter known as ABCC1 may confer

[91]Koletsis EN, Prokakis C, Karanikolas M, Apostolakis E, Dougenis D. Current role of surgery in small cell lung carcinoma. J. Cardiothorac. Surg. 2009;4:30.

[92]O'Brien C, Cavet G, Pandita A, et al. Functional genomics identifies ABCC3 as a mediator of taxane resistance in HER2-amplified breast cancer. Cancer Res. 2008;68:5380−9.

[93]Burtness BA, Manola J, Axelrod R, et al. A randomized phase II study of ixabepilone (BMS-247550) given daily x5 days every 3 weeks or weekly in patients with metastatic or recurrent squamous cell cancer of the head and neck: an Eastern Cooperative Oncology Group study. Ann. Oncol. 2008;19:977−83.

[94]Elliott AM, Al-Hajj MA. ABCB8 mediates doxorubicin resistance in melanoma cells by protecting the mitochondrial genome. Mol. Cancer Res. 2009;7:79−87.

[95]Zhou SF, Wang LL, Di YM, Xue CC, Duan W, Li CG, Li Y. Substrates and inhibitors of human multidrug resistance associated proteins and the implications in drug development. Curr. Med. Chem. 2008;15:1981−2039.

[96]Hembruff SL, Laberge ML, Villeneuve DJ, et al. Role of drug transporters and drug accumulation in the temporal acquisition of drug resistance. BMC Cancer 2008;8:318.

[97]Deeley RG, Cole SP. Substrate recognition and transport by multidrug resistance protein 1 (ABCC1). FEBS Lett. 2006;580:1103−11.

resistance to doxorubicin, daunorubicin, vincristine, etoposide, epirubicin, chlorambucil, methotrexate (98, 99), melphalan, and paclitaxel, ABCC2 may confer resistance to doxorubicin, etoposide, methotrexate, irinotecan (SN-38), vincristine, vinblastine, camptothecin, paclitaxel, docetaxel, etoposide, and cisplatin, and ABCC4 may confer resistance to rubitecan and irinotecan.

b. Biology of Cross-Resistance

Cross-resistance refers to the situation where treating a patient with a first drug confers changes in the physiology of the tumor that reduce the efficacy of a second, unrelated drug that may be administered at a later time (100).

Cross-resistance can result from the situation where the first drug induces expression of one of the ABC transporters, and where this particular ABC transporter pumps the first drug out of the tumor cell, and also pumps a second drug out of the tumor cell, for example, a second drug administered at some later time in a clinical trial.

In making clinical decisions on the administration of different sequences of drugs, caution should be used when faced with information revealing that a first drug induces resistance to a second drug, by way of stimulating the activity of a drug transporter. Also, caution should be used in the situation where the first drug is hydrophilic and the second drug is hydrophobic, and caution should be used where the first drug is a large molecule and the second drug is a small molecule (101).

Also, greater credence should be given to a well-controlled study of drug resistance in actual human subjects, than to a well-controlled study with cultured cells. The ultimate arbiter of appropriate trial design is whether the therapy actually works—many attempts to use drug sequences that were configured to avoid resistance have often failed to be effective (102).

c. A Tumor's Genetic Expression Can Provide Guidance on Drug Resistance

Gene expression data from a tumor can determine whether the tumor is likely to be resistant to a given drug (103, 104).

[98]Maeno K, Nakajima A, Conseil G, Rothnie A, Deeley RG, Cole SP. Molecular basis for reduced estrone sulfate transport and altered modulator sensitivity of transmembrane helix (TM) 6 and TM17 mutants of multidrug resistance protein 1 (ABCC1). Drug Metab. Dispos. 2009;37:1411−20.

[99]Yang HH, Ma MH, Vescio RA, Berenson JR. Overcoming drug resistance in multiple myeloma: the emergence of therapeutic approaches to induce apoptosis. J. Clin. Oncol. 2003;21:4239−47.

[100]Giai M, Biglia N, Sismondi P. Chemoresistance in breast tumors. Eur. J. Gynaecol. Oncol. 1991;12:359−73.

[101]Norris MD. E-mail of October 4, 2010.

[102]Esteva FJ, Hortobagyi GN. Can early response assessment guide neoadjuvant chemotherapy in early-stage breast cancer? J. Natl. Cancer Inst. 2008;100:521−13.

[103]Falgreen S, Dybbkaer K, Young KH, et al. Predicting response to multidrug regimens in cancer patients using cell line experiments and regularised regression models. BMC Cancer 2015;15:235. doi:10.1186/s12885015-1237−6 (15 pages).

[104]Minna JD, Girard L, Xie Y. Tumor mRNA expression profiles predict responses to chemotherapy. J. Clin. Oncol. 2007;25:4329−36.

- *Doxorubicin.* According to Munoz et al. (105), Grant et al. (106), and Di Nicolantionio et al. (107), doxorubicin induces the expression of ABCC1, a multidrug transporter that transports doxorubicin and methotrexate. Hence, it might be expected that, where patients receive doxorubicin, and where their tumors respond by up-regulating ABCC1, the tumors will acquire resistance to both doxorubicin and methotrexate. Doxorubicin is in the anthracycline class of drugs. This drug targets an enzyme used for DNA metabolism, namely, topoisomerase II.

- *Paclitaxel.* Paclitaxel is in the taxane class of drugs. Taxanes can also be eliminated from tumors, by way of the ABC drug transporters, ABCB1 or ABCB4 (108). Where a cancer patient is treated with a taxane, and where the tumors acquire resistance, for example, by overexpression of ABCB1 or ABCB4, the physician can change the drug. For example, tumors of breast cancer patients treated with taxanes often develop resistance to this drug. In this context, the FDA has specifically approved switching to another drug, namely, ixabepilone (109), In a clinical study of breast cancer, Thomas et al. (110) stated that taxane-resistant tumors did not show cross-resistance to ixabepilone. This statement is useful for the situation where a first clinical study uses taxane, and a second clinical study uses ixabepilone. Consistently, Buzdar (111) stated that breast tumors frequently develop resistance to anthracyclines and taxanes by way of overexpression of the *MDR1* gene and *MRP* gene while, in contrast, ixabepitone does not induce these genes.

- *Tamoxifen.* Drug resistance can be acquired by genetic mutations. Chemotherapy of breast cancer with tamoxifen is frequently met with drug resistance by tumors (112). Tamoxifen targets estrogen receptor. The estrogen receptor is part of a cell-signaling pathway that promotes growth of the breast cancer tumor (113). Patients with breast cancer tumors that express estrogen

[105]Munoz M, Henderson M, Haber M, Norris M. Role of the MRP1/ABCC1 multidrug transporter protein in cancer. IUBMB Life. 2007;59:752−7.

[106]Grant CE, Gao M, DeGorter MK, Cole SP, Deeley RG. Structural determinants of substrate specificity differences between human multidrug resistance protein (MRP) 1 (ABCC1) and MRP3 (ABCC3). Drug Metab Dispos. 2008;36:2571−8.

[107]Di Nicolantonio F, Mercer SJ, Knight LA, et al. Cancer cell adaptation to chemotherapy. BMC Cancer 2005;5:78.

[108]Duan Z, Brakora KA, Seiden MV. Inhibition of ABCB1 (MDR1) and ABCB4 (MDR3) expression by small interfering RNA and reversal of paclitaxel resistance in human ovarian cancer cells. Mol. Cancer Ther. 2004;3:833−8.

[109]Yardley DA. Activity of ixabepilone in patients with metastatic breast cancer with primary resistance to taxanes. Clin. Breast Cancer 2008;8:487−92.

[110]Thomas E, Tabernero J, Fornier M, et al. Phase II clinical trial of ixabepilone (BMS-247550), an epothilone B analog, in patients with taxane-resistant metastatic breast cancer. J. Clin. Oncol. 2007;25:3399−406.

[111]Buzdar AU. Preoperative chemotherapy treatment of breast cancer—a review. Cancer 2007;110:2394−407.

[112]Bernard-Marty C, Cardoso F, Piccart MJ. Facts and controversies in systemic treatment of metastatic breast cancer. Oncologist 2004;9:617−32.

[113]Miller TW, Pérez-Torres M, Narasanna A, et al. Loss of phosphatase and tensin homologue deleted on chromosome 10 engages ErbB3 and insulin-like growth factor-I receptor signaling to promote antiestrogen resistance in breast cancer. Cancer Res. 2009;69:4192−201.

receptor are candidates for treatment with this drug (114). A high percentage of ER-positive breast cancers that respond to initial tamoxifen treatment subsequently develop resistance. Sustained tamoxifen resistance continues to be a major problem in managing advanced breast cancer (115). Miller et al. (116) and Fan et al. (117) describe mechanisms by which estrogen receptor acquires resistance to tamoxifen. These include mutations in the tumor's genome that lead to increased activity of the tumor's phosphatidylinositol 3-kinase (PI3K) and can lead to resistance against tamoxifen. Also, tamoxifen resistance can result from reduced expression of TGF-beta receptor type 2, and from increased expression of ABCG2 multidrug resistance protein (118).

Imatinib. c-KIT is a kinase that mediates cell-signaling in normal and cancer cells. But in some tumor cells, c-KIT acquires a mutation that is responsible for the transformation of a normal host cell to a tumor cell (119). Imatinib, which inhibits c-KIT, is used to treat patients with tumors where c-KIT is responsible for this transformation. Mutations in c-KIT that result in drug resistance should be distinguished from mutations in c-KIT that result in the conversion of normal c-KIT into an oncogene (120). Normally, c-KIT is used for erythropoiesis and melanin formation, but mutations can result in this conversion (121). But with imatinib, 50% of patients develop resistance due to additional mutations in c-KIT. Therefore, second-line treatment is with another drug, sunitinib. Sunitinib has been approved for use in cancer, after failure of imatinib due to the tumor's resistance to imatinib (122). Hence, where a clinical study is to be conducted with imatinib, it is reasonable that the Clinical Study Protocol mandate that the subjects be treatment-naive with regard to imatinib, to ensure that the tumors in the subjects are not resistant to imatinib.

[114]Higgins MJ, Stearns V. Understanding resistance to tamoxifen in hormone receptor-positive breast cancer. Clin. Chem. 2009;55:1453−5.

[115]Kumar R, Zhang H, Holm C, Vadlamudi RK, Landberg G, Rayala SK. Extranuclear coactivator signaling confers insensitivity to tamoxifen. Clin. Cancer Res. 2009;15:4123−30.

[116]Miller TW, Pérez-Torres M, Narasanna A, et al. Loss of phosphatase and tensin homologue deleted on chromosome 10 engages ErbB3 and insulin-like growth factor-I receptor signaling to promote antiestrogen resistance in breast cancer. Cancer Res. 2009;69:4192−201.

[117]Fan P, Yue W, Wang JP, et al. Mechanisms of resistance to structurally diverse antiestrogens differ under premenopausal and postmenopausal conditions: evidence from in vitro breast cancer cell models. Endocrinology. 2009;150:2036−45.

[118]Busch S, et al. Loss of TGFbeta receptor type 2 expression impairs estrogen response and confers tamoxifen resistance. Cancer Res. 2015;75:1457−69.

[119]Roberts KG, Smith AM, McDougall F, et al. Essential requirement for PP2A inhibition by the oncogenic receptor c-KIT suggests PP2A reactivation as a strategy to treat c-KIT + cancers. Cancer Res. 2010;70:5438−47.

[120]Bamba S, Hirota S, Inatomi O, et al. Familial and multiple gastrointestinal stromal tumors with fair response to a half-dose of imatinib. Intern. Med. 2015;54:759−64.

[121]Oriss TB, et al. Dendritic cell c-kit signaling and adaptive immunity: implications for the upper airways. Curr. Opin. Allergy Clin. Immunol. 2014;14:7−12.

[122]Gajiwala KS, Wu JC, Christensen J, et al. KIT kinase mutants show unique mechanisms of drug resistance to imatinib and sunitinib in gastrointestinal stromal tumor patients. Proc. Natl. Acad. Sci. USA 2009;106:1542−7.

d. Prior Treatment with Hormones as a Basis for Exclusion

Prostate-specific antigen (PSA) is a biomarker used in clinical trials (123) for prostate cancer, and it is used in routine screening of the general public for prostate cancer. Where men are treated with testosterone (for any reason), the result can be an increased expression of PSA (124). Collette et al. (125) point out that expression of PSA is controlled, at the genetic level, where control is mediated by an androgen-responsive element. Alterations of serum androgen levels can provoke changes in PSA expression, where these changes are totally independent of burden of prostate tumors.

An increase in PSA that occurs by this mechanism does not indicate any increase in risk for prostate cancer.

Moreover, in men diagnosed with metastatic prostate cancer, men are treated with leuprolide or goserelin, which reduce testosterone expression (126). Leuprolide is an oligopeptide that is a hormone analog (127). A consequence of this reduced expression of testosterone is reduced expression of PSA. Because of the fact that hormones (and hormone analogs) can alter the expression of PSA, clinical trials for prostate cancer may exclude men who had been receiving hormones, or may stratify men into those who had been receiving hormones, and those who had not been receiving hormones (128). Another reason for excluding or stratifying men who had reduced testosterone levels, is that reduced testosterone can impair the general quality of life of the men (thereby causing the study subjects to have two disorders, the prostate cancer and the testosterone-induced reduction in life quality) (129).

e. Immune Status for Exclusion Criteria

Immune status is a particular issue for clinical trials on vaccines or on drugs that modulate the immune system, for example, drugs that are cytokines. Where a subject had earlier been vaccinated, the typical result is long-term immune memory. Where a subject had earlier been exposed to an immune adjuvant, such as a cytokine or a TLR-agonist, long-term immune memory may also result. The question of whether to include or exclude subjects who had earlier been treated with a vaccine or immune adjuvant must be addressed on a case-by-case basis. The term "TLR-agonist" refers to a drug that is a stimulant (agonist) of a class of immune proteins in the body called, toll-like receptors (TLRs).

Immune memory is described. Memory immune response allows the immune system to respond more vigorously to pathogens that

[123]Collette L. Prostate-specific antigen (PSA) as a surrogate end point for survival in prostate cancer clinical trials. Eur. Urol. 2008;53:6−9.

[124]Gore J, Rajfer J. Rising PSA during testosterone replacement therapy. Rev. Urol. 2004;6 (Suppl. 6):S41−3.

[125]Collette L, Burzykowski T, Carroll KJ, et al. Is prostate-specific antigen a valid surrogate end point for survival in hormonally treated patients with metastatic prostate cancer? Joint research of the European Organisation for Research and Treatment of Cancer, the Limburgs Universitair Centrum, and AstraZeneca Pharmaceuticals. J. Clin. Oncol. 2005;23:6139−48.

[126]D'Amico AV, Renshaw AA, Loffredo B, Chen MH. Duration of testosterone suppression and the risk of death from prostate cancer in men treated using radiation and 6 months of hormone therapy. Cancer 2007;110:1723−8.

[127]Okada H, Sakura Y, Kawaji H, Yashiki T, Mima H. Regression of rat mammary tumors by a potent luteinizing hormone-releasing hormone analogue (leuprolide) administered vaginally. Cancer Res. 1983;43:1869−74.

[128]Prestidge BR. E-mail of September 27, 2010.

[129]Prestidge BR. E-mail of September 27, 2010.

were previously encountered (130). Upon primary activation by an antigen, $CD8^+$ T cells follow a program of proliferation and differentiation. After this expansion phase, the majority of antigen-specific $CD8^+$ T cells undergo programmed cell death. But a rapid and vigorous recall response is possible because of residual $CD8^+$ T cells in the body.

Prior treatment with a vaccine can interfere with efficacy of a later-administered vaccine. The earlier-administered vaccine can reduce the efficacy of the later vaccine by two different mechanisms. These two mechanisms are immune tolerance (131, 132) and immunodominance (133). Immune tolerance can involve a scenario where a patient receives a vaccine, and where the vaccine provokes immune tolerance, thereby reducing immune response against an antigen of a particular pathogen, or against a particular tumor antigen.

f. Example of Earlier Vaccination as an Inclusion Criterion

A requirement for an earlier vaccination is found in clinical studies on booster vaccinations. Typically, vaccinations take the form of a prime vaccine and a boost vaccine. These two vaccines may be given a few weeks apart or even many years apart. The following concerns vaccination with *Mycobacterium bovis*

Bacille Calmette–Guerin (BCG). This vaccine is used for treating tuberculosis. A number of clinical trials have addressed the efficacy of BCG vaccination given in childhood, followed by a second BCG vaccination given in adulthood. This type of prime-boost scheme is called a BCG-BCG vaccination.

Whelan et al. (134) studied 14 healthy volunteer subjects enrolled in a BCG-BCG clinical trial. All subjects had previously been vaccinated with BCG, in childhood, where the present clinical trial involved an additional BCG vaccination. Following the adulthood vaccination, adult study subjects were monitored at intervals of 1, 2, 4, 8, 24, and 52 weeks. This particular clinical trial required prior treatment with BCG. The basis for this requirement was that the efficacy of the boost BCG vaccination was dependent on the earlier prime BCG vaccination. Prior treatment with BCG was an inclusion criterion.

III. FDA's WARNING LETTERS AND INCLUSION/EXCLUSION CRITERIA

The FDA issues Form 483 notices and Warning Letters to a Sponsor. The contents of the Form 483 notices and Warning Letters reveal the potential consequences of failing to comply with FDA regulations, such as the requirements to comply with the Clinical

---

[130]Cush SS, Anderson KM, Ravneberg DH, Weslow-Schmidt JL, Flaño E. Memory generation and maintenance of $CD8^+$ T cell function during viral persistence. J. Immunol. 2007;179:141–53.

[131]Muraoka D, Kato T, Wang L, et al. Peptide vaccine induces enhanced tumor growth associated with apoptosis induction in $CD8^+$ T cells. J. Immunol. 2010;185:3768–76.

[132]Ichino M, Mor G, Conover J, et al. Factors associated with the development of neonatal tolerance after the administration of a plasmid DNA vaccine. J. Immunol. 1999;162:3814–8.

[133]Riedl P, Wieland A, Lamberth K, et al. Elimination of immunodominant epitopes from multispecific DNA-based vaccines allows induction of CD8 T cells that have a striking antiviral potential. J. Immunol. 2009;183:370–80.

[134]Whelan KT, Pathan AA, Sander CR, et al. Safety and immunogenicity of boosting BCG vaccinated subjects with BCG: comparison with boosting with a new TB vaccine, MVA85A. PLoS One 2009;4:e5934.

Study Protocol. This provides an example of a Form 483 notice, and a subsequent Warning Letter that concerned the inclusion/exclusion criteria in the Protocol.

Inspections by FDA employees can uncover failures to adhere to the Clinical Study Protocol, for example, failures of subjects to comply with the inclusion/exclusion criteria.

This reveals a paper trail that began with FDA's inspection of the Sponsor's facility, which was followed by FDA's issuance of an "establishment inspection report" together with FDA's Form FDA 483, an exchange of letters between the Sponsor and the FDA, and ultimately FDA's issuance of a Warning Letter. The Warning Letter (135) complained about the fact that some of the subjects in the clinical trial were not in compliance with the inclusion/exclusion criteria. To this point, the Warning Letter stated:

> You failed to conduct the studies or to ensure they were conducted according to the investigational plans … [t]he following protocol violations were noted for Protocol … [t]he protocol inclusion criteria specified that … the subject was to have a mean of at least three readings for seated systolic blood pressure (SeSBP) of >140 mm Hg and <180 mm Hg and for seated diastolic blood pressure (SeDBP) of >90 mm Hg and <110 mm Hg … [s]ubject did not meet the inclusion criterion at either Visit P2, when the SeDBP was 85, or Visit P3, when the SeDBP was 87, but nevertheless was enrolled into the study … [f]ailure to adequately and promptly explain the violations noted above may result in regulatory action without further notice.

FDA's Form 483 and FDA's Warning Letters are different procedures that warn a Sponsor about violations. Form 483, "is issued by one or more FDA investigators at the conclusion of a site inspection, and usually is not reviewed by a compliance officer, district director, or an official in FDA's headquarters before it is issued. An FDA Warning Letter, on the other hand, is issued by a district director or headquarters official of similar seniority, and only after review by FDA's Office of Chief Counsel" (136).

IV. SUBGROUPS AND SUBGROUP ANALYSIS

a. Introduction

Typically, subgroup analysis serves to establish a new hypothesis which then has to be proven in a new prospective study (137). A general observation on how subgroup analysis has influenced subsequent courses of action is as follows. Where a phase II trial has shown a drug to have efficacy in one particular subgroup, but not in other subgroups, the investigator can subsequently conduct a phase III trial, where the phase III trial contains only subjects having the characteristics in that one, particular subgroup (138).

Regulatory approval can be granted in the event that statistically significant efficacy is shown for one particular subgroup. The subgroup would need to be predefined by the Clinical Study Protocol. The type 1 error applying to this subgroup would need to be restricted, eg, to 0.05. FDA is very concerned about appropriately defining and restricting

---

[135]Warning Letter Ref. #: 09-HFD-45-01-02, dated February 2, 2009, to Family Practice Associates from Dr. T. Purohit-Sheth, MD, Branch Chief, CDER, FDA.

[136]Cooper RM, Fleder JR. Responding to a Form 483 Warning Letter: a practical guide. Food Drug Law J. 2005;60:479—93.

[137]Dr. Israel Rios. E-mail dated September 26, 2010.

[138]Dr. John Quiring. Personal communication of November 10, 2010.

the false-positive rate (139). In other words, the greater the number of subgroups that are defined by the Clinical Study Protocol, the greater the probability that the study data will provide a false positive. It is this type of false positive that FDA seeks to prevent. Another regulatory body, the European Medicines Agency (EMA), has also cautioned about the over-use of subgroup analysis, writing that, "[a] common misuse of subgroup analysis is to rescue a trial which, formally fails based on the pre-specified primary analysis in the full analysis set" (140). Patsopoulos et al. (141) provide a thorough account of misleading subgroup analyses, involving the subgroups of male versus female, that were based on insufficient and spurious documentation. Examples of subgroups are shown below.

b. Subgroup of Non-Elderly Subjects and Subgroup of Elderly Subjects

In a study of breast cancer, Roché et al. (142) included subgroups of women under 50 years old, and greater or equal to 50 years old. The authors discovered that, "[w]omen age 50 years or older derived significant benefit in DFS from treatment with FEC-D ($P = 0.001$), but this advantage was not found in younger women ($P = 0.65$)." DFS refers to the endpoint of disease-free survival. FEC-D refers to a combination of drugs, namely, fluorouracil, epirubicin, and cyclophosphamide (FEC) followed by docetaxel (D).

This type of discovery, that is, the discovery by Roche et al. (143) that women of age 50 or older derived benefit, is concrete and easy to put into practice in the context of routine patient care. In other words, in treating breast cancer patients, it is easy to determine the patient's age, and it is easy to make a go/no-go decision to administer a particular drug. Both things are easy to do.

The following more broadly concerns the subgroup of elderly subjects and geriatric subjects. In a review of the influence of old age on risk for adverse drug reactions, Shah (144) disclosed that old age, that is, age of 70 years or older, increases the risk for adverse reactions to benoxaprofen. Benoxaprofen is an anti-inflammatory drug with the adverse drug reactions of photosensitivity and hepatotoxicity. Halsey and Cardoe (145) report that benoxaprofen's adverse effects increase greatly in persons over 70 years of age. Shah (146) also documents a few differences in the pharmacokinetics of

---

[139]Rubinstein L. E-mail of October 12, 2010.

[140]European Medicines Agency. Concept paper on the need for a guideline on the use of subgroup analyses in randomised controlled trials. April 22, 2010.

[141]Patsopoulos NA, et al. Claims of sex differences: an empirical assessment in genetic associations. J. Am. Med. Assoc. 2007;298:880−93.

[142]Roché H, Fumoleau P, Spielmann M, et al. Sequential adjuvant epirubicin-based and docetaxel chemotherapy for node-positive breast cancer patients: the FNCLCC PACS 01 trial. J. Clin. Oncol. 2006;24:5664−71.

[143]Roché H, Fumoleau P, Spielmann M, et al. Sequential adjuvant epirubicin-based and docetaxel chemotherapy for node-positive breast cancer patients: the FNCLCC PACS 01 trial. J. Clin. Oncol. 2006;24:5664−71.

[144]Shah RR. Drug development and use in the elderly: search for the right dose and dosing regimen (Parts I and II). Br. J. Clin. Pharmacol. 2004;58:452−69.

[145]Halsey JP, Cardoe N. Benoxaprofen: side-effect profile in 300 patients. Br. Med. J. (Clin. Res. Ed.). 1982;284:1365−8.

[146]Shah RR. Drug development and use in the elderly: search for the right dose and dosing regimen (Parts I and II). Br. J. Clin. Pharmacol. 2004;58:452−69.

various drugs and in the expression of drug-catabolizing enzymes, that is, cytochromes, in the elderly. Although old age appears not to have an effect on the pharmacokinetics of most drugs, the examples set forth by Shah (147) provide a concrete basis for establishing the elderly as a subgroup, or in excluding the elderly, when designing clinical trials.

According to the ICH Guidelines on geriatrics (148), "[t]he geriatric population is arbitrarily defined, for the purpose of this guideline, as comprising patients aged 65 years or older. It is important, however, to seek patients in the older age range, 75 and above, to the extent possible. Protocols should not ordinarily include arbitrary upper age cutoffs." Moreover, the ICH Guidelines provide the advice that, "[p]atients entering clinical trials should be reasonably representative of the population that will be later treated by the drug" (149), and further warn that, "[i]t is important to determine whether or not the pharmacokinetic behavior of the drug in elderly subjects or patients is different from that in younger adults and to characterize the effects of influences, such as abnormal renal or hepatic function, that are more common in the elderly" (150).

c. Subgroup of Subjects with No Metastasis and Subgroup of Subjects with Metastasis

The oncology trial of Grier et al. (151) included two study arms, as indicated:

- *Arm A.* Standard drugs.
- *Arm B.* Standard drugs plus two other drugs, ifosfamide and etopside.

The study population was stratified into two subgroups. The two subgroups were patients with metastasis (at baseline) and those without metastasis (at baseline). The results demonstrated no difference between arm A and arm B, with analysis of the subgroup having metastasis at baseline. However, the results demonstrated a striking and dramatic difference in efficacy in the arm B group, for the subgroup having no metastasis at baseline. To view the data, one of the endpoints was that of 5-year overall survival. Five-year overall survival refers to the percent of all of the subjects, for a given study arm, still alive at the 5-year time point. For the subgroup of non-metastatic subjects, the value for 5-year overall survival for the standard therapy group was 61%, while that for the experimental group was greater, 71% ($P = 0.01$). But for the subgroup of metastatic subjects, no significant difference in 5-year overall survival was detected between the two study arms—there was a slight difference, but this difference was not significant ($P = 0.81$). P values are explained further in this textbook in Chapter 9.

This result is concrete and easy to put into practice in the context of routine patient care. In other words, it is a routine task to determine whether a patient's cancer is metastatic, and to provide the appropriate drugs.

[147]Shah RR. Drug development and use in the elderly: search for the right dose and dosing regimen (Parts I and II). Br. J. Clin. Pharmacol. 2004;58:452−69.

[148]ICH Harmonised Tripartite Guideline. Studies in support of special populations:geriatrics. Step 4 version, June 1993, 4 pages.

[149]ICH Harmonised Tripartite Guideline. Studies in support of special populations:geriatrics. Step 4 version, June 1993, 4 pages.

[150]ICH Harmonised Tripartite Guideline. Studies in support of special populations:geriatrics. Step 4 version, June 1993, 4 pages.

[151]Grier HE, Krailo MD, Tarbell NJ, et al. Addition of ifosfamide and etoposide to standard chemotherapy for Ewing's sarcoma and primitive neuroectodermal tumor of bone. N. Engl. J. Med. 2003;348:694−701.

d. Subgroup of Smokers and Subgroup of Non-Smokers

The oncology study of Miller et al. (152) addressed the efficacy of gefinitinib for treating non-small-cell lung cancer (NSCLC). Gefitinib inhibits the kinase activity of epidermal growth factor receptor (EFGR). The patients in this clinical trial were divided into the following subgroups:

- Whether the patient was a smoker (smoked cigarettes)
- Stage of the cancer
- Age of patient
- Gender
- Whether there was metastasis of the cancer to the bone
- Whether there was prior chemotherapy, before gefitinib.

The study found that 13 of 36 never-smokers experienced objective regressions of tumors as compared with eight of 104 smokers (36% vs 8%; $P = 0.001$). In comments about the response of NSCLC to gefitinib, the authors concluded that, "smoking status ... emerges as a powerful and independent predictor of response." The utility of this study's focus on subgroups is as follows. Physicians will be able to counsel patients being treated with gefitinib that, if they had never smoked cigarettes, their likelihood of success of the chemotherapy is greater.

e. Subgroups Set Forth in a Clinical Study Protocol Can Be Used as a Basis for FDA Approval

One benefit of using the Clinical Study Protocol to define subgroups is to provide guidance for future, better-defined clinical trials. But, for any pharmaceutical company, a better and more immediate reason for defining subgroups is to ensure FDA-approval. The following provides an example of FDA-approval for a drug, based on efficacy results from one particular subgroup in a clinical trial.

Hydralazine and isosorbide dinitrate are each vasodilator drugs (153). The combination of these two drugs is used for treating heart disease. In a clinical study of one particular drug combination, currently marketed as BiDil®, the drugs showed little or no effect on reducing mortality on Caucasians. But BiDil did show significant efficacy on African Americans.

The most relevant clinical trial is the African American Heart Failure Trials (A-HeFT), which included a total of 344 black people and a total of 898 white people (154). Prior to FDA-approval, the two independent drugs had been on the market for about 30 years (155). What was approved by the FDA was a fixed combination of the two drugs, where the approval, as indicated by the package insert, was specifically addressed to African Americans.

[152]Miller VA, Kris MG, Shah N, et al. Bronchioloalveolar pathologic subtype and smoking history predict sensitivity to gefitinib in advanced non-small-cell lung cancer. J. Clin. Oncol. 2004;22:1103–9.

[153]Cohn JN, Johnson G, Ziesche S, et al. A comparison of enalapril with hydralazine-isosorbide dinitrate in the treatment of chronic congestive heart failure. N. Engl. J. Med. 1991;325:303–10.

[154]Temple R, Stockbridge NL. BiDil for heart failure in black patients: The U.S. Food and Drug Administration perspective. Ann. Intern. Med. 2007;146:57–62.

[155]Colvin-Adams M, Taylor AL. Isosorbide dinitrate-hydralazine improves outcomes in African Americans with heart failure. Cleve. Clin. J. Med. 2007;74:227–34.

It is well established that African Americans have a greater prevalence of heart failure (3% in African American men and women, vs 2% in the general population), that African Americans present with heart failure at a younger age, and that African Americans are more likely to have hypertension (than coronary artery disease) as a cause of heart failure. The treatment of hypertension by drugs and diet, as well as the increased risks for hypertension found in African Americans, has been reviewed (156).

The package insert (157) for BiDil refers to the A-HeFT clinical trial, by mentioning that the data are "suggesting an effect on survival in black patients, but showing little evidence of an effect in the white population ..." Moreover, the indication that is stated on the package insert reads, in part, "BiDil is indicated for the treatment of heart failure as an adjunct to standard therapy in self-identified black patients to improve survival, to prolong time to hospitalization for heart failure, and to improve patient-reported functional status." This provides a concrete example showing the value of including subgroups in clinical trials.

f. Subgroup Analysis Enables Recommendations for a Specific Course of Treatment

In a study of head and neck cancer, Pacagnella et al. (158) stratified subjects into the subgroups of:

- Subgroup A. Operable subjects
- Subgroup B. Inoperable subjects.

The clinical trial involved two different treatments. The study found benefit only for the inoperable subjects.

The authors found that, "there were no significant differences in the two treatment strategies in loco-regional failure or in disease-free or overall survival, although the development of distant metastases was reduced ... [f]or inoperable patients, neoadjuvant chemotherapy improved local control, decreased the incidence of distant metastases, and improved the complete remission rate and overall survival."

Thus, a benefit was observed and reported for one subgroup of subjects, that is, those that were inoperable.

In observing the benefits of subgroup analysis from the Pacagnella study, Jacobs (159) reiterated the fact that patients were stratified into inoperable subjects and operable subjects. Jacobs wrote, "these exciting results come from a subgroup analysis of inoperable patients in a trial which included operable patients and which, as a whole, only demonstrated a statistically significant decrease in distant metastases."

Jacobs further implied that this type of discovery, which took advantage of subgroup analysis, could result in a change in standard for therapy of head and neck cancer, "[a]s the authors acknowledge, this trial alone would not be grounds for changing standard treatment, but it lends support to the conclusion that chemotherapy can improve results from radiotherapy in patients with unresectable cancers."

[156]Brody T. Nutritional biochemistry. San Diego, CA: Academic Press; 1999. p. 702–30.

[157]BiDil® package insert (June 23, 2005). Lexington, MA: NitroMed, Inc.

[158]Paccagnella A, Orlando A, Marchiori C, et al. Phase III trial of initial chemotherapy in stage III or IV head and neck cancers: a study by the Gruppo di Studio sui Tumori della Testa e del Collo. J. Natl. Cancer Inst. 1994;86:265–72.

[159]Jacobs C. Head and neck cancer in 1994: a change in the standard of care. J. Natl. Cancer Inst. 1994;86:250–2.

g. Subgroup Analysis Provides Prognostic Factors

In a clinical trial of gastrointestinal (GI) cancer, Van Glabbeke et al. (160) defined several subgroups, including:

- Age
- Gender
- Primary site of disease (abdominal, stomach, small bowel)
- Prior treatments for GI cancer (surgery, radiotherapy, and chemotherapy)
- Size of lesions (diameter of the largest lesion) at the time of trial inclusion
- Baseline hematologic and biologic parameters (white blood cells, granulocytes, platelets, hemoglobin, creatinine, bilirubin, and albumin).

A goal of the clinical trial was to identify subgroups where the drug was less effective. Low efficacy was evident where, during chemotherapy, tumor size or number increased early on, that is, during the first 3 months of chemotherapy. The study determined a subgroup where the drug was less effective. This was the subgroup of patients with *high granulocyte count at baseline*. Based on this finding, the authors recommended increasing the amount of dose of the drug (imatinib) for this particular subgroup, as follows. "In particular, imatinib resistance can be delayed by increasing the initial dose in patients with high granulocyte counts" (161).

h. Recommending Dropping One Subgroup from the Trial, Rather Than Stopping the Entire Trial

Where one particular subgroup in a trial is experiencing severe adverse drug reactions, such as death, the investigator can drop that particular subgroup from the trial (162). Dropping one subgroup from a trial is preferable to stopping the entire trial. Hence, in configuring the subgroups in the study population, the investigator or medical writer should contemplate various risk factors that might be expected in the study population, and for each risk factor, and include in the Clinical Study Protocol criteria that can be used to identify subjects as high, moderate, and low risk. An example of dropping one particular subgroup from a clinical trial can be found in a study of emphysema (163). Further information on dropping a subgroup from a clinical trial appears in this textbook, in the Drug Safety chapter, Chapter 25.

V. FDA's DECISION-MAKING PROCESSES IN EVALUATING STRATIFICATION AND SUBGROUPS

a. Introduction

FDA's comments in its *Medical Reviews* provide guidance for stratification and for

[160]Van Glabbeke M, Verweij J, Casali PG, et al. Initial and late resistance to imatinib in advanced gastrointestinal stromal tumors are predicted by different prognostic factors: a European Organisation for Research and Treatment of Cancer—Italian Sarcoma Group—Australasian Gastrointestinal Trials Group study. J. Clin. Oncol. 2005;23:5795—804.

[161]Van Glabbeke M, Verweij J, Casali PG, et al. Initial and late resistance to imatinib in advanced gastrointestinal stromal tumors are predicted by different prognostic factors: a European Organisation for Research and Treatment of Cancer—Italian Sarcoma Group—Australasian Gastrointestinal Trials Group study. J. Clin. Oncol. 2005;23:5795—804.

[162]DeMets DL, Furberg CD, Friedman LM. Data Monitoring in Clinical Trials. New York, NY: Springer; 2006.

[163]National Emphysema Treatment Trial Research Group. Patients at high risk of death after lung-volume-reduction surgery. N. Engl. J. Med. 2001;345:1075—83.

subgroup analysis. The goal of stratification is to ensure that equal numbers of subjects having a particular characteristic are randomized to the study drug arm and to the control arm, during the process of randomization. The fact that subjects were stratified according to a given factor does imply that this factor was a subgroup of the study subjects, but it is not necessarily the case that the Sponsor conducted any analysis of the efficacy and safety results, according to this subgroup.

b. Where Subjects Are Stratified According to a Certain Factor, It Is Not Necessarily the Case That Subgroup Analysis of Efficacy and Safety Take into Account That Factor

In a clinical trial on *cetuximab* for colorectal cancer, all of the subjects were stratified according to study site, meaning that, for each site, the study design ensured that equal numbers were apportioned into the study drug arm and control arm. This information is from BLA 125084, on March 2015 of FDA's website. The Sponsor refrained from conducting any subgroup analysis based on study site. The reason for not doing subgroup analysis based on the study site was that a large number of sites were used, and that only a small number of subjects were enrolled at each site. The reviewer commented on the fact that subgroup analysis did not take into account the study sites, writing that, "[w]hile the analysis excluded study center … a stratification variable for randomization … this was acceptable because the **large number of centers would create many small or unfilled cells.**"

c. Subgroup Analysis According to Biomarkers

The following subgroup analysis resulted in a recommendation that drug dosing levels be lower for one particular subgroup of patients. Also, the subgroup analysis addressed the number of dose modifications that were made during the course of the clinical trial. Moreover, the subgroup analysis resulted in a warning on the package insert of the marketed product.

This concerns a clinical trial for *lenalidomide* (Revlimid®), for treating anemia in patients with a type of cancer, myelodysplastic syndromes (MDS). The information is from the *Medical Review* for NDA 21880 from November 2013 of FDA's website. This concerns subgroups with and without an abnormality in chromosome 5. The abnormality was "deletion 5q." Regarding this deletion, "loss of all or part of the long arm of chromosome 5, del(5q), is a hallmark of myelodysplastic syndrome" (164).

Sallman et al. (165) commented on hematological disorders that are associated with this deletion, writing that, "[m]yelodysplastic syndromes … represent a hematologically diverse group of myeloid neoplasms, however, one subtype characterized by an isolated deletion of chromosome 5q [del(5q)] is pathologically and clinically distinct. Patients with del(5q) … [have] hypoplastic anemia and unique sensitivity to treatment with lenalidomide."

The clinical trials that were used in support of this submission to FDA included subjects with and without the deletion. According to the *Medical Review*, for one of the clinical trials, "[a] total of 45 subjects were enrolled … with or without an associated del 5." For another of

---

[164]Liu TX, et al. Evolutionary conservation of zebrafish linkage group 14 with frequently deleted regions of human chromosome 5 in myeloid malignancies. Proc. Natl. Acad. Sci. 2002;99:6136–41.

[165]Sallman DA, et al. PP2A: the Achiles heal in MDS with 5q deletion. Front. Oncol. 2014;4:264 (7 pages).

the clinical trials, which involved 95 subjects, 46 of the subjects had del 5.

The FDA reviewer commented on adverse events of the del q subgroup, writing that, "[t]he del 5q MDS population had about double the number of subjects with **neutropenia and thrombocytopenia** ... [t]here was also a doubling in infectious events, including pneumonias, in the del 5q population compared to the non-del population."

In view of this subgroup analysis, the FDA reviewer made the following recommendation, regarding drug administration, "[t]he above findings suggest that lenalidomide starting dose, while possibly appropriate for the non-del 5q MDS population, is clearly too high for the del 5q MDS population."

The FDA reviewer also commented on the dose modifications (dose reductions; dose interruptions) that had been made during the course of the clinical trial, writing that, "[t]he increased sensitivity to lenalidomide in the del 5q population may account for the much greater need for dose reductions and dose interruption of the 10 mg/day starting dose ... in the del 5q population compared to the non-del 5q population ... [t]hese data suggest that the starting dose of lenalidomide is too high for the del 5q population."

As a consequence, the package insert included a *Black Box Warning* that referred to the neutropenia and thrombocytopenia, associated with the study drug (lenalidomide; Revlimid®) (166). The *Black Box Warning* read:

Hematologic Toxicity (Neutropenia and Thrombocytopenia). REVLIMID can cause significant **neutropenia and thrombocytopenia**. Eighty percent of patients with del 5q myelodysplastic syndromes had to have a dose delay/reduction during the major study. Thirty-four percent of patients had to have a second dose delay/reduction ... [p]atients on therapy for del 5q myelodysplastic syndromes

should have their complete blood counts monitored weekly for the first 8 weeks of therapy and at least monthly thereafter. Patients may require dose interruption and/or reduction.

The take-home lesson is that subgroup analysis can facilitate acquisition of information for including in the *Warnings* section of the package insert.

d. Subgroup Analysis According to a Disorder That Is Concurrent with the Disease Under Investigation

This is from the *Medical Review* of *dimethyl fumarate*, a drug for multiple sclerosis. The information is from NDA 204063, available at March 2013 on FDA's website.

The following concerns concurrent GI disorders and diabetes. These disorders occurred in a clinical trial for multiple sclerosis, and they were classified as adverse events.

Analysis by subgroups was used with the goal of explaining the adverse event of elevated urinary ketones. Please note that urinary levels of ketones, usually known as "ketone bodies," are elevated in conditions such as diabetes, fasting, and starvation (167). In exploring the cause for the increased urinary ketones, the Sponsor considered the possibility that the subset of subjects with GI disorders was the subset with increased ketones. The result was that this subset was negative, that is, that this subset was not characterized by increased ketones. Also, the Sponsor explored the possibility that the subset of subjects with diabetes was the subset with increased ketones. Again, the analysis was negative. The *Medical Review* reveals that FDA asked the Sponsor "to explain why a higher percentage of [study drug] ... patients had positive tests for urinary ketones."

[166]Package insert for REVLIMID [lenalidomide] capsules, for oral use. February 2015 (36 pages).

[167]Brody T. Nutritional biochemistry. San Diego, CA: Elsevier/Academic Press, 1999. p. 236–45.

The Sponsor (Biogen) replied:

> Biogen ... proposed, but rejected, that increased ketones may be due to the GI AEs [adverse events] of ... [study drug], which could result in decreased oral intake, diarrhea, and vomiting, and ultimately, starvation ketoses. Biogen analyzed ... urinary ketones for the subgroups of subjects with and without a GI tolerability event ... Biogen did not find an increased incidence of ketonuria in ... subjects with GI tolerability events ... Biogen compared ketonuria in patients with a history of diabetes to those without ... Biogen concluded that the etiology of the increased incidence of ketonuria observed ... relative to placebo is unknown and that this finding does not have clinically meaningful implications.

The FDA reviewer concluded that, "Biogen should further evaluate the finding of elevated urinary ketone results observed in the MS trials. Because Biogen proposed that the observed elevated urinary ketones possibly represent false positive results, they should evaluate this hypothesis." The take-home lesson is that safety analysis should include an analysis of subgroups of study subjects having a concurrent disorder or condition. This type of analysis facilitates the generation of information for the package insert. Please note that the package insert, as eventually published, did not mention urinary ketones, as an adverse event associated with the study drug.

e. Subgroup Analysis According to Location of Study Site—Zanamivir

Of about 125,000 studies listed on the registry known as, www.ClinicalTrials.gov, about 90% of the studies involved only one country. The remaining studies were multinational trials. Clinical trials have become increasingly globalized, and include study sites in non-traditional locations, such as those in central and eastern Europe, Latin America, and Asia (168).

This concerns *zanamivir*, in a clinical trial on influenza virus infections. The information is from the *Medical Review* for NDA 21036, on December 2011 of FDA's website. The FDA reviewer stated that, "[i]n general, FDA accepts foreign studies and may approve a drug based solely on their results provided that the data are clinically generalizable to the target population in the United States and the trials are conducted in a manner consistent with good clinical trial practice."

The FDA reviewer further commented on the fact that some of the study sites were in Europe and in South America, writing that, "[i]n this circumstance, the results of the European and Southern Hemisphere trials are applicable to approvability for the United States, because there is no biological ... reason to believe that drug-response in patients infected with similar types of influenza will differ between countries."

The take-home lessons are as follows. Where a clinical trial involves more than one study site and, in particular, study sites in various countries, the Sponsor should identify characteristics of the study population, such as genetic background, and of the disease, such as genotype of the infecting virus, in order to facilitate communications with FDA.

f. Subgroup Analysis According to Location of Study Site—Fingolimod

This concerns *fingolimod* for multiple sclerosis. The information is from the *Medical Review* for NDA 22527, on July 2011 of FDA's website. The issue was the use of study sites in the United States, as well as in other countries. The non-US study sites were located in Australia, Belgium, Canada, Czech Republic, Estonia, Finland, France, Germany, Greece, Hungary, Ireland, Israel, Netherlands, Poland,

---

[168]Richter, TA. Clinical research: a globalized network. PLoS One 2014;9:e115063 (12 pages).

Romania, Russia, Slovakia, South Africa, Sweden, Switzerland, Turkey, and the United Kingdom.

According to the *Medical Review*, the Sponsor argued that the enrollment of subjects from many countries should not have an adverse influence on FDA's approval process for a drug to be marketed in the United States. The Sponsor argued that:

> MS [multiple sclerosis] is not a disease that has known **geographical differences** in terms of clinical phenotype or severity and that the demographics and disease characteristics of patients from the US … MS practice patterns are homogeneous around the world.

The FDA reviewer also pointed out that, for other drugs that had earlier been FDA-approved for multiple sclerosis, it was the case that the clinical trials for these drugs also involved mainly overseas subjects, and relatively few subjects in the United States. To this point, the reviewer stated that:

> [a]lthough the number of US patients included in the fingolimod trials were … small … many other marketed products for MS had equally small numbers of US patients at the time of marketing approval.

This included the clinical trial for Mitoxanthrone, which did not have any US subjects at all. Finally, the FDA reviewer referred to an agreement with FDA, stating that,

> [a]t a meeting with the sponsor, FDA agreed that … although … only 15% or less of the patients would be from the US in this marketing application this would probably be acceptable.

The take-home lessons are as follows. Where many study sites are in non-US countries, the Sponsor should consider formulating reasons why the results from the non-US subjects would be applicable to a submission for marketing in the United States. These reasons include geographical homogeneity for characteristics of the disease, geographic homogeneity for clinical practices in treating the disease, and the fact that other products approved for the same disease also involved non-US study sites.

The issue of non-US study sites is a recurring concern. For example, in another clinical trial, the FDA reviewer complained that, "[e]xcept for one patient from Canada, the study population is European. It is unclear how this study population correlates with a heterogeneous American population who develops lung cancer." This information is from NDA 20981, available from October 2011 on FDA's website, which was a clinical trial on topotecan for small-cell lung cancer. Again, the take-home lesson is that the Sponsor should be prepared to argue that data on efficacy and safety, from non-US subjects, are applicable to patients in the United States.

g. Stratification by a Multiple Number of Factors—Vemurafenib

This is from a clinical trial on *vemurafenib* for the indication of melanoma. The information is from NDA 202429, on July 2013 of the FDA's website. In this example, study subjects were stratified to each of a multiple number of factors. The *Medical Review* stated that:

"[t]he treatment allocation was based on a minimization algorithm using the following balancing factors:

- Geographic region (North America, Western Europe, Australia/New Zealand, others);
- Eastern Cooperative Oncology Group (ECOG) performance status (0 vs 1);
- Metastatic classification (unresectable Stage IIIC, M1a, M1b, and M1c);
- Serum lactate dehydrogenase (LDH) normal versus LDH elevated."

The Clinical Study Protocol required that all of the subjects have a mutation in the *BRAF* gene, where this mutation was required to be at valine-600. This mutation was required for all of the subjects enrolled in the clinical trial, that is, it was not merely a stratification factor. The *Medical Review* detailed the biology behind this mutation, as quoted in footnote (169).

The stratification factors took into account whether the subject lived in a climate associated with greater sunshine or lesser sunshine, if the subject was in good health (ECOG status of 0) or in impaired health (ECOG score of 1), the stage of the melanoma, and the status of a biomarker (LDH).

Regarding the stratification element LDH in melanoma trials, Eggermont (170) stated that, "characteristics . . . were well balanced between the treatment arms. Stratification involved the following: lactate dehydrogenase (LDH), site of metastases, and Eastern Cooperative Oncology Group performance status." Eggermont (171) further stated that the medical community has "identified **LDH as the most important and simplest stratification** factor" for melanoma clinical trials.

Referring to stratification by geography, the FDA reviewer wrote that, "[p]atients were appropriately enrolled in geographic regions of **high sun exposure**." Regarding sun exposure the FDA reviewer also wrote that, "[s]un exposure, use of tanning beds, fair skin, history of sunburns and immunosuppression all have been associated with an increased risk of melanoma." Other researchers have also documented the association of sun exposure and melanoma (172).

VI. CONCLUDING REMARKS

This chapter provides a selection of topics relating to inclusion/exclusion criteria, defining subgroups, and using the defined subgroups as a basis for stratification, and as a basis for exploratory studies relating to predicting efficacy of a given drug.

Initially, this chapter introduced the Clinical Study Protocol, and described how inclusion/exclusion criteria are identified in the title of the Protocol, in the synopsis, and in the study schema. Following this, the goals of stratification were then outlined, for example, the goal of equal balancing of human subjects in the study drug arm and in the control treatment arm. Then, the chapter disclosed the warning that subgroups should be defined before, rather than after, conducting the clinical study. The forest plot was identified as the most effective way to summarize data on efficacy and safety, for each and every one of the subgroups defined for a particular clinical trial. The topic of inclusion/exclusion criteria was then detailed, in an accounting of the biochemistry of drug resistance by tumors. The topic of inclusion/exclusion criteria was further developed, with short narratives devoted to subgroups relating to the elderly, smokers, racial groups, and to granulocyte levels.

[169]"mutations in BRAF have been identified in melanoma and have a reported frequency of about 40−60%. The most common alteration that occurs is the codon 600 valine to glutamate (V600E) mutation, which represents about 90% of BRAF mutations. The next most common mutation is the codon 600 valine to lysine (V600K) followed by the valine to arginine mutation (V600R). Currently it is hypothesized that V600 mutations constitutively activate BRAF kinase activity leading to ERK activation and aberrant and uncontrolled cell proliferation and survival."

[170]Eggermont AM. Reaching first base in the treatment of metastatic melanoma. J. Clin. Oncol. 2006;24:4673−4.

[171]Eggermont AM. Reaching first base in the treatment of metastatic melanoma. J. Clin. Oncol. 2006;24:4673−4.

[172]Swerdlow AJ. Incidence of malignant melanoma of the skin in England and Wales and its relationship to sunshine. Br. Med. J. 1979;2:1324−7.

5

Inclusion/Exclusion Criteria, Stratification, and Subgroups—Part II

I. INTRODUCTION

The inclusion criteria for subjects enrolling in oncology clinical trials can involve the staging of the cancer. This chapter outlines the tumor node metastasis (TNM) classification of cancers, the physiology of the lymphatic system and of metastasis, examples of staging systems used for two types of cancers (colorectal cancer; breast cancer), and the *Will Rogers phenomenon*. This phenomenon, which can arise when diagnosing most disorders (not just cancer), results when staging systems are revised, or when the sensitivity of diagnostic tools improves over the course of years. Failure to take note of this phenomenon can result in interpretations of data that contain artifacts.

II. STAGING

The TNM classification of cancers describes the anatomic extent of the cancer. The TNM system is a staging system with various uses (1).

First, it can guide choice of treatment. Second, it can serve as a prognostic factor, giving the physician and patient an indication of the chance of survival. Third, it is useful as an inclusion criterion in clinical trials, to ensure uniformity among study subjects. And fourth, it can ensure reasonable comparisons, when comparing results from separate published clinical trials on the same type of cancer.

T means extent of the primary tumor, N means involvement of lymph nodes, and M means metastasis. The primary tumor may be staged from stage I (the least advanced) to stage IV (the most advanced). Lymph node involvement, if any, can be staged from stage I (the least advanced) to stage IV (the most advanced). Metastasis, if any, can be assigned stage I (the least advanced) to stage IV (the most advanced). Some stages are subdivided with letters, in addition to Roman numerals.

Tumors can be classified before treatment, that is, clinical staging (cTNM), and after surgical intervention, that is, pathologic staging (pTNM). Where a particular cancer patient is

[1]Greene FL, Sobin LH. The staging of cancer: a retrospective and prospective appraisal. CA Cancer J. Clin. 2008;58:180−90.

not treated with surgery, pathological staging is not possible. For example, surgery of liver cancer patients is infrequent. Thus, data on pathological staging are not often available from liver cancer patients (2).

a. History of Tumor Staging

The early history of cancer staging is as follows. According to Singletary and Connolly (3), in 1904 Steinthal proposed the division of breast cancer into three prognostic stages: small tumors that were localized to the breast (stage I), larger tumors that involved the axillary lymph nodes (stage II), and tumors that had invaded tissues around the breast (stage III). The four-stage Columbia Clinical Classification System for breast cancer, with stages A through C corresponding to Steinthal's stages was introduced in 1956 by Haagensen and Stout. The TNM system was developed by Denoix starting in 1942, where cancer was classified based on the morphological attributes of malignant tumors that were thought to influence disease prognosis: size of the primary tumor (T), presence and extent of regional lymph node (RLN) involvement (N), and presence of distant metastases (M).

b. Revising Staging Systems

After establishing a given staging system, the system may be updated or revised from time. According to one commentator, "strategies for improving the TNM staging system for patients with colorectal cancer is a subject of intense debate" (4). According to another commentator, "[a]s a consequence of the recommendations for changes in the T and M components of classifications of lung cancer, changes were also suggested for the stage grouping" (5). Regarding updating traditional criteria for staging, Jeruss et al. (6), proposed that, "the scoring systems proposed in this study move beyond the traditional American Joint Committee on Cancer (AJCC) (7) staging system to incorporate biological factors that can further aide in determining the prognosis of patients treated with neoadjuvant therapy."

The fact that staging systems are altered, from time to time, is made explicit by a document from the AJCC, which compares two versions of staging that are used for various types of cancer, an earlier version effective before January 2003, and a replacement version effective on January 2003 (8).

The fact that staging systems are revised from time to time requires a warning about

[2]Marrero JA, Kudo M, Bronowicki JP. The challenge of prognosis and staging for hepatocellular carcinoma. Oncologist 2010;15(Suppl. 4):23–33.

[3]Singletary SE, Connolly JL. Breast cancer staging: working with the sixth edition of the AJCC Cancer Staging Manual. CA Cancer J. Clin. 2006;56:37–47.

[4]Zlobec I, Baker K, Minoo P, Hayashi S, Terracciano L, Lugli A. Tumor border configuration added to TNM staging better stratifies stage II colorectal cancer patients into prognostic subgroups. Cancer 2009;115:4021–9.

[5]Rami-Porta R, Crowley JJ, Goldstraw P. The revised TNM staging system for lung cancer. Ann. Thorac. Cardiovasc. Surg. 2009;15:4–9.

[6]Jeruss JS, Mittendorf EA, Tucker SL, et al. Staging of breast cancer in the neoadjuvant setting. Cancer Res. 2008;68:6477–81.

[7]AJCC periodically updates the tumor node metastasis (TNM) staging system for cancer. AJCC publishes the Cancer Staging Manual and the Cancer Staging Atlas.

[8]American Joint Committee on Cancer. AJCC comparison guide: cancer staging manual fifth versus sixth edition; January 2003 (32 pp.).

the Will Rogers phenomenon. This issue is detailed at the end of this chapter.

c. Biology of Tumors

The biology of tumors is outlined below, using the example of breast cancer. Tumor initiation, growth, and metastasis, generally occur over a prolonged period (9). Mammography has shown that primary breast tumors have an average doubling time of 157 days. Thus, the growth of a tumor from initiation to a size of 1 cm, which is the lower limit of detection by imaging tools, requires an average of 12 years. A tumor of this size (1 cm) contains about ten billion cells and has undergone at least 30 doublings from tumor initiation to diagnosis. A lethal tumor burden is a tumor volume of 1000 cubic centimeters.

The following more generally concerns tumor histology. Tumors contain a mixture of tumor cells and host cells (10). These host cells can include epithelial cells, fibroblasts, endothelial cells, and infiltrating white blood cells. Tumors are heterogeneous, and contain subpopulations of tumor cells, most of which might be able to complete some of the steps in the metastatic process, but not all. Expression of genes required any given tumor cells for the processes of proliferation, angiogenesis, cohesion, motility, and invasion vary among different regions of the tumor.

d. Biology of the Lymphatic System

Because the TNM staging system involves the lymphatics, it is necessary to outline a few aspects of the lymphatic system. In the intestines, the lymphatic system collects fluids from the vicinity of the gut mucosal cells, where the goal that is served is collection of lipid nutrients, and transport of the lipid nutrients to the bloodstream, for eventual processing by the liver. The lumenal surface of the gastrointestinal tract, called the gut mucosa, contains lymphatic capillaries that end in structures called lacteals (11). The lacteals constitute dead ends in the lymphatic capillaries. The function of the lacteals is to collect absorbed dietary lipids. These capillaries coalesce and eventually deliver their contents to a large lymphatic vessel called the thoracic duct. The lymph collected from other parts of the body is also transferred to the thoracic duct. The thoracic duct, in turn, transfers the lymph to the bloodstream. The lymphatic system serves to collect any interstitial fluids that had leaked out of the circulatory system.

As reviewed by Nathanson (12), lymphatic vessels act as a one-way transport system for fluid, proteins, particles, and cells. The initial, or terminal, lymphatics are blind-ended structures that are optimally suited for the uptake of fluids, particles, and cells, including tumor cells. The lumen is the hollow area inside the capillary. Lymphatic capillaries are distinguished by a lumen that is irregular and wide, while the lumen of blood vessel capillaries is regular and narrow. The endothelial cells of lymphatic capillaries are distinguished by the fact that they overlap each other, and do not have much cytoplasm, while the endothelial cells of blood vessel capillaries have endothelial cells that do not overlap and that have an abundant cytoplasm.

---

[9]Talmadge JE, Fidler IJ. AACR centennial series: the biology of cancer metastasis: historical perspective. Cancer Res. 2010;70:5649−69.

[10]Talmadge JE, Fidler IJ. AACR centennial series: the biology of cancer metastasis: historical perspective. Cancer Res. 2010;70:5649−69.

[11]Brody T. Nutritional biochemistry. San Diego, CA: Academic Press; 1999. p. 98.

[12]Nathanson SD. Insights into the mechanisms of lymph node metastasis. Cancer 2003;98:413−23.

e. Relation Between the Tumors and the Lymphatic System

According to Ma and Waxman (13), "[t]umors shed millions of cells into blood and lymphatic circulation in a process that requires penetration through a multi-layer barrier comprised of pericytes, base membrane and endothelial cells." When individual tumor cells leave a tumor, they may encounter the lymphatic capillaries, and move along the external surface of the endothelium, and eventually migrate through the layers of epithelial cells, and invade the lumen of the lymphatic capillary (14). Once in the lumen, tumor cells can migrate through the lymphatic capillaries, where they eventually encounter lymph nodes.

Once residing in a lymph node, the tumor cell may proliferate and create a small tumor. Alternatively, some tumor cells do not reach the sentinel lymph node, but instead adhere to the endothelial cells of the lymphatic capillary, while in transit, where they proliferate and form an "in transit" tumor in the wall of the lymphatic vessel (15).

In-transit tumors can also form in between a tumor and a lymph node, following shedding of cancer cells from a tumor. Tumors arising in this way occur in melanoma and, occasionally, with cutaneous malignancies (16).

A desirable aspect of lymph node physiology, as far as the cancer patient is concerned, is that the event of antigen presentation that occurs in lymph nodes. Tumors in various parts of the body may release tumor antigens. These antigens are picked up by dendritic cells. The dendritic cells then migrate to lymph nodes. Once in a lymph node, the dendritic cells present an epitope from the tumor antigen to T cells (lymphocytes). When the dendritic cells present tumor antigen to T cells, the result is that the T cells are specifically activated. Then, the T cells leave the lymph node, and travel through the body, where they eventually destroy tumor cells. The eventual destruction of tumors by the immune system requires the following steps: uptake of tumor antigens by dendritic cells, activation of the dendritic cells, for example, by an immune adjuvant, presentation of antigen by dendritic cells to T cells, and eventual destruction of tumor cells by $CD8^+$ T cells.

f. Metastasis of Tumors

The "seed and soil" hypothesis proposed by the English surgeon Stephan Paget in 1889 held that specific tumors (seeds) have preferential sites for metastasis (soil) (17,18,19).

[13]Ma J, Waxman DJ. Combination of antiangiogenesis with chemotherapy for more effective cancer treatment. Mol. Cancer Ther. 2008;7:3670−84.

[14]Nathanson SD. Insights into the mechanisms of lymph node metastasis. Cancer 2003;98:413−23.

[15]Nathanson SD. Insights into the mechanisms of lymph node metastasis. Cancer 2003;98:413−23.

[16]Kocaturk E, et al. In-transit metastasis from primary cutaneous squamous cell carcinoma in a nonimmunosuppressed patient. J. Cutan. Med. Surg. 2015;19:167−70.

[17]Talmadge JE, Fidler IJ. AACR centennial series: the biology of cancer metastasis: historical perspective. Cancer Res. 2010;70:5649−69.

[18]Fokas E, Engenhart-Cabillic R, Daniilidis K, Rose F, An HX. Metastasis: the seed and soil theory gains identity. Cancer Metastasis Rev. 2007;26:705−15.

[19]Fidler IJ. The pathogenesis of cancer metastasis: the "seed and soil" hypothesis revisited. Nat. Rev. Cancer 2003;3:453−8.

In 1829, Recamier (20,21) devised the term "metastasis." Typically, cells from primary breast cancer tumors metastasize to the bone or liver. Cells from colorectal cancer metastasize to the liver. Cells from melanoma metastasize to the lungs, liver, gastrointestinal tract, or brain.

Figure 5.1 outlines the process of tumor metastasis. This process includes the following steps:

Step 1. Exit of tumor cell from tumor
Step 2. Tumor cell encounters lymphatic capillary

Step 3. Tumor cell migrates through the wall of the lymphatic to the lumen
Step 4. Once inside the lumen, the tumor cell grows
Step 5. Tumor cells leave the lymph node for the circulatory system. A small fraction of these form metastatic tumors in various organs of the body.

As reviewed by Hirakawa (22), evidence suggests that primary tumors induce new lymphatic vessel growth within draining lymph nodes before the tumors actually metastasize.

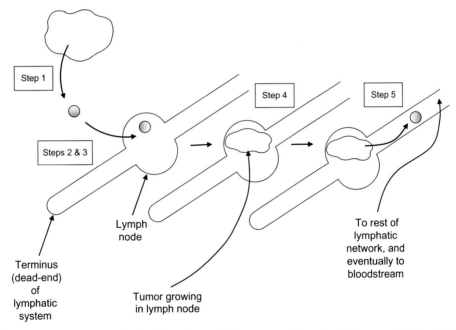

FIGURE 5.1   Tumor metastasis. The drawing shows a single tumor cell leaving the tumor, migrating to the lymphatic system, settling down in the lymph node where the cell forms a new tumor, and finally metastasizing again, where another single tumor cell passes through the lymphatics to the bloodstream. The drawing shows only a single tumor cell for the sake of clarity, and not to imply that the event of metastasis involves only one tumor cell.

[20]Recamier JCA. L'histoire de le Meme Maladie. Gabor 1829;2:110.

[21]Cohen SJ, Punt CJ, Iannotti N, Saidman BH, et al. Relationship of circulating tumor cells to tumor response, progression-free survival, and overall survival in patients with metastatic colorectal cancer. J. Clin. Oncol. 2008;26:3213−21.

[22]Hirakawa S. From tumor lymphangiogenesis to lymphvascular niche. Cancer Sci. 2009;100:983−9.

This means that primary tumors can actively modify future metastatic sites for preferential relocation. Primary tumors appear to alter nearby lymph nodes (draining lymph nodes) by inducing the growth of new blood vessels (angiogenesis). Nutrients from the new blood vessels nourish the tumor cells that metastasize to the lymph nodes. A number of drugs target and prevent angiogenesis, and thereby serve as anticancer agents. These drugs include those that prevent vascular endothelial growth factor (VEGF) from binding to VEGF receptor.

Although tumor metastasis can occur early in tumor progression when the primary tumor is small or even undetectable, most occur later when the primary tumor is larger. This pattern is supported by the observation that surgical excision of smaller lesions often cures the patient of the cancer. Following metastasis, tumor cells may reside in lymph nodes for many years in a dormant phase, before progressing to form metastatic tumors (23).

g. The Sentinal Node and Distant Lymph Nodes

An early step of certain malignant tumors is metastasis to the regional lymph nodes (Fig. 5.1). Where tumors are found in the regional lymph nodes, this indicates a greater risk. The first regional lymph node to which tumors migrate and reside is called the sentinel lymph node. Thus, an early step in metastasis is the exit of tumor cells from the primary tumor, through the lymphatics, to the sentinel lymph node and other lymph nodes, and then to the circulatory system (bloodstream). The event where a tumor cell leaves the tumor is called epithelial—mesenchymal transition (24).

Where a tumor contains epithelial cells, from the primary tumor, some epithelial cells can lose their cell—cell adhesion and become motile mesenchymal cells. The mesenchymal cells can move as single cells or as cell clusters. When present as cell clusters, they are a mixture of epithelial and mesenchymal cells (25). In general, the transition from epithelial cell to mesenchymal cells involves the down-regulation of E-cadherin, and the up-regulation of N-cadherin, vimentin, and metalloproteinase-2 (26). To provide an example of the mechanism of this transition, a study of lung cancer metastasis revealed that the NANOS3 gene is overexpressed in invasive lung cancer cells. NANOS3 controls expression of proteins that mediate cell-to-cell adhesion, such as E-cadherin, while increasing NANOS3 expression in lung cancer cells enhances their invasiveness (27). Dotan et al. (28) reviewed the use of circulating tumor cells as a prognostic factor.

Most tumor cells in a tumor do not metastasize. Others metastasize and travel to the

[23]Röcken M. Early tumor dissemination, but late metastasis: insights into tumor dormancy. J. Clin. Invest. 2010;120:1800−3.

[24]Dotan E, Cohen SJ, Alpaugh KR, Meropol NJ. Circulating tumor cells: evolving evidence and future challenges. Oncologist 2009;14:1070−82.

[25]Barriere G, et al. Epithelial mesenchymal transition: a double-edged sword. Clin. Transl. Med. 2015;14:14. doi:10.1186/s40169-015-0055-4.

[26]Tania M, et al. Epithelial to mesenchymal transition inducing transcription factors and metastatic cancer. Tumour Biol. 2014;35:7335−42.

[27]Grelet S, Andries V, Polette M, et al. The human NANOS3 gene contributes to lung tumour invasion by inducing epithelial-mesenchymal transition. J. Pathol. 2015. doi:10.1002/path.4549.

[28]Dotan E, Cohen SJ, Alpaugh KR, Meropol NJ. Circulating tumor cells: evolving evidence and future challenges. Oncologist 2009;14:1070−82.

sentinel lymph node, while other tumor cells pass through the sentinel lymph node and go into other lymph nodes, or into the bloodstream. And some tumor cells stay in the sentinel lymph node and form a tumor in the node (29). Where tumor cells from a primary tumor leave, and later find residence in a nearby lymph node, the regional lymph nodes can be used for staging, to predict survival, and to assess risk of recurrence (30). Tobler and Detmar (31) and Röcken (32) provide color diagrams, showing the relationships between a tumor, sentinel lymph node, distant lymph nodes, and the circulatory system.

III. STAGING SYSTEMS FOR VARIOUS CANCERS

a. Colorectal Cancer

Colorectal cancer is the third most common cancer in men and women in the United States (33). If diagnosed and surgically removed at an early stage, the prognosis is excellent. However, once disease extends outside the bowel, the prognosis worsens. The liver is the most common site of metastases. If colorectal cancer is left untreated, survival for 5 years or longer is near zero (34).

Computed tomography and ultrasonography are used for staging colorectal cancer. Endoscopic sonography is used to assess the depth of cancer invasion and lymph node metastasis (35). The presence of tumor cells in regional lymph nodes is the most important prognostic marker in staging patients with colorectal cancer. Cancer cells in lymph nodes are associated with a poorer prognosis (36). The number of tumors found in lymph nodes is used to predict the rate of recurrence of colorectal cancer, that is, recurrence following surgery and chemotherapy. In a nutshell, the rate of recurrence of colorectal cancer (following treatment) is 25% of patients with no tumors in lymph nodes, and 60% in patients with four or more lymph nodes harboring metastases (37). The results from staging of colorectal cancer dictate the treatment. Chemotherapy, following surgery, is recommended for all patients with stage III colon cancer. But for patients with

[29]Nathanson SD. Insights into the mechanisms of lymph node metastasis. Cancer 2003;98:413–23.

[30]Hammer C, Fanning A, Crowe J. Overview of breast cancer staging and surgical treatment options. Cleve. Clin. J. Med. 2008;75(Suppl. 1):S10–6.

[31]Tobler NE, Detmar M. Tumor and lymph node lymphangiogenesis—impact on cancer metastasis. J. Leukoc. Biol. 2006;80:691–6.

[32]Röcken M. Early tumor dissemination, but late metastasis: insights into tumor dormancy. J. Clin. Invest. 2010;120:1800–3.

[33]Kukreja SS, Esteban-Agusti E, Velasco JM, Hieken TJ. Increased lymph node evaluation with colorectal cancer resection: does it improve detection of stage III disease? Arch. Surg. 2009;144:612–7.

[34]Robertson DJ, Stukel TA, Gottlieb DJ, Sutherland JM, Fisher ES. Survival after hepatic resection of colorectal cancer metastases: a national experience. Cancer 2009;115:752–9.

[35]Yamada I, Yoshino N, Tetsumura A, et al. Colorectal carcinoma: local tumor staging and assessment of lymph node metastasis by high-resolution MR imaging in surgical specimens. Int. J. Biomed. Imaging 2009;2009:659836.

[36]Mejia A, Schulz S, Hyslop T, Weinberg DS, Waldman SA. GUCY2C reverse transcriptase PCR to stage pN0 colorectal cancer patients. Expert Rev. Mol. Diagn. 2009;9:777–85.

[37]Waldman SA, Terzic A. Therapeutic burden in cancer revealed by molecular staging. Biomark. Med. 2008;2:1–3.

stage II cancer, what is generally recommended is surgery only (38).

b. TNM Definitions for Colorectal Cancer

The following table and text provide definitions for the TNM staging scheme, as it applies to colorectal cancer (Table 5.1).

1. Stage 0

Tis, N0, M0: The cancer is in the earliest stage. It has not grown beyond the inner layer (mucosa) of the colon or rectum. This stage is also known as *carcinoma in situ* or *intramucosal carcinoma*.

2. Stage I

T1—T2, N0, M0: The cancer has grown through the muscularis mucosa into the

TABLE 5.1   Colorectal Definitions for T, N, M[a]

T Primary Tumor

Tis	**Tis:** The cancer is in the earliest stage (in situ). It involves only the mucosa. It has not grown beyond the muscularis mucosa (inner muscle layer)
T1	**T1:** The cancer has grown through the muscularis mucosa and extends into the submucosa
T2	**T2:** The cancer has grown through the submucosa and extends into the muscularis propria (thick outer muscle layer)
T3	**T3:** The cancer has grown through the muscularis propria and into the outermost layers of the colon or rectum but not through them. It has not reached any nearby organs or tissues
T4	**T4a:** The cancer has grown through the serosa (also known as the visceral peritoneum), the outermost lining of the intestines. **T4b:** The cancer has grown through the wall of the colon or rectum and is attached to or invades into nearby tissues or organs

N Regional Lymph Nodes. N categories indicate whether or not the cancer has spread to nearby lymph nodes and, if so, how many lymph nodes are involved. To get an accurate idea about lymph node involvement, most doctors recommend that at least 12 lymph nodes be removed during surgery and looked at under a microscope

N0	No cancer to nearby lymph nodes
N1	**N1a.** Cancer cells are found in 1 nearby lymph node. **N1b.** Cancer cells are found in two to three nearby lymph nodes
N2	**N2a.** Cancer cells are found in four to six nearby lymph nodes. **N2b.** Cancer cells are found in seven or more nearby lymph nodes

M Categories. M categories indicate whether or not the cancer has spread (metastasized) to distant organs, such as the liver, lungs, or distant lymph nodes

M0	No regional lymph node metastasis histologically, no additional examination for isolated tumor cells
M1a	The cancer has spread to one distant organ or set of distant lymph nodes
M1b	The cancer has spread to more than one distant organ or set of distant lymph nodes, or it has spread to distant parts of the peritoneum (the lining of the abdominal cavity)

[a]*American Cancer Society (Revised August 9, 2010) http://www.cancer.org/Cancer/ColonandRectumCancer/DetailedGuide/colorectal-cancer-staged*

[38]Govindarajan A, Baxter NN. Lymph node evaluation in early-stage colon cancer. Clin. Colorectal Cancer 2008;7:240—6.

submucosa (T1) *or* it may also have grown into the muscularis propria (T2). It has not spread to nearby lymph nodes or distant sites.

3. *Stage IIA*

T3, N0, M0: The cancer has grown into the outermost layers of the colon or rectum but has not gone through them. It has not reached nearby organs. It has not yet spread to the nearby lymph nodes or distant sites.

4. *Stage IIB*

T4a, N0, M0: The cancer has grown through the wall of the colon or rectum but has not grown into other nearby tissues or organs. It has not yet spread to the nearby lymph nodes or distant sites.

5. *Stage IIC*

T4b, N0, M0: The cancer has grown through the wall of the colon or rectum and is attached to or has grown into other nearby tissues or organs. It has not yet spread to the nearby lymph nodes or distant sites.

6. *Stage IIIA*

One of the following applies.

T1−T2, N1, M0: The cancer has grown through the mucosa into the submucosa (T1) or it may also have grown into the muscularis propria (T2). It has spread to one to three nearby lymph nodes (N1a/N1b) or into areas of fat near the lymph nodes but not the nodes themselves (N1c). It has not spread to distant sites.

T1, N2a, M0: The cancer has grown through the mucosa into the submucosa. It has spread to four to six nearby lymph nodes. It has not spread to distant sites.

7. *Stage IIIB*

One of the following applies.

T3−T4a, N1, M0: The cancer has grown into the outermost layers of the colon or rectum (T3) or through the visceral peritoneum (T4a)

but has not reached nearby organs. It has spread to one to three nearby lymph nodes (N1a/N1b) or into areas of fat near the lymph nodes but not the nodes themselves (N1c). It has not spread to distant sites.

T2−T3, N2a, M0: The cancer has grown into the muscularis propria (T2) or into the outermost layers of the colon or rectum (T3). It has spread to four to six nearby lymph nodes. It has not spread to distant sites.

T1−T2, N2b, M0: The cancer has grown through the mucosa into the submucosa (T1) or it may also have grown into the muscularis propria (T2). It has spread to seven or more nearby lymph nodes. It has not spread to distant sites.

8. *Stage IIIC*

One of the following applies.

T4a, N2a, M0: The cancer has grown through the wall of the colon or rectum (including the visceral peritoneum) but has not reached nearby organs. It has spread to four to six nearby lymph nodes. It has not spread to distant sites.

T3−T4a, N2b, M0: The cancer has grown into the outermost layers of the colon or rectum (T3) or through the visceral peritoneum (T4a) but has not reached nearby organs. It has spread to seven or more nearby lymph nodes. It has not spread to distant sites.

T4b, N1−N2, M0: The cancer has grown through the wall of the colon or rectum and is attached to or has grown into other nearby tissues or organs. It has spread to one or more nearby lymph nodes or into areas of fat near the lymph nodes. It has not spread to distant sites.

9. *Stage IVA*

Any T, Any N, M1a: The cancer may or may not have grown through the wall of the colon or rectum, and it may or may not have spread to nearby lymph nodes. It has spread to one distant organ (such as the liver or lung) or set of lymph nodes.

10. *Stage IVB*

Any T, Any N, M1b: The cancer may or may not have grown through the wall of the colon or rectum, and it may or may not have spread to nearby lymph nodes. It has spread to more than one distant organ (such as the liver or lung) or set of lymph nodes, or it has spread to distant parts of the peritoneum (the lining of the abdominal cavity).

c. Breast Cancer

The following provides the example of TNM staging of breast cancer. Breast cancer takes a number of forms, as outlined below (39).

d. Breast Cancer In Situ (DCIS and LCIS)

Many breast cancers detected early, typically by mammography, are classified as breast cancer in situ. Two types of breast cancer in situ are: (1) ductal carcinoma in situ (DCIS) and (2) lobular carcinoma in situ (LCIS), as outlined below. Raju et al. (40) provide color photographs comparing the histology of DCIS and LCIS. Sullivan et al. (41) highlight the importance of a correct interpretation of the

histology, as the two types of cancer are subject to different types of treatment. DCIS can be managed with surgery plus radiation, while LCIS, which tends to resist radiation, is treated with methods other than radiation.

- *DCIS*. DCIS means that abnormal cells are found only in the lining of a milk duct of the breast. These abnormal cells have not spread outside the duct. There are several types of DCIS. If not removed, some may change over time and become invasive cancers, while others may not. DCIS is the fourth most common form of cancer in women in the United States (42). Although DCIS is a noninvasive or preinvasive lesion characterized by cancerous ductal cells confined to the duct lumen, if surgery alone is used to remove cancerous tissue, about 12% of patients experience a recurrence within 5 years (43). Hence, the preferred treatment is surgery in combination with radiation or chemotherapy.
- *LCIS*. LCIS means that abnormal cells are found in the lining of a milk lobule. Although LCIS is not considered to be actual breast cancer at this noninvasive stage, it is a warning sign of an increased risk of developing invasive cancer. LCIS is sometimes found in a biopsy for another lump or unusual change detected on a mammogram.

---

[39]http://www.ucsfhealth.org/adult/medical_services/cancer/breast/conditions/breastcancer/signs.html; May 8, 2007; University of California at San Francisco).

[40]Raju U, Mei L, Seema S, Hina Q, Wolman SR, Worsham MJ. Molecular classification of breast carcinoma in situ. Curr. Genom. 2006;7:523−32.

[41]Sullivan ME, Khan SA, Sullu Y, Schiller C, Susnik B. Lobular carcinoma in situ variants in breast cores: potential for misdiagnosis, upgrade rates at surgical excision, and practical implications. Arch. Pathol. Lab. Med. 2010;134:1024−8.

[42]Kuerer HM, Albarracin CT, Yang WT, et al. Ductal carcinoma in situ: state of the science and roadmap to advance the field. J. Clin. Oncol. 2009; 27:279−88.

[43]Wong JS, Kaelin CM, Troyan SL, et al. Prospective study of wide excision alone for ductal carcinoma in situ of the breast. J. Clin. Oncol. 2006;24:1031−6.

e. Invasive Breast Cancer

Invasive cancer cells form in the ducts or the milk lobules and spread to the breast tissue around them. Tumors can be found during a breast exam or through screening, such as a mammogram. The size of the tumor, appearance under the microscope, and whether it has spread to the lymph nodes determine the severity of the cancer and therapy.

- *Metastatic breast cancer.* Metastatic cancer begins in the breast, but spreads outside the breast through the blood or lymph system to other organs. Women usually develop metastatic disease in the months or years following the diagnosis of breast cancer. This cancer most commonly spreads beyond the breast to the bones, lungs, liver, and brain.
- *Locally advanced breast cancer, including inflammatory breast cancer.* Inflammatory breast cancer, which is a subtype of locally advanced breast cancer, is a very aggressive type of breast cancer. The breast looks red and feels warm. The skin is red because of increased vascularization. Inflammatory breast cancer represents about 5% of all breast cancers (44).

f. Definitions for Breast Cancer

The following table and text provide definitions for the TNM staging scheme, as it applies to breast cancer. Following these definitions are descriptions of each breast cancer stage (Table 5.2).

g. Breast Cancer Staging

Stage 0: Tis, N0, M0: This is DCIS, the earliest form of breast cancer. In DCIS, cancer cells are still within a duct and have not invaded deeper into the surrounding fatty breast tissue. LCIS is sometimes also classified as stage 0 breast cancer, but most oncologists believe it is not a true breast cancer. In LCIS, abnormal cells grow within the lobules or milk-producing glands, but they do not penetrate through the wall of these lobules. Paget disease of the nipple (without an underlying tumor mass) is also stage 0. In all cases the cancer has not spread to lymph nodes or distant sites.

Stage IA: T1, N0, M0: The tumor is 2 cm (about 3/4 of an inch) or less across (T1) and has not spread to lymph nodes (N0) or distant sites (M0).

Stage IB: T0 or T1, N1mi, M0: The tumor is 2 cm or less across (or is not found) (T0 or T1) with micrometastases in one to three axillary lymph nodes (the cancer in the lymph nodes is greater than 0.2 mm across and/or more than 200 cells but is not larger than 2 mm) (N1mi). The cancer has not spread to distant sites (M0).

Stage IIA: One of the following applies.

T0 or T1, N1 (but not N1mi), M0: The tumor is 2 cm or less across (or is not found) (T1 or T0) and either:

- It has spread to one to three axillary lymph nodes, with the cancer in the lymph nodes larger than 2 mm across (N1a), OR
- Tiny amounts of cancer are found in internal mammary lymph nodes on sentinel lymph node biopsy (N1b), OR
- It has spread to one to three lymph nodes under the arm and to internal mammary lymph nodes (found on sentinel lymph node biopsy) (N1c).

OR

T2, N0, M0: The tumor is larger than 2 cm across and less than 5 cm (T2) but has not spread to the lymph nodes (N0).

---

[44]Wedam SB, Low JA, Yang SX, et al. Antiangiogenic and antitumor effects of bevacizumab in patients with inflammatory and locally advanced breast cancer. J. Clin. Oncol. 2006;24:769–77.

TABLE 5.2 Breast Cancer Definitions for T, N, M[a]

T Primary Tumor Definitions

T0	No evidence of primary tumor
Tis	Carcinoma in situ
T1	Tumor is 2 cm (3/4 of an inch) or less across
T2	Tumor is more than 2 cm but not more than 5 cm (2 inch) across
T3	Tumor is more than 5 cm across
T4	Tumor of any size growing into the chest wall or skin. This includes inflammatory breast cancer

N Lymph Node Definitions

N0   Cancer has not spread to nearby lymph nodes

N1   **N1**: Cancer has spread to one to three axillary (underarm) lymph node(s), and/or tiny amounts of cancer are found in internal mammary lymph nodes (those near the breast bone) on sentinel lymph node biopsy

N1mi: Micrometastases (tiny areas of cancer spread) in one to three lymph nodes under the arm. The areas of cancer spread in the lymph nodes are 2 mm or less across (but at least 200 cancer cells or 0.2 mm across)

N1a: Cancer has spread to one to three lymph nodes under the arm with at least one area of cancer spread greater than 2 mm across

N1b: Cancer has spread to internal mammary lymph nodes, but this spread could only be found on sentinel lymph node biopsy (it did not cause the lymph nodes to become enlarged)

N1c: Both N1a and N1b apply

N2   **N2**: Cancer has spread to four to nine lymph nodes under the arm, or cancer has enlarged the internal mammary lymph nodes (either N2a or N2b, but not both)

N2a: Cancer has spread to four to nine lymph nodes under the arm, with at least one area of cancer spread larger than 2 mm

N2b: Cancer has spread to one or more internal mammary lymph nodes, causing them to become enlarged

N3   **N3**: Any of the following:
N3a: either

- Cancer has spread to 10 or more axillary lymph nodes, with at least one area of cancer spread greater than 2 mm, OR

- Cancer has spread to the lymph nodes under the clavicle (collar bone), with at least one area of cancer spread greater than 2 mm

N3b: either

- Cancer is found in at least one axillary lymph node (with at least one area of cancer spread greater than 2 mm) and has enlarged the internal mammary lymph nodes, OR

- Cancer involves four or more axillary lymph nodes (with at least one area of cancer spread greater than 2 mm), and tiny amounts of cancer are found in internal mammary lymph nodes on sentinel lymph node biopsy

N3c: Cancer has spread to the lymph nodes above the clavicle with at least one area of cancer spread greater than 2 mm

(Continued)

TABLE 5.2   (Continued)

Regional Lymph Nodes (pN) Definitions[b]

pN0	No regional lymph node metastasis histologically, no additional examination for isolated tumor cells
pN1	Metastasis in one to three axillary lymph nodes, and/or in internal mammary nodes with microscopic disease detected by sentinel lymph node dissection but not clinically apparent
pN1mi	Micrometastasis (>0.2 mm, none >2.0 mm)
pN1a	Metastasis in one to three axillary lymph nodes
pN1b	Metastasis in internal mammary nodes with microscopic disease detected by sentinel lymph node dissection but not clinically apparent
pN1c	Metastasis in one to three axillary lymph nodes and in internal mammary lymph nodes with microscopic disease detected by sentinel lymph node dissection but not clinically apparent

Metastasis (M) Definitions

M0	No distant spread is found on X-rays (or other imaging procedures) or by physical exam
cM0 (i+)	Small numbers of cancer cells are found in blood or bone marrow (found only by special tests), or tiny areas of cancer spread (no larger than 0.2 mm) are found in lymph nodes away from the breast
M1	Spread to distant organs is present. (The most common sites are bone, lung, brain, and liver)

[a]http://www.cancer.org/acs/groups/cid/documents/webcontent/003090-pdf.pdf (Revised September 17, 2010 by American Cancer Society).
[b]Singletary SE, Connolly JL. Breast cancer staging: working with the sixth edition of the AJCC Cancer Staging Manual. CA Cancer J. Clin. 2006; 56:37–47.

The cancer has not spread to distant sites (M0).

Stage IIB: One of the following applies.

T2, N1, M0: The tumor is larger than 2 cm and less than 5 cm across (T2). It has spread to one to three axillary lymph nodes and/or tiny amounts of cancer are found in internal mammary lymph nodes on sentinel lymph node biopsy (N1). The cancer has not spread to distant sites (M0).

OR

T3, N0, M0: The tumor is larger than 5 cm across but does not grow into the chest wall or skin and has not spread to lymph nodes (T3, N0). The cancer has not spread to distant sites (M0).

Stage IIIA: One of the following applies.

T0–T2, N2, M0: The tumor is not more than 5 cm across (or cannot be found) (T0 to T2). It has spread to four to nine axillary lymph nodes, or it has enlarged the internal mammary lymph nodes (N2). The cancer has not spread to distant sites (M0).

OR

T3, N1 or N2, M0: The tumor is larger than 5 cm across but does not grow into the chest wall or skin (T3). It has spread to one to nine axillary nodes, or to internal mammary nodes (N1 or N2). The cancer has not spread to distant sites (M0).

Stage IIIB: T4, N0–N2, M0: The tumor has grown into the chest wall or skin (T4), and one of the following applies:

- It has not spread to the lymph nodes (N0).
- It has spread to one to three axillary lymph nodes and/or tiny amounts of cancer are found in internal mammary lymph nodes on sentinel lymph node biopsy (N1).
- It has spread to four to nine axillary lymph nodes, or it has enlarged the internal mammary lymph nodes (N2).

The cancer has not spread to distant sites (M0).

Inflammatory breast cancer is classified as T4 and is stage IIIB unless it has spread to distant lymph nodes or organs, in which case it would be stage IV.

Stage IIIC: any T, N3, M0: The tumor is any size (or cannot be found), and one of the following applies:

- Cancer has spread to 10 or more axillary lymph nodes (N3).
- Cancer has spread to the lymph nodes under the clavicle (collar bone) (N3).
- Cancer has spread to the lymph nodes above the clavicle (N3).
- Cancer involves axillary lymph nodes and has enlarged the internal mammary lymph nodes (N3).
- Cancer has spread to four or more axillary lymph nodes, and tiny amounts of cancer are found in internal mammary lymph nodes on sentinel lymph node biopsy (N3).

The cancer has not spread to distant sites (M0).

Stage IV: any T, any N, M1: The cancer can be any size (any T) and may or may not have spread to nearby lymph nodes (any N). It has spread to distant organs or to lymph nodes far from the breast (M1). The most common sites of spread are the bone, liver, brain, or lung. In addition to staging, the diagnosis of breast cancer, and formulating the strategy for treatment, also involves expression or genes and proteins. Gene expression can be analyzed by techniques based on hybridization or on the polymerase chain reaction, while protein expression is analyzed using antibodies. The relevant genes and proteins include estrogen receptor, progesterone receptor, and human epidermal growth factor receptor-2 (HER-2) (45,46). Overexpressed or amplified HER-2 is a relatively weak prognostic factor in untreated patients, but it is a strong predictive factor for responsiveness to trastuzumab, an antibody also known as Herceptin[®]. As a general proposition, applicable to almost any disease, one should ask if a given marker is relevant only to prognosis of the untreated disease, or alternatively, if the marker is relevant only to the efficacy of a given drug.

h. Summary

TNM staging systems have been established for many of the solid tumor cancers. These staging systems can be used for cancer diagnosis, for defining the inclusion criteria, for defining strata in the study population, for defining study groups for the purpose of an exploratory analysis after collecting all the study data, in formulating the prognosis, and in guiding the best therapy. Thus, TNM staging has many uses. What is separate from TNM staging are other types of criteria, including the assessment of clinical features, such as Eastern Cooperative Oncology Group (ECOG) performance status, and objective criteria, such as the expression of biomarkers.

IV. THE WILL ROGERS PHENOMENON

a. Introduction

The *Will Rogers phenomenon* refers to an artifact where there is an apparent change in distribution or prevalence of a particular disease, but where this change does not result from any biological change. This artifact results from changes or revisions in disease staging, or from improvements in the sensitivity of diagnostic instruments, such

---

[45]Allred DC. The utility of conventional and molecular pathology in managing breast cancer. Breast Cancer Res. 2008;10(Suppl. 4):S4.

[46]Peppercorn J, Partridge AH. Breast cancer in young women: a new color or a different shade of pink? J. Clin. Oncol. 2008;26:3303−5.

as in tumor-detection technologies (47). The term arises from one of the quotations of Will Rogers, namely, "When the Okies left Oklahoma and moved to California, they raised the average intelligence level in both states" (48).

This phenomenon has been expressly recognized by statements from oncologists, for example, "[s]tage migration is an evolutionary hazard in oncology . . . the use of novel imaging techniques to detect occult metastases . . . shifted patients with early-stage lung cancer into higher stages and artificially inflated survival rates . . . [t]hus the survival rates rise in each group with no actual improvement in individual outcomes. This was coined the Will Rogers phenomenon" (49), "[a]mong patients included in our analysis, we found that more LNs [lymph nodes] were examined in newer- versus old-era trials, resulting in stage migration through the Will Rogers phenomenon" (50), and "[w]e also observed increases in stage-specific survival, which we attributed to a well-known artifact of stage migration sometimes termed the Will Rogers Phenomenon" (51).

b. Will Rogers Phenomenon for Prostate Cancer

In a study of data from tumor registries, Albertsen et al. (52,53) discovered that there was a change, over a number of years, in the distribution of stages of prostate cancer. The researchers studied a prostate tumor registry, and found that the reported incidence of low-grade prostate cancer had declined over the course of years. The researchers concluded that this decline did not reflect any biological phenomenon, but that it was an artifact due to a change in the scoring system (Gleason score) for prostate cancer.

c. Will Rogers Phenomenon for Nonsmall Lung Cancer

In a survey of imaging data for nonsmall-cell lung cancer, Chee et al. (54) reviewed data from an era before widespread use of positron emission tomography (PET) (1994−98), and in the years after the introduction of PET (1999−2004). The researchers found a 5.4%

[47]Feinstein AR, Sosin DM, Wells CK. The Will Rogers phenomenon. Stage migration and new diagnostic techniques as a source of misleading statistics for survival in cancer. New Engl. J. Med. 1985;312:1604−8.

[48]Chee KG, Nguyen DV, Brown M, Gandara DR, Wun T, Lara Jr PN. Positron emission tomography and improved survival in patients with lung cancer: the Will Rogers phenomenon revisited. Arch. Intern. Med. 2008;168:1541−9.

[49]Leighl NB. Positron emission tomography use and stage migration in lung cancer: a false sense of accomplishment? J. Clin. Oncol. 2012;30:2710−1.

[50]Shi Q, Andre T, Grothey A, et al. Comparison of outcomes after fluorouracil-based adjuvant therapy for stages II and III colon cancer between 1978 to 1995 and 1996 to 2007: evidence of stage migration from the ACCENT database. J. Clin. Oncol. 2013;31:3656−63.

[51]Dinan MA, et al. Reply to M.S. Hoffman et al. J. Clin. Oncol. 2013;820. doi:10.1200.

[52]Albertsen PC, Hanley JA, Barrows GH, et al. Prostate cancer and the Will Rogers phenomenon. J. Natl Cancer Inst. 2005;97:1248−53.

[53]Thompson IM, Canby-Hagino E, Lucia MS. Stage migration and grade inflation in prostate cancer: Will Rogers meets Garrison Keillor. J. Natl Cancer Inst. 2005;97:1236−7.

[54]Chee KG, Nguyen DV, Brown M, Gandara DR, Wun T, Lara Jr PN. Positron emission tomography and improved survival in patients with lung cancer: the Will Rogers phenomenon revisited. Arch. Intern. Med. 2008;168:1541−9.

decline in the number of patients with stage III disease and an 8.4% increase in the number of patients with stage IV disease, during the later interval of time, as compared to the earlier interval. The authors attributed this to the Will Rogers phenomenon, where the PET scan use had "up-staged" patients who might otherwise be diagnosed as having stage III disease to stage IV, by detecting distant metastatic disease not visualized by other routine imaging studies.

d. Will Rogers Phenomenon for Rectal Cancer

In a study of rectal cancer, Folkesson et al. (55) attributed the success of their study to the Will Rogers phenomenon, where a conclusion regarding the benefit of radiation for stage I rectal cancer may have resulted from a change in their surgical technique. The new technique was "total mesorectal excision." Although the Folkesson trial used this new technique, at that time most hospitals had not adopted this new method. The new method was first used in 1982 (56,57) and later became widely adopted (58).

e. Will Rogers Phenomenon for Multiple Sclerosis

Clinical trials on multiple sclerosis were subjected to the Will Rogers phenomenon, beginning with the introduction of magnetic resonance imaging (MRI) for use in conjunction with the McDonald criteria. MRI and the McDonald criteria replaced the earlier Poser diagnostic criteria (59). Given the five-fold greater sensitivity of MRI, in comparison for earlier methods, for detecting disease activity, the McDonald criteria are expected to allow an earlier diagnosis of multiple sclerosis. In stepping back to view the historical picture, one can see that stage migration has occurred, in the transition from the earlier Poser criteria to the later McDonald criteria.

Sormani et al. (60) conducted a side-by-side comparison using the earlier Poser scale with the later McDonald scale. These investigators found that the prevalence of this disease was 16%, according to the older Poser scale, and 44%, according to the more recent McDonald scale. Sormani et al. (61,62) also provided a general warning regarding all clinical trials that

[55] Folkesson J, Birgisson H, Pahlman L, Cedermark B, Glimelius B, Gunnarsson U. Swedish rectal cancer trial: long lasting benefits from radiotherapy on survival and local recurrence rate. J. Clin. Oncol. 2005;23:5644–50.

[56] Zolfaghari S, Williams LJ, Moloo H, Boushey RP. Rectal cancer: current surgical management. Minerva Chir. 2010;65:197–211.

[57] Maughan NJ, Quirke P. Modern management of colorectal cancer—a pathologist's view. Scand. J. Surg. 2003;92:11–9.

[58] Glynne-Jones R, Mawdsley S, Pearce T, Buyse M. Alternative clinical end points in rectal cancer—are we getting closer? Ann. Oncol. 2006;17:1239–48.

[59] Gafson A, et al. The diagnostic criteria for multiple sclerosis: from Charcot to McDonald. Mult. Scler. Relat. Disord. 2012;1:9–14.

[60] Sormani MP, Tintorè M, Rovaris M, et al. Will Rogers phenomenon in multiple sclerosis. Ann. Neurol. 2008;64:428–33.

[61] Sormani MP. The Will Rogers phenomenon: the effect of different diagnostic criteria. J. Neurol. Sci. 2009;287 (Suppl. 1):S46–9.

[62] Sormani MP, Tintorè M, Rovaris M, et al. Will Rogers phenomenon in multiple sclerosis. Ann. Neurol. 2008;64:428–33.

do not have a control arm, but instead employ a historical control. This warning applies to all diseases where there exists a standard staging scale, for example, cancer, immune disorders such as multiple sclerosis, and infections.

V. OTHER SOURCES OF ARTIFACTS IN DATA FROM CLINICAL TRIALS

Artifacts in clinical trials can also arise when clinical trials are conducted in various far-flung parts of the world, for example, in China, India, and Russia. Carrato (63) has observed different polymorphisms in Eastern and Western patient populations may account for the different efficacy profiles, and different profiles, that have been observed.

Another source of artifacts is that the nature of the disease itself may change over the course of decades. Ardalan et al. (64) observed, in the context of esophageal cancer that, during the 1970s and 1980s, squamous cell cancer dominated, but after the 1990s, adenocarcinoma dominated, in the Western world. Interestingly, the epidemiologists reporting on this phenomenon considered the possibility that the Will Rogers phenomenon as being responsible, but then rejected it (65).

VI. CONCLUDING REMARKS

When planning a clinical trial, or when comparing data from published clinical trials, it is necessary to determine the staging system that was used. Where data from two different clinical trials are being compared, but where the two trials used different staging systems, the result is that the extent and details of conclusions that might be made will likely be impaired or constrained. Moreover, when data from two different clinical trials are being compared, and where the same staging system is used, but where different technologies are used to detect the disease, again the result is that the extent and details of conclusions will likely be impaired. From time to time, standards for tumor staging are changed.

A perplexing situation arises where a tumor staging scheme, or where a standard for measuring objective tumor response, is changed half-way through the course of a clinical trial. Mitchell et al. (66), Freyer et al. (67),

[63]Carrato A. Adjuvant treatment of colorectal cancer. Gastrointest. Cancer Res. 2008;2(4 Suppl.):S42−6.

[64]Ardalan B, Spector SA, Livingstone AS, et al. Neoadjuvant, surgery and adjuvant chemotherapy without radiation for esophageal cancer. Jpn J. Clin. Oncol. 2007;37:590−6.

[65]Devesa SS, Blot WJ, Fraumeni Jr JF. Changing patterns in the incidence of esophageal and gastric carcinoma in the United States. Cancer 1998;83:2049−53.

[66]Mitchell MS, Abrams J, Thompson JA, et al. Randomized trial of an allogeneic melanoma lysate vaccine with low-dose interferon Alfa-2b compared with high-dose interferon Alfa-2b for resected stage III cutaneous melanoma. J. Clin. Oncol. 2007;25:2078−85.

[67]Freyer G, Delozier T, Lichinister M, et al. Phase II study of oral vinorelbine in first-line advanced breast cancer chemotherapy. J. Clin. Oncol. 2003;21:35−40.

Grothey et al. (68), Pérez-Soler et al. (69), Rustin et al. (70), and Kaufmann et al. (71) represent studies where the investigators were aware of a revision in standards for measuring tumors resulting in a new standard, and/or of the existence of two different standards that were both accepted by the medical community, and where the investigators took steps to prevent conflicts from being introduced into their data.

[68]Grothey A, Hedrick EE, Mass RD, et al. Response-independent survival benefit in metastatic colorectal cancer: a comparative analysis of N9741 and AVF2107. J. Clin. Oncol. 2008;26:183–9.

[69]Pérez-Soler R, Chachoua A, Hammond LA, et al. Determinants of tumor response and survival with erlotinib in patients with non-small-cell lung cancer. J. Clin. Oncol. 2004;22:3238–47.

[70]Rustin GJ, Timmers P, Nelstrop A, et al. Comparison of CA-125 and standard definitions of progression of ovarian cancer in the intergroup trial of cisplatin and paclitaxel versus cisplatin and cyclophosphamide. J. Clin. Oncol. 2006;24:45–51.

[71]Kaufmann R, Spieth K, Leiter U, et al. Temozolomide in combination with interferon-alfa versus temozolomide alone in patients with advanced metastatic melanoma: a randomized, phase III, multicenter study from the Dermatologic Cooperative Oncology Group. J. Clin. Oncol. 2005;23:9001–7.

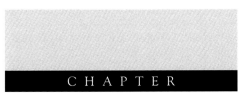

CHAPTER

6

Blinding, Randomization, and Allocation

I. INTRODUCTION

For any clinical trial, subjects must first be recruited and enrolled. Recruitment is the first step in a study subject's involvement in a clinical trial. Recruiting may involve an interview by a physician or by a clinical research associate (CRA). In a study of subjects enrolling in clinical trials, Wright et al. (1) administered a questionnaire and determined the reasons that motivate subjects to enroll. The most frequent reasons were the beliefs that, "clinical trials are important for future patients," "overall I have a favorable impression of my doctor," and because, "overall I have a favorable impression of the CRA."

Clinical trial design, at least in randomized double-blinded trials, involves randomization, allocation, blinding, and unblinding. The *open-label trial*, another type of trial design,

does not involve blinding. In an open-label trial, the fact of whether any given subject receives the drug or control treatment is not shielded from study subjects and is not shielded from clinicians. Yet another type of trial, the *single-arm trial*, is distinguished by the fact that the study design involves only one arm, and not two or more arms, and does not involve randomization. Nonrandomized clinical trials involving two or more arms may also be conducted. But Llovet et al. (2) describe the likely consequence of conducting a nonrandomized study. This consequence is evidence (data) that is not robust, not sufficient to change the existing standard of care, and not sufficient to warrant drug approval.

The events of recruitment, randomization, allocation, drug administration, and unblinding, are indicated in the following time line:

[1]Wright JR, Whelan TJ, Schiff S, et al. Why cancer patients enter randomized clinical trials: exploring the factors that influence their decision. J. Clin. Oncol. 2004;22:4312−8.

[2]Llovet JM, Di Bisceglie AM, Bruix J, et al. Design and endpoints of clinical trials in hepatocellular carcinoma. J. Natl Cancer Inst. 2008;100:698−711.

Clinical Trials.
DOI: http://dx.doi.org/10.1016/B978-0-12-804217-5.00006-0

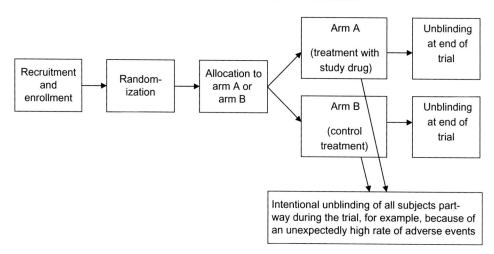

The following definitions provide a context for this chapter.

- *Open-label study.* All parties are aware of treatment being received after randomization. Open-label studies are not blinded.
- *Single-blind study.* The study subject is not aware of the treatment assignment, but the investigator is aware of the treatment assigned to every subject.
- *Double-blind study.* Both the study subject and the investigator are unaware of the treatment assigned to any individual subject.
- *Double-dummy design.* When there is a study drug group, and an active control drug (active comparator drug), blinding can be ensured by the double-dummy design. This design involves two different placebos, one placebo to serve as a control for the study drug, and another placebo to serve as a control for the active comparator drug. The trial involves two active drugs and two matching placebos. For example, in comparing two agents, one in a blue capsule and the other in a red capsule, the investigators would acquire blue placebo capsules and red placebo capsules. Then every subject in the study drug group receives a blue and a red capsule, one active and one inactive. And every subject in the active control group receives a blue and a red capsule.

- *Blinding.* Blinding refers to various features of clinical trial design that, when taken together, prevent the study subjects and most (but not all) study personnel from gaining access to the knowledge over whether any given study subject is receiving the study drug or control. There does not exist any particular moment in a clinical trial that is called "blinding" or that is called a "blinding step."
- *Unblinding.* The disclosure, planned or unintended, of the allocation of one study subject, one group of subjects, or all subjects. Unblinding can take place at a distinct moment, that is, at the moment when information is revealed about whether one or more subjects had received the study drug or control.

Blinding is desired for a number of reasons. Schulz et al. (3) divided these reasons into behaviors of the investigators and behaviors of the study subjects. The term *investigators* encompasses a variety of personnel, including trial designers, physicians and nurses, clerks who enroll study subjects, clerks who randomize the study subjects, and data collectors. Pildal et al. (4) report that there is no uniform standard as to the list of investigator personnel who must be blinded in a double-blind study.

Where unblinding occurs, or is not implemented in the first place, this can influence how the patient reports the disease. For example, if a patient believes that she is in the study drug arm, she may tend to report that she is recovering. If a subject learns that he or she is receiving the study drug, and not placebo, the subject may try to please the doctor by exaggerating the improvement, and conversely, a subject learning that he is in the placebo group may tend to view their experiences more negatively, as he may feel deprived of treatment (5). Unblinding can also influence how the patient conforms to the study protocol. For example, if a patient believes (rightly or wrongly) that he is in the placebo group, he may fail to take his drugs on time. Unblinding can also influence the tendency of a subject to drop out of the study. If a subject believes that she is in the placebo group, she may be tempted to drop out of the study. Unblinding can also influence the tendency to become lost to follow-up. If a subject believes that she was in the placebo group, she may fail to provide information to the investigator, in the years following the study. If a study subject learns that he has been assigned to the placebo group, he may be more willing to drop out of the clinical trial, once it is underway (6). Disproportionate dropout rates from one study arm, relative to another study arm, can influence the interpretation and outcome of clinical trials.

According to International Conference on Harmonization (ICH) Guidelines (7), blinding can prevent the following sources of bias:

(1) Subjects on active drug might report more favorable outcomes because they expect a benefit or might be more likely to stay in a study if they knew they were on active drug.

(2) Observers might be less likely to identify and report treatment responses in a no-treatment group or might be more sensitive to a favorable outcome or adverse event in patients receiving active drug.

(3) Knowledge of treatment assignment could affect vigor of attempts to obtain on-study or follow-up data.

(4) Knowledge of treatment assignment could affect decisions about whether a subject should remain on treatment or receive concomitant medications or other ancillary therapy.

(5) Knowledge of treatment assignment could affect decisions as to whether a given subject's results should be included in an analysis.

[3]Schulz KF, Chalmers I, Altman DG. The landscape and lexicon of blinding in randomized trials. Ann. Intern. Med. 2002;136:254−9.

[4]Pildal J, Hróbjartsson A, Jørgensen KJ, Hilden J, Altman DG, Gøtzsche PC. Impact of allocation concealment on conclusions drawn from meta-analyses of randomized trials. Int. J. Epidemiol. 2007;36:847−57.

[5]Krogsbøll LT, Hróbjartsson A, Gøtzsche PC. Spontaneous improvement in randomised clinical trials: meta-analysis of three-armed trials comparing no treatment, placebo and active intervention. BMC Med. Res. Methodol. 2009;9:1.

[6]Forder PM, Gebski VJ, Keech AC. Allocation concealment and blinding: when ignorance is bliss. Med. J. Aust. 2005;182:87−9.

[7]ICH Harmonised Tripartite Guideline. Choice of control group and related issues in clinical trials E10. (Step 4 version); July 2000 (33 pp.).

In observing the uneven quality of reporting on methods for allocation and blinding, as has occurred in publications of clinical trials, D.C. Bauer (8) an editor of a journal, mandated that the CONSORT guidelines for reporting clinical trials be used in his journal. The CONSORT guidelines (9) provide a reasonable list of parameters for including in publications relating to clinical trials.

Where side effects specifically associated with the study drug are known by the subjects or by clinical trial personnel, the presentation of these side effects can result in unintentional unblinding. Masking of these side effects can be undertaken, before the study, by using a placebo that causes the same type of side effects. As discussed in Chapter 7, an active placebo is a placebo with properties that mimic side effects such as dry mouth, or sweating, that might otherwise reveal that a subject is in the study drug group or placebo group (10,11). Another approach for preventing unblinding caused by known side effects of the study drug is shown by the following example. In a clinical trial on spironolactone, which produces the adverse drug reaction of feminization (of male subjects), the investigators maintained blinding by mandating that this, and other, adverse events by represented by letters of the alphabet (12).

Unintentional unblinding can also occur where the study drug requires continual dose adjustments during the course of the trial. Thus, physicians who are compelled to adjust the doses of some subjects, but not of other subjects, may be able to guess that the adjusted subjects are in the study drug arm, and that nonadjusted subjects are in the placebo arm. This type of unblinding can be prevented by requiring some of the placebo subjects to have adjustments of placebo (13,14,15).

II. LOGISTICS OF KEEPING TRACK OF STUDY SUBJECTS

An excerpt from a Clinical Study Protocol on an anticancer drug provides concrete guidance on how to keep track of study subjects. Proper accounting of each study subjects was ensured by way of a number that identifies the

[8]Bauer DC. Randomized trial reporting in general endocrine journals: the good, the bad, and the ugly. J. Clin. Endocrinol. Metab. 2008;93:3733—4.

[9]Schulz KF, Altman DG, Moher D; CONSORT Group. CONSORT 2010 statement: updated guidelines for reporting parallel group randomised trials. PLoS Med. 2010;7(3):e1000251.

[10]Schulz KF, Chalmers I, Altman DG. The landscape and lexicon of blinding in randomized trials. Ann. Intern. Med. 2002;136:254—9.

[11]Moncrieff J, Wessely S, Hardy R. Active placebos versus antidepressants for depression. Cochrane database of systematic reviews; 2004, Issue 1. Art. No.: CD003012. http://dx.doi.org/10.1002/14651858.CD003012.pub2.

[12]DeMets DL, Furbert CD, Friedman LM. Data monitoring in clinical trials. New York: Springer; 2006. p. 150—1.

[13]Hertzberg V, Chimowitz M, Lynn M, et al. Use of dose modification schedules is effective for blinding trials of warfarin: evidence from the WASID study. Clin. Trials 2008;5:25—30.

[14]Coumadin Aspirin Reinfarction Study (CARS) Investigators. Randomised double-blind trial of fixed low-dose warfarin with aspirin after myocardial infarction. Lancet 2008;350:389—96.

[15]Friedman LM, Furberg CD, DeMets DL. Fundamentals of clinical trials. 4th ed. New York: Springer; 2010. p. 123.

study site and the subject. The instructions in the Protocol read (16):

> **Patient numbering and screening.** Patients … will be asked to sign a study informed consent before a patient number will be assigned and before any study specific testing is performed for the purpose of determining a patient's eligibility for this study. Each patient in the study is uniquely identified by a **9-digit patient number** which is a combination of his/her **4-digit center number** and **5-digit subject number** … [t]he procedures for subject numbering and cohort coordination between the sites involved will be provided in a separate document before study start. Upon signing the informed consent form, the patient is assigned a subject number by the investigator or his/her designee. Once assigned to a patient, a patient number will not be reused.

a. Allocation and Allocation Concealment

Allocation refers to the act, decision-making process, or automated process, of assigning each subject to one of the study arms. In short, allocation means the act of connecting a given subject to a given treatment. Allocation is not the same thing as randomization. Allocation can either be random or nonrandom. According to Schulz (17), "[t]o ensure unpredictability of that allocation sequence, investigators should generate it by a random process (e.g., computer generated numbers, random number tables, or coin flipping)."

Allocation concealment seeks to prevent selection bias, and protects the allocation sequence before and until assignment to one of the study arms. Without the protection provided by allocation concealment, investigators have been known to change who gets assigned to a particular treatment, for example, who gets assigned to the study drug arm or placebo arm (18). To provide a hypothetic example, where there is no allocation concealment, the clerk who admits participants could ascertain the upcoming treatment allocations and then route participants with better prognoses to the experimental group and those with poorer prognoses to the control group, where the clerk's goal is to make the study drug appear to have greater efficacy. Allocation concealment is not the same thing as blinding. In contrast to allocation concealment, blinding seeks to prevent the introduction of bias after allocation.

As explained by Poolman et al. (19), "[a]llocation in a trial is concealed when investigators cannot beforehand determine the allocated treatment of the next patient enrolled into their study. Allocation concealment is necessary to prevent selection bias, whereas blinding is important to prevent detection bias, i.e., a biased assessment of outcome."

Schulz et al. (20) distinguish between allocation concealment and blinding by way of an example. This example is a clinical study that involves surgery. In a hypothetical clinical

[16]Oncology Clinical Trial Protocol CLDK378X2101. A phase I, multicenter, open-label dose escalation study of LDK378, administered orally in adult patients with tumors characterized by genetic abnormalities in anaplastic lymphoma kinase (ALK); August 19, 2010.

[17]Schulz KF. Assessing allocation concealment and blinding in randomised controlled trials: why bother? Evid. Based Nurs. 2001;4:4−6.

[18]Schulz KF. Assessing allocation concealment and blinding in randomised controlled trials: why bother? Evid. Based Nurs. 2001;4:4−6.

[19]Poolman RW, Struijs PA, Krips R, et al. Reporting of outcomes in orthopaedic randomized trials: does blinding of outcome assessors matter? J. Bone Joint Surg. Am. 2007;89:550−558.

[20]Schulz KF, Chalmers I, Altman DG. The landscape and lexicon of blinding in randomized trials. Ann. Intern. Med. 2002;136:254−9.

trial that compares *a new type of knee surgery technique* for sports injuries (arm A) with *an established knee surgery technique* for sports injuries (arm B), a goal will be to use randomization techniques that ensure that arm A does not consist mainly of people with arthritis. Allocation concealment prevents study personnel from secretly putting all of the arthritic people in arm B. But in this particular hypothetical, blinding is impossible (at least as it applies to blinding of the physician), because the physician will know which of the two types of surgery she is required to perform. In comments about allocation concealment, Rios et al. (21) found that lack of allocation concealment can permit selective assignment of the clinical study design, thereby destroying the purpose of randomization. Thus, in this hypothetical, we do have allocation concealment, but we do not have blinding.

Vickers (22) provides a concrete example of how an investigator can inadvertently subvert a clinical trial:

> Say that, on a given day, the surgeon has seen the randomization list and knows that the next patient will be randomly assigned to the surgery group. In walks a patient who meets the eligibility criteria for the trial but who the surgeon feels, on balance, is probably not going to do that well. Accordingly, the surgeon advises against surgery and does not raise the study with the patient; the next patient, however, is a great candidate for

surgery, and although he is rather wary of research, the surgeon pressures him to consent. In other words, the surgeon is able to subvert randomization and select which patients get which treatment, the very problem randomization was designed to avoid.

Viera and Bangdiwala (23) provide another example of the dangers of allocation schemes that do not involve allocation concealment. In a hypothetical example involving an antiobesity drug, called *Slimmenow*, these authors wrote:

> If the referring health care provider is aware of the next allocation, he … may (even unknowingly) influence enrollment or selection of participating subjects. For example, if the referring health care provider knows the next subject will be allocated to *Slimmenow*, he … may be inclined to try to help a certain patient he/she thinks may benefit more. Or perhaps knowing the next subject is to be allocated to placebo, he/she refers someone who really does not need to lose much weight.

Pildal et al. (24) characterized the failure to conceal allocation as, "[w]ithout concealment the person in charge of enrolment might channel patients with a better prognosis into his … preferred treatment."

Schulz (25) described a number of intentional attempts to subvert allocation, thereby resulting in unblinding of clinical trials. These include attempts to obtain the master randomization list, and using X-rays to screen sealed envelopes containing the patient's allocation to drug or placebo. In another publication, Schulz et al. (26),

[21]Rios LP, Odueyungbo A, Moitri MO, Rahman MO, Thabane L. Quality of reporting of randomized controlled trials in general endocrinology literature. J. Clin. Endocrinol. Metab. 2008;93:3810–6.

[22]Vickers AJ. How to randomize. J. Soc. Integr. Oncol. 2006;4:194–8.

[23]Viera AJ, Bangdiwala SI. Eliminating bias in randomized controlled trials: importance of allocation concealment and masking. Fam. Med. 2007;39:132–7.

[24]Pildal J, Hróbjartsson A, Jørgensen KJ, Hilden J, Altman DG, Gøtzsche PC. Impact of allocation concealment on conclusions drawn from meta-analyses of randomized trials. Int. J. Epidemiol. 2007;36:847–57.

[25]Schulz KF. Subverting randomization in controlled trials. J. Am. Med. Assoc. 1995;274:1456–8.

[26]Schulz KF, Chalmers I, Hayes RJ, Altman DG. Empirical evidence of bias. Dimensions of methodological quality associated with estimates of treatment effects in controlled trials. J. Am. Med. Assoc. 1995;273:408–12.

identified a few clinical studies where allocation was poorly controlled, and where there appeared to be consequent bias in the results.

According to Torgerson and Roberts (27), "[a] trial which has had its randomisation compromised may apparently show a treatment effect that is entirely due to biased allocation. The results of such a study are more damaging than an explicitly unrandomised study, as bias in the latter is acknowledged."

Randomization is a consequence of proper allocation. The reverse circumstance is not the case. According to Gluud (28), "[a]dequate randomization requires that the allocation of the next patient be unpredictable."

b. Simple Randomization

Simple randomization refers to the act of flipping a coin for each person enrolling in the trial, and using the coin flip to allocate the person to Treatment A or Treatment B. But according to Schulz and Grimes (29), this method of randomization can lead to errors, especially when the total number of people enrolling in the trial is small. For a clinical trial containing only 16 subjects, where eight are men and eight are women, the ideal clinical trial is one where four men and four women receive Treatment A, and four men and four women receive Treatment B. But it is intuitively obvious that imbalances are expected. The laws of probability inform us that it is quite possible for the coin-flipping technique to assign most, or even all, of the subjects to Treatment B. Other methods of simple randomization, for example, taking note of the subject's birth date (even-numbered birth date vs odd-numbered birth date) may be correlated in some way with some aspect of the subject's medical history, and therefore are not be truly random (30).

c. Stratification

Stratification refers to the act of classifying subjects according to subgroups, and equal allocation of the various subgroups to each of the study arms. In designing a clinical trial, investigators often divide the population into various subgroups. This activity is called stratification. Typically, stratification involves classifying each study subject according to gender, age (over 65 years vs under 65 years), stage of the disease (stage II vs stage III), and so on (31).

Vickers (32) provides a hypothetical example of stratification for a clinical trial on an antipain drug. Prior to enrollment, potential enrollees had two types of pain, for example, *bone pain* and *neuropathic pain*. Allocation according to subgroups might work in the following manner. Imagine that the first subject enrolling in the pain trial had *bone pain*. This subject is allocated to the treatment arm (not the placebo arm). The second subject to enroll has *bone pain*, and is allocated to the placebo arm. The third subject also has *bone pain*, and is allocated to the treatment arm. The fourth

[27]Torgerson DJ, Roberts C. Understanding controlled trials. Randomisation methods: concealment. Br. Med. J. 1999;319:375−6.

[28]Gluud LL. Bias in clinical intervention research. Am. J. Epidemiol. 2006;163:493−501.

[29]Schulz KF, Grimes DA. Generation of allocation sequences in randomised trials: chance, not choice. Lancet 2002;359:515−9.

[30]Berger VW, Weinstein S. Ensuring the comparability of comparison groups: is randomization enough? Control Clin. Trials 2004;25:515−24.

[31]Kundt G, Glass A. Evaluation of imbalance in stratified blocked randomization. Methods Inf. Med. 2012;51:55−62.

[32]Vickers AJ. How to randomize. J. Soc. Integr. Oncol. 2006;4:194−8.

subject presents with *neuropathic pain*, so this subject is randomized to the treatment arm. The goal of stratification and allocation is to ensure that roughly equal numbers of subjects with a particular characteristic end up in the treatment arm and in the placebo arm.

Where the design of the clinical trial also contains the subgroups of male and female, prospective subjects are randomized into different blocks, that is, men with bone pain, men with neuropathic pain, women with bone pain, and women with neuropathic pain.

In a clinical trial where study design does not have subgroups, subjects entering the trial are allocated by a random order, for example, arm A, arm A, arm B, arm A, arm B, arm A, arm A, arm A, arm B, arm B, and so on. But where stratification is included in the study design, the allocation procedure attempts to ensure that arm A and arm B contain the same proportion of subjects with *bone pain*, the same proportion of subjects who have *neuropathic pain*, the same proportion of subjects who are *male*, and the same proportion of subjects who are *female*.

d. Manual Technique for Allocation

A straightforward technique for allocation utilizes sealed, opaque sequentially numbered envelopes (SNOSE technique) (33,34,35,36). An understanding of this manual technique has the utility of teaching the goal of computerized allocation.

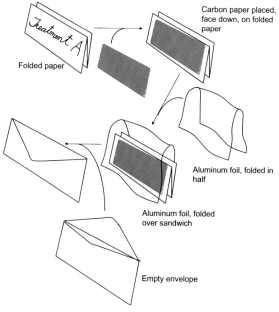

FIGURE 6.1 Sealed envelope technique for allocation and randomization. The sealed envelope technique accomplishes the task of establishing the association of each study subject to one of the study arms.

The following provides materials for allocating subjects for a typical 50-patient trial (Fig. 6.1). The allocation kit requires 50 opaque, letter-sized envelopes, 50 sheets of standard size paper, and 50 sheets of carbon paper. The kit also requires 50 sheets of aluminum foil, cut in rectangles that are as wide as the envelope, but twice as high. The carbon paper should have the same dimensions as the envelope.

[33]Doig GS, Simpson F. Randomization and allocation concealment: a practical guide for researchers. J. Crit. Care 2005;20:187−93.

[34]Quirke M, et al. Oral flucloxacillin and phenoxymethylpenicillin versus flucloxacillin alone for the emergency department outpatient treatment of cellulitis: study protocol for a randomised controlled trial. Trials 2013;14: 164 (6 pp.).

[35]Galli TT, et al. Effects of transcutaneous electrical nerve stimulation on pain, walking function, respiratory muscle strength and vital capacity in kidney donors: a protocol of a randomized controlled trial. BMC Nephrol. 2013;14:7 (6 pp.).

[36]Liebano RE, et al. Transcutaneous electrical nerve stimulation and conditioned pain modulation influence the perception of pain in humans. Eur. J. Pain. 2013;17:1539−46.

On 25 of the paper sheets, print "Treatment A" and on the other 25 paper sheets, write, "Treatment B." (Do not print "study drug." Do not print "placebo.")

Now, make sandwiches for the Treatment A group (Fig. 6.1). The sandwiches consist of the letter paper, carbon paper, and aluminum foil, as shown in the following diagram. First, fold the paper marked "Treatment A" so that it can fit inside the envelope. Then, place a carbon paper against the folded paper, ink-side of the carbon paper facing the folded paper. Then, fold the aluminum foil over both sides of the carbon paper/letter paper sandwich. Finally, after the aluminum foil has been folded over the sandwich, the completed big sandwich is placed inside the envelope. The foil will prevent people from holding the envelope up to the light, and seeing if the paper reads, "Treatment A" or "Treatment B."

If the carbon paper is positioned properly, writing on the front of the envelope will be transferred to the treatment allocation paper inside (Fig. 6.1). The carbon paper serves to establish an audit trail that can be used to monitor violations of allocation concealment. Complete all 25 Treatment A envelopes and seal each envelope.

Prepare the Treatment B envelopes as above (Fig. 6.1). When Treatment B envelopes are finished, there should be one pile of 25 sealed Treatment A envelopes and a second pile of 25 sealed Treatment B envelopes. Combine the 25 sealed Treatment A envelopes with the 25 sealed Treatment B envelopes and shuffle as you would a deck of cards. Then, with a firm hand, mark a unique number on the front of each envelope, sequentially from 1 to 50, in pen. The carbon paper inside the envelope will transfer this number to the allocation paper inside. At this point in time, the paper inside bears writing that reads, "Treatment A" or "Treatment B," and also bears the unique number. Place these envelopes into the plastic container, in numerical order, ready for use.

To use the kit, write the patient's study identifier number on the front of the envelope. The carbon paper inside the envelope will transfer the patient identifier to the treatment allocation paper inside (Fig. 6.1).

In practice, potential study subjects never see the envelope and never touch the envelope. The envelopes may be prepared entirely by a party independent of the investigator. The envelopes help to guarantee only that allocation of each study subject is concealed. The envelopes have no bearing on accidental or unwanted unblinding of study subjects, once the trial is underway. What helps guarantee blinding of study subjects, once the study is underway, is secret codes on labels of study drug and placebo. These codes are known only to an independent group, called the Investigational Drug Service (IDS) [37].

The need to use sealed envelopes for allocating study subjects is critical for the following reasons. First, most clinical trials enroll subjects, not all at once, but over the course of weeks or months. If paper slips showing the patient's identification number and their treatment (Treatment A vs Treatment B) were not sealed, this would tempt study personnel (over the course of time) to guess which subjects were to receive the study drug or placebo. Second, many clinical trials take place at several sites. Hence, the creation of 50 sealed envelopes (for 50 subjects in this hypothetical example), all at once, solves the problem of using a different randomization scheme at each study center. The envelope technique also requires that each person who contributes any writing, add their signature to the outside of the sealed envelope. In this way, an audit trail is created, which lends a degree of security to the method.

[37]Viera A. E-mail of October 13, 2010.

Internet-based systems of allocation and randomization are also available, for example, a vendor called, Sealed Envelope, Ltd, located in London, England. Clinical trials that have used this vendor are cited in footnotes (38,39,40). Swingler and Zwarenstein (41) describe a technique similar to the above-described envelope technique, but it is not as secure. Their method uses sealed envelopes, but no carbon paper. Berger and Weinstein (42) document a number of clinical trials where the sealed envelopes were tampered with, for example, by holding the envelopes up to the light. Use of aluminum foil can prevent this particular tampering problem.

Clinical trials on human subjects may include an independent organization, called an IDS, whose members are the only ones to receive and know the study arm assignment. In other words, the IDS is the only party that opens the envelope. Bottles of pills or vials are coded with symbols that only the IDS understands, that is, the bottles of pills would not be labeled as, "Treatment A" and "Treatment B." Study investigators, physicians taking care of patients, statisticians, monitoring boards, would have no information about what arm a participant is in, until there is a formal decision to unblind specific subjects, subgroups, or the entire study population.

A pharmacist can be informed of patient assignment by code in order to dispense placebo or the appropriate dose of study drug to each subject, as used, for example, in the cited study (43).

e. Allocation by Coin-Toss Versus Allocation by Sealed Envelope

While enrolling subjects in a clinical trial, it is possible to allocate each subject, as they are enrolled, to either Treatment A or Treatment B, by flipping a penny. Heads means Treatment A, while tails means Treatment B. As mentioned above, a problem with this technique, is that it is statistically possible to have all subjects allocated to receive Treatment A (and none receiving Treatment B). Thus, the coin-toss method must not be used. Allocation by sealed envelope absolutely ensures that equal numbers of subjects receive Treatment A and Treatment B.

III. BLOCKED RANDOMIZATION

For most clinical trials, subjects are enrolled one by one, over the course of many months. The simplest allocation procedure is complete randomization (analogous to repeated coin-tossing in the case of two arms), where each

---

[38]Kapoor R, Furby J, Hayton T, et al. Lamotrigine for neuroprotection in secondary progressive multiple sclerosis: a randomised, double-blind, placebo-controlled, parallel-group trial. Lancet Neurol. 2010;9:681–8.

[39]Beardsall K, Vanhaesebrouck S, Ogilvy-Stuart AL, et al. Early insulin therapy in very-low-birth-weight infants. New Engl. J. Med. 2008;359:1873–84.

[40]Brady AR, Gibbs JS, Greenhalgh RM, et al. Perioperative beta-blockade (POBBLE) for patients undergoing infrarenal vascular surgery: results of a randomized double-blind controlled trial. J. Vasc. Surg. 2005;4:602–9.

[41]Swingler GH, Zwarenstein M. An effectiveness trial of a diagnostic test in a busy outpatients department in a developing country: issues around allocation concealment and envelope randomization. J. Clin. Epidemiol. 2000;53:702–6.

[42]Berger VW, Weinstein S. Ensuring the comparability of comparison groups: is randomization enough? Control Clin. Trials 2004;25:515–24.

[43]Romine JS, Sipe JC, Koziol JA, Zyroff J, Beutler E. A double-blind, placebo-controlled, randomized trial of cladribine in relapsing-remitting multiple sclerosis. Proc. Assoc. Am. Physicians 1999;111:35–44.

allocation is made completely at random (44). Let us assume that allocation is accomplished by using a hat containing 50 red balls and 50 green balls. Each person that enters the enrollment office puts a hand into the hat, takes out a ball, and takes it to the pharmacy to receive Treatment A or Treatment B. With use of this method, it is possible for the first 30 or subjects to receive only Treatment A (none receiving Treatment B). It is only after every single ball is taken from the hat, can we be assured that equal numbers of subjects are receiving Treatment A and Treatment B (45). But a reality of clinical trials, is that efficacy and safety are continually monitored. Please contemplate the following hypothetical. Assume that the trial is still in its early phases, and only 30 balls have been taken from the hat, and that nearly all of the subjects are receiving Treatment A. Let us further assume, that Treatment A is an active control, for example, methotrexate (a very toxic anticancer agent), and let us assume that Treatment B is the antibody, trastuzumab (not particularly toxic). Now, returning to the hypothetical, it can be seen that most of the subjects in the early phases of the clinical trial may be experiencing severe toxic reactions, due to the methotrexate. As a consequence of the high prevalence of toxic reactions, the study investigators will request that the subjects be unblinded, and the nature of the treatments revealed, and the available data analyzed. In view of the high prevalence of toxic reactions, the investigators may also bring the trial to a temporary halt, and stop enrolling any more subjects. The

above problem can be solved by blocked randomization.

Allocation and randomization by the technique of blocked randomization ensures that roughly equal proportions of subjects are allocated to Treatment A and Treatment B, from the earliest stages of the trial, on through the clinical trial, and as long as new subjects are being enrolled (46).

The following example is with blocks of 4 (four-unit blocks) (47). In this example, each block has a constant size of four subjects. In blocked randomization, the first four subjects are allocated to receive Treatment A or Treatment B, in this order: BBAA. The next four subjects receive Treatment A or Treatment B in this respective order: ABBA. And the next four subjects, respectively, receive Treatments A or B in the order: BBAA. In this way, the allocation is randomized. Also, by using the blocked randomization technique, balance between the number of subjects receiving Treatment A or Treatment B is ensured, from the very start of the trial.

Each block has a defined sequence, that is, AABB, BBAA, ABAB, BABA, ABBA, and BAAB. The particular order in which the blocks are utilized for allocating subjects is totally random. These blocks are four units long. But blocks of other sizes are used in clinical trials, for example, six-unit blocks. The agency conducting allocation does not reveal the block size to the investigator or to the subjects. Moreover, any given trial can use a mixture of 4-unit blocks, 6-unit blocks, or 10-unit blocks, for example. The effectiveness of

[44]Kundt G, Glass A. Evaluation of imbalance in stratified blocked randomization. Methods Inf. Med. 2012;51:55−62.

[45]Schulz KF, Grimes DA. Generation of allocation sequences in randomised trials: chance, not choice. Lancet 2002;359:515−9.

[46]Efird J. Block randomization with randomly selected block sizes. Int. J. Environ. Res. Publ. Health 2011;8:15−20.

[47]Matts JP, Lachin JM. Properties of permuted-block randomization in clinical trials. Control Clin. Trials 1988;9:327−44.

stratified blocked randomization can be reduced, when the number of strata is large, or the block sizes are too large in relation to the number of patients enrolled (48).

IV. CLINICAL STUDY PROTOCOL RANDOMIZATION INSTRUCTIONS

This provides examples of randomization instructions from two Clinical Study Protocols. The Protocols were published as supplements to articles appearing in the *New England Journal of Medicine*.

a. Randomization Procedure From a Clinical Study Protocol for a COPD Study

This provides an example of randomization instructions from a Clinical Study Protocol. The Protocol concerned chronic obstructive pulmonary disease (COPD). The study drug was the antibiotic, *azithromycin*. The excerpt states that the user inputs information at a website. The user chooses a study site. The website's software stratifies study subjects by study sites, that is, study sites that are within a given clinical center. The software responds by providing a "treatment assignment number." This number, in turn, is coupled with a "schedule" that is kept at a pharmacy. The excerpt from the Protocol reads (49):

> Randomization will be carried out by linking to the Data Coordinating Center through a website, (http://www.copdcrn.org) using a . . . User ID and

password. After securing entry a menu listing the clinical sites appears. The user must choose one of these . . . [clinical sites] . . . Randomization is stratified by each designated site in each clinical center. As an example, the Minneapolis clinical center has three sites: the VA Hospital in Minneapolis, Health Partners, and the Mayo Clinic . . . If all eligibility criteria are met the randomization program will issue a treatment assignment number such as '113'. This number matches a schedule that is retained in each site's clinical pharmacy, where separate supplies of capsules containing the active drug and the placebo are also kept. The only person knowing this schedule will be the pharmacist and the DCC. When the clinic coordinator requests pills for treatment assignment #113, the pharmacist will check the schedule and distribute the assigned drug from the appropriate pharmacy supply. The actual assignment will only be revealed in cases of emergencies.

b. Randomization Procedure From Clinical Study Protocol for an Arthritis Study

This provides another example of a randomization procedure from a Clinical Study Protocol. The clinical trial concerned *tofacitinib* for treating rheumatoid arthritis. The procedure refers to the fact that the potential subject visits the investigative site for screening, and that during the visit, an employee at the site contacts an automated randomization system. The procedure states that information on the subject is inputted, and that the system responds by providing a "Patient ID number." The procedure also refers to a subsequent visit to the investigative site (the "Baseline Visit"), where the subject gets assigned a code that corresponds to a drug, for example, the study drug or a placebo. The procedure read (50):

[48]Kundt G, Glass A. Evaluation of imbalance in stratified blocked randomization. Methods Inf. Med. 2013;51:55–62.

[49]Albert RK, Connett J, Bailey WC, et al. Azithromycin for prevention of exacerbations of COPD. New Engl. J. Med. 2011;365:689–98.

[50]Phase 3 randomized, double-blind study of the efficacy and safety of 2 doses of CP690,550 compared to methotrexate in methotrexate-naive patients with rheumatoid arthritis. Compound Name: tofacitinib. US IND No: 70,903. Protocol No: A3921069; November 2012.

Approximately 900 patients will be randomized in a 2:2:1 ratio to Treatment Arm 1, Treatment Arm 2, or Treatment Arm 3, respectively. Randomization will be accomplished using Impala (an automated web/telephone randomization system provided by the sponsor) … At the Screening Visit, the investigative site will contact Impala (online or by telephone call). The site will enroll the patient into the Impala by indicating minimal information sufficient to distinguish one patient from another (e.g., date of birth and initials) and receive the Patient ID number. At the Baseline Visit, the system will associate that patient with the next available treatment on the randomization schedule and provide the randomization number. The system will then give the investigative site a code which corresponds to study drug that was previously shipped to the site and is in the site's inventory ready to be dispensed. This code corresponds to the study drug of that period in the treatment sequence in which the patient has just been randomized.

V. INSTRUCTIONS FOR UNBLINDING

a. Introduction

In addition to instructions on randomization and blinding, the Clinical Study Protocol can include instructions for unblinding. ICH Guidelines (51) specifically recommend that the sponsor identify methods of randomization, and situations where it is permissible to break the code:

A description of the specific procedures used to carry out blinding should be provided (e.g., how bottles were labeled, labels that reveal blind-breakage, sealed code list/envelopes, double dummy techniques), including the circumstances in which the blind would be broken for an individual or for all patients, e.g., for serious adverse events, the procedures used and who had access to patient codes.

The following excerpts from a variety of Clinical Study Protocols provide instructions on randomization codes, persons possessing the randomization code, and conditions under which the code may be broken. The "[XXXX]" indicates the redacted name of the sponsor.

b. When to Break the Randomization Code—Clinical Study Protocol for Trial on Alzheimer's Disease (52)

Patients participating in the trial will be assigned a sequential trial number. The computer-generated list of trial numbers is linked to a randomized list with medication numbers, equivalent to 80 batches of indomethacin and 80 batches of placebo. The participating pharmacist will retain the randomization code.

In case of an adverse event with a possible causal relationship to the use of indomethacin, the medical attendant (e.g. family physician, physician) will discontinue the trial medication. The trial ends, however the trial code will not be broken and the patient's data will be analyzed. The medical attendant will be asked to report this decision to the investigators as soon as possible.

The medical attendant is allowed to lower the dose of the study medication, in case of a dubious causal relationship between the adverse event and the study medication. The trial code will not be broken and the patient will be considered a normal participator of the trial.

In case of a serious adverse event, the patient's medical attendant will ask the pharmacist to announce the nature of trial medication. The code will then be broken, the medication will be discontinued and the patient's data will not be included in the analysis of the final outcome measures. However, the data of patients discontinuing the trial will analyzed according to the intention to treat" principle.

[51]ICH Harmonised Tripartite Guideline. Structure and content of clinical study reports E3. Step 4 version; November 1995. 43 pp.

[52]Clinical Study Protocol. Effect of indomethacin on the progression of Alzheimer's disease. A randomized double blind, placebo-controlled, multicenter clinical trial. Kremer HPH, Jansen RWMM. Radboud University Medical Center Nijmegen.

c. When to Break the Randomization Code—Clinical Study Protocol for Trial on Malaria Vaccine (53)

Code break envelopes, for each study enrolled subject and associating each treatment number with a specific vaccine, will be kept by the Local Safety Monitor in Gabon as well as by Central Safety at [XXXX], Rixensart in a safe and locked place with no access for unauthorized personnel. If deemed necessary for reasons such as safety, the Local Safety Monitor in Gabon as well as [XXXX] Central Safety will unblind the specific enrolled subject without revealing the study blind to the investigators.

d. When to Break the Randomization Code—Clinical Study Protocol for Trial Typhoid Vaccine (54)

The code for a particular subject can be broken in a medical emergency if knowing the identity of the treatment allocation would influence the treatment of the subject. Whenever a code is broken, the person breaking the code must record the time, date and reason as well as their initials in the source documents. If the site needs to break the code, the sponsor should, if possible, be contacted prior to breaking the code. In all cases, the Study Monitor must be notified within 24 hours after the code has been broken. All code break (whether broken or not) must be kept throughout the study period. Codes will be checked for integrity and collected by the Study Monitor at study site closure.

e. When to Break the Randomization Code—Clinical Study Protocol for Trial on Lung Cancer (55)

The treatment group (nitroglycerin or placebo) is determined by the patient number. The randomisation list is generated by a computer programme. Randomisation will be balanced (1:1) within blocks. Patients belonging to the same block will be treated in one centre. The treatment assignment of an individual patient will be documented in a sealed envelope carrying the patient number which may be opened in case of an emergency. If the envelope is opened, date and reason for opening must be documented. Not opened envelopes must be returned at the end of the trial.

f. When to Break the Randomization Code—Clinical Study Protocol for Trial on Sepsis (56)

Individual treatment codes will be available via IVRS. Only the pharmacist at each study centre will be unblinded to treatment. Investigators and other study centre staff will remain blinded to treatment. The treatment code must not be broken by blinded staff except in medical emergencies when the appropriate management of the patient necessitates knowledge of the treatment randomisation. The investigator(s) must document and report to the Medical Monitor any breaking of the treatment code. The investigator should notify the Medical Monitor prior to contacting IVRS to obtain the treatment code. All calls resulting in an unblinding event

[53]Clinical Study Protocol. A Phase II randomized, double-blind bridging study of the safety and immunogenicity of [XXXX] candidate *Plasmodium falciparum* malaria vaccine RTS,S/AS01E (0.5 mL dose) to RTS,S/AS02D (0.5 mL dose) administered IM according to a 0-, 1-, 2-month vaccination schedule in children aged 18 months to 4 years living in Gabon; December 7, 2005.

[54]Clinical Study Protocol. A placebo controlled, single-blind, single oral dose study to determine the safety and immunogenicity of M01ZH09 typhoid vaccine (oral live *S. typhi* (Ty2 *aroC ssaV*) ZH9) in healthy paediatric subjects, aged 5 to 14 years inclusive, of Vietnamese origin; January 2007.

[55]Clinical Study Protocol. Randomized, double-blind phase II study to compare nitroglycerin plus oral vinorelbine plus cisplatin with oral vinorelbine plus cisplatin alone in patients with stage IIIB/IV non-small cell lung cancer (NSCLC); May 2007.

[56]Clinical Study Protocol. A placebo-controlled, double-blind, dose-escalating study to assess the safety, tolerability, and pharmacokinetics and pharmacodynamics of single and multiple intravenous infusions of [XXXX] in patients with severe sepsis; September 2008.

will be recorded and reported by the IVRS to the Medical Monitor. [XXXX] retains the right to break the code for SAEs that are unexpected and are suspected to be causally related to an investigational product and that potentially require expedited reporting to regulatory authorities. If the blind is broken, the date, time and reason must be recorded in the patient's eCRF, and any associated AE report. If a patient's study treatment is unblinded by the investigator or designee, the patient will be withdrawn from study treatment as described in Section 3.3.5.

g. When to Break the Randomization Code—Clinical Study Protocol for Trial on Melanoma (57)

Under normal circumstances, the blind should not be broken until all subjects have completed the study and the database is locked. If specific emergency treatment for a subject requires knowledge of the treatment assignment or if subsequent therapy requires it, the Investigator will call the IVRS to identify the treatment code for that one subject (see Study Manual). The Investigator will be allowed to break the treatment code only when a serious adverse event occurs and knowledge of the treatment by the Investigator is deemed useful as to the subject's safety or the need for subsequent treatment.

h. When to Break the Randomization Code—Clinical Study Protocol for Trial on Multiple Sclerosis (58)

The treatment randomization will be produced by [XXXX]. The biostatistician and supporting programmers are the only individuals with access to the randomization codes, with the exception of the drug packaging and labeling department which also

has one copy of the code to use in the labeling and packaging of drug.

Emergency Unmasking for Medical Reasons. A sealed envelope containing the identification of the study medation for each patient will be provided to the study center. These sealed envelopes must be kept in a secure area to be available for monitoring.

In an emergency, the investigator will first contact the [XXXX] CRA or medical monitor prior to revealing the code for a particular patient. If the [XXXX] CRA or medical monitor cannot be reached, the treating physician or designee may break the double-masked code by opening the envelope and revealing the code for that particular patient. The person breaking the code must not reveal the information to the evaluating physician. The person breaking the code will note the date, time and reason for unmasking, and document the procedure with his/her signature. This information will be noted on the envelope in the section provided and the envelope will be resealed. All sealed and unsealed envelopes will be returned to [XXXX] to verify that masking was maintained.

VI. SUMMARY OF UNBLINDING

A serious adverse event or an emergency in a particular study subject can trigger the decision to unblind that subject. Clinical Study Protocols differ in their disclosure of which persons will receive information on the unblinded subject, that is, should only the safety monitor receive unblinded information, or should the sponsor also receive unblinded information. Another concept is that only selected personnel, for example, a pharmacist, possess the randomization code. To understand the event that can trigger unblinding, namely, the *serious adverse event*, the reader may review Chapter 25.

[57]Clinical Study Protocol. A prospective, randomized, double-blind, parallel, multicenter, Phase 3 study of dacarbazine plus [XXXX] compared to dacarbazine plus placebo in chemo-naive subjects with state IV melanoma and baseline LCH ≤ 1.2 times the upper limit of normal; September 2008.

[58]Clinical Study Protocol. Phase III, double-masked, placebo-controlled study to evaluate the safety and efficacy of two doses of betaseron in patients with secondary-progressive multiple sclerosis; August 19, 1997.

VII. FDA WARNING LETTERS

a. Blinding Oversights During a Clinical Trial

FDA's Warning Letters provide guidance for selected features of clinical trials, most frequently, about the need to adhere to instructions in the Clinical Study Protocol, and to the responsibilities of the Institutional Review Board (IRB). The following Warning Letter concerns one of the instructions in a Protocol, that relating to blinding. The letter referred to 21 CFR §312.50, and complained about failure to follow instructions regarding the need for nurses to be blinded as to the treatment versus control [59]:

> [s]tudy monitors failed to ensure that planned study blinding procedures were correctly followed for Study [redacted] at Site #063. This study was to be conducted in a double-blind fashion. According to the Protocol … "the unblinded pharmacist will be responsible for preparing the study medication for each subject in such a way that investigators and staff remain blinded to the medication being administered" … study nurses, rather than the unblinded pharmacist, were responsible for completing drug dissolution and reconstitution, as well as administering study drug infusions and caring for the subjects. Therefore, nursing personnel caring for subjects … were not blinded to study treatment, as specified by the protocol.

The letter further complained that, "nursing notes were viewed by clinical investigators at the site. Although it appears that the nurses used correction fluid to cover writing, in some cases the covered writing could still be read."

b. Sponsor Made Claims About the Study Drug in Advertisements, but the Advertisements Contained Information From Poorly Designed Clinical Trials That Were Not Blinded

In addition to regulating the design and conduct of clinical trials, the FDA also regulates the information on package labels of the marketed drug, as well as any promotions and advertisements. The following Warning Letter complained about a promotion that was considered to be misleading, because the promotion made use of poorly designed clinical trials that were not blinded. The drug was *dexmethylphenidate* (Focalin XR®) for treating hyperactivity in children [60]. Please note the letter's use of the term "open-label" to refer to clinical trials that lack blinding. The letter complained that [61]:

> [t]he slide deck presents numerous claims about the long-term effectiveness and safety of Focalin XR … [t]hese presentations misleadingly imply that Focalin XR is effective for long-term use when this has not been demonstrated by substantial evidence or substantial clinical experience … [i]n fact, no well-controlled trial supports long-term effectiveness, and the reference in slides 25–27 refers to an **open-label**, not concurrently controlled study that would not be considered substantial evidence of long-term effectiveness.

The Warning Letter specifically addressed the fact that, in general, subjective data must be acquired or captured using a blinded trial design. By subjective data, what is meant is data on feelings and emotions of the study subjects. This type of data is usually captured

[59]Warning Letter No. 09-HFD-45-0702. From Dr. Leslie K. Ball, MD, Office of Compliance, CDER, U.S. Food and Drug Administration; August 10, 2009.

[60]Seif E, Carlson J. The prevalance of medication use in head start preschool sample. Dialog 2015;17:83–98.

[61]Warning letter to Sue Duvall (no letter no.). From Robert Dean, Division of Drug Marketing, Advertising, and Communications, U.S. Food and Drug Administration; September 25, 2008.

using questionnaires. The questionnaire for this clinical trial captured data using a scale for measuring severity of hyperactivity. The letter complained that (62):

> [a]n open-label **(nonblinded)** study is not an appropriate study design to evaluate subjective end-points, such as those measured by the Attention Deficit/Hyperactivity Disorder Rating Scale ... **[b] linding** is intended to minimize potential biases resulting from differences in management, treatment, or assessment of patients, or interpretation of results that could arise as a result of subject or investigator knowledge of the assigned treatment. Thus, because the study was not **blinded**, the findings for Focalin XR are not unbiased and the study can not be relied upon as substantial evidence in support of the claims.

c. FDA's Warning Letters About Randomization

The following Warning Letter describes the bizarre situation where an investigator had performed randomization after (not before) performing a medical procedure on the study subjects. The letter reminded the investigator that the Clinical Study Protocol required randomization before performing the medical procedure. Citing 21 CFR §312.60, the letter complained that (63):

> [y]ou failed to ensure that the investigation was conducted according to the investigational plan ... [s]ubjects were randomized postoperatively, as opposed to preoperatively, in violation of the protocol ... randomization was to take place following screening on Day 0, a day prior to surgery ... [i]n your June 3, 2009 written response, you stated that

this violation occurred due to a misunderstanding of the protocol.

Another Warning Letter issued the same complaint. The letter reveals that the Clinical Study Protocol appropriately required randomization before (not after) surgery, as is evident from the comment about the "Protocol Deviation." It is likely that this letter and the following letter were from the same clinical trial because, although the letters were issued to different physicians, both letters were issued to physicians living in Alabama, and the letters were dated about 1 week apart from each other. The letter complained that (64):

> [y]ou failed to ensure that the investigation was conducted according to the investigational plan ... [t]he protocol required that randomization take place following screening on Day 0, one day prior to surgery. However, subjects at your site were randomized postoperatively, as opposed to preoperatively, in violation of the protocol. In a Protocol Deviations report dated May 30, 2007, your site notified the Institutional Review Board (IRB) that subjects 5001 through 5139 were randomized post-surgery.

VIII. INTERACTIVE VOICE RESPONSE SYSTEMS

An Interactive Voice Response System (IVRS) can be used to screen and register study subjects, to ensure that only persons signing the consent form are registered, and for managing data from study subjects during the entire clinical trial. IVRSs enable remote site

---

[62]Warning letter to Sue Duvall (no letter no.). Rrom Robert Dean, Division of Drug Marketing, Advertising, and Communications, U.S. Food and Drug Administration; September 25, 2008.

[63]Warning Letter No. 10-HFD-45-11-03. From Dr. Leslie K. Ball, MD, Office of Compliance, CDER, U.S. Food and Drug Administration; November 24, 2009.

[64]Warning Letter No. 10-HFD-45-12-01. From Dr. Leslie K. Ball, MD, Office of Compliance, CDER, U.S. Food and Drug Administration; December 3, 2009.

randomization of new subjects. IVRSs are a tool where the telephone, or internet, is used to input information. In subject recruitment through an IVRS, potential subjects can telephone a toll-free number, and answer a series of questions to determine their potential eligibility, for example, questions on demographics (65). The user listens to prerecorded prompts that list the various options available or that request responses to particular questions (66). If the IVRS finds the subject is eligible then it records subject details and stores the information in the database, while those failing may be given information about how to seek further advice for their condition. Then the IVRS generates an automatic alert to inform the study site or trained telephone caller to contact the subject. To reiterate, IVRSs enable the screening of subjects according to a list of inclusion/exclusion criteria, stratification and randomization of treatment assignments, and the collection of patient-reported outcomes (67). IVRSs can be used for obtaining informed consent, registering subjects, randomizing study subjects, managing patient diaries, and keeping track of the number of enrolled subjects (68).

A vivid and instructive account of how an IVRS can be used is found in the following report of a clinical trial in oncology. Thus, "simple stratified randomization with permuted blocks of size 4 was used by the sponsor to create a prospective randomization schedule that was provided to the vendor for the telephone-based interactive voice recognition system (IVRS). Random assignment of eligible patients was performed by designated personnel at each participating site using the IVRS in a double-blind fashion such that the investigator, sponsor, and patient did not know the treatment assignment" (69).

In addition to use for screening study subjects, enrollment, and randomization, IVRSs are used to provide up-to-the-minute information on the number of subjects randomized, picking up medication, withdrawing from the study, completing the study (70), monitoring adverse events, medication compliance, emergency code breaking, and managing the study medication supply chain (71).

The following concerns interactions between the IVRS and study subjects. IVRSs accommodate both incoming and outgoing calls (72,73). This concerns outgoing calls initiated by study subjects. Participants call a telephone number that directs them to a prerecorded survey, and they respond to each survey question by

[65]Stone J. Conducting clinical research: a practical guide for physicians, nurses, study coordinators, and investigators. 2nd ed. Cumberland, MD: Mountainside MD Press; 2010. p. 156, 517.

[66]Byrom B. Using IVRS in clinical trial management. Appl. Clin. Trials 2002;36–42.

[67]Syntellect, Inc., 16610 North Black Canyon Highway, Phoenix, AZ.

[68]Premier Research, Centre Square West, Philadelphia, PA.

[69]McDermott DF, Sosman JA, Gonzalez R, et al. Double-blind randomized phase II study of the combination of sorafenib and dacarbazine in patients with advanced melanoma: a report from the 11715 Study Group. J. Clin. Oncol. 2008;26:2178–85.

[70]Byrom B. Using IVRS in clinical trial management. Appl. Clin. Trials 2002;36–42.

[71]Abu-Hasaballah K, James A, Aseltine Jr RH. Lessons and pitfalls of interactive voice response in medical research. Contemp. Clin. Trials 2007;28:593–602.

[72]Lee H, Friedman ME, Cukor P, Ahern D. Interactive voice response system (IVRS) in health care services. Nurs. Outlook 2003;51:277–83.

[73]Abu-Hasaballah K, James A, Aseltine Jr RH. Lessons and pitfalls of interactive voice response in medical research. Contemp. Clin. Trials 2007;28:593–602.

pressing a number on the telephone keypad or giving voice responses that are recorded. Study participants dialing a local or toll-free number that has been assigned to the IVRS can initiate incoming calls. The system may respond to an incoming call by administering a survey. In some studies, access to the script is restricted to only those participants who supply a valid pass code. But in the recruitment phase of a study, the IVRS can be programmed to collect information to uniquely identify the participant through the combination of a zip code, last four digits of social security number, and birth date, to create a unique subject identifier (74). An interesting observation regarding use of IVRS by study subjects, is that subjects using an IVRS have been found to provide more honest answers when disclosing sensitive information, such as alcohol and drug use, sexual function, and psychological function, as compared to calls to a live interviewer (75).

Outgoing calls are initiated by the IVRS, which automatically calls participants' telephone numbers according to a predetermined schedule. Outgoing calls are used to support the study protocol and enhance compliance.

For example, the IVRS can call study participants and remind them to take study drugs, or to call the IVRS to take their scheduled interview (76).

A side-by-side study of diaries kept by study subjects, comparing paper diaries and diaries kept by IVRS, revealed lack of bias (for either type of data collection) and that data collected by both methods was highly correlated ($P < 0.001$) (77). In a study of health-related quality-of-life information collected in an oncology clinical trial, Lundy et al. (78), found data collected by a paper form and by IVRS to be equivalent. In a clinical study collecting data on health-related quality of life, Moore et al. (79) determined that IVRS telephone calls required an average of about 4 min to complete. It is interesting to note, however, that in an allergy clinical trial that collected data by paper forms (diary card) and by IVRS, Weiler et al. (80) determined that study subjects overwhelmingly preferred using the paper forms. One reason is that they can be filled out while waiting in an automobile.

Another issue relating to recruitment, as well as to the entire clinical trial, is confidentiality. Clinical trials conducted in the United

[74]Abu-Hasaballah K, James A, Aseltine Jr RH. Lessons and pitfalls of interactive voice response in medical research. Contemp. Clin. Trials 2007;28:593–602.

[75]Lee H, Friedman ME, Cukor P, Ahern D. Interactive voice response system (IVRS) in health care services. Nurs. Outlook 2003;51:277–83.

[76]Abu-Hasaballah K, James A, Aseltine Jr RH. Lessons and pitfalls of interactive voice response in medical research. Contemp. Clin. Trials 2007;28:593–602.

[77]Kelly MD, Young DY, Lane NM, Shames RS. Validation of electronic versus paper subject diaries. J. Allergy Clin. Immunol. 2004;113(Suppl.):S320 (abstract).

[78]Lundy JJ, Coons SJ, Aaronson NK. Testing the measurement equivalence of paper and interactive voice response (IVR) versions of the EORTC QLQ-C30. Abstract PCN85. ISPOR 11th Annual European Congress. November 8–11, 2008, Athens, Greece.

[79]Moore HK, Wohlreich MM, Wilson MG, et al. Using daily interactive voice response assessments: to measure onset of symptom improvement with duloxetine. Psychiatry (Edgmont) 2007;4:30–8.

[80]Weiler K, Christ AM, Woodworth GG, Weiler RL, Weiler JM. Quality of patient-reported outcome data captured using paper and interactive voice response diaries in an allergic rhinitis study: is electronic data capture really better? Ann. Allergy Asthma Immunol. 2004;92:335–9.

States are subject to the Health Insurance Portability and Accountability Act (HIPAA), which provides privacy and security safeguards to protect the confidentiality of personal health information of study subjects (81).

The following concerns use of IVRS to manage the supply chain. Kuznetsova (82) described use of IVRS to distribute drugs in a clinical trial, that is, in studies where drug bottles are labeled with unique drug codes, where codes refer, for example, to placebo, 1 mg active drug tablets, and 2 mg active drug tablets. Labeling the bottles with the codes allows appropriate bottles to be sent to any subject for any visit when this type of drug is supposed to be dispensed. IVRS can be used to dispense medication packs to subjects, and to maintain appropriate stock levels at the drug distribution depot, that is, at a pharmaceutical company or at an external packing and distribution agency, and at the study site (83). The IVR system dispenses the medication packs, identifies when the stock at the site for that treatment has fallen to a predefined minimum, and sends a request to the drug distribution depot for additional supplies to be sent to the site. An IVRS can be used to allocate kit numbers to subjects, to allow for stock subtractions to be made and monitor inventories of all medications remaining at each study site (84). In managing clinical supplies, the IVRS also keeps track of drug expiration dates (85). These tasks allows for conducting the trial with a minimum supply of medicines, avoiding overstocking, and for resupplying drugs on a just-in-time basis (86). Additional types of information that can be captured by an IVRS include rate of site initiation (percentage of sites that have initial supplies requested, sites per month initiated), rate of recruitment (over the study to date, over each previous month, by country and by study), screening failure rate, and tracking of end points that have been reached, for example, number of deaths, number of successful completers (87).

The following excerpt from a Clinical Study Protocol on prostate cancer outlines part of the enrollment procedure for study subjects that includes use of an IVRS. The excerpt reveals the steps of screening, completing a randomization authorization form, using an IVRS for doing the randomization, and assigning a drug

[81]Hathaway CR, Manthei JR, Haas JB, Scherer CA. Looking abroad: clinical drug trials. Food Rug Law J. 2008;63:673−81.

[82]Kuznetsova OM. Why permutation is even more important in IVRS drug codes schedule generation than in patient randomization schedule generation. Control. Clin. Trials 2001;22:69−71.

[83]Byrom B. Using IVRS in clinical trial management. Appl. Clin. Trials 2002;36−42.

[84]Clinical Trial Services. Improving clinical trial supply using existing tools. Almac Group, Ltd., 20 Seagoe Industrial Estate, Craigavon, UK.

[85]Premier Research, Centre Square West, Philadelphia, PA.

[86]Clinical Trial Services. Improving clinical trial supply using existing tools. Almac Group, Ltd., 20 Seagoe Industrial Estate, Craigavon, UK.

[87]Futcher A. Qualitative and quantitative benefits of IVR and IWR clinical trials. Pharmaceutical Visions, Highbury House Communications PLC, London (date and volume not available), p. 51−54.

bottle number and patient ID number to the subjects (88,89):

> After a patient is screened and the Investigator determines that the patient is eligible for enrollment, the site staff will complete the Randomization Authorization Form and fax it to [Sponsor] or designee. [Sponsor] or designee will approve the patient's enrollment in writing. Once the site has approval, the patient may undergo his Day 1 visit. After confirming that all inclusion criteria and no exclusion criteria are met on Day 1, the site will randomize the patient to treatment by using the Interactive Voice/Web Recognition Service (IVRS/IWRS) during the patient's Day 1 visit. The IVRS/IWRS will assign the patient a study drug bottle number available at the site according to the randomization code. The IVRS/IWRS will also assign the Patient ID Number.

IX. CONCLUDING REMARKS

This chapter focuses on methodological aspects of clinical trials, rather than on medical or scientific aspects. Proper study design of the most common type of clinical trial, that is, the randomized, double-blinded clinical trial, requires a knowledge of techniques used for enrolling and screening study subjects, allocation, randomization, and ensuring allocation concealment and ensuring that blinding is maintained. It might also be prudent to include, in the Clinical Study Protocol, guidance on how to respond when a subject is inadvertently unblinded, and guidance on how to unblind a subject when the subject experiences a serious adverse event.

---

[88]Clinical Research Protocol. Study Title: PREVAIL: A Multinational Phase 3, Randomized, Double-Blind, Placebo-Controlled Efficacy and Safety Study of Oral MDV3100 in Chemotherapy-Naïve Patients withProgressive Metastatic Prostate Cancer Who Have Failed Androgen Deprivation Therapy Protocol No: MDV3100-03.

[89]Clinical Study Protocol available as supplement to, Beer TM, Armstrong AJ, Rathkopf DE, et al. Enzalutamide in metastatic prostate cancer before chemotherapy. New Engl. J. Med. 2014;371:424–33.

Placebo Arm as Part of Clinical Trial Design

I. INTRODUCTION

The topic of trial design was initiated in this textbook by descriptions of the schema. This topic was continued by an account of specialized features of the schema, such as the run-in period and stratification. This chapter concerns yet another specialized feature of trial design, namely, the placebo arm. Placebo group and the "standard of care" are concepts that each raise ethical issues, and for this reason "standard of care" is defined in this chapter. The term "standard of care" is widely used in US Food and Drug Administration (FDA) submissions and in medical publications.

Clinical trials may be designed as single-arm studies, or as two-arm studies, where one arm is the study drug arm and the other is the control arm. In single-arm studies, each patient serves as his own control. Alternatively, a single-arm study can be one where the control is a population of study subjects that serves as a historical control. Where there is a separate control arm, the control treatment may take

the form of an active control, a placebo, or no treatment.

Where the goal of a clinical study is to compare a new drug with an existing drug, for example, to show that the new drug has greater efficacy, a better safety profile, or both, then the appropriate control arm is one that contains an active control, that is, a comparator drug.

But there are many reasons to use a placebo and not use an active control drug. Use of an active control arm introduces elements of uncertainty into the clinical trial. First, the course of the disease, in its untreated state, is inherently uncertain, and differs somewhat from subject to subject. Use of an active control drug adds another layer of uncertainty. Daugherty et al. (1) emphasize the point that a placebo group is especially important for clinical trials on disorders that fluctuate in intensity, that is, spontaneously wax and wane, or where the disorder is characterized by an unpredictable outcome. Disorders of this type include a type of multiple sclerosis (MS) called

---

[1]Daugherty CK, Ratain MJ, Emanuel EJ, Farrell AT, Schilsky RL. Ethical, scientific, and regulatory perspectives regarding the use of placebos in cancer clinical trials. J. Clin. Oncol. 2008;26:1371—8.

Clinical Trials.
DOI: http://dx.doi.org/10.1016/B978-0-12-804217-5.00007-2

relapsing—remitting MS, and chemotherapy-induced nausea and vomiting. Second, the compliance of various study subjects with the active drug may differ from subject to subject. Third, the response of the disease to the active control drug will differ somewhat, from subject to subject. Moreover, where there does not exist a suitable comparator drug, the clinical trial may be compelled to use a placebo.

Placebos may be associated with a placebo-effect. Placebo-effect refers to the situation where the act of taking the placebo (and not the chemicals in the placebo) has efficacy against a disorder. Placebo effects have been documented for disorders such as pain, asthma, and hypertension, but the statistical significance of these effects is slight (2,3).

Tumor response in the placebo arm is sometimes found in clinical trials on renal cancer, because this particular type of cancer can spontaneously go into remission (4). Where the goal of an oncology clinical trial is to assess the efficacy of drugs that prevent nausea or vomiting (antiemetics) or to prevent pain, placebos can have a slight effect (5). However, in oncology clinical trials, there cannot be any placebo effect on the rate of tumor growth (6). Temple (7) finds that, in the context of oncology clinical trials, there is little or no placebo effect in terms of endpoints such as pain, appetite, or performance status.

II. HAWTHORNE EFFECT

A phenomenon related to the placebo effect is the Hawthorne effect. The Hawthorne effect refers to responses, in study subjects, to mere attention paid by clinical trial personnel to study subjects (8,9). Mere attention can take the form of telephone calls from clinical personnel to study subjects. The placebo effect and the Hawthorne effect may influence the subject's responses to health-related quality-of-life (HRQoL) tools. HRQoL tools are questionnaires that are used in clinical trials in oncology and other chronic diseases, and that measure a variety of subjective parameters. The chapters on HRQoL tools reveal that, where a clinical trial compares study drug and an active control, and where the efficacy responses for both study arms are identical or nearly identical, results from HRQoL can tip the scale, in persuading the FDA that the study drug is superior to the established standard of care.

It is interesting to point out that a Clinical Study Protocol mentioned the Hawthorne effect. This mention occurred in the Protocol, in a discussion of methods for ensuring that study subjects complied with the Protocol's instructions for taking their medication. The Protocol stated that, "Finally, all monitoring methods are susceptible to the Hawthorne effect, i.e., compliance being improved because

[2]Hróbjartsson A, Gøtzsche PC. Is the placebo powerless? An analysis of clinical trials comparing placebo with no treatment. New Engl. J. Med. 2001;344:1594−602.

[3]Hróbjartsson A, Gøtzsche PC. Is the placebo powerless? Update of a systematic review with 52 new randomized trials comparing placebo with no treatment. J. Intern. Med. 2004;256:91−100.

[4]Chvetzoff G, Tannock IF. Placebo effects in oncology. J. Natl Cancer Inst. 2003;95:19−29.

[5]Chvetzoff G, Tannock IF. Placebo effects in oncology. J. Natl Cancer Inst. 2003;95:19−29.

[6]Wang L. In clinical trials and in the clinic, what is the placebo's effect? J. Natl Cancer Inst. 2003;95:6−7.

[7]Temple RJ. Implications of effects in placebo groups. J. Natl Cancer Inst. 2003;95:2−3.

[8]Johansson B, Brandberg Y, Hellbom M, et al. Health-related quality of life and distress in cancer patients: results from a large randomised study. Br. J. Cancer 2008;99:1975−83.

[9]de Craen AJM, Kaptchuk TH, Tijssen JG, Kleijnen J. Placebos and placebo effects in medicine: historical overview. J. R. Soc. Med. 1999;92:511−5.

the patients know that their drug use is being monitored." The Protocol was published as a supplement to a medical journal article (10).

III. THE NO-TREATMENT ARM

Clinical trials sometimes include a no-treatment arm, that is, an arm where subjects do not receive study drug and do not receive any placebo. No-treatment arms are required for a unique type of clinical study, that is, studies that characterize the placebo effect. Clinical trial that is configured to study the placebo effect can use three arms: (1) study drug arm, (2) placebo arm, and (3) no-treatment arm. In a survey of three-arm clinical studies of this type, Krogsbøll et al. (11) arrived at the conclusion that, at least for some disorders, it might be erroneous to ascribe improvement to a "placebo effect." This conclusion is supported by the fact that, at least for some disorders, the degree of improvement in the placebo arm and no-treatment arm, were similar to each other. Disorders where spontaneous improvement (no-treatment arm) and improvement in the placebo arm were similar, are nausea, depression, acute pain, cigarette smoking, and phobia. Nausea, depression, and pain are common adverse events in oncology clinical trials. Hence, in evaluating data on these adverse events, the medical writer might consider refraining from concluding that there was a "placebo effect."

IV. PHYSICAL ASPECTS OF THE PLACEBO

Where the study drug is a pill, liquid, powder, solution, slurry, suspension, suppository, topical cream, aerosol, and the like, the placebo (or active control drug) should always be manufactured in a way that impairs the ability of the patient, medical personnel, and clerical personnel, from telling the difference between the study drug, active control drug, and placebo. This statement also applies to degradation products of the drug and placebo. With storage over the course of many months, the study drug or placebo may acquire an altered color or physical characteristic. In a study of pills, including placebo pills, Camarco et al. (12) discloses the properties of mouth feel and friability. Mouth feel encompasses a gritty feeling resulting from large particles used to manufacture the pill, and a gummy feeling resulting from a gel-like consistency upon contact of the pill with water.

The placebo and study drug should be indistinguishable in terms of packaging, labels, size, shape, opacity, coatings, viscosity, color, smell, flavor, and route of administration (13). Where the study drug or active control are commercially available, it is not likely that a corresponding placebo will also be available, since pharmaceutical companies have little incentive to manufacture placebos on the small quantity required by clinical trials (14). Because of the need to ensure blinding, the

[10]Albert RK, Connett J, Bailey WC, et al. Azithromycin for prevention of exacerbations of COPD. New Engl. J. Med. 2011;365:689−98.

[11]Krogsbøll LT, Hróbjartsson A, Gøtzsche PC. Spontaneous improvement in randomised clinical trials: meta-analysis of three-armed trials comparing no treatment, placebo and active intervention. BMC Med. Res. Methodol. 2009;9:1.

[12]Camarco W, Ray D, Druffner A. Selecting superdisintegrants for orally disintegrating tablet formulations. Pharm. Technol. 2006;(Oct. Suppl.):5 pp.

[13]Monkhouse DC, Rhodes CT. Drug products for clinical trials: an international guide to formulation, production, quality control. New York: Marcel Dekker, Inc.; 1998.

[14]Wan M, et al. Blinding in pharmacological trials: the devil is in the details. Arch. Dis. Child. 2013;98:656−9.

Sponsor might also need to custom-manufacture the formulation of the study drug or active control drug, for example, by using a new excipient to mask the taste of the drug. The technique of over-encapsulation is sometimes use to ensure that the study drug and control both have the same shape and size. Over-encapsulation is hiding a tablet or capsule inside an opaque capsule shell (often involving the addition of a backfilled excipient to prevent rattling), so that the contents are concealed, producing products that are visually identical. A potential problem is that over-encapsulation can increase the size of the drug, to the extent that it impairs swallowing (15).

V. ACTIVE PLACEBO

Some drugs have obvious side effects. Thus, where an investigator or study subject has some knowledge of the expected side effects, it will be easy to guess whether the administered material is a drug or a placebo. For this reason, the pharmaceutical community has devised the *active placebo*. An active placebo is a placebo with properties that mimic the symptoms or side effects, for example, dry mouth or sweating, that might otherwise reveal whether any given subject is in the study drug group or placebo group (16,17).

VI. SUBJECTS IN THE PLACEBO ARM MAY RECEIVE BEST SUPPORTIVE CARE OR PALLIATIVE CARE

Best supportive care (BSC) and palliative care are treatments used in the context of clinical trials, as well as outside of clinical trials, for example, in a hospice. Typically, BSC and palliative care include pain control, emotional support, and efforts to maximize HRQoL. These types of care may include treatments intended to maximize quality of life, pain control, antibiotics, analgesics, antiemetics, and treatment of coughs (18).

The National Consensus Project for Quality Palliative Care, an organization that devotes itself to promoting palliative care, defines palliative care. This definition, in part, is: "Palliative care is operationalized through effective management of pain and other distressing symptoms, while incorporating psychosocial and spiritual care with consideration of patient/family needs, preferences, values, beliefs, and culture" (19). The above organization focuses its efforts on disorders, such as Alzheimer disease, Parkinson disease, dyspnea, MS, heart failure, and cancer, in the context of people in the final months or weeks of life.

The definitions of BSC and of palliative care are sometimes not clearly set forth in medical

[15]Wan M, et al. Blinding in pharmacological trials: the devil is in the details. Arch. Dis. Child. 2013;98:656–9.

[16]Schulz KF, Chalmers I, Altman DG. The landscape and lexicon of blinding in randomized trials. Ann. Intern. Med. 2002;136:254–9.

[17]Moncrieff J, Wessely S, Hardy R. Active placebos versus antidepressants for depression. Cochrane database of systematic reviews 2004, Issue 1. Art. No.: CD003012. 10.1002/14651858.CD003012.pub2.

[18]Zafar SY, Currow D, Abernethy AP. Defining best supportive care. J. Clin. Oncol. 2008;26:5139–40.

[19]National Consensus Project for Quality Palliative Care. Clinical practice guidelines for quality. 2nd ed. Pittsburgh, PA: Palliative Care; 2009.

publications. Zafar et al. (20,21) suggest that the medical writers ensure that these types of care be detailed in any publications or reports. Prof. R.L. Schilsky (22) finds that:

> [m]ost palliative care experts feel that PC [palliative care] is a component of cancer care from the time of diagnosis until death, and encompasses essentially all aspects of medical and psychological management directed at symptom control and improving QoL. Best supportive care does the same but the term often refers to palliative care applied primarily when active anti-cancer treatment is no longer being applied. Thus while newly diagnosed patients being treated with curative intent should receive appropriate palliative care as a component of the their overall treatment, patients who have exhausted all known treatment options and choose to participate in a clinical trial of an unproven new agent might be randomized to receive best supportive care. Admittedly a very fine distinction between the two.

BSC has been the sole treatment for trial in a number of clinical trials in oncology, as documented below. Unfortunately, the following also demonstrates that the nature of BSC is sometimes not disclosed.

In a trial of *lung cancer* by Shepherd et al. (23), subjects in the control arm received only BSC. BSC was disclosed as "[p]atients randomized to the BSC arm were treated with whichever therapy was judged to be appropriate by the treating physician. This treatment could have included treatment with antibiotics, analgesic drugs, transfusions, and palliative radiotherapy."

In a clinical trial on *mesothelioma* by Jassem et al. (24), subjects in the control arm received only BSC, where this took the form of:

> Patients on the BSC arm received treatment administered with the intent to maximize quality of life without a specific antineoplastic regimen. This included antibiotics, analgesics, antiemetics, thoracentesis, pleurodesis, blood transfusions, nutritional support, and focal external-beam radiation for control of pain, cough, dyspnea, or hemoptysis. BSC excluded surgery, immunotherapy, anticancer hormonal therapy, systemic chemotherapy, and radiotherapy (except palliative).

In a study of *glioblastoma*, Keime-Guibert et al. (25), provided the control group with supportive care only, where supportive care was defined as, "[s]upportive care consisted of treatment with corticosteroids and anticonvulsant agents, physical and psychological support, and management by a palliative care team."

In a trial of *urothelial tract cancer* by Bellmunt et al. (26), subjects in the control arm

---

[20]Zafar SY, Currow D, Abernethy AP. Defining best supportive care. J. Clin. Oncol. 2008;26:5139−40.

[21]Cherny NI, Abernethy AP, Strasser F, Sapir R, Currow D, Zafar SY. Improving the methodologic and ethical validity of best supportive care studies in oncology: lessons from a systematic review. J. Clin. Oncol. 2009;27:5476−86.

[22]Schilsky RL. E-mail of October 10, 2010.

[23]Shepherd FA, Dancey J, Ramlau R, et al. Prospective randomized trial of docetaxel versus best supportive care in patients with non-small-cell lung cancer previously treated with platinum-based chemotherapy. J. Clin. Oncol. 2000;18:2095−103.

[24]Jassem J, Ramlau R, Santoro A, et al. Phase III trial of pemetrexed plus best supportive care compared with best supportive care in previously treated patients with advanced malignant pleural mesothelioma. J. Clin. Oncol. 2008;26:1698−704.

[25]Keime-Guibert F, Chinot O, Taillandier L, et al. Radiotherapy for glioblastoma in the elderly. New Engl. J. Med. 2007;356:1527−35.

[26]Bellmunt J, Théodore C, Demkov T, et al. Phase III trial of vinflunine plus best supportive care compared with best supportive care alone after a platinum-containing regimen in patients with advanced transitional cell carcinoma of the urothelial tract. J. Clin. Oncol. 2009;27:4454−61.

received only BSC, where this was described as, "BSC was administered according to institutional standards (including palliative radiotherapy, antibiotics, analgesics, corticosteroids, and transfusion)."

The above reports provide concrete statements, regarding what was BSC. In contrast, other disclosures of BSC are characterized by little or no detail, as is evident from the following.

In a study of *colorectal cancer* by Van Cutsem et al. (27), subjects in the control arm received only BSC, where this care was described as, "BSC was defined as the best palliative care per investigator excluding antineoplastic agents."

In a study of *liver cancer* by Barbare et al. (28), subjects in the control arm received only BSC, as described, "[a]ll patients in the study group and in the control group received best supportive care and appropriate management of the liver disease as usually practiced in the individual centers."

survival, and HRQoL. Where HRQoL is one of the endpoints, and where the control arm receives only BSC, it is critical that the study drug arm also receives BSC. To provide an instructive example, in a study of pancreatic cancer, Glimelius et al. (29) used HRQoL as one of their endpoints. The control arm received BSC only. These authors were careful to state that both study arms had received BSC, that is, the study drug arm and also the control arm received BSC. Interference of BSC with the endpoint of HRQoL has been documented in the clinical trial of Smith et al. (30), "[o]ur data did not show improved quality of life associated with ... therapy, possibly owing to the high proportion of patients with advanced disease receiving palliative care." Data collected on quality of life can be a deciding factor, in comparing efficacy and safety of the study drug group and control group (31).

VII. CLASH BETWEEN BSC AND THE ENDPOINT OF HRQoL

Typically, clinical trials in oncology include the endpoints of objective response, overall

VIII. ETHICS OF PLACEBOS

The following provides a context, when contemplating the ethics of placebos. In a classic book on study design, E.B. Wilson (32) wrote that, "[t]he use of controls in medical and other researches introduces serious moral

[27]Van Cutsem E, Peeters M, Siena S, et al. Open-label phase III trial of panitumumab plus best supportive care compared with best supportive care alone in patients with chemotherapy-refractory metastatic colorectal cancer. J. Clin. Oncol. 2007;25:1658–64.

[28]Barbare JC, Bouché O, Bonnetain F, et al. Randomized controlled trial of tamoxifen in advanced hepatocellular carcinoma. J. Clin. Oncol. 2005;23:4338–46.

[29]Glimelius B, Hoffman K, Sjödén PO, et al. Chemotherapy improves survival and quality of life in advanced pancreatic and biliary cancer. Ann. Oncol. 1996;7:593–600.

[30]Smith Jr RE, Aapro MS, Ludwig H, et al. Darbepoetin alpha for the treatment of anemia in patients with active cancer not receiving chemotherapy or radiotherapy: results of a phase III, multicenter, randomized, double-blind, placebo-controlled study. J. Clin. Oncol. 2008;26:1040–50.

[31]Efficace F, Bottomley A, Osoba D, et al. Beyond the development of health-related quality-of-life (HRQOL) measures: a checklist for evaluating HRQOL outcomes in cancer clinical trials—does HRQOL evaluation in prostate cancer research inform clinical decision making? J. Clin. Oncol. 2003;21:3502–11.

[32]Wilson EB. An introduction to scientific research. New York: Dover Publications, Inc.; 1952. p. 40.

questions. It may be questioned whether it is right to decide by the toss of a coin whether to use one treatment or another on a given patients." In continuing, the author further found that, "the history of medicine is full of fallacious or actually dangerous treatments firmly believed in … and then discarded … because of the gradual realization that the original treatment was ineffective" (33).

The following bullet points disclose reasons for considering a placebo group to be ethical:

- Without a suitable control group, such as a placebo group, it might not be possible to determine efficacy and safety of the drug, not be possible to acquire approval, and not be possible to provide patients with an approved drug. The term *approval* refers to a drug approved by the FDA, the Council for International Organization of Medical Sciences (CIOMS), or the European Medicines Agency (EMA). Without regulatory approval, it will not be possible for the public to have access to a new type of drug.
- According to the FDA's Guidance for Industry, "In cases where an available treatment is known to *prevent* serious harm, such as death or irreversible morbidity in the study population, it is generally inappropriate to use a placebo control … [i]n other situations, where there is no serious harm, it is generally considered ethical to ask patients to participate in a placebo-controlled trial, even if they may experience discomfort as a result, provided the setting is

non-coercive and patients are fully informed about available therapies and the consequences of delaying treatment" (34,35). This account from the FDA identifies situations where a placebo may be unethical, and also situations where a placebo may be ethical.

- Including a placebo group ensures that the investigator has a firm grounding or an anchor to determine assay sensitivity. In other words, if the clinical trial has two arms, the study drug arm and an active control arm, the following situation sometimes occurs. The situation is that the study drug fails to work, and the active control fails to work. When this situation occurs, the investigator will likely conclude that the study drug works about as well as the active control drug. But this conclusion will be in error. To avoid this error, the FDA recommends that a placebo group be included. In other words, in the situation where it is expected that the active control drug will fail for the entire population of control subjects, for example in clinical trials on antidepressants, a placebo is ethically justified (36).
- Clinical studies are voluntary, in contrast, for example, to certain vaccines (37) or to military service. The study subjects signed a consent form that disclosed the risks of the study, including the fact that the subject might be in the placebo arm. The consent forms set forth the condition that signing

[33]Wilson EB. An Introduction to scientific research. New York: Dover Publications, Inc.; 1952. p. 40.

[34]U.S. Department of Health and Human Services. Food and Drug Administration. Guidance for industry. Non-inferiority clinical trials; March 2010.

[35]International Conference on Harmonization (ICH) guidance E10. Choice of control group and related issues in clinical trials.

[36]U.S. Department of Health and Human Services. Food and Drug Administration. Guidance for industry. Non-inferiority clinical trials; March 2010.

[37]Pickering LK, Baker CJ, Freed GL, et al. Immunization programs for infants, children, adolescents, and adults: clinical practice guidelines by the Infectious Diseases Society of America. Clin. Infect. Dis. 2009;49:817−40.

the form and participating in the clinical trial are entirely voluntary (38,39,40,41).

- The consent form is reviewed and approved by an independent ethics committee, that is, the Institutional Review Board (IRB) (42,43). In other words, the fact that a body of experts that is independent from the study sponsor considers the clinical trial to be ethical, lends support to the specific argument that the placebo is ethical. Consent forms must also comply with the standards set forth in standards, such as those set forth by the Nuremberg Code (44), the Declaration of Helsinki (45,46), and the Belmont Report (47).
- Placebo groups are not without any kind of treatment. Placebo groups may receive treatment in the form of BSC or palliative care. In commentary about oncology clinical trials, Daugherty et al. (48) wrote that, "[f]or the trial to be ethical, patients assigned to the placebo arm must also receive best supportive care ... clinical trials that include best supportive care should carefully delineate the elements of such care, including consultation with appropriate experts."
- Placebos do not have toxic effects because they are manufactured from inert ingredients (49). In contrast, study drugs often produce adverse drug reactions.
- The FDA has recognized a clinical trial study design that includes an *early escape* (50). Clinical trials in oncology, for example, have a number of endpoints, such as disease progression and survival time. Disease

[38]Paasche-Orlow MK, Taylor HA, Brancati FL. Readability standards for informed-consent forms as compared with actual readability. New Engl. J. Med. 2003;348:721−6.

[39]Simon CM, Siminoff LA, Kodish ED, Burant C. Comparison of the informed consent process for randomized clinical trials in pediatric and adult oncology. J. Clin. Oncol. 2004;22:2708−17.

[40]Russell FM, Carapetis JR, Liddle H, Edwards T, Ruff TA, Devitt J. A pilot study of the quality of informed consent materials for Aboriginal participants in clinical trials. J. Med. Ethics 2005;31:490−4.

[41]Daugherty CK. Impact of therapeutic research on informed consent and the ethics of clinical trials: a medical oncology perspective. J. Clin. Oncol. 1999;17:1601−17.

[42]Sansone RA, McDonald S, Hanley P, Sellbom M, Gaither GA. The stipulations of one Institutional Review Board: a five year review. J. Med. Ethics 2004;30:308−10.

[43]Whitney SN, Alcser K, Schneider C, McCullough LB, McGuire AL, Volk RJ. Principal investigator views of the IRB system. Int. J. Med. Sci. 2008;5:68−72.

[44]Hutton JL, Eccles MP, Grimshaw JM. Ethical issues in implementation research: a discussion of the problems in achieving informed consent. Implement Sci. 2008;3:52.

[45]Luce JM. Informed consent for clinical research involving patients with chest disease in the United States. Chest 2009;135:1061−8.

[46]Carlson RV, Boyd KM, Webb DJ. The revision of the Declaration of Helsinki: past, present and future. Br. J. Clin. Pharmacol. 2004;57:695−713.

[47]Rice TW. The historical, ethical, and legal background of human-subjects research. Respir. Care 2008;53:1325−9.

[48]Daugherty CK, Ratain MJ, Emanuel EJ, Farrell AT, Schilsky RL. Ethical, scientific, and regulatory perspectives regarding the use of placebos in cancer clinical trials. J. Clin. Oncol. 2008;26:1371−8.

[49]Lichtenberg P, Heresco-Levy U, Nitzan U. The ethics of the placebo in clinical practice. J. Med. Ethics 2004;30:551−4.

[50]U.S. Department of Health and Human Services. Food and Drug Administration. Guidance for industry. Non-inferiority clinical trials; March 2010.

progression refers to a particular day, during the course of the clinical trial, when tumors increase beyond a prespecified size and number. This prespecified number is set forth by a set of criteria called the RECIST criteria. The ethical nature of a placebo in clinical trials is supported by the fact that the *early escape* trial design specifically allows subjects experiencing disease progression to discontinue placebo, and to begin taking an active drug. In this way, the *early escape* design allows study subjects to halt the placebo, and to take, instead, the study drug or the standard of care (51).

Early escape is sometimes an element in the study design. The following provides an example, from a clinical trial for infliximab, a drug used for treating an immune disorder. Specifically, this drug is used to treat Crohn disease. According to one of the FDA's paper trails used for approving this drug, "Patients who did not respond at 4 weeks after the initial blinded infusion were offered an open-label infusion of 10 mg/kg cA2 to be administered within 2 weeks of the 4 week evaluation visit" (52). (cA2 is an abbreviation for the study drug.)

- Clinical trials in oncology are designed with a number of endpoints, including surrogate endpoints that have potential use in predicting whether the drug actually works in improving survival. Clinical trials of all types, including those that involve a placebo arm, can be designed so that placebo subjects who meet one of the endpoints can convert to an active drug (53). This kind of trial design may be called a *cross-over* design. Use of a surrogate endpoint with a cross-over design can ethically justify use of a placebo.

- Where a clinical trial concerns a condition that is of a cosmetic nature, or a condition that presents only a mild threat to health and only mild discomfort (if untreated), the issue of placebo ethics is a mild or nonexistent issue. Temple and Ellenberg (54) listed the examples of clinical trials for baldness, or for short-term studies of allergic rhinitis, insomnia, anxiety, dermatoses, heartburn, or headaches.

- This is about lack of deception when the clinical trial evaluates a drug. In the context of medical treatments that are drugs (pills, injections), the physician will not be put into the position of deceiving any patient, and will not be in the position of deceiving the patients as a whole. This is in contrast to medical treatments that involve surgery. According to Horng and Miller (55), "[u]nlike pharmacologic placebos, sham procedures and surgery sometimes require that an investigator actively mislead participants into believing that the active intervention is being performed in order to maintain the blind and control for the

[51]Daugherty CK, Ratain MJ, Emanuel EJ, Farrell AT, Schilsky RL. Ethical, scientific, and regulatory perspectives regarding the use of placebos in cancer clinical trials. J. Clin. Oncol. 2008;26:1371−8.

[52]Matthews BG. Review of BLA submission 98-0012. Chimeric (human-murine) monoclonal antibody (cA2) to tumor necrosis factor for infiammatory bowel disease (Infliximab, Remicade™); July 10, 1998.

[53]Daugherty CK, Ratain MJ, Emanuel EJ, Farrell AT, Schilsky RL. Ethical, scientific, and regulatory perspectives regarding the use of placebos in cancer clinical trials. J. Clin. Oncol. 2008;26:1371−8.

[54]Temple R, Ellenberg SS. Placebo-controlled trials and active-control trials in the evaluation of new treatments. Part 1: Ethical and scientific issues. Ann. Intern. Med. 2000;133:455−63.

[55]Horng SH, Miller FG. Placebo-controlled procedural trials for neurological conditions. Neurotherapeutics 2007;4:531−6.

placebo effect." This particular example constitutes an argument that placebos in drug trials are not unethical.

The following summarizes reasons for doubting that a placebo group is ethical:

- Physicians are bound by the Hippocratic oath (56). This oath places the patient's best interests above the interests of the physician. It places the patient's interests above the interests of the sponsor of the clinical trial. In contrast, when contributing to a clinical trial, physicians are required to serve the interests of the sponsor, that is, a drug company. In this regard, physicians contributing to clinical trials have been called double agents (57).
- "In cases where an available treatment is known to prevent serious harm, such as death or irreversible morbidity in the study population, it is generally inappropriate to use a placebo control. Thus the use of placebos or untreated controls is nearly always unethical when therapy exists that has been shown to improve survival or decrease serious morbidity" (58).
- Many patients do not have enough scientific background to understand what is a placebo (59).
- Many people reading and signing a consent form are not likely to understand much of what is on the form. In view of the consistent findings of surveys that consent forms need to be written at the level of a 12-year-old, clinical trials managers have continued to issue consent forms written at a more advanced level (60,61,62,63,64,65).
- Where a clinical trial involves a new technique of surgery, the placebo will necessarily take the form of sham surgery. According to Horng and Miller (66), "sham surgery typically exposes subjects to the risk of an invasive procedure ... which may include hemorrhage and/or infection."
- Where a suitable active control is available, the FDA recommends against using a

[56] Coller BS. The physician-scientist, the state, and the oath: thoughts for our times. J. Clin. Invest. 2006;116:2567–70.

[57] Levine RJ. Clinical trials and physicians as double agents. Yale J. Biol. Med. 1992;65:65–74.

[58] Daugherty CK, Ratain MJ, Emanuel EJ, Farrell AT, Schilsky RL. Ethical, scientific, and regulatory perspectives regarding the use of placebos in cancer clinical trials. J. Clin. Oncol. 2008;26:1371–8.

[59] De Deyn PP, D'Hooge R. Placebos in clinical practice and research. J. Med. Ethics 1996;22:140–6.

[60] Davis TC, Holcombe RF, Berkel HJ, Pramanik S, Divers SG. Informed consent for clinical trials: a comparative study of standard versus simplified forms. J. Natl Cancer Inst. 1998;90:668–74.

[61] Flory J, Emanuel E. Interventions to improve research participants' understanding in informed consent for research: a systematic review. J. Am. Med. Assoc. 2004;292:1593–601.

[62] Stead M, Eadie D, Gordon D, Angus K. "Hello, hello—it's English I speak!": a qualitative exploration of patients' understanding of the science of clinical trials. J. Med. Ethics 2005;31:664–9.

[63] Paasche-Orlow MK, Taylor HA, Brancati FL. Readability standards for informed-consent forms as compared with actual readability. New Engl. J. Med. 2003;348:721–6.

[64] Beardsley E, Jefford M, Mileshkin L. Longer consent forms for clinical trials compromise patient understanding: so why are they lengthening? J. Clin. Oncol. 2007;25:e13–4.

[65] Coyne CA, Xu R, Raich P, et al. Randomized, controlled trial of an easy-to-read informed consent statement for clinical trial participation: a study of the Eastern Cooperative Oncology Group. J. Clin. Oncol. 2003;21:836–42.

[66] Horng SH, Miller FG. Placebo-controlled procedural trials for neurological conditions. Neurotherapeutics 2007;4:531–6.

placebo. In the FDA's Guidance for Industry for rheumatoid arthritis, what is recommended is that, "the availability of effective RA therapies and the shifting paradigm in the treatment of both early and established RA with a focus on early control of disease activity ... have provided a rationale for limiting the exposure of patients to placebo" (67).

To conclude, the issue of whether a placebo is appropriate for a given clinical trial needs to be decided on a case-by-case basis, and not on a per se basis.

IX. FDA's DECISION-MAKING PROCESS IN EVALUATING THE PLACEBO ARM

a. Introduction

At the time that the FDA provides its Approval Letter, the FDA also publishes its *Medical Reviews*, *Pharmacology Reviews*, and other reviews of the Sponsor's NDA or BLA. These reviews provide an accurate picture of the FDA's decision-making process. Guidance for using or interpreting placebos is provided by the following *Medical Reviews*.

b. Everolimus for Astrocytoma

This concerns a clinical trial that had a placebo control arm. The study drug was *everolimus* for astrocytoma, a type of brain cancer. This information is from NDA 203985, available on November 2015 on FDA's website. The *Medical Review* provides some very insightful comments as to the acceptability of the placebo control group. The most interesting of the reasons for ethical acceptability is that the cancer is a slow-growing tumor, and that the trial

design *permitted patients to crossover from placebo to the study drug*, at the first sign that the tumors were growing beyond a prespecified size. This prespecified size was established by way of the conventional meaning of the term "progression."

In the FDA reviewer's own words, the placebo was ethical for the following reasons:

- "The study protocol excluded enrollment of patients that required immediate surgical intervention."
- "Surgery was not considered an appropriate control arm in this population due to the potential for surgical morbidity."
- "There was no active pharmacologic comparator that had been shown benefit to patients ... at the time this study was initiated."
- "SEGA [subependymal giant cell astrocytoma] are slow-growing tumors, and [the clinical trial] ... permitted [placebo] patients to crossover at the first radiologic sign of progression."

c. Dasafinib for Chronic Myeloid Leukemia

This concerns a clinical trial on patients with chronic myeloid leukemia (CML). The following discloses the situation where there does not exist a suitable comparator drug, for use as an active-control, and where use of a *placebo would have been unethical*. When faced with this situation, the Sponsor may use a *single-arm study*, that is, a study design where there is no control arm. The information is from NDA 21986, from January 2015 of FDA's website. To view the detail of suitable comparator drugs, imatinib might be considered to be a suitable comparator, but all of the subjects enrolled in the dasafinib trial

[67]U.S. Department of Health and Human Services. Food and Drug Administration. Guidance for industry. Rheumatoid arthritis: developing drug products for treatment; May 2013 (11 pp.).

had already been found to be resistant to or intolerant to imatinib.

In the *Medical Review*, the FDA reviewer stated that the clinical trials "were uncontrolled single-arm studies, because there is no effective comparator drug, and because a placebo control is deemed to be unethical." The reviewer explained that "a *placebo control would be unethical*, because "patients with advanced stages of CML ... are known to not have spontaneous cytogenic or hematologic responses and *generally have short survival*."

In comments about single-arm clinical trials, Daugherty et al. (68) state that, "[i]n diseases where spontaneous remission ... are not observed, single-arm trials may be useful. A response rate (tumor size reduction) is considered a direct effect of the treatment as it is not usually observed in the untreated natural history of the disease."

d. Telbividine for Hepatitis B Virus

The following discloses the Sponsor's decision tree in deciding not to use a placebo arm, but instead to use an active-control arm. The following also reveals how the Sponsor chose among the candidate drugs for the active-control arm.

Although the statistical design of the clinical trial was that of a noninferiority trial, the Sponsor hoped to find that its drug was noninferior, and also superior, with respect to the active control drug. The information is from NDA 22011, from December 2013 of the FDA's website.

Design of the control arm was raised in the *Medical Review* of *telbivudine*, a drug for hepatitis B virus. The FDA reviewer provided the following timeline:

- *Lamivudine* for hepatitis B virus was FDA-approved in 1998.
- The Sponsor's meeting with FDA, conducted after the end of its phase II clinical trial, and before the phase III clinical trial on *telbivudine* for hepatitis B virus, was held on June 17, 2002.
- Another drug against hepatitis B virus (*adefovir*) was approved shortly after the end-of-phase II meeting, where this approval was granted on June 20, 2001.

The FDA reviewer stated that there were "difficulties associated with a placebo-control design" and that the Sponsor "agreed that an active-control design was acceptable." (Details on these difficulties were not disclosed in the *Medical Review*.) The reviewer pointed out that the only available active control was lamivudine, because of the fact that at the time of the end-of-phase II meeting, adefovir was not yet FDA approved.

In short, the trial design that was decided upon was a noninferiority trial, where the Sponsor's goal was to demonstrate that telbivudine was no worse than lamivudine by a prespecified noninferiority margin.

Evans (69) discloses two situations where use of a placebo may be unethical. The first is where a single-arm study is preferred over one with a placebo arm, and this is for clinical trials where, "spontaneous improvement in participants is not expected." The second situation, is for a noninferiority trial, where "a placebo is unethical due to the availability of a proven effective therapy."

Actually, placebos were, in fact, used in the clinical trial on telbivudine. Because the study drug arm received large pills (600 mg telbuvidine) and the active control arm received small pills (100 mg), it was the case

---

[68]Daugherty CK, et al. Ethical, scientific, and regulatory perspectives regarding the use of placebos in cancer clinical trials. J. Clin. Oncol. 2008;26:1371–8.

[69]Evans SR. Clinical trial structures. J. Exp. Stroke Transl. Med. 2010;3:8–18.

that the telbuvidine-treated subjects received telbuvidine plus a placebo resembling the active-control pill, and the active-control arm subjects received active-control pills plus a placebo resembling the telbuvidine pill. This type of trial design is called "double dummy." The desired effect of using the "double-dummy" technique was allocation concealment.

e. Correcting for the Placebo Effect—Aliskirin for Hypertension

This is from a clinical trial on *aliskirin* for hypertension. The information is from the *Medical Review* for NDA 21985, available from March 2015 on the FDA's website.

The primary endpoint in this clinical trial is *diastolic blood pressure* (DBP). The data included a figure (Fig. 7.1) (Fig. 12 in the *Medical Review*) and a table (Table 7.1) (Table 13 in the *Medical Review*). According to the FDA's *Medical Review*, the reductions in blood pressure were typically seen after 2 weeks of therapy, and maximal reductions in blood pressure occurred at 4 weeks of therapy. This time-course is evident in the figure (Fig. 7.1). Data from the placebo arm are in the top line (open diamonds). Data with the highest dose of the study drug (aliskiren) are the lowest line (open squares). The two intermediate lines are from the intermediate doses of study drug (150 and 300 mg).

The placebo effect is evident from the reductions in blood pressure occurring in the placebo arm of the various clinical trials, that were included in the NDA submission.

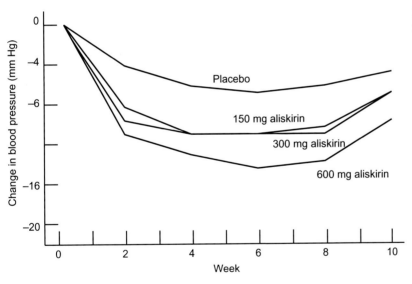

FIGURE 7.1 Sponsor's change from baseline in DBP.

TABLE 7.1 Reviewer's Placebo-Subtracted Changes from Baseline in Seated Trough Cuff DBP in the Five Pivotol Studies

Study	Median Group *n*	Placebo	Placebo-Subtracted DBP Change		
			150	300	600
2308	169 subjects	−4.9	−5.4	−6.2	−7.6

The FDA reviewer referred to placebo effects, writing that, "[p]lacebo effect may vary among subgroups as well as among studies." The reviewer referred to various clinical studies that were numbered, study 1201 [−3.2], study 2201 [−6.5], study 2203 [−8.4], study 2204 [−7.0], and study 2308 [−4.8]. The placebo effect on blood pressure is indicated by the bracketed number. The reviewer stated that, "[t]here do appear to be substantial differences in placebo effect by study."

In addition to pointing out differences in placebo effect in different studies, the reviewer referred to gender subgroups and racial subgroups. To these points, the reviewer wrote that, "[s]ome studies, but not all, show a substantial difference in placebo effect by gender." The FDA reviewer concluded that, "[h]ence it seems reasonable to me to do placebo correction by both study and gender." Regarding race, the FDA reviewer wrote, "[o]verall whites showed a higher placebo effect than blacks and Asians showed the lowest … estimates of placebo effects for blacks and Asians … were highly variable, likely the result of insufficient numbers of these racial groups."

Thus, for all data on the study drug's influence on blood pressure, the FDA reviewer made corrections for the placebo effects, prior to arriving at conclusions on efficacy.

f. Risks for Mistakes When Using the Double-Dummy Technique

This is from a clinical trial on *apixaban*, for preventing stroke and embolisms. The information is from NDA 202155, on March 2015 of the FDA's website.

The study drug arm received apixaban plus a dummy for the active control, warfarin. The control arm received the active comparator (warfarin) plus a dummy for the study drug.

A problem was that a small number of subjects were given two bottles, one containing

apixaban and the other containing warfarin. Another problem was that some subjects were given two bottles, each containing a placebo, where the first bottle had the apixaban placebo and the second bottle had the warfarin placebo. The FDA reviewer commented that, "thus, medication errors could conceivably result in a patient concomitantly … two different active products (Warfarin and apixaban) … [or] … two placebos."

Fortunately for the Sponsor, few of these errors occurred, and the FDA concluded that, "the Applicant's response to our … letter … convinced us that the likelihood that the trial results were confounded by … medication errors was acceptably low." The take-home lesson is that medication errors are a real possibility for any clinical trial, where the risk for errors may increase with use of the double-dummy technique.

g. Need to Ensure That Study Subjects, as Well as Clinical Trial Personnel, Are Blinded as to Study Drug Versus Placebo

This is from a clinical trial on *apixaban*, for preventing stroke and embolisms, as described immediately above. The information is from the same NDA as described immediately above, namely, NDA 202155, on March 2015 of the FDA's website. The problem was a difference in size of the pill providing the study drug, and the pill providing the placebo version of that drug. Regarding the fact that the casual observer could have seen the difference between the drug and placebo, the FDA reviewer stated:

> Following a discussion of this issue with the Applicant, we received a submission that downplayed the importance of the **difference in thickness** between the **placebo** and **active 5 mg apixaban tablets**, but acknowledged its existence. The Applicant argued that individual patients would be exposed only to **active** or **placebo** … and would

ordinarily never have the opportunity to appreciated the difference.

The FDA reviewer went on to explain why the study drug and placebo must be indistinguishable from each other. The reviewer wrote:

> Applicant argued that individual **patients** would be exposed only to active or placebo ... and would ... never have the opportunity to appreciated the difference. While this might be true, **site personnel** handled active drug and placebo tablets ... [s]ite personnel could have become aware of a **difference in thickness** ... [i]f for some reason the results ... became known, the site might become completely unblinded to the assignment of all patients at the site.

h. Poor Design of the Placebo Capsules, Enabled Easy Unblinding

The issue of unblinding, as a result of a poorly designed placebo, was raised in a clinical trial on *ticagrelor*, a drug for preventing thrombosis. The information is from NDA 22433, from March 2015 of the FDA's website. The study drug was ticagrelor, and the active control was clopidogrel.

The problem was inadequate design of the placebo version of clopidogrel. The problem is that, in the FDA reviewer's words, "[t]he clopidogel formulation used was a clopidogrel tablet cut into two and stuffed into a capsule. The dummy was identical in appearance. However, the sites could unblind any patient by breaking one of the patient's clopidogrel/dummy capsules and examining its contents." The FDA reviewer went on to explain that, "[t]hat being said, it would have been possible to unblind the study drug by opening the overencapsulated clopidogrel

tablet, since the clopidogrel placebo capsule would have been empty."

X. STANDARD OF CARE

a. Example from Melanoma Clinical Trial

The term "standard of care" (SOC) is sometimes used in FDA-submissions to refer to an active comparator drug, that is, to a drug administered to a control group. Standard of care is described in this placebo chapter because the concepts of standard of care and of placebo each raises ethical issues. One ethical issue is that study subjects typically receive an experimental drug that has not been recognized, at the time of the study, as the standard of care (70).

The following provides an exemplary account of the use of the term, standard of care. This is an exemplary account because it establishes that at any given time, there may be more than one type of standard of care, because it establishes that the standard of care is distinguished from the experimental drug being tested in the clinical trial, and because it refers to the fact that the standard of care may change over the course of years.

The example is from a clinical trial on melanoma, where subjects in the control arm received an antibody (the study drug) and a small molecule (active comparator drug). In this example, subjects in the control arm were actually given one of two different small-molecule drugs, where each was referred to as the "standard of care." To quote from the report (71), "[p]atients randomly assigned to the standard-of-care arm received either single-agent DTIC ... or single-agent temozolomide ... orally on days 1 to 5 of a

[70]Nardini C. The ethics of clinical trials. Ecancer 2014;8:387. http://dx.doi.org/10.3332/ecancer.2014.387.

[71]Ribas A, Kefford R, Marshall MA, et al. Phase III randomized clinical trial comparing tremelimumab with standard-of-care chemotherapy in patients with advanced melanoma. J. Clin. Oncol. 2013;31:616—22.

28-day cycle." To repeat, the standard of care drug was either dacarbazine (DTIC) or temozolomide.

The melanoma study included a rationale, explaining why DTIC and temozolomide each were considered to be "the standard of care." One rationale was that DTIC was "standard reference therapy." The other rationale was that temozolomide was "commonly used," even though not FDA-approved for melanoma. The melanoma study read (72), "[a]t the time of design of our study, dacarbazine (DTIC) was the **standard reference therapy** for patients with metastatic melanoma. Oral temozolomide and ... DTIC are both prodrugs for the same active antitumor metabolite. Although temozolomide is not approved for patients with melanoma, it was **commonly used** for this indication in some countries." The melanoma study also disclosed that the standard of care for melanoma had changed, that is, from a small molecule to an antibody (ipilimumab) and to a new type of small molecule (vemurafenib). Referring to this change, the melanoma study stated that, "[s]ince the trial described in this report was initiated, the **standard of care for melanoma has changed**. Ipilimumab ... a CTLA4-blocking ... monoclonal antibody, and ... vemurafenib ... have recently been approved in several countries, including the United States."

To summarize, the exemplary account from the melanoma study demonstrates that the term "standard of care" can be simultaneously defined in more than one way (standard reference therapy; commonly used), and that the meaning of the term can change over the course of years, for example, when the FDA grants approval to a new drug.

b. Coexisting Multiplicity of Definitions for Standard of Care

The melanoma study provides a good reference point when reviewing published comments on the uses and definitions of "standard of care." Consistent with the two different definitions for standard of care, as set forth in the melanoma study, Miller and Silverman (73) commented that, "the medical standard of care is used in two different senses ... it refers to prevailing or routine practice patterns within a given medical community ... [and] it refers to what is regarded as 'best' practice in view of current scientific knowledge and expert opinion." Guidance that is more concrete is provided by Strauss and Thomas (74) as well as Bramwell (75), who point out that the standard of care for any disease is published by various medical associations, for example, in "practice guidelines." Strauss and Thomas (76) caution that publications describing the standard of care for a given

[72]Ribas A, Kefford R, Marshall MA, et al. Phase III randomized clinical trial comparing tremelimumab with standard-of-care chemotherapy in patients with advanced melanoma. J. Clin. Oncol. 2013;31:616–22.

[73]Miller FG, Silverman HJ. The ethical relevance of the standard of care in the design of clinical trials. Am. J. Respir. Crit. Care Med. 2004;169:562–4.

[74]Strauss DC, Thomas JM. What does the medical profession mean by "standard of care?" J. Clin. Oncol. 2009;27: e192–3.

[75]Bramwell VH. Adjuvant chemotherapy for adult soft tissue sarcoma: is there a standard of care? J. Clin. Oncol. 2001;19:1235–7.

[76]Strauss DC, Thomas JM. What does the medical profession mean by "standard of care?" J. Clin. Oncol. 2009;27: e192–3.

disease may actually take the form of self-promoting opinions, and thus should not, in fact, be taken as any "standard of care."

c. Ethics of the Standard of Care in Clinical Trials Distinguished from Ethics in Everyday Medical Practice

Regarding ethics, Miller and Silverman (77) comment on the "ethical significance of the medical standard of care for the design of clinical research." In a nutshell, the standard of care treatment is not provided to all subjects in clinical trials, because of the necessity for an arm that receives an experimental drug (not the standard of care), because of the use in some clinical trials of a placebo (not the standard of care), and because the Clinical Study Protocol typically requires restrictions, such as restrictions on concomitant medications because of the need "to produce valid data." Miller and Silverman (78) conclude that, "[i]t follows from these differences that the ethical principles that govern clinical research are not the same as those that primarily apply to medical care."

The following distinguishes the meaning of standard of care, as it applies to clinical trials, from standard of care, as it applies to everyday medical practice. De Ville and Brigham (79) point out that, "physician-researchers cannot be held ... to the traditional medical malpractice 'standard of care' and the duty to act in the best interests of their patients ... much of clinical research does not conform to medical standard of care." Miller and Silverman (80) describe the legal use of the term, standard of care, as applied to malpractice lawsuits relating to ordinary medical practice, writing that, "the concept of the standard of care ... derives from the law relating to medical malpractice. The traditional legal understanding of the standard of care to which physicians are held accountable refers to the typical or customary practice of physicians in the professional community, as evidenced by the testimony of expert witnesses." Further concerning the concept that "standard of care" is a legal term, Strauss and Thomas (81) state that the term is a legal term that is defined as, "the caution that a reasonable person in similar circumstances would exercise in providing care to a patient." According to Moffett and Moore (82), a commonly used legal definition in present day use is, "what a minimally competent physician in the same field would do in the same situation, with the same resources." Thus, although many courtroom opinions provide definitions of the standard of care, and provide guidance on how to identify the standard of care for a given disease (eg, using

[77]Miller FG, Silverman HJ. The ethical relevance of the standard of care in the design of clinical trials. Am. J. Respir. Crit. Care Med. 2004;169:562−4.

[78]Miller FG, Silverman HJ. The ethical relevance of the standard of care in the design of clinical trials. Am. J. Respir. Crit. Care Med. 2004;169:562−4.

[79]De Ville KA, Brigham D. Chapter 9. Liability in clinical trials research in medical malpractice survival handbook. Mosby, Inc. p. 91−110.

[80]Miller FG, Silverman HJ. The ethical relevance of the standard of care in the design of clinical trials. Am. J. Respir. Crit. Care Med. 2004;169:562−4.

[81]Strauss DC, Thomas JM. What does the medical profession mean by "standard of care?" J. Clin. Oncol. 2009;27: e192−3.

[82]Moffett P, Moore G. The standard of care: legal history and definitions: the bad and good news. Western J. Emergency Med. 2011;12:109−12.

expert witnesses), writings from courtroom opinions that concern everyday medical practice are not necessarily relevant to the term "standard of care," as applied to clinical trials. As applied to clinical trials, the term "standard of care" typically refers to a study arm where subjects receive the same drug that is considered to be the standard of care (in the nonresearch setting), and does not necessarily mean that study subjects additionally receive further types of therapy or further diagnostic tests, as might be provided in everyday medical practice.

d. Conclusions

To conclude, clinical trial design often includes a study arm where subjects are treated with a drug referred to as, the "standard of care." This author recommends that medical writers using the term "standard of care" should identify a publication that establishes that the treatment is, in fact, the "standard of care." The publication may be from, for example, a medical association, the FDA, or the EMA. The National Comprehensive Cancer Network (NCCN), for example, provides information on the standard of care for various cancers. For melanoma, NCCN states that (83), "surgical

excision remains the standard of care for in situ melanoma." For CML, the NCCN states that (84), "TKI [tyrosine kinase inhibitor] therapy has become the standard of care for patients with CML." Another organization, the European Society for Medical Oncology (ESMO), provides various Clinical Practice Guidelines, and states that all of these guidelines (85), "are intended to provide … recommendations for the best standards of cancer care." The Clinical Practice Guidelines for melanoma (86) and for chronic myeloid leukemia (CML) (87) are available, as cited. The ESMO's Clinical Practice Guidelines for CML provide an account of the changing standard of care over the years, "[i]nterferon-alpha … became the gold standard in the 90s and for a decade, before the introduction of tyrosine kinase inhibitors (TKI) … [i]matinib was the first TKI to be used and is still the gold standard of first-line treatment worldwide." The ESMO's statement about tyrosine kinase inhibitors is consistent with the NCCN's statement regarding CML.

Also note that FDA's Guidance for Industry publications provides brief comments on the standard of care for clinical trials on systemic lupus erythematosus (88), skin wounds (89), influenza virus (90), and obesity (91).

[83]National Comprehensive Cancer Network. NCCN clinical practice guidelines in oncology (NCCN Guidelines®) Melanoma. Ver. 3.2015; March 11, 2015 (75 pp.).

[84]National Comprehensive Cancer Network. NCCN clinical practice guidelines in oncology (NCCN Guidelines®) Chronic Myelogenous Leukemia. Ver. 1.2015; August 28, 2014 (101 pp.).

[85]Website of European Society for Medical Oncology (ESMO) Switzerland, www.esmo.org [accessed 18.08.15].

[86]Dummer R, Hauschild A, Guggenheim M, et al. Cutaneous melanoma: ESMO clinical practice guidelines for diagnosis, treatment and follow-up. Ann. Oncol. 2012;23(Suppl. 7):vii86–vii91.

[87]Baccani M, Pileri S, Steegmann J-L, et al. Chronic myeloid leukemia: ESMO clinical practice guidelines for diagnosis, treatment and follow-up. Ann. Oncol. 2012;23(Suppl. 7):vii72–vii77.

[88]Guidance for Industry. Systemic lupus erythematosus—developing medical products for treatment; June 2010 (15 pp.).

[89]Guidance for Industry. Chronic cutaneous ulcer and burn wounds—developing products for treatment; June 2006 (18 pp.).

[90]Guidance for Industry. Influenza: developing drugs for treatment and/or prophylaxis; April 2011 (30 pp.).

[91]Guidance for Industry. Developing products for weight management; February 2007 (16 pp.).

8

Intent-to-Treat Analysis Versus Per Protocol Analysis

I. INTRODUCTION

The concepts of *intent-to-treat* and *per protocol* are relevant to study design and to statistics. Therefore, this chapter resides between the chapters on study design and the statistics chapter. In the term *per protocol*, the word "protocol" refers to the Clinical Study Protocol.

a. Definition of Intent-to-Treat Analysis

Intent-to-treat (ITT), also known as *intention-to-treat*, refers to the population of subjects enrolled in a clinical trial. The ITT population includes all enrolled subjects, and encompasses those (at the time of enrollment) who were believed to meet all the inclusion/exclusion criteria, and those who, some time after enrollment, were found not to have actually met these criteria on the enrollment date. Moreover, the ITT population includes all subjects who complied with the terms of the Clinical Study Protocol through the duration of the clinical trial, as well as subjects who deviated from the Clinical Study Protocol. Typical deviations include failure to sign the consent form, failure to take the study drug or control according to the required schedule, failure to make all the scheduled assessment visits, and dropping out of the trial.

According to the ICH Guidelines (1), the ITT principle is defined as:

> The principle that asserts that the effect of a treatment policy can be best assessed by evaluating on the basis of the intention to treat a subject (i.e. the planned treatment regimen) rather than the actual treatment given. It has the consequence that subjects allocated to a treatment group should be followed up, assessed and analysed as members of that group irrespective of their compliance to the planned course of treatment.

FDA has used the same definition in its Guidance for Industry documents (2).

[1] ICH Guidelines, Statistical Principles for Clinical Trials E9; February 1998.

[2] U.S. Department of Health and Human Services, Food and Drug Administration. Guidance for Industry. Developing medical imaging drug and biological products, Part 3: design, analysis, and interpretation of clinical studies; June 2004.

Clinical Trials.
DOI: http://dx.doi.org/10.1016/B978-0-12-804217-5.00008-4

Consistently, but in more succinct terms, the FDA has defined the ITT group as, "all patients who were randomized" (3).

According to a review by Heritier et al. (4), analysis by ITT is a strategy that compares the study groups in terms of the treatment to which they were randomly allocated, irrespective of the treatment they actually received. An analysis that excludes noncompliant subjects, or subjects who had been treated according to a deviation from the clinical study protocol, is not an ITT analysis.

ITT analysis prevents introduction of various biases, for example, attrition bias. According to Nüesch et al. (5), deviations from the protocol and losses to follow-up can result in some subjects being excluded from the analysis. These excluded subjects are not likely to be representative of patients remaining in the trial. For example, subjects may not be available for follow-up because they have severe side effects. And subjects who had deviated from the directions in the Clinical Study Protocol may have a worse prognosis than subjects adhering to the protocol. Thus, ITT analysis ensures that the study drug group and control group are comparable.

ITT analysis requires including data from subjects who are noncompliers and drop-outs in the analyses of efficacy and safety. While the exact approach taken, in using these types of data, requires the dedicated expertise of a statistician, the FDA has provided a layperson's description of a common approach. FDA's Guidance for Industry (6) recommends that:

> The effects of dropouts should be addressed in all trial analyses to demonstrate that the conclusion is robust. One trial design approach is following all patients, including dropouts, to the planned trial endpoint, even if postdropout information is confounded by new therapy, and performing an analysis including these patients. Another approach involves the worst case rule: assigning the best possible score to all postdropout placebo patients and the worst score to all postdropout treatment patients, then performing an analysis including these scores.

Regarding the goal of preventing dropouts and other failures, Friedman et al. (7) suggest that study staff remind subjects of upcoming clinic visits by way of postcards, telephone calls, or e-mail messages.

b. Deviations and Inconsistencies

The concept of ITT analysis might best be taught by documenting errors in study design, as it applies to ITT analysis, and by contrasting ITT analysis with per protocol (PP) analysis. Errors in reporting clinical trials can take the form of inconsistent start date for calculating endpoints, use of HRQoL questionnaires during the clinical trial but failure to obtain baseline HRQoL data, and failure to disclose the method of allocation. These particular inconsistencies are documented elsewhere in this

---

[3]U.S. Department of Health and Human Services, Food and Drug Administration. Guidance for Industry. Community-acquired bacterial pneumonia: developing drugs for treatment; March 2009.

[4]Heritier SR, Gebski VL, Keech AC. Inclusion of patients in clinical trial analysis: the intention-to-treat principle. Med. J. Aust. 2003;179:438−40.

[5]Nüesch E, Trelle S, Reichenbach S, et al. The effects of excluding patients from the analysis in randomised controlled trials: meta-epidemiological study. Brit. Med. J. 2009;339:b3244.

[6]U.S. Department of Health and Human Services, Food and Drug Administration. Guidance for Industry. Clinical development programs for drugs, devices, and biological products for the treatment of rheumatoid arthritis (RA); March 1998.

[7]Friedman LM, Furberg CD, DeMets DL. Fundamentals of clinical trials. 4th ed. Munich: Springer; 2010. p. 259.

book. Another inconsistency is failure to comply with the definitions of ITT that are set forth by the FDA or by the ICH Guidelines.

Auerbach et al. (8) defined the ITT group as, "[f]or safety data, the intent-to-treat (ITT) population was analyzed. This population was defined as all patients who received at least one dose of study drug." But this definition is incorrect, because it deviates from those set forth by the ICH Guidelines and by the FDA's Guidance for Industry.

Krainick-Strobel et al. (9) defined the ITT group as, "[i]n view of the primary objective of the trial, this efficacy population was modified a posteriori to exclude both untreated patients and those who took study medication for less than 4 months." But this definition is also incorrect, because it also deviates from those set forth by the ICH Guidelines and by the FDA's Guidance for Industry. Instead, the authors should have used the term, modified ITT analysis.

Vazquez et al. (10), defined ITT group as, "[s]afety analyses were performed on the intent-to-treat population (ITT), which included all participants with diagnoses of OPC or EC who received at least 1 dose of study drug." Caraceni et al. (11) defined the ITT group as, "[t]he main analysis was performed on the intent-to-treat (ITT) population (all patients who received at least one study medication)." Pichichero et al. (12) defined the ITT group as, "all patients who received at least one dose of study drug and who had at least one postbaseline clinical safety assessment." File et al. (13) defined the ITT group as, "intent to-treat population comprised all randomized patients who took at least one dose of study medication." Vahdat et al. (14) defined the ITT group as, "[t]he intent-to-treat (ITT) population consisted of all patients who had received at least one dose of eribulin." But all of these

[8]Auerbach M, Ballard H, Trout JR, et al. Intravenous iron optimizes the response to recombinant human erythropoietin in cancer patients with chemotherapy-related anemia: a multicenter, open-label, randomized trial. J. Clin. Oncol. 2004;22:1301−7.

[9]Krainick-Strobel UE, Lichtenegger W, Wallwiener D, et al. Neoadjuvant letrozole in postmenopausal estrogen and/or progesterone receptor positive breast cancer: a phase IIb/III trial to investigate optimal duration of preoperative endocrine therapy. BMC Cancer 2008;8:62−72.

[10]Vazquez JA, Skiest DJ, Tissot-Dupont H, Lennox JL, Boparai, MS, Isaacs R. Safety and efficacy of posaconazole in the long-term treatment of azole-refractory oropharyngeal and esophageal candidiasis in patients with HIV infection. HIV Clin. Trials 2007;8:86−97.

[11]Caraceni A, Zecca E, Bonezzi C. Gabapentin for neuropathic cancer pain: a randomized controlled trial from the gabapentin cancer pain study group. J. Clin. Oncol. 2004;22:2909−17.

[12]Pichichero ME, Casey JR, Block SL, et al. Pharmacodynamic analysis and clinical trial of amoxicillin sprinkle administered once daily for 7 days compared to penicillin V potassium administered four times daily for 10 days in the treatment of tonsillopharyngitis due to Streptococcus pyogenes in children. Antimicrob. Agents Chemother. 2008;52:2512−20.

[13]File TM, Lode H, Kurz H, Kozak R, Xie H, Berkowitz E. Double-blind, randomized study of the efficacy and safety of oral pharmacokinetically enhanced amoxicillin-clavulanate (2,000/125 milligrams) versus those of amoxicillin-clavulanate (875/125 milligrams), both given twice daily for 7 days, in treatment of bacterial community-acquired pneumonia in adults. Antimicrob. Agents Chemother. 2004;48:3323−31.

[14]Vahdat LT, Pruitt B, Fabian CJ, et al. Phase II study of eribulin mesylate, a halichondrin B analog, in patients with metastatic breast cancer previously treated with an anthracycline and a taxane. J. Clin. Oncol. 2009; 27:2954−61.

definitions are incorrect. The term that should have been used is modified ITT analysis.

To repeat, all of these definitions deviate from those set forth by the ICH Guidelines and by FDA's Guidance for Industry.

A survey of published clinical trials by Altman et al. (15) distinguishes between ITT analysis and PP analysis. According to these authors, of 119 reports stating that all participants were included in the analysis in the groups to which they were originally assigned, 15 (13%) failed to include all of the allocated patients in the analysis. Furthermore, according to these authors, excluding a subject after randomization, for the reason of failing to meet the inclusion/exclusion criteria, is "contrary to the intent to treat principle." The resulting analysis is properly classified as PP analysis.

In a survey by Gravel et al. (16) of 249 clinical trials that reported using ITT analysis, 7% of these (17 trials) actually used PP analysis. Gravel et al. (17) concluded that these 17 trials clearly violated the requirements of ITT analysis. In a survey of 81 published studies on arthritis clinical trials, Baron et al. (18) found that ITT analysis was performed in only 6 of the studies, and PP analysis was performed in 48 of the studies.

In reviewing clinical trial design, the medical writer needs to distinguish between data from an ITT population, modified ITT population, and per protocol population. By distinguishing between these three populations, the reader will better be able to interpret efficacy data and to detect sources of bias, and will better be able to interpret safety data and to detect sources of bias in the data.

II. ITT ANALYSIS CONTRASTED WITH PP ANALYSIS

Per protocol (PP) analysis means including, in the analysis, only subjects who were enrolled in the clinical trial, and who actually complied with all of the substantive instructions set forth in the Clinical Study Protocol. In one of its Guidance for Industry documents, FDA defines PP analysis as, "[t]he set of data generated by the subset of subjects who complied with the protocol sufficiently to ensure that these data would be likely to exhibit the effects of treatment according to the underlying scientific model. Compliance covers such considerations as exposure to treatment, availability of measurements, and absence of major protocol violations" (19).

[15]Altman DG, Schulz KF, Moher D, et al. The revised CONSORT statement for reporting randomized trials: explanation and elaboration. Ann. Intern. Med. 2001;134:663−94.

[16]Gravel J, Opatrny L, Shapiro S. The intention-to-treat approach in randomized controlled trials: are authors saying what they do and doing what they say? Clin. Trials 2007;4:350−6.

[17]Gravel J, Opatrny L, Shapiro S. The intention-to-treat approach in randomized controlled trials: are authors saying what they do and doing what they say? Clin. Trials 2007;4:350−6.

[18]Baron G, Boutron I, Giraudeau B, Ravaud P. Violation of the intent-to-treat principle and rate of missing data in superiority trials assessing structural outcomes in rheumatic diseases. Arthritis Rheum. 2005;52:1858−65.

[19]U.S. Department of Health and Human Services, Food and Drug Administration. Guidance for Industry. Coronary drug-eluting stents—nonclinical and clinical studies; March 2008.

Le Henanff et al. (20) defined PP analysis, and distinguished it from ITT analysis, as follows. According to these authors, ITT analysis includes all subjects, regardless of their compliance with the entry criteria, treatment actually received, withdrawal from treatment, or deviation from the protocol while, in contrast, PP analysis includes only subjects who satisfied the entry criteria of the trial and who completed the treatment as defined in the Clinical Study Protocol.

The appeal of performing PP analysis is intuitive, and easy for any layperson to understand. According to the European Medicines Agency (EMA) (21), Per protocol analysis can maximize the opportunity for a new treatment to show additional efficacy in the analysis. PP analysis most closely reflects the scientific basis underlying the study design for the clinical trial.

However, the EMA (22) cautions that, regarding the use of PP analysis, "[h]owever, the corresponding test of the hypothesis and estimate of the treatment effect may or may not be conservative depending on the trial; the bias, which may be severe, arises from the fact that adherence to the study protocol may be related to treatment and outcome. The problems that lead to the exclusion of subjects to create the PP set, and other protocol violations, should be fully identified and summarised."

Per protocol analysis can result in bias as follows. If a subject experiences severe adverse events, and refuses to comply with the dosing protocol, or is not able to comply with an appointment at the clinic, exclusion of this subject from the trial's analysis will prevent the trial from accomplishing it goal of detecting adverse events. In this way, PP analysis can make a study drug appear safer than it really is.

a. ITT Analysis Versus PP Analysis— The Molina Study

In a clinical trial on *Trypanosoma cruzi* infections, Molina et al. (23) used both ITT analysis and PP analysis. The group used for PP analysis was defined as all enrolled patients, but excluding "patients who were lost to follow-up, those who dropped out owing to adverse events," as well as patients where the drug actually failed in treating the infection, as determined by measuring the trypanosomal DNA in the bloodstream. The clinical trial was actually on patients with Chagas' disease, which is caused by *T. cruzi*.

This clinical trial is unusual, in that the results from ITT analysis and PP analysis were dramatically different. The following explores the results only from the active control group, which used a drug that was established as effective, namely, benznidazole. In the ITT group, the active control was shown to be effective in 61.6% of the patients, while in the PP group, the active control worked in 94.4% of the patients. This difference is notable, in view of the author's finding that in most clinical trials that include both ITT analysis and PP

[20]Le Henanff AL, Giraudeau B, Baron G, Ravaud P. Quality of reporting of noninferiority and equivalence randomized trials. J. Am. Med. Assoc. 2006;295:1147−51.

[21]European Medicines Agency (EMEA) ICH Topic E9 Statistical Principles for Clinical Trials; September 1998.

[22]European Medicines Agency (EMEA) ICH Topic E9 Statistical Principles for Clinical Trials; September 1998.

[23]Molina I, Prat J, Salvador F, et al. Randomized trial of posaconazole and benznidazloe for chronic Chagas' disease. New Engl. J. Med. 2014;370:1899−908.

analysis, the efficacy results are similar to each other.

Why was the efficacy of the active control greater in the PP group than in the ITT group? Efficacy was measured by the parameter of "treatment failure" which, in turn, was defined as the summation of, "patients who were lost to follow-up, those who dropped out owing to adverse events," and those with actual disease according to analysis of trypanosomal DNA in the blood. A large proportion (one-third) of the patients had treatment failure. Of the 26 patients in the study drug group, 9 had treatment failure, where 5 of these withdrew because of adverse events and 4 were lost to follow-up.

The take-home lesson is as follows. If a *large proportion* of the subjects enrolled in a clinical trial is excluded from the PP analysis group (and included in the ITT analysis group), and where the most prevalent reason for exclusion was for lack of "efficacy," then it will likely be the case that efficacy results from the PP group and ITT group will be different.

b. ITT Analysis Versus PP Analysis— The Sethi Study

In a study of bronchitis infections, Sethi et al. (24) used both ITT analysis and PP analysis, and defined the PP population to exclude patients who violated any aspect of the study protocol to a degree that might affect assessment of treatment efficacy. Protocol violations that might affect assessment were determined

prior to beginning the study and included violation of exclusion criteria (including age), serious or complicating infection or disease, active alcohol or drug abuse, use of prohibited concomitant medication, compromising adverse event, medication or visit noncompliance, failure to meet the inclusion criterion of acute exacerbations of chronic bronchitis, and an outcome of "unable to determine."

c. ITT Analysis Versus PP Analysis— The Abrial Study

In a study of chemotherapy for breast cancer, Abrial et al. (25) used both ITT analysis and PP analysis. Per protocol analysis was conducted because a large fraction of the study subjects did not receive the entire treatment. Eight subjects out of 50 did not receive the entire treatment because of allergy or toxicity. Hence, the clinical results and data from mammograms and ultrasound were calculated on both an ITT basis (50 subjects) and PP basis (42 subjects).

Data from PP analysis were somewhat more favorable than with ITT analysis. Regarding clinical evaluation of efficacy, complete response was found in 26% of the ITT subjects and in 31% of the PP subjects. Regarding the objective evaluation of efficacy (mammograms), complete response was found in 18% of the ITT subjects, while complete response was found in 21.4% of the PP subjects. ITT analysis and PP analysis showed similar efficacy results.

[24]Sethi S, Breton J, Wynne B. Efficacy and safety of pharmacokinetically enhanced amoxicillin-clavulanate at 2,000/125 milligrams twice daily for 5 days versus amoxicillin-clavulanate at 875/125 milligrams twice daily for 7 days in the treatment of acute exacerbations of chronic bronchitis. Antimicrob. Agents Chemother. 2005;49:153—60.

[25]Abrial C, van Praagh I, Delva R, et al. Pathological and clinical response of a primary chemotherapy regimen combining vinorelbine, epirubicin, and paclitaxel as neoadjuvant treatment in patients with operable breast cancer. Oncologist 2005;10:242—9.

d. ITT Analysis Versus PP Analysis— The Berthold Study

In a study of a natural product tested for lowering cholesterol, Berthold et al. (26) defined the PP population. Patients were classified as nonadherent if they failed to take at least 80% or took more than 120% of the prescribed dose. Adherence was checked by pill count at visit four (day 0) for the placebo run-in phase and at visit five (6 weeks) and visit six (12 weeks) for the treatment phase. Patients found not to have adhered to the clinical trial regimen at visits five or six were not included in the PP analysis. One hundred and forty-three subjects were used for the ITT analysis, while 129 were used for the PP analysis. The authors found no differences in the results, with either analysis.

e. ITT Analysis Versus PP Analysis— The Geddes Study

Geddes et al. (27) defined PP analysis as all treated subjects with clinical signs and symptoms of sepsis and proven infection, excluding major protocol violators. Major protocol violators, who were not included in the PP population, were subjects with incorrect entry diagnosis, incorrect treatment duration, antibiotic pretreatment, or a missing posttreatment clinical evaluation. The investigators conducted both ITT analysis and PP analysis in their clinical study of two different antibiotic treatments. According to ITT analysis, the cure rate for levofloxacin (77%) was higher than that for imipenem/cilastatin (68%). According to PP analysis, the cure rate for levofloxacin (89%) was similar to that for imipenem/cilastatin (85%). Thus, the Geddes study documents an example where ITT analysis and PP analysis resulted in different conclusions regarding efficacy.

III. DISADVANTAGES OF ITT ANALYSIS

Most comments regarding ITT analysis versus PP analysis dwell on biases that occur with use of PP analysis. But biases can also result when ITT analysis is used. According to Nüesch et al. (28), ITT analysis can introduce bias into the analysis of the clinical trial, as follows. Trials without exclusions more often report imputations of missing data than those with exclusions. In other words, missing values were replaced by the last value observed. This method is popular for imputation of missing data, but leads to overly precise estimates and to bias.

Also, as detailed later in this chapter, ITT analysis can be misleading where subjects are enrolled on an emergency basis before it can be confirmed that the study subject actually has the suspected disease.

[26]Berthold HK, Unverdorben S, Degenhardt R, Bulitta M, Gouni-Berthold I. Effect of policosanol on lipid levels among patients with hypercholesterolemia or combined hyperlipidemia. J. Am. Med. Assoc. 2006;295:2262–9.

[27]Geddes A, Thaler M, Schonwald S, Härkönen M, Jacobs F, Nowotny I. Levofloxacin in the empirical treatment of patients with suspected bacteraemia/sepsis: comparison with imipenem/cilastatin in an open, randomized trial. J. Antimicrob. Chemother. 1999;44:799–810.

[28]Nüesch E, Trelle S, Reichenbach S, et al. The effects of excluding patients from the analysis in randomised controlled trials: meta-epidemiological study. Brit. Med. J. 2009;339:b3244.

IV. RUN-IN PERIOD, AS PART OF THE STUDY DESIGN, IS RELEVANT TO ITT ANALYSIS AND PP ANALYSIS

Montori and Guyatt (29) teach that the bias introduced when using a PP analysis can be overcome where the schema of a clinical trial uses a run-in period. According to these authors, this type of study design ensures maximal adherence, in the time period following the start date. A run-in period can identify nonadherent subjects or noncompliant subjects, so they can be excluded before randomization. With this type of study design, only subjects successfully adhering to the requirements set forth during the run-in period are included in the ITT population.

a. Run-In Period Specifically Used to Determine Diagnosis

One form of study design, which takes the form of a run-in period, is to identify potential subjects for enrolling in a clinical trial, to initiate drug treatment, and to order time-consuming diagnostic tests. Once the time-consuming diagnostic tests have been completed, the subjects are then formally enrolled in the clinical trial. Using this form of study design, the investigators can refer to their analysis as ITT analysis (while avoiding using the term, *modified ITT analysis*). This form of study design was used by Schutz et al. (30), in a study of leukemia, where the time-consuming diagnostic test involved chromosomal analysis. The time-consuming test took the form of histological techniques to identify the Philadelphia chromosome, a conventional diagnostic test for acute lymphoblastic leukemia. Chemotherapy was initiated with all potential study subjects, followed by starting work on the time-consuming histological tests. Only those potential study subjects proven to bear the Philadelphia chromosome were actually enrolled in the trial, and were considered to be part of the ITT population. The chemotherapy that was administered during the run-in period was vincristine, asparaginase, and prednisone or dexamethasone (31).

V. SUMMARY

Intent-to-treat analysis is the gold standard for randomized clinical trials (32). In ITT analysis, data from all subjects initially enrolled in a clinical trial are used for the analysis of efficacy and safety. In view of the fact that the collected data may be incomplete, and in view of the fact that some subjects may have deviated somewhat from the instructions in the Clinical

---

[29]Montori VM, Guyatt GH. Intention-to-treat principle. Can. Med. Assoc. J. 2001;165:1339−41.

[30]Schultz KR, Bowman WP, Aledo A, et al. Improved early event-free survival with imatinib in Philadelphia chromosome-positive acute lymphoblastic leukemia: a children's oncology group study. J. Clin. Oncol. 2009;27:5175−81.

[31]Schultz KR, Bowman WP, Aledo A, et al. Improved early event-free survival with imatinib in Philadelphia chromosome-positive acute lymphoblastic leukemia: a children's oncology group study. J. Clin. Oncol. 2009;27:5175−81.

[32]Tillmann HC, Sharpe N, Sponer G, Wehling M. Does intention-to-treat analysis answer all questions in long-term mortality trials? Considerations on the basis of the ANZ trial. Int. J. Clin. Pharmacol. Ther. 2001;39:205−12.

Study Protocol, it is tempting to perform the analysis using only data from "perfect" subjects, where this analysis is called, PP analysis. Intent-to-treat analysis and PP analysis can each introduce different biases into the conclusions, regarding safety and efficacy. For this reason, investigators typically conduct both types of analysis.

VI. HYPOTHETICAL EXAMPLE WHERE STUDY DRUG AND CONTROL DRUG HAVE THE SAME EFFICACY

Brittain and Lin (33) provide a hypothetical example where ITT analysis produces an incorrect conclusion (an artifact), whereas PP analysis produces a correct conclusion. This hypothetical involves a study design where the study drug is compared with a control drug, that is, an active control drug. In this hypothetical, the study drug and the control drug have exactly the same efficacy. They are equally effective in treating the disease. Of course, for either arm of this study, where a subject drops out of the study, the drug can no longer be effective because the subject no longer receives the drug. Now, in this hypothetical please imagine that one of the two drugs produces unbearable adverse drug reactions and causes many subjects to drop out of the study.

In this hypothetical, *ITT analysis of efficacy* will favor the study arm where patients stayed with the drug for a greater length of time, and thus will compel the conclusion that the less toxic drug has greater efficacy. But *PP analysis of efficacy* will provide the correct answer. The correct answer is that both drugs have the same efficacy.

The take-home lesson is that the investigator needs to take into account differences in drop-out rates between the two arms of a clinical trial. This warning is relevant where the study design involves study drug versus active control drug, and also the study design involves study drug versus placebo. The concern is that, where ITT analysis is used, drop-outs among the study population can dilute the true difference between the two study arms. In contrast, where PP analysis is used, drop-outs among the study population will not dilute the true difference between the two study arms.

VII. MODIFIED ITT ANALYSIS

a. Introduction

Modified intent-to-treat (modified ITT, mITT) analysis includes fewer subjects than ITT analysis, and more subjects than PP analysis. In a survey, Abraha and Montedori (34) report that about half of clinical trials use a modified ITT analysis. Modified ITT excludes specific subjects from the statistical analysis, for example, subjects who were enrolled in the trial but later found not to satisfy the inclusion or exclusion criteria, subjects not taking all scheduled study drugs, or subjects with

[33]Brittain E, Lin D. A comparison of intent-to-treat and per-protocol results in antibiotic non-inferiority trials. Stat. Med. 2005;24:1–10.

[34]Abraha I, Montedori A. Modified intention to treat reporting in randomised controlled trials: systematic review. Brit. Med. J. 2010;340:c2697. http://dx.doi.org/10.1136/bmj.c2697 (8 pp.).

missing data, subjects who did not receive the entire treatment course, subjects who were enrolled and randomized before information on eligibility was obtained, and subjects who died before receiving treatment.

A clinical trial on a bacterial infection provides an example of modified ITT analysis. In a study of *Helicobacter pylori* infections, Vaira et al. (35) compared eradication using standard drug treatment with sequential drug treatment. ITT analysis included all subjects (300 subjects in all). The Clinical Study Protocol required daily doses for 10 days.

Subjects that were in the ITT group, but were left out of the modified ITT group, were these five subjects. The reasons they were left out were due to failure to meet inclusion criteria; failure to receive any study drugs as a result of severe abdominal pain; the discovery that a patient was pregnant; the fact that a subject decided not to take drugs; and because a subject moved out of the country.

FDA's Guidance for Industry provides this recommendation for ITT analysis, modified ITT analysis, and PP analysis, for clinical trials on *H. pylori* (36):

> Sponsors should perform efficacy analyses on two specific populations: MITT and per-protocol … [i]n addition, a third population, the intent-to-treat (ITT) population, which can also be called the safety population, should be defined as all patients who

took at least one dose of trial medication, regardless of baseline infection status.

FDA's Guidance for Industry defines the mITT population as:

- *Helicobacter pylori* infection is documented by UBT or endoscopy before treatment.
- At least one dose of trial medication is taken.
- An active duodenal ulcer with a diameter between 3 and 25 mm is documented at the baseline endoscopy or a history of duodenal ulcer within the previous 5 years is documented (by endoscopy or radiograph) before enrollment.

According to an FDA official, sponsors of clinical trials for antimicrobials sometimes ensure that efficacy data include PP analysis, for the following reason: "PP rates continue to appear in newer antimicrobial drug labels … is for comparability between newer and older drugs. Since many of the older drugs have PP rates, and ITT rates are generally lower than PP rates, the newer drug may appear less effective than the older drug unless the PP results are retained in the label" (37). An example of a package label with efficacy data on ITT and PP populations, for an antimicrobial drug, is that for clarithromycin, which has a table entitled, "Per-Protocol and Intent-to-Treat *H. Pylori* Eradication Rates" (38).

[35]Vaira D, Zullo A, MD, Vakil N. Sequential therapy versus standard triple-drug therapy for *Helicobacter pylori* eradication. Ann. Intern. Med. 2007;146:556–63.

[36]U.S. Dept. of Health and Human Services. Food and Drug Administration. Guidance for Industry. *Helicobacter pylori*-associated duodenal ulcer disease in adults: developing drugs for treatment; October 2009 (15 pp.).

[37]Kind thanks to Dr Joette M. Meyer, PharmD of FDA. E-mail of July 14, 2010.

[38]Package insert for BIAXIN®Filmtab® (clarithromycin tablets, USP) January 2015. AbbVie, Inc., North Chicago, IL (49 pp.).

b. Flow Chart Showing Subjects Included in the ITT Analysis, Modified ITT Analysis, and PP Analysis

Modified ITT analysis is clearly documented by flow charts appearing in many published accounts of clinical trials (Fig. 8.1). This type of flow chart is not a study schema. This kind of flow chart is totally different from the schema. Flow charts of the same type, which identify the number of subjects in the ITT group, modified ITT group, and PP group,

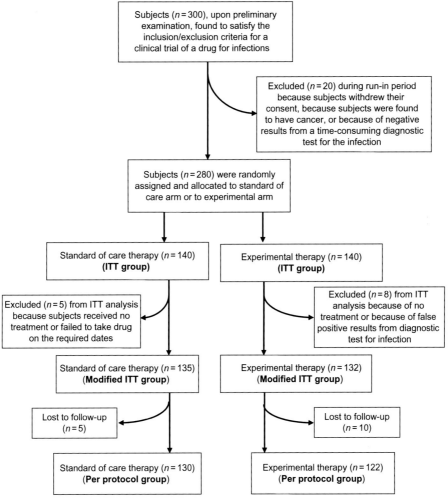

FIGURE 8.1 Flow chart showing milestones in a typical pharmacology clinical trial. The chart contains a run-in period, and includes the numbers of subjects enrolled in the ITT group, in the modified ITT group, and in the per protocol group, and provides the different reasons for excluding certain subjects from these groups. The flow chart is a composite from publications of various clinical trials.

can be found in reports for many other clinical trials, as indicated in the footnotes (39,40,41,42,43,44,45,46,47,48,49,50,51,52,53). This type of flow chart is recommended, for inclusion

[39]Chiasson JL, Josse RG, Gomis R, et al. Acarbose treatment and the risk of cardiovascular disease and hypertension in patients with impaired glucose tolerance: the STOP-NIDDM trial. J. Am. Med. Assoc. 2003;290:486−94.

[40]Emery P, Fleischmann RM, Moreland LW, et al. Golimumab, a human anti-tumor necrosis factor alpha monoclonal antibody, injected subcutaneously every four weeks in methotrexate-naive patients with active rheumatoid arthritis: twenty-four-week results of a phase III, multicenter, randomized, double-blind, placebo-controlled study of golimumab before methotrexate as first-line therapy for early-onset rheumatoid arthritis. Arthritis Rheum. 2009;60:2272−83.

[41]Hesketh PJ, Grunberg SM, Gralla RJ, et al. The oral neurokinin-1 antagonist aprepitant for the prevention of chemotherapy-induced nausea and vomiting: a multinational, randomized, double-blind, placebo-controlled trial in patients receiving high-dose cisplatin—the Aprepitant Protocol 052 Study Group. J. Clin. Oncol. 2003;21:4112−9.

[42]Manegold C, Gravenor D, Woytowitz D, et al. Randomized phase II trial of a toll-like receptor 9 agonist oligodeoxynucleotide, PF-3512676, in combination with first-line taxane plus platinum chemotherapy for advanced-stage non-small-cell lung cancer. J. Clin. Oncol. 2008;26:3979−86.

[43]Rijnders BJ, Van Wijngaerden E, Vandecasteele SJ, Stas M, Peetermans WE. Treatment of long-term intravascular catheter-related bacteraemia with antibiotic lock: randomized, placebo-controlled trial. J. Antimicrob. Chemother. 2005;55:90−4.

[44]Strasser F, Demmer R, Böhme C, et al. Prevention of docetaxel- or paclitaxel-associated taste alterations in cancer patients with oral glutamine: a randomized, placebo-controlled, double-blind study. Oncologist 2008;13:337−46.

[45]Waltzman R, Croot C, Justice GR, Fesen MR, Charu V, Williams D. Randomized comparison of epoetin alfa (40,000 U weekly) and darbepoetin alfa (200 microg every 2 weeks) in anemic patients with cancer receiving chemotherapy. Oncologist 2005;10:642−50.

[46]Warr DG, Hesketh PJ, Gralla RJ, et al. Efficacy and tolerability of aprepitant for the prevention of chemotherapy-induced nausea and vomiting in patients with breast cancer after moderately emetogenic chemotherapy. J. Clin. Oncol. 2005;23:2822−30.

[47]Cohen JA, Barkhof F, Comi G, et al. Oral fingolimod or intramuscular interferon for relapsing multiple sclerosis. New Engl. J. Med. 2010;362:402−15.

[48]Haldar P, Brightling CE, Hargadon B, et al. Mepolizumab and exacerbations of refractory eosinophilic asthma. New Engl. J. Med. 2009;360:973−84.

[49]Jonas MM, Mizerski J, Badia IB, et al. Clinical trial of lamivudine in children with chronic hepatitis B. New Engl. J. Med. 2002;346:1706−13.

[50]Shiffman ML, Suter F, Bacon BR, et al. Peginterferon alfa-2a and ribavirin for 16 or 24 weeks in HCV genotype 2 or 3. New Engl. J. Med. 2007;357:124−34.

[51]Leroy O, Saux P, Bédos JP, Caulin E. Comparison of levofloxacin and cefotaxime combined with ofloxacin for ICU patients with community-acquired pneumonia who do not require vasopressors. Chest 2005;128:172−83.

[52]Kreijkamp-Kaspers S, Kok L, Grobbee DE, et al. Effect of soy protein containing isoflavones on cognitive function, bone mineral density, and plasma lipids in postmenopausal women: a randomized controlled trial. J. Am. Med. Assoc. 2004;292:65−74.

[53]Vaira D, Zullo A, Vakil N, et al. Sequential therapy versus standard triple-drug therapy for *Helicobacter pylori* eradication. Ann. Intern. Med. 2007;146:556−63.

in medical publications, by the CONSORT 2010 Statement (54). This type of flow chart may be called a CONSORT diagram. CONSORT means Consolidated Standards of Reporting Trials. Toerien et al. (55), Paccagnella et al. (56), and Wee et al. (57), provide excellent examples of CONSORT diagrams. This type of flow chart is also called a disposition diagram (58).

The CONSORT Statement, which has been revised every few years, is the product of a group which describes itself as an international group of managers of clinical trials and medical journal editors (59). The CONSORT statement, which consists of a checklist of items to be addressed, was developed to improve poor reporting in the context of clinical trials.

c. Reasons for Using Modified ITT Analysis

The following bullet points outline reasons for defining a modified ITT group, and for using modified ITT analysis. As compared to the ITT group, the modified ITT group can exclude study subjects who:

- Withdrew their consent
- Failed to receive any study drug
- Met the definition of a certain subgroup

- Dropped out because of toxicity of the study drug
- Were given the wrong treatment by the healthcare provider
- Failed to receive study drug long enough to have a measurable effect
- Violated certain aspects of the Clinical Study Protocol, for example, by taking prohibited drugs
- Were determined, after enrollment, not to have met the inclusion criteria or exclusion criteria.

d. Listing of All Reasons for Excluding Subjects From Modified ITT Analysis, and Further Reasons for Excluding Subjects From PP Analysis—The Jindani Study

This shows how to define populations of subjects to be used for modified ITT analysis and PP analysis. In a clinical trial on *Mycobacterium tuberculosis* infections, Jindani et al. (60) used both modified ITT analysis and PP analysis. (ITT analysis was not reported.) This publication is distinguished, in that it provides a list of reasons for excluding subjects from the modified ITT analysis, and a second list for excluding additional subjects from the PP analysis. The number of enrolled subjects,

[54]Schulz KF, Altman DG, Moher D, CONSORT Group. CONSORT 2010 statement: updated guidelines for reporting parallel group randomised trials. PLoS Med. 2010;7(3):e1000251.

[55]Toerien M, Brookes ST, Metcalfe C, et al. A review of reporting of participant recruitment and retention in RCTs in six major journals. Trials 2009;10:52.

[56]Paccagnella A, Oniga F, Bearz A, et al. Adding gemcitabine to paclitaxel/carboplatin combination increases survival in advanced non-small-cell lung cancer: results of a phase II-III study. J. Clin. Oncol. 2006;24:681−7.

[57]Wee J, Tan EH, Tai BC, et al. Randomized trial of radiotherapy versus concurrent chemoradiotherapy followed by adjuvant chemotherapy in patients with American Joint Committee on Cancer/International Union against cancer stage III and IV nasopharyngeal cancer of the endemic variety. J. Clin. Oncol. 2005;23:6730−8.

[58]Fidias PM, Dakhil SR, Lyss AP, et al. Phase III study of immediate compared with delayed docetaxel after front-line therapy with gemcitabine plus carboplatin in advanced non-small-cell lung cancer. J. Clin. Oncol. 2009;27:591−8.

[59]www.consort-statement.org (quotation acquired on February 27, 2011).

[60]Jindani A, Harrison TS, Nunn AJ, et al. High-dose rifapentine with moxifloxacin for pulmonary tuberculosis. New Engl. J. Med. 2014;371:1599−608.

which ordinarily would have been used for ITT analysis, was 827 subjects. The first list was:

- Had bacterial culture taken too early
- Had missing bacterial culture result
- Had contaminated culture
- Subject was lost to follow-up
- Subject died for reason unrelated to tuberculosis
- Subject had a reinfection
- Did not produce sputum
- Withdrawn from the clinical trial because of pregnancy.

For the PP analysis, subjects were excluded for the above reasons, and also for the additional reason of failing to complete an adequate course of treatment. The above exclusion reasons took the format of a CONSORT diagram, a format that is recommended by the *New England Journal of Medicine*, and other journals (61).

e. Excluding Subjects Who Failed to Meet Inclusion or Exclusion Criteria, or Who Failed to Receive Study Drug—The Vaira Study

In a study of *Helicobacter* infections by Vaira et al. (62), modified ITT analysis was used to exclude 5 subjects, out of the 300 subjects enrolled in the study. One of the subjects was found not to meet the criteria for *Helicobacter* infection at baseline, while four did not receive any study medication. These patients did not receive study medication because one patient developed severe abdominal pain and had cholecystectomy the day after the baseline visit, one patient discovered that she was pregnant before commencing therapy, one patient elected not to take study medications after randomization, and one patient moved out of the country and forgot to take the medications. PP analysis was also conducted, and this PP analysis mandated further exclusions. For PP analysis, the above five patients were excluded, and an additional six patients were excluded (five were lost to follow-up and one discontinued therapy after 1 day because of side effects).

Helicobacter is a bacterium that has acquired notoriety for being a cause of stomach ulcers. The standard test for *Helicobacter* infections, which is a breath test, occasionally provides false-positive results (63,64,65,66,67). After conducting the breath test, false positives from the breath test generally can be detected by using a bacterial culture test.

---

[61]*New England Journal of Medicine* recommends that, "authors may provide a flow diagram in CONSORT format and all of the information required by the CONSORT checklist . . . [t]he CONSORT statement, checklist, and flow diagram are available on the CONSORT website." (NEJM instructions to authors accessed on May 6, 2015.)

[62]Vaira D, Zullo A, Vakil N, et al. Sequential therapy versus standard triple-drug therapy for *Helicobacter pylori* eradication. Ann. Intern. Med. 2007;146:556–63.

[63]Cardinali LC, Rocha GA, Rocha AM, et al. Evaluation of [^{13}C]urea breath test and *Helicobacter pylori* stool antigen test for diagnosis of *H. pylori* infection in children from a developing country. J. Clin. Microbiol. 2003;41:3334–5.

[64]Kindermann A, Demmelmair H, Koletzko B, Krauss-Etschmann S, Wiebecke B, Koletzko S. Influence of age on ^{13}C-urea breath test results in children. J. Pediatr. Gastroenterol. Nutr. 2000;30:85–91.

[65]Mauro M, Radovic V, Zhou P, et al. ^{13}C urea breath test for *Helicobacter pylori*: determination of the optimal cutoff point in a Canadian community population. Can. J. Gasteoenterol. 2006;20:770–4.

[66]Osaki T, Mabe K, Hanawa T, Kamiya S. Urease-positive bacteria in the stomach induce a false-positive reaction in a urea breath test for diagnosis of *Helicobacter pylori* infection. J. Med. Microbiol. 2008;57:814–9.

[67]Abraha I, Alessandro Montedori A. Modified intention to treat reporting in randomised controlled trials: systematic review. Brit. Med. J. 2010;340:c2697.

f. Excluding Subjects Who Failed to Meet Inclusion or Exclusion Criteria— The Weigelt Study

In a study of soft tissue infections, Weigelt et al. (68) analyzed efficacy by ITT analysis as well as by modified ITT analysis. The ITT population included all randomized patients who received one or more doses of study medication. But the modified ITT population included only ITT patients who had a culture-confirmed Gram-positive pathogen at baseline. The basis for this modified ITT group was that the inclusion criteria required only that a Gram-positive infection be "presumed," and did not require the availability of actual laboratory data for enrollment in the clinical trial. Of the patients completing the study, the ITT group consisted of 930 patients, while the modified ITT group consisted of 664 patients. By "patients completing the study," what is meant is the number of patients evaluated 7 days after drug treatment was completed. This demonstrates that the percentage of patients in failing to have a confirmed Gram-positive bacterial infection was significant and dramatic.

g. Excluding Subjects Who Failed to Meet Inclusion or Exclusion Criteria— The Pinchichero Study

In a study of bacterial infections treated with antibiotics by Pichichero et al. (69),

patients were screened for *Streptococcus pyogenes* by way of a rapid test (immunoassay), where a positive result constituted one of the inclusion criteria. At the time of the rapid test, a second biological sample was taken, and then used for a slower test (bacterial culture assay), where the result was made available at a later time. All subjects satisfying the rapid test were part of the ITT group, but subjects satisfying the rapid test and failing the slower test, were excluded from the modified ITT analysis. The percentage of subjects failing the subsequent test was under 5% (70).

Four different populations were used for the statistical analysis, not just the ITT population and modified ITT population, as disclosed below. It might be noted that the ITT group fails to conform to the definition set forth by the ICH Guidelines.

1. Intent-to-treat (ITT)/safety, all patients who received at least one dose of study drug and who had at least one postbaseline clinical safety assessment.
2. Modified intent-to-treat, all ITT/safety patients with a baseline throat swab culture that was positive for *S. pyogenes*. The percentage of all patients, who initially screened positive by the rapid-screening immunoassay test for *S. pyogenes*, but were found later by the laboratory swab culture test not to be infected with *S. pyogenes*, was less than 5% (71).

---

[68]Weigelt J, Itani K, Stevens D, Lau W, Dryden M, Knirsch C. Linezolid versus vancomycin in treatment of complicated skin and soft tissue infections. Antimicrob. Agents Chemother. 2005;49:2260–6.

[69]Pichichero ME, Casey JR, Block SL, et al. Pharmacodynamic analysis and clinical trial of amoxicillin sprinkle administered once daily for 7 days compared to penicillin V potassium administered four times daily for 10 days in the treatment of tonsillopharyngitis due to *Streptococcus pyogenes* in children. Antimicrob. Agents Chemother. 2008;52:2512–20.

[70]Pichichero ME. E-mail of August 16, 2010.

[71]Pichichero ME. E-mail of August 13, 2010.

3. Per-protocol clinical (PPc), all ITT/safety patients with either a rapid *Streptococcus* A test at baseline or a baseline throat swab culture that was positive for *S. pyogenes*, excluding those with major protocol violations and those who did not have a clinical assessment at the TOC visit.

4. Per-protocol bacteriological (PPb), the primary efficacy population, which consisted of all PPc patients with a baseline throat swab culture positive for *S. pyogenes* and with throat swab culture results available at the TOC visit. Efficacy results for clinical failures that withdrew early from the study and started a new antimicrobial for tonsillitis and/or pharyngitis due to tonsillitis and/or pharyngitis were included in the PPb analyses.

Pichichero et al. (72), demonstrates that definitions of groups used for the statistical analysis can be custom-made to track specific characteristics of the study subjects, for example, availability of various diagnostic tests used for determining eligibility.

h. Excluding Subjects Who Failed to Meet Inclusion or Exclusion Criteria—The Leroy Study

When subjects are enrolled in clinical trial for anti-antibacterial drugs, it is typical that the subject is enrolled on the basis of preliminary tests, but before conclusive laboratory tests are available. Patients are enrolled in anti-infective trials when presenting with appropriate symptoms, and it might take too long to get a culture result back before treating them. Later, the culture might show they did not have the type of infection the drug was intended to treat, and they may be excluded from the primary efficacy analysis (73). This is in contrast to the situation in oncology clinical trials, where analysis of a tumor biopsy is required for enrollment. Moreover, it should be pointed out that bacterial infections sometimes take the form of a medical emergency, in contrast to the situation with cancer.

In a study of pneumonia treated with either monotherapy (levofloxacin) or combination therapy (cefotaxamine plus ofloxacin), Leroy et al. (74) conducted a modified ITT analysis and PP analysis. The ITT group contained 398 randomized patients. The modified ITT group (308 patients) excluded patients where the infection had been misdiagnosed. In all, 62 patients had been misdiagnosed. The PP group (271 patients), which excluded patients with major protocol violations, required that a causative pathogen for pneumonia was isolated on study inclusion. A number of misdiagnosed subjects, excluded from the modified ITT group, had been admitted to an intensive care unit on an emergency basis, where misdiagnosis was due to pulmonary embolism or heart failure, which can mimic the symptoms of pneumonia (75).

---

[72]Pichichero ME, Casey JR, Block SL, et al. Pharmacodynamic analysis and clinical trial of amoxicillin sprinkle administered once daily for 7 days compared to penicillin V potassium administered four times daily for 10 days in the treatment of tonsillopharyngitis due to *Streptococcus pyogenes* in children. Antimicrob. Agents Chemother. 2008;52:2512–20.

[73]Bittman R. E-mail of July 14, 2010.

[74]Leroy O, Saux P, Bédos JP, Caulin E. Comparison of levofloxacin and cefotaxime combined with ofloxacin for ICU patients with community-acquired pneumonia who do not require vasopressors. Chest 2005;128:172–83.

[75]Leroy O. E-mail of August 31, 2010.

i. Exclusion of Study Subjects Because of Failure to Satisfy the Inclusion Criteria, and for Withdrawing Consent—The Dupont Study

In a study of antibiotic treatment against peritonitis, Dupont et al. (76) conducted an ITT analysis, modified ITT analysis, and PP analysis. ITT analysis was conducted on 227 subjects.

For modified ITT analysis, subjects where infection was not proven were later excluded. Twenty-three subjects were excluded. Also, 14 patients of the subjects in the randomized group were excluded from the ITT group, after they withdrew their consent.

PP analysis excluded subjects who had major deviations from the clinical study protocol. For the PP analysis, 45 more subjects were excluded.

j. Exclusion of Study Subjects Because of Failure to Satisfy the Inclusion Criteria—The Florescu Study

In a study of antibiotic treatment of *Staphylococcus aureus*, Florescu et al. (77) described the ITT group, modified ITT group, and a "microbiological evaluable group." The ITT group consisted of all randomized subjects. The modified ITT group consisted of all subjects who received at least one dose of study drug. The "microbiologically evaluable group" was defined as subjects who met inclusion/exclusion criteria, received no more than one dose of therapy for methicillin-resistant *Staphylococcus aureus* (MRSA) or vancomycin-resistant enterococci (VRE) infection after the first dose of the study drug, and exhibited a pretherapy culture containing MRSA or VRE that was susceptible to both of the study drugs. This study demonstrates the fact-pattern where the investigator can configure specific definitions of the modified ITT group in order to suit the needs of a specific clinical trial.

k. Excluding Subjects Who Took Prohibited Drugs During the Clinical Trial, or Who Withdrew Consent—The Manegold Study

In a study of lung cancer reported by Manegold et al. (78), the ITT group contained 117 subjects, but for the modified ITT analysis, the group contained fewer subjects (111 subjects). Thus, six subjects were excluded. The six subjects were excluded for various issues occurring after randomization. These were, taking drugs that were prohibited by the study protocol, declining Karnofsky Performance Status (79), and withdrawal of consent.

[76]Dupont H, Carbon C, Carlet J. Monotherapy with a broad-spectrum beta-lactam is as effective as its combination with an aminoglycoside in treatment of severe generalized peritonitis: a multicenter randomized controlled trial. Antimicrob. Agents Chemother. 2000;44:2028–33.

[77]Florescu I, Beuran M, Dimov R, et al. Efficacy and safety of tigecycline compared with vancomycin or linezolid for treatment of serious infections with methicillin-resistant *Staphylococcus aureus* or vancomycin-resistant enterococci: a Phase 3, multicentre, double-blind, randomized study. J. Antimicrob. Chemother. 2008;62(Suppl. 1): i17–i28.

[78]Manegold C, Gravenor D, Woytowitz D, et al. Randomized phase II trial of a toll-like receptor 9 agonist oligodeoxynucleotide, PF-3512676, in combination with first-line taxane plus platinum chemotherapy for advanced-stage non-small-cell lung cancer. J. Clin. Oncol. 2008;26:3979–86.

[79]Schag CC, Heinrich RL, Ganz PA. Karnofsky performance status revisited: reliability, validity, and guidelines. J. Clin. Oncol. 1984;2:187–93.

l. Excluding Subjects Who Failed to Receive the Assigned Treatment Because of a Mistake by the Healthcare Provider—The Berek Study

In a study of ovarian cancer, Berek et al. (80) analyzed the data by modified ITT analysis. Modified ITT analysis was conducted only on subjects who received at least one dose of study treatment. Thus, subjects not exposed to any treatment were excluded from the analysis. According to the authors, the study was blinded using a third-party pharmacist who prepared the treatment infusion bags. A few of the subjects were incorrectly started on and completed a full series of the opposite treatment than assigned. This incorrect treatment was only identified during the audit procedures of the pharmacy after the blind was broken (81).

m. Exclusion of Study Subjects Who Failed to Take Drug Long Enough to Have the Expected Efficacy—The Krainick-Strobel Study

In study of breast cancer with letrozole, Krainick-Strobel et al. (82) used a modified ITT analysis and PP analysis. The modified ITT analysis excluded both untreated patients and those who took study medication for less than 4 months, which was the minimum treatment duration for clinically sound assessment of tumor shrinkage. The authors stated that a valid assessment of letrozole efficacy, in terms

of tumor shrinkage, required at least 4 months of treatment. The PP analysis excluded all patients with major protocol violations, these being defined as: (1) an interval of more than 30 days between the last dose of letrozole and breast surgery; (2) the patient's refusal to undergo surgery; (3) deviation from clinically relevant selection criteria; and (4) any treatment with prohibited medication.

The Krainick-Strobel study is distinguished in that the subjects evaluated for efficacy were defined separately to the subjects evaluated for safety. In other words, all subjects receiving study drugs (no matter the duration) were evaluated for safety (32 subjects), whereas subjects evaluated for efficacy were 29 subjects (modified ITT group) and 25 subjects (PP group).

n. Excluding Subject Who Dropped Out Because of Adverse Events, and Because of the Bad Flavor of the Study Drug—The Kreijkamp-Kaspers Study

In a study of plant estrogen supplements on bone mineral density, Kreijkamp-Kaspers et al. (83) used both modified ITT analysis and PP analysis. The ITT population was 202 subjects. The modified ITT population was fewer, namely, 175 subjects, and these were subjects who received an analysis at baseline, and at least one additional analysis. The PP population were even fewer, and consisted of the 153 subjects who had completed the entire treatment protocol. Thus, following randomization,

[80]Berek JS, Taylor PT, Gordon A, et al. Randomized, placebo-controlled study of oregovomab for consolidation of clinical remission in patients with advanced ovarian cancer. J. Clin. Oncol. 2004;22:3507−16.

[81]Berek JS. E-mail of August 10, 2010.

[82]Krainick-Strobel UE, Lichtenegger W, Wallwiener D, et al. Neoadjuvant letrozole in postmenopausal estrogen and/or progesterone receptor positive breast cancer: a phase IIb/III trial to investigate optimal duration of preoperative endocrine therapy. BMC Cancer 2008;8:62.

[83]Kreijkamp-Kaspers S, Kok L, Grobbee DE, et al. Effect of soy protein containing isoflavones on cognitive function, bone mineral density, and plasma lipids in postmenopausal women: a randomized controlled trial. J. Am. Med. Assoc. 2004;292:65−74.

the steady dropout of subjects due to gastrointestinal distress, aversion to the taste of the study drug, had the consequence that the modified ITT group was only 175 subjects, and the PP group was only 153 subjects.

o. Excluding Subjects Who Failed to Receive the Assigned Treatment Because of Adverse Events—The Caraceni Study

In a study of neuropathic pain, Caraceni et al. (84) analyzed the data by ITT analysis and by modified ITT analysis.

The ITT population consisted of all subjects with at least one administration of gabapentin or placebo. The modified ITT population consisted of 115 patients, where the inclusion criterion for this analysis was at least 3 days of pain assessments. Reasons for withdrawing patients from the trial were adverse events in six patients (7.6%) receiving gabapentin and in three patients receiving placebo (7.3%). Five patients (two in the placebo group and three in the gabapentin group) had less than 3 days of follow-up.

Analysis of the ITT population (120 subjects) showed a significant difference of average pain intensity between gabapentin and placebo group ($P = 0.0250$). Modified ITT analysis also demonstrated a significant difference in pain intensity between the gabapentin group and placebo group ($P = 0.0257$).

p. Modified ITT Group Based on a Subgroup of Study Subjects—The Gralla Study

In a study of chemotherapy-induced vomiting, Gralla et al. (85) provided patients with a control antiemetic regimen, or with an antiemetic regimen that included an additional drug, namely, aprepitant. There were 1043 study subjects in all. Aprepitant is a small organic molecule. A modified ITT approach was used to analyze the data, and included all patients who received cisplatin, took study drug, and had at least one posttreatment assessment.

The criterion for receiving posttreatment assessment was that the patient receive only the most emetogenic (vomiting-inducing) combination of chemotherapeutic drugs. This combination involved doxorubicin and cyclophosphamide.

This criterion resulted in only 142 study subjects (out of 1043 subjects) being included in the modified ITT analysis.

Results from the ITT group, and from the modified ITT group, showed that including aprepitant was effective in reducing vomiting, where a more dramatic result came from analysis of the modified ITT group. Gralla referred to this group as, "A modified intent-to-treat approach."

The Gralla study provides an example where the definition of the modified ITT group was not based on the usual criterion of compliance with the Clinical Study Protocol. Instead, the modified ITT group was based on a predetermined subgroup of the study population. To view the big picture, it is almost always the case that clinical trials stratify the study population into various subgroups, such as by age, gender, or location of the clinic. In the Gralla study, subgroups were defined, not during the event of stratification, but according to a criterion that was applicable only after therapy had commenced, where this criterion was the need

[84]Caraceni A, Zecca E, Bonezzi C, et al. Gabapentin for neuropathic cancer pain: a randomized controlled trial from the Gabapentin Cancer Pain Study Group. J. Clin. Oncol. 2004;22:2909–17.

[85]Gralla RJ, de Wit R, Herrstedt J. Antiemetic efficacy of the neurokinin-1 antagonist, aprepitant, plus a 5HT3 antagonist and a corticosteroid in patients receiving anthracyclines or cyclophosphamide in addition to high-dose cisplatin. Cancer 2005;104:864–8.

to administer doxorubicin or cyclophospha-mide. For subgroups defined by any technique, or for subgroups defined either before or after initiation of the clinical trial, analysis by this subgroup will fall under the category of modified ITT analysis or PP analysis.

q. Drafting the Clinical Study Protocol to Account for Deviations

The Clinical Study Protocol can be drafted so that it takes into account deviations that might occur during the course of the trial. In providing a decision-tree that applies to these deviations, the Sponsor can prevent the loss of otherwise valid data for safety and efficacy analysis, using the ITT population. The following provides an example of a decision-tree from a Clinical Study Protocol for a drug for cystic fibrosis. The decision-tree provides instructions for slight delays in dosing. The instructions are down-to-earth, and refer to the possibility that a subject may "forget to take his dose" (86):

> **Missed Doses.** If subjects miss a dose and recall the missed dose within 6 hours, they should take their dose with food. If more than 6 hours have elapsed after their usual dosing time, they should skip that dose and resume their normal schedule for the following dose. For example, if the morning dose of study drug should have been taken at approximately 08:00, and the subject remembers at 12:00 that he/she forgot to take his/her dose, he/she should take the dose with food as soon as possible. If the morning dose of study drug should have been taken at approximately 08:00, and greater than

6 hours have elapsed beyond the scheduled dosing time (i.e., the time is past 14:00), the subject would resume dosing with the evening dose at approximately 20:00.

VIII. START DATE FOR ENDPOINTS IN CLINICAL TRIALS

In a survey, Mathoulin-Pelissier et al. (87) revealed that published clinical studies often fail to define the start date, or fail to provide a clear definition of an endpoint. These particular problems encumber at least a quarter of published clinical studies. Deviations from the proper start date, as set forth by ICH Guidelines (date of randomization), are documented below.

Endpoints have a start date and a date of measurement, where what is measured can be an objective endpoint such as tumor number, a biochemical parameter, or a clinical endpoint such as change in performance status score. As documented below, the start dates may vary in different studies. The start date may be the date of diagnosis, the date of randomization, the date of surgery, or a date that is exactly 6 months after surgery (88). Hence, the medical writer needs to be vigilant, not only in ensuring that the start date is identified in regulatory submissions and manuscripts, but also when comparing publications on clinical trials.

The most usual start date is the date of randomization. For example, the date of randomization was used as the start date in studies of

---

[86]Clinical Study Protocol A Phase 3, Randomized, Double-Blind, Placebo-Controlled, Parallel-Group Study to Evaluate the Efficacy and Safety of Lumacaftor in Combination With Ivacaftor in Subjects Aged 12 Years and Older With Cystic Fibrosis, Homozygous for the F508del-CFTR Mutation Vertex Study Number: VX12-809-103 Lumacaftor IND No: 79,521 Ivacaftor IND No: 74,633 EUDRACT No: 2012-003989-40.

[87]Mathoulin-Pelissier S, Gourgou-Bourgade S, Bonnetain F, Kramar A. Survival end point reporting in randomized cancer clinical trials: a review of major journals. J. Clin. Oncol. 2008;26:3721–6.

[88]Allum WH, Stenning SP, Bancewicz J, Clark PI, Langley RE. Long-term results of a randomized trial of surgery with or without preoperative chemotherapy in esophageal cancer. J. Clin. Oncol. 2009;27:5062–7.

colon cancer by van Geelan et al. (89) and by Gill et al. (90), studies of breast cancer by Goss et al. (91), by Schmid et al. (92), and by Dirix et al. (93), and a study of prostate cancer by Roach et al. (94). Date of diagnosis likely occurs only shortly before date of randomization. The *diagnosis date* was used to begin various time periods, in a study of breast cancer by DiGiovanna et al. (95). In the DiGiovanna study, *diagnosis date* was used for calculating various endpoints. In Ferrier et al. (96), the starting date was the *date of registration* in the clinical trial. Similarly, Betticher et al. (97) used *date of enrollment* for calculating various endpoints.

Date of surgery has also been used as a start date for endpoint calculations. In studies of colon cancer by Berger et al. (98), by Mitry et al. (99), and by Lembersky et al. (100), *the date of surgery* was used as the start date for calculating various endpoints. In studies of breast cancer by Merlo et al. (101), Colleoni

[89]van Geelen CM, Westra JL, de Vries EG, et al. Prognostic significance of tumor necrosis factor-related apoptosis-inducing ligand and its receptors in adjuvantly treated stage III colon cancer patients. J. Clin. Oncol. 2006;24:4998–5004.

[90]Gill S, Charles L, Loprinzi CL, Sargent DJ, et al. Pooled analysis of fluorouracil-based adjuvant therapy for stage II and III colon cancer: who benefits and by how much? J. Clin. Oncol. 2004;22:1797–806.

[91]Goss PE, Ingle JN, Martino S, et al. Efficacy of letrozole extended adjuvant therapy according to estrogen receptor and progesterone receptor status of the primary tumor: National Cancer Institute of Canada Clinical Trials Group MA.17. J. Clin. Oncol. 2007;25:2006–11.

[92]Schmid P, Untch M, Kossé V, et al. Leuprorelin acetate every-3-months depot versus cyclophosphamide, methotrexate, and fluorouracil as adjuvant treatment in premenopausal patients with node-positive breast cancer: the TABLE Study. J. Clin. Oncol. 2007;25:2509–15.

[93]Dirix LY, Ignacio J, Nag S, Bapsy P, et al. Treatment of advanced hormone-sensitive breast cancer in postmenopausal women with exemestane alone or in combination with celecoxib. J. Clin. Oncol. 2008;26:1253–9.

[94]Roach M, Bae K, Speight J, et al. Short-term neoadjuvant androgen deprivation therapy and external-beam radiotherapy for locally advanced prostate cancer: long-term results of RTOG 8610. J. Clin. Oncol. 2008;26:585–91.

[95]DiGiovanna MP, Stern DF, Edgerton SM, Whalen SG, Moore D, Thor AD. Relationship of epidermal growth factor receptor expression to ErbB-2 signaling activity and prognosis in breast cancer patients. J. Clin. Oncol. 2005;23:1152–60.

[96]Ferrier CM, Suciu S, van Geloof WL, et al. High tPA-expression in primary melanoma of the limb correlates with good prognosis. Br. J. Cancer 2000;83:1351–9.

[97]Betticher DC, Schmitz SH, Totsch M, et al. Mediastinal lymph node clearance after docetaxel-cisplatin neoadjuvant chemotherapy is prognostic of survival in patients with stage IIIA pN2 non-small-cell lung cancer: a multicenter phase II trial. J. Clin. Oncol. 2003;21:1752–9.

[98]Berger AC, Sigurdson ER, LeVoyer T, et al. Colon cancer survival is associated with decreasing ratio of metastatic to examined lymph nodes. J. Clin. Oncol. 23:8706–12.

[99]Mitry E, Fields AL, Bleiberg H, et al. Adjuvant chemotherapy after potentially curative resection of metastases from colorectal cancer: a pooled analysis of two randomized trials. J. Clin. Oncol. 2008;26:4906–11.

[100]Lembersky BC, Wieand HS, Petrelli NJ, et al. Oral uracil and tegafur plus leucovorin compared with intravenous fluorouracil and leucovorin in stage II and III carcinoma of the colon: results from National Surgical Adjuvant Breast and Bowel Project Protocol C-06. J. Clin. Oncol. 2006;24:2059–64.

[101]Merlo A, Casalini P, Carcangiu ML, et al. FOXP3 expression and overall survival in breast cancer. J. Clin. Oncol. 2009;27:1746–52.

et al. (102), and Bilimoria et al. (103), endpoints were calculated from the *date of surgery*. In a clinical trial of esophageal surgery, Allum et al. (104) used a date occurring at *6 months after surgery* as the start date. Where date of surgery is used as the start date, this method for endpoint calculation (for the endpoint of DFS) prevents the particular inconsistency detailed earlier in this textbook in the chapter on disease-free survival.

IX. FDA'S DECISION-MAKING PROCESSES, RELATING TO ITT ANALYSIS AND PP ANALYSIS

a. Introduction

FDA's decision-making process, as it applies to ITT analysis and PP analysis is illustrated by quotations from FDA's *Medical Reviews*, *Statistical Reviews*, and other reviews published with the FDA's Approval Letter.

The following examples should be compared with the FDA's definition of per protocol analysis. To reiterate the definition, PP analysis is, "[t]he set of data generated by the subset of subjects who complied with the protocol sufficiently to ensure that these data would be likely to exhibit the effects of treatment according to the underlying scientific

model. Compliance covers such considerations as exposure to treatment, availability of measurements, and absence of major protocol violations" (105,106). Thus, it is the case that PP analysis requires that the subjects comply with the Clinical Study Protocol to the degree that effects of the drug are likely to have been exhibited.

The following narrative concerns violations of the Clinical Study Protocol, where the consequence is that the data from violating study subjects be used only for ITT analysis, and not for PP analysis.

The following examples are from two independent FDA submissions, one for cetuximab and the other for ibrutinib. FDA's reviews of NDA and BLA submissions can be acquired from FDA's website by the footnoted procedure (107).

b. FDA's Decision-Making Process for Clinical Trials on Antibiotics

For clinical trials on some types of infections, subjects are enrolled and randomized based on suspected infection, where confirmation of the infection of interest occurs several days after randomization. Hence, the use of modified ITT (mITT) or per protocol (PP) analysis makes more sense than ITT analysis,

[102]Colleoni M, Rotmensz N, Peruzzotti G, et al. Size of breast cancer metastases in axillary lymph nodes: clinical relevance of minimal lymph node involvement. J. Clin. Oncol. 2005;23:1379–89.

[103]Bilimoria KY, Bentrem DJ, Hansen NM, et al. Comparison of sentinel lymph node biopsy alone and completion axillary lymph node dissection for node-positive breast cancer. J. Clin. Oncol. 2009;27:2946–53.

[104]Allum WH, Stenning SP, Bancewicz J, Clark PI, Langley RE. Long-term results of a randomized trial of surgery with or without preoperative chemotherapy in esophageal cancer. J. Clin. Oncol. 2009;27:5062–7.

[105]U.S. Dept. of Health and Human Services. Food and Drug Administration. Guidance for Industry. E9. Statistical principles for clinical trials; September 1998 (43 pp.).

[106]U.S. Dept. of Health and Human Services. Food and Drug Administration. Guidance for Industry. Coronary drug-eluting stents—nonclinical and clinical studies; May 2008 (84 pp.).

[107]On the FDA's website, under DRUGS, click on, "Search Drug Approvals by Month Using Drugs@FDA." Then, select the month and year. What is provided is the Approval Letter, Medical Review, Pharmacological Review, Statistical Review, and other reviews, that are published at the time FDA grants approval to a NDA or to a BLA.

where the ITT population includes many subjects not having the infection.

This example is from a clinical trial on antibiotic (*azithromycin*) eye drops versus placebo eye drops. The information is from the *Medical Review* and *Statistical Review* of NDA 050810, at April 2007 of the FDA's website. In a section of the *Medical Review* entitled, "Intent to Treat (i.e., not necessarily culture positive," the FDA reviewer stated that, "[t]he Intent-to-Treat population included patients who were suspected to have bacterial conjunctivitis but did not meet the criteria needed to confirm bacterial conjunctivitis" (108).

The *ITT group* had 683 subjects, the *modified ITT group* had 283 subjects, and the *PP group* had 279 subjects.

The FDA reviewer provided a definition of the modified ITT group, which was, "all randomized subjects who received at least one drop of the study medication, had baseline cultures indicating pathogenic bacterial levels." The PP group was defined as, "all randomized subjects who received at least one drop of the study medication, had baseline cultures indicating pathogenic bacterial levels and had at least one post-first-dose efficacy measurement."

FDA granted approval to the study drug, and stated that results from the ITT group were not necessary, writing, "[a]lthough not necessary to support approval, AzaSite [study drug] was superior to its vehicle [control] in the Intent-to-Treat population."

Thus, in contrast to clinical trials on chronic conditions, such as cancer, chronic viral infections, and autoimmune disorders, it is the case that for some bacterial infections, enrollment and randomization must take place before it is time to confirm the suspected identity of the bacterium. In this situation, mITT and PP analysis are preferred as the primary basis for FDA approval.

c. FDA's Decision-Making Process in Evaluating Efficacy Data Based on the ITT Population Versus the Modified ITT Population

This concerns *ceftolozane* plus *tazobactam* for urinary tract infections. The information is from the *Statistical Review* of NDA 206829 at December 2014 of the FDA's website.

The FDA reviewer complained that the modified ITT population might be stratified in a way that was not consistent with that of the ITT population, that is, the population of subjects as originally randomized. The reviewer cautions that any analysis based on the modified ITT population might give misleading results, writing that, "[f]or example, although the initial randomization of ITT subjects … was stratified by study site, some imbalances in the MITT population were observed for the region variable."

The reviewer further cautioned that this could lead to confounding results, but proceeded and compared analyses using both ITT and modified ITT analysis, adding that, "[a]lthough this can lead to potential confounding in the primary analysis, findings from Reviewer sensitivity analyses which adjusted for major risk factors (eg, stratification factors) showed findings which were similar to those of the primary analysis."

The Sponsor's main analysis was not on the ITT population, but on a subset of this group, called the "modified microbiological intention-to-treat (mMITT) population." The Sponsor defined two subsets of the ITT population, and these were the MTT population, which was all randomized subjects who received any amount of study drug, and the mMITT population, which was all randomized subjects who received any amount of study drug and had a microbiologically confirmed infection from

---

[108]Page 17 of 38-page pdf file containing the Medical Review, of NDA 050810 (April 2007 of FDA website).

a specimen taken prior to study drug administration.

The take-home lesson is the same for all Sponsors that perform efficacy or safety analysis on a subset of the ITT population, namely, that the Sponsor should take into account that equal stratification was lost, when defining any subset.

d. Protocol Violations That Distinguish Between the ITT Population and the PP Population—Example of Ibrutinib

The following information concerns an FDA submission for *ibrutinib*. This information is from NDA 205552, at November 2013 on the FDA's website.

The FDA reviewer provided an exemplary table (Table 8.1), listing the protocol violations that had accumulated during the course of the clinical trial. The table, which is from the FDA's *Medical Review*, is reproduced below.

Table 8.1 describes each violation in terms of "Category" and in terms of a more detailed "Description" of the violation. Where the category of violation is an inclusion or exclusion criterion, the table refers to the Clinical Study Protocol's list of inclusion/exclusion criteria by using a number.

The comments from the FDA reviewer track the FDA's definition of per protocol analysis, in its reference to "patient safety or trial endpoints," and that the comments indicate that PP analysis is appropriate for the entire population of subjects. In fact, the FDA reviewer stated that the protocol violations "did not impact patient safety or the trial endpoints" (109).

Table 8.1 also discloses a number of concepts that are described in other chapters in this book, namely the fact that inclusion criteria may require that subjects be "treatment-naive" or, alternatively, may require that the subjects had required previous treatment with another drug.

TABLE 8.1 Significant Protocol Violations of Eligibility Criteria

Subject ID	Category of Violation	Description	FDA Reviewer Comments
032-001	Prohibited Medication	Received neupogen Cycle 1, Days 18–20	No significant impact on patient safety or trial endpoints
032-011	Exclusion Criterion #8	Past medical history of subtotal colectomy	No significant impact on patient safety or trial endpoints
200-001	Inclusion Criterion #5b	Prior exposure to bortezomib	Protocol Amendment #1 permitted enrollment of patients with prior bortezomib exposure
200-003	Baseline Disease Assessment	Bone marrow biopsy and aspirate were obtained >30 days after start of treatment and during prior treatment regimen	Unsure whether disease was present in bone marrow at start of ibrutinib therapy
200-009	Informed Consent	Subject did not consent to optional laboratory testing, but sample was obtained; lab was notified and destroyed sample	No significant impact on patient safety or trial endpoint

[109]Pages 25–26 of 87-page pdf file containing the Medical Review, for NDA 205552.

e. Protocol Violations That Can Separate Subjects in the ITT Population From Those in the PP Population, and That Can Also Result in a Refuse to File Notice

Clinical trials typically involve protocol violations that are low in number or severity, and merely compel the conclusion that data from the violating subjects can be included in ITT analysis, but not used for PP analysis. But protocol violations that are great in number, and that are severe, may have an additional consequence of a *Refuse to File* (RTF) notice.

The following is from a clinical trial on cetuximab, an antibody drug against cancer. As part of the study design, *cetuximab* was used in combination with another drug, *irinotecan*. The information is from BLA 125084, available at March 2015 of the FDA's website.

The *Medical Review* focuses on an earlier clinical trial, the 9923 trial, which the FDA called a "supporting trial," and a later clinical trial, the 62202-007 trial, which the FDA called the "pivotal trial." The earlier trial had major protocol deviations that were so severe and great in number, that the FDA issued a *Refuse to File* notice. The later trial also had some major and minor protocol deviations, but these did not dissuade the FDA from granting approval to the drug. The locations, in the *Medical Review*, of the FDA's comments, are identified in footnote (110).

1. The Earlier (No. 9923) "Supporting" Clinical Trial, Which Resulted in the FDA Issuing a Refuse to File

This discloses the protocol violations of the earlier of two clinical trials that were part of BLA 12504 for *cetuximab* (Erbitux®). This also includes the unfavorable comments from the FDA reviewer.

The *Medical Review* divided the Protocol violations into those that were Protocol Eligibility Violations and Protocol Deviations During the Study. These are shown in Tables 8.2 and 8.3.

TABLE 8.2 Protocol Eligibility Violations

	Percent of Patients
INCLUSION CRITERION	
Bidimensionally measurable disease; index lesions not previously irradiated	2.9
Signed informed consent after enrollment	2.9
Hematological function	4.3
Hepatic function	25.9
Renal function	6.5
EXCLUSION CRITERION	
Prior murine Ab or cetuximab therapy	1.4
Surgery within 1 month of study entry	1.4
Chemotherapy for colorectal cancer between irinotecan regimen and enrollment	0.7
History of clinical significant cardiac disease, arrhythmias, or conduction abnormalities	0.7

[110]Study 62202-007, the later trial which the FDA called "pivotal," is described on pages 36–50 of the first 50-page pdf file and on pages 1–13 of the second 50-page pdf file. Study 9932, which the FDA called "supporting," and which inspired the FDA to issue a Refuse to File, is described on pages 19–20 of the second 50-page pdf file, that is part of the FDA's Medical Review. This Medical Review has three pdf files.

TABLE 8.3　Protocol Deviations During Study

	Percent of Patients
Absent/inappropriate cetuximab treatment alterations due to grade 3/4 adverse events	5.8
Absent/inappropriate irinotecan treatment alterations due to grade 3/4 adverse events	0.7
On-study cetuximab dose discrepancies from planned dose	36.2
On-study irinotecan dose discrepancies from planned dose	28.3
On-study hematology determinations missing/incorrect	11.6
On-study chemistry determinations missing/incorrect	18.8
Urinalysis determinations missing/incorrect	31.2
Diagnostic tests missing/incorrect	29.0
Diphenhydramine hydrochloride administration for test dose missing/incorrect	1.4

The FDA reviewer complained that, "the large number and severity of protocol violations and deviations place in question the integrity and safety data derived from this study. Most disconcerting are the large number of … dose discrepancies … and the absent/inappropriate treatment alterations due to severe adverse events" (111).

2. The Later (No. 62202-007) Pivotal Clinical Trial, Which Led to FDA Approval

This discloses the Protocol violations of the later of two clinical trials that were part of BLA 12504 for *cetuximab* (Erbitux). This also includes the favorable comments from the FDA reviewer, which led to FDA approval of the drug.

The following is an excerpt of the list of *major protocol violations*:

"Major violations were prespecified in the protocol and are defined as:

• No evidence of metastatic colorectal cancer at baseline
• Lack of the least one unidimensionally measurable index lesion

• Additional nonpermitted chemotherapy under treatment
• Randomization failure (ie, incorrect treatment group allocation).

There were three major violations … [o]ne patient in each treatment group had no evidence of positive EGFr expression … and one patient in the monotherapy had no evidence of metastatic colorectal cancer at baseline."

The following is an excerpt of the list of *minor protocol violations*. With each type of minor protocol violation, the FDA reviewer notated the number of applicable subjects and the percentage of total enrolled subjects. The term "uln" means, upper limit of normal:

"Minor protocol deviations … are as follow [sic]:

1. Inclusion/exclusion violations
   • Patient did not provide 2 signed consents: 1 (0.3%)
   • Neutrophils not $>1.5 \times 109/L$ or platelets not $>100 \times 109$ or Hb not >9 g/L: 5 (1.5%)

[111]Page 22 of 50-page pdf file, second pdf file of three pdf files containing the Medical Review, for BLA 125084.

- Bilirubin either not normal and not <1.5 xuln: 3 (0.9%)
- Surgery or radiation within 4 weeks prior to study entry: 1 (0.3%)
2. Post randomization violation
   - >7 days between randomization and start of treatment: 14 (4.3%)"

Regarding the *minor protocol violations*, the reviewer wrote that, "[t]hese minor violations did not impact on efficacy or safety analysis and were similar in both arms." Regarding the *major protocol violations*, the FDA reviewer commented that, "[t]he number of patients with major violations was small and did not impact the efficacy or safety analysis."

f. Refuse to File—Example of Cetuximab

FDA describes the *Refuse to File* notice in its Good Review Practice document (112). In a narrative on the FDA's *Refuse to File* notices, including the *Refuse to File* that was issued for the cetuximab (Erbitux) BLA, Scheindlin (113) wrote:

> Review of the NDA is done by an interdisciplinary group of scientists ... including pharmacologists, physicians, statisticians, pharmacists, and chemists. The first step is a cursory yet complete scan of the application, to see if all the "pieces" mandated by the regulations are there. If the NDA is deemed incomplete at this stage, the FDA may refuse to file it ... [t]he deficiency may be relatively minor, in which case the firm is able to make corrections quickly; or it may involve a major flaw, causing repercussions ... [o]nce the filing hurdle is cleared, the substantive review of the NDA begins.

One of the FDA's reviews, the *Administrative Documents* review, published with the approval of cetuximab, includes a memo mentioning the *Refuse to File*.

In the memo, the FDA reviewer stated that, "[t]he review team identified ... deviations from Good Clinical Practices ... of the clinical protocols, missing data and inconsistencies in reported data for efficacy and adverse events ... inadequate justification for the proposed dose and schedule ... [t]he totality of the deficiencies rendered the application unacceptable for filing and a *Refuse to File* letter was issued."

In the *Statistical Review*, the FDA reviewer commented on the scope of a *Refuse to File*, and expressed hope that the Sponsor could correct the deficiencies set forth in the *Refuse to File*. The reviewer stated that it, "may be relatively minor, in which case the firm is able to make corrections quickly, or it may involve a major flaw ... as ... for example [was the case with] Erbitux®."

To conclude, the *Medical Review* and other reviews that were published at the time of FDA approval, provide concrete data regarding protocol violations that occur at a relatively minor frequency, and where the only consequence is that the subjects with the violations are excluded from any PP analysis. Also, these Reviews provide clear-cut information, as to the nature and frequency of protocol violations that might inspire the FDA to issue a *Refuse to File*. Moreover, the Review provides an exemplary account of violations that are protocol eligibility violations, and those that are protocol deviations that occur during the study. Additionally, the BLA is a good example of the fact that most NDAs and BLAs are based on data from two or more clinical trials, not just one.

---

[112]U.S. Dept. of Health and Human Services. Food and Drug Administration. Manual of Policies and Procedures. Good Review Practice: Refuse to File; October 11, 2013 (21 pp.).

[113]Scheindlin S. Demystifying the New Drug Application. Mol. Interv. 2004;4:188–91.

g. Protocol Violations Can Result in a Warning Letter from the FDA

1. FDA's Warning Letters and Clinical Trials on Diseases That Are Medical Emergencies

As stated above, patient enrollment for medical emergencies may need to enroll study subjects and initiate randomization and treatment, prior to confirming that the subject had the disease in question. This raises the issue that the FDA may issue Warning Letters against the Sponsor, where the clinical trial involved protocol violations.

A Warning Letter (114) issued to a Sponsor engaged in a clinical trial of acute infections complained about protocol violations relating to tests needed at the time of enrollment. The letter complained about failure to identify the infectious organism, failure to ensure subjects had the required white blood cell count, and failure to take a complete medical history that acquired information about respiratory illnesses and smoking.

The Sponsor replied to this complaint, by explaining that the study concerned a medical emergency, namely, acute infections. The Sponsor's explanation is documented in the FDA's Warning Letter, which stated (115), "[i]n your September 18, 2007, written response, you noted that patients coming into the office with an acute infection need to be treated quickly. You further stated that study

participants had to be screened, enrolled and randomized in a manner that is typically much faster than for other types of noninfectious disease clinical trials." Unfortunately for the Sponsor, the FDA complained that, "[t]his answer is inadequate. FDA regulations require that clinical investigators ... help ensure the reliability of data collected during the study and that the rights, safety and welfare ... are protected."

X. CONCLUDING REMARKS

ITT analysis is the gold standard for clinical trials. Although PP analysis intuitively seems the best method of analysis, PP analysis can be a source of various biases. Modified ITT analysis is commonly used in clinical trials on infections, where subjects present as medical emergencies, and where subjects must be enrolled in the clinical trial before time is available for a conclusive identification of the infection. Infections presenting as medical emergencies are described by Leroy et al. (116), where one quarter of the subjects initially enrolled were excluded from the modified ITT analysis, once the time-consuming full diagnosis had been performed. Time-consuming diagnostic tests are also disclosed by Schutz et al. (117), in a study of leukemia.

---

[114]Warning Letter No. 08-HFD-45-0204 from Dr Leslie K. Ball, MD, Office of Compliance, CDER, U.S. Food and Drug Administration; May 8, 2001.

[115]Warning Letter No. 08-HFD-45-0204 from Dr Leslie K. Ball, MD, Office of Compliance, CDER, U.S. Food and Drug Administration; May 8, 2001.

[116]Leroy O, Saux P, Bédos JP, Caulin E. Comparison of levofloxacin and cefotaxime combined with ofloxacin for ICU patients with community-acquired pneumonia who do not require vasopressors. Chest 2005;128:172–83.

[117]Schultz KR, Bowman WP, Aledo A, et al. Improved early event-free survival with imatinib in Philadelphia chromosome-positive acute lymphoblastic leukemia: a children's oncology group study. J. Clin. Oncol. 2009;27:5175–81.

The issue of using ITT analysis versus PP analysis is also an issue when the following topic in statistics arises. This statistical topic is that of analysis by noninferiority analysis versus superiority analysis (118,119,120).

[118]Piaggio G, Elbourne DR, Altman DG, Pocock SJ, Evans SJ, CONSORT Group. Reporting of noninferiority and equivalence randomized trials: an extension of the CONSORT statement. J. Am. Med. Assoc. 2006;295:1152−60.

[119]Tuma RS. Trend toward noninferiority trials mean more difficult interpretation of trial results. J. Natl. Cancer Inst. 2007;99:1746−8.

[120]Eyawo O, Lee CW, Rachlis B, Mills EJ. Reporting of noninferiority and equivalence randomized trials for major prostaglandins: a systematic survey of the ophthalmology literature. Trials 2008;9:69.

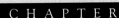

C H A P T E R

9

Biostatistics—Part I

I. INTRODUCTION

Statisticians contribute an essential intellectual component to most clinical trials [1,2]. This introduces statistical formulas, such as the Kaplan−Meier plot, the Z statistic, the t statistic, P values, the hazard ratio (HR), and the concept of *sample group* versus *population group*, and the concept of *superiority analysis* versus *noninferiority* analysis.

a. Kaplan−Meier Plot

Kaplan−Meier plots are usually used to represent deaths occurring during the course of clinical trials in oncology, and hence are often called survival plots [3]. Kaplan−Meier plots are also used to represent other types of events in clinical trials, such as time to metastasis, time to a nonfatal heart attack, time to disappearance of pain in studies of arthritis drugs, and time to recovery from an infection after antibiotic treatment [4,5].

A Kaplan−Meier plot is a curve or, more accurately, a step-function. In this curve, the x axis is time and the y axis is the *cumulative proportion* of study subjects experiencing the event of interest at any given time. In clinical trials in oncology the event of interest is often death. Where a study subject dies, this death is shown by a downward (vertical) step in the

[1]The author thanks Dr Harvey Motulsky, MD, of GraphPad Software, Inc., La Jolla, CA, for reviewing the draft chapter and for responding with perceptive suggestions.

[2]The author thanks Dr Jenna Elder, PhD, of PharPoint Research, Inc., Wilmington, NC, for reviewing the draft chapter and for providing insightful suggestions.

[3]Kaplan EL, Meier P. Nonparametric estimation from incomplete observations. J. Am. Stat. Assoc. 1958;53:457−81.

[4]Duerden M. What are hazard ratios? What is . . . ? series. Hayward Medical Communications, Hayward Group, Ltd.; 2009. p. 8.

[5]Machin D, Gardner MJ. Calculating confidence intervals for survival time analyses. Brit. Med. J. 1988; 296:1369−71.

curve. Intervals of time, during the clinical trial where there are no deaths, are shown by horizontal lines (no downward steps). In other words, for any interval in time where none of the subjects die, the line in the plot just travels from left to right, that is, horizontally. Typically, horizontal components of the plot are shorter near the beginning of the clinical trial, because many, many subjects are participating in the trial (they have not yet died) and thus many subjects are at risk for triggering the event of interest, while horizontal components of the plot are longer near the end of the clinical trial, because relatively few subjects are still participating in the trial, and deaths are encountered only now and then (6).

In Kaplan—Meier plots, the event must be a one-time event. In other words, if relief from arthritis pain is found at 2 months into the trial, and found again in the same subject at 3 months into the trial, the event is only counted once (only the relief from pain occurring at 2 months is counted). Alternatively, where the event of interest is "relief from pain without relapse," and where relief is first detected at a scheduled assessment at 2 months, and where relief is again detected at a scheduled assessment at 3 months, then relief at both of these scheduled endpoints is mandated to trigger the endpoint (7). Where the goal of the investigator is to make a graph of events of a recurring nature, Kaplan—Meier plots are not used (8).

Where the Kaplan—Meier plot contains two curves, data used for plotting these curves are also used for calculating the P value and the hazard ratio (HR).

b. Examples of Kaplan—Meier Plots—The Holm Study

Holm et al. (9) conducted a clinical trial on breast cancer patients. The trial enrolled 564 subjects. All of the subjects received surgery followed by radiation in an attempt to eliminate the cancer. Of these, 276 subjects were then enrolled in arm A of the clinical trial and received tamoxifen, while 288 subjects were enrolled in arm B and received only placebo. The two arms are summarized below:

- **Arm A**: Tamoxifen.
- **Arm B**: Placebo.

Tamoxifen and placebo were administered for a period of 2 years. Subjects were observed for 15 years in all, starting from the day of assignment to arm A or arm B. During these years, subjects were periodically tested for recurrence of the cancer. Data that were collected took the form of an endpoint called recurrence-free survival.

For each of the subjects, the event of recurrence of the breast cancer, or the event of death from recurrence of the breast cancer, triggered this endpoint.

For each subject, when the event was triggered, the investigators placed a point on the survival curve, also known as the Kaplan—Meier plot (Fig. 9.1). This plot includes two survival curves, one for arm A and the other for arm B. The dots on the curves represent subjects who were censored. Each dot represents one subject. The Kaplan—Meier plot shown in Fig. 9.1 was simplified somewhat from the

[6]Kirkwood BR, Sterne JA. Essential medical statistics. 2nd ed. Malden, MA: Blackwell Science Ltd.; 2003. p. 278.

[7]The author thanks Dr Jenna Elder for this suggestion.

[8]Motulsky H. Intuitive biostatistics. New York, NY: Oxford Univerity Press; 1995. p. 54.

[9]Holm C, Rayala S, Jirström K, Stål O, Kumar R, Landberg G. Association between Pak1 expression and subcellular localization and tamoxifen resistance in breast cancer patients. J. Natl. Cancer Inst. 2006;98:671—80.

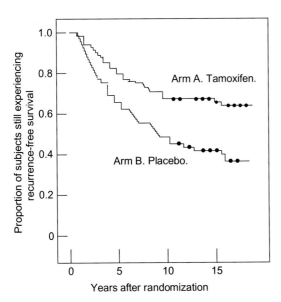

FIGURE 9.1 Kaplan–Meier plot from Holm study. The Kaplan–Meier plot contains two curves enabling the comparison of events experienced by subjects in two study arms over the course of time. The degree of separation of the two curves is measured by the hazard ratio, and the significance of this separation is measured by the P value.

original diagram, for clarity in presentation. Subjects who are censored are usually represented by dots or tick marks, though some investigators choose not to indicate censored subjects. Censoring is defined below.

Visual inspection of the separation between the two curves can indicate the efficacy of the experimental treatment relative to the control treatment. While it is hoped that the experimental treatment results in better survival than the control treatment, it is often the case that there is no discernible difference, and sometimes the case that the experimental treatment reduces survival relative to the control. A measure of the difference in efficacy of the experimental and control treatments is conventionally expressed, in numbers, by way of the hazard ratio. Statisticians define the hazard ratio as the hazard rate of the event of interest in arm A, compared to the hazard rate of the same event in arm B (10). In clinical trials in oncology, an event that is typically plotted on the Kaplan–Meier plot is an increase in tumor burden beyond a predetermined standard. This increase is called "progression." Another event typically plotted on Kaplan–Meier plots is the event of death. In clinical trials on other disorders, the event can be the occurrence of an eye disorder (macular degeneration) (11), occurrence of relapse in patients with multiple sclerosis (12), appearance of a bacterial infection in patients with cirrhosis (13), or a heart attack in patients with atherosclerosis (14). Where a Kaplan–Meier plot is used, it provides information on two things, the cumulative percentage of subjects experiencing the event, and timing of the event.

For the Kaplan–Meier plot from the cancer study of Holm et al. (15), the hazard ratio was

[10]Dawson B, Trapp RG. Basic and clinical biostatistics. 4th ed. New York, NY: Lange Medical Books; 2004. pp. 229–35.

[11]Cukras C, Agrón E, Klein ML, et al. Natural history of drusenoid pigment epithelial detachment in age-related macular degeneration: Age-Related Eye Disease Study Report No. 28. Ophthalmology. 2010;117:489–99.

[12]Kappos L, Radue EW, O'Connor P, et al. A placebo-controlled trial of oral fingolimod in relapsing multiple sclerosis. N. Engl. J. Med. 2010;362:387–401.

[13]Papp M, Norman GL, Vitalis Z, et al. Presence of anti-microbial antibodies in liver cirrhosis—a tell-tale sign of compromised immunity? PLoS One. 2010;5:e12957.

[14]Stone GW, Maehara A, Lansky AJ, et al. A prospective natural-history study of coronary atherosclerosis. N. Engl. J. Med. 2011;364:226–35.

[15]Holm C, Rayala S, Jirström K, Stål O, Kumar R, Landberg G. Association between Pak1 expression and subcellular localization and tamoxifen resistance in breast cancer patients. J. Natl. Cancer Inst. 2006;98:671–80.

0.502. In calculating the hazard ratio, it is always the case that HR = 1.0 means that there is no difference in the underlying hazard rates of the two groups.

The P value corresponding to the significance of separation of the curves from arm A and arm B, from this particular Kaplan–Meier plot was $P = 0.001$. The P value is applied for interpreting the experiment as follows. It means that the probability of observing a result as extreme as, or more extreme than, the one actually observed from chance alone is one in one thousand. If the P value had been 0.01, it would have meant that the probability of observing a result as extreme as, or more extreme than, the one actually observed from chance alone is one in 100. Because the value of 0.001 is less than 0.05, this means that we can reject the null hypothesis. Holm et al. (16) expressly stated that, "$P < 0.05$ was considered statistically significant." By convention, in the context of handling P values, this number (0.05) is called the *alpha value*.

c. Censoring Data

Data on any given subject are "censored" when a subject drops out of the clinical trial. Data on any subjects still alive when a clinical trial on cancer has come to its end, and when the clinical trial has been formally concluded, are also censored. For subjects still alive at the end of an oncology clinical trial, the event that is usually of interest (death) has not occurred, and for this reason the subject is censored.

The term censored means that the exact date of the subject's death is not marked by a downward step on the Kaplan–Meier plot, and is not used for calculating the fraction of surviving study subjects. Where a study subject is censored, this may be indicated on the Kaplan–Meier plot by way of a tick mark or dot. Bland and Altman (17) described the Kaplan–Meier plot as, "the 'curve' is a step function, with sudden changes in the estimated probability corresponding to times at which an event was observed. The times of the censored data are indicated by short vertical lines." Where a subject is censored, a tick mark or dot is shown on the graph.

Generally, subjects are censored when they are lost to the study, but it is not advisable to censor subjects for problems that are less severe, for example, failure to adhere to the drug schedule. If a subject is too ill to travel to the clinic for an infusion of an anticancer drug, and if that subject is censored, the act of censoring that particular subject may introduce bias into the calculations and analysis. Please consider the following hypothetical. In this hypothetical, an experimental drug is ineffective against breast cancer, except for a minority of people in the general population with a rare mutation in the epidermal growth factor gene. Now, please imagine that the health of most of the study subjects deteriorates to the point where they can no longer come to the clinic, and where the investigator decides to censor data from the subjects. In this hypothetical, only a fraction of the subjects—perhaps 5% of the total subjects enrolled in the study—having the rare mutation will feel good enough to come to the clinical for more treatment. In this hypothetical, the subset of study subjects with the rare mutation generally feel good enough to travel to the clinic for scheduled tests and drug doses. The result of the censoring will be as follows. The result will be that the drug is discovered to be dramatically effective against breast cancer. But this will be a misleading and artifactual result because, in fact, the drug is only effective in 5% of the subjects (the subjects with the mutation).

[16]Holm C, Rayala S, Jirström K, Stål O, Kumar R, Landberg G. Association between Pak1 expression and subcellular localization and tamoxifen resistance in breast cancer patients. J. Natl. Cancer Inst. 2006;98:671–80.

[17]Bland JM, Altman DG. Survival probabilities (the Kaplan–Meier method). Brit. Med. J. 1998;317:1572.

In reviewing data from a clinical trial, the statistician can analyze the data from the total population of study subjects, as well as from specific subgroups. These subgroups typically include subjects between 18 and 65 years of age versus subjects over 65 years, subjects previously treated with chemotherapy versus those who are treatment-naive, and subjects with wild-type gene, for example, epidermal growth factor gene versus those with a mutated gene. If there is reason to suspect that expression of a given gene is relevant to response to a study drug, or that a mutation in the gene is relevant to response, then subgroup analysis can be performed when the study is completed, and when all of the data are collected. Dr Harvey Motulsky [18] has emphasized that good methodology in study design requires the definition of subgroups before initiating the clinical trial, and not after the clinical trial when the data are available, and that defining subgroups after the clinical trial can raise the issue of "data mining." Data mining has been described as, "data dredging or fishing and ... the process of trawling through data in the hope of identifying patterns" [19].

d. Hazard Ratio

The hazard ratio is the ratio of (chance of an event occurring in the treatment arm)/(chance of an event occurring in the control arm) [20]. The HR has also been defined as, the ratio of (risk of outcome in one group)/(risk of outcome in another group), occurring at a given interval of time [21]. In the situation where the hazard for an outcome is exactly twice in Group A than in Group B, the value of the hazard ratio can be either 2.0 or 0.5. The result of the calculation (whether HR = 2.0 or 0.5) depends on whether the investigator chooses to calculate the ratio of hazards for (Group A)/(Group B) or, alternatively, to calculate the ratio of hazards for (Group B)/(Group A) [22,23].

The term "hazard" refers to the probability that an individual, under observation in a clinical trial at time t, has an event at that time [24]. It represents the instantaneous event rate for an individual who has already survived to the time "t."

The two arms of a clinical trial can be compared by way of the hazard ratio and the P value. The following serves as a starting point for defining hazard ratio and P value, as it applies to two curves in a Kaplan–Meier plot. The hazard ratio is a measure of the magnitude of the difference between the two curves in the Kaplan–Meier plot, while the P value measures the statistical significance of this difference. These two definitions serve only as starting points for our present goal in arriving at accurate, correct definitions. The following are the correct definitions. The numerical value of the hazard ratio expresses the relative hazard reduction achieved by the study drug compared to

[18]Motulsky H. E-mail of May 9, 2011.

[19]Hand DJ. Data mining: statistics and more? The American Statistician. 1998;52:112–18.

[20]Duerden M. What are hazard ratios? What is ... ? series. Hayward Medical Communications, Hayward Group, Ltd., 2009. p. 8.

[21]Dawson B, Trapp RG. Basic and clinical biostatistics. 4th ed. New York, NY: Lange Medical Books; 2004, p. 407.

[22]Machin D, Cheung YB. Survival analysis: a practical approach. 2nd ed. Hoboken, NJ: John Wiley & Sons, Inc.; 2006. p. 62.

[23]Crowley J. Handbook of statistics in clinical oncology. New York, NY: Marcel Dekker; 2001. p. 541.

[24]Duerden M. What are hazard ratios? What is ... ? series. Hayward Medical Communications, Hayward Group, Ltd. 2009. p. 8.

the hazard reduction by the control treatment. The numerical value can be a fraction of 1.0 or it can be greater than 1.0. For example, a hazard ratio of 0.70 means that the study drug provides 30% risk reduction compared to the control treatment [25]. A hazard ratio of exactly 1.0 means that the study drug provides zero risk reduction, compared to the control treatment. The P value gives the probability of observing an event by chance alone, if the null hypothesis is true. The P value expresses the probability of observing a difference as extreme as that observed, if in fact the null hypothesis is true [26]. If the P value from the study results is smaller than the alpha value, it is concluded that the observed difference is unlikely to be from chance, and that it arose from the treatment used in the clinical trial.

A Kaplan—Meier plot can be used to plot results from only one group. The Kaplan—Meier plot can also be used to plot results from two groups, for example, study drug group and control group. The Kaplan—Meier plot can also be used for data from more than two groups. But an hazard ratio is used to represent the relative difference between only two groups. Please also note that when the hazard ratio is used as a measure for the difference between two survival curves (on one Kaplan—Meier plot), the hazard ratio can be calculated from data collected from the entire study period or, alternatively, from an early time interval or from a late time interval [27]. According to Dr Harvey Motulsky [28], the hazard ratio is only meaningful if you assume that the hazard ratio is the same at all time points.

II. DEFINITIONS AND FORMULAS

The following definitions and formulas are used to calculate the hazard ratio [29].

O_1 is the observed number of deaths at time t, for group 1.

O_2 is the observed number of deaths at time t, for group 2.

E_1 is the expected number of deaths at time t, for group 1, where this expectation is based on the number of deaths occurring in this group for the immediately previous time point (the time just before time t).

E_2 is the expected number of deaths at time t, for group 2, where this expectation is based on the number of deaths occurring in this group for the immediately previous time point (the time just before time t).

E_1 is calculated from the following formula (Eqn (9.1)):

$$E_1 = \sum \left[\frac{(r_{1i})(d_i)}{r_i} \right] \qquad (9.1)$$

E_2 is calculated from the following formula (Eqn (9.2)):

$$E_2 = \sum \left[\frac{(r_{2i})(d_i)}{r_i} \right] \qquad (9.2)$$

The term r_{1i} is the number of subjects alive and not censored in group 1, just before time t_i.

The term r_{2i} is the number of subjects alive and not censored in group 2, just before time t_i.

[25]Kane RC. The clinical significance of statistical significance. The Oncologist. 2008;13:1129−1133.

[26]Kane RC. The clinical significance of statistical significance. The Oncologist. 2008;13:1129−1133.

[27]Kestenbaum B. Epidemiology and biostatistics: an introduction to clinical research. New York, NY: Springer; 2009. p. 227−28.

[28]Motulsky H. E-mail of May 9, 2011.

[29]Machin D, Gardner MJ. Calculating confidence intervals for survival time analyses. Brit. Med. J. 1988;296: 1369−71.

The term r_i, which appears in the denominator, means: $r_{1i} + r_{2i}$. In other words, r_i is the total number of subjects alive in both groups and not censored, just before time t.

The term d_i is the total number of subjects who died at time t_i, in both groups combined. In other words, $d_i = d_{1i} + d_{2i}$.

The symbol $\sum$ (summation sign) indicates the addition over each time of death up to and including time t. The summation sign indicates that the following calculation must be made. Please assume that the clinical study has six time periods. This type of clinical study can be represented by a Kaplan–Meier plot where each curve has six points.

The hazard ratio is calculated from the following formula (Eqn (9.3)) (30):

$$h = \frac{O_1/E_1}{O_2/E_2} \qquad (9.3)$$

III. DATA FROM THE STUDY OF MACHIN AND GARDNER

Machin and Gardner (31) provide an example of data from a clinical study of 49 subjects with colorectal cancer. Twenty-five of the subjects were treated with study drug, while 24 were controls. The following table discloses the times when a subject died, and times when a subject was censored. The time a subject died is the "survival time."

The raw data provided were as follows:

Events of death: Subjects died on the following months. Repeated numbers mean that more than one subject died on that month. In Group 1, subjects died on months: 6, 6, 10, 10, 12, 12, 12, 12, 24, and 32. In Group 2, subjects died on months: 6, 6, 6, 6, 8, 8, 12, 12, 20, 24, 30, and 42.

Censored subjects: Subjects were censored on the following months. Repeated numbers mean that more than one subject was censored on that month. In Group 1, subjects were censored on month: 1, 5, 9, 10, 12, 13, 15, 16, 20, 24, 27, 34, 36, 36, 44. In Group 2, subjects were censored on month: 3, 12, 15, 16, 18, 18, 22, 28, 28, 28, 30, 33.

In all cases, a subject experiencing the event of interest (death) was a different human being than a subject who was censored. Events and censoring are entered into the calculations, but at different points in the mathematical formulas.

The following table provides numbers (r_{1i}, r_{2i}, and d_i) that occur as intermediates in the calculation of the hazard ratio (Table 9.1).

In approaching the conclusion of the calculation of the hazard ratio, it is found that $O_1 = 10$, $E_1 = 11.37$, $O_2 = 12$, and $E_2 = 10.63$. In arriving at the conclusion of this calculation, it is seen that the HR is as follows (Eqn (9.4)):

$$\text{Hazard ratio} = \frac{O_1/E_1}{O_2/E_2} = \frac{10/11.37}{12/10.63} = 0.78 \quad (9.4)$$

This means that treatment with the study drug is associated with a reduction in deaths to 78% of that found with the control treatment. Dawson and Trapp (32) provide another example of calculating the hazard ratio, along with intermediate numbers that were used during the course of the calculation.

---

[30]Machin D, Gardner MJ. Calculating confidence intervals for survival time analyses. Brit. Med. J. 1988;296: 1369–71.

[31]Machin D, Gardner MJ. Calculating confidence intervals for survival time analyses. Brit. Med. J. 1988;296: 1369–71.

[32]Dawson B, Trapp RG. Basic and clinical biostatistics. 4th ed. New York, NY: Lange Medical Books; 2004. pp. 229–235.

TABLE 9.1　Data From a Clinical Trial for Calculating the Hazard Ratio[a]

Months (i)	Group 1 (Study Drug) r_{1i} (r_{1i} is number of subjects alive and not censored, just before time t_i)	Group 2 (Control) r_{2i} (r_{2i} is number of subjects alive and not censored, just before time t_i)	d_i Total Deaths at Time t_i
1	25	24	0
3	24	24	0
5	24	23	0
6	23	23	6
8	21	19	2
9	21	17	0
10	20	17	2
12	17	17	6
13	13	14	0
15	11	14	0
16	10	13	0
18	9	12	0
20	9	10	1
22	8	9	0
24	8	8	2
27	6	7	0
28	5	7	0
30	5	4	1
32	5	2	1
33	4	2	0
34	4	1	0
36	3	1	0
42	1	1	1
44	1	0	0

[a]Machin D, Gardner MJ. Calculating confidence intervals for survival time analyses. Brit. Med. J. 1988;296:1369–71.

IV. DATA USED FOR CONSTRUCTING THE KAPLAN–MEIER PLOT ARE FROM SUBJECTS ENROLLING AT DIFFERENT TIMES

In a typical clinical trial, the sequence of events for each subject involves responding to an advertisement, contacting the sponsor, and undergoing screening and enrollment.

It is usually *not the case* that the sponsor enrolls the desired number of subjects, and then administers the study drug or control treatment to all of the subjects *on exactly the same day*. What is indicated at "day 0" on the Kaplan–Meier plot may correspond, in actuality, to hundreds of different days spread out over the course of a year. The fact that study drug and control treatments are started for each subject, shortly after the subject becomes available and immediately after the subject is properly enrolled in the trial, has prompted some investigators to compare differences in the subjects' baseline characteristics, for subjects enrolled early in the trial with subjects enrolled late in the trial. Jacobs et al. (33) provide a good example of this comparison.

In nutritional studies, all of the enrolled subjects are typically started on experimental and control treatments on exactly the same day. The ample supply of healthy subjects willing to participate in a nutritional study enables this kind of study design. Moreover, the requirement for keeping nutritional study subjects confined in a "metabolic unit" during the course of the study, to prevent subjects from consuming nonstudy foods, necessitates that all subjects begin the trial on the same date (34).

[33]Jacobs LD, Cookfair DL, Rudick RA, et al. Intramuscular interferon beta-1a for disease progression in relapsing multiple sclerosis. The Multiple Sclerosis Collaborative Research Group (MSCRG). Ann. Neurol. 1996;39:285–94.

[34]Margen S, Chu JY, Kaufmann NA, Calloway DH. Studies in calcium metabolism. I. The calciuretic effect of dietary protein. Am. J. Clin. Nutr. 1974;27:584–89.

It is also the case that some clinical trials are concluded before the event of interest has occurred in every single one of the subjects. This situation can lead to bias, where the physiological properties of patients enrolled early in the trial differ from those enrolled late in the trial. As articulated by Bland and Altman (35), "we assume that the survival probabilities are the same for subjects recruited early and late in the study. In a long term observational study of patients with cancer, for example, the case mix may change over the period of recruitment."

V. SAMPLE VERSUS POPULATION

The terms *sample* and *population* are standard terms in statistics. The term *sample* refers to data acquired by actual measurements. The investigator has the option of testing one sample, taken from a population, or of testing more than one sample, taken from the population. In discussions of statistics, it is the case that the term *sample* refers to a group of objects, for example, 50 drug tablets, while the term *population* refers to the entire batch of 10,000 drug tablets that was manufactured. In statistics, it is the case that the term *sample* refers to 100 subjects enrolled in a clinical trial, while the term *population* refers to the entire world's population of people with the disease of interest. The sample needs to be representative of the population.

The term *population* can refer to a hypothesized, underlying value or to an imaginary, idealized value. In some situations, it is possible for the researcher to measure a parameter of interest from all members of the population. But often, it is impractical or impossible to measure the parameter in all members of the population. Data acquired by analyzing a sample are subject to variations in the properties of the sample and to variations in the techniques used by the investigator. For example, in a study of 50 human subjects, 15 of the subjects may have a mutation in a growth factor receptor gene, while the other 35 subjects have the wild-type gene. Or, in a study of 50 human subjects, five of the subjects may have forgotten to take two of their drug doses, while 45 of the subjects had remembered to take all of the drug doses. But data acquired by analyzing a population take into account these and all other variations. But data acquired by analyzing only a 15-person sample taken from this population of 50 human subjects may be drastically biased, for example, where all of the subjects in the 15-person sample have the genetic mutation.

Researchers may be interested in measuring a parameter from a sample, where the goal is to predict the same parameter in the entire population, that is, where it is not practical or not possible to determine that parameter in the population. An example can be found in the manufacture of tablets or pills. Where the goal is to determine the weight of the tablets, and to determine whether the range of weights is within manufacturing specifications, the analyst can measure the weights of 100 tablets, taken from a population of 1 million tablets that was manufactured in a specific batch. In this situation, the 100 tablets constitute a "sample," while the 1 million tablets manufactured in a specific batch constitute the "population." Batchwise manufacture is distinguished in that each component has a specific lot number, and by the fact that the machinery was cleaned and calibrated specifically for the manufacture of that batch.

In this scenario, the various statistical parameters of the sample (mean; standard deviation) are known, and the statistical parameters of the population (mean; standard deviation) are also known. Instead of measuring a parameter of 1 million tablets, the researcher can refer to standards set forth by the pharmaceutical industry. These standards may relate to mean weight and standard deviation.

---

[35]Bland JM, Altman DG. Survival probabilities (the Kaplan—Meier method). Brit. Med. J. 1998;317:1572.

Researchers may also want to compare a parameter from a *first sample* with the same parameter of a *second sample*. This situation occurs in clinical trials where there are two study arms, that is, an experimental drug group and a control group. In the context of a clinical trial, the relevant parameters (mean value of death rate; standard deviation) are collected from the two *samples*. But the relevant *population* parameters (mean value of death rate; standard deviation) would usually be impossible to collect, because this *population* would consist of all of the people in the world having the disease of interest, and satisfying the particular inclusion criteria and exclusion criteria mandated by the trial design.

VI. WHAT CAN BE COMPARED

Tests in drug manufacturing, or comparisons made in clinical trials, often take one of the following three forms (36). First, the mean value from a sample can be compared with a hypothetical value. The hypothetical value can be a standard (manufacturing specification) set forth by the manufacturing industry. The hypothetical can be a value from a census, or from an epidemiological study, involving every person in a country. For this type of study, there is one sample group and one population group.

A second type of comparison can involve paired data. For each subject, a parameter is measured before treatment and after treatment.

Thus, each subject serves as his own control. For this type of study, there are two samples (but no population group). The statistical analysis compares the mean value of the "before" measurements, with the mean value of the "after" measurements. Disis et al. (37) provide an excellent example of the statistical analysis of paired data, where immune response in cancer patients was measured before and after vaccination.

Third, the mean value from a first sample can be compared with the mean value of a second sample. With this type of comparison, in the context of clinical trials, the human subjects in the first sample are not the same people as the human subjects in the second sample. This third type of comparison is the most common trial design that is used in randomized clinical trials.

VII. ONE-TAILED TEST VERSUS TWO-TAILED TEST

The terms one-tailed test and two-tailed test are encountered, for example, when conducting analytical studies on manufactured tablets and when conducting clinical trials. When doing calculations, these terms are encountered when plugging a Z-value into a table of areas under the standard normal curve, and acquiring a P value. A one-tailed test is also called a one-sided test, and a two-tailed test is also called a two-sided test.

This standard table has been called, "Standard Normal Distribution Areas" (38),

---

[36]Whitley E, Bell J. Statistics review 5: comparison of means. Critical Care. 2002;6:424–28.

[37]Disis ML, Wallace DR, Gooley TA, et al. Concurrent trastuzumab and HER2/neu-specific vaccination in patients with metastatic breast cancer. J. Clin. Oncol. 2009;27:4685–92.

[38]Durham TA, Turner JR. Introduction to statistics in pharmaceutical clinical trials. PhP Pharmaceutical Press, Chicago, 2008. pp. 195–203.

"Areas in Tail of the Standard Normal Distribution" (39), and "Areas Under the Standard Normal Curve" (40).

The heading of the table of areas under the standard normal curve typically directs the reader to one column of numbers, which is to be used for one-tailed tests, and to another column of numbers, which is to be used for two-tailed tests (41).

A one-tailed test is used to determine whether the mean of group 1 is greater than the mean of group 2, while a two-tailed test is used to determine whether the mean of group 1 is different than the mean of group 2 (42). By "different," what is meant here is whether there is a statistically significant difference. More accurately, by "different," what is meant is if the difference is plausible within an acceptable degree of error (43). As explained by Dawson and Trapp (44), the one-tailed test is a directional test, while the two-tailed test is a nondirectional test.

A one-tailed test should be used where the goal is to determine whether the value of a mean of a sample is significantly greater than the value of the mean for the corresponding population. The one-tailed test is also used where the goal is to determine whether the value of a mean of a sample is significantly greater than the value of the mean of another sample.

Thus, a one-tailed test is used where the goal is to determine whether a new, improved pill dissolves faster in water than an older formulation of the pill. Also, a one-tailed test is used where the goal is to determine whether a drug having expected curative properties results in a better cure than an inactive placebo.

To provide another example, a one-tailed test is used where the goal is to determine whether vials containing a vaccine are contaminated with 10 or more bacteria (45). In this case, the analyst is only interested in whether the vials contain 10 or more bacteria, in view of industry-wide specifications requiring that vials must contain less than 10 bacteria. Generally, the one-tailed test is used to determine whether sample A is significantly greater than sample B, in the situation where it would not be reasonable to expect sample A to be significantly less than sample B.

But a two-tailed test should be used where the goal is to determine the percentage of tablet weights that are greater or lesser (the sum of the percentage of tablets that are greater plus the sum of the percentage of tablets that are lesser) than the required specification, when comparing tablets made by manufacturer 1 with tablets made by manufacturer 2. Two-tailed tests are more widely used in clinical trials than the one-tailed test, in view of the

[39]Kirkwood BR, Sterne JA. Essential medical statistics. 2nd ed. Malden, MA: Blackwell Science Ltd.; 2003. pp. 470–71.

[40]Dawson B, Trapp RG. Basic and clinical biostatistics. 4th ed. New York, NY: Lange Medical Books/McGraw-Hill; 2004. pp. 364–65.

[41]Dawson B, Trapp RG. Basic and clinical biostatistics. 4th ed. New York, NY: Lange Medical Books/McGraw-Hill; 2004. pp. 364–65.

[42]Norman GR, Streiner DL. Biostatistics. 3rd ed. Hamilton, Ontario: B.C. Decker, Inc.; 2008. p. 56.

[43]Elder J. E-mail of May 12, 2011.

[44]Dawson B, Trapp RG. Basic and clinical biostatistics. 4th ed. New York, NY: Lange Medical Books/McGraw-Hill; 2004. p. 104.

[45]Example derived from page 108 of Jones D. Pharmaceutical statistics. Pharmaceutical Press: Chicago, IL; 2002.

fact that the two-tailed test is more stringent and more conservative (46,47).

VIII. P VALUE

The *P* value is used in a procedure called *hypothesis testing*. *P*, which stands for probability, can be any number between 0.0 and 1.0. According to Whitley and Ball (48), "values close to 0 indicate that the observed difference is unlikely to be due to chance, whereas a *P* value close to 1 suggests there is no difference between groups other than that due to random variation." According to Motulsky (49), "*P* value is simply a probability that answers the following question: If the null hypothesis were true … what is the probability that random sampling … would result in a difference as big or bigger than the one observed?"

Whitley and Ball (50) explain why hypothesis testing is needed, using the example of a drug (nitrate) for preventing deaths from heart disease. Even if there is no real effect of nitrate on mortality, sampling variation makes it unlikely that exactly the same proportion of patients in each group will die. Thus, any observed difference between the two groups may be due to the treatment or it may simply be due to chance. The aim of hypothesis testing is to establish which of these two explanations, treatment versus chance, is more likely.

Hypothesis testing can involve asking whether the mean of a sample has a statistically significant difference from the mean of a population (51). The question of whether there is any difference takes the form of the "null hypothesis." The null hypothesis is that there is no statistically significant difference between the sample and the population.

Where a clinical study involves comparing a study drug group and a placebo group (or study drug sample group and an entire population), the null hypothesis is that there is no statistically significant difference between the study drug group and the placebo group (or no difference between the study drug sample group and the entire population).

The sample mean from the study drug group and the population mean (or the sample mean from the study drug group and the sample mean from the placebo group) can be used to calculate a *P* value. This *P* value is then applied to the null hypothesis.

In hypothesis testing that involves the *null hypothesis*, the researcher does not ask, "Does the study drug work better than the placebo?"

The *null hypothesis* only asks, "Does the study drug work the same as the placebo?"

The question asked by the null hypothesis is the more conservative of these two questions. According to a number of authors (52,53) the null hypothesis is a "straw man" hypothesis.

---

[46]Norman GR, Streiner DL. Biostatistics. 3rd ed. Hamilton, Ontario: B.C. Decker, Inc.; 2008. p. 56.

[47]Motulsky H. Intuitive biostatistics: A nonmathematical guide to statistical thinking. 2nd ed. New York, NY: Oxford University Press; 2010. p. 99.

[48]Whitley E, Ball J. Statistics review 3: hypothesis testing and *P* values. Critical Care. 2002;6:222—25.

[49]Motulsky H. Intuitive biostatistics: A nonmathematical guide to statistical thinking. 2nd ed. New York, NY: Oxford University Press; 2010. p. 104.

[50]Whitley E, Ball J. Statistics review 3: hypothesis testing and *P* values. Critical Care. 2002;6:222—25.

[51]Jones D. Pharmaceutical statistics. Pharmaceutical Press: Chicago, IL; 2002. pp. 154—6.

[52]Durham TA, Turner JR. Introduction to statistics in pharmaceutical clinical trials. PhP Pharmaceutical Press, Chicago, IL; 2008. p. 76.

[53]Hulley SB, Cummings SR, Browner WS, Grady DG, Newman TB. Designing Clinical Research, 3rd ed. Lippincott, Williams, and Wilkins, New York, NY, 2006. p. 58.

Failure to reject the null hypothesis can arise from several sources, including: (1) random scatter or noise in the data; (2) use of too few subjects in the clinical trial; (3) lack of a true, underlying difference between efficacy of the study drug and efficacy of the control treatment. Random scatter can arise from several sources. These include failure of study subjects to take pills according to the required schedule, genetic variability of the infecting virus in clinical trials on antiviral drugs, genetic variability of the tumor in clinical trials using anticancer drugs, and genetic variability of normal tissues in study subjects. Genetic variability of study subjects includes differences in cytochrome P-450 (54) and differences in a component of the immune system called major histocompatibility complex (MHC) (55,56). Cytochrome P-450 is a class of enzymes capable of degrading and inactivating a wide variety of drugs. MHC is a membrane-bound protein of white blood cells that is required for antigen presentation.

After the P value is calculated, the researcher compares it with 0.05. This value (0.05) is called the *alpha value*. In making this comparison, if it is evident that P is equal to or less than 0.05, then the difference between the sample group and the population group (or the study drug group and the control group) is considered significant (and the null hypothesis is rejected).

According to the editorial board of the *American Journal of Physiology*, if the achieved significance level P is less than the critical significance level alpha value then the experimental effect is likely to be real. Most researchers define alpha to be 0.05. Where a researcher chooses an alpha of 0.05, this means that 5% of the time the researcher is willing to declare than an effect exists when (in fact) the effect does not exist (57). The statistician decides upon the alpha value to use before any data are collected.

Thus, according to this editorial, the number 0.05 is used, by researchers, for comparing the P value derived from their calculations. Researchers can choose other alpha values, for example, an alpha value of 0.01 or an alpha value of 0.001. Using an alpha value of 0.01 provides a more stringent test of statistical significance. An alpha value of 0.0001 provides an even more stringent test.

Regarding the alpha value of 0.05, Healy (58) finds that, the "issue is where to draw the line between significant and non-significant. No such line exists and any distinction of this kind is completely arbitrary. A convention has grown up which places the dividing line at a significance level of 0.05." In the instances where a smaller alpha value is used, these tend to involve experiments that are more under the control of the investigator (when compared to clinical trials on human subjects),

[54]De Gregori M, Allegri M, De Gregori S, et al. How and why to screen for CYP2D6 interindividual variability in patients under pharmacological treatments. Curr. Drug Metab. 2010;11:276–82.

[55]Sidney J, Steen A, Moore C, et al. Divergent motifs but overlapping binding repertoires of six HLA-DQ molecules frequently expressed in the worldwide human population. J. Immunol. 2010;185:4189–98.

[56]de Araujo Souza PS, Sichero L, Maciag PC. HPV variants and HLA polymorphisms: the role of variability on the risk of cervical cancer. Future Oncol. 2009;5:359–70.

[57]Curran-Everett D, Benos DJ. Guidelines for reporting statistics in journals published by the American Physiological Socieity. 2004;287:E189–91.

[58]Healy MJR. Significance tests. Arch. Dis. Childhood. 1991;66:1457–8.

such as experiments in bacteriology (59) or genetics (60,61,62). In these cited articles, alpha values of 0.001 were used.

Statistical significance needs to be distinguished from clinical significance. Kaul and Diamond (63), Kane (64), Bhardwaj et al. (65), and Houle and Stump (66), warn of the situation where data are statistically significant but are not clinically significant and have no real-world value. A number of publications have reported that a parameter was statistically significant, but not clinically significant, for example, Jeffrey et al. (67), and van Maldegem et al. (68). Fethney (69) pointed out that the P value on its own provides no information about the overall importance or meaning of the results to clinical practice.

IX. CALCULATING THE P VALUE—A WORKING EXAMPLE

The following table lists the parameters needed for calculating the P value (Table 9.2).

Only one example will be shown for calculating the P value. This example involves comparing the mean of a first sample (study drug group) with the mean of a second sample (control group). The data are from Machin and Gardner (70).

In Group 1 (study drug group), subjects died on months: 6, 6, 10, 10, 12, 12, 12, 12, 24, and 32.

In Group 0 (control group), subjects died on months: 6, 6, 6, 6, 8, 8, 12, 12, 20, 24, 30, and 42.

When faced with the need to calculate a P value, the researcher must choose between various different statistical tests. One of these

[59]Kinder SA, Holt SC. Characterization of coaggregation between *Bacteroides gingivalis* T22 and *Fusobacterium nucleatum* T18. Infect. Immun. 1989;57:3425–33.

[60]Mutch DM, Simmering R, Donnicola D, et al. Impact of commensal microbiota on murine gastrointestinal tract gene ontologies. Physiol. Genomics. 2004;19:22–31.

[61]Travers SA, Tully DC, McCormack GP, Fares MA. A study of the coevolutionary patterns operating within the env gene of the HIV-1 group M subtypes. Mol. Biol. Evol. 2007;24:2787–801.

[62]Znaidi S, Weber S, Al-Abdin OZ, et al. Genomewide location analysis of *Candida albicans* Upc2p, a regulator of sterol metabolism and azole drug resistance. Eukaryot. Cell. 2008;7:836–47.

[63]Kaul S, Diamond GA. Trial and error. How to avoid commonly encountered limitations of published clinical trials. J. Am. Coll. Cardiol. 2010;55:15–427.

[64]Kane RC. The clinical significance of statistical significance. Oncologist. 2008;13:1129–33.

[65]Bhardwaj SS, Camacho F, Derrow A, Fleischer Jr AB, Feldman SR. Statistical significance and clinical relevance: the importance of power in clinical trials in dermatology. Arch Dermatol. 2004;140:1520–23.

[66]Houle TT, Stump DA. Statistical significance versus clinical significance. Semin. Cardiothorac. Vasc. Anesth. 2008;12:5–6.

[67]Jeffery NN, Douek N, Guo DY, Patel MI. Discrepancy between radiological and pathological size of renal masses. BMC Urol. 2011;11:2 (9 pages).

[68]van Maldegem BT, Duran M, Wanders RJ, et al. Clinical, biochemical, and genetic heterogeneity in short-chain acyl-coenzyme A dehydrogenase deficiency. J. Am. Med. Assoc. 2006;296:943–52.

[69]Fethney J. Statistical and clinical significance, and how to use confidence intervals to help interpret both. Aust. Crit. Care. 2010;23:93–7.

[70]Machin D, Gardner MJ. Calculating confidence intervals for survival time analyses. Brit. Med. J. 1988;296:1369–71.

TABLE 9.2 Definitions and Formulas

	Symbol	Equation	Formula or Definition
Sample number	n		This is the number of individuals in a given sample. This can be the number of tablets taken for sampling from a larger, defined manufacturing batch. This can also be the number of people (meeting enrollment criteria) with a specific disease who are actually enrolled in a clinical trial, and allocated to a specific arm of the trial
Population number	N		This can be the total number of tablets in a large, defined manufacturing batch. This can also be the number of people (meeting enrollment criteria) with a specific disease, in the entire world
Sample mean (pronounced "*x*-bar")[a]	$\bar{x}$	Eqn (9.5)	$\bar{x} = (1/n) \sum x_i$
Population mean	μ	Eqn (9.6)	$\mu = (1/N) \sum x_i$
Sample standard deviation[a,b]	s	Eqn (9.7)	$s = \sqrt{\sum (x_j - \bar{x})^2 / (n-1)}$
Population standard deviation[b]	σ	Eqn (9.8)	$\sigma = \sqrt{\sum (x_j - \bar{x})^2 / N}$
Square root	$\sqrt{}$		The $\sqrt{}$ symbol requires taking the square root of everything occurring to the right of the symbol
Z-score (calculated using population standard deviation)[c]	Z	Eqn (9.9)	$Z = (\bar{x} - \mu)/\sigma$
Z-score used when comparing two samples (study drug group and control group).[c] $\bar{x}_1$ is the mean of the parameter of interest from the study drug group, while $\bar{x}_0$ is the mean of the corresponding parameter of interest from the control group[c]	Z	Eqn (9.10)	Where σ is known: $Z = (\bar{x}_1 - \bar{x}_0)/\sqrt{(\sigma_1^2/n_1) + (\sigma_0^2/n_0)}$
		Eqn (9.11)	Where σ is not known:[d] $Z = (\bar{x}_1 - \bar{x}_0)/\sqrt{(s_1^2/n_1) + (s_0^2/n_0)}$

[a]*Whitley E, Ball J. Statistics review 1: presenting and summarising data. Critical Care. 2002;6:66–71.*
[b]*Jones D. Pharmaceutical statistics. Pharmaceutical Press: Chicago, IL; 2002. p. 21.*
[c]*Kirkwood BR, Sterne JA. Essential medical statistics. 2nd ed. Malden, MA: Blackwell Science Ltd.; 2003. pp. 39, 45, 51, 53–4, 58, 61–2.*
[d]*Where the value of the population standard deviation (σ) is not known, the value of the sample standard deviation (s) may be used instead (Kirkwood BR, Sterne JA. Essential medical statistics. 2nd ed. Malden, MA: Blackwell Science Ltd.; 2003. p. 39; Norman GR, Streiner DL. Biostatistics. 3rd ed. Hamilton, Ontario: B.C. Decker, Inc.; 2008. p. 50).*

tests involves an intermediate step where the *Z* statistic is calculated, while another commonly used test has an intermediate step where the *t* statistic is calculated. According to Pocock (71) the simplest test is the one using the *Z* statistic. But it should be noted that calculations using the *Z* statistic may be misleading when analyzing small samples, and that the *t* statistic is

[71]Pocock SJ. The simplest statistical test: how to check for a difference between treatments. Brit. Med. J. 2006; 332:1256–8.

more appropriate with small samples [72]. With large samples the t statistic and Z statistic are equivalent to each other [73].

The relevant formulas are from the above table (Table 9.2). These formulas are as follows.

- Sample standard deviation (Eqn (9.12)):

$$s = \sqrt{\frac{\sum (x_j - \bar{x})^2}{n-1}} \qquad (9.12)$$

- Z value when comparing two samples: study drug (group 1) and control (group 0) (Eqn (9.13)):

$$Z = \frac{\bar{x}_1 - \bar{x}_0}{\sqrt{(s_1^2/n_1) + (s_0^2/n_0)}} \qquad (9.13)$$

Intermediate steps in making the calculation appear in Table 9.3. Table 9.3 shows the calculation of sample standard deviation for the two samples (study drug group; control group), for goal of determining Z value, and for eventual goal of determining P value.

The following continues with the calculations (Eqn (9.14)):

$$Z = \frac{\bar{x}_1 - \bar{x}_0}{\sqrt{(s_1^2/n_1) + (s_0^2/n_0)}}$$

$$= \frac{13.6 - 15.0}{\sqrt{(66.49/10) + (136.35/12)}} \qquad (9.14)$$

$$= \frac{-1.4}{\sqrt{6.649 + 11.36}} = -0.330$$

Plugging $Z = -0.330$ into a standard table (Table 9.4) that converts Z values to probabilities (to areas under a normal curve) results in $P = 0.3707$. The relevant numbers are shown in bold in Table 9.4. This probability is a one-tailed P value. As mentioned above, this standard table has names, such as, "Standard Normal Distribution Areas" [74], "Areas in Tail of the Standard Normal Distribution" [75], and "Areas Under the Standard Normal Curve" [76]. Comments on the nature of this table appear in footnotes [77,78]. The y-axis (left border) shows the number immediately before the decimal, and immediately after the decimal, for the Z

---

[72]Motulsky H. E-mail of May 9, 2011.

[73]Motulsky H. E-mail of May 9, 2011.

[74]Durham TA, Turner JR. Introduction to statistics in pharmaceutical clinical trials. PhP Pharmaceutical Press, Chicago, 2008. pp. 195–203.

[75]Kirkwood BR, Sterne JA. Essential medical statistics. 2nd ed. Malden, MA: Blackwell Science Ltd.; 2003. pp. 470–71.

[76]Dawson B, Trapp RG. Basic and clinical biostatistics. 4th ed. New York, NY: Lange Medical Books/McGraw-Hill; 2004. pp. 364–65.

[77]http://www.stat.lsu.edu/exstweb/statlab/Tables/TABLES98-Z.html.

[78]This table, which was from Louisiana State University, has numbers that are rounded off differently from, but contains numbers that are essentially identical to, corresponding tables in Kirkwood BR, Sterne JA. Essential medical statistics. 2nd ed. Malden, MA: Blackwell Science Ltd.; 2003. pp. 470–71, Dawson B, Trapp RG. Basic and clinical biostatistics. 4th ed. New York, NY: Lange Medical Books/McGraw-Hill; 2004. pp. 364–65, and Durham TA, Turner JR. Introduction to statistics in pharmaceutical clinical trials. PhP Pharmaceutical Press, Chicago, 2008. pp. 195–203.

TABLE 9.3 Steps for Calculating the Z Value

Column 1 Study Drug Group 1 (Survival Time, months)	Column 2 Survival Time Minus Mean (Mean = 13.6 months)	Column 3 Squared Value From Column 2	Column 4 Sum of All Squared Values	Column 5 Sample Standard Deviation (n = 10; n − 1 = 9)	Column 6 Control group Group 0 (survival time, months)	Column 7 Survival time minus mean (mean = 15.0 months)	Column 8 Squared value from column 7	Column 9 Sum of all squared values	Column 10 Sample standard deviation (n = 12; n − 1 = 11)
6	−7.6	57.76	598.4	8.154 months	6	−9	81	1500	11.677 months
6	−7.6	57.76			6	−9	81		
10	−3.6	12.96			6	−9	81		
10	−3.6	12.96			6	−9	81		
12	−1.6	2.56			8	−7	49		
12	−1.6	2.56			8	−7	49		
12	−1.6	2.56			12	−3	9		
12	−1.6	2.56			12	−3	9		
24	10.4	108.16			20	5	25		
32	18.4	338.56			24	9	81		
					30	15	225		
					42	27	729		

TABLE 9.4 Areas in Tail of the Standard Normal Distribution (Right-Tail Areas From Z to Infinity)

Z Value	0.00	0.01	0.02	**0.03**	0.04	0.05	0.06	0.07	0.08	0.09
0.00	0.5000	0.4960	0.4920	0.4880	0.4840	0.4801	0.4761	0.4721	0.4681	0.4641
0.10	0.4602	0.4562	0.4522	0.4483	0.4443	0.4404	0.4364	0.4325	0.4286	0.4247
0.20	0.4207	0.4168	0.4129	0.4090	0.4052	0.4013	0.3974	0.3936	0.3897	0.3859
0.30	0.3821	0.3783	0.3745	**0.3707**	0.3669	0.3632	0.3594	0.3557	0.3520	0.3483
0.40	0.3446	0.3409	0.3372	0.3336	0.3300	0.3264	0.3228	0.3192	0.3156	0.3121
0.50	0.3085	0.3050	0.3015	0.2981	0.2946	0.2912	0.2877	0.2843	0.2810	0.2776
0.60	0.2743	0.2709	0.2676	0.2643	0.2611	0.2578	0.2546	0.2514	0.2483	0.2451
0.70	0.2420	0.2389	0.2358	0.2327	0.2296	0.2266	0.2236	0.2206	0.2177	0.2148
0.80	0.2119	0.2090	0.2061	0.2033	0.2005	0.1977	0.1949	0.1922	0.1894	0.1867
0.90	0.1841	0.1814	0.1788	0.1762	0.1736	0.1711	0.1685	0.1660	0.1635	0.1611
1.00	0.1587	0.1562	0.1539	0.1515	0.1492	0.1469	0.1446	0.1423	0.1401	0.1379
1.10	0.1357	0.1335	0.1314	0.1292	0.1271	0.1251	0.1230	0.1210	0.1190	0.1170
1.20	0.1151	0.1131	0.1112	0.1093	0.1075	0.1056	0.1038	0.1020	0.1003	0.0985
1.30	0.0968	0.0951	0.0934	0.0918	0.0901	0.0885	0.0869	0.0853	0.0838	0.0823
1.40	0.0808	0.0793	0.0778	0.0764	0.0749	0.0735	0.0721	0.0708	0.0694	0.0681
1.50	0.0668	0.0655	0.0643	0.0630	0.0618	0.0606	0.0594	0.0582	0.0571	0.0559
1.60	0.0548	0.0537	0.0526	0.0516	0.0505	0.0495	0.0485	0.0475	0.0465	0.0455
1.70	0.0446	0.0436	0.0427	0.0418	0.0409	0.0401	0.0392	0.0384	0.0375	0.0367
1.80	0.0359	0.0351	0.0344	0.0336	0.0329	0.0322	0.0314	0.0307	0.0301	0.0294
1.90	0.0287	0.0281	0.0274	0.0268	0.0262	0.0256	0.0250	0.0244	0.0239	0.0233
2.00	0.0228	0.0222	0.0217	0.0212	0.0207	0.0202	0.0197	0.0192	0.0188	0.0183
2.10	0.0179	0.0174	0.0170	0.0166	0.0162	0.0158	0.0154	0.0150	0.0146	0.0143
2.20	0.0139	0.0136	0.0132	0.0129	0.0125	0.0122	0.0119	0.0116	0.0113	0.0110
2.30	0.0107	0.0104	0.0102	0.0099	0.0096	0.0094	0.0091	0.0089	0.0087	0.0084
2.40	0.0082	0.0080	0.0078	0.0075	0.0073	0.0071	0.0069	0.0068	0.0066	0.0064
2.50	0.0062	0.0060	0.0059	0.0057	0.0055	0.0054	0.0052	0.0051	0.0049	0.0048
2.60	0.0047	0.0045	0.0044	0.0043	0.0041	0.0040	0.0039	0.0038	0.0037	0.0036
2.70	0.0035	0.0034	0.0033	0.0032	0.0031	0.0030	0.0029	0.0028	0.0027	0.0026
2.80	0.0026	0.0025	0.0024	0.0023	0.0023	0.0022	0.0021	0.0021	0.0020	0.0019
2.90	0.0019	0.0018	0.0018	0.0017	0.0016	0.0016	0.0015	0.0015	0.0014	0.0014
3.00	0.0013	0.0013	0.0013	0.0012	0.0012	0.0011	0.0011	0.0011	0.0010	0.0010

(*Continued*)

TABLE 9.4 (Continued)

3.10	0.0010	0.0009	0.0009	0.0009	0.0008	0.0008	0.0008	0.0008	0.0007	0.0007
3.20	0.0007	0.0007	0.0006	0.0006	0.0006	0.0006	0.0006	0.0005	0.0005	0.0005
3.30	0.0005	0.0005	0.0005	0.0004	0.0004	0.0004	0.0004	0.0004	0.0004	0.0003
3.40	0.0003	0.0003	0.0003	0.0003	0.0003	0.0003	0.0003	0.0003	0.0003	0.0002
3.50	0.0002	0.0002	0.0002	0.0002	0.0002	0.0002	0.0002	0.0002	0.0002	0.0002
3.60	0.0002	0.0002	0.0001	0.0001	0.0001	0.0001	0.0001	0.0001	0.0001	0.0001
3.70	0.0001	0.0001	0.0001	0.0001	0.0001	0.0001	0.0001	0.0001	0.0001	0.0001
3.80	0.0001	0.0001	0.0001	0.0001	0.0001	0.0001	0.0001	0.0001	0.0001	0.0001
3.90	0.0000	0.0000	0.0000	0.0000	0.0000	0.0000	0.0000	0.0000	0.0000	0.0000
4.00	0.0000	0.0000	0.0000	0.0000	0.0000	0.0000	0.0000	0.0000	0.0000	0.0000

value. The x-axis (top border) shows the second decimal place number of the Z value. The body of the table (Table 9.4) shows the P values (probabilities; areas).

Because 0.3707 is greater than 0.05, it is concluded that the difference between Group 1 and Group 0 is not statistically significant. Because the difference between Group 1 and Group 0 is not significant, the null hypothesis is accepted.

The reader needs to use extreme caution before using the standard table because the format is not particularly standard. Depending on the statistics book, different formats are used. Norman and Streiner (79), expressly warn that one should be careful reading tables of the normal curve in statistics books. The problem is that in some books, the area equivalent to $Z = 0.0$ is assigned as being 0.5, while in other books, the area equivalent to $Z = 0.0$ is assigned as 0.0. In using these tables, the reader needs to determine if the area (the probability) corresponds to the area above the Z value, or to the area below the Z value.

Kirkwood and Sterne (80) provide the same sort of calculation in an example involving two samples. The first sample is an experimental group (Group 1; 36 smokers), while the second sample is a control group (Group 0; 64 nonsmokers). In this example, the mean value (lung volume) for the smokers was $\bar{x}_1 = 4.7$ liters, while the mean value (lung volume) for the nonsmokers was $\bar{x}_0 = 5.0$ liters. The standard deviations for the two groups were s_1 (smokers) $= 0.6$ and s_0 (nonsmokers) $= 0.6$. (It was only a coincidence that the standard deviations were both the same.) In working through the calculations, one finds that (Eq. (9.15)):

$$Z = \frac{\bar{x}_1 - \bar{x}_0}{\sqrt{(s_1^2/n_1) + (s_0^2/n_0)}} = \frac{-0.3}{0.125} = -2.4 \quad (9.15)$$

Plugging the Z value of -2.4 into the standard table, provides $P = 0.0082$. This probability is a one-tailed P value. Since 0.0082 is less than 0.05, the difference is found to be

[79]Norman GR, Streiner DL. Biostatistics. 3rd ed. Hamilton, Ontario: B.C. Decker, Inc.; 2008. p. 35.

[80]Kirkwood BR, Sterne JA. Essential medical statistics. 2nd ed. Malden, MA: Blackwell Science Ltd.; 2003. pp. 61−3.

significant, and the null hypothesis is rejected. What is rejected is the notion that smoking does not significantly influence lung volume.

In configuring the smoking study, the statistician can ask, "Does smoking significantly reduce lung volume?" This involves using a one-sided P value. Alternatively, the statistician can ask, "Does smoking significantly change lung volume?" This involves using a two-sided P value. The value of the two-sided P value is twice 0.0082, that is, $P = 0.0164$.

Please note the negative sign in the above Z value, that is, $Z = -2.4$. For the purposes of plugging in the Z value and obtaining a probability, the negative sign can be ignored. In the words of Norman and Streiner (81), "what we do is ignore the sign, but keep it in our minds."

Pocock (82) provides additional examples from actual clinical trials. What is provided are numbers for plugging into the formula, $Z = (\bar{x}_1 - \bar{x}_0)/\left[\sqrt{(s_1^2/n_1) + (s_0^2/n_0)}\right]$, the calculated number for the Z value, instructions on plugging the Z value into the standard table, the value for P that was determined from this table, and instructions for interpreting the P value.

X. SUMMARY

To calculate the P value, the investigator starts with data, regarding an event of interest, from a first sample, and data, regarding the same event but from a second sample. From these data, the investigator then calculates the means, standard deviations, and the Z value. The Z value is then plugged into a standard table with numbers corresponding to areas under a normal distribution curve. In plugging in the Z value, the investigator then arrives at the P value. This particular routine is used where the distribution of values in the first sample (study drug) follows a normal distribution, and where the distribution in the second sample (control treatment) also follows a normal distribution. Where the distribution of values is not normal, that is, where the distribution is skewed or contains two peaks, the investigator should use a different statistical tool, that is, a statistical tool that is a nonparametric test.

Daniel (83) provides a flow chart (decision tree) for determining which statistical formula to use. The decision tree asks whether the population is normally distributed, if the sample is large or if the sample is small, and if the population variance (or standard deviation) is known or unknown. Depending on the answers, the researcher may need to use, or may prefer to use, the Z statistic, the t statistic, or a nonparametric test such as the Wilcoxon rank sum test.

XI. THEORY BEHIND THE Z VALUE AND THE TABLE OF AREAS IN TAIL OF THE STANDARD NORMAL DISTRIBUTION

In brief, calculating the Z value converts the raw data into a normalized value. The normalized value, when plugged into the standard table, provides an area under a curve that depicts the normal distribution. This area is, in effect, identical with the probability (P value). The goal of this chapter is to serve as a starting point in biostatistics, and to provide a reference point for use in navigating through textbooks on biostatistics.

[81]Norman GR, Streiner DL. Biostatistics. 3rd ed. Hamilton, Ontario: B.C. Decker, Inc.; 2008. p. 35.

[82]Pocock SJ. The simplest statistical test:how to check for a difference between treatments. Brit. Med. J. 2006;332:1256−58.

[83]Daniel WW. Biostatistics. 9th ed. Hoboken, NJ: John Wiley & Sons, Inc.; 2009. p. 176.

XII. STATISTICAL ANALYSIS BY SUPERIORITY ANALYSIS VERSUS BY NONINFERIORITY ANALYSIS

The two arms found in a typical Kaplan–Meier plot can be compared or analyzed by various statistical methods, including superiority analysis and noninferiority analysis. Where the study drug is compared to a placebo, superiority analysis is used. But where the study drug is compared with an active control drug, or with the standard or traditional treatment, both superiority analysis and noninferiority analysis are used (84).

While sponsors and investigators prefer that their drug be superior to the control treatment, the difference in efficacy may be insignificant. Where the difference is insignificant, the clinical trial can be rescued, at least in some situations, by noninferiority analysis.

Following the clinical trial, the statistician analyzes the results to determine whether the study drug is superior to the active control drug. The statistician also analyzes the results to determine whether the study drug is not significantly inferior to the active control.

With noninferiority analysis, the goal of the investigator is to prove that the efficacy of the study drug is better than, equivalent to, or only trivially worse than the active control, in terms of efficacy (85). D'Agostino et al. (86),

emphasize that, in designing a noninferiority clinical trial, the comparator drug should be the *best available* comparator drug.

In addition to the superiority trial design, and the noninferiority trial design, another type of trial design is the equivalence trial. The goal of this type of trial is to demonstrate that the study drug is both insignificantly better than and insignificantly worse than an active control drug. Paggio et al. (87), document the fact that published reports of clinical trials frequently confuse the concepts of noninferiority and equivalence.

In conducting a clinical trial, the sponsor prefers to show that its study drug is superior to an active control drug, in terms of efficacy. However, if superiority in terms of efficacy cannot be shown, and where the investigator is not willing to scrap the results from the clinical trial, the results can be salvaged by using noninferiority analysis. In practice, statisticians conduct the noninferiority analysis first, and once this is complete, they conduct the superiority analysis (88). The following situation concerns a finding of noninferiority where the efficacy of the study drug is found to be not statistically better than that of the active control drug (comparator drug). In this case, regulatory approval can be granted based on the fact that the study drug is safer, cheaper to produce, easier to administer (injected vs oral),

[84]US Department of Health and Human Services. Food and Drug Administration. Guidance for Industry. Non-inferiority clinical trials. 2010 (66 pages).

[85]Piaggio G, Elbourne DR, Altman DG, Pocock SJ, Evans SJ; CONSORT Group. Reporting of noninferiority and equivalence randomized trials: an extension of the CONSORT statement. J. Am. Med. Assoc. 2006;295:1152–60.

[86]D'Agostino RB Sr, Massaro JM, Sullivan LM. Non-inferiority trials: design concepts and issues—the encounters of academic consultants in statistics. Stat. Med. 2003;22:169–86.

[87]Piaggio G, Elbourne DR, Altman DG, Pocock SJ, Evans SJ; CONSORT Group. Reporting of noninferiority and equivalence randomized trials: an extension of the CONSORT statement. J. Am. Med. Assoc. 2006;295:1152–60.

[88]The author thanks Dr Jenna Elder for this fact.

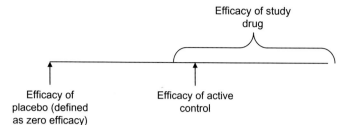

FIGURE 9.2 Noninferiority trial. In a noninferiority trial, the efficacy of the study drug must not be significantly less than the efficacy of the active control, and it also must be significantly greater than the apparent efficacy of the placebo group. The open-ended bracket indicates the range of what is significantly greater.

or where compliance by patients outside of the clinical trial is expected to be better (89,90). Better compliance, for example, will occur with a pill taken once a day compared with a pill that must be taken three times per day at strictly timed intervals.

Noninferiority analysis is relevant only where the study design compares study drug with an active control drug (comparator drug). This type of analysis is not relevant and not appropriate where the study design compares study drug with placebo (91).

Where the investigator foresees performing a noninferiority analysis of the efficacy results, the best trial design is a three-arm study, involving study drug, active control drug (comparator drug), and placebo. According to the ICH Guidelines, "non-inferiority trials may also incorporate a placebo, thus pursuing multiple goals in one trial; for example, they may establish superiority to placebo and hence validate the trial design and simultaneously evaluate the degree of similarity of efficacy and safety to the active comparator" (92).

D'Agostino et al. (93), provide a diagram with tick-marks showing efficacy of various treatments, where the distance between tick-marks represents statistically significant differences and statistically insignificant differences. The take-home lesson of this diagram is as follows. To arrive at a conclusion that the study drug is noninferior to an active control drug, the efficacy of the study drug (which takes the form of a range called the confidence interval) must be greater than the efficacy of the placebo (defined as zero efficacy). Also, the efficacy of the study drug must reside in an open-ended range, where the lower end of the range is defined as insignificantly less than the efficacy of the active control, and the upper range is defined as being greater than the efficacy of the active control. Fig. 9.2 shows this diagram.

For comparison, what is then shown is a diagram of a superiority analysis (Fig. 9.3).

Noninferiority trials are different from superiority trials in terms of how the data are analyzed, but also in terms of study design. Noninferiority trials require more study

[89]Lesaffre E. Superiority, equivalence, and non-inferiority trials. Bulletin NYU Hospital for Joint Diseases. 2008;66:150−4.

[90]Durham TA, Turner JR. Introduction to statistics in pharmaceutical clinical trials. PhP Pharmaceutical Press, Chicago, IL, 2008. pp. 28, 130−31.

[91]Durham TA, Turner JR. Introduction to statistics in pharmaceutical clinical trials. PhP Pharmaceutical Press, Chicago, IL; 2008. p. 187.

[92]European Medicines Agency (EMEA) ICH Topic E9. Statistical principles for clinical trials. 1998 (37 pages).

[93]D'Agostino RB Sr, Massaro JM, Sullivan LM. Non-inferiority trials: design concepts and issues—the encounters of academic consultants in statistics. Stat. Med. 2003;22:169−86.

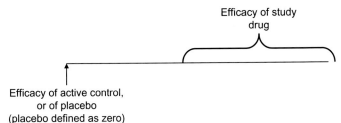

Efficacy of study drug

Efficacy of active control, or of placebo (placebo defined as zero)

FIGURE 9.3 Superiority trial. In a superiority trial, the efficacy of the study drug must be significantly greater than the efficacy of the active control (or placebo). The open-ended bracket indicates the range of what is significantly greater.

subjects. In the words of one commentator, "because the acceptable difference between the two arms is typically smaller by half than what was gained moving from a placebo to a standard treatment, the number of patients required to maintain the same statistical power increases substantially. On average, fourfold more patients are required for a non-inferiority design than for a superiority one" (94).

Le Henanff et al. (95), provide guidance on designing and reporting of noninferiority trials. For example, it was recommended that, "it is surely preferable to use standard vocabulary such as treatment A 'is not inferior to' … treatment B 'with regard to the margin prespecified at Δ' rather than stating a treatment is 'not substantially lower than' … a control treatment" (96). For reporting the results of noninferiority trials, these authors also recommend disclosing the results from PP analysis,

as well as from intent-to-treat (ITT) analysis, and reporting the confidence interval. For noninferiority trials, PP analysis is preferred, while ITT analysis is secondary (97,98). In the context of a noninferiority trial, PP analysis may provide conclusions that are more conservative or careful, than conclusions provided by ITT analysis (99,100).

The confidence interval defines the difference between the efficacy of the study drug and the active control drug. Moreover, these authors recommend reporting the number of subjects dropping out of the trial.

In view of the fact that noninferiority trials are conducted with the expectation that efficacy of the study drug and active control drug are the same, Dignam (101) has warned against the early termination of clinical trials where the available data implicate the study drug as superior to the active control. Thus,

[94]Tuma RS. Trend toward noninferiority trials mean more difficult interpretation of trial results. J. Natl. Cancer Inst. 2007;99:1746−8.

[95]Le Henanff A, Giraudeau B, Baron G, Ravaud P. Quality of reporting of noninferiority and equivalence randomized trials. J. Am. Med. Assoc. 2006;295:1147−51.

[96]Le Henanff A, Giraudeau B, Baron G, Ravaud P. Quality of reporting of noninferiority and equivalence randomized trials. J. Am. Med. Assoc. 2006;295:1147−51.

[97]Sanjay Mitter, personal communication of May 13, 2011.

[98]The author thanks Dr Jenna Elder for this advice.

[99]Matsuyama Y. A comparison of the results of intent-to-treat, per-protocol, and g-estimation in the presence of non-random treatment changes in a time-to-event non-inferiority trial. Stat. Med. 2010;29:2107−16.

[100]Matilde Sanchez M, Chen X. Choosing the analysis population in non-inferiority studies: per protocol or intent-to-treat. Stat. Med. 2006;25:1169−81.

[101]Dignam JJ. Early viewing of noninferiority trials in progress. J. Clin. Oncol. 2005;23:5461−3.

during the early phases of any clinical trial, the available data may show that the study drug clearly works better than the control treatment. But often, data available during the first weeks or months of a clinical trial are of a sporadic nature, that is, early indications of remarkable efficacy or unusual toxicity typically disappear as more and more data are collected. Thus, in the context of a noninferiority trial, where there is an expectation of no difference in efficacy, investigators should refrain from deciding that the study drug is more effective than the active control, where the clinical trial is only partly completed.

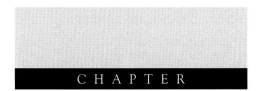

C H A P T E R

10

Biostatistics—Part II

Dr. Jennifer Elder, Ph.D.

Chief Scientific Officer, PharPoint Research, Inc., Durham, NC

I. INTRODUCTION

A question commonly asked of statisticians in clinical trials is, "How many subjects do I need for this study?" This question is not easily answered as it depends on a number of practical and statistical considerations. In general, the sample size should be large enough to provide a reasonable answer to the underlying research objective of the study, but must be reasonably set based on the total patient population under investigation, the available study budget, or the length of time available for study evaluation. Wittes (1) stated that, "[t]he sample size of a trial must be large enough to allow a reasonable chance of answering the question posed but not so large that continuing randomization past the point of near-certainty will lead to ethical discomfort."

II. DISCUSSIONS THAT IMPACT SAMPLE SIZE DETERMINATION

The assumptions necessary for defining the sample size should be listed in the Clinical Study Protocol. These assumptions are often comprised from answers to the following questions:

- What is the primary objective of the study?
- What measure will be used to determine this outcome for a given subject?
- What is the clinically meaningful difference?
- What treatment effect is expected?
- What data analysis technique is appropriate for determining a difference between treatments?
- What degree of certainty is expected or required for ascertaining treatment difference?

[1]Wittes J. Sample size calculations for randomized controlled trials. Epidemiol. Rev. 2002;24(1).

Clinical Trials.
DOI: http://dx.doi.org/10.1016/B978-0-12-804217-5.00010-2

A statistician can translate the responses to these questions into statistical assumptions which can be utilized to determine a sample size or a range of sample sizes that could be considered for the trial based on statistical principles. These values are then reviewed with the clinical trial design team to set the sample size for the study. For this reason, it is important to have a basic understanding of these terms to ensure productive conversations around sample size determination.

a. What Is the Primary Objective of the Study?

Clinical trial objectives are concise statements of the major and minor questions that the trial is designed to answer. Statement of the objective should include specific details about the purpose of the trial (2). The primary objective of the study is typically related to the assessment of efficacy. For example, CEL-SCI initiated a phase III, open-label, randomized, controlled, multicenter study to evaluate the effects of Multikine Plus Standard of Care (Surgery + Radiotherapy or Surgery + Concurrent Chemoradiotherapy) in Subjects with Advanced Primary Squamous Cell Carcinoma of the Oral Cavity and Soft Palate Versus Standard of Care Only. The Clinical Study Protocol stated primary objective is, "to evaluate the efficacy of peri-tumoral and peri-lymphatic injection of the investigational Multikine therapy given prior to Standard of Care (SOC) (as currently defined by the NCCN Guidelines)." For this study, efficacy will be evaluated using overall survival (3). It should be

noted that primary objectives of clinical trials can be related to the determination of safety or a combination of multiple endpoints. In these cases, the required sample size may be larger than would have been required for the primary efficacy objective alone (4). The concept of "Standard of Care" is defined in Chapter 7.

b. What Measure Will be Used to Determine This Outcome for a Given Subject?

The measure used to determine the primary objective is often referred to as the primary endpoint. This measurement should be accepted as clinically relevant or exhibiting important treatment benefit in the subject population under evaluation. It should be a measurement that can be obtained or observed for each subject participating in the clinical trial. Using the Multikine study discussed earlier, the primary efficacy endpoint is overall survival. Here, each subject will be observed for the duration of the study and overall survival recorded.

c. What Is the Clinically Meaningful Difference?

The clinically meaningful difference is the difference generally regarded as clinically important or meaningful to a patient or clinician. The determination of clinically meaningful differences is an evolving science, specifically in the development of patient-reported outcomes. For objective measurements of response (ie, survival, changes in

---

[2]Spilker B. Guide to clinical trials. Philadelphia, PA: Lippincott Williams & Wilkins; 1991.

[3]CelSci Corporation, Vienna, VA. http://www.cel-sci.com/multikine_phase_3_clinical_trial_design.html [accessed 28.07.15].

[4]Stenger M. ASCO Committee defines clinically meaningful goals for clinical trials in pancreas, breast, lung, and colorectal cancers. The ASCO Post. May 15, 2014, vol. 5, issue 8, Harborside Press. http://www.ascopost.com/issues/may-15,-2014/asco-committee-defines-clinically-meaningful-goals-for-clinical-trials-in-pancreas,-breast,-lung,-and-colorectal-cancers.aspx [accessed 28.07.15].

blood pressure, reduction in HIV-1 RNA levels), clinically meaningful differences are based on evaluation of published data and discussion through research working groups and other committees tasked with evaluating results from clinical trials. For example, the American Society of Clinical Oncology (ASCO) working group on pancreatic cancer recently suggested that a clinically meaningful survival benefit for a new treatment in folfirinox-eligible pancreatic cancer patients may be 4–5 months (4). It is important to understand what constitutes a clinically meaningful difference as there are situations where a very small, but clinically trivial difference can be detected using statistical techniques. Recall that to establish effectiveness, a trial must provide, "highly reliable and statistically strong evidence of an important clinical benefit" (5).

d. What Treatment Effect Is Expected?

Treatment effect is the effect or benefit of getting one treatment over another. In preliminary trials, the treatment effect in humans may not be known. For later-phase studies, assumptions of treatment effect are normally based on the results of previously completed studies, if available. In the absence of data from an earlier trial, researchers are tasked with the problem of how to estimate the treatment effect. Typically, one of two common approaches are used: estimate treatment effect according to available information with the clinically meaningful difference or using available published data from similar studies to provide a best guess of treatment effect. For example, in phase I trials for anti-HIV compounds, it is commonly expected that at least a 1 $\log_{10}$ copies/mL drop in HIV-1 RNA is expected following a 14-day treatment in HIV-infected subjects. Given that the size of trial is inversely related to the treatment effect size, it is easy to see the importance of making informed assumptions of treatment effect in the process of calculating sample sizes.

e. What Data Analysis Technique Is Appropriate for Determining a Difference Between Treatments?

The data analysis technique utilized will depend on the design of the study and the type of endpoint being utilized for the measure of the primary objective, and, potentially, regulatory precedence. Common data analysis techniques are tests of proportions for differences in binary data, t-tests, Wilcoxon rank sum tests, and analysis of variance models for the assessment of differences in continuous endpoints, and logrank tests for differences in time to event data. Most often the data analysis technique will be determined by a statistician during preliminary planning of the Protocol.

f. What Degree of Certainty Is Expected or Required for Ascertaining Treatment Difference?

The degree of certainty or power is defined as the probability of detecting the stated treatment effect, if such an effect truly exists. Commonly, power is set at 80% or 90%, but setting power as 95% or 99% may be advisable in cases where a single study may constitute the evidence of effectiveness for a drug candidate.

---

[5]U.S. Department of Health and Human Services. Food and Drug Administration. Guidance for industry. Providing clinical evidence of effectiveness for human drug and biological products; May 1998 (23 pp.).

III. STATISTICAL TERMS COMMONLY USED IN SAMPLE SIZE CALCULATIONS

As stated previously, a statistician can translate the discussions surrounding the six questions posed previously into sample size calculations. In order to demonstrate this process, it is important to introduce a few statistical concepts and their relationship to the questions above.

IV. NULL AND ALTERNATIVE HYPOTHESES

In the case of the CEL-SCI Multikine study discussed earlier, the primary research question to be tested is "Is the survival rate of subjects treated with Multikine plus SOC ($p_{Muilikine+SOC}$) better than the survival rate of subjects treated with SOC only (p_{SOC})?" This statement in statistical terms would be, "Is $p_{Muilikine+SOC} > p_{SOC}$?" Certainly, the company believes that it is, or it would not be initiating a large phase III study. In statistics, hypotheses are constructed to evaluate the likelihood of such statements. These hypotheses can then be tested using statistical techniques. Each hypothesis test requires the statement of a null hypothesis (H_0) and the alternative hypothesis (H_1). These hypotheses are opposites of one another. The null hypothesis is the statement of what a researcher believes to be untrue and is commonly stated in terms including equality. In our example, the null hypothesis could be stated as H_0: $p_{Muilikine+SOC} \leq p_{SOC}$. The alternative hypothesis is a statement of what a researcher believes to be true. For our

example, the alternative hypothesis is H_1: $p_{Muilikine+SOC} > p_{SOC}$. It is worth noting that this example is of a one-sided set of hypotheses. Here, the researcher is only interested if the new treatment is better than SOC. In regulatory settings, we typically are concerned with two-sided hypotheses. Here, the two-sided statement of this same example would be: H_0: $p_{Muilikine+SOC} = p_{SOC}$ and H_1: $p_{Muilikine+SOC} \neq p_{SOC}$.

Statistical methods commonly utilized in clinical trials test these hypotheses using an appropriate statistical technique. The outcome of this test can be either to reject the null hypothesis or fail to reject the null hypothesis. It should be noted that failing to reject the null hypothesis is not the same as accepting the null hypothesis. That is to say, in our two-sided example above, if we fail to reject the null hypothesis, H_0: $p_{Muilikine+SOC} = p_{SOC}$, we have not proved that the survival rate of subjects treated with Multikine + SOC is the same as the survival rate of subjects treated with SOC (standard of care) alone. Instead, we do not have conclusive evidence to support that the survival rate of subjects treated with Multikine + SOC is different than that of subjects treated with SOC alone. Similarly, if we reject the null hypothesis, we accept the alternative hypothesis. This does not represent proof of the alternative hypothesis, but rather provides evidence supporting the alternative hypothesis. As stated above, Standard of Care is defined in Chapter 7 (6,7).

The rationale for this distinction is grounded in the discussion of degree of certainty which can be visualized using Table 10.1.

[6]Moffet P, Moore G. The standard of care: legal history and definitions: the bad and good news. Western J. Emergency Med. 2011;7:109–12.

[7]Straus DC, Thomas JM. What does the medical profession mean by "standard of care?" J. Clin. Oncol. 2009;27: e192–3.

TABLE 10.1   Degree of Certainty.

Statistical Decision	Truth	
	H_0 Is True	H_1 Is True
Fail to reject H_0	Correct decision	Type II error (beta, β)
Reject H_0 (accept H_1)	Type I error (alpha, α)	Correct decision

V. DEGREE OF CERTAINTY: ALPHA (α) AND BETA (β)

In reality (truth), the null hypothesis is either true or false. The statistical decision process is set up so that it either rejects the null hypothesis or fails to reject the null hypothesis. This leaves four possibilities of the outcome of our statistical testing. In two of the four possibilities, we will make the correct decision. However, there are two possibilities where we will make an error in our decision process. The type I error, commonly referred to as the alpha (α) value, is the probability of incorrectly rejecting the null hypothesis or the false-positive rate. From a society perspective, this type of error is to be minimized, as it would not be acceptable to have products on the market that do not work. Commonly, the type I error rate is set to 5% or less. However, the actual type I error rate has to be determined based on the design of the study. Studies with more than one objective being tested (ie, more than one hypothesis test constructed) may need to adjust the α level to preserve the true probability of observing a significant result. Additional factors that could impact the alpha (α) level include a study that has more than two treatment arms or that includes interim analyses of the data. These items lead to what are commonly referred to as multiplicity problems. If we test a single set of hypotheses then the type I error rate is maintained at the level we set. However, if we test more than one set of hypotheses, the type I error rate is inflated, and for at least one test is larger than we set.

The second type of error, type II error or the beta (β) value, is the probability of failing to reject the null hypothesis when the alternative hypothesis is true. It is a false-negative result and represents risk from the researcher's standpoint. Here, while the alternative hypothesis is true, it is not confirmed by mistake. As such, a truly effective treatment may be overlooked or discounted due to the finding. Here, researchers want to keep this value small, typically in the 10–20% range. A related concept to type II error is power, which is calculated as $1-\beta$ in proportion or $100-\beta$ if we are using percentages. Hence, if $\beta = 10\%$, then power is 90%.

VI. STATISTICAL METHODS FOR DETERMINING TRIAL SIZE

A variety of statistical analysis techniques can be applied to the statistical problems encountered in clinical trials. For each of these techniques, there is an appropriate method for determining sample size appropriate for use in that setting. This section provides a starting point for calculating sample sizes appropriate when utilizing the most commonly encountered data analysis techniques.

VII. CONTINUOUS VARIABLES: TESTING THE DIFFERENCE BETWEEN TWO MEANS

Clinical trials commonly have endpoints which can be measured on a continuous numeric scale, such as changes from baseline in HIV-1 RNA for studies of HIV subjects or changes in FEV_1 for studies in subjects with chronic obstructive pulmonary disease. While sophisticated statistical modeling techniques could be applied, it is often the case that determining the difference, if any, of the means of two groups for a continuous variable is of critical importance. In this case, a simple formula derived from the formula for the z-test statistic can be used to compute sample size for a two-sided set of hypotheses when type II error (β), α level, size of difference in means (called the treatment difference), and variability are specified:

$$n = \frac{2\sigma^2 \left(z_{1-(\alpha/2)} + z_{1-\beta}\right)^2}{(\mu_1 - \mu_2)^2}$$

where n is the sample size per group, μ_1 is the mean in group 1, μ_2 is the mean in group 2, σ^2 represents the variance (ie, σ is the standard deviation), α is the type I error rate under evaluation, β is the type II error rate, $z_{1-(\alpha/2)}$ and $z_{1-\beta}$ are critical values from a standard normal distribution. Values for the quantity $(z_{1-(\alpha/2)} + z_{1-\beta})$ can be obtained from Table 10.2 for commonly chosen values of α and β. For values of α and β not represented in Table 10.2, the critical values may be obtained from standard statistical software packages such as SAS® or R or from reference books containing statistical tables, such as Geigy (8), and used to calculate the quantity

$(z_{1-(\alpha/2)} + z_{1-\beta})$. For the sample size formula represented here to be valid, the following assumptions have to hold:

1. The responses represent independent observations. Generally speaking this means that each observation is taken from a single patient.
2. The data are normally distributed or the sample size is large enough to be able to utilize the central limit theorem. In general, a sample size of 30 subjects or more in each arm is reasonable enough to rely on the central limit theorem.
3. The variance, σ^2, is known and the same for both treatment groups.
4. The number of subjects in each group is the same.

Should the validity of any of these assumptions be suspect, sample size should be calculated with a different formula. However, this formula can be used as a "back of the napkin" starting place for planning trial sizes.

a. Example 1: Sample Size Calculation for the Difference Between Two Means With a Known Standard Deviation

Suppose that a drug candidate for pain relief of osteoarthritis of the knee is to be tested to see if it improves pain as measured on the Western Ontario and McMaster Universities OA Index (WOMAC) A pain subscale. Based on previous studies, the mean difference in the change from baseline to 12 weeks between the new drug candidate and the active control is 0.8 units, with a standard deviation of 2 units. If the drug company would like to plan a new study with power ($100 - \beta$) of 90% and a type I error rate (α) of 5%, what sample size would be needed? To calculate the sample size, we

TABLE 10.2 Values for the Quantity $(z_{1-(\alpha/2)} + z_{1-\beta})^2$ Based on Choices for α (Alpha) and β (Beta)

α (Type I Error)	β (Type II Error)			
	0.01	0.05	0.1	0.2
0.01	24.0	17.8	14.9	11.7
0.02	21.6	15.8	13.0	10.0
0.05	18.4	13.0	10.5	7.8
0.1	15.8	10.8	8.6	6.2

[8]Lentner C, editors. Geigy scientific tables. 8th edition. Vol 2: Introduction to statistics, statistical tables, mathematical formulae. Basle: Ciba-Gigy; 1982. ISBN 0-914168-51-7.

can map the information from the assumptions into the sample size formula as $\sigma = 2$ (ie, the standard deviation is 2), $\mu_1 - \mu_2 = 0.08$ (ie, the mean difference in the change from baseline to 12 weeks between the new drug candidate and the active control is 0.8), and the value of the quantity $(z_{1-(\alpha/2)} + z_{1-\beta})$ is obtained from Table 10.2 corresponding to $\alpha = 0.05$ and $\beta = 0.10$ (ie, 10.5). Plugging these values into the our sample size formula, we see that:

$$n = \frac{2(2)^2(10.5)}{(0.8)^2} = 131.25$$

Here, 132 subjects would be needed for each treatment group or the total size of the trial should be 264 subjects. If the drug company opted to utilize 80% power instead, the sample size per group required would be:

$$n = \frac{2(2)^2(7.8)}{(0.8)^2} = 97.5$$

The total size of the study would be 196 subjects. Hence, changing the power assumption from 80% to 90% requires an increase of the sample size by almost 35%.

b. Example 2: Sample Size Calculation for the Difference Between Two Means Using Available Information from a Confidence Interval

Suppose that a drug candidate for relief of symptoms from allergic rhinitis was to be assessed in a placebo-controlled trial. Additionally, suppose that the difference from placebo in mean change from baseline in the 2-week reflective total nasal symptom score (TNSS) from a previously conducted study was reported as -0.5 with a two-sided 95% confidence interval of $(-0.9, -0.1)$. The sample size from the previous study was 50 subjects in total. If the drug company would like to

plan a new study with power $(100 - \beta)$ of 80% and a type I error rate (α) of 5%, what sample size would be needed?

To calculate the sample size, we can map the information from the assumptions into the sample size formula as $\mu_1 - \mu_2 = -0.5$ (ie, the mean difference in the change from baseline in the 2-week reflective TNSS between the new drug candidate and placebo is -0.5), and the value of the quantity $(z_{1-(\alpha/2)} + z_{1-\beta})$ is obtained from Table 10.2 corresponding to $\alpha = 0.05$ and $\beta = 0.20$ (ie, 7.8). However, it appears that the information about the standard deviation (σ) necessary to complete the formula is missing. While this information is not directly stated in the information above, it is available, indirectly, through the use of the information available about the confidence interval and sample size from the previous study. The two-sided $(1 - \alpha)$ confidence interval for the mean for normally distributed data when the variance is known is given by the formula:

$$\bar{x} \pm z_{1-(\alpha/2)} \frac{\sigma}{\sqrt{n}}$$

where $\bar{x}$ is the estimate of the mean, α (alpha) is the type I error rate, $z_{1-(\alpha/2)}$ is the critical value from the standard normal distribution, σ (sigma) is the standard deviation, and n is the sample size. In our example, the confidence interval is reported as -0.5 ± 0.4 (ie, $-0.5 - 0.4 = -0.9$ and $-0.5 + 0.4 = -0.1$ which are the reported lower and upper limits of the two-sided 95% confidence interval). This indicates that $z_{1-(\alpha/2)}\sigma/\sqrt{n} = 0.4$. We know or can easily obtain the values of n and $z_{1-(\alpha/2)}$ from the information given in the example. The sample size (n) was reported as 50. The confidence interval is reported as 95%, the overall type I error rate is 5% (ie, $\alpha = 0.05$). The corresponding critical value, $z_{1-(\alpha/2)}$, can be obtained from standard statistical software packages such as SAS or R or from reference books containing statistical tables, such as

TABLE 10.3 Common Critical Values From the Standard Normal Distribution ($z_{1-(\alpha/2)}$ or $z_{1-\beta}$) Based on Choices for α (Alpha) or β (Beta)

α (Type I Error)	β (Type II Error)	$z_{1-(\alpha/2)}$ or $z_{1-\beta}$
0.01	0.005	2.58
0.02	0.01	2.33
0.05	0.025	1.96
0.1	0.05	1.64
0.2	0.1	1.28
0.4	0.2	0.84
0.9	0.45	0.13

Geigy (9). Critical values based on various commonly utilized values of α are reported in Table 10.3. Using this table, we see that when α (alpha) is 0.05 the critical value, $z_{1-(\alpha/2)}$, is 1.96. Plugging in the pieces of information that we have into our formula we have:

$$1.96\frac{\sigma}{\sqrt{50}} = 0.4$$

With some algebraic manipulation, we have:

$$1.96\frac{\sigma}{7.07} = 0.4, \quad 0.28\sigma = 0.4, \quad \sigma = \frac{0.4}{0.28}, \quad \sigma = 1.43$$

Now, we have all the information to calculate the sample size for the new study with the stated requirements for power. Plugging these values into our sample size formula, we see that the required sample size per group is:

$$n = \frac{2(1.43)^2(7.8)}{(-0.5)^2} = 127.60$$

Here, 128 subjects would be needed for each treatment group or the total size of the trial should be 256 subjects.

Suppose the drug company was concerned about the assumption of the mean difference between the treatment groups not being exactly as observed from the previous study. In this case, the company may want to consider a range of reasonable values. Certainly, it would be reasonable to consider the lower and upper limits of the two-sided 95% confidence interval about the mean difference from placebo, $(-0.9, -0.1)$ as plausible values for the value of $\mu_1 - \mu_2$. Using the value of the lower limit of the confidence interval, -0.9, as the value of $\mu_1 - \mu_2$ and holding the other assumptions as before, yields a sample size per group of:

$$n = \frac{2(1.43)^2(7.8)}{(-0.9)^2} = 39.38$$

Similarly, substituting the value of the upper limit of the confidence interval, -0.1, as the value of $\mu_1 - \mu_2$ and holding the other assumptions as before, yields a sample size per group of:

$$n = \frac{2(1.43)^2(7.8)}{(-0.1)^2} = 3190.04$$

VIII. CHANGES IN SAMPLE SIZE ASSUMPTIONS CAN YIELD DRAMATIC CHANGES TO SAMPLE SIZE

It is clear from the examples presented in this section that seemingly small changes in any of the assumptions can lead to very large changes in the sample size necessary to achieve the required power for a trial. The choices of α and β are controlled by the individual or individuals who are initiating the study, and can be varied according to the needs or requirements of the clinical program.

[9]Lentner C, editors. Geigy scientific tables. 8th edition. Vol 2: Introduction to statistics, statistical tables, mathematical formulae. Basle: Ciba-Gigy; 1982. ISBN 0-914168-51-7.

The assumptions surrounding the values of $\mu_1 - \mu_2$ and σ, however, are certainly beyond control, and quite often, very uncertain. In these cases, it is very practical to consider a range of plausible values when determining the sample size to be utilized in a given study. It should be noted that the sample size formula can be rewritten as:

$$n = 2\left(\frac{1}{\theta}\right)^2 \left(z_{1-(\alpha/2)} + z_{1-\beta}\right)^2$$

where $\theta = (\mu_1 - \mu_2)/\sigma$. The value of θ is sometimes referred to as the population effect size, which is the standardized mean difference between two populations. Given that the formula is multiplicative in $1/\theta$ and $(z_{1-(\alpha/2)} + z_{1-\beta})$, it is clear that increases in the value of $(z_{1-(\alpha/2)} + z_{1-\beta})$ while holding $1/\theta$ constant will lead to increases in sample size. Similarly, decreases in the value of $(z_{1-(\alpha/2)} + z_{1-\beta})$ while holding $1/\theta$ constant will lead to decreases in sample size. When considering changes to the population effect size, θ, it should be noted that larger values of θ will yield smaller values of $1/\theta$. Hence, increasing the effect size while holding $(z_{1-(\alpha/2)} + z_{1-\beta})$ constant, will yield smaller sample sizes (as $1/\theta$ will be smaller), and decreasing the effect size while holding $(z_{1-(\alpha/2)} + z_{1-\beta})$ constant, will yield larger sample sizes (as $1/\theta$ will be larger).

IX. CHANGING ASSUMPTIONS ABOUT ALPHA (α) OR BETA (β)

Consider the following, suppose a company is considering study design A with an effect size of θ, $1-\beta_a$ power, and type I error of α_a and study design B has an effect size of θ, $1-\beta_b$ power, and type I error of α_b. The relative size difference between the two designs can then be written as the ratio of the two sample sizes:

$$\frac{n_A}{n_B} = \frac{2(1/\theta)^2 \left(z_{1-(\alpha_a/2)} + z_{1-\alpha_a}\right)^2}{2(1/\theta)^2 \left(z_{1-(\alpha_b/2)} + z_{1-\alpha_b}\right)^2}$$

After reducing the fraction by removing common terms, the equation becomes simply a ratio of quantities that can be obtained from Table 10.2, as:

$$\frac{n_A}{n_B} = \frac{\left(z_{1-(\alpha_a/2)} + z_{1-\alpha_a}\right)^2}{\left(z_{1-(\alpha_b/2)} + z_{1-\alpha_b}\right)^2}$$

For example, if study design A has 90% power and a type I error rate of 5% and study design B has 80% power and a type I error rate of 5%, the equation becomes:

$$\frac{n_A}{n_B} = \frac{\left(z_{1-(0.05/2)} + z_{1-0.1}\right)^2}{\left(z_{1-(0.05/2)} + z_{1-0.2}\right)^2}$$

$$\frac{n_A}{n_B} = \frac{10.5}{7.8} = 1.35$$

Here, we see that the size difference for these two designs is 35%. Recall in Example 1 of this section, the calculated sample sizes per group were 131.5 and 97.5 for 90% and 80% power, respectively. Taking the ratio of these two values verifies the calculation above:

$$\frac{n_A}{n_B} = \frac{131.5}{97.5} = 1.35$$

Given this relationship, it is easy to transform the values in Table 10.2 to relative efficiencies of two designs with the same effect size, but varying values of α and β. This can be done by choosing a reference design, say $\alpha = 0.05$ and $\beta = 0.2$, and then dividing each value of the quantity $(z_{1-(\alpha/2)} + z_{1-\beta})^2$ contained in the table by the corresponding value of $(z_{1-(\alpha/2)} + z_{1-\beta})^2$ for the reference design, here, 7.8. These values are presented in Table 10.4.

For example, if the effect size is the same, the sample size for a study with 95% power and 1% type I error rate is 2.3 times the sample size for the same study with 80% power and a 5% type I error rate. This can be represented visually through the use of power curves. Power curves are just line graphs of the values of the sample size per treatment relative to power $(1 - \beta)$ for the varying values of α for a given effect size. These curves are very useful when trying to visualize the differences in sample size and power for various assumptions. Fig. 10.1 represents the power curves for

Example 1 when mimicking the values of α and β used in Table 10.2. Here, we see the sample size varies directly with changes to α and $1 - \beta$ (power).

X. CHANGING ASSUMPTIONS ABOUT THETA (θ)

In this section, changing assumptions about the population effect size, θ, are considered. Here, the study design parameters of α and β are considered constant, and only changes to θ are of interest. If two values of θ are possible, called θ_1 and θ_2, the sample sizes between the two scenarios can be represented as:

$$\frac{n_1}{n_2} = \frac{2(1/\theta_1)^2 (z_{1-(\alpha/2)} + z_{1-\beta})^2}{2(1/\theta_2)^2 (z_{1-(\alpha/2)} + z_{1-\beta})^2}$$

After reducing the fraction by removing common terms, the equation becomes:

$$\frac{n_1}{n_2} = \frac{(1/\theta_1)^2}{(1/\theta_2)^2}$$

TABLE 10.4 Efficiency of Sample Size Relative to a Reference Study With $\alpha = 0.05$ when $\beta = 0.20$ When Effect Size Is Constant

α (Type I Error)	β (Type II Error)			
	0.01	0.05	0.1	0.2
0.01	3.1	2.3	1.9	1.5
0.02	2.8	2.0	1.7	1.3
0.05	2.4	1.7	1.3	1
0.1	2.0	1.4	1.1	0.8

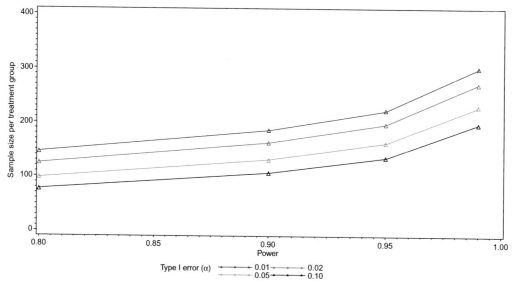

FIGURE 10.1 Power curves corresponding to Example 1.

After rearranging the terms, we have:

$$\frac{n_1}{n_2} = \frac{\theta_2^2}{\theta_1^2} = \left(\frac{\theta_2}{\theta_1}\right)^2$$

Here, we see that the size difference is inversely related to the squared ratio of the effect size. This indicates that if the effect size of scenario 1 is larger than the effect size of scenario 2, the sample size corresponding to scenario 1 is less than the sample size of scenario 2 and vice versa. Power curves corresponding to various effect sizes are presented in Fig. 10.2. Here, it is very clear that increases to effect size yield lower sample sizes and decreasing values of effect size require larger sample sizes. From a practical viewpoint, this is quite reasonable given that smaller differences should be more difficult to uncover and, hence, require a larger sample size to show evidence of a positive result.

XI. BINARY VARIABLES: TESTING THE DIFFERENCE BETWEEN TWO PROPORTIONS

Qualitative endpoints are often utilized in clinical trials. When these endpoints are dichotomous in nature, they are referred to as binary endpoints. Binary endpoints are used where the subject's outcome can be classified as a "success" or "failure." Examples include having undetectable HIV-1 RNA at 48 weeks in studies of HIV-infected subjects or being free of bacteria at the test of cure visit in trials of antibiotics. The sample size formula for testing the difference of two proportions is derived from that used for difference in two means due to the fact that for large samples, the binomial distribution is approximated by the normal distribution through the use of the central limit theorem. Here, we find that:

$$n = \frac{(p_1(1-p_1) + p_2(1-p_2))\left(z_{1-(\alpha/2)} + z_{1-\beta}\right)^2}{(p_1 - p_2)^2}$$

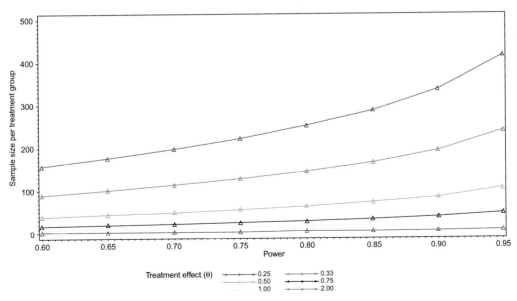

FIGURE 10.2   Power curves corresponding to various effect sizes, θ (theta), when $\alpha = 0.05$.

where n is the sample size per group, p_1 is the proportion of subjects with "success" in group 1, p_2 is the proportion of subjects with "success" in group 2, α is the type I error rate under evaluation, β is the type II error rate, $z_{1-(\alpha/2)}$ and $z_{1-\beta}$ are critical values from a standard normal distribution. As before, values for the quantity $(z_{1-(\alpha/2)}+z_{1-\beta})^2$ can be obtained from Table 10.2 for commonly chosen values of α and β. For the sample size formula represented here to be valid, the following assumptions have to hold:

- The responses represent independent observations. Generally speaking this means that each observation is taken from a single patient.
- The number of subjects in each group is the same.

a. Example 3: Sample Size Calculation for the Difference Between Two Proportions

Suppose that a drug candidate for the treatment of HIV in naive subjects is expected to have 90% of subjects with HIV-1 RNA below the lower limit of detection at 48 weeks when added to standard of care. The standard of care will have 80% of subjects with HIV-1 RNA below the lower limit of detection at the same time point. If the drug company would like to plan a new study with power $(100 - \beta)$ of 95% and a type I error rate (α) of 5%, what sample size would be needed? To calculate the sample size, we can translate the request into the sample size formula as $p_1 = 0.9$, $p_2 = 0.80$, $(p_1 - p_2) = 0.1$, and the value of the quantity $(z_{1-(\alpha/2)}+z_{1-\beta})^2$ is obtained from Table 10.2 corresponding to $\alpha = 0.05$ and $\beta = 0.05$ (ie, 13.0). Plugging these values into our sample size formula, we see that:

$$n = \frac{(0.9(1 - 0.9) + 0.8(1 - 0.8))(13.0)}{(0.1)^2} = 325$$

Here, 325 subjects would be needed for each treatment group or the total size of the trial should be 650 subjects.

b. Example 4: Estimating Power for a Given Sample Size and Testing the Difference Between Two Proportions

Often there are practical limitations for sample sizes. For example, in an orphan drug indication, there can be a limited number of subjects which can be studied. Another example can be when a company has to have a result in a set timeframe. In such cases, the sample size may be capped at a certain value to ensure the study is completed in the required timeframe. In these cases, the sample size is known, but the corresponding power of the study may be of interest if only to advise the research community of the likelihood of a successful result under the stated assumptions. Consider as an example where a company is conducting an early phase trial in a rare form of cancer. For the type of cancer under investigation, the response rate under the standard of care treatment is expected to be 30% and for the experimental treatment, 50%. Since the cancer is rare, the company can only expect to enroll 50 subjects per group in a reasonable timeframe. The Chief Medical Officer would like to know the power of this planned study. Assuming that a 5% type I error rate is reasonable for this study, the power can be determined using the sample size formula, by rearranging the terms to solve for β:

$$n = \frac{(p_1(1 - p_1) + p_2(1 - p_2))(z_{1-(\alpha/2)}+z_{1-\beta})^2}{(p_1 - p_2)^2},$$

$$\frac{n(p_1 - p_2)^2}{(p_1(1 - p_1) + p_2(1 - p_2))} = (z_{1-(\alpha/2)}+z_{1-\beta})^2,$$

$$\sqrt{\frac{n(p_1 - p_2)^2}{(p_1(1 - p_1) + p_2(1 - p_2))}} = (z_{1-(\alpha/2)} + z_{1-\beta}),$$

$$\sqrt{\frac{n(p_1 - p_2)^2}{(p_1(1 - p_1) + p_2(1 - p_2))}} - z_{1-(\alpha/2)} = z_{1-\beta}$$

Plugging in the values for $p_1 = 0.5$, $p_2 = 0.3$, $n = 50$, and obtaining the value for

$z_{1-(\alpha/2)} = 1.96$ from Table 10.3, the formula reduces to:

$$z_{1-\beta} = \sqrt{\frac{50(0.5-0.3)^2}{(0.5(1-0.5)+0.3(1-0.3))}} - 1.96,$$

$$z_{1-\beta} = \sqrt{\frac{50(0.2)^2}{(0.5(0.5)+0.3(0.7))}} - 1.96,$$

$$z_{1-\beta} = \sqrt{\frac{2}{0.46}} - 1.96,$$

$$z_{1-\beta} = \sqrt{4.35} - 1.96,$$

$$z_{1-\beta} = 0.125$$

A standard computing program or a statistical table can be used to obtain the value of β corresponding to a critical value of 0.125, which may be rounded to 0.13. Using Table 10.3, we see that the critical value of 0.13 corresponds to $z_{1-\beta}$ where β is 0.45. Given that power is calculated as $1-\beta = 1-0.45 = 0.55$, we see that power is just over 50% for this study. With the probability of showing a successful result nearing that of a coin-flip, the Chief Medical Officer may decide to put the study on hold until sufficient time can be devoted to obtain a more reasonable number of subjects or she may choose to evaluate single-arm study options which may be reasonable in this indication.

XII. TIME TO EVENT VARIABLES: TESTING FOR DIFFERENCES BETWEEN TWO GROUPS USING THE LOGRANK TEST

In certain clinical studies, the primary endpoint is based on the length of time until an event occurs, such as death or progression, in an oncology study or until symptoms alleviate, as in a study of influenza. For these studies, subjects are followed for either a set study period or for varying lengths of time. There is the possibility that the subject may never experience the event, and the response would have to be censored in some way. The logrank test is commonly used to assess differences between two groups with a time to event endpoint. Here, there are two sample sizes that have to be established: the number of events to be observed and the number of subjects. Following the work of Schoenfeld (10), the total number of events required to be observed during the study is given by the formula:

$$n_{Events} = 4 \frac{\left(z_{1-(\alpha/2)} + z_{1-\beta}\right)^2}{(\ln(h))^2}$$

and the number of subjects required in each treatment group to be able to see the required number of events is given by:

$$n = \left(\frac{4}{(p_1 + p_2)}\right)\left(\frac{\left(z_{1-(\alpha/2)} + z_{1-\beta}\right)^2}{(\ln(h))^2}\right)$$

where p_1 is the proportion of subjects in group 1 who will experience the event at any time in the study, p_2 is the proportion of group 2 who will experience the event at any time in the study, h is the hazard ratio, which is defined as $\ln(1-p_1)/\ln(1-p_2)$, α is the type I error rate under evaluation, β is the type II error rate, $z_{1-(\alpha/2)}$ and $z_{1-\beta}$ are critical values from a standard normal distribution. As before, values for the quantity $(z_{1-(\alpha/2)} + z_{1-\beta})^2$ can be obtained from Table 10.2 for commonly chosen values of α and β. It should be noted that the formula for the number of events is for the total number of events between both treatment groups, whereas the formula for the number of subjects is for the number of subjects in each treatment group. To get the total number of subjects required, the number of subjects per group should be multiplied by two.

---

[10]Schoenfeld D. The asymptotic properties of nonparametric tests for comparing survival distributions. Biometrika 1981;68:316−9.

For the sample size formula represented here to be valid, the following assumptions have to hold:

1. The number of subjects in each treatment group has to be the same.
2. The event rate is such that within each of the two groups every participant in a given treatment group has approximately the same probability of experiencing an event.
3. There is no loss to follow-up (ie, no subject withdraws from the study prior to either the study ending or the subject experiencing the event).

a. Example 5: Sample Size Calculation for the Difference Between Two Groups Using the Logrank Test

Suppose that there is a drug candidate for the treatment of folfirinox-eligible pancreatic cancer. It is estimated that 50% of subjects with the drug candidate + standard of care will die during the study period, whereas 63% of subjects taken with the standard of care will die during the study period. If the drug company would like to plan a new study with power $(100 - \beta)$ of 95% and a type I error rate (α) of 1%, what sample size would be needed? To calculate the number of events and the number of subjects necessary, we first need to translate the request into the components of each calculation. Here, the components can be mapped as:

$p_1 = 0.5$, $p_2 = 0.63$, $h = \ln(1 - p_1)/\ln(1 - p_2) = 0.697$, $\ln(h) = -0.361$, and the value of the quantity $(z_{1-(\alpha/2)} + z_{1-\beta})^2$ is obtained from Table 10.2 corresponding to $\alpha = 0.01$ and $\beta = 0.05$ (ie, 17.8). Plugging these values into the our sample size formula, we see that:

$$n_{Events} = 4 \frac{17.8}{(-0.361)^2} = 546.343$$

and

$$n = \left(\frac{4}{(0.5 + 0.63)} \right) \left(\frac{17.8}{(-0.361)^2} \right) = 483.49$$

Here, 484 subjects per treatment group (ie, 968 total) are required in order to observe a minimum of 547 events during the study.

b. Example 6: Evaluating a Sample Size for a Difference Between Two Groups Using the Logrank Test

Suppose that a project manager is reviewing a Clinical Study Protocol for a promising new treatment in gallbladder cancer. The statistical section of the Protocol states that a minimum of 234 progression-free survival events provides 90% power to detect the target hazard ratio of 0.6 based on a logrank test and a one-sided overall significance level of 0.005. Is the stated sample size reasonable?

Here, it is reasonable to use the number of events formula, with $h = 0.6$, $\beta = 0.10$, and $\alpha = 0.01$. Note that α (alpha) is adjusted to be 0.01 as the formula for events is based on a two-sided test. The example Protocol specifies that a one-sided test rather than a two-sided test is utilized. As such, we have to adjust for this in our formula accordingly. If $\alpha = 0.01$ then $\alpha/2 = 0.005$, indicating that we have 0.005 of the overall α in one side of our two-sided test. Using these values in the number of events formula, we have $\ln(h) = -0.511$, and the value of the quantity $(z_{1-(\alpha/2)} + z_{1-\beta})^2$ is obtained from Table 10.2 corresponding to $\alpha = 0.01$ and $\beta = 0.1$ (ie, 14.9).

$$n_{Events} = 4 \frac{14.9}{(-0.511)^2} = 228.247.$$

This estimate of 229 events is very close to the Protocol stated estimate of 234 events, and the slight difference could be explained by rounding differences or slight differences used in available calculations. At any rate, the sample size for the

TABLE 10.5 Calculated Sample Sizes Per Treatment Group for Example 6 for Estimated Values of p_2, When the Hazard Ratio, h, Is 0.6 and $\alpha = 0.01$ and $\beta = 0.1$

p_2	$p_1 = 1 - \exp(h(\ln(1 - p_2)))$	$n = \left(\dfrac{4}{(p_1 + p_2)}\right)\left(\dfrac{(z_{1-(\alpha/2)} + z_{1-\beta})^2}{(\ln(h))^2}\right)$
0.3	$p_1 = 1 - \exp(0.6(\ln(1 - 0.3))) = 0.19$	$n = \left(\dfrac{4}{(0.3 + 0.19)}\right)\left(\dfrac{14.9}{(-0.511)^2}\right) = 465.81$
0.4	$p_1 = 1 - \exp(0.6(\ln(1 - 0.4))) = 0.26$	$n = \left(\dfrac{4}{(0.4 + 0.26)}\right)\left(\dfrac{14.9}{(-0.511)^2}\right) = 345.83$
0.5	$p_1 = 1 - \exp(0.6(\ln(1 - 0.5))) = 0.34$	$n = \left(\dfrac{4}{(0.5 + 0.34)}\right)\left(\dfrac{14.9}{(-0.511)^2}\right) = 271.72$
0.6	$p_1 = 1 - \exp(0.6(\ln(1 - 0.6))) = 0.42$	$n = \left(\dfrac{4}{(0.6 + 0.42)}\right)\left(\dfrac{14.9}{(-0.511)^2}\right) = 223.77$
0.7	$p_1 = 1 - \exp(0.6(\ln(1 - 0.7))) = 0.51$	$n = \left(\dfrac{4}{(0.7 + 0.51)}\right)\left(\dfrac{14.9}{(-0.511)^2}\right) = 188.63$

number of events stated in the Protocol appears reasonable based on the assumptions provided. It should be noted, however, that the number of subjects per treatment cannot be determined based on the information provided. The Protocol section only states the target hazard ratio of 0.6, but does not state the expected proportion of subjects experiencing progression-free survival occurring in either treatment group. Without this information, it is not possible to calculate the sample size per group. It is possible to estimate the required sample size by using a range of values for the expected proportion of subjects experiencing progression-free survival occurring in one of the two groups and using the relationship between the hazard ratio and the proportion of subjects experiencing progression-free survival for each of the two groups. This can be demonstrated as follows:

$$h = \frac{\ln(1 - p_1)}{\ln(1 - p_2)}$$

Solving for one of the necessary proportions, say p_1, we find that:

$$h(\ln(1 - p_2)) = \ln(1 - p_1),$$
$$\exp(h(\ln(1 - p_2))) = (1 - p_1),$$
$$p_1 = 1 - \exp(h(\ln(1 - p_2)))$$

Using various values of p_2 and the specified value of the hazard ratio, we can estimate corresponding values of p_1, and then calculate the sample size per group. Using values of p_2 ranging from 0.3 to 0.7 by 0.1, calculated sample sizes are presented in Table 10.5.

Examining the values from Table 10.5, it is clear that the proportion of subjects experiencing progression-free survival is an important assumption in setting the sample size for the given study. As such, this would be important information to include in the sample size section of the Protocol.

XIII. BINARY VARIABLE: TESTING FOR EQUIVALENCE OF TWO PROPORTIONS

To this point, the sample size calculations have all corresponded to tests of superiority. By this, we want to assess whether the two treatments are different from one another. What if, however, we want to show that the two treatments are not different from one another? The objective of an equivalence trial is to provide evidence that the two treatments provide the same or nearly the same clinical benefit. This can be seen in the case where a drug candidate may not outperform an already approved product with regard to efficacy, but could still provide benefit to patients because it has a superior safety profile or the mechanism of action is unique in some way. We choose to accept that two treatments are equivalent if their treatment effect does not differ by some given amount, typically referred to as the equivalence margin. Clearly, analyzing the data as a superiority test would not work, as we cannot simply assume equality if we fail to reject the null hypothesis, so special consideration is necessary when approaching these types of problems. Typically, the sample size of an equivalence trial is based on the concept of generating a confidence interval for the treatment difference that shows that the treatments differ at most by a clinically acceptable difference. Makuch and Simon (11) described a very simple formula for determining the sample size necessary to generate a upper $100 (1 - \alpha)\%$ confidence limit for the difference in two proportions that should not exceed a clinically acceptable difference, d, with probability $1 - \beta$. This formula is:

$$n = \frac{(2p(1 - p))\left(z_{1-(\alpha/2)} + z_{1-\beta}\right)^2}{d^2}$$

where p is the proportion of successes expected to occur, d is the clinically acceptable difference, α (alpha) is the type I error rate under evaluation, β (beta) is the type II error rate, $z_{1-(\alpha/2)}$ and $z_{1-\beta}$ are critical values from a standard normal distribution. As before, values for the quantity $(z_{1-(\alpha/2)} + z_{1-\beta})^2$

can be obtained from Table 10.2 for commonly chosen values of α and β.

For this formula to be valid, the following assumptions have to hold:

1. The responses represent independent observations. Generally speaking this means that each observation is taken from a single patient.
2. The number of subjects in each group is the same.
3. The underlying difference between the two groups is zero.

It should be noted that this last assumption is particularly troublesome. As noted in ICH E9 (12), if the true difference is assumed to be zero, the sample size necessary to provide the stated level of power will be underestimated if the test product response rate is lower than that of the active control product. As such, caution should be exercised when evaluating sample sizes using the stated formula. Also, the choice of an appropriate clinically acceptable difference should be justified in any sample size calculation. The procedure for how to determine this difference is a subject of much debate, but is most often reliably done by reviewing available data from placebo-controlled trials in the therapeutic area and determining what is best described as a small portion of the treatment/no treatment difference (13).

a. Example 7: Sample Size Calculation for Equivalence of Two Proportions

Suppose that a drug candidate for the treatment of HIV in naive subjects is expected to

[11]Makuch R, Simon R. Sample size requirements for evaluating a conservative therapy. Cancer Treat. Rep. 62:1037−40.

[12]ICH Harmonised Tripartite Guideline. Statistical principles for clinical trials E9; September 1998 (12 pp.).

[13]U.S. Department of Health and Human Services. Food and Drug Administration. Guidance for industry. Non-inferiority clinical trials; March 2010 (66 pp.).

have 80% of subjects with HIV-1 RNA below the lower limit of detection at 48 weeks. If a drug company would like to plan a new study with power $(100 - \beta)$ of 90% and a type I error rate (α) of 5%, what sample size would be needed to establish the equivalence of a new drug candidate if the clinically acceptable difference is 10%? To calculate the sample size, we can translate the request into the sample size formula as $p = 0.8$, $d = 0.1$, and the value of the quantity $(z_{1-(\alpha/2)} + z_{1-\beta})^2$ is obtained from Table 10.2 corresponding to $\alpha = 0.05$ and $\beta = 0.1$ (ie, 10.5). Plugging these values into the our sample size formula, we see that:

$$n = \frac{2(0.8)(0.2)(10.5)}{(0.1)^2} = 336.$$

Here, 336 subjects would be needed for each treatment group or the total size of the trial should be 672 subjects.

b. Example 8: Sample Size Calculation for Equivalence of Two Proportions

Consider a drug candidate for the treatment of HIV in naive subjects that is expected to have 85% of subjects with HIV-1 RNA below the lower limit of detection at 48 weeks. If a drug company would like to plan a new study with power $(100 - \beta)$ of 90% and a type I error rate (α) of 1%, what sample size would be needed to establish the equivalence of a new drug candidate if the clinically acceptable difference is 12%? To calculate the sample size, we can translate the request into the sample size formula as $p = 0.85$, $d = 0.12$, and the value of the quantity $(z_{1-(\alpha/2)} + z_{1-\beta})^2$ is obtained from Table 10.2 corresponding to $\alpha = 0.01$ and $\beta = 0.1$ (ie, 14.9). Plugging these values into the our sample size formula, we see that:

$$n = \frac{2(0.85)(0.15)(14.9)}{(0.12)^2} = 263.85$$

Here, 264 subjects would be needed for each treatment group or the total size of the trial should be 528 subjects.

XIV. OTHER HELPFUL CONSIDERATIONS

Sample size calculations should refer to the number of subjects required for the primary analysis. If the number of subjects in the primary analysis will deviate from the number of subjects randomized, then the sample size will need to be adjusted accordingly. For instance, certain studies are allowed to make use of a modified intent-to-treat population (mITT) defined as all subjects randomized who receive at least one dose of study drug and have at least one postbaseline measurement. The sample size calculation for such studies should calculate the number of subjects needed for the mITT population, not the number of subjects to be randomized. If it is expected that roughly 10% of the subjects randomized will fail to meet the criterion for inclusion in the mITT population, the numbers from the sample size calculation would need to be adjusted accordingly to yield the appropriate number of subjects to be randomized. In the case of the pain study discussed earlier, if the sample size calculation indicates a total of 264 subjects in the mITT population are necessary to detect the 0.8 unit difference at 90% power, then we would need to randomize at least 294 subjects in order to obtain the 264 subjects necessary for our primary analysis.

As a reminder, the sample size calculations presented in this chapter represent simple formulas which can be applied when certain assumptions are met. There are a number of considerations common in clinical trials which could necessitate the use of more sophisticated statistical methods. These include, but are not limited to, having unknown or unequal variances, inclusion of interim analyses, use of stratification variables, use of more than two treatment groups, missing data, differential follow-up times in studies utilizing a time-to-event variable as the primary endpoint. Methods are available to address each of these issues as well as countless other issues encountered in clinical trials. However, many of these methods may require someone formally trained in statistics to successfully determine and implement the proper method for a given situation.

It is worth stating that even in the statistical community, sample size calculations are viewed as an art backed by science. Given the sensitivity of calculations to seemingly modest changes in assumptions, it is very important to investigate the sample sizes necessary for a reasonable range of values for the expected treatment effect or variance. This exercise will provide a review of the risk/benefit of choosing a particular sample size over another. While this review can sometimes be painful, it is most often enlightening, as it is best to set the trial size armed with the most information available rather than for it to be arbitrarily picked using only scant information. In the case that there are little to no good data on which to base sample size calculations, it is possible to include procedures to reestimate the sample size during the conduct of the study. These methods, called sample size reestimation techniques, use interim data to recalculate the sample size, while preserving the type I error rate of the study. The FDA issued draft guidance on adaptive designs which included its current thinking on sample size reestimation (14). Methods which are focused on reestimation using blinded data are available and have been successfully utilized in clinical studies.

After the conduct of a study and review of the results, statisticians are sometimes asked "What was the power of the study based on the treatment differences that were observed in the study?" In essence, the investigator is asking for a post-hoc analysis of power. As stated previously, power is the probability of correctly rejecting the null hypothesis. From a statistical perspective, once the study has been conducted, the power as related to that study is either 100% (ie, the null hypothesis was correctly rejected) or 0% (ie, the null hypothesis was not correctly rejected). With that said, evaluating power for a future study based on the observed effects from the given study may be a valuable tool for researchers as they evaluate the future development of the drug candidate. For these post-hoc analyses of power, the formulas as presented in this chapter may be applied using the observed treatment differences or treatment effect, as appropriate. If it is found that the revised assumptions would have required a larger sample size, then these estimates should be considered when planning future studies.

XV. WRITING A SAMPLE SIZE SECTION OF A CLINICAL STUDY PROTOCOL

Every Clinical Study Protocol should include some justification of the sample size utilized in the study. The justification should include the following information: the primary endpoint, the null and alternative hypotheses being tested, the test statistic, the type I and type II error rates, estimates of treatment effect and/or variability, and any other information that would be helpful should someone need to reproduce the calculation. An example of a sample size justification which could be included in a Protocol is as follows.

---

[14] U.S. Department of Health and Human Services. Food and Drug Administration. Guidance for industry. Adaptive design clinical trials for drugs and biologics; February 2010 (50 pp.).

For this phase III, randomized, multicenter study of HIV-infected subjects, the null hypothesis (H_0) is that the proportion of subjects who have HIV-1 RNA below the lower limit of detection at 48 weeks when taking a drug candidate added to standard of care is the same as the proportion of subjects who have HIV-1 RNA below the lower limit of detection at 48 weeks when taking standard of care alone. From review of the available literature, the standard of care will have 80% of subjects with HIV-1 RNA below the lower limit of detection at 48 weeks. Based on the results of the recently completed phase II study, it is expected that this proportion will be 90% in subjects receiving the drug candidate added to standard of care. Based on these assumptions and using a z-test statistic, 325 subjects per group (650 total subjects) in the ITT analysis is sufficient to detect a 10% difference in the proportion of subjects with HIV-1 RNA below the lower limit of detection at 48 weeks with 95% power and a 5% type I error rate.

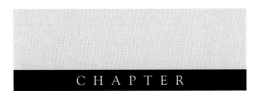

11

Introduction to Endpoints

I. FDA's GUIDANCE FOR INDUSTRY

Endpoints in clinical trials are used to assess the efficacy and safety of a drug or medical device. Clinical trial design typically includes primary endpoints, secondary endpoints, and exploratory endpoints. As explained by FDA's Guidance for Industry (1), clinical trial design includes a:

> hierarchy of endpoints ... determined by the trial's stated objectives and the clinical relevance and importance of each specific measure independently and in relationship to each other. We consider any endpoints that are not part of the prespecified hierarchy of primary and key secondary endpoints to be exploratory. Endpoints included for economic evaluation that are not intended for labeling claims should be designated as such, and will be regarded as exploratory.

Additionally, the FDA states that (2):

> primary and secondary efficacy endpoints should be chosen based on the drug's putative mechanism of action and the proposed indication ... [s]econdary efficacy endpoints can provide useful information on the effect of the treatment and ... provide support to the primary efficacy endpoint. Secondary efficacy endpoints also can explore other effects of the drug on the disease. Commonly used secondary efficacy endpoints include ... symptom scores, activity scales, and health-related quality-of-life instruments. Biomarkers can, in some cases, also provide support of efficacy.

FDA considers safety endpoints to be secondary endpoints (3). A publication from FDA officials provided a distinction between primary endpoints and secondary endpoints, "In considering approval or nonapproval of an application of a product ... the results from

[1]U.S. Department of Health and Human Services. Food and Drug Administration. Guidance for industry. Patient-reported outcome measures: use in medical product development to support labeling claim; December 2009 (39 pp.).

[2]U.S. Department of Health and Human Services. Food and Drug Administration. Guidance for industry. Chronic obstructive pulmonary disease: developing drugs for treatment; November 2009 (17 pp.).

[3]U.S. Department of Health and Human Services. Food and Drug Administration. Safety reporting requirements for INDs and BA/BE studies; December 2012 (29 pp.).

Clinical Trials.
DOI: http://dx.doi.org/10.1016/B978-0-12-804217-5.00011-4

single studies should be highly statistically significant and the drug being evaluated should have a clinically meaningful superior treatment effect based on the primary endpoint of the study and **corroborative treatment effect must be observed** in secondary endpoints" (4).

a. Phase I Clinical Trial Endpoints

Phase I clinical trials are primarily conducted for arriving at an optimal dose, for use in phase II and III clinical trials, but only secondarily, if at all, for acquiring data on efficacy. In comments about phase I trials in the context of oncology, Llovet et al. (5), find that, "[i]n current oncological practice, phase I studies are intended to define appropriate dosage by using endpoints such as dose-limiting toxicity, maximum tolerated dose, pharmacokinetic profile, and pharmacodynamic profile. The primary endpoint of these studies is the safety profile or change in measures that reflect relevant biologic processes."

b. Clinical Endpoints

The endpoints that are most relevant to the study subject are events of which the study subject is aware or afraid of, such as death, a heart attack, loss of vision, or the arising need for a liver transplant due to viral infection (6). These endpoints are classified as *clinical*

endpoints. In clinical trials on life-threatening disorders, the most common clinical endpoint is overall survival (OS). But, according to Le Tourneau et al. (7), "[t]he main drawback of overall survival is that it usually requires larger patient numbers and longer follow-up than surrogate time-to-event end points."

c. Surrogate Endpoints

Another class of endpoints is *surrogate endpoints*. Where the natural time course of a particular disease is extremely long, or where the window of drug therapy is extremely long, trial design may include one or more surrogate endpoints. When included in trial design, surrogate endpoints can reduce the cost and duration of the trial. According to Fleming and DeMets (8), a surrogate endpoint is a laboratory measurement or a clinical sign used as a substitute for a clinically meaningful endpoint. The surrogate endpoint measures how a patient functions, survives, or feels. The surrogate endpoint is supposed to operate as follows. Changes induced by a therapy on the surrogate endpoint reflect changes in the clinically meaningful endpoint.

Examples of surrogate endpoints include tumor size and number, or time to detection of tumor metastasis in clinical trials in oncology, LDL-cholesterol in clinical trials with drugs for atherosclerosis, and reduction in brain lesions in

---

[4]Sridhara R, et al. Review of oncology and hematology drug product approvals at the US Food and Drug Administration between July 2005 and December 2007. J. Natl Cancer Inst. 2010;102:222−35.

[5]Llovet JM, Di Bisceglie AM, Bruix J, et al. Design and endpoints of clinical trials in hepatocellular carcinoma. J. Natl Cancer Inst. 2008;100:698−711.

[6]Fleming RT, DeMets DL. Surrogate end points in clinical trials: are we being misled? Ann. Intern. Med. 1996;125:605−13.

[7]Le Tourneau C, Michiels S, Gan HK, Siu LL. Reporting of time-to-event end points and tracking of failures in randomized trials of radiotherapy with or without any concomitant anticancer agent for locally advanced head and neck cancer. J. Clin. Oncol. 2009;27:5965−71.

[8]Fleming RT, DeMets DL. Surrogate end points in clinical trials: are we being misled? Ann. Intern. Med. 1996;125:605−13.

clinical trials on multiple sclerosis. In the context of clinical trials on infections, Smith et al. (9) expressly categorized endpoints as clinical endpoints (relates to signs and symptoms of the infection) and as bacteriological endpoints (measures the titer of the infecting agent).

The proper place of surrogate endpoints in trial design has been reviewed by Dhani et al. (10), Gill and Sargent (11), Pazdur (12), McKee et al. (13), Allegra et al. (14), Hoos et al. (15), Soria et al. (16), Lamborn et al. (17), and Armstrong and Febbo (18).

While surrogate endpoints may be included in the list of endpoints for any clinical trial, surrogate endpoints are of increased importance for the FDA's accelerated drug approval program. According to one of FDA's Guidance for Industry documents, surrogate endpoints may be a basis for FDA approval for drugs used to treat serious or life-threatening diseases, and "[i]n this setting, FDA may grant approval based on an effect on a surrogate endpoint that is *reasonably likely* to predict clinical benefit" (19).

d. Relatively Objective Endpoints Versus Relatively Subjective Endpoints

The next few chapters in this book concern endpoints used in clinical trials on solid tumors, hematological cancers, immune disorders, and infections. Following these accounts are chapters on another type of endpoint, health-related quality of life (HRQoL). HRQoL refers to subjective information collected from study subjects by way of questionnaires. HRQoL data may be used, as an endpoint, in efforts to gain FDA approval for various drugs and medical devices.

[9]Smith C, Burley C, Ireson M, et al. Clinical trials of antibacterial agents: a practical guide to design and analysis. Statisticians in the Pharmaceutical Industry Working Party. J. Antimicrob. Chemother. 1998;41:467−80.

[10]Dhani N, Tu D, Sargent DJ, Seymour L, Moore MJ. Alternate endpoints for screening phase II studies. Clin. Cancer Res. 2009;15:1873−82.

[11]Gill S, Sargent D. End points for adjuvant therapy trials: has the time come to accept disease-free survival as a surrogate end point for overall survival? Oncologist 2006;11:624−9.

[12]Pazdur R. Endpoints for assessing drug activity in clinical trials. The Oncologist 2008;13(Suppl. 2):19−21.

[13]McKee AE, Farrell AT, Pazdur R, Woodcock J. The role of the U.S. Food and Drug Administration review process: clinical trial endpoints in oncology. Oncologist 2010;15(Suppl. 1):13−18.

[14]Allegra C, Blanke C, Buyse M, et al. End points in advanced colon cancer clinical trials: a review and proposal. J. Clin. Oncol. 2007; 25:3572−5.

[15]Hoos A, Eggermont AM, Janetzki S, et al. Improved endpoints for cancer immunotherapy trials. J. Natl Cancer Inst. 2010;102:1388−97.

[16]Soria JC, Massard C, Le Chevalier T. Should progression-free survival be the primary measure of efficacy for advanced NSCLC therapy? Ann. Oncol. 2010;21:2324−32.

[17]Lamborn KR, Yung WK, Chang SM, et al. Progression-free survival: an important end point in evaluating therapy for recurrent high-grade gliomas. Neuro. Oncol. 2008;10:162−70.

[18]Armstrong AJ, Febbo PG. Using surrogate biomarkers to predict clinical benefit in men with castration-resistant prostate cancer: an update and review of the literature. Oncologist 2009;14:816−27.

[19]U.S. Department of Health and Human Services. Food and Drug Administration. Guidance for industry. Clinical trial endpoints for the approval of cancer drugs and biologics; 2005 (23 pp.).

Publications that systematically address the utility and reliability of HRQoL questionnaires describe HRQoL questionnaires in clinical trials on cancer, including breast cancer (20), colorectal cancer (21), lung cancer (22), melanoma (23), and liver cancer (24), as well as for diseases that are not cancer, such as hepatitis C virus (25), tuberculosis (26,27), multiple sclerosis (28,29), and asthma (30).

At the objective end of the endpoint spectrum, is OS (death), while at the subjective end of the spectrum is HRQoL. Regarding survival, Slamon et al. (31) refer to this as "an end point free of ascertainment bias."

Endpoints that reside at intermediate points in this spectrum include endpoints that rely on tumor size and number. Even though tumor size and number seem straightforward, these are often determined by measurements by an independent radiologist, and by the investigator's radiologist, and they are often determined at a given time point, and then confirmed at a later time point. Other endpoints can reside in-between the far-objective and far-subjective ends of the spectrum. For patient-reported outcomes (PRO) (32,33) the question of objectivity and subjectivity depends on the exact outcome that is being measured. The PRO of migraine

[20]Twelves CJ, Miles DW, Hall A. Quality of life in women with advanced breast cancer treated with docetaxel. Clin. Breast Cancer 2004;5:216−22.

[21]Cornish D, Holterhues C, van de Poll-Franse LV, Coebergh JW, Nijsten T. A systematic review of health-related quality of life in cutaneous melanoma. Ann. Oncol. 2009;20(Suppl. 6):51−8.

[22]Gridelli C, Ardizzoni A, Le Chevalier T, et al. Treatment of advanced non-small-cell lung cancer patients with ECOG performance status 2: results of an European Experts Panel. Ann. Oncol. 2004;15:419−26.

[23]Cornish D, Holterhues C, van de Poll-Franse LV, Coebergh JW, Nijsten T. A systematic review of health-related quality of life in cutaneous melanoma. Ann. Oncol. 2009;20(Suppl. 6):51−8.

[24]Yeo W, Mo FK, Koh J, et al. Quality of life is predictive of survival in patients with unresectable hepatocellular carcinoma. Ann. Oncol. 2006;17:1083−9.

[25]Gutteling JJ, de Man RA, Busschbach JJ, Darlington AS. Overview of research on health-related quality of life in patients with chronic liver disease. Neth. J. Med. 2007;65:227−34.

[26]Guo N, Marra F, Marra CA. Measuring health-related quality of life in tuberculosis: a systematic review. Health Qual. Life Outcomes 2009;7:14.

[27]Marra CA, Marra F, Colley L, Moadebi S, Elwood RK, Fitzgerald JM. Health-related quality of life trajectories among adults with tuberculosis: differences between latent and active infection. Chest 2008;133:396−403.

[28]Ramp M, Khan F, Misajon RA, Pallant JF. Rasch analysis of the Multiple Sclerosis Impact Scale MSIS-29. Health Qual Life Outcomes 2009;7:58.

[29]Mowry EM, Beheshtian A, Waubant E, et al. Quality of life in multiple sclerosis is associated with lesion burden and brain volume measures. Neurology 2009;72:1760−5.

[30]Ehrs PO, Nokela M, Ställberg B, Hjemdahl P, Wikström Jonsson E. Brief questionnaires for patient-reported outcomes in asthma: validation and usefulness in a primary care setting. Chest 2006;129:925−32.

[31]Slamon DJ, Leyland-Jones B, Shak S, et al. Use of chemotherapy plus a monoclonal antibody against HER2 for metastatic breast cancer that overexpresses HER2. New Engl. J. Med. 2001;344:783−92.

[32]U.S. Department of Health and Human Services. Food and Drug Administration. Guidance for industry. Patient-reported outcome measures: use in medical product development to support labeling claims; December 2009.

[33]Bharmal M, Viswanathan S. Late-phase patient reported outcomes. Appl. Clin. Trials 2009;18:5 pp.

headaches (34), hot flashes (35), and tinnitus (36), are relatively objective. But the PRO of fatigue or depression are relatively subjective.

For oncology clinical trials, various scales and questionnaires that are used include Eastern Cooperative Oncology Group (ECOG) performance status, Karnofsky performance status, and HRQoL.

e. Using Multiple Endpoints, and Choosing the Endpoint on Which to Base Conclusions

The International Conference Harmonization (ICH) Guidelines provides a general warning, applicable to many diseases, regarding endpoint choice. According to the ICH Guidelines (37):

> When two treatments are used for the same disease or condition, they may differentially affect various outcomes of interest in that disease, particularly if they represent different classes or modalities of treatment. Therefore, when comparing them in a clinical trial, the choice and timing of endpoints may favor one treatment or the other. For example, thrombolytics in patients with acute myocardial infarction can reduce mortality but increase hemorrhagic stroke risk. If a new, more pharmacologically active, thrombolytic were compared with an older thrombolytic, the more active treatment might look better if the endpoint were mortality, but worse if the endpoint were a composite of mortality and disabling stroke. Similarly, in comparing two analgesics in the management of dental pain, assigning a particularly heavy weight to pain at early time points would favor the drug with more rapid onset of effect, while assigning more weight to later time points would favor a drug with a longer duration of effect.

While any give drug may have three distinct benefits, and where each benefit can be measured at three different time points, failure to be aware of these variables can result in artifactual conclusions from the clinical trial. The next few chapters detail the endpoints used in clinical trials of oncology, clinical trials in multiple sclerosis, and clinical trials on hepatitis C virus. The chapters on oncology endpoints provide guidance on deciding which endpoints to include in the clinical trial, for example, objective response, progression-free survival, time to progression, disease-free survival, and OS. These chapters document the fact, for example, that reduction in tumor size and number, as measured by the Response Evaluation Criteria in Solid Tumors (RECIST) criteria, do not necessarily correlate with long-term survival to the cancer.

f. In Choosing Endpoints Keep in Mind the Eventual Goals of the Clinical Trial

For any given parameter collected during a clinical trial, the sponsor of the trial needs to determine whether the parameter is properly used as an endpoint in the clinical trial, and whether FDA will accept data on that particular parameter for:

- Regulatory approval of the drug,
- Including in the package insert for the drug, and
- Use in advertising to the public, that is, promotional claims.

[34]Acquadro C, Berzon R, Dubois D, et al. Incorporating the patient's perspective into drug development and communication: an ad hoc task force report of the Patient-Reported Outcomes (PRO) Harmonization Group meeting at the Food and Drug Administration, February 16, 2001. Value Health 2003;6:522−31.

[35]Freedman RR. Patient satisfaction with miniature, ambulatory, postmenopausal hot flash recorder. Open Med. Device J. 2009;1:1−2.

[36]Meikle MB, Stewart BJ, Griest SE, Henry JA. Tinnitus outcomes assessment. Trends Amplif. 2008;223−35.

[37]ICH Harmonised Tripartite Guideline. Choice of control group and related issues in clinical trials E10. Step 4 version, July 2000 (33 pp.).

A document, used by pharmaceutical companies and called the target product profile (TPP) can be used to keep track of these goals (38,39). The TPP lists the essential attributes required for a drug to be a clinically successful product. The TPP defines the target patient population, desired levels of efficacy and safety, the dosing route and schedule, the drug formulation, and acceptable cost of the formulated drug (40). Moreover, the TPP constrains or determines the actions of scientists developing the formulation. Thus, the TPP's information on route of administration, dosage form and size, maximum and minimum doses, and patient population (pediatric formulations may require chewable tablets or a suspension), provides a guide for formulation development (41).

[38]U.S. Department of Health and Human Services. Food and Drug Administration. Guidance for industry. Target product profile—a strategic development process tool; March 2007 (25 pp.).

[39]Lambert WJ. Considerations in developing a target product profile for parenteral pharmaceutical products. AAPS PharmSciTech. 2010;11:1476–81.

[40]Wyatt PG, et al. Target validation: linking target and chemical properties to desired product profile. Curr. Top. Med. Chem. 2011;11:1275–83.

[41]Lionberger RA, et al. Quality by design: concepts for ANDAs. AAPS J. 2008;10:268–76.

12

Oncology Endpoint—Objective Response

I. INTRODUCTION TO ENDPOINTS IN ONCOLOGY CLINICAL TRIALS

Survival, as it applies to an individual study subject, and overall survival (OS), as it applies to a population of study subjects, are clinical endpoints for oncology trials. Survival and OS are used in clinical trials on solid tumors and on trials for the hematological cancers.

Oncology clinical trials also use a number of endpoints that serve as a surrogate for survival. These surrogate endpoints are intended to correlate with survival and are intended to predict OS. Surrogate endpoints in clinical trials on solid tumors include objective response, progression-free survival (PFS), time to progression (TTP),

disease-free survival (DFS), and time to distant metastasis (TDM) (1). Examples of biomarkers used in oncology clinical trials include epidermal growth factor receptor for nonsmall-cell lung cancer (2), BRAF for colorectal cancer (3), and prostate-specific antigen for prostate cancer (4). BRAF refers to an oncogene that encodes a kinase.

For use with populations of subjects, endpoints relating to PFS include median PFS, 6-month PFS, 2-year PFS, 5-year PFS, as well as the statistical parameter known as the hazard ratio. Please note that it is impossible to calculate a "median" unless there exists a plurality of numbers.

For populations of subjects, endpoints that relate specifically to survival time include the endpoints of median OS, 6-month OS, 2-year OS and 5-year OS.

[1]Kelloff GJ, Bast Jr RC, Coffey DS, et al. Biomarkers, surrogate end points, and the acceleration of drug development for cancer prevention and treatment: an update prologue. Clin. Cancer Res. 2004;10:3881−4.

[2]Murray N. The challenge of using biomarkers and molecularly targeted drugs to improve cure rate in early stage non-small cell lung cancer. Thorac. Dis. 2015;7:230−4.

[3]Dienstmann R, et al. Personalizing colon cancer adjuvant therapy: selecting optimal treatments for individual patients. J. Clin. Oncol. 2015;pii:JCO.2014.60.0213.

[4]Bryant RJ, Sjoberg DD, Vickers AJ, et al. Predicting high-grade cancer at ten—core prostate biopsy using four kallikrein markers measured in blood in the ProtecT study. J. Natl Cancer Inst. 107. pii: djv095. http://dx.doi.org/10.1093/jnci/djv095 (6 pp.).

Clinical Trials.
DOI: http://dx.doi.org/10.1016/B978-0-12-804217-5.00012-6

Median PFS and *median* OS refer to the average value from all study subjects or, at least, a number of subjects that is sufficient to provide the median value. Endpoints keyed to a specific time, such as 2-year PFS, refer not to any average value, but to the percent of all study subjects (in the entire study) experiencing that endpoint by the 2-year timepoint.

The following bullet points provide a context showing how this chapter fits into the next few chapters. While all of these are endpoints used in oncology, an understanding of these will enable a better understanding of endpoints used in other disorders, for example, immune diseases, infections, and metabolic diseases. This chapter concerns objective response, as indicated by the check mark.

- Objective response✓
- Overall survival
- Progression-free survival
- Time to progression
- Disease-free survival
- Time to distant metastasis

Dhani et al. (5), Pazdur (6), Yothers (7), Mathoulin-Pelissier et al. (8), Saad and Katz (9), and Beckman (10), provide additional guidance on endpoints used in oncology clinical trials.

a. Objective Response

In a general statement about oncology, Grothey et al. (11) teach that the efficacy of a new oncology drug traditionally has been assessed by its ability to shrink existing tumors and to prolong OS. Reliable data on tumor shrinkage can be obtained by small or large clinical trials, while reliable data on OS generally can only be obtained from large clinical trials. Tumor shrinkage can be easily measured in small trials, thus justifying further testing of the drug in a large clinical trial. In clinical practice, the observation of a tumor shrinkage, also called "response," may convince the patient and the oncologist that the selected therapy is active against the cancer.

Objective response is an endpoint used in clinical trials on solid tumors. The term *objective response* refers to the size and number of the subject's tumors. The earliest attempts to standardize tumor measurements were conducted

[5]Dhani N, Tu D, Sargent DJ, Seymour L, Moore MJ. Alternate endpoints for screening phase II studies. Clin. Cancer Res. 2009;15:1873—82.

[6]Pazdur R. Endpoints for assessing drug activity in clinical trials. Oncologist 2008;13(Suppl. 2):19—21.

[7]Yothers G. Toward progression-free survival as a primary end point in advanced colorectal cancer. J. Clin. Oncol. 2007;25:5153—4.

[8]Mathoulin-Pelissier S, Gourgou-Bourgade S, Bonnetain F, Kramar A. Survival end point reporting in randomized cancer clinical trials: a review of major journals. J. Clin. Oncol. 2008;26:3721—6.

[9]Saad ED, Katz A. Progression-free survival and time to progression as primary end points in advanced breast cancer: often used, sometimes loosely defined. Ann. Oncol. 2009;20:460—4.

[10]Beckman M. More clinical cancer treatments judged by progression-free rather than overall survival. J. Natl Cancer Inst. 99:1068—9.

[11]Grothey A, Hedrick EE, Mass RD, Sarkar S, Suzuki S, Ramanathan RK, et al. Response-independent survival benefit in metastatic colorectal cancer: a comparative analysis of N9741 and AVF2107. J. Clin. Oncol. 2008;26:183—9.

by Moertel and Hanley during the 1960s and 1970s (12). At that time, palpitation and X-rays were used to assess tumor size. Since that time, more accurate imaging methods have been introduced and adopted, including, computed tomography (CT), positron emission tomography (PET), and magnetic resonance imaging (MRI) (13).

The criteria for measuring tumor size and numbers are available from the World Health Organization (WHO) and the European Organization for Research and Treatment of Cancer (EORTC). In 1979, imaging was adopted for lesion measurement in the WHO criteria. However, because of some limitations to the WHO criteria, Response Evaluation Criteria in Solid Tumors (RECIST) was introduced in 2000. For reporting results from clinical trials, or for publications, the response of tumors to therapy, in terms of tumor size and number, can be expressed by the RECIST criteria (14–16), as well as by the earlier set of criteria, the WHO response criteria (17,18). The RECIST criteria were created by the EORTC (19).

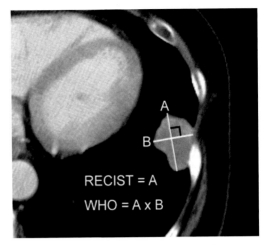

FIGURE 12.1 Radiologic image. Methods of tumor measurement according to the RECIST and WHO criteria. With the WHO criteria, the longest diameter (A) and the longest perpendicular diameter (B) are obtained and multiplied (2D measurement). With RECIST, only the longest diameter (A) is obtained (uni- or one-dimensional [1D] measurement).

Figure 12.1 introduces the differences between the WHO criteria and the RECIST criteria (20). With the WHO criteria, a two-dimensional (2D)

[12]Wahl RL, Jacene H, Kasamon Y, Lodge MA. From RECIST to PERCIST: evolving considerations for PET response criteria in solid tumors. J. Nucl. Med. 2009;50(Suppl. 1):122S–50S.

[13]van Persijn van Meerten EL, Gelderblom H, Bloem JL. RECIST revised: implications for the radiologist. A review article on the modified RECIST guideline. Eur. Radiol. 2010;20:1456–67.

[14]Eisenhauer EA, Therasse P, Bogaerts J, et al. New response evaluation criteria in solid tumours: revised RECIST guideline (version 1.1). Eur. J. Cancer 2009;45:228–47.

[15]Therasse P, Arbuck SG, Eisenhauer EA, et al. New guidelines to evaluate the response to treatment in solid tumors. European Organization for Research and Treatment of Cancer, National Cancer Institute of the United States, National Cancer Institute of Canada. J. Natl Cancer Inst. 2000;92:205–16.

[16]Schwartz LH, Bogaerts J, Ford R, et al. Evaluation of lymph nodes with RECIST 1.1. Eur. J. Cancer 2009;45:261–7.

[17]World Health Organization. Handbook for reporting results of cancer treatment. Geneva: World Health Organization; 1979, publication 48.

[18]Park JO, Lee SI, Song SY, et al. Measuring response in solid tumors: comparison of RECIST and WHO response criteria. Jpn J. Clin. Oncol. 2003;33:533–7.

[19]Suzuki C, Jacobsson H, Hatschek T, et al. Radiologic measurements of tumor response to treatment: practical approaches and limitations. Radiographics 2008;28:329–44.

[20]Suzuki C, Jacobsson H, Hatschek T, et al. Radiologic measurements of tumor response to treatment: practical approaches and limitations. Radiographics 2008;28:329–44.

measurement is used. The longest diameter (A) and the longest perpendicular diameter (B) are obtained and multiplied. With RECIST criteria, only the longest diameter (A) is obtained. This is a one-dimensional (1D) measurement.

This provides further perspective regarding the endpoint of objective response. According to Rubinstein et al. (21), in the era before RECIST criteria, the typical endpoint of the phase II trials in oncology was objective tumor response (change in size and number of tumors). Unfortunately, for many diseases, such as lung, colon, breast, and renal cancers, objective tumor response failed to predict survival benefit (22). For other cancers, such as glioblastoma and prostate cancer, tumor response has proven difficult to measure. Hence, it is recognized that it is by no means automatic that objective response is the most appropriate endpoint for an oncology clinical trial.

In comments about clinical trials on melanoma, Korn et al. (23) found it has generally not been the case that objective response is correlated with survival. Korn et al. (24), as well as

Dy et al. (25), also point out that objective response is not a particularly sensitive reflection of the therapeutic effect of a class of drugs known as cytostatic drugs. Cytostatic drugs tend to result only in stabilization of the tumors. As a consequence, these authors concluded that OS and PFS are better endpoints than objective response in trials of cytostatic drugs. This point was reiterated by Grothey et al. (26), who found that although objective change in tumor size is an important criterion for the treatment of solid tumors, this criterion may be more relevant as surrogate markers of drug efficacy for *cytotoxic* chemotherapy than for drugs that tend to have a more *cytostatic* effect.

Objective response is often used with drugs that are cytotoxic agents (27). Rixe and Fojo (28), as well as Fleming et al. (29), describe how the efficacy of a cytotoxic agent, which by its nature causes both tumor shrinkage and tumor stasis, is more easily detected by objective response, while efficacy of a cytotoxic agent, which by its nature causes mainly

[21]Rubinstein L, Crowley J, Ivy P, Leblanc M, Sargent D. Randomized phase II designs. Clin. Cancer Res. 2009;15:1883−90.

[22]Rubinstein L, Crowley J, Ivy P, Leblanc M, Sargent D. Randomized phase II designs. Clin. Cancer Res. 2009;15:1883−90.

[23]Korn EL, Liu PY, Lee SJ, Chapman JA, et al. Meta-analysis of phase II cooperative group trials in metastatic stage IV melanoma to determine progression-free and overall survival benchmarks for future phase II trials. J. Clin. Oncol. 2008;26:527−34.

[24]Korn EL, Liu PY, Lee SJ, Chapman JA, et al. Meta-analysis of phase II cooperative group trials in metastatic stage IV melanoma to determine progression-free and overall survival benchmarks for future phase II trials. J. Clin. Oncol. 2008;26:527−34.

[25]Dy GK, Miller AA, Mandrekar SJ, et al. A phase II trial of imatinib (ST1571) in patients with c-kit expressing relapsed small-cell lung cancer: a CALGB and NCCTG study. Ann. Oncol. 2005;16:1811−6.

[26]Grothey A, Hedrick EE, Mass RD, et al. Response-independent survival benefit in metastatic colorectal cancer: a comparative analysis of N9741 and AVF2107. J. Clin. Oncol. 2008;26:183−9.

[27]Rubinstein, L. E-mail of August 21, 2010.

[28]Rixe O, Fojo T. Is cell death a critical end point for anticancer therapies or is cytostasis sufficient? Clin. Cancer Res. 2007;13:7280−7.

[29]Fleming TR, Rothmann MD, Lu HL. Issues in using progression-free survival when evaluating oncology products. J. Clin. Oncol. 2009;27:2874−80.

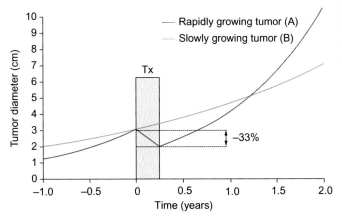

FIGURE 12.2 Tumor size versus years. This hypothetical diagram of tumor growth shows growth of a rapidly growing tumor (A) and growth of a slow-growing tumor (B). *Tx* means treatment.

tumor stasis, is less easily detected by objective response. Cisplatin, and other drugs that disrupt DNA metabolism, tend to be more *cytotoxic*, while sorafenib and flavopiridol may have properties that are more *cytostatic* (30).

The layperson may find it intuitively obvious that measuring tumor size and number is the best way to determine efficacy of a drug, and for predicting long-term survival. Unfortunately, attempts to find a correlation between objective response and OS, in the realm of solid tumors, are typically met with disappointment.

Figure 12.2 demonstrates some of the shortcomings of using objective response as a measure of drug efficacy. In the following hypothetical example, provided by Weber (31), a rapidly growing tumor (red) shrinks with therapy. But another tumor, a slowly growing tumor (green), continues to grow. At this point in time, the physician might conclude that the drug is effective against the rapidly growing tumor. However, as far as the patient is concerned, the drug provides no long-term benefit, because the rapidly growing tumor recovers from the toxic effects of the drug, and

eventually is much larger than before. This hypothetical demonstrates why, for many oncology clinical trials, the endpoints of PFS and OS are typically chosen as primary endpoints, while objective response is used only as a secondary endpoint.

The next few quotations provide a context for introducing the RECIST criteria. The examples are from breast cancer, colorectal cancer, lung cancer, and cancer of the head and neck. Endpoints that are objective responses are *bolded*. Definitions of the indicated subsets of objective response will then be disclosed.

In a study of breast cancer by Geyer et al. (32), the list of endpoints included objective response, where this was classed as a secondary endpoint:

> The primary end point was the time to progression, defined as the time from randomization to disease progression or death due to breast cancer. Secondary end points were progression-free survival, defined as the time from randomization to disease progression or death due to any cause; overall survival; **the overall response rate;** ... **complete response, partial response, or stable disease** for at least 6 months.

[30]Rixe O, Fojo T. Is cell death a critical end point for anticancer therapies or is cytostasis sufficient? Clin. Cancer Res. 2007;13:7280–7.

[31]Weber WA. Assessing tumor response to therapy. J. Nucl. Med. 2009;50:1S–10S.

[32]Geyer CE, Forster J, Lindquist D, et al. Lapatinib plus capecitabine for HER2-positive advanced breast cancer. New Engl. J. Med. 2006;355:2733–43.

In a study of colorectal cancer by Van Cutsem et al. (33), the list of endpoints included objective response, where this was classed as a secondary endpoint:

> The primary end point was progression-free survival time, defined as the time from randomization to disease progression or death from any cause within 60 days after the last tumor assessment or after randomization. Secondary end points included the overall survival time, the ... **complete response or partial response**, defined as a response persisting for at least 28 days.

In a study of lung cancer, Shepherd et al. (34) included a list of primary endpoints and secondary endpoints:

> The primary end point was overall survival. Secondary end points included progression-free survival, **overall response rate (complete and partial)**, duration of response, toxic effects, and quality of life. Responses were assessed with the use of the Response Evaluation Criteria in Solid Tumors (RECIST) criteria.

In a study of cancer of the head and neck, Vermorken et al. (35) provided an extensive list of endpoints, where the secondary endpoints included objective response:

> The primary end point was overall survival, defined as the time from randomization to death. Secondary end points were progression-free survival (the time from randomization to the first radiologic confirmation of disease progression, or death from any cause within 60 days after the last assessment or randomization, whichever came first) ... **a complete

response, a partial response, or stable disease**), the time to treatment failure (the time from randomization until the date of the first occurrence of one of the events specified in the protocol as constituting treatment failure).

Now, let is turn to the actual RECIST criteria. The RECIST criteria include the following subsets (36):

1. Complete response (CR): Disappearance of all target lesions.
2. Partial response (PR): At least a 30% decrease in the sum of diameters of target lesions, taking as reference the baseline sum diameters.
3. Progressive disease (PD): At least a 20% increase in the sum of diameters of target lesions, taking as reference the smallest sum on study (this includes the baseline sum if that is the smallest on study). In addition to the relative increase of 20%, the sum must also demonstrate an absolute increase of at least 5 mm. The appearance of one or more new lesions is also considered progression.
4. Stable disease (SD): Neither sufficient shrinkage to qualify for PR nor sufficient increase to qualify for PD, taking as reference the smallest sum diameters while on study.

b. Objective Response—Demetri's Example of PR

The clinical trial of Demetri et al. (37) concerned gastrointestinal stromal tumors (GIST).

---

[33]Van Cutsem E, Köhne CH, Hitre E, et al. Cetuximab and chemotherapy as initial treatment for metastatic colorectal cancer. New Engl. J. Med. 2009;360:1408–17.

[34]Shepherd FA, Rodrigues Pereira J, Ciuleanu T, et al. Erlotinib in previously treated non-small-cell lung cancer. New Engl. J. Med. 2005;353:123–32.

[35]Vermorken JB, Mesia R, Rivera F, et al. Platinum-based chemotherapy plus cetuximab in head and neck cancer. New Engl. J. Med. 2008;359:1116–27.

[36]Eisenhauer EA, Therasse P, Bogaerts J, et al. New response evaluation criteria in solid tumours: revised RECIST guideline (version 1.1). Eur. J. Cancer 2009;45:228–47.

[37]Demetri GD, von Mehren M, Blanke CD, et al. Efficacy and safety of imatinib mesylate in advanced gastrointestinal stromal tumors. New Engl. J. Med. 2002;347:472–80.

Patients received *imatinib*, a small molecule that inhibits a small group of related tyrosine kinases, including the KIT receptor tyrosine kinase. The clinical trial contained two arms, where patients in arm A received 400 mg imatinib daily, and arm B received 600 mg imatinib daily.

There was no control group, but data from earlier clinical trials demonstrated that responses of this type of cancer to standard forms of chemotherapy were low. The documented objective response rate was 5%, and the OS in unresectable patients was less than 12 months (38). Subsequent clinical trials assessing the safety and efficacy of imatinib for GIST also did not contain any control group, for example, the clinical trial of Heinrich et al. (39).

This provides background information regarding GIST. Most GISTs result from activating mutations in the KIT receptor tyrosine kinase, where this activating mutation is the mechanism responsible for about 85% of GIST patients. For about 8% of GIST patients, the mechanism responsible for the cancer is an activating mutation in a related enzyme, namely, platelet-derived growth factor receptor-alpha (PDGFRA) (40). The survival of metastatic GIST patients is dramatically improved by treatment with the KIT and PDGFRA inhibitor imatinib, a small molecule that inhibits KIT and PDGFRA. Unfortunately, tumors eventually acquire resistance to imatinib due to evolution of mutations in these two enzymes (41).

The response of GIST to chemotherapy can be measured by imaging techniques, such as PET or CT. PET works better in the context of GIST clinical trials. For PET imaging, the patient receives an infusion of [^{18}F]fluoro-2-deoxyglucose. Objective response is according to the standard set forth by the Eastern Cooperative Oncology Group (ECOG). These guidelines state that a 25% reduction in the maximum standardized uptake value should be considered as the threshold for definition of PR (42). These guidelines are not the same as the RECIST guidelines, but they are used in a similar manner. Interestingly, it has been found that when the RECIST criteria are used, the result does not predict the outcome of survival in response to chemotherapy while, in contrast, when the ECOG criteria are used, objective response does correlate with survival outcome (43). Another publication, entitled, "We Should Desist Using RECIST, at Least in GIST," directly addressed the fact that the

[38]von Mehren M. E-mail of May 2, 2011.

[39]Heinrich MC, Owzar K, Corless CL, et al. Correlation of kinase genotype and clinical outcome in the North American Intergroup Phase III Trial of imatinib mesylate for treatment of advanced gastrointestinal stromal tumor: CALGB 150105 Study by Cancer and Leukemia Group B and Southwest Oncology Group. J. Clin. Oncol. 2008;26:5360−7.

[40]Demetri GD, Heinrich MC, Fletcher JA, et al. Molecular target modulation, imaging, and clinical evaluation of gastrointestinal stromal tumor patients treated with sunitinib malate after imatinib failure. Clin. Cancer Res. 2009;15:5902−9.

[41]Demetri GD, Heinrich MC, Fletcher JA, et al. Molecular target modulation, imaging, and clinical evaluation of gastrointestinal stromal tumor patients treated with sunitinib malate after imatinib failure. Clin. Cancer Res. 2009;15:5902−9.

[42]Holdsworth CH, Badawi RD, Manola JB. CT and PET: early prognostic indicators of response to imatinib mesylate in patients with gastrointestinal stromal tumor. Am. J. Roentgenol. 2007;189:W324−30.

[43]Holdsworth CH, Badawi RD, Manola JB. CT and PET: early prognostic indicators of response to imatinib mesylate in patients with gastrointestinal stromal tumor. Am. J. Roentgenol. 2007;189:W324−30.

TABLE 12.1 The Demitri Study of Gastrointestinal Stromal Tumors

	Nature of Objective Response (% of Subjects)	
	400 mg Imatinib	600 mg Imatinib
Complete response	0	0
Partial response	49.3	58.1
Stable disease	31.5	24.3
Progressive disease	16.4	10.8
Could not be evaluated	2.7	6.8

RECIST criteria result in poor correlations of objective response with survival (44).

The results from the clinical trial of Demetri et al. (45) are indicated in Table 12.1. The responses were assessed by PET scanning, followed by a confirmatory scan at least 28 days later. There results demonstrate that about half the subjects showed a PR (partial shrinkage) while about a quarter of the subjects showed SD. Only about 14% of the subjects experienced increases in tumor size. There were no significant differences in objective response between the two doses of imatinib. Figure 12.3 discloses representative PET scans (raw data) from one particular subject, where scans were taken at baseline, after 1 month of imatinib treatment, and after 16 months of imatinib treatment. The figure reveals a dramatic reduction and near-disappearance of the pelvic-level signal arising from the tumors.

c. Objective Response—van Meerten's Example of PR

In a description of lung tumors, occurring with the metastasis of uterine cancer, van Persijn van Meerten et al. (46) provide images of tumors assessed by objective response, according to the RECIST criteria. In Fig. 12.4, panels a and b show CT scans *before chemotherapy* (baseline data), while panels c and d show scans *after chemotherapy*. The arrows in panels a and c point to target lesions, while the arrows in b and d point to nontarget lesions. The term "target lesions" refers to specific tumors that the investigator has decided to measure repeatedly during the course of the study.

All of the images are of lung tumors from the same woman being treated for uterine cancer. In comparing a and c, it is easy to see that the target lesion (arrow) has shrunk but has not disappeared. In comparing b and d, it is easy to see that one of the nontarget lesions (arrow) has actually increased in size. The patient's response was classified as PR. In other words, the patient's response was not classified as CR or as SD, but instead it was classed as PR.

d. Objective Response—Example of PD

The data in Fig. 12.5 are used to illustrate the endpoint of PD, also known as disease progression. This provides a clear-cut example of the application of the RECIST criteria to the endpoint of PD. In a description of a man with rectal cancer, Suzuki et al. (47) provide images of tumors that have metastasized to the lungs

[44]Benjamin RS, Choi H, Macapinlac HA, et al. We should desist using RECIST, at least in GIST. J. Clin. Oncol. 2007;25:1760–4.

[45]Demetri GD, von Mehren M, Blanke CD, et al. Efficacy and safety of imatinib mesylate in advanced gastrointestinal stromal tumors. New Engl. J. Med. 2002;347:472–80.

[46]van Persijn van Meerten EL, Gelderblom H, Bloem JL. RECIST revised: implications for the radiologist. A review article on the modified RECIST guideline. Eur. Radiol. 2010;20:1456–67.

[47]Suzuki C, Jacobsson H, Hatschek T, et al. Radiologic measurements of tumor response to treatment: practical approaches and limitations. Radiographics 2008;28:329–44.

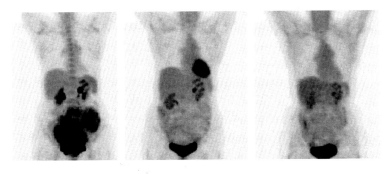

FIGURE 12.3 PET scan of a subject with GIST, during the course of treatment with imatinib. Baseline (*left figure*); 1 month chemotherapy (*central figure*); 16 months chemotherapy (*right figure*).

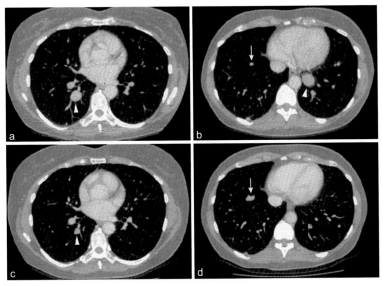

FIGURE 12.4 Computed tomography. Images of tumors are shown before (a, b) and after (c, d) chemotherapy. The images are from 50-year-old woman with a uterus sarcoma.

and adrenal gland. The top panels (Fig. 12.5a,b) depict images of the *lungs*, before and after chemotherapy, respectively. An identical white arrow appears in the before and after images of the lungs, demonstrating shrinkage of a lung tumor. The lower panels (Fig. 12.5c,d) show images of the *abdomen*, which includes the adrenal gland, before and after chemotherapy, respectively. In the images of the abdomen, a black arrow is shown, indicating a new tumor that materialized after chemotherapy. The objective response shown by the tumors in the adrenal gland was classified as PD.

Suzuki et al. (48) provide a warning about indiscriminate use of the endpoint of PD, and caution that, "WHO criteria ... were based on bi- or two-dimensional (2D) measurements because it was not possible to measure tumor volume with the imaging technology available at that time ... [t]hese criteria were based on the assumption that the tumor is spherical and has a circular cross section ... [t]hese criteria have received wide acceptance and have become known as the WHO criteria for reporting the results of cancer treatment ... [h]owever, WHO criteria

[48]Suzuki C, Jacobsson H, Hatschek T, et al. Radiologic measurements of tumor response to treatment: practical approaches and limitations. Radiographics 2008;28:329–44.

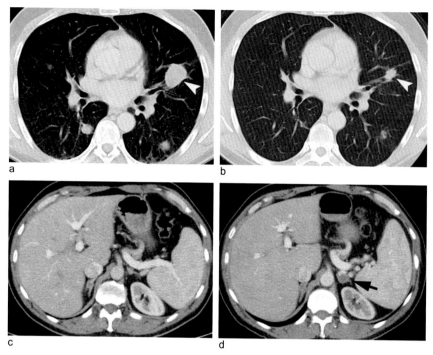

FIGURE 12.5 Objective response that is PD. Images of lungs where rectal cancer has metastasized to the lungs (a, b) and to the adrenal gland (c, d). CT scans (lung window) obtained before (a) and after (b) treatment show multiple lung metastases. The target lesion (*arrowhead*) and many other lesions decreased in size after treatment. CT scans of the abdomen, obtained before (c) and after (d) treatment, show a new lesion in the adrenal gland after treatment (*arrow* in d).

do not mention the minimum lesion size or the number of lesions to be selected in patients with multiple lesions. Nor do the WHO criteria consider the type of imaging modality that should be used. Progressive disease (PD), originally defined as a 25% increase in the product of 2D diameters, was defined by some investigators as the increase in the sum of all lesions and by others as the increase in any one lesion." Suzuki et al. (49), in its entirety, provides an exemplary account of how to use objective endpoints, including the endpoint of PD.

II. STUDIES CHARACTERIZING AN ASSOCIATION BETWEEN OBJECTIVE RESPONSE AND SURVIVAL

As detailed in the colorectal cancer study of Grothey et al. (50), the magnitude of objective

[49]Suzuki C, Jacobsson H, Hatschek T, et al. Radiologic measurements of tumor response to treatment: practical approaches and limitations. Radiographics 2008;28:329—44.

[50]Grothey A, Hedrick EE, Mass RD, Sarkar S, Suzuki S, Ramanathan RK, et al. Response-independent survival benefit in metastatic colorectal cancer: a comparative analysis of N9741 and AVF2107. J. Clin. Oncol. 2008;26:183—9.

response may be correlated, at least to some extent, with the magnitude of OS. Buyse et al. (51) also reported a moderately good correlation between objective response and survival, for colorectal cancer. According to a personal communication from Dr A. Grothey (52) a stronger correlation between objective response and OS can be found from studies of testicular cancer. Also, excellent correlations between objective response and OS occur with hematological cancers, for example, the leukemias (53). Moreover, according to Benjamin et al. (54), objective response may be correlated with survival for GIST.

However, unfortunately, objective tumor response has generally been a poor surrogate for survival in most solid tumors (55). According to Sargent (56), improvements in objective response do not necessarily translate to OS benefit. And conversely, it has been shown that, for example, patients with colon cancer still receive a benefit, in terms of OS, from a more effective treatment even if they do not show objective response (57).

III. AVOIDING CONFUSION WHEN USING OBJECTIVE RESPONSE AS AN ENDPOINT

The endpoint of objective response is potentially confusing, for the reasons listed below. These sources of confusion also apply to endpoints that require data on objective response, that is, the endpoints of PFS and TTP.

a. Date for Beginning Objective Response Measurements in Two Study Arms, Relative to Start Date of Treatment

When a clinical trial contains two study arms, confusion can result when assessments of objective response (in both arms) are not initiated on the same date (relative to the date of initiating drug treatment).

For example, consider the example of a cancer clinical trial involving two study arms, one receiving study drug and the other a control treatment. Let us say that the start date for assessing objective response of the study drug is delayed by 2 weeks, that is, delayed 2 weeks after the corresponding date for the control treatment.

For the sake of this hypothetical, assume that the true efficacies of both treatments (study drug; control treatment) are about the same. But in the situation where assessments of objective response for the study drug are delayed, for example, by 2 weeks, the clinical trial will conclude that the study drug works better than the control treatment.

This particular situation was actually described, in a study of melanoma comparing efficacy of temozolomide (study drug) and

[51]Buyse M, Thirion P, Carlson RW, et al. Relation between tumour response to first-line chemotherapy and survival in advanced colorectal cancer: a meta-analysis. The Lancet 2000;356:373–8.

[52]Grothey A. E-mail of August 25, 2010.

[53]Hedrick EE. Personal communication, March 2, 2011.

[54]Benjamin RS, Choi H, Macapinlac HA, et al. We should desist using RECIST, at least in GIST. J. Clin. Oncol. 2007;25:1760–4.

[55]Sargent, DJ. E-mail of August 31, 2010.

[56]Sargent D. General and statistical hierarchy of appropriate biologic endpoints. Oncology 2006;20(6 Suppl. 5):5–9.

[57]Sargent D. General and statistical hierarchy of appropriate biologic endpoints. Oncology 2006;20(6 Suppl. 5):5–9.

dacarbazine (control treatment) (58). Timing of objective response assessments in the two arms was initiated on different dates, relative to the start date for initiating treatment. Assessments of temozolomide efficacy were delayed by 2 weeks.

The efficacy of the study drug (temozolomide) appeared to be slightly better than the efficacy of the active control (dacarbazine; DTIC). (The difference in start date for measuring objective response was not proven to be the source of this difference, but was only suggested as a cause.)

In the words of the authors, "DTIC treated patients underwent the first formal assessment for disease progression 2 weeks earlier than did temozolomide treated patients, which may have contributed to the difference observed in PFS" (59).

b. Where Multiple Measurements of Objective Response Are Taken, Which Measurement Is Used for Analysis of Efficacy?

Where duplicate measurements of objective response are taken, ambiguity can result where the publication does not clearly state which value, that is, which data collection, had been used for triggering the event of objective response. Typically, the second of the two measurements is confirmatory.

For example, in a clinical trial of melanoma, objective response (for every subject) was measured at two different time points. A personal communication from the investigator settled the issue, revealing that the value reported in the publication was that from the second time point (60,61).

In another study of melanoma, multiple readings of objective response were taken, but the paper did not expressly state which reading from any given study subject was used for reporting objective response for that particular subject. Readings were taken after every 8-week cycle of therapy (62). A personal communication from the principal investigator revealed that the reading providing the best result, for example, greatest tumor shrinkage, was used for statistical analysis and for reporting in the publication, that is, "The object response rate is calculated based on the 'best response' of each individual patient. CRs are often durable, but partial responses are often not" (63,64). Thus, the reading that gave the best response was the reading used for assessing efficacy.

[58]Middleton MR, Grob JJ, Aaronson N, et al. Randomized phase III study of temozolomide versus dacarbazine in the treatment of patients with advanced metastatic malignant melanoma. J. Clin. Oncol. 2000;18:158−66.

[59]Middleton MR, Grob JJ, Aaronson N, et al. Randomized phase III study of temozolomide versus dacarbazine in the treatment of patients with advanced metastatic malignant melanoma. J. Clin. Oncol. 2000;18:158−66.

[60]Tarhini AA, Kirkwood JM, Gooding WE, Cai C, Agarwala SS. Durable complete responses with high-dose bolus interleukin-2 in patients with metastatic melanoma who have experienced progression after biochemotherapy. J. Clin. Oncol. 2007;25:3802−7.

[61]Agarwala SS. E-mail of September 8, 2010.

[62]Hwu WJ, Krown SE, Menell JH, et al. Phase II study of temozolomide plus thalidomide for the treatment of metastatic melanoma. J. Clin. Oncol. 2003;21:3351−6.

[63]Hwu WJ, Krown SE, Menell JH, et al. Phase II study of temozolomide plus thalidomide for the treatment of metastatic melanoma. J. Clin. Oncol. 2003;21:3351−6.

[64]Hwu WJ. E-mail of September 10, 2010.

c. How Is It Possible to Obtain a Meaningful Value for Objective Response, or for Endpoints (PFS; TTP) That Comprise Objective Response?

In assessing efficacy of an anticancer drug or radiation therapy, it might be expected that tumors begin to grow shortly after treatment. Hence, how is it logically possible for a typical clinical trial to report that the value for PFS was, for example, 3 months or perhaps 5 months? The answer is that objective response is measured according to the RECIST criteria, or a similar standard, which mandates that objective response (and endpoints that comprise objective response) is not triggered until there a specific increase in tumor size or number has occurred.

d. Objective Response Is Reported in Terms of a "Rate" and Also as a "Percent"

Oncology journal articles use the term "objective response rate" in the text, when referring to data on tumor size and number. But in the tables in the same journal articles, this "rate" has the unit "percent." This practice is potentially confusing, in view of the fact that the term "rate," as it is used in chemistry and physics, entails the unit of time. But in oncology, the term "objective response rate" does not entail the unit of time. Instead, the term "objective response rate" means proportion or percent (65). To repeat, in published reports on clinical trials, the term "rate" is usually not used for referring to any rate, but instead the term "rate" refers to percent.

e. Drugs That Are Cytostatic and Not Cytotoxic may Provide Misleading Results, Where the Endpoint of Objective Response Is Used

In a review of oncology endpoints, Dhani et al. (66) warned that, in the case of certain drugs, the failure of the drug to provide an impressive objective response may give a misleading impression of eventual OS. The term RR means response rate, which is a subset of objective response. These authors referred to drugs having a very modest response rate, resulting in prolongation of PFS or OS, suggesting that tumor stabilization rather than shrinkage may still result in clinical benefit. Dhani et al. (67) found that using response rate as a "go/no go" criterion may lead to inappropriate termination of pursuit of the drug in question. A striking example is the putative Raf kinase and antivascular agent sorafenib in renal cell carcinoma and hepatocellular cancer, where response rates using the RECIST criteria were under 10%, conventionally a signal to abandon further development. Fortunately, however, subsequent clinical trials showed significant prolongation of both PFS and OS.

f. Use of Different Criteria (Standards) for Objective Response, and the Availability of Updated Criteria

Yet another potential source of confusion, which can occur when comparing drug efficacies from different clinical trials, is the use of different standards for assessing objective response. As noted above, the available standards include the WHO criteria, and different,

---

[65]Eisenhauer E. E-mail of September 12, 2010.

[66]Dhani N, Tu D, Sargent DJ, Seymour L, Moore MJ. Alternate endpoints for screening phase II studies. Clin. Cancer Res. 2009;15:1873−82.

[67]Dhani N, Tu D, Sargent DJ, Seymour L, Moore MJ. Alternate endpoints for screening phase II studies. Clin. Cancer Res. 2009;15:1873−82.

updated versions of the RECIST criteria. Potential confusion can also result when, during the course of a clinical trial, a new set of standards is issued, and where the investigators contemplate switching to the new standards. Yet another source of confusion is where more sensitive methods of tumor imaging become available. A more sensitive method of tumor imaging will have a direct effect on the ability to detect tumor progression. This issue is developed elsewhere in this textbook, in the material on the *Will Rogers phenomenon.*

IV. FDA'S DECISION-MAKING PROCESS IN EVALUATING OBJECTIVE RESPONSE

a. Introduction

This concerns a drug for treating glioma, a type of brain cancer. The drug was *temozolomide*, and the Sponsor's submission was for approval of this drug for treating two different kinds of gliomas, *glioblastoma multiforme* and *anaplastic astrocytoma*. The Sponsor submitted two different NDAs, NDA 21050 for glioblastoma multiforme and NDA 21029 for anaplastic astrocytoma. The information is from June 2011 on the FDA's website.

b. Irregular Shape of Glioma Tumors

The main issue in FDA's review was the irregular shape of glioma tumors and, in particular, the irregular shape of glioblastoma multiforme tumors. Researchers have documented the fact that the irregular shape of glioma tumors can impair accurate measurements of tumor size, in response to anticancer drugs (68,69).

c. Objective Response

For all gliomas, objective response was determined by MRI, and what was measured was area of a cross-section. Tumor volume was not measured. As is the case with most other clinical trials on solid tumors, the parameters of objective response included CR, PR, PD, and SD. PD, for example, was defined as greater or equal to a 25% increase in the product of the largest perpendicular diameters of any lesion or any new tumor. The FDA defines the rate of objective response, in a study population, as "the proportion of patients with tumor size reduction of a predefined amount and for a minimum time period. Response duration usually is measured from the time of initial response until documented tumor progression. Generally, the FDA has defined ORR [objective response rate] as the sum of partial responses plus complete responses" (70).

d. Overestimation and Underestimation of Tumor Size

Unfortunately for the Sponsor, the FDA reviewer commented on the fact that some of the imaging in the *glioblastoma* study resulted in tumor size that was "overestimated" or "underestimated." In detail, the reviewer stated that, "[i]n the 9 recurrent GMB [glioblastoma multiforme] cases the 20 ... images underestimated lesion size (6 images), overestimated tumor size (5 images) or correctly identified lesion size (9 images)."

[68]van den Bent MJ, et al. End point assessment in gliomas: novel treatments limit usefulness of classical Macdonald's criteria. J. Clin. Oncol. 2009;27:2905–8.

[69]Upadhyay N, Waldman AD. Conventional MRI evaluation of gliomas. Br. J. Radiol. 2011;84:S107–11.

[70]U.S. Department of Health and Human Services. Food and Drug Administration. Guidance for industry. Clinical trial endpoints for the approval of cancer drugs and biologics; May 2007 (19 pp.).

In contrast, imaging for *astrocytoma* was more accurate, and the reviewer stated that, "[a]ccuracy was better for untreated AA [anaplastic astrocytoma] where 7 of 8 images were accurate and one was underestimated."

In comments on the Sponsor's data on glioblastoma, the FDA reviewer referred to the problem that, "FDA and its outside experts do not believe that tumor shrinkage or increase can be adequately assessed ... because of their irregular configuration. Thus tumor response and tumor progression cannot be used as the principal basis for approval."

At this point, the take-home lesson is that, when conducting a clinical trial on a solid tumor that has an irregular shape, the Sponsor should consider using, as a primary endpoint, an endpoint that does not require measurements of tumor area or tumor volume.

e. FDA Approves Drug for Indication of Astrocytoma, but Refused to Approve Drug for Indication of Glioblastoma

The *Medical Review* stated that, "[t]he FDA reviewers did not believe that accurate tumor measurements could be obtained in ... glioma [glioblastoma multiforme] patients thus confounding determination of progression free survival ... [b]ased on these considerations the FDA review team believed that Temozolomide should not be approved for the treatment of ... Glioblastoma Multiforme patients."

In contrast, the FDA granted approval for temozolomide for treating astrocytoma. To this point, the *Medical Review* stated, "[t]he applicant is requesting ... approval based on objective tumor response rate in patients ... FDA reviewers

felt that these response rates and response durations ... along with a satisfactory safety profile where sufficient to grant ... approval."

f. Unreliability of Objective Response, Where Tumor Size Measurements Are Not Accurate

FDA officials have warned about the problem of basing a clinical trial on objective tumor response, in the situation where tumor size measurements are not accurate. McKee et al. (71) warn that, "[t]he uncertainty of radiographic tumor assessment may make radiographic-based endpoints, such as response rate ... unreliable. Advanced mesotheliomas, gastric cancers, and locally advanced pancreatic cancers are examples of tumors for which radiographic assessments of the tumor are unreliable and an assessment of OS [overall survival] is necessary."

With regard to measuring the size of glioblastoma tumors, FDA officials acknowledged that, "GBMs are morphologically heterogeneous tumors with varying amounts of edema, necrosis ... [b]ecause of the infiltrating nature of GBMs, the **accurate measurement of tumor diameters** on MRI poses problems, as was evident in the current trial, in which the **concordance of MRI readings by two neuroradiologists was only about 50%**" (72).

g. Accelerated Approval

Please note that the Sponsor's clinical trials for both types of glioma (glioblastoma, astrocytoma) were submitted by way of the FDA's accelerated approval pathway. Accelerated

---

[71]McKee AE, et al. The role of U.S. Food and Drug Administration review process: clinical trial endpoints in oncology. The Oncologist 2010;15(Suppl. 1):13−18.

[72]Cohen MH, et al. FDA drug approval summary: bevacizumab (Avastin®) as treatment of recurrent glioblastoma multiforme. The Oncologist 2009;14:1131−8.

approval permits a Sponsor to win FDA approval for marketing a drug, based on objective tumor response, without data showing increased survival. Thus, the Sponsor's use of the accelerated approval procedure increased the burden on the Sponsor for demonstrating that the study drug resulted in a convincing objective response. The FDA's accelerated approval procedure is detailed in Chapter 33.

V. CONCLUDING REMARKS

To conclude, where objective response (tumor size and number) is used as a primary endpoint in a clinical trial for an anticancer drug, the Sponsor should ensure tumor size can be accurately measured, and that the nature of the data in the FDA submission is sufficient to convince reviewers that the tumor size measurements are accurate.

13

Oncology Endpoints: Overall Survival and Progression-Free Survival

I. INTRODUCTION

This chapter continues with the topic of oncology endpoints, and covers the second and third of the topics indicated by the check marks.

- Objective response
- Overall survival (OS) ✓
- Progression-free survival (PFS) ✓
- Time to progression (TTP)

- Disease-free survival (DFS)
- Time to distant metastasis.

Overall survival (OS) is recognized by the US Food and Drug Administration (FDA) and the European Medicines Agency (EMA) as the gold standard for clinical benefit in oncology clinical trials (1,2). Overall survival has been called the gold standard for oncology clinical trials in general (3,4,5,6) as well as specifically for colorectal cancer (7), prostate cancer (8,9), cancer of the

[1]Bergmann L, Berns B, Dalgleish AG, et al. Investigator-initiated trials of targeted oncology agents: why independent research is at risk? Ann. Oncol. 2010;21:1573–8.

[2]Pazdur R. Endpoints for assessing drug activity in clinical trials. Oncologist 2008;13(Suppl. 2):19–21.

[3]Johnson JR, Williams G, Pazdur R. End points and United States Food and Drug Administration approval of oncology drugs. J. Clin. Oncol. 2003;21:1404–11.

[4]Steensma DP, Loprinzi CL. Erythropoietin use in cancer patients: a matter of life and death? J. Clin. Oncol. 2005;23:5865–8.

[5]Wolff SN. Applying sensitivity analysis to overall survival in cancer clinical trials. J. Clin. Oncol. 2010;28:1147.

[6]Montagnani F, Migali C, Fiorentini G. Progression-free survival in bevacizumab-based first-line treatment for patients with metastatic colorectal cancer: is it a really good end point? J. Clin. Oncol. 2009;27:e132–3.

[7]Allegra C, Blanke C, Buyse M, et al. End points in advanced colon cancer clinical trials: a review and proposal. J. Clin. Oncol. 2007;25:3572–5.

[8]Halabi S, Vogelzang NJ, Ou SS, Owzar K, Archer L, Small EJ. Progression-free survival as a predictor of overall survival in men with castrate-resistant prostate cancer. J. Clin. Oncol. 2009;27:2766–71.

[9]Hussain M, Goldman B, Tangen C, et al. Prostate-specific antigen progression predicts overall survival in patients with metastatic prostate cancer: data from Southwest Oncology Group Trials 9346 (Intergroup Study 0162) and 9916. J. Clin. Oncol. 2009;27:2450–6.

head and neck (10), and gastric cancer (11). This endpoint is triggered by only one event, death from any cause. Overall survival is the most common endpoint in oncology clinical trials, followed by PFS, TTP, and DFS (12).

FDA's Guidance for Industry (13) defines PFS as the time from randomization until objective response or death. PFS is an endpoint that, for any given individual subject, may be reached before the endpoint of overall survival is reached. PFS is triggered by two events, the event of progression, and the event of death from any cause. In other words, for any given study subject, where tumors grow beyond a predetermined limit, this counts as the event of PFS. Also, for any given study subject, where the subject dies for any reason, this also counts as an event of PFS. If a study subject dies, and is also found to have tumors that grew beyond the predetermined limit, this counts as only one event of PFS (not as two events).

a. Review of Objective Response

The predetermined limit mentioned above is that of *objective response*. Objective response is gauged by a conventional standard of tumor measurement, such as the Response Evaluation Criteria in Solid Tumors (RECIST) criteria or the WHO criteria. The following provides a concrete example where objective response is defined. Freidlin et al. (14) refer to objective response as, "[b]y this, we mean the time that the tumor has grown enough so to satisfy the radiologic criteria for progression (e.g., 20% increase in the longest maximum dimension)."

b. Contrast Between PFS and TTP

This contrasts PFS with TTP. TTP is defined as the time from randomization until objective tumor progression. TTP does not include deaths. In analysis involving the endpoint of TTP, deaths are censored and are not included in the value of time. According to Bergmann et al. (15), the date of progression should be assigned based on the time of the first evidence of objective progression or recurrence, regardless of violations, discontinuation of study drug, or change of therapy. According to Llovet et al. (16), "regulatory agencies prefer progression free survival to time to progression for drug approval because the former endpoint may be better correlated with overall survival."

[10]Le Tourneau C, Michiels S, Gan HK, Siu LL. Reporting of time-to-event end points and tracking of failures in randomized trials of radiotherapy with or without any concomitant anticancer agent for locally advanced head and neck cancer. J. Clin. Oncol. 2009;27:5965−71.

[11]Methy N, Bedenne L, Bonnetain F. Surrogate endpoints for overall survival in digestive oncology trials: which candidates? A questionnaires survey among clinicians and methodologists. BMC Cancer 2010;10:277.

[12]Mathoulin-Pelissier S, Gourgou-Bourgade S, Bonnetain F, Kramar A. Survival end point reporting in randomized cancer clinical trials: a review of major journals. J. Clin. Oncol. 2008;26:3721−6.

[13]U.S. Department of Health and Human Services. Food and Drug Administration. Guidance for industry. Clinical trial endpoints for the approval of cancer drugs and biologics; April 2005.

[14]Freidlin B, Korn EL, Hunsberger S, Gray R, Saxman S, Zujewski JA. Proposal for the use of progression-free survival in unblinded randomized trials. J. Clin. Oncol. 2007;25:2122−6.

[15]Bergmann L, Berns B, Dalgleish AG, et al. Investigator-initiated trials of targeted oncology agents: why independent research is at risk? Ann. Oncol. 2010;21:1573−8.

[16]Llovet JM, Di Bisceglie AM, Bruix J, et al. Design and endpoints of clinical trials in hepatocellular carcinoma. J. Natl Cancer Inst. 2008;100:698−711.

c. Excellence of PFS as an Endpoint

To understand why PFS is an excellent endpoint, let us first contemplate why a given endpoint might be a poor endpoint. Fleming and DeMets (17) describe several reasons why a surrogate endpoint may fail (18):

- The surrogate is not in the causal pathway of the disease process.
- The intervention influences only the pathway mediated through the surrogate but does not affect other important causal pathways.
- The surrogate is insensitive to the treatment effect or is not in the pathway of the treatment's effect.
- The treatment has mechanisms of action independent of the disease process.

According to Prentice (19), a surrogate marker must be both correlated with the true end point and fully capture the net effect of treatment on the true endpoint. As reiterated by Methy et al. (20), the fact that a certain parameter might be "correlated" with the rate of survival, does not mean that the parameter is a prognostic factor for that rate. The layperson can appreciate the fact that, in collecting data on study subjects, it is possible to find a correlation between the color of the subject's clothing, on the first day of the trial, and the subsequent rate of tumor metastasis.

The endpoint of PFS likely satisfies the above criteria. First of all, the value of PFS (by definition) will have some correlation with the value for overall survival. This is because PFS includes deaths. Thus, PFS is connected with, and will be ensured to have some correlation with the endpoint of overall survival. Secondly, PFS is triggered by objective response, that is, growth or increase in the number of tumors. It is self-evident that growth or increase in number of tumors is part of the causal pathway of cancer that leads to death. Prentice (21) recommends that, for a surrogate endpoint to be a valid endpoint, the event that is used as the surrogate should be part of the pathway that leads to death (or to some other feature of the disease that impairs the life of the patient).

According to one of FDA's Guidance for Industry documents (22):

> PFS has desirable qualities of a surrogate endpoint because it reflects tumor growth (a phenomenon likely to be on the causal pathway for cancer-associated morbidity and death), can be assessed prior to demonstration of a survival benefit, and is not subject to the potential confounding impact of subsequent therapy.

[17]Fleming TR, DeMets DL. Surrogate end points in clinical trials: are we being misled? Ann. Intern. Med. 1996;125:605–13.

[18]Gill S, Sargent D. End points for adjuvant therapy trials: has the time come to accept disease-free survival as a surrogate end point for overall survival? Oncologist 2006;11:624–9.

[19]Prentice RL. Surrogate endpoints in clinical trials: definition and operational criteria. Stat. Med. 1989;8:431–40.

[20]Methy N, Bedenne L, Bonnetain F. Surrogate endpoints for overall survival in digestive oncology trials: which candidates? A questionnaires survey among clinicians and methodologists. BMC Cancer 2010;10:277.

[21]Prentice RL. Surrogate endpoints in clinical trials: definition and operational criteria. Stat. Med. 1989;8:431–40.

[22]U.S. Department of Health and Human Services. Food and Drug Administration. Guidance for industry. Clinical trial endpoints for the approval of cancer drugs and biologics; April 2005.

II. ADVANTAGES OF PFS OVER OVERALL SURVIVAL

a. Introduction

PFS has some advantages, as an endpoint, over the endpoint of overall survival. These relative advantages arise from:

- Confusion from effects of nonstudy drugs given to subjects who leave the trial.
- Collecting data on overall survival may require an extended follow-up period.
- Confusion from the multiplicity of causes of death.
- Ethical reasons.
- Need for premature halt of the trial, where the halt allows collection of data on PFS, but not collection of data on overall survival.
- Conclusions arising from data on overall survival may be redundant with conclusions made from data on PFS.

b. Confusion From Effects of Nonstudy Drugs Given to Subjects Who Leave the Trial

Overall survival can be unreliable, in the situation where patients completing the trial begin taking a drug that is not part of the study [23]. In this case, efforts to acquire survival data in the follow-up period could be confounded by the second drug. According to Van Cutsem et al. [24], "[t]reatment added after the conclusion of a study can confound the analysis of overall survival, and in this study, approximately two thirds of patients in each group received subsequent chemotherapy after completion of the study." Similarly, Sobrero et al. [25] found that, "[p]ost-protocol treatment may have affected survival, given the substantial proportion (46.9%) of initial irinotecan patients who subsequently received a cetuximab-based regimen, an effective standard treatment after irinotecan failure."

c. Collecting Data on Overall Survival may Require an Extended Follow-Up Period

Hudis et al. [26] and Gill and Sargent [27] describe yet another advantage of using the endpoint of PFS. For any given patient, OS might not be triggered until many years after the clinical trial has started. Cancers with a time course that takes many years until death require an extended follow-up period, thereby prolonging the drug-approval process. In contrast, the event of disease progression, which is a component of PFS, usually occurs earlier than death.

[23]Burzykowski T, Buyse M, Yothers G, Sakamoto J, Sargent D. Exploring and validating surrogate endpoints in colorectal cancer. Lifetime Data Anal. 2008;14:54–64.

[24]Van Cutsem E, Köhne CH, Hitre E, et al. Cetuximab and chemotherapy as initial treatment for metastatic colorectal cancer. New Engl. J. Med. 2009;360:1408–17.

[25]Sobrero AF, Maurel J, Fehrenbacher L, et al. EPIC: phase III trial of cetuximab plus irinotecan after fluoropyrimidine and oxaliplatin failure in patients with metastatic colorectal cancer. J. Clin. Oncol. 2008;26:2311–9.

[26]Hudis CA, Barlow WE, Costantino JP, et al. Proposal for standardized definitions for efficacy end points in adjuvant breast cancer trials: the STEEP system. J. Clin. Oncol. 2007;25:2127–32.

[27]Gill S, Sargent D. End points for adjuvant therapy trials: has the time come to accept disease-free survival as a surrogate end point for overall survival? Oncologist 2006;11:624–9.

d. Weakened Conclusions, Regarding Efficacy of Study Drug, When the Endpoint Is Keyed to a Longer Timeframe

This concerns endpoints that are keyed to a particular interval of time, for example, 6-month PFS, 2-year PFS, 5-year PFS, and 10-year PFS, or 6-month OS, 2-year OS, 5-year OS, and 10-year OS. While the longer timeframe endpoints are not often used in oncology clinical trials, they tend to be used for some hematological cancers, apparently because of their high cure rate. Allum et al. (28), provide guidance for selecting the timeframe, by warning that the values for 10-year survival, for the study drug group and control group, may be nearly equal to each other. The reason for this is that, for both groups, most of the subjects will likely have died by 10 years.

According to Allum et al. (29), the original analysis showed a hazard ratio for OS of 0.79 in favor of the group receiving cisplatin plus surgery. The data showed slightly weaker beneficial hazard ratio of 0.84 after longer follow-up. This hazard ratio showing weaker benefit than was expected, because survival curves will naturally become closer as time passes and the proportion of survivors falls towards zero (30). The term *original analysis* means analysis of data acquired from an earlier time point in the clinical trial. The clinical trial compared cisplatin plus surgery versus surgery alone.

To view a hypothetical, any endpoint that is calculated after a follow-up time of 200 years is useless, because all of the study subjects, in both the study drug arm and control treatment arm, have perished. To view a more realistic example, where a follow-up time of 15 years is used, arm A of the trial may have a 5% OS and arm B may have a 6% OS. This kind of result does not permit a conclusion as to which treatment was better (arm A vs arm B). This problem can be alleviated by using the endpoint of PFS, by expressing OS data in terms of 2-year survival (2 years is usually not long enough to permit most of the subjects in arm A and arm B to die), or by expressing OS data in terms of median OS.

e. Confusion From the Multiplicity of Causes of Death

For any individual subject, PFS may be triggered at a time point that triggers OS. The reason is that PFS may be triggered within a few months after the trial begins, while OS may be triggered a few years after the trial begins. During these years, the study subject may die from a cause unrelated to the disease, for example, from a car accident, where time to death from this unrelated cause is collected and used for the statistical analysis of the trial. Yothers (31) wrote, "[i]f we follow patients long enough, they will all experience an event. Hypothetically, a patient could experience progression at 6 months, die as a passenger in a car accident at 8 months—totally unrelated to CRC or treatment." Please note that progression is an event that triggers PFS. CRC refers to colorectal cancer.

[28]Allum WH, Stenning SP, Bancewicz J, Clark PI, Langley RE. Long-term results of a randomized trial of surgery with or without preoperative chemotherapy in esophageal cancer. J. Clin. Oncol. 2009;27:5062−7.

[29]Allum WH, Stenning SP, Bancewicz J, Clark PI, Langley RE. Long-term results of a randomized trial of surgery with or without preoperative chemotherapy in esophageal cancer. J. Clin. Oncol. 2009;27:5062−7.

[30]Allum WH, Stenning SP, Bancewicz J, Clark PI, Langley RE. Long-term results of a randomized trial of surgery with or without preoperative chemotherapy in esophageal cancer. J. Clin. Oncol. 2009;27:5062−7.

[31]Yothers G. Toward progression-free survival as a primary end point in advanced colorectal cancer. J. Clin. Oncol. 2007;25:5153−4.

f. Ethical Reasons

The endpoint of PFS is also advantageous, where study subjects wish to leave the trial, in order to stop taking placebo and to start taking the standard of care, or to stop taking the study drug and to start taking the standard of care.

g. Need for Premature Halt of the Trial, Where the Halt Allows Collection of Data on PFS, but Prevents Collection of Data on Overall Survival

As an endpoint in a clinical trial, PFS can be advantageous in the situation where patient accrual is slow. As a result of slow accrual, the trial may need to be terminated early (32).

A related issue is the need to submit data to a regulatory agency, or to publish the data, where sufficient data on OS are not available. Grever et al. (33) provide an example of one study where the researchers wanted to publish their results as soon as convincing data on PFS became available, and where the researchers did not want to wait for the availability of sufficient data on OS. In these author's words, "[a]t the time of this analysis, OS data are immature. However, PFS survival data are mature based on the large number of reported clinical events." Another example can be found in Gradishar et al. (34), who reported a

clinical trial that disclosed PFS, but failed to disclose OS. In the words of these investigators, "[p]atient survival data were not mature at the time of data cutoff for this publication."

h. Conclusions Arising From Data on Overall Survival may be Redundant with Conclusions Made From Data on PFS

Tang et al. (35) reviewed a large number of published clinical trials, and found that, in about 80% of the trials, the results from PFS (or from the endpoint of TTP) were not significantly different from the results from OS. In only 20% of the trials, were the results for PFS (or TTP) and OS significantly different from each other.

III. ADVANTAGES OF OVERALL SURVIVAL OVER PFS

The endpoint of OS provides some advantages over the endpoint of PFS, as outlined.

a. Overall Survival Is the Gold Standard

According to the FDA, OS "is considered the most reliable cancer endpoint ... [t]his endpoint is precise and easy to measure, documented by the data of death. Bias is not a factor in endpoint measurement" (36).

---

[32]Petrelli NJ. Perioperative or adjuvant therapy for resectable colorectal hepatic metastases. J. Clin. Oncol. 2008;26:4862–3.

[33]Grever MR, Lucas DM, Dewald GW, et al. Comprehensive assessment of genetic and molecular features predicting outcome in patients with chronic lymphocytic leukemia: results from the US Intergroup Phase III Trial E2997. J. Clin. Oncol. 2007;25:799–804.

[34]Gradishar WJ, Krasnojon D, Cheporov S, et al. Significantly longer progression-free survival with nab-paclitaxel compared with docetaxel as first-line therapy for metastatic breast cancer. J. Clin. Oncol. 2009;27:3611–9.

[35]Tang PA, Bentzen SM, Chen EX, Siu LL. Surrogate end points for median overall survival in metastatic colorectal cancer: literature-based analysis from 39 randomized controlled trials of first-line chemotherapy. J. Clin. Oncol. 2007;25:4562–8.

[36]U.S. Department of Health and Human Services. Food and Drug Administration. Guidance for industry. Clinical trial endpoints for the approval of cancer drugs and biologics; May 2007.

According to one commentator (37), "[o]verall survival (OS) has been the gold standard for demonstrating clinical benefit for cancer drugs. It is 100% accurate for the event and time, it is assessed daily, its importance is unquestioned, and it addresses both safety and efficacy."

b. The Date of the Event That Triggers PFS may be Ambiguous, While the Date That Triggers Overall Survival is Not Ambiguous

According to Stone et al. (38), the exact time a patient progresses, unlike death, is never actually observed. The event of progression is recorded as having occurred in an interval between two visits. Pangeas et al. (39) pointed out that PFS can be expressed in three different ways, where this ambiguity arises from the fact that "progression" of the tumor is not measured on a daily basis, but only at times that are scheduled and set forth by the clinical study protocol. The three ways of measuring PFS are shown by the following bullet points:

• The date that progression was detected by a tumor scan.
• The date of the tumor scan before the one at which progression was identified.
• In terms of the date half-way between these two dates.

When writing a Clinical Study Protocol, the medical writer should be sure to state when tumor imaging is to be performed. Thus, according to Freidlin et al. (40), "because patients will not be seen at exactly a specified date, the protocol should specify the range of dates acceptable for a scheduled scan time (eg, 6 months +/−2 weeks after the randomization date)."

The date used for basing PFS measurements can influence how the final outcome of the study is interpreted. Dancey et al. (41) find that a higher frequency of tumor assessments is more likely to provide a difference between the study drug group and the control group. In other words, if the interval of time between tumor assessments is lengthy, the study design of the clinical will be less likely to result in a detected difference in PFS between the two arms of the clinical trial, that is, the study drug arm and the control arm.

IV. GUIDANCE FROM CLINICAL TRIALS ON USING ENDPOINTS

Before contemplating data from a number of clinical trials, please consider these technical details on the term "rate" and on the utility of an endpoint that is tied to a specific interval of time, such as, 6 months.

[37]Zhuang SH, Xiu L, Elsayed YA. Overall survival: a gold standard in search of a surrogate: the value of progression-free survival and time to progression as end points of drug efficacy. Cancer J. 2009;15:395−400.

[38]Stone A, Wheeler C, Carroll K, Barge A. et al. Optimizing randomized phase II trials assessing tumor progression. Contemp. Clin. Trials 2007;28:146−52.

[39]Pangeas KS, Ben-Porat L, Dickler MN, Chapman PB, Schrag D. When you look matters: the effect of assessment schedule on progression-free survival. J. Natl Cancer Inst. 2007;99:428−32.

[40]Freidlin B, Korn EL, Hunsberger S, Gray R, Saxman S, Zujewski JA. Proposal for the use of progression-free survival in unblinded randomized trials. J. Clin. Oncol. 2007;25:2122−6.

[41]Dancey JE, Dodd LE, Ford R, et al. Recommendations for the assessment of progression in randomised cancer treatment trials. Eur. J. Cancer 2009;45:281−9.

a. Use of the Word "Rate"

As mentioned in Chapter 12, the term "rate" is often used when reporting objective response, PFS, and other endpoints. This is potentially confusing because in general, as in the fields of chemistry, physics, and physiology (42), the word rate always refers to the ratio of [events]/[unit of time]. The unit of objective response is not a rate, or at least, it is not the same kind of rate as used in chemistry, physics, and physiology. In clinical trial reporting, the word "rate," as it applies to endpoints, actually refers to "percent" or "proportion" (43).

b. Endpoint Keyed to One Specific Time Point—6-Month PFS

When reporting data from clinical trials, PFS can be expressed in terms of "median PFS," which is the data when exactly half of the subjects have experienced this endpoint. The unit for this time point is months. Alternatively, PFS can be expressed in terms of a specific date, such as "6-month PFS." Six-month PFS means the percent of all of the study subjects who have experienced PFS by the 6-month time point in the clinical trial. The unit for this time point is percent.

Lamborn et al. (44) point out an advantage of using PFS that is tied to a specific time point, "[w]hen PFS is used as the primary efficacy end point, a fixed time point (in this case 6 months) reduces time-dependent assessment bias, such as that caused by visit or imaging frequency."

c. Data on PFS may be More Significant Than Data on Overall Survival—The Maemondo Study

In a study on nonsmall-cell lung cancer (NSCLC), Maemondo et al. (45) divided study subjects into two arms:

- Arm A. Gefitinib (study drug).
- Arm B. Carboplatin plus paclitaxel combination (standard treatment).

Chemotherapy was for 9 weeks and, in some cases longer, and following chemotherapy subjects were followed for about 42 months. During this follow-up period, the response of the tumors to chemotherapy was assessed by computed tomography at 2-month intervals. Analysis by computed tomography enabled the measurement of size and number of lung tumors, and comparison of the size and number with the RECIST criteria. In conducting this comparison, the researchers classified the objective response as partial response, complete response, stable disease, or progressive disease.

The endpoints in the Maemondo study included objective response, PFS, and OS. The results for objective response are shown in Table 13.1. These results demonstrate that geftinib worked better than the carboplatin–paclitaxel combination, in terms of all of the parameters. For example, the percent of subjects experiencing partial reponse was about twice as great in the geftinib arm as in the carboplatin plus paclitaxel arm. The percent of subjects experiencing progressive disease

---

[42]Reaction rate, heart rate, blood cell sedimentation rate.

[43]Eisenhauer EA. E-mail of September 11, 2010.

[44]Lamborn KR, Yung WK, Chang SM, et al. Progression-free survival: an important end point in evaluating therapy for recurrent high-grade gliomas. Neuro. Oncol. 2008;10:162–70.

[45]Maemondo M, Inoue A, Kobayashi K, et al. Gefitinib or chemotherapy for non-small-cell lung cancer with mutated EGFR. New Engl. J. Med. 2010;362:2380–8.

was about 50% greater in the carboplatin plus paclitaxel arm than in the geftinib arm.

PFS is shown in the following Kaplan–Meier plot (Fig. 13.1). Visual inspection of this plot reveals that the endpoint of PFS was triggered at earlier time points by subjects receiving carboplatin plus paclitaxel (standard treatment), and triggered at later time points in subjects receiving geftinib. In other words, with standard treatment tumors progressed at an earlier time, and deaths occurred at an earlier time.

TABLE 13.1 Objective Response for Subjects Enrolled in the Maemondo Study

Objective Response	Geftinib Arm (% of Subjects)	Carboplatin Plus Paclitaxel Arm (% of Subjects)
Complete response	4.4	0
Partial response	69.3	30.7
Stable disease	15.8	49.1
Progressive disease	9.6	14.0

The data used to construct this plot were used to calculate the hazard ratio, which was HR = 0.30. The significance of the difference between the two curves on the Kaplan–Meier plot was $P < 0.001$. The hazard ratio is a measure of the separation of the two curves, where HR = 1.0 means that there is no separation. In general, a P value of 0.05 or less means that the separation between the two curves is significant.

PFS was calculated in another way, namely, by finding the median. Median PFS was 10.8 months with geftinib versus 5.4 months with carboplatin plus paclitaxel ($P < 0.001$). Again, the results show well-separated efficacy between the two study arms, and that the separation was significant.

Unfortunately, data on OS were not as persuasive as those on PFS. The following Kaplan–Meier plot shows data on OS (Fig. 13.2). Visual inspection of this plot reveals that the endpoint of overall was triggered at the same frequency, during the first 20 months of the study, in arm A and arm B. At later times, that is, from about 20 months until 40 months, the endpoint of OS was triggered at a somewhat greater frequency in arm B than in arm A. Thus, at least from the survival data

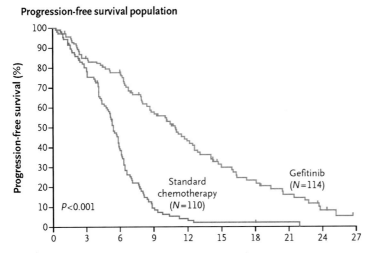

Progression-free survival population

FIGURE 13.1 Kaplan–Meier plot of PFS. The *upper curve* represents PFS data from subjects receiving geftinib, while the *lower curve* represents PFS data from subjects receiving carboplatin plus paclitaxel.

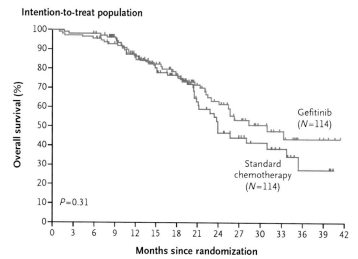

Intention-to-treat population

FIGURE 13.2   Kaplan–Meier plot of overall survival. The *upper curve* represents OS data from subjects receiving geftinib, while the *lower curve* represents OS data from subjects receiving carboplatin plus paclitaxel.

produced later on in the trial, it might be concluded that geftinib had superior efficacy to carboplatin plus paclitaxel. But when all the data are taken into account, the difference between the two study arms was not significant ($P = 0.31$).

The difference in OS was also measured by the parameter of median OS. The median survival time was 30.5 months for the geftinib group, and 23.6 months for the carboplatin plus paclitaxel group. According to this parameter, geftinib had superior efficacy to carboplatin plus paclitaxel.

To view the big picture, the data on objective response, PFS as measured by the hazard ratio, median PFS, and OS, all show that gefitinib has superior efficacy to carboplatin plus paclitaxel.

As in all clinical trials, roughly equal emphasis was placed on collecting efficacy data and safety data. The Maemondo study revealed that geftinib was less toxic, producing diarrhea and rash, while the combination of carboplatin plus paclitaxel was more toxic, producing hematologic and neurologic toxic effects. Thus, the superior efficacy data for gefitinib, in terms of the PFS endpoint, together with gefitinib's lesser toxicity, recommends getitinib as a preferred chemotherapy for NSCLC. According to more recent review articles, the preferred treatments for NSCLC include gefitinib, cisplatin, or carboplatin, depending on the characteristics of the patient (46,47).

d. Methodology Tip—Shapes of Kaplan–Meier Plots in the Maemondo Study

Wittes (48) made an observation regarding Kaplan–Meier plots where two curves, for example, representing study drug arm versus

[46]de Marinis F, Rossi A, Di Maio M, Ricciardi S, Gridelli C. Treatment of advanced non-small-cell lung cancer: Italian Association of Thoracic Oncology (AIOT) clinical practice guidelines. Lung Cancer. Mar 24, 2011 [Epub ahead of print].

[47]Keedy VL, Temin S, Somerfield MR, et al. American Society of Clinical Oncology provisional clinical opinion: epidermal growth factor receptor (EGFR) mutation testing for patients with advanced non-small-cell lung cancer considering first-line EGFR tyrosine kinase inhibitor therapy. J. Clin. Oncol. April 11, 2011 [Epub ahead of print].

[48]Wittes J. Times to event: why are they hard to visualize? J. Natl Cancer Inst. 2008;100:80–1.

placebo arm, closely track each other during most of the course of the clinical trial, but where the two curves separate distinctly from each other towards the end of the clinical trial. This situation can be found, for example, in the Kaplan–Meier plot of survival, disclosed above, for the clinical trial by Maemondo et al. (49) (Fig. 13.2). In a general comment applicable to clinical trials for any disease or with any treatment, Wittes observed that the, "large white space between the two curves does not mean a dramatic benefit (or harm) of treatment if one waits long enough but, rather, likely reflects variability arising from the small sample sizes available for analysis at the end of the study" (50). For this reason, investigators noticing a remarkable separation between two study arms that materializes towards the end of a clinical trial should take care to observe the significance (P value) of the separation between the two curves.

e. Methodology Tips—Independent Radiology Assessments in the Gradishar Study

In a study of breast cancer, Gradishar et al. (51), divided the subjects into four arms, as shown below. Paclitaxel and docetaxel are both classed as taxanes (52).

- Arm 1. Paclitaxel at 300 mg/m^2, every 3 weeks;
- Arm 2. Paclitaxel at 100 mg/m^2, weekly;
- Arm 3. Paclitaxel at 150 mg/m^2, weekly; or
- Arm 4. Docetaxel at 100 mg/m^2, every 3 weeks.

Objective response, that is, tumor size and number as measured by the RECIST criteria, was assessed by the investigator's radiologist and also by an independent radiologist. Data on tumor size and number were used for calculating data on the endpoint of objective response, as well as for calculating data for the endpoint of PFS.

The Gradishar study is distinguished from almost all other oncology clinical trials, in that the authors published separate Kaplan–Meier plots, one representing data collected by the investigator's radiologist, and the other representing data from the independent radiologist. A related issue is as follows. The same radiologist may make duplicate measurements of tumor size and number, where the measurements are spaced about 2 weeks apart. The approach of using a first examination and a confirmatory examination was used by Bedikian et al. (53) and by Tarhini et al. (54), for example. The principal investigator of the Tarhini study stated that only data from the second examination were reported, where these data served to confirm data from the first examination (55).

[49]Maemondo M, Inoue A, Kobayashi K, et al. Gefitinib or chemotherapy for non-small-cell lung cancer with mutated EGFR. New Engl. J. Med. 2010;362:2380–8.

[50]Wittes J. Times to event: why are they hard to visualize? J. Natl Cancer Inst. 2008;100:80–1.

[51]Gradishar WJ, Krasnojon D, Cheporov S, et al. Significantly longer progression-free survival with nab-paclitaxel compared with docetaxel as first-line therapy for metastatic breast cancer. J. Clin. Oncol. 2009;27:3611–19.

[52]Woodward EJ, Twelves C. Scheduling of taxanes: a review. Curr. Clin. Pharmacol. 2010;5:226–31.

[53]Bedikian AY, Millward M, Pehamberger H, et al. Bcl-2 antisense (oblimersen sodium) plus dacarbazine in patients with advanced melanoma: the Oblimersen Melanoma Study Group. J. Clin. Oncol. 2006;24:4738–45.

[54]Tarhini AA, Kirkwood JM, Gooding WE, Cai C, Agarwala SS. Durable complete responses with high-dose bolus interleukin-2 in patients with metastatic melanoma who have experienced progression after biochemotherapy. J. Clin. Oncol. 2007;25:3802–7.

[55]Agarwala SS. E-mail of September 8, 2010.

Another methodological point is as follows. This concerns the relationship between the endpoints of PFS and OS. According to Gradishar et al. (56), "[p]atient survival data were not mature at the time of data cutoff for this publication." This statement reveals an advantage of endpoints such as PFS, TTP, and DFS, over the endpoint of OS. The advantage is that PFS, TTP, and DFS can be calculated long before enough data are available for calculating OS. Progression of a tumor, or a corresponding parameter in clinical trials on fatal infections, can occur long before the event (death) used for calculating the endpoint of OS. Investigators might not have enough information to calculate OS because study subjects continue to live beyond the timeframe originally expected by the investigators, because of the need to terminate the trial early due to a dwindling supply of potential enrollees, or because of a need for immediate publication in a journal. For all of these reasons, the endpoints of PFS, TTP, and DFS, are advantageous over the endpoint of OS.

f. Agreement Between Objective Response and Median PFS—The Robert Study

In a clinical trial on melanoma, reported by Robert et al. (57), agreement was found between objective response and PFS. This study is an exemplary account where the endpoint of objective response, as measured by RECIST criteria, agrees with the clinical endpoint of median PFS.

The Robert clinical trial had acquired endpoint data for a sufficient time to calculate the endpoint of median PFS, and here, the median PFS for the pembrolizumab arm was 4.1–5.5 months, and for the ipilimumab arm, median PFS was substantially less, only 2.8 months.

Pembroluzumab's objective response was better than ipilimumab's objective response, and pembrolizumab's median PFS was better than ipilimuab's median PFS. The data are shown in the following bullet points:

- Pembrolizumab: objective response 33%; median PFS of 5.5–4.1 months.
- Ipilimumab: objective response only 11.9%; median PFS of only 2.8 months.

This contrasts from the issue, mentioned earlier in this chapter, of lack of agreement in objective response with clinical endpoints, such as PFS or OS.

The Robert trial is exemplary, in that objective response and median PFS agreed with each other, and also because the trial was conducted long enough to collect data for calculating median PFS. Failure to continue the trial long enough to calculate, for example, median PFS or median OS, is illustrated by the Postow clinical trial on melanoma (58).

In the Postow clinical trial data were analyzed and published before the time point when median PFS was reached (to calculate median PFS, half of the subjects need to satisfy the criteria for this endpoint). The researchers reported that, "the median progression free survival was not reached with the combination therapy."

[56]Gradishar WJ, Krasnojon D, Cheporov S, et al. Significantly longer progression-free survival with nab-paclitaxel compared with docetaxel as first-line therapy for metastatic breast cancer. J. Clin. Oncol. 2009;27:3611–19.

[57]Robert C, Schacter J, Long GV, et al. Pembrolizumab versus ipilimumab in advanced melanoma. New Engl. J. Med. 2015. http://dx.doi.org/10.1056/NEJMoa1503093 (12 pp.).

[58]Postow MA, Chesney J, Pavlick AC, et al. Nivolumab and ipilimumab versus ipilimumab in untreated melanoma. New Engl. J. Med. 2015. http://dx.doi.org/10.1065/NEJMoa1414428.

g. Antibodies Against PD-1, Against PD-L1, or Against CTLA-4 for Treating Melanoma

The Robert trial and the Postow trial, along with another trial, the Weber trial, should be contemplated a bit further, because of the dramatic efficacy of the study drugs in melanoma clinical trials. Although it was mentioned above that "the median progression free survival was not reached" in one of the study arms, this was not because the trial was discontinued due to severe drug toxicity. Instead, the results of the clinical trial were analyzed and published prior to reaching median PFS, because it was obvious, at the early point in the trial, that the drug was working.

Dramatic efficacy was found in the following melanoma trials:

* *Weber trial.* Chemotherapy arm versus antibody arm [dacarbazine chemotherapy versus novilumab (anti-PD-1)] (59).
* *Robert trial.* First antibody arm versus second antibody arm [pembrolizumab (anti-PD-1) vs ipilimumab (anti-CTLA-4)] (60).
* *Postow trial.* Antibody monotherapy arm versus combination arm with two antibodies (ipilimumab vs ipilimumab plus nivolumab) (61).

Pembrolizumab is an anti-PD-1 antibody. Nivolumab is also an anti-PD-1 antibody. Ipilimumab is an anti-CTLA-4 antibody. It is self-evident that nivolumab and ipilimumab

have different mechanisms of action, because they bind to different targets. Also, it might be expected that administering the combination of both antibodies to a melanoma patient will have an additive effect.

In the Weber trial—*chemotherapy* versus *antibody (anti-PD-1 antibody)*—objective response rate with chemotherapy was only 11%, while that with nivolumab was 32%.

In the Robert trial—*pembrolizumab* (anti-PD-1) versus *ipilimumab (anti-CTLA-4)*—that is, where each antibody bound to a different target, pembrolizumab had greater efficacy and produced an objective response rate of about 33% while, in contrast, ipilimumab was less effective, and produced an objective response rate of only 11.9%.

In the Postow trial—combination of *nivolumab plus ipilimumab* versus *ipilimumab only*—the combination had a greater efficacy, providing an objective response of 61%, and the ipilimumab monotherapy resulted in an objective response of only 11% (62).

Thus, it can be seen that in the three melanoma trials, chemotherapy was least effective, and the combination of nivolumab plus ipilimumab was the most effective.

h. Data on PFS can Present Earlier, and can be More Dramatic, Than Data on OS—The Slamon Study

In a clinical trial on breast cancer, Slamon et al. (63), treated women with surgery. After surgery, HER2 expression was measured on

[59]Weber JS, D'Angelo SP, Minor D, et al. Nivolumab versus chemotherapy in patients with advanced melanoma who progressed after anti-CTLA-4 treatment (CheckMate 037): a randomised, controlled, open-label, phase 3 trial. Lancet Oncol. 2015;16:375–84.

[60]Robert C, Schacter J, Long GV, et al. Pembrolizumab versus ipilimumab in advanced melanoma. New Engl. J. Med. 2015. http://dx.doi.org/10.1056/NEJMoa1503093 (12 pp.).

[61]Postow MA, Chesney J, Pavlick AC, et al. Nivolumab and ipilimumab versus ipilimumab in untreated melanoma. New Engl. J. Med. 2015. http://dx.doi.org/10.1065/NEJMoa1414428.

[62]Postow MA, Chesney J, Pavlick AC, et al. Nivolumab and ipilimumab versus ipilimumab in untreated melanoma. New Engl. J. Med. 2015. http://dx.doi.org/10.1065/NEJMoa1414428.

[63]Slamon DJ, Leyland-Jones B, Shak S, et al. Use of chemotherapy plus a monoclonal antibody against HER2 for metastatic breast cancer that overexpresses HER2. New Engl. J. Med. 2001;344:783–92.

tumor samples. Only women bearing tumors that overexpressed HER2 were included in the clinical trial. For a patient to be eligible for the clinical trial, overexpression needed to be at the level of at least plus 2 over the entire tumor membrane, or at the level of plus 3 in more than 10% of the tumor cells.

After surgery and screening for HER2 expression, patients received either:

- Arm A. Chemotherapy, or
- Arm B. Chemotherapy plus trastuzumab.

Chemotherapy took the form of various combinations of doxorubicin, epirubicin, cyclophosphamide, and paclitaxel. The endpoints that were used are indicated by the following bullet points:

- objective response,
- progression-free survival,
- overall survival.

Data used for calculating the objective response and PFS were acquired by measuring tumors at baseline, and at week 8, week 20, and then at 12-week intervals. Objective response encompassed the categories of complete response and partial response. Complete response was defined as the disappearance of all tumor on the basis of radiographic evidence, visual inspection, or both.

The results for objective response are show in Table 13.2. The results demonstrated that response was more favorable in arm B.

A Kaplan–Meier plot showing PFS is shown in Fig. 13.3 (64), while a Kaplan–Meier plot showing OS appears in Fig. 13.4. Both plots

TABLE 13.2 Objective Response in the Slamon Study

	Complete Response (%)	Partial Response (%)
Arm A. Chemotherapy only	3	28
Arm B. Chemotherapy plus trastuzumab	8	43

demonstrate superior efficacy for arm B. In other words, trastuzumab is an effective add-on, when combined with chemotherapy. Trastuzumab was effective, as determined by visual inspection of the Kaplan–Meier plots, and also as determined by values for median PFS and for median OS. Median PFS was 4.6 months (arm A) and 7.4 months (arm B), while median survival was 20.3 months (arm A) and 25.1 months (arm B). The authors concluded that trastuzumab, when added to conventional chemotherapy, can benefit patients with metastatic breast cancer that overexpresses HER2. As with many clinical trials, efficacy was demonstrated by PFS a couple of months before survival data were able to demonstrate efficacy.

The principal investigator of this study, Dr Dennis J. Slamon, is the subject of a movie called, *Living Proof* (65). The movie documented his efforts in developing and testing the antibody.

i. PFS and Subgroup Analysis—The Van Cutsem Study

The clinical trial of colorectal cancer by Van Cutsem et al. (66) contained two arms, as

[64]According to the statistician who analyzed the data from the Slamon study, the figure may have contained a typographical error. Although the figure in the published study reads, progression-free survival, this may have been a typographical error, and the figure probably should actually read, time to progression. Fleming T. E-mail of April 6, 2011. However, it should be noted that, when the question is directly addressed in clinical trials, Kaplan–Meier curves that follow progression-free survival are often essentially identical to curves that follow time to progression.

[65]Living Proof. Sony Pictures Television, 2008.

[66]Van Cutsem E, Köhne CH, Hitre E, et al. Cetuximab and chemotherapy as initial treatment for metastatic colorectal cancer. New Engl. J. Med. 2009;360:1408–17.

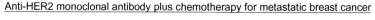

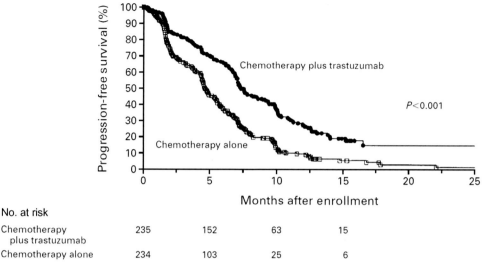

FIGURE 13.3 Kaplan–Meier plot of PFS from the Slamon study. The survival curves show PFS for the study drug arm and control arm.

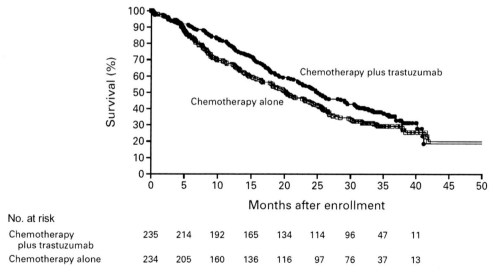

FIGURE 13.4 Kaplan–Meier plot of overall survival from the Slamon study. The survival curves show overall survival for the study drug arm and control arm.

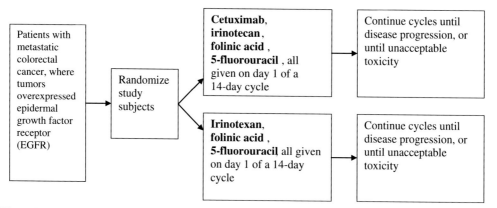

FIGURE 13.5 Study schema from the Van Cutsem study. The design was an "add-on" study, where cetuximab was the drug that was added on.

shown by the bullet points below. The study drug was cetuximab, an antibody.

- Arm A. Cetuximab, irinotecan, folinic acid, and 5-fluorouracil.
- Arm B. Irinotecan, folinic acid, and 5-fluorouracil.

Cetuximab, used for colorectal cancer, is an antibody targeting the epidermal growth factor receptor. This drug is approved as monotherapy in patients with disease progression after treatment with irinotecan or oxaliplatin and in patients intolerant to irinotecan (67). Cetuximab is also approved in combination with irinotecan for irinotecan-resistant patients.

The following narrative reiterates some of the concepts from Chapter 2, regarding the study schema. The study schema for the Van Cutsem study is shown below (Fig. 13.5). The schema identifies each drug, the doses, and the dosing schedules. The schema also identifies the randomization period, and the criteria for terminating the drug treatment schedule for any given patient.

FOLFIRI refers to therapy using FOLinic acid, Fluorouracil, and IRInotecan. Folinic acid, which is 5-formyl-tetrahydrofolic acid (leucovorin), is administered in conjunction with antifolate chemotherapy. Folinic acid rescues normal host cells from the toxic effects of antifolate drugs.

The endpoints included objective response, PFS, and OS. Objective response (reduction in tumor size and number) was determined by radiologic imaging using the WHO criteria (68).

Objective response was found in 38.7% of patients (no antibody; arm B), and this increased to 46.9% in the arm receiving the antibody (arm A). Median PFS was 8.0 months (no antibody), and this increased to 8.9 months in the arm receiving the antibody. Median OS was 18.6 months (no antibody) and this increased to 19.9 months in the arm receiving the antibody.

[67]Hess GP, Wang PF, Quach D, Barber B, Zhao Z. Systemic therapy for metastatic colorectal cancer: patterns of chemotherapy and biologic therapy use in US medical oncology practice. J. Oncol. Pract. 2010;6:301−7.

[68]World Health Organization. WHO handbook for reporting results of cancer treatment. Geneva: World Health Organization, Offset Publication 48; 1979.

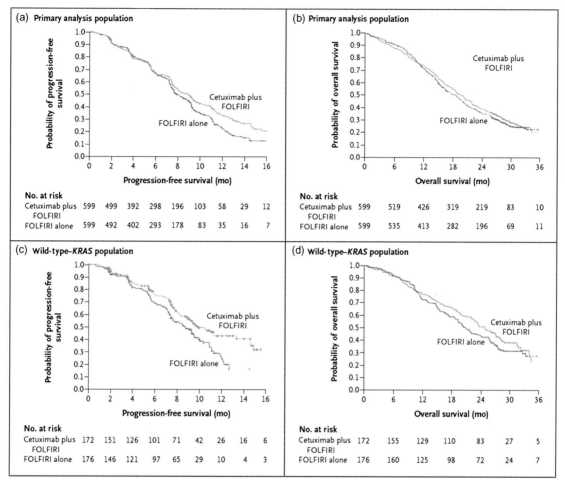

FIGURE 13.6 Kaplan–Meier plots from the Van Cutsem study. (a) PFS from the entire study population (1198 subjects); (b) Overall survival for entire study population (1198 subjects); (c) PFS for subgroup with non-mutated KRAS (348 subjects); and (d) OS in the subgroup with non-mutated KRAS (348 subjects).

The Kaplan–Meier plots shown below reveal PFS in the entire study population (Fig. 13.6a), PFS in the subgroup with non-mutated KRAS (Fig. 13.6b), OS in the entire population (Fig. 13.6c), and OS in the subgroup with nonmutated KRAS (Fig. 13.6d). Visual inspection of these plots reveals that the antibody was somewhat effective in improving PFS, particularly for the subgroup having nonmutated KRAS, and that the antibody was not particularly effective in improving OS.

Van Cutsem et al. (69) attempted to find correlations between mutation status of the KRAS gene and the efficacy endpoints. KRAS, also called Ki-RAS or Kirsten-RAS, was named

---

[69]Van Cutsem E, Köhne CH, Hitre E, et al. Cetuximab and chemotherapy as initial treatment for metastatic colorectal cancer. New Engl. J. Med. 2009;360:1408–17.

after Werner Kirsten (70,71). Oncogenic mutations in KRAS occur in about 40% of colorectal cancers. Further details of the utility of the KRAS biomarker are provided, in this textbook, in Chapter 19. Tumor samples were obtained at baseline and were used for analysis of the sequence of the KRAS gene. Two-thirds (64.4%) of the subjects had wild-type KRAS, while one-third (35.6%) had a mutated KRAS gene.

Efficacy, using the endpoint of PFS, can be expressed in terms of median PFS for arm A and median PFS for arm B. Efficacy using PFS can also be expressed as the hazard ratio, a parameter that compares arm A to arm B. The hazard ratio for the overall population was $HR = 0.85$ ($P = 0.048$), indicating that the antibody was somewhat effective. The P value of $P = 0.048$ shows that the difference was significant. The hazard ratio for the subgroup of subjects containing tumors having nonmutated KRAS was $HR = 0.68$ ($P = 0.02$), again indicating that the antibody was effective, and that it was more effective than for the population as a whole. The P value of $P = 0.02$ means that the difference was significant. The hazard ratio data show that the antibody is more effective for the subgroup than for the population as a whole. This result has been confirmed by other studies showing that cetuximab is more effective where tumors contain wild-type KRAS, and less effective where tumors contain mutated KRAS (72,73).

Published comments about the study reiterated the finding that the antibody did not result in significant improvement in OS (74). However, it should be noted that the same investigators subsequently used genetic analysis to identify subgroups of patients that are more responsive to the antibody (75,76).

The Van Cutsem (77) study contains an exemplary presentation that shows Kaplan–Meier curves for the entire study population, along with Kaplan–Meier curves for a subgroup within this population. This type of presentation is a frequent theme in reporting clinical trials in oncology, as well as for immune disorders, infections, metabolic diseases, and other disorders.

[70]Russo A, Bazan V, Agnese V, Rodolico V, Gebbia N. Prognostic and predictive factors in colorectal cancer: Kirsten Ras in CRC (RASCAL) and TP53CRC collaborative studies. Ann. Oncol. 2005;16(Suppl. 4):iv 44–9.

[71]Kirsten WH, Schauf V, McCoy J. Properties of a murine sarcoma virus. Bibl. Haematol. 1970;36:246–9.

[72]Van Cutsem E, Köhne CH, Láng I, et al. Cetuximab plus irinotecan, fluorouracil, and leucovorin as first-line treatment for metastatic colorectal cancer: updated analysis of overall survival according to tumor KRAS and BRAF mutation status. J. Clin. Oncol. April 18, 2011 [Epub ahead of print].

[73]De Roock W, Claes B, Bernasconi D, et al. Effects of KRAS, BRAF, NRAS, and PIK3CA mutations on the efficacy of cetuximab plus chemotherapy in chemotherapy-refractory metastatic colorectal cancer: a retrospective consortium analysis. Lancet Oncol. 2010;11:753–62.

[74]Garattini S, Valter Torri V, Floriani I. To the editor. New Engl. J. Med. 2009;361:95–7.

[75]Van Cutsem E, Köhne CH, Láng I, et al. Cetuximab plus irinotecan, fluorouracil, and leucovorin as first-line treatment for metastatic colorectal cancer: updated analysis of overall survival according to tumor KRAS and BRAF mutation status. J. Clin. Oncol. April 18, 2011 [Epub ahead of print].

[76]De Roock W, Claes B, Bernasconi D, et al. Effects of KRAS, BRAF, NRAS, and PIK3CA mutations on the efficacy of cetuximab plus chemotherapy in chemotherapy-refractory metastatic colorectal cancer: a retrospective consortium analysis. Lancet Oncol. 2010;11:753–62.

[77]Van Cutsem E, Köhne CH, Hitre E, et al. Cetuximab and chemotherapy as initial treatment for metastatic colorectal cancer. New Engl. J. Med. 2009;360:1408–17.

j. FDA's Decision-Making Process in Evaluating Clinical Trials Based on OS and PFS

This illustrates a problem that arises in clinical trials on some types of cancer, where the trial relies on OS as a primary endpoint. This concerns *vendetanib* for the indication of medullary thyroid cancer. The information is from NDA 22405, on July 2013 of FDA's website. Patients with medullary thyroid cancer have a long survival time. This type of cancer has been described as being "indolent," a term meaning slow to develop (78).

The primary endpoint for the clinical trial was PFS, while the secondary endpoint was OS. The FDA granted approval of the drug, based on data from PFS. The date that FDA completed its *Medical Review* was March 2011. However, at this time, the available data on OS failed to show any efficacy, as stated by the FDA reviewer:

> [o]verall survival was a key secondary endpoint, however at the time of the data cutoff, no significant difference between the vandetanib arm and the placebo arm was seen. It is important to note that only 15% of the events have occurred ... a final analysis of this endpoint will occur at 50% of events which currently is anticipated to be in 2012.

In addition to complaining that data on OS were not available, the FDA reviewer complained that, in general, for this type of cancer (medullary thyroid cancer), PFS is a poor surrogate for OS, because it is not practical to expect to obtain OS data. Regarding the impractical nature of OS data in clinical trials for this type of cancer, the reviewer wrote:

> Conducting a trial with overall survival as the primary endpoint in this patient population would be very difficult to do. Given the long natural

history of this disease, it is difficult to determine the clinical benefit of the primary endpoint of progression free survival. In prior meetings, the applicant and the FDA have come to agree that PFS can be used for full approval, provided that the risk/benefit profile favored treatment with vandetanib.

The take-home lesson is that the Sponsor should scrutinize each endpoint, and assess whether it may not be practical or possible to acquire sufficient data for each endpoint, by the time that it expects to write its NDA or BLA. The *Medical Review* also reveals that PFS can serve as a basis for FDA-approval of a drug, even where the Sponsor had not taken advantage of the pathway of accelerated approval. The accelerated approval pathway is described in Chapter 33.

V. CONCLUDING REMARKS

The Maemondo trial demonstrated that efficacy of the study drug, as well as the control drug, can first be detected at an earlier time, during the course of a clinical trial, with the endpoint of PFS, when compared to the endpoint of OS.

The Gradishar trial also demonstrates that efficacy of a drug can be evaluated at an earlier time using the endpoint of PFS, as compared to use of the endpoint of OS. This study also demonstrates the utility of reviewing the same radiological data twice, by two separate radiologists.

The Robert trial agreement between *objective response* and *median PFS*, as can be seen from the general trends, where for pembrolizumab: objective response 33%, median PFS of 5.5−4.1 months, and for ipilimumab: objective response only 11.9%, median PFS of only 2.8 months.

---

[78]de Groot JW, et al. Determinants of life expectancy in medullary thyroid cancer: age does not matter. Clin. Endocrinol. 2006;65:729−36.

The Slamon trial demonstrates that superior efficacy of a study drug may be seen at an earlier time with the endpoint of PFS, when compared to OS, and that the significance of this superior efficacy may be greater when using PFS, as compared to OS.

The Van Cutsem trial demonstrates that data on the endpoint of PFS may provide a more convincing story for efficacy than data from OS. This study demonstrates the utility of subgroup analysis, where the subgroup was defined by mutations in the KRAS gene of tumor cells.

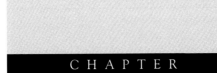

C H A P T E R

14

Oncology Endpoints: Time to Progression

I. INTRODUCTION

This chapter continues with oncology endpoints, and covers the fourth topic, as indicated by the check mark.

- Objective response
- Overall survival
- Progression-free survival (PFS)
- Time to progression (TTP)✓
- Disease-free survival (DFS)
- Time to distant metastasis.

Time to progression (TTP), also known as *time to disease progression*, is a common endpoint in oncology clinical trials. TTP and PFS are defined by FDA's Guidance for Industry (1), as follows:

TTP and PFS have served as primary endpoints for drug approval. TTP is defined as the time from randomization until objective tumor progression; TTP does not include deaths. PFS is defined as the time from randomization until objective tumor progression or death. The precise definition of tumor progression is important and should be carefully detailed in the protocol.

But the values for TTP and PFS are often almost identical, as revealed in the following examples from several clinical trials of breast cancer (2). In one of these trials, the values of TTP and PFS, for one particular arm, were both 5.5 months (3). In another trial, the values for TTP and PFS, for one of the arms, were both 6.7 months (4). In yet another trial, the values for TTP and PFS for one of the arms were identical,

[1]U.S. Department of Health and Human Services. Food and Drug Administration. Guidance for industry. Clinical trial endpoints for the approval of cancer drugs and biologics; April 2005.

[2]Burzykowski T, Buyse M, Piccart-Gebhart MJ, et al. Evaluation of tumor response, disease control, progression-free survival, and time to progression as potential surrogate end points in metastatic breast cancer. J. Clin. Oncol. 2008;26:1987–92.

[3]Bonneterre J, Dieras V, Tubiana-Hulin M, et al. Phase II multicenter randomized study of deocetaxel plus epirubicin versus fluorouracil plus epirubicin and cyclophosphamide in metastatic breast cancer. Br. J. Cancer 2004;91:1466–71.

[4]Bontenbal M, Creemers GJ, Braun HJ, et al. Phase II to III study comparing doxorubicin and docetaxel with fluorouracil, doxorubicin, and cyclophosphamide as first-line chemotherapy in patients with metastatic breast cancer: results of a Dutch community setting trial for the clinical trial group of the Comprehensive Cancer Centre. J. Clin. Oncol. 2005;23:7081–8.

TABLE 14.1   The Paccagnella Study

	Arm A (PC Arm) (Paclitaxel + Carboplatin)	Arm B (PCG Arm) (Paclitaxel + Carboplatin + Gemcitabine)	Significance of Difference Between the Two Study Arms
Objective response	20.2%	43.6%	$P < 0.0001$
TTP	5.1 months	7.6 months	$P = 0.012$
Overall survival	8.3 months	10.8 months	$P = 0.032$

7.4 months (5). Moreover, in another trial the values for PFS and TTP were both 18.4 weeks (6). Please note that TTP does not, but PFS does, use survival time as a trigger for the endpoint.

As a matter of first impression, it might be asked, "What is the use of having both types of endpoints?"

II. AGREEMENT OF RESULTS FROM OBJECTIVE RESPONSE, TTP, AND OVERALL SURVIVAL—THE PACCAGNELLA STUDY

The following clinical trial provides a straightforward account of various endpoints.

In a clinical trial of nonsmall-cell lung cancer (NSCLC), Paccagnella et al. (7) used three endpoints, objective response, TTP, and overall survival. The trial had two arms, as indicated in Table 14.1.

- *Arm A.* Paclitaxel and carboplatin (PC).
- *Arm B.* Paclitaxel, carboplatin, and gemcitabine (PCG).

The results are straightforward (Table 14.1). The triple-drug combination was superior, in terms of objective response (WHO criteria), median TTP, and median overall survival. It might be pointed out that the significance (*P* value) was greater for the endpoint of TTP than for overall survival, indicating an advantage in using TTP as an endpoint.

III. CAN THE VALUE FOR PFS BE LESS THAN THE VALUE FOR TTP?

PFS and TTP often have values that are nearly identical. Hence, it might be asked what might cause these values to differ, for example, what might cause the value of PFS to be less than TTP. The situation where PFS is less than the value for TTP is one where deaths due to drug toxicity (but not from the cancer) occur early on in the trial. This is, "when deaths due to the disease are rare, but those due to the drug are not" (8). Examples of this are likely to

---

[5]Paridaens R, Biganzoli L, Bruning P, et al. Paclitaxel versus doxorubicin as first-line singleagent chemotherapy for metastatic breast cancer: a European Organization for Research and Treatment of Cancer randomized study with cross-over. J. Clin. Oncol. 2000;18:724-33.

[6]Brandes AA, Basso U, Reni M, et al. First-line chemotherapy with cisplatin plus fractionated temozolomide in recurrent glioblastoma multiforme: a phase II study of the Gruppo Italiano Cooperativo di Neuro-Oncologia. J. Clin. Oncol. 2004;22:1598–604.

[7]Paccagnella A, Oniga F, Bearz A, et al. Adding gemcitabine to paclitaxel/carboplatin combination increases survival in advanced non-small-cell lung cancer: results of a phase II-III study. J. Clin. Oncol. 2006;24:681–7.

[8]Burzykowski T. E-mail of September 12, 2010.

be found in clinical trials on the elderly, especially where radiation therapy is followed by chemotherapy (9).

It might also be asked when will the value for PFS likely be equal to the value for TTP. PFS will likely be equal to TTP when, at early times in the clinical trial, the tumors in most patients grow to the point where they trigger the Response Evaluation Criteria in Solid Tumors (RECIST) criteria for tumor progression, but where the rate of patient deaths, due to any cause, is low.

IV. DATA ON THE ENDPOINT OF TTP CAN BE USED TO GAIN FDA-APPROVAL

A clinical trial on olaparib (Lynparza®) for ovarian cancer illustrates the fact that TTP data can help persuade the FDA to grant approval to a drug. TTP is a measure of objective response, not of clinical response. The fact of this persuasion is dramatically demonstrated by the writing on the package insert, "[t]he indication is approved ... based on objective response rate."

The package insert (10), the corresponding *Medical Review* by the FDA (11), and the report in *New England Journal of Medicine* (12), are cited.

The objective response rate took the form of "time to progression according to the RECIST guidelines or CA-125 level, whichever showed earlier progression" (13). To compare the numbers for the study drug arm and the placebo arm, it was the case that TTP was "significantly longer in the olaparib group than in the placebo group ... 8.3 months vs. 3.7 months" (14).

A fine point is noted regarding the information used to trigger the TTP endpoint. This endpoint was keyed to two forms of objective response, tumor size and number according to RECIST and the biomarker CA-125. The CA-125 levels were defined according to the Gynecological Cancer InterGroup criteria (15).

V. TTP MAY BE THE PREFERRED ENDPOINT WHERE, ONCE THE TRIAL IS CONCLUDED, PATIENTS RECEIVE ADDITIONAL CHEMOTHERAPY—THE PARK STUDY

In a clinical trial of NSCLC, Park et al. (16) used the endpoints of objective response, TTP, overall survival, as well as endpoints set forth in health-related quality-of-life questionnaires.

[9]Buyse M. E-mail of September 12, 2010.

[10]Package insert for LYNPARZA™ (olaparib) capsules, for oral use; December 2014 (4 pp.).

[11]*Medical Review* for olaparib (Lynparza®) for NDA 206162, from December 2014 on FDA's website.

[12]Ledermann J, Harter P, Gourley C, et al. Olaparib maintenance therapy in platinum-sensitive relapsed ovarian cancer. New Engl. J. Med. 2012;366:1382−92.

[13]Ledermann J, Harter P, Gourley C, et al. Olaparib maintenance therapy in platinum-sensitive relapsed ovarian cancer. New Engl. J. Med. 2012;366:1382-92.

[14]Ledermann J, Harter P, Gourley C, et al. Olaparib maintenance therapy in platinum-sensitive relapsed ovarian cancer. New Engl. J. Med. 2012;366:1382−92.

[15]Ledermann J, Harter P, Gourley C, et al. Olaparib maintenance therapy in platinum-sensitive relapsed ovarian cancer. New Engl. J. Med. 2012;366:1382−92.

[16]Park JO, Kim SW, Ahn JS, et al. Phase III trial of two versus four additional cycles in patients who are nonprogressive after two cycles of platinum-based chemotherapy in non small-cell lung cancer. J. Clin. Oncol. 2007;25:5233−9.

The objective response was determined by the WHO criteria. Before randomizing the subjects, all subjects were treated with two cycles of chemotherapy in a run-in period. Only subjects not showing disease progression were randomized to the two arms. Regarding the run-in period, the investigators stated that one reason for including the run-in was to enrich the study with a more homogeneous patient population. This particular rationale is further described in Chapter 3.

The Park study had two arms, as follows:

• *Arm A.* Six cycles of chemotherapy.
• *Arm B.* Four cycles of chemotherapy.

Patients were monitored for a total of 18 months. Objective response was measured at 3-month intervals by computed tomography. According to TTP, arm A fared better than arm B, as shown in Table 14.2. According to overall survival, there was no significant difference between arms A and B.

The investigators were careful to describe reasons for leaving the trial, writing that "[t]reatment was continued until the maximum of four or six cycles was completed, depending on random assignment, unless disease progression or unacceptable toxicity occurred or unless the patient refused further chemotherapy." Where tumor size or number increased to the point where the endpoint of progression was triggered, treatment with study drugs was discontinued, and the subjects had the option

of second-line therapy. As stated, "[s]econd-line chemotherapy was considered at the discretion of the treating oncologist after documentation of progression."

To clarify this point, it is often the case in trial design, that where the subject experiences progression (the tumor size or number reaches or passes a limit set for by the RECIST or WHO criteria), treatment with study drug or control is halted, and the subject has the option of receiving second-line treatment.

At this point, it is intuitively obvious that this second-line chemotherapy cannot influence the date of progression (for any given patient), but it can influence the survival time. Regarding the finding that the six-cycle group fared better than the four-cycle group, in terms of the TTP endpoint, but that there was little difference in the endpoints of overall survival, the authors believed that this discrepancy was likely due to confounding of the survival times by the second-line therapy. In the author's words, "[t]he main reason why the TTP benefit did not translate into the survival benefit probably involved the dilution effect of the second-line chemotherapy." The take-home lesson is that clinical trials should include the endpoint of TTP, where it is expected that many patients will be receiving second-line treatments.

VI. THE ENDPOINT OF TTP MAY BE PREFERRED OVER SURVIVAL ENDPOINTS, WHERE DEATHS RESULT FROM CAUSES OTHER THAN CANCER—THE LLOVET STUDY

TTP may be the preferred endpoint, over an endpoint that takes into account survival data, such as the endpoints of PFS, DFS, or overall survival. This type of preference for TTP is the case where the major cause of death, during the course of the clinical trial, is unrelated to the cancer.

TABLE 14.2 The Park Study

	TTP (Months; Median Value)	Overall Survival (Months; Median Value)
Arm A (six cycles)	6.2 months	14.9 months
Arm B (four cycles)	4.6 months	15.9 months
Significance of difference between arms A and B	$P = 0.001$	$P = 0.461$

The following provides the example of liver cancer, that is, hepatocellular carcinoma (HCC). According to Llovet et al. (17), "although disease- and progression-free survival are appropriate endpoints in other solid tumors, they are particularly unreliable endpoints in HCC research because death resulting from the natural history of cirrhosis might confound detection of potential benefits from effective drugs. That is, a type II error might result from using progression-free survival as an endpoint in a suboptimal population in early phases of drug development."

Consistently, Dancey et al. (18) stated that, "deaths prior to disease progression are not correlated with progression. In situations where many deaths are unrelated to cancer or treatment, TTP can be an acceptable and preferred end-point."

The term, type II error, refers to the conclusion that the drug does not work, when in fact, it actually does work (19). The term type I error, refers to the conclusion that the drug works when, in fact, it really fails to work.

A related problem is that, during the course of a clinical trial, the cause of death is often not reliably collected or documented. Typically, deaths occurring after disease progression are considered malignant, while all deaths occurring prior to disease progression are considered nonmalignant (20). The distinction between drug-induced deaths and disease-induced deaths is not often made.

In the context of liver cancer, the endpoint of overall survival is expected to be reliable, where examination of study subjects show that cirrhosis is not a problem. Thus, "[i]n the exceptional circumstances in which these [survival] endpoints are applied, a restrictive selection of patients with well-preserved liver function is recommended to minimize the impact of death unrelated with tumor progression" (21).

In a study of HCC, Llovet et al. (22) treated subjects with either sorafenib or placebo. The study was designed to capture information on drug efficacy while confounding the effects of deaths unrelated to cancer. Since HCC occurs mainly in patients with cirrhosis, the inclusion/exclusion criteria required that subjects have well-preserved liver function. However, it was still the case that endpoints tied to survival, such as PFS, might be suboptimal because of the confusing effect of the cirrhosis. Thus, the Llovet study provides a general lesson regarding the selection of inclusion/exclusion criteria.

[17]Llovet JM, Di Bisceglie AM, Bruix J, et al. Design and endpoints of clinical trials in hepatocellular carcinoma. J. Natl Cancer Inst. 2008;100:698—711.

[18]Dancey JE, Dodd LE, Ford R, et al. Recommendations for the assessment of progression in randomised cancer treatment trials. Eur. J. Cancer 2009;45:281—9.

[19]Type I error is rejecting the null hypothesis when it is true and type II error is accepting the null hypothesis when it is false. See, for example, Biau DJ, Jolles BM, Porcher R. P value and the theory of hypothesis testing: an explanation for new researchers. Clin. Orthop. Relat. Res. 2010;468:885—92.

[20]Buyse M. E-mail of September 20, 2010.

[21]Llovet JM, Di Bisceglie AM, Bruix J, et al. Design and endpoints of clinical trials in hepatocellular carcinoma. J. Natl Cancer Inst. 2008;100:698—711.

[22]Llovet JM, Ricci S, Mazzaferro V, et al. Sorafenib in advanced hepatocellular carcinoma. New Engl. J. Med. 2008;359:378—90.

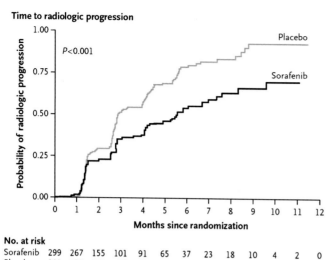

Time to radiologic progression

No. at risk

Sorafenib	299	267	155	101	91	65	37	23	18	10	4	2	0
Placebo	303	275	142	78	62	41	21	11	10	3	1	1	0

FIGURE 14.1 Kaplan–Meier plot of TTP. Progression was defined by the RECIST criteria. A comparison of arm A (sorafenib) and arm B (placebo) reveals that the study drug was effective against the cancer. Median TTP was 5.5 months (arm A) and 2.8 months (arm B).

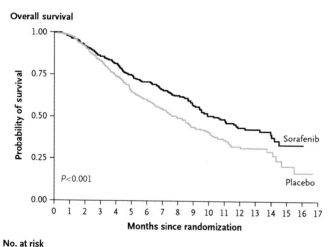

Overall survival

No. at risk

Sorafenib	299	290	270	249	234	213	200	172	140	111	89	68	48	37	24	7	1	0
Placebo	303	295	272	243	217	189	174	143	108	83	69	47	31	23	14	6	3	0

FIGURE 14.2 Kaplan–Meier plot of overall survival. A comparison of arm A (sorafenib) and arm B (placebo) reveals that the study drug was effective against the cancer. Median overall survival was 10.7 months (arm A) and 7.9 months (arm B).

In the sorafenib group, seven patients (2%) had a partial response and 211 (71%) had stable disease (according to RECIST), whereas in the placebo group, two patients (1%) had a partial response and 204 (67%) had stable disease. There were no complete responses in either group.

Median TTP was 5.5 months in the sorafenib arm and 2.8 months in the placebo arm (HR = 0.58; $P < 0.001$), while median overall survival was 10.7 months in the sorafenib arm and 7.9 months in the placebo arm (HR = 0.69; $P < 0.001$). This demonstrable efficacy of sorafenib was considered to be a therapeutic breakthrough, in view of the inevitably fatal outcome of this type of cancer, and lack of any effective treatment (Figs. 14.1, 14.2).

VII. THE ENDPOINT OF OVERALL SURVIVAL MAY BE PREFERRED OVER OBJECTIVE RESPONSE OR OVER TTP, WHERE THE DRUG IS CLASSED AS A CYTOSTATIC DRUG—THE LLOVET STUDY

Llovet et al. (23) provide a lesson regarding the utility, or actually lack thereof, of objective response, where the drug is cytostatic, rather than cytotoxic. The Llovet study compares the endpoint of objective response with the endpoint of overall survival. The study drug, sorafenib, inhibits angiogenesis and delays the progression of liver tumors in HCC. In the Llovet study, response consisted of complete response, partial response, or stable disease, according to the RECIST criteria.

Where a drug is classed as a cytostatic drug, endpoints that rely entirely on tumor size or number, such as objective response and TTP, might not give due justice to the survival benefit of the drug. With a cytostatic drug, a more reasonable assessment of the drug's efficacy might be acquired by using endpoints that rely partially or entirely on survival time. In the words of Llovet et al. (24), "current targeted agents may act as cytostatic agents … and possibly improve survival with no measurable change in tumor size." Thus overall survival might be a better endpoint than endpoints that are derived from objective response, such as the endpoint of objective response itself, or the endpoint of TTP, when the drug is classified as one that is cytostatic (not cytotoxic).

The Llovet study on sorafenib concluded that the incidence of objective response was relatively low, and the effects on overall survival were high. Consistent with this interpretation, a review article observed that sorafenib does not commonly improve objective response, though it does stabilize cancer and enhances survival (25). Regarding cytostatic drugs, Fleming et al. (26) reiterated the point that endpoints of objective response and TTP are relatively insensitive to the effects of cytostatic drugs, and that the efficacy of this class of drugs can more effectively be captured by the endpoint of PFS or overall survival. Another way around the problem of objective response, is to change the technology used for measuring objective response. Instead of just using techniques that measure the dimensions of tumors, techniques of functional imaging, such as positron emission tomography, can be used to assess the metabolism of existing tumors (27,28,29).

[23]Llovet JM, Ricci S, Mazzaferro V, et al. Sorafenib in advanced hepatocellular carcinoma. New Engl. J. Med. 2008;359:378−90.

[24]Llovet JM, Di Bisceglie AM, Bruix J, et al. Design and endpoints of clinical trials in hepatocellular carcinoma. J. Natl Cancer Inst. 2008;100:698−711.

[25]Almhanna K, Philip PA. Safety and efficacy of sorafenib in the treatment of hepatocellular carcinoma. Onco. Targets Ther. 2009;2:261−7.

[26]Fleming TR, Rothmann MD, Lu HL. Issues in using progression-free survival when evaluating oncology products. J. Clin. Oncol. 2009;27:2874−80.

[27]Avril N, Propper D. Functional PET imaging in cancer drug development. Future Oncol. 2007;3:215−28.

[28]Kyle F, Spicer J. Targeted therapies in non-small cell lung cancer. Cancer Imaging 2008;8:199−205.

[29]Weber WA. Positron emission tomography as an imaging biomarker. J. Clin. Oncol. 2006;24:3282−92.

TABLE 14.3 The McDermott Study

	Arm A. Placebo	Arm B. Sorafenib	Hazard Ratio	P Value
TTP	11.7 weeks	21.1 weeks	0.619	0.03
PFS	11.7 weeks	21.1 weeks	0.665	0.068
Overall survival	45.6	51.3	1.022	0.927

VIII. TTP MAY SHOW EFFICACY, WHERE THE ENDPOINT OF OVERALL SURVIVAL FAILS TO SHOW EFFICACY, WHERE THE NUMBER OF SUBJECTS IS SMALL—THE MCDERMOTT STUDY

The melanoma study by McDermott et al. (30) used the endpoints of objective response (RECIST criteria), TTP, PFS, and overall survival.

There were two study arms. This study used an *add-on design*. In other words, subjects in one arm received dacarbazine plus placebo, while subjects in the other arm received dacarbazine plus sorafenib. At the time of the clinical trial, dacarbazine was the most commonly used drug for melanoma. In part for ethical reasons, both study arms received dacarbazine. Sorafenib was the add-on drug.

- *Arm A*. Dacarbazine plus placebo.
- *Arm B*. Dacarbazine plus sorafenib.

The results are shown in Table 14.3. The study drug worked better than the placebo, as measured by the endpoints of TTP and PFS.

However, there were no differences in terms of the endpoints of overall survival. The data provide an instructive account of the use of hazard ratio. The authors stated that, in terms of overall survival, there was "no difference." The "no difference" result has a hazard ratio of 1.022, which is consistent with the teachings in Chapter 9. Spruance et al. (31) remind us that the hazard ratio can be greater than 1.0, or less than 1.0, depending on whether it is asked if treatment A works better than treatment B, or if treatment B works better than treatment A.

The authors pointed out that the study drug was better than placebo, according to the endpoints of TTP and PFS, but explained the lack of effect in overall survival, by referring to the small number of subjects. In the words of the authors, "[r]andomized phase II clinical trials are often limited by their small sample sizes to detect true treatment differences between the study arms. In this study, we observed improvements in PFS and TTP ... however, these findings did not translate into an improvement in OS" (32).

[30]McDermott DF, Sosman JA, Gonzalez R, et al. Double-blind randomized phase II study of the combination of sorafenib and dacarbazine in patients with advanced melanoma: a report from the 11715 Study Group. J. Clin. Oncol. 2008;26:2178–85.

[31]Spruance SL, Reid JE, Grace M, Samore M. Hazard ratio in clinical trials. Antimicrob. Agents Chemother. 2004;48:2787–92.

[32]McDermott DF, Sosman JA, Gonzalez R, et al. Double-blind randomized phase II study of the combination of sorafenib and dacarbazine in patients with advanced melanoma: a report from the 11715 Study Group. J. Clin. Oncol. 2008;26:2178–85.

TABLE 14.4   The Cappuzzo Study

	Patients with EGFR-Positive Tumors	Patients with EGFR-Negative Tumors	Significance of Difference of Endpoint, Comparing EGFR + and EGFR− Patients
Objective response	68.0%	9.1%	$P < 0.001$
TTP	7.6 months	2.7 months	$P = 0.02$
Overall survival	Median survival not reached	7.4 months	—

IX. TTP MAY SHOW EFFICACY, WHERE THE ENDPOINT OF OVERALL SURVIVAL FAILED TO SHOW EFFICACY, WHERE THE DURATION OF THE TRIAL WAS TOO SHORT—THE CAPPUZZO STUDY

The following study on non-small cell lung cancer (NSCLC) used the endpoints of objective response, TTP, and overall survival. Cappuzzo et al. (33) administered the same drug (gefitinib) to all study subjects. Gefitinib inhibits enzymatic activity of a particular kinase, namely, epidermal growth factor receptor (EGFR) tyrosine kinase. Cytogenetic assays were conducted on all study subjects prior to administering drug, to determine the number of EGFR genes in tumor cells. Tumor cells were acquired via biopsies, and the number of copies of the EGFR gene in a sampling of tumor cells was determined by way of the fluorescent in situ hybridization (FISH) technique.

Twenty-five of the patients were FISH-positive for EGFR. Eleven patients were FISH-negative for EGFR. "FISH-positive" was defined as tumor cells carrying four or more copies of EGFR gene, in 40% of the tumor cells.

"FISH-negative" was defined as tumor cells carrying four or more copies of EGFR gene, in less than 40% of the tumor cells.

Table 14.4 demonstrates the greater efficacy of gefitinib in patients bearing EGFR-positive tumor cells (as compared to patients with EGFR-negative tumor cells). This greater efficacy was demonstrated with the endpoints of objective response and TTP.

The Cappuzzo study provides the take-home lesson that, to forestall data acquisition problems due to short follow-up times, it is wise to include endpoints that can be fully captured early in the clinical trial. Suitable endpoints that can be captured early in the trial include objective response (RECIST criteria) and TTP.

A schematic representation of the Kaplan–Meier plot demonstrates the striking differences in TTP that were associated with the change in EGFR gene copy number (Fig. 14.3). The authors concluded that EGFR FISH analysis is an accurate predictor for efficacy with gefitinib therapy against lung cancer. To conclude, the Cappuzzo study demonstrates that EGFR is a useful biomarker. Other biomarkers, such as HER2 and KRAS, are described in Chapter 19.

---

[33]Cappuzzo F, Ligorio C, Jänne PA, et al. Prospective study of gefitinib in epidermal growth factor receptor fluorescence in situ hybridization-positive/phospho-Akt-positive or never smoker patients with advanced non-small-cell lung cancer: the ONCOBELL trial. J. Clin. Oncol. 2007;25:2248–55.

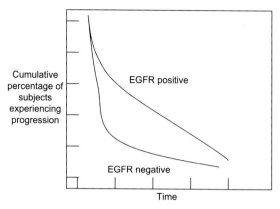

FIGURE 14.3 Schematic representation of a Kaplan–Meier plot. This was a one-arm study. All patients received gefitinib. The two *curves* show TTP for the subgroup of 25 patients with high EGFR (FISH-positive), and TTP for the subgroup of 11 patients with low EGFR (FISH-negative).

survival, but not be too short to calculate median TTP. The following concerns the median and the mean, which are statistical parameters used for calculating an average. Calculating the mean requires acquisition of all data points. Thus, in the context of a clinical trial, *mean* survival time calculations could require waiting decades until all subjects die. In contrast, *median* survival time calculations only require waiting until half of the subjects have reached the endpoint in question. The median is the middle observation, that is, the point at which half the observations are smaller and half are larger (35). In general, median TTP is reached at an earlier time in oncology clinical trials than median survival, because tumor progression is usually a prerequisite for death.

X. METHODOLOGY TIP— ADVANTAGE OF USING AN ENDPOINT THAT INCORPORATES A "MEDIAN" TIME

The data of Cappuzzo et al. (34), as disclosed above, were incomplete for the endpoint of overall survival, as indicated in Table 14.4. As explained by the authors, "the median follow-up time was too short ... for significant tests of differences in survival outcomes."

But one might ask how can a clinical trial be too short to calculate results of median overall

XI. SUMMARY

To summarize the material presented so far, the Cappuzzo (36) study reveals that TTP may have an advantage over the endpoint of overall survival, where the trial has a relatively short duration. The McDermott (37) study indicates that TTP may have an advantage over overall survival, in the situation where the number of subjects is small. The comments of Llovet (38) reveal that TTP may

[34]Cappuzzo F, Ligorio C, Jänne PA, et al. Prospective study of gefitinib in epidermal growth factor receptor fluorescence in situ hybridization-positive/phospho-Akt-positive or never smoker patients with advanced non-small-cell lung cancer: the ONCOBELL trial. J. Clin. Oncol. 2007;25:2248–55.

[35]Dawson B, Trapp RG. Basic and clinical biostatistics. 4th ed. New York: Lange Medical Books; 2004. p. 28.

[36]Cappuzzo F, Ligorio C, Jänne PA, et al. Prospective study of gefitinib in epidermal growth factor receptor fluorescence in situ hybridization-positive/phospho-Akt-positive or never smoker patients with advanced non-small-cell lung cancer: the ONCOBELL trial. J. Clin. Oncol. 2007;25:2248–55.

[37]McDermott DF, Sosman JA, Gonzalez R, et al. Double-blind randomized phase II study of the combination of sorafenib and dacarbazine in patients with advanced melanoma: a report from the 11715 Study Group. J. Clin. Oncol. 2008;26:2178–85.

[38]Llovet JM, Di Bisceglie AM, Bruix J, et al. Design and endpoints of clinical trials in hepatocellular carcinoma. J. Natl Cancer Inst. 2008;100:698–711.

have an advantage over the endpoint of overall survival, in the situation where deaths result from health factors other than the cancer. The Park (39) study demonstrates the fact-pattern where TTP may have an advantage over the endpoint of overall survival, in the situation where subjects receive second-line treatment.

XII. THYMIDINE PHOSPHORYLASE AS A BIOMARKER FOR SURVIVAL—THE MEROPOL STUDY

In a study of colorectal cancer, Meropol et al. (40) administered the same chemotherapy to all patients. The treatment was irinotecan plus cepecitabine. Cepecitabine is distinguished in that it is converted in the cell to 5-fluorouracil. This conversion is catalyzed by *thymidine phosphorylase*. This enzyme is preferentially expressed by colorectal cancer cells, thus lending specificity of cepecitabine's toxic effects to the cancer cells, rather than to normal tissues. The efficacy of capecitabine is similar to that of 5-fluorouracil. The toxicity of capecitabine is less than the toxicity of bolus 5-fluorouracil, but similar to that with infusional 5-fluorouracil (41).

The goal of the study was to assess the possible correlation of *thymidine phosphorylase* expression with outcome. Thus, this was a study of a predictive biomarker. The difference between a "predictive biomarker" and a "prognostic biomarker" is detailed in Chapter 19.

TABLE 14.5   The Meropol Study

	Biopsy Positive (+) for Thymidine Phosphorylase	Biopsy Negative (−) for Thymidine Phosphorylase
TTP		
Primary tumor	8.7 months	6.0 months
Metastatic tumor	8.7 months	5.4 months
OVERALL SURVIVAL		
Primary tumor	28.2 months	14.9 months
Metastatic tumor	26.2 months	9.8 months

The data demonstrated that increased expression of *thymidine phosphorylase* is an excellent predictor of increased TTP (Table 14.5). Also, the data demonstrated that increased expression was an excellent predictor of increased overall survival.

The data on overall survival were especially dramatic.

All 52 patients provided biopsies of primary tumors. But at the time of diagnosis, only 30 of these patients had metastatic tumors. Most of the metastatic colorectal cancer tumors were located in the liver, lung, and lymph nodes. Hence, data from only 30 patients are available for correlating the biomarker expressing on metastatic tumors with the endpoints.

Regarding the predictive value of *thymidine phosphorylase* found in the Meropol study, it has been suggested that the medical community

[39]Park JO, Kim SW, Ahn JS, et al. Phase III trial of two versus four additional cycles in patients who are nonprogressive after two cycles of platinum-based chemotherapy in non small-cell lung cancer. J. Clin. Oncol. 2007;25:5233−9.

[40]Meropol NJ, Gold PJ, Diasio RB, et al. Thymidine phosphorylase expression is associated with response to capecitabine plus irinotecan in patients with metastatic colorectal cancer. J. Clin. Oncol. 2006;24:4069−77.

[41]O'Neil BH, McLeod HL. Thymidine phosphorylase and capecitabine: a predictive marker for therapy selection? J Clin. Oncol. 2006;24:4051−3.

should select capecitabine versus 5-fluorouracil rationally based on analysis of tumor *thymidine phosphorylase* levels using a simple test for enzyme expression, for example, by measuring RNA levels by a PCR-based method, or protein levels, by an antibody-based method (42).

XIII. DRUG COMBINATIONS THAT INCLUDE CAPECITABINE

The Meropol et al. (43) study administered a combination of irinotecan and cepecitabine in a clinical study of colorectal cancer. In a different clinical trial on colorectal cancer, using a different drug combination (capecitabine plus oxiplatin), Petrioli et al. (44) also found that higher expression of *thymidine phosphorylase* is associated with a more favorable clinical response. The common use of drug combinations in oncology, and the frequent decision to change one of the drugs used in a two-drug combination therapy, raises the issue of synergy. In this context, synergy refers to an effect that is more than additive, as it applies to efficacy, and an effect that is more than additive,

as it applies to toxicity. Aprile et al. (45) report that taxane drugs stimulate the expression of *thymidine phosphorylase*, and that this effect accounts for the increased antitumor activity of the combination of capecitabine and taxane. Kikuno et al. (46) report the induction of this enzyme, with use of the taxane, paclitaxel. Paclitaxel is distinguished in that it is a natural product isolated from the Western yew tree.

XIV. METHODOLOGY TIP—DO CHANGES IN mRNA EXPRESSION RESULT IN CORRESPONDING CHANGES IN EXPRESSION OF POLYPEPTIDE?

Meropol et al. (47) measured the expression of thymidine phosphorylase with immunological assays sensitive to the polypeptide, and with PCR-based assays sensitive to the expressed mRNA. As a general proposition, it is hoped that changes in mRNA expression correlate with changes in the polypeptide. But it must not be assumed that an increase in mRNA results in a corresponding increase in protein. Pennica et al.

[42]O'Neil BH, McLeod HL. Thymidine phosphorylase and capecitabine: a predictive marker for therapy selection? J Clin. Oncol. 2006;24:4051–3.

[43]Meropol NJ, Gold PJ, Diasio RB, et al. Thymidine phosphorylase expression is associated with response to capecitabine plus irinotecan in patients with metastatic colorectal cancer. J. Clin. Oncol. 2006;24:4069–77.

[44]Petrioli R, Bargagli G, Lazzi S, et al. Thymidine phosphorylase expression in metastatic sites is predictive for response in patients with colorectal cancer treated with continuous oral capecitabine and biweekly oxaliplatin. Anticancer Drugs 2010;21:313–9.

[45]Aprile G, Mazzer M, Moroso S, Puglisi F. Pharmacology and therapeutic efficacy of capecitabine: focus on breast and colorectal cancer. Anticancer Drugs 2009;20:217–29.

[46]Kikuno N, Moriyama-Gonda N, Yoshino T, et al. Blockade of paclitaxel-induced thymidine phosphorylase expression can accelerate apoptosis in human prostate cancer cells. Cancer Res. 2004;64:7526–32.

[47]Meropol NJ, Gold PJ, Diasio RB, et al. Thymidine phosphorylase expression is associated with response to capecitabine plus irinotecan in patients with metastatic colorectal cancer. J. Clin. Oncol. 2006;24:4069–77.

(48), Haynes et al. (49), Hu et al. (50), Oh et al. (51), Schantz and Pegg (52), and Anderson and Seilhamer (53), all address the issue of whether or not increased expression of polypeptide correlates with increased mRNA expression. Fu et al. (54), for example, demonstrate the scenario where there is no correlation at all. These publications can be used as a basis for arguing that increased mRNA will likely lead to an increase in protein or, conversely, for arguing that increased mRNA does not necessarily lead to an increase in protein (55).

XV. CONCLUDING REMARKS

The endpoint of TTP does not take into account the survival time. TTP is not a measure of survival for any given subject, or for the study population as a whole. As an endpoint, TTP has advantages over endpoints that take survival time into account. An advantage is that data on TTP can be captured at a time earlier than data on overall survival, thus enabling the investigator to arrive at conclusions regarding efficacy before the trial is formally concluded. This advantage is especially important where a significant number of subjects drop out of the trial before they trigger the endpoint of survival (death). A related advantage occurs in the situation where study subjects leaving the trial receive second-line therapy Similarly, use of TTP as an endpoint, rather than survival, is advantageous where death arises from noncancer-related causes, such as liver cirrhosis. Also note that it is better for a clinical trial to include more endpoints than fewer endpoints, as it cannot be known ahead of time which endpoint will give the most statistically significant results.

[48]Pennica D, Swanson TA, Welsh JW, et al. WISP genes are members of the connective tissue growth factor family that are up-regulated in wnt-1-transformed cells and aberrantly expressed in human colon tumors. Proc. Natl Acad. Sci. USA 1998;95:14717−22.

[49]Haynes PA, Gygi SP, Figeys D, Aebersold R. Proteome analysis: biological assay or data archive? Electrophoresis 1998;19:1862−71.

[50]Hu Y, Hines LM, Weng H, Zuo D, Rivera M, Richardson A, LaBaer J. Analysis of genomic and proteomic data using advanced literature mining. J. Proteome Res. 2003;2:405−12.

[51]Oh JM, Brichory F, Puravs E, et al. A database of protein expression in lung cancer. Proteomics 2001;1:1303−19.

[52]Shantz LM, Pegg AE. Translational regulation of ornithine decarboxylase and other enzymes of the polyamine pathway. Int. J. Biochem. Cell Biol. 1999;31:107−22.

[53]Anderson L, Seilhamer J. A comparison of selected mRNA and protein abundances in human liver. Electrophoresis 1997;18:533−7.

[54]Fu L, Minden MD, Benchimol S. Translational regulation of human p53 gene expression. EMBO J. 1996;15:4392−401.

[55]See, for example, file histories of U.S. Patent Nos. 7,008,799; 7,144,990; and 7,230,076. These file histories contain the arguments by researchers, and are available from the PUBLIC PAIR device found at www.uspto.gov. The term "file history" refers to the collection of rejections against the claims imposed by the patent examiner and the rebuttals submitted by the inventor or by the inventor's attorney.

15

Oncology Endpoint: Disease-Free Survival

I. INTRODUCTION

This chapter further develops the topic of oncology endpoints, and covers the fifth topic, as indicated by the check mark.

- Objective response
- Overall survival
- Progression-free survival (PFS)
- Time to progression
- Disease-free survival (DFS) ✓
- Time to distant metastasis

FDA's Guidance for Industry recognizes the endpoint of DFS, writing, "DFS is defined as the time from randomization until recurrence of tumor or death from any cause" (1). Moreover, this particular FDA document (2) also informs us that, "[t]he most frequent use of this endpoint is in the adjuvant setting after definitive surgery or radiotherapy. Disease-free survival also can be an important endpoint when a large percentage of patients achieve *complete responses* with chemotherapy."

Disease-free survival takes into account the timeframe starting when a subject is rendered free of disease following therapy, until the cancer returns or until the subject dies. However, it is typically the case that the value for DFS is the timeframe from the date of randomization, through the treatment phase of the clinical trial, until relapse following primary treatment.

Regarding the event that tolls the endpoint of DFS, Wee et al. (3) state that, "[i]n the analysis of DFS, a patient was considered to have had an event if he relapsed after the completion of all primary treatment." Regarding the

[1]U.S. Department of Health and Human Services. Food and Drug Administration. Guidance for industry. Clinical trial endpoints for the approval of cancer drugs and biologics; April 2005.

[2]U.S. Department of Health and Human Services. Food and Drug Administration. Guidance for industry. Clinical trial endpoints for the approval of cancer drugs and biologics; April 2005.

[3]Wee J, Tan EH, Tai BC, et al. Randomized trial of radiotherapy versus concurrent chemoradiotherapy followed by adjuvant chemotherapy in patients with American Joint Committee on Cancer/International Union against cancer stage III and IV nasopharyngeal cancer of the endemic variety. J. Clin. Oncol. 2005;23:6730—8.

actual time that is measured by DFS, Wee et al. (4) further state that, "[t]he starting point for DFS was the date of random assignment, and the terminating point was the date when a relapse first occurred or, in the case of persistent disease and other causes of deaths."

Where data establish that a drug results in DFS of several years, the question arises whether it can be concluded that the patient has actually been cured. Commentary from Pui (5) provides the following perspective to this issue. Where a drug results in DFS of 3 years in about 90% of the study subjects, it is reasonable to require a follow-up time of several more years to establish that a cure had been effected.

II. DIFFERENCE BETWEEN DFS AND PFS

Where a patient's cancer is completely removed by surgery, as part of the clinical study protocol, the physician may wonder whether PFS or DFS is the better endpoint to use. In this situation, these two endpoints are likely to be identical, since immediately after surgery, all subjects are considered to be disease-free, and all subjects are in a state where the physician is awaiting the moment when progression is detected (6).

But PFS has a different meaning from DFS. Usually, the endpoint of PFS is used in the context of advanced disease, that is, when the primary treatment failed to lead to complete remission, when tumors still linger, and where these tumors are destined to progress (7). PFS implies that detectable disease was present at baseline, whereas DFS (or the endpoint of relapse-free survival) have traditionally been used for patients without evidence of disease at baseline (8). Both terms enable the investigator to mark the time from intervention until detectable worsening of the disease. Published reports of PFS describe patients with metastatic disease, whereas published reports of DFS are likely to focus on early-stage patients (9).

Disease-free survival is the usual primary endpoint of adjuvant breast cancer trials, since it is considered a good surrogate for the ultimate endpoint, overall survival (10). In breast cancer, DFS is composed of distant and local/regional metastases. According to Dr Miguel Martin, the endpoint of PFS should be reserved for metastatic breast cancer trials, that is, for trials where subjects have advanced cancer at baseline (11).

III. AMBIGUITY IN THE NAME OF THE ENDPOINT, "DFS"

Typically, endpoints in clinical trials are calculated from the date of randomization. The issue of disclosing the endpoint, and the occasional failure to identify this endpoint, is documented in Chapter 8. Where the endpoint

---

[4]Wee J, Tan EH, Tai BC, et al. Randomized trial of radiotherapy versus concurrent chemoradiotherapy followed by adjuvant chemotherapy in patients with American Joint Committee on Cancer/International Union against cancer stage III and IV nasopharyngeal cancer of the endemic variety. J. Clin. Oncol. 2005;23:6730–8.

[5]Pui C-H. Toward a total cure for acute lymphoblastic leukemia. J. Clin. Oncol. 2009;27:5121–3.

[6]Bepler G. E-mail of August 19, 2010.

[7]Bepler G. E-mail of August 19, 2010.

[8]Hudis CA. E-mail of August 19, 2010.

[9]Hudis CA. E-mail of August 19, 2010.

[10]Martin M. E-mail of August 18, 2010.

[11]Martin M. E-mail of August 18, 2010.

of DFS is calculated from the date of randomization, the result appears to present a contradiction. In short, when subjects are enrolled, they are typically not disease-free. If they were disease-free at the time of enrollment, they would not meet the inclusion criteria for the trial. They can only be considered "disease-free" after, for example, surgery that is performed at the beginning of the study. According to Dr Sally Stenning, "[s]trictly disease-free survival can only apply to patients who are free from disease at your time origin, so for example it would be an appropriate outcome measure for patients in adjuvant therapy trials who are free from disease after surgery" (12). In any trial where patients are macroscopically free of disease at entry, for example, adjuvant therapy trials in breast or colorectal cancer, DFS dated from randomization is accurate and appropriate as an endpoint (13).

This slight contradiction might not make much difference if the interval between enrollment and surgery is short and where also the time from enrollment to the first endpoint is long.

At any rate, to avoid any contradiction, investigators should use a start date that resides after surgery, when calculating DFS. This is exactly what was done by Allum et al. (14), in designing a clinical trial of esophageal cancer. The actual motivation for using a start date set at 6 months after surgery was not really to avoid this contradiction, but instead to allow for a difference in timing of the surgery between the arms of the clinical trial. The following quotation reveals that overall survival was calculated by the conventional start date (randomization) but that DFS was calculated from a later date.

Allum et al. (15), wrote, "[o]verall survival was calculated from the date of random assignment to date of death from any cause and surviving patients were censored at the date they were last known to be alive. Disease-free survival was calculated from a landmark time of 6 months from random assignment to allow for the difference in timing of surgery between the two groups."

Consistently, Rothmann et al. (16), wrote, "[f]or resected disease, a frequently used approval endpoint is disease-free survival (DFS). For unresected disease an important endpoint that has been used for accelerated or regular approval is progression-free survival (PFS)."

IV. DISEASE-FREE SURVIVAL PROVIDES EARLIER RESULTS ON EFFICACY THAN OVERALL SURVIVAL—THE ADD-ON BREAST CANCER STUDY OF ROMOND

In a study of breast cancer, Romond et al. (17) treated women with surgery, and assayed tumor samples for expression of the biomarker, HER2. Only women with overexpressed HER2

---

[12]Stenning S. E-mail of March 30, 2011.

[13]Stenning S. E-mail of March 31, 2011.

[14]Allum WH, Stenning SP, Bancewicz J, Clark PI, Langley RE. Long-term results of a randomized trial of surgery with or without preoperative chemotherapy in esophageal cancer. J. Clin. Oncol. 2009;27:5062–7.

[15]Allum WH, Stenning SP, Bancewicz J, Clark PI, Langley RE. Long-term results of a randomized trial of surgery with or without preoperative chemotherapy in esophageal cancer. J. Clin. Oncol. 2009;27:5062–7.

[16]Rothmann MD, Koti K, Lee KY, Lu HL, Shen YL. Missing data in biologic oncology products. J. Biopharm. Stat. 2009;19:1074–84.

[17]Romond EH, Perez EA, Bryant J, et al. Trastuzumab plus adjuvant chemotherapy for operable HER2-positive breast cancer. New Engl. J. Med. 2005;353:1673–84.

were enrolled. These were randomized into two arms, as indicated.

- *Arm A.* Doxorubicin and cyclophosophamide, followed by paclitaxel.
- *Arm B.* Doxorubicin and cyclophosophamide followed by paclitaxel and concurrent trastuzumab.

To be enrolled in the trial, patients were required to have breast cancer that was surgically treated, where surgery resulted in complete resection of the primary tumor. Potential subjects with metastasis were not permitted to enroll in the trial.

The endpoints included DFS and overall survival. The endpoint of DFS was tolled as follows. Events determining DFS were local, regional, and distant recurrence; contralateral breast cancer, including ductal carcinoma in situ; other second primary cancers; and death before recurrence or a second primary cancer. It should be noted that the value for DFS was expressed as the value

found at the 3-year time point, and that the value was not expressed in terms of median DFS.

The results for both endpoints, that is, DFS and overall survival, appear in Table 15.1. The results demonstrate the advantage of including the antibody in the treatment scheme.

Disease-free survival for the trastuzumab arm and control arm is shown in the first Kaplan–Meier plot (Fig. 15.1a). This plot

TABLE 15.1   The Romond Study

	Arm A. Control (%)	Arm B. Trastuzumab (%)	Hazard Ratio	Significance
DFS at 3 years	75.4	87.1	HR=0.48	P<0.0001
Overall survival at 3 years	91.7	94.3	HR=0.67	P=0.015

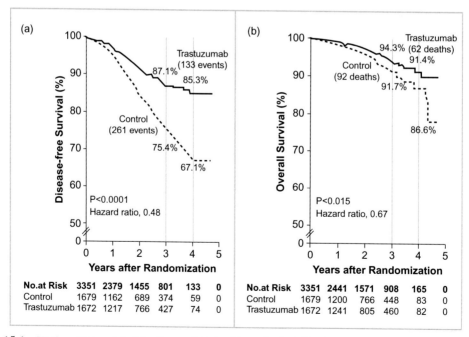

FIGURE 15.1   Kaplan–Meier plot of the Romond study: (a) results for DFS; (b) results for overall survival.

shows that trastuzumab provides a dramatic early advantage over the control treatment.

Overall survival for the trastuzumab arm and control arm is shown in the second Kaplan–Meier plot (Fig. 15.1b). This plot shows that trastuzumab also provides a dramatic advantage over the control treatment. But according to this endpoint, this advantage is not evident until 4 years have passed.

V. DISEASE-FREE SURVIVAL AS AN ENDPOINT IN THE ANALYSIS OF SUBGROUPS—THE ADD-ON BREAST CANCER STUDY OF HAYES

In a clinical trial of breast cancer by Hayes et al. (18) using the add-on drug of paclitaxel, patients received either doxorubicin plus cyclophosphamide (Arm A) or doxorubicin plus cyclophosphamide followed by paclitaxel (Arm B). This might be contrasted with the above-described study of breast cancer of Romond et al. (19), which also used an add-on study design. But in the case of the Romond study, the added drug was trastuzumab.

The Hayes study of breast cancer included patients with tumor biopsies that were HER2-positive and HER2-negative. All patients had completed surgery before starting the clinical trial and hence were considered to be free of disease. Tissue samples were considered to be HER2-positive if 50% or greater of the cancer cells stained with anti-HER2 antibody, and if the staining was of a 3+ intensity.

The endpoints included DFS and overall survival, where the events triggering the endpoint of DFS were the first local or distant recurrence of breast cancer, or death from any cause. The following Kaplan–Meier plots (Fig. 15.2a,b) show DFS versus time, where Fig. 15.2a is for the subgroup of patients where tumors were HER2-negative, and Fig. 15.2b is for the subgroup of patients where tumors were HER2-positive. The first Kaplan–Meier plot (Fig. 15.2a) shows that both curves closely track each other, but are not quite identical to each other. The second Kaplan–Meier plot (Fig. 15.2b) shows a dramatic separation, demonstrating that paclitaxel shows remarkable efficacy as an add-on drug. Other investigators have also noted that HER2-positive status

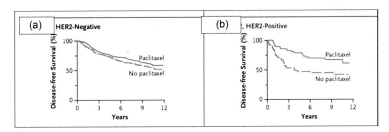

FIGURE 15.2   Kaplan–Meier plot showing efficacy of adding paclitaxel to chemotherapy with doxorubicin plus cyclophosphamide: (a) adding paclitaxel results in a slight improvement in the DFS; (b) adding paclitaxel produces a remarkable improvement in DFS.

[18]Hayes DF, Thor AD, Dressler LG, et al. HER2 and response to paclitaxel in node-positive breast cancer. New Engl. J. Med. 2007;357:1496–506.

[19]Romond EH, Perez EA, Bryant J, et al. Trastuzumab plus adjuvant chemotherapy for operable HER2-positive breast cancer. New Engl. J. Med. 2005;353:1673–84.

can be associated with a better response to paclitaxel (20,21).

The Hayes study then probed deeper into subgroup analysis. In viewing only the DFS data from HER2-negative subjects (the subjects that failed to respond much to paclitaxel), the researchers then separated the data into those where biopsies were negative for estrogen receptor, and those where biopsies were positive for estrogen receptor. Again, the results were dramatic. In performing this more detailed subgroup analysis, it became apparent that paclitaxel had a significant ($P = 0.002$) effect of improving DFS, where this benefit was found only in the estrogen receptor-negative subgroup. In striking contrast, paclitaxel had no significant effect ($P = 0.71$) in the estrogen receptor-positive subgroup.

The take-home lessons are as follows. First, DFS is used as an endpoint where all subjects are considered to be free of disease at the start of the clinical trial. Second, the identification of subgroups that fail to respond to paclitaxel constitute an important subgroup, because physicians can then spare patients with the relevant criteria from being exposed to a toxic drug (paclitaxel). In short, the Hayes study provides guidance to physicians, that paclitaxel should not be given where tumors are negative in HER2 and positive in estrogen receptor. Third, it can reasonably be asked whether the efficacy of a small molecule, such as paclitaxel, depends on the expression level of HER2, even though HER2 is not expected to be directly targeted by paclitaxel.

VI. NEOADJUVANT THERAPY VERSUS ADJUVANT THERAPY FOR RECTAL CANCER—THE ROH STUDY

In a study of rectal cancer, Roh et al. (22) treated subjects with chemotherapy before surgery (preoperative chemotherapy; neoadjuvant) or with surgery followed by chemotherapy (postoperative chemotherapy; adjuvant). The two study arms are shown below:

- *Arm A. Neoadjuvant treatment (preoperative).* 5-Fluorouracil, then radiation plus 5-fluorouracil, followed by surgery, and finally 5-fluorouracil.
- *Arm B. Adjuvant treatment (postoperative).* Surgery, then 5-fluorouracil, followed by radiation plus 5-fluorouracil, and finally 5-fluorouracil.

DFS was defined as the time from random assignment to recurrence, second primary cancer (excluding basal cell carcinomas of the skin and carcinoma in situ of the cervix), or death without evidence of recurrence or second primary cancer.

The timepoint of DFS had its start at the time of assignment. The patients had rectal cancer at the time of the study and were not free of disease (23). But this situation is only a matter of semantics, and has no bearing on the interpretation of the results.

Data on DFS and overall survival were expressed in terms of the hazard ratio. Disease, as well as survival, for each individual subject

[20]Bedard PL, Di Leo A, Piccart-Gebhart MJ. Taxanes: optimizing adjuvant chemotherapy for early-stage breast cancer. Nat. Rev. Clin. Oncol. 2010;7:22–36.

[21]Kimura M, Sano M, Fujimori M, et al. Neoadjuvant paclitaxel for operable breast cancer: multicenter phase II trial with clinical outcomes. Anticancer Res. 2008;28(2B):1239–44.

[22]Roh MS, Colangelo LH, O'Connell MJ, et al. Preoperative multimodality therapy improves disease-free survival in patients with carcinoma of the rectum: NSABP R-03. J. Clin. Oncol. 2009;27:5124–30.

[23]Colangelo L. E-mail of May 3, 2011.

was followed over the course of 7 years. Kaplan—Meier plots, not shown here, were constructed by connecting data points acquired from each individual subject, where each datum was produced whenever a subject triggered an endpoint. Regarding the endpoint of DFS, the hazard ratio was HR = 0.629 ($P = 0.011$), demonstrating a benefit for preoperative therapy.

The following concerns overall survival. The hazard ratio comparing preoperative with postoperative patients was HR = 0.693 ($P = 0.065$), suggesting a possible survival benefit for preoperative therapy. Taken together, the results demonstrate that preoperative chemoradiation works better than postoperative chemoradiation.

The results for DFS were more dramatic than with overall survival, demonstrating the advantage of including a multiplicity of endpoints in any given clinical trial, in addition to the gold standard endpoint of overall survival.

VII. WHERE EFFICACY OF TWO DIFFERENT TREATMENTS IS THE SAME, CHOICE OF TREATMENT SHIFTS TO THE TREATMENT THAT IMPROVES QUALITY OF LIFE—THE RING STUDY

In a study of breast cancer, Ring et al. (24) used the endpoints of DFS and overall survival. The study had two arms, as indicated below.

- *Arm A.* Chemotherapy followed by surgery.
- *Arm B.* Chemotherapy (no surgery).

The results are shown in Table 15.2.

TABLE 15.2   The Ring Study

	Disease-Free Survival	
	5-Year DFS (%)	10-Year DFS ($P=0.7$) (%)
Chemotherapy, then surgery	64	52
Chemotherapy (no surgery)	61	46

	Overall Surgery	
	5-Year Overall Survival (%)	10-Year Overall Survival ($P=0.9$) (%)
Chemotherapy, then surgery	74	60
Chemotherapy (no surgery)	76	70

The study found no significant difference in DFS between the two groups. Also, the study found no significant difference in overall survival between the groups. The large P values mean that the significance of the difference was low. In other words, it is possible for a study to result in a slight difference in two study arms, where this slight difference had a tiny P value, meaning that the slight difference was very convincing. But in this study, there were slight differences in the values for 5-year DFS and 5-year overall survival, and these sight differences were convincing.

The investigators arrived at the following useful result. The result is that women can be reasonably counseled on the benefits of treatment with no surgery. In the words of Ring et al. (25), "[t]he avoidance of surgery altogether would eliminate common postoperative

[24]Ring A, Webb A, Ashley S, et al. Is surgery necessary after complete clinical remission following neoadjuvant chemotherapy for early breast cancer? J. Clin. Oncol. 2003;21:4540–5.

[25]Ring A, Webb A, Ashley S, et al. Is surgery necessary after complete clinical remission following neoadjuvant chemotherapy for early breast cancer? J. Clin. Oncol. 2003;21:4540–5.

problems including chronic arm morbidity, pain, seroma formation, and wound infections. In addition, some of the psychological and cosmetic impact of surgery might be avoided. Rare anesthetic problems and complications such as thromboembolic disease would also not occur, and considerable inpatient resource savings would be made." Seroma is a frequent complication after breast cancer surgery (26).

In general, where a clinical trial fails to show that treatment A has a different efficacy than treatment B, the decision-making process then shifts to the safety profile and to the quality-of-life profile. If safety or quality of life for treatment A is superior, then the investigators may be justified in recommending that treatment A be used.

VIII. DFS AND OVERALL SURVIVAL ARE USEFUL TOOLS FOR TESTING AND VALIDATING PROGNOSTIC BIOMARKERS—THE BEPLER STUDY

This demonstrates the utility of the *RRM1* gene and *PTEN* gene as prognostic markers. Bepler et al. (27) acquired two sets of frozen lung tumor samples. The first set was the *exploratory set*, while the second set was the *validation set*. The exploratory tissue samples were acquired from a tissue procurement facility. The validation set was from 77 patients enrolled in the Bepler study. Tissue samples were all frozen within 20 min after collection, according to a standard procedure, and stored at −80°C. Essentially all of the patients used for the exploratory tissue set were treated with surgery only (no chemotherapy, no radiation). The use of surgery only totally eliminates the possibility that any radiation or drugs would influence gene expression.

Analysis of gene expression in the exploratory tissue set showed increased expression of the *RRM1* gene was significantly associated with increased overall survival ($P = 0.013$), and that increased expression of the *PTEN* gene was also significantly associated with increased overall survival ($P = 0.011$). Survival was longer for patients whose tumors expressed high levels of the respective gene compared with low levels (median survival time of 52 months vs 24 months for *RRM1*, and 62 months vs 23 months for *PTEN*).

The results from the prospective study were as follows. As seen from the published Kaplan–Meier plots of the DFS endpoint and the overall survival endpoint, the results were striking and dramatic. In viewing the DFS data, a clear separation between high-gene-expressing patients and low-gene-expressing patients could be seen by 10 months into the clinical trial. But with the overall survival data, a clear separation could not be seen until about 20 months. Data on DFS and overall survival were collected until about 100 months.

The hazard ratios were disclosed for the endpoint of overall survival. In dividing the patients into high-*RRM1*-expressing tumors, and into low-*RRM1*-expressing tumors, and drawing two curves corresponding to overall survival for the high-*RRP1*-expressers and the low-*RRP1*-expressers, the resulting hazard ratio was HR = 0.452.

Hazard ratio data also showed an association between expression (high vs low) with survival, for the *PTEN* marker. The hazard ratios were disclosed for the endpoint of overall survival. In dividing the patients into high-*PTEN*-expressing tumors, and into

---

26Hashemi E, Kaviani A, Najafi M, Ebrahimi M, Hooshmand H, Montazeri A. Seroma formation after surgery for breast cancer. World J. Surg. Oncol. 2004;2:44–9.

27Bepler G, Sharma S, Cantor A, et al. *RRM1* and *PTEN* as prognostic parameters for overall and disease-free survival in patients with non-small-cell lung cancer. J. Clin. Oncol. 2004;22:1878–85.

low-*PTEN*-expressing tumors, and drawing two curves corresponding to overall survival for the high-*PTEN*-expressers and the low-*PTEN*-expressers, the resulting hazard ratio was HR = 0.469.

The authors concluded, "we confirmed this strong association between *RRM1* and *PTEN* expression in two separate datasets and show that *RRM1* expression seems to be marginally better in predicting clinical outcome than *PTEN* expression." The authors concluded with the recommendation that, "[f]uture randomized trials in *NSCLC* should stratify patients based on *RRM1* and/or *PTEN* expression because tumors with high levels of expression have an intrinsically less malignant phenotype" (28).

Interest in the *RRM1* gene and *PTEN* gene had the following origins (29). Data showed an association between chromosome 11p15.5 allele loss and metastasis formation and poor survival in patients with lung cancer. One of the genes in the deleted region is *RRM1*. Interest in the *PTEN* gene began as follows. *PTEN* was originally identified as occurring in a region of frequent allele loss on chromosome 10q23 in breast and brain tumors.

IX. FDA'S DECISION-MAKING PROCESS IN EVALUATING THE ENDPOINT OF DFS

This concerns a clinical trial on trastuzumab (Herceptin®) for treating breast cancer. The information is from BLA 103792, from May 22, 2008 of the FDA's website.

The primary endpoint was DFS and the secondary endpoint was overall survival. The unit of DFS is a period of time. According to FDA's Guidance for Industry, "[g]enerally, DFS is defined as the time from randomization until recurrence of tumor or death from any cause" (30).

FDA granted approval of the drug, and the fact that FDA's approval was based on data from DFS (and not based on overall survival) is evident from comments by the FDA reviewer that analysis of "the anthracycline containing arm (Herceptin concurrently with docetaxel) demonstrated . . . longer disease-free survival, as compared to the [active control] . . . treatment arm. Follow-up was too short for . . . comparison of survival."

The FDA reviewer complained about the fact that the Sponsor's definition of DFS included the parameter of, the "date of second primary cancer." Regarding this parameter, the reviewer complained that secondary primary cancers are considered unrelated to the primary breast cancer and therefore cannot be accepted as an event for DFS. The FDA reviewer then recalculated the efficacy results, using its own definition of DFS, and arrived at its own conclusions on efficacy. The following quotation from the *Medical Review* reveals the definition of DFS that was used by the FDA reviewer. Please note that FDA refers to DFS as a composite endpoint:

> FDA does not agree with the protocol's definition of disease-free survival: 'the interval from the

---

[28]Bepler G, Sharma S, Cantor A, et al. *RRM1* and *PTEN* as prognostic parameters for overall and disease-free survival in patients with non-small-cell lung cancer. J. Clin. Oncol. 2004;22:1878–85.

[29]Gautam A, Li ZR, Bepler G. RRM1-induced metastasis suppression through PTEN-regulated pathways. Oncogene 2003;22:2135–42.

[30]U.S. Department of Health and Human Services. Food and Drug Administration. Guidance for industry. Clinical trial endpoints for the approval of cancer drugs and biologics; May 2007 (19 pp.).

date of randomization to the date of local, regional or metastatic relapse or the **date of second primary cancer** or death from any cause, whichever occurs first'. Currently there is no standard definition of disease free survival. However, FDA had accepted in previous applications the following components of this composite endpoint: local recurrence, distal recurrence . . . and unrelated deaths. Second primary cancers are considered unrelated to breast cancer and therefore cannot be accepted as an event for disease-free survival.

The quotation reveals this difference between the Sponsor's calculations and FDA's calculations:

> Patients who had events due to second primary malignancy were not counted as events except except [sic] 8 patients . . . who had another breast primary tumor and who were counted as DFS events and patients who died who were counted as death events.

Consistent with the above remarks, the *Medical Review* revealed that the FDA reviewer had "decided that the definition of DFS events should exclude non-breast cancer related secondary primary tumor. The results shown in this analysis are close to the sponsor's proposed results."

The take-home lesson is that the Sponsor should ensure that FDA will accept the proposed endpoints for the clinical trial, before actually conducting the clinical trial. This *Medical Review* provides a clear-cut example of the fact that FDA reviewers will contemplate the Sponsor's data, perform its own calculations, and arrive at its own independent conclusions. Any given review may contain comments from different FDA employees (31).

X. SUMMARY

The Romond study provides a straightforward example showing that the study drug (trastuzumab) works better than the control, where DFS provides dramatic efficacy results long before overall survival data provide dramatic results.

The Roh study, which compared neoadjuvant therapy with adjuvant therapy, demonstrated that neoadjuvant chemoradiation works better than adjuvant chemoradiation, where the results were more dramatic with DFS than with overall survival.

In the Ring breast cancer study the DFS data and the overall survival data failed to show a significant difference between either of the two treatments. But since one of the treatments involved surgery, the results justified counseling patients to use the nonsurgical treatment, in order to avoid complications associated with surgery.

The Bepler study concerned two biomarkers, the *RRM1* gene and *PTEN* gene. Expression of either of these markers, that is, low expression versus high expression, proved to have prognostic value for the endpoints of DFS and overall survival.

---

[31]"Note that there may be differences among reviewers since the FDA review divisions and teams operate slightly differently from one another." Response by RL, Drug Information Specialist, Division of Drug Information, Center for Drug Evaluation and Research, FDA. E-mail response dated March 2, 2015.

16

Oncology Endpoint: Time to Distant Metastasis

I. INTRODUCTION

This chapter further details the topic of oncology endpoints, and covers the last topic indicated by the check mark.

- Objective response
- Overall survival
- Progression-free survival
- Time to progression (TTP)
- Disease-free survival
- Time to distant metastasis (TDM) ✓

Time to distant metastasis is an endpoint used in oncology clinical trials. This endpoint is measured from the date of random assignment to the date of occurrence of distant metastasis (1,2). TDM is a preferred endpoint for cancers where the event of metastasis is invariably followed by mortality. Hence, TDM is a preferred endpoint for breast cancer that has metastasized, in view of the fact that metastatic breast cancer is incurable (3,4). For breast cancer, once metastasis is detected, the metastasis is a highly reliable prognostic factor for death. In other words, TDM can be an excellent surrogate for the gold standard endpoint of *overall survival*. In contrast, TDM is not a particularly practical

[1] Roach M, Bae K, Speight J, et al. Short-term neoadjuvant androgen deprivation therapy and external-beam radiotherapy for locally advanced prostate cancer: long-term results of RTOG 8610. J. Clin. Oncol. 2008;26:585–91.

[2] Wee J, Tan EH, Tai BC, et al. Randomized trial of radiotherapy versus concurrent chemoradiotherapy followed by adjuvant chemotherapy in patients with American Joint Committee on Cancer/International Union against cancer stage III and IV nasopharyngeal cancer of the endemic variety. J. Clin. Oncol. 2005;23:6730–8.

[3] Wong ST, Goodin S. Overcoming drug resistance in patients with metastatic breast cancer. Pharmacotherapy 2009;29:954–65.

[4] Barnett CM. Survival data of patients with anthracycline- or taxane-pretreated or resistant metastatic breast cancer. Pharmacotherapy 2009;29:1482–90.

endpoint for clinical trials on basal cell carcinoma (nonmelanoma skin cancer) (5,6,7) or fibromatosis (8), because these types of cancer rarely metastasize. A benefit of using the endpoint of TDM is that data can be acquired at an earlier time than with the endpoint of overall survival.

II. TDM DATA ARE ACQUIRED BEFORE OVERALL SURVIVAL DATA ARE ACQUIRED—THE WEE STUDY

The clinical trial of Wee et al. (9) concerned nasopharyngeal cancer. Nasopharyngeal cancer is distinguished by the high success rate of radiation therapy, where the result is 75% survival at 5 years after radiotherapy. The Wee study improved on this success rate by using the combination of radiation and chemotherapy. The endpoints included TDM and overall survival.

The study had two arms, as indicated:

- Arm A. Radiation only.
- Arm B. Radiation plus cisplatin and 5-fluorouracil.

The radiotherapy group contained 110 subjects, while the radiochemotherapy group contained 111 subjects. Over the course of the 6-year study, subjects in the radiotherapy group had 38 distant relapses, while subjects

in the chemoradiotherapy group had 18 distant relapses. Regarding local relapses, the radiotherapy group had 10 local relapses, and the chemoradiotherapy group had 9 local relapses. The endpoint of TDM takes into account only the distant relapses.

The results were as follows. Typically, results from oncology clinical trials are expressed in terms of median TTP, median TDM, or median overall survival. But sometimes, results are expressed in terms of cumulative events that occurred, during the course of a trial, until a specific time, for example, until the 2-year time point. That was the case in the Wee study. The 2-year TDM was 30% in the radiotherapy group, and 13% in the chemoradiotherapy group. A plot of the raw data is shown in Fig. 16.1. The results are dramatic and demonstrate a distinct separation in the two study arms by the 2-year time point, where this separation is maintained until at least the 6-year time point.

A schematic representation of the Kaplan–Meier plot of the survival data is shown in Fig. 16.2. The magnitude of the difference between the two curves is shown by hazard ratio of $HR = 0.51$, where the significance of this difference is shown by the P value ($P = 0.0061$). It can be concluded that the combination of radiation plus chemotherapy provides greater overall survival, as compared to radiation alone.

[5]Selvin GJ. Basal cell and squamous cell carcinomas. Optom. Clin. 1993;3:17–28.

[6]Ozgediz D, Smith EB, Zheng J, Otero J, Tabatabai ZL, Corvera CU. Basal cell carcinoma does metastasize. Dermatol. Online J. 2008;14:5.

[7]Ting PT, Kasper R, Arlette JP. Metastatic basal cell carcinoma: report of two cases and literature review. J. Cutan. Med. Surg. 2005;9:10–5.

[8]O'Dwyer HM, Keogh CF, O'Connell JX, Munk PL. A case report of synchronous osteoblastoma and fibromatosis. Br. J. Radiol. 2008;81:e68–71.

[9]Wee J, Tan EH, Tai BC, et al. Randomized trial of radiotherapy versus concurrent chemoradiotherapy followed by adjuvant chemotherapy in patients with American Joint Committee on Cancer/International Union against cancer stage III and IV nasopharyngeal cancer of the endemic variety. J. Clin. Oncol. 2005;23:6730–8.

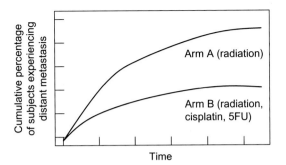

FIGURE 16.1 Schematic diagram of Kaplan–Meier plot showing TDM. The *Y*-axis has the unit of percentage of subjects triggering the endpoint of distant metastasis, at the indicated time (years). The plot shows two curves, one curve corresponding to subjects receiving radiation only (*upper curve*), and the other corresponding to subjects receiving the combination of radiation and chemotherapy (*lower curve*). The difference between two curves was significant (*P* = 0.0029).

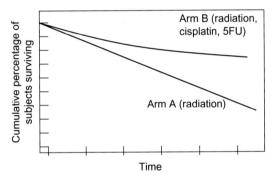

FIGURE 16.2 Schematic of Kaplan–Meier plot of overall survival. The *Y*-axis has the unit of percentage of subjects triggering the endpoint of overall survival, at the indicated time. The plot shows two curves, one curve corresponding to subjects receiving radiation only (*lower curve*), and the other corresponding to subjects receiving the combination of radiation and chemotherapy (*upper curve*). The magnitude of the difference between the two curves is shown by hazard ratio of HR = 0.51, where the significance of this difference is shown by the *P* value (*P* = 0.0061).

Regarding choice of endpoints, it is evident that TDM has the advantage over the endpoint of overall survival, in that a distinction between the two study arms can present at an earlier time.

The survival data were also expressed in terms of the unit of 2-year survival. The 2-year survival value for the radiotherapy arm was 78%, and that for the chemoradiotherapy arm was 85%. This difference is only slight. But with an additional year of data collection, the difference became obvious. The 3-year survival value was 65% for the radiotherapy group and 80% for the chemoradiotherapy group. Again, it is evident that TDM has the advantage over the endpoint of overall survival, in that a distinction can be detected at an earlier time with TDM.

III. TIME TO DISTANT METASTASIS DATA CAN REVEAL A DRAMATIC ADVANTAGE OF THE STUDY DRUG, IN A SITUATION WHERE OVERALL SURVIVAL FAILS TO SHOW ANY ADVANTAGE—THE ROACH STUDY

In a study of prostate cancer, Roach et al. (10) used the endpoints of TDM and overall survival. The study had two arms:

- Arm A. Radiation plus goserelin and flutamidine.
- Arm B. Radiation only.

Goserelin and flutamidine are hormones. Goserelin causes "chemical castration" and reduces testosterone, while flutamide is an antiandrogen compound (11). Administering the combination of goserelin and flutamidine is called *androgen deprivation therapy* (ADT)

[10]Roach M, Bae K, Speight J, et al. Short-term neoadjuvant androgen deprivation therapy and external-beam radiotherapy for locally advanced prostate cancer: long-term results of RTOG 8610. J. Clin. Oncol. 2008;26:585–91.

[11]Tyrrell CJ. Controversies in the management of advanced prostate cancer. Br. J. Cancer 1999;79:146–55.

(12). The ADT was given before radiation, and thus was classified as neoadjuvant therapy. Concurrent androgen therapy was also administered, and this was not classified as neoadjuvant therapy or as adjuvant therapy.

TDM was measured from the time of randomization to the date of occurrence of distant metastasis. When TDM is used as an endpoint, the endpoint can be expressed in terms of *median TDM*, that is the average (median) value of TDM for all study subjects.

Median TDM has been used as an endpoint in many studies, for example, in the studies of Andre et al. (13), Chagpar et al. (14), Coen et al. (15), Gomez-Fernandez et al. (16), Jeremic et al. (17), and Specenier et al. (18).

But in the Roach study, the TDM results, as well as the overall survival results, were expressed by using the hazard ratio (HR). The authors provided a Kaplan—Meier plot (not reproduced here) showing the percentage of subjects triggering the endpoint of TDM over the course of 15 years. The hazard ratio for

TDM was HR = 1.52 (P = 0.006), which indicates a moderate separation between arm A and arm B.

The authors provided an additional, different Kaplan—Meier plot showing the percentage of subjects triggering the endpoint of survival (dying), over the course of 15 years. The hazard ratio for overall survival was only HR = 1.18 (P = 0.12), indicating almost no separation between the study arms.

The investigators were pleased with the improvement in TDM found in arm A, writing that the delayed time for 40% of patients to develop metastasis by 8 years with the addition of just 4 months of neoadjuvant ADT with EBRT was "remarkable" (19). The term ADT refers to androgen deprivation therapy, while EBRT refers to radiotherapy.

Thus, the Roach study shows the utility of using the endpoint of TDM, in that a clear separation between study arms may be reached prior to separation with the endpoint of overall survival. Also, the utility of TDM may be that

[12]Ray ME, Bae K, Hussain MH, Hanks GE, Shipley WU, Sandler HM. Potential surrogate endpoints for prostate cancer survival: analysis of a phase III randomized trial. J. Natl Cancer Inst. 2009;101:228—36.

[13]Andre F, Xia W, Conforti R, Wei Y, et al. CXCR4 expression in early breast cancer and risk of distant recurrence. Oncologist 2009;14:1182—8.

[14]Chagpar AB, McMasters KM, Martin RC, et al. Determinants of early distant metastatic disease in elderly patients with breast cancer. Am. J. Surg. 2006;192:317—21.

[15]Coen JJ, Zietman AL, Thakral H, Shipley WU. Radical radiation for localized prostate cancer: local persistence of disease results in a late wave of metastases. J. Clin. Oncol. 2002;20:3199—205.

[16]Gomez-Fernandez C, Daneshbod Y, Nassiri M, Milikowski C, Alvarez C, Nadji M. Immunohistochemically determined estrogen receptor phenotype remains stable in recurrent and metastatic breast cancer. Am. J. Clin. Pathol. 2008;130:879—82.

[17]Jeremic B, Milicic B, Acimovic L, Milisavljevic S. Concurrent hyperfractionated radiotherapy and low-dose daily carboplatin and paclitaxel in patients with stage III non-small-cell lung cancer: long-term results of a phase II study. J. Clin. Oncol. 2005;23:1144—51.

[18]Specenier PM, Van Den Brande J, Schrijvers D, et al. Docetaxel, ifosfamide and cisplatin (DIP) in squamous cell carcinoma of the head and neck. Anticancer Res. 2009;29:5137—42.

[19]Roach M, Bae K, Speight J, et al. Short-term neoadjuvant androgen deprivation therapy and external-beam radiotherapy for locally advanced prostate cancer: long-term results of RTOG 8610. J. Clin. Oncol. 2008;26:585—91.

study arms using the endpoint of TDM may be clearly separated, but that clear separation between study arms may never be reached with the endpoint of overall survival.

IV. USE OF A GENE ARRAY AS A PROGNOSTIC FACTOR FOR BREAST CANCER PATIENTS, USING THE ENDPOINT OF TDM—THE LOI STUDY

In a study of breast cancer, Loi et al. (20) analyzed biopsies from 417 breast cancer patients. Only patients where tumors were ER-positive were included in the study.

All breast cancer biopsies were ER-positive. The patients had received surgery, but no systemic chemotherapy. ER means estrogen receptor.

Gene expression from each tumor biopsy was measured using a microarray sensitive to 97 genes. These 97 genes are identified by Sotiriou et al. (21). As a matter of introduction to the genes included in this set, it was found that the top overexpressed genes included *UBE2C*, *KPNA2*, *TPX2*, *FOXM1*, *STK6*, *CCNA2*, *BIRC5*, and *MYBL2*. The trivial names for all of these genes, as well as the nucleotide sequences of these genes, can easily be found on the world wide web at ncbi.nlm.nih.gov.

Gene expression was used to provide a score, namely, the *Gene expression Grade Index* (GGI). The score was either low or high, that is, high-grade GGI or low-grade GGI. Gene expression from biopsies of all patients provided individual scores from each biopsy. These two groups, high GGI versus low GGI, represented two subgroups of the study population. A Kaplan—Meier plot was used to present the data, where the plot had two different curves. One curve corresponded to high-GGI patients experiencing distant metastasis, while the other curve corresponded to low-GGI patients experiencing distant metastasis. The results demonstrated that a low-GGI score is prognostic for good outcome, while a high-GGI score is prognostic for poor outcome.

An eventual goal of the researchers was to use the 97-gene microarray for guidance in choosing the best treatment for breast cancer patients.

V. USE OF MICRO-RNA EXPRESSION DATA AS A PROGNOSTIC FACTOR FOR BREAST CANCER PATIENTS—THE FOEKENS STUDY

In a study of breast cancer patients, Foekens et al. (22) examined gene expression by tumor biopsies, and attempted to find correlations between gene expression and the endpoint of TDM. All of the genes were in the class micro-RNA (miRNA). All of the biopsies were from tumors that were ER-positive (ER+). A gene array consisting of 249 different miRNA sequences was used, and a comparison of expression versus TDM revealed a specific group of genes, showing a large expression difference in patients with a poor TDM versus in patients with a favorable TDM. This specific group of genes included, *miR-7*, *miR-22*, *miR-34b*, *miR-128a*, *miR-145*, *miR-151*, *miR-193b*, *miR-205*, *miR-210*, *miR-449*, *miR-489*, and *miR-516—3p*.

[20]Loi S, Haibe-Kains B, Desmedt C, et al. Definition of clinically distinct molecular subtypes in estrogen receptor-positive breast carcinomas through genomic grade. J. Clin. Oncol. 2007;25:1239—46.

[21]Sotiriou C, Wirapati P, Loi S, et al. Gene expression profiling in breast cancer: understanding the molecular basis of histologic grade to improve prognosis. J. Natl Cancer Inst. 2006;98:262—72.

[22]Foekens JA, Sieuwerts AM, Smid M, et al. Four miRNAs associated with aggressiveness of lymph node-negative, estrogen receptor-positive human breast cancer. Proc. Natl Acad. Sci. USA 2008;105:13021—6.

These were the most differentially expressed miRNAs, as determined by comparing biopsy expression data from patients having an early TDM versus patients with a late TDM.

In an exploration of possible associations of these miRNAs with characteristics of the tumors, the researchers found a positive association of *miR-7*, *miR-34b*, and *miR-151* with *tumor size* ($P < 0.05$), and the association of *miR-7*, *miR-210*, *miR-489*, and *miR-516–3p* with *pathological grade* ($P < 0.01$). Further analysis of the 249 genes revealed one group of miRNA (cluster 1) that was associated with good prognosis, that is, a greater value for TDM, and another group of miRNA (cluster 3) that was associated with poor prognosis, that is, a small value for TDM.

To summarize, the study found that specific miRNA sequences were differentially expressed, when comparing poor TDM patients with favorable TDM patients. Moreover, the study found that specific miRNA sequences were correlated with tumor size. Also, certain miRNA sequences were associated with pathological grade. In view of the identification of miRNAs associated with poor prognosis, the authors proposed designing drugs that could target and silence these particular miRNAs.

VI. BIOLOGY OF miRNA

miRNAs are small 19–25-nucleotide noncoding RNAs that can modulate gene expression by hybridizing to complementary target mRNAs, resulting in either inhibition of translation inhibition or in the degradation of the mRNA (23). miRNA is believed to be used for the regulation of a large proportion, perhaps 30–50%, of all human genes (24,25).

miRNAs are transcribed by RNA polymerase II or RNA polymerase III as longer primary miRNAs termed pri-miRNA (26). This molecule is subsequently cleaved into smaller segments by RNAse III. At this point, what is formed is a precursor that is about 60–70 nucleotides, which is exported to the cytoplasm and modified by another enzyme, RNAse II, to form miRNA. In turn, the miRNA is loaded onto the RNA-induced silencing complex, where it is then able to either cleave mRNA targets or to repress translation of the mRNA, dependent upon its complementarity to the target mRNA.

Regarding cancer, several miRNAs have been identified that are either proangiogenic or antiangiogenic. The antiangiogenic miRNAs include miR-221/222, which regulate the expression of the c-kit and cyclin G1 genes. The proangiogenic miRNAs include miR-126 and miR-378, which regulate expression of the *VEGF* gene. Experiments that knockout miR-126, for example, have the consequence of reducing angiogenesis.

This concerns metastasis. Detachment of cancer cells from tumors, followed by migration, invasion, and expression of enzymes that break down the extracellular matrix, are activities of cancer cells during migation and invasion in early stages of tumor progression.

[23]Le XF, Merchant O, Bast RC, Calin GA. The roles of microRNAs in the cancer invasion-metastasis cascade. Cancer Microenviron. 2010;3:137–47.

[24]Junker A, Hohlfeld R, Meinl E. The emerging role of microRNAs in multiple sclerosis. Nat. Rev. Neurol. 2011;7:56–9.

[25]Qin S, Zhang C. MicroRNAs in vascular disease. J. Cardiovasc. Pharmacol. 2011;57:8–12.

[26]Budhu A, Ji J, Wang XW. The clinical potential of microRNAs. J. Hematol. Oncol. 2010;3:37 (7 pp.).

The miRNA, miR-21, is elevated in many tumors and promotes cancer cell proliferation, migration, detachment, and invasion, while suppressing apoptosis.

Still other types of miRNA modulate the final step of tumor metastasis, namely, the establishment of macroscopic tumors at distant sites. These include the miR-34 family (miR-34a, miR-34b, and miR-34c).

A variety of studies demonstrate that miRNA is likely suitable for classifying subtypes of any given cancer, and for serving as a prognostic factor (27). miRNA also plays a role in the etiology of immune disorders, such as multiple sclerosis (28,29), as well as diabetes (30), atherosclerosis (31), viral infections (32), and mental disorders, such as depression (33).

VII. CONCLUDING REMARKS

Time to distant metastasis is an excellent surrogate endpoint for the endpoint of overall survival for cancers where distant metastasis is almost always followed by death. The Wee study showed that TDM has the advantage over the endpoint of overall survival, in that a distinction between the two study arms can appear at an earlier time. The Roach study demonstrated that the endpoint of TDM could have an advantage over the endpoint of overall survival, where efficacy is apparent from TDM data, but where efficacy is not at all shown by overall survival data. The Loi study and the Foekens study demonstrate that gene expression data can be used as a prognostic marker, where the endpoint is TDM.

[27]Gusev Y, Brackett DJ. MicroRNA expression profiling in cancer from a bioinformatics prospective. Expert Rev. Mol. Diagn. 2007;7:787–92.

[28]Dai R, Ahmed SA. MicroRNA, a new paradigm for understanding immunoregulation, inflammation, and autoimmune diseases. Transl Res. 2011;157:163–79.

[29]Junker A, Hohlfeld R, Meinl E. The emerging role of microRNAs in multiple sclerosis. Nat. Rev. Neurol. 2011;7:56–9.

[30]Guay C, Roggli E, Nesca V, Jacovetti C, Regazzi R. Diabetes mellitus, a microRNA-related disease? Transl. Res. 2011;157:253–64.

[31]Qin S, Zhang C. MicroRNAs in vascular disease. J. Cardiovasc. Pharmacol. 2011;57:8–12.

[32]Li YP, Gottwein JM, Scheel TK, Jensen TB, Bukh J. MicroRNA-122 antagonism against hepatitis C virus genotypes 1–6 and reduced efficacy by host RNA insertion or mutations in the HCV 5′ UTR. Proc. Natl Acad. Sci. USA 2011;108:4991–6.

[33]Baudry A, Mouillet-Richard S, Schneider B, Launay JM, Kellermann O. miR-16 targets the serotonin transporter: a new facet for adaptive responses to antidepressants. Science 2010;329:1537–41.

17

Neoadjuvant Therapy Versus Adjuvant Therapy

Neoadjuvant therapy, also called induction therapy, refers to chemotherapy or radiation that is administered *before* surgical removal of tumors. Adjuvant therapy refers to chemotherapy or radiation that is administered *after* surgical removal of tumors. This chapter concerns a form of oncology study design involving two distinct steps, namely, a chemotherapy step and a surgery step. A similar concept occurs in study design and treatment for some autoimmune disorders, where this concept is that of an induction step and a maintenance step.

The use of an induction step and maintenance step is also described in this chapter.

Neoadjuvant therapy (1) and adjuvant therapy are more often used for solid tumors, and are less often issues for the hematological malignancies. When the term "adjuvant" occurs in articles on the hematological cancers, it is almost always the case that it refers to the following unfortunate adverse event. This adverse event is where previous adjuvant therapy for a solid tumor has the consequence of causing a hematological cancer, such as

---

[1]In a search in *Journal of Clinical Oncology* (2000–11), 1612 articles contained the term "neoadjuvant." But of these, zero articles contained the term, in the title/abstract, "acute lymphoblastic," "acute myeloid," "chronic lymphocytic," or "chronic lymphoblastic" (search conducted March 22, 2011).

leukemia or myelodysplastic syndrome, as documented elsewhere (2,3,4,5,6,7,8).

Chemotherapy and radiation therapy can take various forms. These forms include single-agent therapy, combination therapy, and sequential treatment (9). Sequential chemotherapy allows each of two different drugs to be administered separately at its maximally tolerable dose (10). Combination therapy may be preferred where the combination of drugs shows synergy or some additive effect, in terms of efficacy. Of course, additive effects of toxicity are not desired. Drug combinations that have a synergistic effect are reported, for example, by Carlomagno et al. (11), Rom et al. (12), Toledano et al. (13), Rodriguez-Galindo et al. (14), Gatzemeier et al. (15), and Tsimberidou et al. (16).

The ultimate goal of choosing neoadjuvant therapy over adjuvant therapy, or vice versa, is to increase patient survival. Chemotherapy can also be administered both before and after

[2]Flaig TW, Tangen CM, Hussain MH, et al. Randomization reveals unexpected acute leukemias in Southwest Oncology Group prostate cancer trial. J. Clin. Oncol. 2008;26:1532–6.

[3]Le Deley MC, Suzan F, Cutuli B, et al. Anthracyclines, mitoxantrone, radiotherapy, and granulocyte colony-stimulating factor: risk factors for leukemia and myelodysplastic syndrome after breast cancer. J. Clin. Oncol. 2007;25:292–300.

[4]Beaumont M, Sanz M, Carli PM, et al. Therapy-related acute promyelocytic leukemia. J. Clin. Oncol. 2003;21:2123–37.

[5]Praga C, Bergh J, Bliss J, et al. Risk of acute myeloid leukemia and myelodysplastic syndrome in trials of adjuvant epirubicin for early breast cancer: correlation with doses of epirubicin and cyclophosphamide. J. Clin. Oncol. 2005;23:4179–91.

[6]Crump M, Tu D, Shepherd L, et al. Risk of acute leukemia following epirubicin-based adjuvant chemotherapy: a report from the National Cancer Institute of Canada Clinical Trials Group. J. Clin. Oncol. 2003;21:3066–71.

[7]Chaplain G, Milan C, Sgro C, Carli PM, Bonithon-Kopp C. Increased risk of acute leukemia after adjuvant chemotherapy for breast cancer: a population-based study. J. Clin. Oncol. 2000;18:2836–42.

[8]Patt DA, Duan Z, Fang S, Hortobagyi GN, Giordano SH. Acute myeloid leukemia after adjuvant breast cancer therapy in older women: understanding risk. J. Clin. Oncol. 2007;25:3871–6.

[9]Buzdar AU. Preoperative chemotherapy treatment of breast cancer—a review. Cancer 2007;110:2394–407.

[10]Buzdar AU. Preoperative chemotherapy treatment of breast cancer—a review. Cancer 2007;110:2394–407.

[11]Carlomagno C, Farella A, Bucci L, et al. Neo-adjuvant treatment of rectal cancer with capecitabine and oxaliplatin in combination with radiotherapy: a phase II study. Ann. Oncol. 2009;20:906–12.

[12]Rom J, von Minckwitz G, Eiermann W, et al. Oblimersen combined with docetaxel, adriamycin and cyclophosphamide as neo-adjuvant systemic treatment in primary breast cancer: final results of a multicentric phase I study. Ann. Oncol. 2008;19:1698–705.

[13]Toledano A, Azria D, Garaud P, et al. Phase III trial of concurrent or sequential adjuvant chemoradiotherapy after conservative surgery for early-stage breast cancer: final results of the ARCOSEIN trial. J. Clin. Oncol. 2007;25:405–10.

[14]Rodriguez-Galindo C, Wilson MW, Haik BG, et al. Treatment of intraocular retinoblastoma with vincristine and carboplatin. J. Clin. Oncol. 2003;21:2019–25.

[15]Gatzemeier U, Pluzanska A, Szczesna A, et al. Phase III study of erlotinib in combination with cisplatin and gemcitabine in advanced non-small-cell lung cancer: the Tarceva Lung Cancer Investigation Trial. J. Clin. Oncol. 2007;25:1545–52.

[16]Tsimberidou AM, Wierda WG, Plunkett W, et al. Phase I-II study of oxaliplatin, fludarabine, cytarabine, and rituximab combination therapy in patients with Richter's syndrome or fludarabine-refractory chronic lymphocytic leukemia. J. Clin. Oncol. 2008;26:196–203.

surgery. Survival is the gold standard endpoint in clinical trials in oncology, however, any comparison of survival results from neoadjuvant versus adjuvant clinical trials should take into account adherence to the chemotherapy. In a review of rectal cancer clinical trials, Boland and Fakih (17) cautioned that, "[w]hile these results are in some ways disappointing, it is important to note the very poor rates of adherence to chemotherapy: 82% preoperatively and just 42.9% postoperatively." Review articles comparing neoadjuvant therapy with adjuvant therapy are available (18,19,20,21,22).

For cancer therapy involving radiation, please note that the unit Gray (Gy) refers to radiation doses. The Gray is defined as, $1\,Gy = 1\,J/kg$. This means that 1 Gy is the energy absorbed by a mass of 1 kg when exposed to ionizing radiation providing 1 J of energy. This unit was named after Louis H. Gray (1905−1965) (23,24).

I. ADVANTAGES OF NEOADJUVANT THERAPY

The advantages of neoadjuvant therapy over adjuvant therapy are listed here.

a. Killing Micrometastases

An advantage of neoadjuvant therapy is that there is no delay before administering therapy that is active against micrometastases, that is, metastases that are not detectable to the naked eye (25,26). Surgery is not effective against micrometastases.

b. Making Surgery Easier

Another advantage of neoadjuvant therapy is that it can down-stage tumors, with the consequence that tumors that could not be effectively removed by surgery, before

[17]Boland PM, Fakih M. The emerging role of neoadjuvant chemotherapy for rectal cancer. J. Gastrointest. Oncol. 2014;5:362−73.

[18]Miller E, Lee HJ, Lulla A, et al. Current treatment of early breast cancer: adjuvant and neoadjuvant therapy. F1000Research. 2014;3:198 (14 pp.).

[19]Schirren R, et al. Adjuvant and/or neoadjuvant thereapy for gastric cancer? A perspective review. Ther. Adv. Med. Oncol. 2015;7:39−48.

[20]Boland PM, Fakih M. The emerging role of neoadjuvant chemotherapy for rectal cancer. J. Gastrointest. Oncol. 2014;5:362−73.

[21]Janni W, von Minckwitz G, Möbus V, Nitz U. Adjuvant and neoadjuvant therapy with lapatinib in ErbB2-overexpressing breast cancer. Breast Care (Basel) 2008;3(s1):17−20.

[22]von Minckwitz G. Preoperative therapy: what, when and for whom? Ann. Oncol. 2008;19(Suppl. 5):113−6.

[23]Conger AD. Louis Harold Gray, M.A., Ph. D.; F.R.S. 1905−1965. Mutat. Res. 1966;3:1−2.

[24]Powers EL. Louis Harold Gray, 1905−1965. Phys. Med. Biol. 1966;11:329−331.

[25]D'Auria G, Ciprotti M, Conte D, et al. Neo-adjuvant and adjuvant chemotherapy in bladder cancer. Ann. Oncol. 2007;18(Suppl. 6):vi162−3.

[26]De Vita F, Giuliani F, Galizia G, et al. Neo-adjuvant and adjuvant chemotherapy of gastric cancer. Ann. Oncol. 2007;18(Suppl. 6):vi120−3.

the neoadjuvant therapy, become more operable after the neoadjuvant therapy (27). Some forms of surgery cannot be easily performed unless neoadjuvant therapy is first used to shrink the tumors (28). The term down-stage refers to standard classification schemes (staging) that are applied to various types of cancers.

A distinct advantage is that, for some cancers, surgery alone is simply not effective. Advanced colorectal cancer, for example, might require treatment with neoadjuvant chemotherapy followed by surgery (29). In the case of liver cancer, some tumors are located next to major blood vessels, and cannot be removed by surgery. In this case, neoadjuvant therapy allows subsequent surgery. In comments about liver cancer, Malik (30) finds that, "the presence of awkwardly placed tumours adjacent to vascular structures can today be regarded as a true test of inoperability."

c. Preserving Functions, or Cosmetic Issues, of Organs

Using chemotherapy to down-stage breast cancer allows the clinician to perform only a lumpectomy, and to avoid a mastectomy (31,32). In an account of advantages of neoadjuvant therapy, Bear et al. (33) state that:

> [n]eoadjuvant chemotherapy has become established as a reasonable alternative to adjuvant chemotherapy for ... breast cancer, since it can increase the rates of breast-conserving surgery and decrease the need for complete axillary lymph-node dissection. Neoadjuvant chemotherapy also offers the potential for rapidly testing regimens that may improve response rates.

Using chemotherapy to down-stage cancer of the larynx can allow the patient to live a life without having to use a tracheostomy tube, or without having impaired speech (34,35). Radiation plus chemotherapy, administered

[27]De Vita F, Giuliani F, Galizia G, et al. Neo-adjuvant and adjuvant chemotherapy of gastric cancer. Ann. Oncol. 2007;18(Suppl 6):vi120−3.

[28]Buzdar AU. Preoperative chemotherapy treatment of breast cancer—a review. Cancer 2007;110:2394−407.

[29]Gosens MJ, Dresen RC, Rutten HJ, et al. Preoperative radiochemotherapy is successful also in patients with locally advanced rectal cancer who have intrinsically high apoptotic tumours. Ann. Oncol. 2008;19:2026−32.

[30]Malik HZ. The case for neo-adjuvant chemotherapy for colorectal liver metastasis. Ann. R. Coll. Surg. Engl. 2008;90:452−4.

[31]White J, DeMichele A. Neoadjuvant therapy for breast cancer: controversies in clinical trial design and standard of care. Am. Soc. Clin. Oncol. Educ. Book 2015;35:e17−23.

[32]Esteva FJ, Hortobagyi GN. Can early response assessment guide neoadjuvant chemotherapy in early-stage breast cancer? J. Natl Cancer Inst. 2008;100:521−3.

[33]Bear HD, Tang G, Rastogi P, et al. Bevacizumab added to neoadjuvant chemotherapy for breast cancer. New Engl. J. Med. 2012;366:310−20.

[34]Worden FP, Kumar B, Lee JS, et al. Chemoselection as a strategy for organ preservation in advanced oropharynx cancer: response and survival positively associated with HPV16 copy number. J. Clin. Oncol. 2008;26:3138−46.

[35]Fung K, Lyden TH, Lee J, et al. Voice and swallowing outcomes of an organ-preservation trial for advanced laryngeal cancer. Int. J. Radiat. Oncol. Biol. Phys. 2005;63:1395−9.

before surgery for rectal cancer, may allow preservation of function of the sphincter (36,37). Glynne-Jones and Harrison (38) reviewed the goal of sphincter-sparing surgery, neoadjuvant chemoradiation versus adjuvant chemoradiation, and concurrent chemotherapy plus radiation versus sequential chemotherapy versus radiation, as it applies to rectal cancer. In this regard, it might be pointed out that the endpoint of *minimizing functional loss of an organ* can be used as one of the endpoints in an oncology clinical trial. However, the endpoint of *minimizing functional loss of an organ* is less important than the endpoint of overall survival (39).

One reason to preserve functions is to maintain an intact vasculature to a tumor, in order to allow efficient delivery of a drug to the tumor. If surgery is performed first, it could sever the blood supply to tumors that remain in the body after surgery, thereby preventing subsequent chemotherapy from reaching these tumors. Regarding this point, Franke et al. (40) state that, "because neoadjuvant therapy is delivered prior to resection, the intact ... blood supply maximizes the delivery of chemotherapy as well as avoids hypoxia (a known cause of tumor radio-resistance) within the target organ."

d. Enabling the Physician to Perform an Experiment That Enables a Decision Regarding Subsequent Therapy

Yet another advantage of neoadjuvant therapy, is that it provides the clinician with an opportunity to evaluate the effects of the chemotherapy on the tumors (41). In the words of Wood and Margulis (42), "presurgical therapy has the potential to provide real-time clinical feedback on the responsiveness of the patient's overall tumor burden to a given systemic therapy before committing the patient to what could be a highly morbid surgical procedure." Thus, an advantage of neoadjuvant therapy is that it allows the clinician to perform a little experiment with the patient, that is, to try one drug, and if that drug does not work, to increase the dose, to use a more prolonged dose, or to try a different drug (43). In a study

[36]Weiser MR, Quah HM, Shia J, et al. Sphincter preservation in low rectal cancer is facilitated by preoperative chemoradiation and intersphincteric dissection. Ann. Surg. 2009;249:236–42.

[37]Leibold T, Guillem JG. The role of neoadjuvant therapy in sphincter-saving surgery for mid and distal rectal cancer. Cancer Invest. 2010;28:259–67.

[38]Glynne-Jones R, Harrison M. Locally advanced rectal cancer: what is the evidence for induction chemoradiation? Oncologist 2007;12:1309–18.

[39]Licitra L, Vermorken JB. Is there still a role for neoadjuvant chemotherapy in head and neck cancer? Ann. Oncol. 2004;15:7–11.

[40]Franke AJ, et al. The role of radiation therapy in pancreatic ductal adenocarcinoma in the neoadjuvant and adjuvant settings. Semin. Oncol. 2015;42:144–62.

[41]D'Auria G, Ciprotti M, Conte D, et al. Neo-adjuvant and adjuvant chemotherapy in bladder cancer. Ann. Oncol. 2007;18(Suppl. 6):vi162–3.

[42]Wood CG, Margulis V. Neoadjuvant (presurgical) therapy for renal cell carcinoma: a new treatment paradigm for locally advanced and metastatic disease. Cancer 2009;115(10 Suppl.):2355–60.

[43]von Minckwitz G, Kümmel S, Vogel P, et al. Intensified neoadjuvant chemotherapy in early-responding breast cancer: phase III randomized GeparTrio study. J. Natl Cancer Inst. 2008;100:552–62.

of oropharynx cancer, Worden et al. (44) provided all patients with chemotherapy. Then, the investigators waited 3 weeks, after which the patients were taken back to the operating room for a direct laryngoscopy to assess the amount of tumor shrinkage, that is, to determine objective response (45). If there was over 50% response (extensive reduction in tumor size), then patients received chemotherapy plus radiation. But if the response was only 50% or less, patients were not given further chemotherapy, but instead received surgery plus radiation. Worden et al. (46) provide a detailed schema of their clinical trial. In a study of cancer of the larynx, Pointreau et al. (47) treated all patients with docetaxel, cisplatin, and 5-fluorouracil, followed by assessing response. Responders were treated with radiation (no surgery), and nonresponders were treated with surgery. The term response refers to objective response (size and number of tumors) as measured by a set of standard criteria, such as the RECIST criteria.

e. Improving Ability of Patient to Tolerate Chemotherapy

Still another advantage of neoadjuvant therapy over adjuvant therapy, is that the patient may have a greater tolerance to the toxic effects of chemotherapy (48). In contrast, in the case of gastric cancer, for example, chemotherapy taking place immediately after surgery may result in an increase in surgery-related adverse effects (49). Adjuvant chemotherapy may not be possible if attempted after surgery, because the adjuvant chemotherapy may need to be interrupted or delayed due to slow recovery from surgery (50).

II. ADVANTAGES OF ADJUVANT THERAPY

The advantages of adjuvant therapy over neoadjuvant therapy include the following.

a. Immediate Surgery and Reduced Risk of Metastasis

An advantage of adjuvant therapy is that there is no delay until surgery (51). Immediate surgery for bladder cancer, for example, will minimize the risk of metastasis during the

[44]Worden FP, Kumar B, Lee JS, et al. Chemoselection as a strategy for organ preservation in advanced oropharynx cancer: response and survival positively associated with HPV16 copy number. J. Clin. Oncol. 2008;26:3138−46.

[45]Worden FP. E-mail of September 8, 2010.

[46]Worden FP, Kumar B, Lee JS, et al. Chemoselection as a strategy for organ preservation in advanced oropharynx cancer: response and survival positively associated with HPV16 copy number. J. Clin. Oncol. 2008;26:3138−46.

[47]Pointreau Y, Garaud P, Chapet S, et al. Randomized trial of induction chemotherapy with cisplatin and 5-fluorouracil with or without docetaxel for larynx preservation. J. Natl Cancer Inst. 2009;101:498−506.

[48]D'Auria G, Ciprotti M, Conte D, et al. Neo-adjuvant and adjuvant chemotherapy in bladder cancer. Ann. Oncol. 2007;18(Suppl. 6):vi162−3.

[49]De Vita F, Giuliani F, Galizia G, et al. Neo-adjuvant and adjuvant chemotherapy of gastric cancer. Ann. Oncol. 2007;18(Suppl. 6):vi120−3.

[50]Teply BA, Kim JJ. Systemic therapy for bladder cancer—a medical oncologist's perspective. J. Solid Tumors 2014;4:25−35.

[51]D'Auria G, Ciprotti M, Conte D, et al. Neo-adjuvant and adjuvant chemotherapy in bladder cancer. Ann. Oncol. 2007;18(Suppl. 6):vi162−3.

time from diagnosis to surgery (52). Black and So (53) and D'Auria et al. (54) point out that if ineffective chemotherapy is delivered, there is a delay in providing surgery. In other words, attempts at providing chemotherapy that prove ineffective can potentially reduce survival.

b. More Accurate Staging

An advantage of adjuvant staging is that it enables more accurate staging of tumors (55,56,57,58). The particular stage of a tumor is routinely assessed for cancer patients, and is used as part of the entry criteria in clinical trials, and may be correlated with specific courses of treatment. However, if patients have been treated with chemotherapy or radiation therapy before surgery, staging of the tumor will not likely be accurate.

c. Drugs That Require Chronic Treatment, for Example, for 5 Years

An advantage of adjuvant therapy over neoadjuvant therapy is where the drug requires chronic administration. In this situation, adjuvant therapy must be used. For example, surgery for breast cancer may be followed by 5 years of administering tamoxifen (59,60,61). In detail, extended adjuvant endocrine therapy (tamoxifen) is recommended for postmenopausal women with endocrine-responsive breast cancers. The reverse type of study design, that is, neoadjuvant therapy for 5 years, followed by surgery, would not make any sense.

III. TWO MEANINGS OF THE WORD ADJUVANT

The term *adjuvant* has two different meanings. One of the meanings, which is the subject of this chapter, means therapy such as chemotherapy or radiotherapy that is given after surgery. The second meaning relates to vaccines. In the context of vaccines, adjuvant refers to a drug that provokes a nonspecific increase in immune response, that is, a specific drug that provokes an increase in immune response

[52]So A. Perioperative chemotherapy: the case for adjuvant chemotherapy for muscle-invasive bladder cancer. Can. Urol. Assoc. J. 2008;2:225–7.

[53]Black P, So A. Perioperative chemotherapy for muscle-invasive bladder cancer. Can. Urol. Assoc. J. 2009;3 (6 Suppl. 4):S223–7.

[54]D'Auria G, Ciprotti M, Conte D, et al. Neo-adjuvant and adjuvant chemotherapy in bladder cancer. Ann. Oncol. 2007;18(Suppl. 6):vi162–3.

[55]Witjes JA, Comperat E, Cowan NC, et al. Guidelines on muscle-invasive and metastatic bladder cancer. European Association of Urology; 2015 (60 pp.).

[56]Lorusso V, Silvestris N. Systemic chemotherapy for patients with advanced and metastatic bladder cancer: current status and future directions. Ann. Oncol. 2005;16(Suppl. 4):iv85–9.

[57]Tsukamoto T, Kitamura H, Takahashi A, Masumori N. Treatment of invasive bladder cancer: lessons from the past and perspective for the future. Jpn J. Clin. Oncol. 2004;34:295–306.

[58]Jacobs BL, Lee CT, Montie JE. Bladder cancer in 2010: how far have we come? CA Cancer J. Clin. 2010;60:244–72.

[59]Kennecke HF, Olivotto IA, Speers C, et al. Late risk of relapse and mortality among postmenopausal women with estrogen responsive early breast cancer after 5 years of tamoxifen. Ann. Oncol. 2007;18:45–51.

[60]Brewster AM, Hortobagyi GN, Broglio KR, et al. Residual risk of breast cancer recurrence 5 years after adjuvant therapy. J. Natl Cancer Inst. 2008;100:1179–83.

[61]Abrial C, Durando X, Mouret-Reynier MA, et al. Role of neo-adjuvant hormonal therapy in the treatment of breast cancer: a review of clinical trials. Int. J. Gen. Med. 2009;2:129–40.

against a wide variety of specific antigens. Immune adjuvants include cytokines, CpG oligonucleotides (62), poly(I:C) (63), imiquimod (64), and Freund's incomplete adjuvant (65). Immune adjuvants can increase the immuno-stimulatory effect of the vaccine (66,67,68).

IV. SUMMARY OF NEOADJUVANT VERSUS ADJUVANT THERAPY IN CANCER

Oncology clinical trial design includes the options of using surgery only, chemotherapy only, the combination of chemotherapy and surgery, and the option of radiation. These choices further compel the need for deciding the ordering of treatments, for example, using neoadjuvant therapy versus adjuvant therapy. It is interesting to note that, when a promising new drug becomes available, such as imatinib, the medical community responds by testing its efficacy in clinical trials that use neoadjuvant design and adjuvant design (69,70).

V. INDUCTION THERAPY VERSUS MAINTENANCE THERAPY IN AUTOIMMUNE DISEASES

a. Introduction to Induction Therapy and Maintenance Therapy

The concepts of sequential pairing of chemotherapy followed by surgery (or surgery followed by chemotherapy) in cancer have a counterpart in treatments for autoimmune diseases. Autoimmune disease treatment may involve induction therapy followed by maintenance therapy. As is the case with chemotherapy followed by surgery (or vice versa), it is the case that induction therapy may be followed by an assessment of response, with a defined interval of time required before initiation of maintenance therapy. The following reveals that induction phases and maintenance phases are used in the treatment of the autoimmune diseases, systemic lupus erythematosus (SLE), rheumatoid arthritis (RA), and psoriasis.

[62]Weiner GJ. CpG oligodeoxynucleotide-based therapy of lymphoid malignancies. Adv. Drug Deliv. Rev. 2009;61:263–7.

[63]Verdeil G, Marquardt K, Surh CD, Sherman LA. Adjuvants targeting innate and adaptive immunity synergize to enhance tumor immunotherapy. Proc. Natl Acad. Sci. USA 2008;105:16683–8.

[64]van den Boorn JG, Konijnenberg D, Tjin EP, et al. Effective melanoma immunotherapy in mice by the skin-depigmenting agent monobenzone and the adjuvants imiquimod and CpG. PLoS One 2010;5:e10626.

[65]Miller LH, Saul A, Mahanty S. Revisiting Freund's incomplete adjuvant for vaccines in the developing world. Trends Parasitol. 2005;21:412–14.

[66]Jahrsdörfer B, Weiner GJ. CpG oligodeoxynucleotides for immune stimulation in cancer immunotherapy. Curr. Opin. Investig. Drugs 2003;4:686–90.

[67]Aoki N, Xing Z. Use of cytokines in infection. Expert Opin. Emerg. Drugs 2004;9:223–36.

[68]Ishii KJ, Akira S. Toll or toll-free adjuvant path toward the optimal vaccine development. J. Clin. Immunol. 2007;27:363–71.

[69]Linch M, et al. Update on imatinib for gastrointestinal stromal tumors: duration of treatment. Onco. Targets Ther. 2013;6:1011–23.

[70]Sicklick JK, Lopez NE. Optimizing surgical and imatinib therapy for the treatment of gastrointestinal stromal tumors. J. Gastrointest. Surg. 2013;17:1997–2006.

b. Induction Phase and Maintenance Phase for Clinical Trials on SLE

A review article of various clinical trials on SLE referred to the use of drugs, in various combinations, for the induction phase and maintenance phase. To this end, Houssiau (71) described the use of cyclophosphamide (induction) and azathioprine (maintenance), or MMF (induction) and MMF (maintenance), or cyclophosphamide (induction) and MMF (maintenance), for the indicated phases. An example of commentary from this review included, "MMF was found to be superior to ... cyclophosphamide at inducting complete remission." MMF is mycophenolate mofetil.

The following Clinical Study Protocol provides a detailed account of the induction and maintenance phases, as applied to SLE (72,73). The study drug was MMF. In the induction phase and in the maintenance phase each used the MMF study drug, but different comparator drugs were used for the control arm.

The Protocol outlined these two phases as, "[a]fter screening assessment and randomization, subjects will return at Week 2, Week 4, and subsequently every 4 weeks until Week 24 of the induction phase. After re-randomization into the maintenance phase, subjects will initially return 3 times in the first 3 months ... [t] hereafter, subjects will return at every 3 months ... until Month 36 of the maintenance phase or study termination."

According to the study design, subjects were randomized and then treated in the induction phase, followed by determining efficacy (responders), followed by randomizing the responders and then treating them in the maintenance phase. Protocol instructed that, "the total sample for the induction phase will be 358 subjects (179 per treatment group) ... [a]pproximately 278 responders from the induction phase are projected to be randomized into the maintenance phase (139 in each treatment group)."

The induction phase had two arms, one arm receiving MMF and the other arm receiving intravenous cyclophosphamide (IVC). The Protocol's instructions included, "**Induction Phase.** MMF 1.5 g BID ... OR IVC 0.5 to 1.0 g/ m^2 in monthly pulses."

The maintenance phase included two arms, the MMF arm and the azithromycin arm. The Protocol's instructions included, "**Maintenance Phase.** MMF: 1 g BID with placebo matching azathioprine 2 mg/kg/day ... OR Azathioprine: 2 mg/kg/day with placebo matching MMF 1 g BID ... This part of the study is double-blind double-dummy. Subjects will take one active treatment (MMF or azathioprine) and the placebo matching the alternative treatment."

The fact that the active comparator drug used in the induction phase was different from the active comparator in the maintenance phase is emphasized by the Protocol's disclosure that, "[t]he active comparator during the induction phase is IV **cyclophosphamide** (0.5 g/m^2 to 1 g/m^2) ... [t]he active comparator during the maintenance phase is **azathioprine** (2 mg/kg/day)."

---

[71]Houssiau FA. Therapy of lupus nephritis: lessons learned from clinical research and daily care of patients. Arthritis Res. Therapy 2012;14:202 (8 pp.).

[72]Clinical Study Protocol. Protocol Number WX17801. Aspreva Lupus Management Study (ALMS) (April 12, 2007).

[73]The Clinical Study Protocol was a supplement to, Dooley MA, Jayne D, Ginzler E, et al. Mycophenolate versus azathioprine as maintenance therapy for lupus nephritis. New Engl. J. Med. 2011;365:1886−95.

c. Induction Phase and Maintenance Phase for Clinical Trials on RA

Bolge et al. (74) reviewed drugs, such as infliximab, that are used in various clinical trials on rheumatoid arthritis (RA), and described the use of induction phases and maintenance phases in these trials. Infliximab is an antibody that binds to tumor necrosis factor-alpha (75).

Commenting on these phases, the Bolge et al. (76) stated that, "Infliximab has been shown to reduce signs and symptoms of RA, inhibit the progression of structural damage, and improve physical function in patients with moderately to severely active RA. For this indication, the US Food and Drug Administration (FDA) recommends that infliximab, in combination with methotrexate, be administered at 3 mg/kg at weeks 0, 2, and 6 (induction period) and every 8 weeks thereafter (maintenance period)."

d. Induction Phase and Maintenance Phase for a Clinical Trial on Psoriasis

In an exemplary account of a clinical trial on the autoimmune disease, psoriasis, Gordon et al. (77) disclose the use of an induction phase and a maintenance phase. The induction phase lasted from weeks 0 to 12, and the maintenance phase was from weeks 12 to 52. The study drug was briakinumab, an antibody that binds to interleukin-23 (IL-23). IL-23 is a cytokine that is highly expressed in psoriasis skin lesions. Initially, the subjects were randomized to the study drug arm (briakinumab) or placebo arm. Then, after completing the induction phase, subjects were rerandomized to a study drug arm or placebo arm. In other words, after the induction phase, subjects from the study drug arm were rerandomized to study drug or placebo, and also subjects from the initial placebo arm were then rerandomized to either study drug or placebo.

VI. CONCLUSIONS

Neoadjuvant therapy and adjuvant therapy are mainstream topics in oncology. These terms refer to the pairing of sequential steps of therapy, that is, chemotherapy followed by surgery, or surgery followed by chemotherapy. Therapy of certain autoimmune diseases also involves sequential steps of treatment. These steps are called induction therapy and maintenance therapy. Because this chapter resides at an early part of this textbook, and because this book's emphasis includes oncology and autoimmune diseases, it is fitting that an account of the sequential steps used in autoimmune diseases be included at this point.

---

[74]Bolge SC, et al. Comparative multidatabase analysis of dosing patterns and infusion intervals for the first 12 infliximab infusions in patients with rheumatoid arthritis. Clin. Ther. 2012;34:2286—92.

[75]Takeuchi T, et al. Prediction of clinical response after 1 year of infliximab therapy in rheumatoid arthritis based on disease activity at 3 months: posthoc analysis of the RISING study. J. Rheumatol. 2015;42:599—607.

[76]Bolge SC, et al. Comparative multidatabase analysis of dosing patterns and infusion intervals for the first 12 infliximab infusions in patients with rheumatoid arthritis. Clin. Ther. 2012;34:2286—92.

[77]Gordon KB, Langley RG, Gottlieb AB, et al. A phase III, randomized, controlled trial of the fully human IL-12/23 mAb briakinumab in moderate-to-severe psoriasis. J. Invest. Dermatol. 2012;132:304—14.

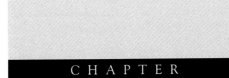

C H A P T E R

18

Hematological Cancers

I. INTRODUCTION

Cancers that are not solid tumors include hematological cancers, such as the leukemias and the myelodysplastic syndromes (MDS). Some of the hematological cancers are listed in Table 18.1 (1). Hematological cancers are sometimes called *liquid tumors* (2,3,4). This chapter concerns only the leukemias and the MDS. Other hematological cancers include multiple myeloma (5) and the lymphomas (6). This chapter explains methods for diagnosing the hematological cancers, as well as staging methods, biomarkers, and endpoints.

Acute lymphocytic leukemia (ALL) can be cured using combination therapy with dexamethasone, vincristine, L-asparaginase, and daunorubicin (7).

Chronic lymphocytic leukemia (CLL) can be cured with the combination of fludarabine, cyclophosphamide, and rituximab (anti-CD20 antibody). *Acute myeloid leukemia* (AML) can be cured with the combination of cytarabine and daunorubicin (or idarubicin). *Chronic myeloid leukemia* (CML), which is diagnosed by Philadelphia chromosome, can be cured with imatinib, dasatinib, or nilotinib (8).

Relapse-free survival (RFS) is an endpoint commonly used for the hematological cancers. In one report of a leukemia clinical trial, this endpoint was defined as, "[r]elapse-free survival (RFS) was determined only for patients who achieved a complete remission, and it was defined as the time from the date of complete remission until relapse, with deaths in

[1]Medinger M, Mross K. Clinical trials with anti-angiogenic agents in hematological malignancies. J. Angiogenesis Res. 2010;2:10.

[2]Hedrick EE. Personal communication, March 2, 2011.

[3]Abel GA, Friese CR, Magazu LS, et al. Delays in referral and diagnosis for chronic hematologic malignancies: a literature review. Leuk. Lymphoma 2008;49:1352—9.

[4]Dias S, Hattori K, Heissig B, et al. Inhibition of both paracrine and autocrine VEGF/VEGFR-2 signaling pathways is essential to induce long-term remission of xenotransplanted human leukemias. Proc. Natl Acad. Sci. USA 2001;98:10857—62.

[5]Szalat R, Munshi NC. Genomic heterogeneity in multiple myeloma. Curr. Opin. Genet. Dev. 2015;30:56—65.

[6]Upadhyay R, et al. Lymphoma: immune evasion strategies. Cancers (Basel) 2015;7:736—62.

[7]Freireich EJ, et al. The leukemias: a half-century of discovery. J. Clin. Oncol. 2014;32:3463—9.

[8]Freireich EJ, et al. The leukemias: a half-century of discovery. J. Clin. Oncol. 2014;32:3463—9.

Clinical Trials.
DOI: http://dx.doi.org/10.1016/B978-0-12-804217-5.00018-7

TABLE 18.1   Hematological Cancers

LYMPHOID CANCERS	
ALL	Acute lymphocytic leukemia; acute lymphoblastic leukemia[a]
CLL	Chronic lymphocytic leukemia; chronic lymphoblastic leukemia[b]
HCL	Hairy cell leukemia
MYELOID CANCERS	
AML	Acute myeloid leukemia; acute myelogenous leukemia
APL	Acute promyelocytic leukemia
CML	Chronic myeloid leukemia; chronic myelogenous leukemia
MDS	Myelodysplastic syndromes

[a]*The term acute lymphoblastic leukemia is 10 times more prevalent than acute lymphocytic leukemia, as determined by searching titles/abstracts, in articles published in 2000–11, in* Journal of Clinical Oncology. *Search conducted Mar. 21, 2011.*

[b]*The term chronic lymphocytic leukemia is 10 times more prevalent than chronic lymphoblastic leukemia, as determined by searching titles/abstracts, in articles published 2000–11, in* Journal of Clinical Oncology. *Search conducted Mar. 21, 2011.*

remission being censored" (9). Utilization of the endpoint of RFS requires a definition of "relapse." Another report of a leukemia clinical trial defined relapse as, "[r]elapse was defined as at least 5% blasts in the BM [bone marrow] or development of extramedullary leukemia" (10).

Solid tumors are sometimes treated in two steps, that is, with neoadjuvant therapy followed by surgery, or with surgery followed by adjuvant therapy. The hematological cancers involve a similar concept, namely, *induction therapy* followed by *consolidation therapy*. Induction therapy produces remission of the cancer, while consolidation is used to reduce any residual disease. Cooper and Brown (11) provide a definition for this relation in their writing that, "remission induction is followed by consolidation, which aims to eradicate the submicroscopic residual disease that remains after a complete remission is obtained." Expanding on this definition, as it applies to ALL, Cooper and Brown further state that, "[r]emission induction is the first block of chemotherapy, lasting 4 to 6 weeks. Patients are usually admitted to the hospital for their initial treatment ... but once any complications have stabilized the patient may be discharged before the completion of this phase with close outpatient follow-up. The goal of this block of therapy is to induce a complete remission by its completion, with approximately 95% of all patients achieving this benchmark." Cooper and Brown then describe consolidation as, "[l]asting approximately 6 to 9 months, it varies in length and intensity among different protocols, with those patients with higher-risk disease receiving

[9]Moorman AV, et al. IGH@ translocations, CRLF2 deregulation, and microdeletions in adolescents and adults with acute lymphoblastic leukemia. J. Clin. Oncol. 2012;30:3100–8.

[10]Chen Y, Cortes J, Estrov Z, et al. Persistence of cytogenetic abnormalities at complete remission after induction in patients with acute myeloid leukemia: prognostic significance and the potential role of allogeneic stem-cell transplantation. J. Clin. Oncol. 2011;29:2507–13.

[11]Cooper SL, Brown PA. Treatment of pediatric acute lymphoblastic leukemia. Pediatr. Clin. North Am. 2015;62:61–73.

longer and more intensive consolidation regimens. Consolidation is usually administered on an outpatient basis." Induction and consolidation are frequently used in therapy for leukemia therapy and MDS, occasionally in breast cancer therapy, but almost never for other types of cancers (12).

a. Classification of Hematological Cancers

Guidance for the classification of hematological cancers is available from the World Health Organization (WHO) (13,14,15). The WHO classification scheme is periodically revised, for example, to add genetic criteria to earlier-existing criteria that mainly rely on morphologic, cytochemical, and histological data. A separate classification scheme, that of the French-American-British (FAB) Cooperate Group, uses data on morphology and from cytochemical stains to classify the acute leukemias (16,17,18,19). The FAB scheme divides the leukemic cells of AML into eight subtypes, that is, M0, M1, M2, M3, M4, M5, M6, and M7. *Acute promyelocytic leukemia* (APL) is designated as subtype M3 (20). As disclosed below, APL is a subset of AML that comprises about 10% of adults with AML (21). Examples of clinical studies that use the FAB classification scheme can be found in the AML studies of Creutzig et al. (22),

[12]The terms induction and consolidation were used in 612 out of 1991 clinical trials on leukemia (one-third of all clinical trials), 41 out of 199 MDS trials (20%), 90 out of 3008 breast cancer trials, 9 out of 722 melanoma trials, 5 out of 715 prostate cancer trials, and only one out of 974 colorectal cancer trials. This search was conducted on the *Journal of Clinical Oncology* website on May 29, 2015 for all articles from 1983 to May 2015, inputting the name of the cancer in the title/abstract query box, and the terms induction and consolidation in the text query box (or omitted from the text query box).

[13]Swerdlow SH, et al., editors. WHO classification of tumours of haematopoietic and lymphoid tissues. 4th ed. Geneva: World Health Organization; 2008.

[14]Jaffe ES, Harris NL, Diebold J, Muller-Hermelink HK. World Health Organization classification of neoplastic diseases of the hematopoietic and lymphoid tissues. A progress report. Am. J. Clin. Pathol. 1999;111(1 Suppl. 1): S8−12.

[15]Vardiman JW, Thiele J, Arber DA, et al. The 2008 revision of the World Health Organization (WHO) classification of myeloid neoplasms and acute leukemia: rationale and important changes. Blood 2009;114:937−51.

[16]Das A, et al. An unusual case of phenotype switch between AML FAB subtypes. Clin. Case Rep. 2015;3:118−20.

[17]Miller DR, Leikin S, Albo V, Sather H, Hammond D. Prognostic importance of morphology (FAB classification) in childhood acute lymphoblastic leukaemia (ALL). Br. J. Haematol. 1981;48:199−206.

[18]Tallman MS. Relevance of pathologic classifications and diagnosis of acute myeloid leukemia to clinical trials and clinical practice. Cancer Treat Res. 2004;121:45−67.

[19]Willman CL. Molecular evaluation of acute myeloid leukemias. Semin. Hematol. 1999;36:390−400.

[20]Gregory TK, Wald D, Chen Y, et al. Molecular prognostic markers for adult acute myeloid leukemia with normal cytogenetics. J. Hematol. Oncol. 2009;2:23 (10 pp.).

[21]Rowe JM. Optimal induction and post-remission therapy for AML in first remission. Hematol. Am. Soc. Hematol. Educ. Program 2009:396−405.

[22]Creutzig U, Zimmermann M, Reinhardt D, et al. Early deaths and treatment-related mortality in children undergoing therapy for acute myeloid leukemia: analysis of the multicenter clinical trials AML-BFM 93 and AML-BFM 98. J. Clin. Oncol. 2004;22:4384−93.

Langebrake et al. (23), Lapillonne et al. (24), and Hess et al. (25). The FAB classification scheme is also used for the MDS (26) but in one specific context, that is, for predicting progression MDS to AML.

Cancerous cells in the various leukemias, and cancer cells in the various MDS, can be distinguished from each other by cytogenetics and by flow cytometry (27). The cytogenetics of ALL (28), CLL (29), AML (30), CML (31), and MDS (32,33), have been reviewed, as cited.

The nomenclature used for identifying the cytogenetics of the hematological malignancies has been standardized, and is periodically revised (34,35). The standard nomenclature is the *International System for Human Cytogenetic Nomenclature* (ISCN).

Flow cytometry, reviewed by Belov et al. (36), uses the CD nomenclature. The CD nomenclature can be used to distinguish between the various hematological cancers. "CD" stands for cluster of differentiation

[23]Langebrake C, Creutzig U, Dworzak M, et al. Residual disease monitoring in childhood acute myeloid leukemia by multiparameter flow cytometry: the MRD-AML-BFM Study Group. J. Clin. Oncol. 2006;24:3686–92.

[24]Lapillonne H, Renneville A, Auvrignon A, et al. High WT1 expression after induction therapy predicts high risk of relapse and death in pediatric acute myeloid leukemia. J. Clin. Oncol. 2006;24:1507–15.

[25]Hess CJ, Berkhof J, Denkers F, et al. Activated intrinsic apoptosis pathway is a key related prognostic parameter in acute myeloid leukemia. J. Clin. Oncol. 2007;25:1209–15.

[26]Haase D, Germing U, Schanz J, et al. New insights into the prognostic impact of the karyotype in MDS and correlation with subtypes: evidence from a core dataset of 2124 patients. Blood 2007;110:4385–95.

[27]Wood BL. Principles of minimal residual disease detection for hematopoietic neoplasms by flow cytometry. Cytometry B Clin. Cytom. 2015. doi:10.1002/ cyto.b.21239.

[28]Wetzler M. Cytogenetics in adult acute lymphocytic leukemia. Hematol. Oncol. Clin. North Am. 2000;14:1237–49.

[29]Higgins RA, Gunn SR, Robetorye RS. Clinical application of array-based comparative genomic hybridization for the identification of prognostically important genetic alterations in chronic lymphocytic leukemia. Mol. Diagn. Ther. 2008;12:271–80.

[30]Gregory TK, Wald D, Chen Y, Vermaat JM, Xiong Y, Tse W. Molecular prognostic markers for adult acute myeloid leukemia with normal cytogenetics. J. Hematol. Oncol. 20092;2:23.

[31]Tefferi A, Dewald GW, Litzow ML, et al. Chronic myeloid leukemia: current application of cytogenetics and molecular testing for diagnosis and treatment. Mayo Clin. Proc. 2005;80:390–402.

[32]Costa D, Valera S, Carrió A, et al. Do we need to do fluorescence in situ hybridization analysis in myelodysplastic syndromes as often as we do? Leuk. Res. 2010;34:1437–41.

[33]Steensma DP, List AF. Genetic testing in the myelodysplastic syndromes: molecular insights into hematologic diversity. Mayo Clin Proc. 2005;80:681–98.

[34]Shaffer LG, Slovak ML, Campbell LJ, editors. ISCN 2009: an International System for Human Cytogenetic Nomenclature (2009): recommendations of the International Standing Committee on Human Cytogenetic Nomenclature, Karger, Switzerland; 2009.

[35]Brothman AR, Persons DL, Shaffer LG. Nomenclature evolution: changes in the ISCN from the 2005 to the 2009 edition. Cytogenet. Genome Res. 2009;127:1–4.

[36]Belov L, de la Vega O, dos Remedios CG, Mulligan SP, Christopherson RI. Immunophenotyping of leukemias using a cluster of differentiation antibody microarray. Cancer Res. 2001;61:4483–9.

(37,38). Examples of the CD terminology include CD3, CD4, and CD8. The same type of CD terminology that is used to designate CD4$^+$ T cells and CD8$^+$ T cells is also used to identify leukemic cells. Flow cytometry has a routine sensitivity of detection of 0.01%, that is, one leukemic cell (blast) in 10,000 normal cells (39).

The earlier oncology chapters in this book focused on endpoints. In these previous chapters, there was little reason to spend time convincing the reader—to give an example—that prostate cancer cells are different from ovarian cancer cells, that prostate cancer and ovarian cancer occupy different organs in the body, or that prostate cancer inflicts only men and that ovarian cancer inflicts only women. It is obvious that prostate cancer occurs in the prostate gland. And it is self-evident that prostate cancer affects males, and that ovarian cancer affects females.

But things are not as clear-cut with the hematological cancers.

Distinguishing between the various leukemias is a subtle task. Thus, the focus of the present chapter is to distinguish the various leukemias, and between the various types of MDS. These distinctions are set forth below by the criteria used for diagnosing these cancers, the methods of treatment, and mechanisms of drug action.

The RECIST criteria are generally not used in clinical trials for leukemia or MDS, though Blum et al. (40) raised the potential utility of the RECIST criteria for monitoring lymph node dimensions, in the context of leukemia. Information on parameters, such as endpoints, inclusion/exclusion criteria, that are needed in Clinical Study Protocols for the hematological cancers, can easily be found on the world wide web at www.clinicaltrials.gov.

b. Secondary Hematological Cancers

The secondary hematological cancers are those that arise from prior chemotherapy for an earlier-existing disease, such as an earlier-existing cancer. Secondary AML (41,42) and secondary ALL (43,44) are well-documented. Secondary CML also occurs, but only on rare

[37]Zola H, Swart B. The human leucocyte differentiation antigens (HLDA) workshops: the evolving role of antibodies in research, diagnosis and therapy. Cell Res. 2005;15:691–4.

[38]Lai L, Alaverdi N, Maltais L, Morse HC. Mouse cell surface antigens: nomenclature and immunophenotyping. J. Immunol. 1998;160:3861–8.

[39]Campana D. Minimal residual disease in acute lymphoblastic leukemia. Hematol. Am. Soc. Hematol. Educ. Program 2010;2010:7–12.

[40]Blum KA, Young D, Broering S, et al. Computed tomography scans do not improve the predictive power of 1996 national cancer institute sponsored working group chronic lymphocytic leukemia response criteria. J. Clin. Oncol. 2007;25:5624–9.

[41]Stone RM, Mazzola E, Neuberg D, et al. Phase III open-label randomized study of cytarabine in combination with amonafide L-malate or daunorubicin as induction therapy for patients with secondary acute myeloid leukemia. J. Clin. Oncol. 2015;33:1252–7.

[42]Kayser S, Döhner K, Krauter J, et al. The impact of therapy-related acute myeloid leukemia (AML) on outcome in 2853 adult patients with newly diagnosed AML. Blood 2011;117:2137–45.

[43]Kelleher N, Olga G, Gallardo D, et al. Incidence, clinical and biological characteristics and outcome of secondary acute lymphoblastic leukemia after solid organ or hematologic malignancy. Leuk. Lymphoma 2015;12:1–6.

[44]Shivakumar R, et al. Biologic features and treatment outcome of secondary acute lymphoblastic leukemia—a review of 101 cases. Ann. Oncol. 2008;19:1634–8.

occasions (45). Secondary MDS (46,47,48) and secondary lymphomas are also well-documented (49). For example, survivors of Hodgkin's lymphoma, that is, after treatment with chemotherapy or radiation, are at risk for developing secondary leukemias, as well as other cancers, such as sarcomas, breast, thyroid, gastrointestinal, and lung carcinoma (50). Most secondary leukemias can be divided in two groups, those secondary to the use of two classes of agents that act on the chromosome: alkylating agents and those associated with topoisomerase inhibitors (51,52). The fact that damage to the chromosome, when left unrepaired, can lead to cancer is one of the most established precepts of biology (53).

c. Hematopoietic Stem Cells Give Rise to the Lymphoid Lineage and Myeloid Lineage

Normal blood cells, as well as neoplastic blood cells, arise from a type of stem cell called the hematopoietic stem cell. Hematopoietic stem cells differentiate into pluripotent stem cells which, in turn, gives rise to two lineages (54). The two lineages are the lymphoid lineage and the myeloid lineage. The lymphoid lineage includes T cells, NK cells, and B cells. The myeloid lineage includes red blood cells, megakaryocytes, macrophages, neutrophils, basophils, and eosinophils. Megakaryocytes are cells that manufacture platelets (55).

[45]Ramanarayanan J, et al. Chronic myeloid leukemia after treatment of lymphoid malignancies: response to imatinib mesylate and favorable outcomes in three patients. Leuk. Res. 2006;30:701—5.

[46]Haase D, Germing U, Schanz J, et al. New insights into the prognostic impact of the karyotype in MDS and correlation with subtypes: evidence from a core dataset of 2124 patients. Blood 2007;110:4385—95.

[47]Lee-Jones L, et al. Characterization of psu dic(6;5)(p21.3;q13) with reverse chromosome painting in a patient with secondary myelodysplastic syndrome following treatment for multiple myeloma. Cancer Genet. Cytogenet. 2004;148:49—54.

[48]Knipp S, et al. Secondary myelodysplastic syndromes following treatment with azathioprine are associated with aberrations of chromosome 7. Haematologica 2005;90:691—3.

[49]Cwynarski K, van Biezen A, de Wreede, et al. Autologous and allogeneic stem-cell transplantation for transformed chronic lymphocytic leukemia (Richter's syndrome): a retrospective analysis from the chronic lymphocytic leukemia subcommittee of the chronic leukemia working party and lymphoma working party of the European Group for Blood and Marrow Transplantation. J. Clin. Oncol. 2012;30:2211—7.

[50]O'Brien MM, et al. Second malignant neoplasms in survivors of pediatric Hodgkin's lymphoma treated with low-dose radiation and chemotherapy. J. Clin. Oncol. 2010; 28:1232—9.

[51]Leone G, et al. Therapy related leukemias: susceptibility, prevention and treatment. Leuk. Lymphoma 2001;41:255—76.

[52]Kantidze OL, Razin SV. Chemotherapy-related secondary leukemias: a role for DNA repair by error-prone non-homologous end joining in topoisomerase II—Induced chromosomal rearrangements. Gene 2007;391:76—9.

[53]Brower V. Tracking chemotherapy's effects on secondary cancers. J. Natl Cancer Inst. 2013;105:1421—2.

[54]Kindler V, Suva D, Soulas C, Chapuis B. Haematopoietic stem cells and mesenchymal stem cells as tools for present and future cellular therapies. Swiss Med. Wkly 2006;136:333—7.

[55]Brody T. Nutritional biochemistry. 2nd ed. San Diego, CA: Academic Press; 1999. p. 512.

Moreover, the lymphoid lineage gives rise to lymphoid neoplasms, while the myeloid lineage produces myeloid neoplasms. Reviews of lymphoid neoplasms (56,57,58,59) and myeloid neoplasms are available (60,61,62). The myelodyplastic syndromes are a subset of myeloid neoplasms (63).

The term "blast cells" is used in publications on leukemia, and hence will be defined. Blast cells are immature precursors of either lymphocytes (lymphoblasts) or granulocytes (myeloblasts). Blast cells normally represent up to 5% of the cells in the bone marrow. They do not normally appear in peripheral blood, but when they do, they can be recognized by their large size and primitive nuclei. When present in blood, blast cells often signify leukemia. Figure 18.1 discloses the existence of two kinds of blasts, myeloblasts (myeloid blasts) and lymphoblasts (lymphoid blasts) (64).

Leukemia involves impaired blast maturation. The leukemias are characterized by an accumulation of immature blast cells that fail to differentiate into functional cells (65). As a general proposition relevant to all cancers, Warner et al. (66) declared that virtually all cancers are clonal and represent the progeny of a single cell, and that leukemia represents a clonal expansion of blasts, where the disease is sustained by the leukemic stem cell (67,68).

[56]Pizzi M, et al. The role of molecular biology in the diagnosis of lymphoid neoplasms. Front. Biosci. (Landmark Ed.) 2014;19:1088−104.

[57]Jaffe ES, Harris NL, Stein H, Isaacson PG. Classification of lymphoid neoplasms: the microscope as a tool for disease discovery. Blood 2008;112:4384−99.

[58]Morton LM, Turner JJ, Cerhan JR, et al. Proposed classification of lymphoid neoplasms for epidemiologic research from the Pathology Working Group of the International Lymphoma Epidemiology Consortium (InterLymph). Blood 2007;110:695−708.

[59]Morton LM, Wang SS, Devesa SS, Hartge P, Weisenburger DD, Linet MS. Lymphoma incidence patterns by WHO subtype in the United States, 1992−2001. Blood 2006;107:265−76.

[60]Kuo FC, Dong F. Next-generation sequencing-based panel testing for myeloid neoplasms. Curr. Hematol. Malig. Rep. 2015;10:104−11.

[61]Vardiman JW, Harris NL, Brunning RD. The World Health Organization (WHO) classification of the myeloid neoplasms. Blood 2002;100:2292−302.

[62]Vardiman JW, Thiele J, Arber DA, et al. The 2008 revision of the World Health Organization (WHO) classification of myeloid neoplasms and acute leukemia: rationale and important changes. Blood 2009;114:937−51.

[63]Ornstein MC, et al. More is better: combination therapies for myelodysplastic syndromes. Best Pract. Res. Clin. Haematol. 2015;28:22−31.

[64]Permission granted by Terese Winslow (2007) Alexandria, VA (703) 836−9121; terese.winslow@mindspring.com.

[65]Warner JK, Wang JC, Hope KJ, Jin L, Dick JE. Concepts of human leukemic development. Oncogene 2004;23:7164−77.

[66]Warner JK, Wang JC, Hope KJ, Jin L, Dick JE. Concepts of human leukemic development. Oncogene 2004;23:7164−77.

[67]Faderl S, O'Brien S, Pui CH, et al. Adult acute lymphoblastic leukemia: concepts and strategies. Cancer 2010;116:1165−76.

[68]Campana D. Minimal residual disease in acute lymphoblastic leukemia. Hematol. Am. Soc. Hematol. Educ. Program 2010;2010:7−12.

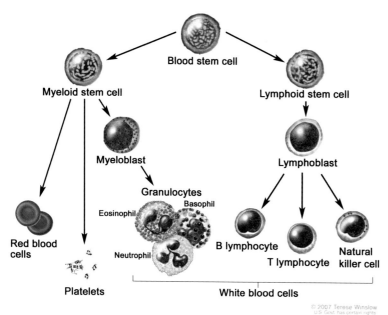

FIGURE 18.1 Normal differentiation pathways for the differentiation of various blood cells. The pathway begins with a stem cell, which becomes a myeloid stem cell or lymphoid stem cell. The myeloid stem cell differentiates into red blood cells, or a type of white blood cell, a neutrophil. The lymphoid stem cell differentiates into T cells, B cells, and NK cells. The leukemias involve a pathological accumulation of immature blasts.

d. Locations of Leukemic Cells in the Body

Leukemia generally arises from bone marrow. Leukemic cells circulate through blood vessels to organs and tissues throughout the body. Sometimes, leukemia can arise from outside of bone marrow, for example, from cells residing in lymph nodes or in a mediastinal mass (69). When the leukemia recurs, recurrence usually arises from a quiescent leukemic cell that was not eradicated by treatment. Depending on the site where the quiescent leukemic cell resides, relapse can occur in any part of the body, generally bone marrow, central nervous system (70), and occasionally the testes. The brain and testes are sanctuary sites, protected from chemotherapy by the blood—brain barrier or by the P-glycoprotein, which pumps drugs out of the cells (71). While relapse can occur in any tissue or organ, oncologists rarely refer to leukemic relapse as "recurrence in a metastatic site" (72). While the leukemias can metastasize to various parts of the body, that is, the liver, spleen, testes, or skin, leukemia causes a diffuse infiltration, rather than a mass (73). Regarding patients with CLL, 3—10% of CLL patients develop

[69]Pui CH. E-mail of January 2, 2011.

[70]Pui CH, Campana D, Pei D, et al. Treating childhood acute lymphoblastic leukemia without cranial irradiation. New Engl. J. Med. 2009;360:2730–41.

[71]Lee CA, Cook JA, Reyner EL, Smith DA. P-glycoprotein related drug interactions: clinical importance and a consideration of disease states. Expert Opin. Drug Metab. Toxicol. 2010;6:603–19.

[72]Pui CH. E-mail of January 2, 2011.

[73]Berg SL. E-mail of January 6, 2011.

what is called Richter syndrome or Richter transformation (74,75,76). This syndrome involves transformation of a leukemic cell to a lymphoma, where the neoplasm can occur in the lymph nodes, central nervous system, gastrointestinal tract, or eye. Lymphomas can be quantitated by a modified form of the RECIST criteria (77).

e. Lymphoid Neoplasms

1. Acute Lymphocytic Leukemia

In the United States, there are over 5000 new cases of ALL per year (78). The terms lymphocyte and lymphoblast refer to the cells that are involved. When normal, the cells are lymphocytes, but in ALL these cells are in a relatively immature state, and are therefore called blasts. For children under 15 years of age, ALL is approximately five times more common than AML, accounting for approximately 76% of all childhood leukemia diagnoses. Leukemia is the most common cancer diagnosis in children under 15 years of age (79). Appelbaum et al. (80) reviewed the endpoints used in clinical trials on ALL.

ALL can be treated by administering the enzyme, asparaginase (81,82). Asparaginase catalyzes the breakdown of extracellular asparagine into aspartic acid and ammonia. Depletion of extracellular asparagine inhibits the growth of lymphocytic leukemic cells. Unlike normal cells, lymphoblasts lack the enzyme that biosynthesizes asparagine, and thus require an exogenous source of this amino acid.

Imatinib (Gleevec®), shown below, is a small molecule that inhibits tyrosine kinase. Specifically, this drug inhibits the tyrosine kinase activity of the fusion protein, BCR-ABL (83). The drug is used for treating hematological disorders where cells contain the Philadelphia chromosome (or express BCR-ABL) (84). These disorders include CML and a subset of cases of AML. Regarding this subset

[74]Hartmann T. E-mail of January 28, 2011.

[75]Tsimberidou AM, Keating MJ. Richter syndrome: biology, incidence, and therapeutic strategies. Cancer 2005;103:216−28.

[76]Omoti CE, Omoti AE. Richter syndrome: a review of clinical, ocular, neurological and other manifestations. Br. J. Haematol. 2008;142:709−16.

[77]Assouline S, Meyer RM, Infante-Rivard C, et al. Development of adapted RECIST criteria to assess response in lymphoma and their comparison to the International Workshop Criteria. Leuk Lymphoma 2007;48:513−20.

[78]National Cancer Institute. What you need to know about leukemia. NIH publication no.08-3775; 2008 (55 pp.).

[79]Deschler B, Lübbert M. Acute myeloid leukemia: epidemiology and etiology. Cancer 2006;107:2099−107.

[80]Appelbaum FR, Rosenblum D, Arceci RJ, et al. End points to establish the efficacy of new agents in the treatment of acute leukemia. Blood 2007;109:1810−6.

[81]Asselin B, Rizzari C. Asparaginase pharmacokinetics and implications of therapeutic drug monitoring. Leuk. Lymphoma 2015;11:1−8.

[82]Masetti R, Pession A. First-line treatment of acute lymphoblastic leukemia with pegasparaginase. Biologics 2009;3:359−68.

[83]Woyach JA, Furman RR, Liu TM, et al. Resistance mechanisms for the Bruton's tyrosine kinase inhibitor ibrutinib. New Engl. J. Med. 2014;370:2286−94.

[84]Kantarjian H, O'Brien S, Cortes J, et al. Therapeutic advances in leukemia and myelodysplastic syndrome over the past 40 years. Cancer 2008;113(7 Suppl.):1933−52.

of ALL, about 20% of adult ALL cases and about 3–5% of childhood cases of ALL contain the Philadelphia chromosome.

The fact that imatinib and asparaginase are both useful drugs against ALL is revealed by the fact that both drugs have been administered to the same ALL patient, as was the case in the clinical trials of Schultz et al. (85) and Raetz et al. (86).

A chromosomal abnormality, known as the *Philadelphia chromosome*, commonly occurs in ALL. Philadelphia chromosome results from a translocation involving chromosomes 9 and 22, that is, t(9;22). As mentioned above, this abnormality is occurs in 3–5% of children and up to 20% of adults with ALL (87). The result is a fusion gene called BCR-ABL, where this fusion gene encodes a fusion protein (BCR-ABL).

BCR means *breakpoint cluster region*, and is a gene residing on chromosome 22q11.2 (88). *ABL* means *Abelson oncogene*, and is a gene residing on chromosome 9q34. The consequence of the translocation is the BCR-ABL fusion oncogene, where expression of this gene is the BCR-ABL fusion protein.

A diagram of the event of translocation, which produces two abnormal chromosomes, is shown below (89). Collectively, both translocation products are called the *Philadelphia chromosome* (90). In translocation, the tip of the long arm of chromosome 9 is joined to the body of chromosome 22, producing the Philadelphia chromosome. Simultaneously, the distal part of the long arm of chromosome 22 is joined to the body of chromosome 9. Philadelphia chromosome contains a fusion gene that consists of the amino part of *BCR* and the carboxyl portion of ABL.

Where the patient's leukemic cells contain Philadelphia chromosome, optimal treatment requires administering a tyrosine kinase inhibitor, such as imatinib (91,92). The decision to administer imatinib is based on the diagnostic test revealing the presence of Philadelphia chromosome (Fig. 18.2).

[85]Schultz KR, Bowman WP, Aledo A, et al. Improved early event-free survival with imatinib in Philadelphia chromosome-positive acute lymphoblastic leukemia: a children's oncology group study. J. Clin. Oncol. 2009;27:5175–81.

[86]Raetz EA, Borowitz MJ, Devidas M, et al. Reinduction platform for children with first marrow relapse of acute lymphoblastic leukemia: a Children's Oncology Group Study. J. Clin. Oncol. 2008;26:3971–8.

[87]Carroll WL, Bhojwani D, Min DJ, et al. Pediatric acute lymphoblastic leukemia. Hematol. Am. Soc. Hematol. Educ. Program 2003:102–31.

[88]Jabbour E, Cortes J, Kantarjian H. Nilotinib for the treatment of chronic myeloid leukemia: an evidence-based review. Core Evid. 2010;4:207–13.

[89]The author is deeply grateful to Prof. Bruce A. Rowe of the University of Oklahoma for providing a modification of my diagram of the Philadelphia chromosome. E-mail dated March 9, 2011.

[90]Fielding AK. E-mail of March 18, 2011.

[91]Apostolidou E, Swords R, Alvarado Y, Giles FJ. Treatment of acute lymphoblastic leukaemia: a new era. Drugs 2007;67:2153–71.

[92]Raetz EA, Borowitz MJ, Devidas M, et al. Reinduction platform for children with first marrow relapse of acute lymphoblastic leukemia: a Children's Oncology Group Study. J. Clin. Oncol. 2008;26:3971–8.

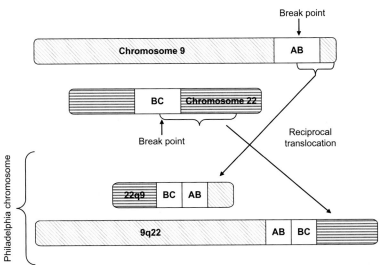

FIGURE 18.2 The Philadelphia chromosome. The Philadelphia chromosome occurs by a genetic event called a reciprocal translocation. The reactants are chromosome 9 and chromosome 22, and the products are collectively referred to as the Philadelphia chromosome. ABL, *Abelson oncogene locus*; BCL, *breakpoint cluster locus*.

2. Chronic Lymphocytic Leukemia

In the United States, there are about 15,000 new cases of CLL per year (93). CLL involves fever without evidence of infection, extreme fatigue, night sweats, weight loss (94,95). The disease also results in anemia or thrombocytopenia due to bone marrow failure. Infections are frequent. The disease also involves a rapidly rising lymphocyte count in peripheral blood, with a doubling time of less than 6 months.

The criteria for response to treatment include blood counts (lymphocytes, platelets, neutrophils), blood hemoglobin, and the number of nodules in the bone marrow, as set forth by the Guidelines from the NCI-sponsored Working Group Response Criteria for CLL (96), as well as progression-free survival (PFS) (97) and time to progression (TPP) (98). The endpoints of PFS and TTP require and depend upon acquiring data as set forth in these Guidelines.

Hallek et al. (99) provide methods for diagnosing CLL, for assessing the course of CLL, for assessing response of CLL to treatment,

[93]National Cancer Institute. What you need to know about leukemia. NIH publication no.08-3775; 2008 (55 pp.).

[94]Montserrat E, Moreno C. Chronic lymphocytic leukaemia: a short overview. Ann. Oncol. 2008;19(Suppl. 7):vii320–5.

[95]Yee KW, O'Brien SM. Chronic lymphocytic leukemia: diagnosis and treatment. Mayo Clin. Proc. 2006;81:1105–29.

[96]Cheson BD, Bennett JM, Grever M, et al. National Cancer Institute-sponsored Working Group guidelines for chronic lymphocytic leukemia: revised guidelines for diagnosis and treatment. Blood 1996;87:4990–7.

[97]Hillmen P, Skotnicki AB, Robak T, et al. Alemtuzumab compared with chlorambucil as first-line therapy for chronic lymphocytic leukemia. J. Clin. Oncol. 2007;25:5616–23.

[98]Elter T, Borchmann P, Schulz H, et al. Fludarabine in combination with alemtuzumab is effective and feasible in patients with relapsed or refractory B-cell chronic lymphocytic leukemia: results of a phase II trial. J. Clin. Oncol. 2005;23:7024–31.

[99]Hallek M, Cheson BD, Catovsky D, et al. Guidelines for the diagnosis and treatment of chronic lymphocytic leukemia: a report from the International Workshop on Chronic Lymphocytic Leukemia updating the National Cancer Institute-Working Group 1996 guidelines. Blood 2008;111:5446–56.

and the relevant endpoints. The diagnosis of CLL requires at least 5000 B lymphocytes per microliter of peripheral blood. The levels of membrane-bound proteins on the surface of the B cells, CD20, and CD79b, are low compared with levels found on normal B cells. Abnormal cytogenetics occur in more than 80% of all CLL cases. The most common deletions are in the long arm of chromosome 13. The relevant cytogenic abnormality is abbreviated as: del(13q14). This deletion occurs in part of chromosome 13. Other cytogenetic abnormalities of CLL include trisomy 12, deletions at 11q22, and deletions at 17p13 (100). These abnormalities can be determined by the fluorescence in situ hybridization (FISH) technique.

Parameters used for assessing the course of CLL and for assessing response include complete remission, partial remission, stable disease, and treatment failure. These parameters are determined by lymphocyte counts, lymph node size, neutrophil counts, platelet counts, and bone marrow cytology. Surrogate endpoints coupled with these parameters include TTP and PFS, while the clinical endpoint is overall survival.

CLL is often treated with fludarabine, though treatment is different for patients that are physically fit and those that are unfit. For physically fit patients, therapy with fludarabine, cyclophosphamide, and rituximab is the standard therapy, while for unfit patients, treatment is with an anti-CD20 antibody (obinutuzumab, rituximab, or ofatumumab) (101). Fludarabine is a purine analog. After entering the cell, it is phosphorylated to produce fludarabine 5′-triphosphate (102). After phosphorylation, the drug causes damage to the chromosome, that is, crosslinking of DNA (103). In turn, the crosslinking of DNA induces apoptosis. The structure of fludarabine is shown below.

Rituximab is an antibody that binds to CD20. CD20 is a membrane-bound protein of B cells. When this antibody binds to the CD20 of malignant B cells, the result is depletion of these cells (104). The mechanisms of action of rituximab in killing cancer cells includes the mechanism of antibody-dependent cell cytotoxicity (ADCC) (105). In a nutshell, in ADCC the antibody serves as an adhesive, that

[100] Alhourani E, et al. Comprehensive chronic lymphocytic leukemia diagnostics by combined multiplex ligation dependent probe amplification (MLPA) and interphase fluorescence in situ hybridization (iFISH). Mol. Cytogenet. 2014;7:79. doi:10.1186/ s13039-014-0079-2.

[101] Hallek M. Chronic lymphocytic leukemia: 2015 Update on diagnosis, risk stratification, and treatment. Am. J. Hematol. 2015;90:446–60.

[102] Gandhi V, Kemena A, Keating MJ, Plunkett W. Fludarabine infusion potentiates arabinosylcytosine metabolism in lymphocytes of patients with chronic lymphocytic leukemia. Cancer Res. 1992;52:897–903.

[103] Li L, Liu X, Glassman AB, et al. Fludarabine triphosphate inhibits nucleotide excision repair of cisplatin-induced DNA adducts in vitro. Cancer Res. 1997;57:1487–94.

[104] Bryan J, Borthakur G. Role of rituximab in first-line treatment of chronic lymphocytic leukemia. Ther. Clin. Risk Manage. 2010;7:1–11.

[105] Weiner GJ. Rituximab: mechanism of action. Semin. Hematol. 2010;47:115–23.

positions a CD8$^+$ T cell in close proximity with a cancer cell, thus ensuring that the CD8$^+$ T cell will kill the cancer cell.

3. Hairy Cell Leukemia

Hairy cell leukemia (HCL) is a rare type of cancer, accounting for about 2% of lymphoid leukemias (106). There are only 500–800 new cases in the United States per year (107). Cladribine (108,109), a drug that kills T cells, is effective in treating at least 80% of patients with HCL. One week of therapy typically results in remissions lasting for a decade (110). Cladiribine lacks the typical side effects of chemotherapy, such as nausea and alopecia, but it can facilitate infections from viruses or from

Pneumocystis jirovecii, a fungus formerly known as *Pneumocystis carinii* (111). Cladribine is distinguished in that it is also used for treating multiple sclerosis, as detailed elsewhere in this book.

f. Myeloid Neoplasms

1. Acute Myeloid Leukemia

In the United States there are about 13,000 new cases of AML per year (112). AML accounts for about 25% of all leukemias in adults (113). The disease presents by fatigue, bruising or bleeding, fever, and infection (114). Cheson et al. (115,116), Feldman et al. (117), and Appelbaum et al. (118), provide some of the endpoints used in clinical trials against AML.

[106]Chen YH, Tallman MS, Goolsby C, Peterson L. Immunophenotypic variations in hairy cell leukemia. Am. J. Clin. Pathol. 2006;125:251–9.

[107]Holzman D. Has success spoiled hairy cell leukemia research? Key questions go unanswered, despite big gains. J. Natl Cancer Inst. 2009;101:370–3.

[108]Freyer CW, et al. Revisiting the role of cladribine in acute myeloid leukemia: an improvement on past accomplishments or more old news? Am. J. Hematol. 2015;90:62–72.

[109]Maevis V, et al. Hairy cell leukemia: short review, today's recommendations and outlook. Blood Cancer J. 2014;4:e184. doi:10.1038/bcj.2014.3.

[110]Sigal DS, Miller HJ, Schram ED, Saven A. Beyond hairy cell: the activity of cladribine in other hematologic malignancies. Blood. 2010;116:2884–96.

[111]Hauser PM, Burdet FX, Cissé OH, et al. Comparative genomics suggests that the fungal pathogen *Pneumocystis* is an obligate parasite scavenging amino acids from its host's lungs. PLoS One 2010;5(12):e15152.

[112]National Cancer Institute. What you need to know about leukemia. NIH publication no.08-3775; 2008 (55 pp.).

[113]Deschler B, Lübbert M. Acute myeloid leukemia: epidemiology and etiology. Cancer 2006;107:2099–107.

[114]Jabbour EJ, Estey E, Kantarjian HM. Adult acute myeloid leukemia. Mayo Clin. Proc. 2006;81:247–60.

[115]Cheson BD, Bennett JM, Kopecky KJ, et al. Revised recommendations of the International Working Group for Diagnosis, Standardization of Response Criteria, Treatment Outcomes, and Reporting Standards for Therapeutic Trials in Acute Myeloid Leukemia. J. Clin. Oncol. 2003;21:4642–9.

[116]Cheson BD, Cassileth PA, Head DR, et al. Report of the National Cancer Institute-sponsored workshop on definitions of diagnosis and response in acute myeloid leukemia. J. Clin. Oncol. 1990;8:813–9.

[117]Feldman EJ, Brandwein J, Stone R, et al. Phase III randomized multicenter study of a humanized anti-CD33 monoclonal antibody, lintuzumab, in combination with chemotherapy, versus chemotherapy alone in patients with refractory or first-relapsed acute myeloid leukemia. J. Clin. Oncol. 2005;23:4110–6.

[118]Appelbaum FR, Rosenblum D, Arceci RJ, et al. End points to establish the efficacy of new agents in the treatment of acute leukemia. Blood 2007;109:1810–6.

AML develops in individuals of all ages, although the incidence increases with advancing age and rises dramatically in patients older than 65 years (119). In spite of therapy for AML, two-thirds of young adults and 90% of older adults still die of their disease (120). (But a rare subtype of AML, known as APL, is easily cured, as indicated below.)

Patients with AML show a heterogeneous response to therapy. The most frequent therapeutic approach is an initial phase (induction) with the combination of cytarabine and an anthracycline, which hopefully provides a remission, followed by postremission chemotherapy (121).

Chromosomal translocations resulting in fusion genes and fusion proteins are a common finding in AML. About half of AML patients have chromosomal abnormalities that involve fusion genes (122). In AML, the fusion genes, and the corresponding expressed fusion proteins,

include PML-RAR-alpha, RUNX1-RUNX1T1 (AML1-ETO), CBFb-MYH11 (123,124), MLL-AF9, and NUP98-HOXA9 (125). PML means *promyelocytic leukemia gene*; MLL means *mixed lineage leukemia*; RAR is *retinoic acid receptor*; CBF is *core binding factor*; NUP refers to *nucleoporin*; and HOX means *homeobox*. The results of these chromosomal abnormalities, which differ depending on the exact genes involved in the fusion product, can be increased self-renewal of the affected cell, increased long-term proliferation of the affected cell, or a block in maturation of the affected cell (126). From the variety of chromosomal rearrangements found in AML, it is obvious that AML is a very heterogeneous type of cancer.

Regarding patient outcome, some of the chromosomal rearrangements in AML are associated with an especially poor prognosis, while others are associated with a relatively good prognosis (127).

[119]Schiffer CA. "I am older, not elderly," said the patient with acute myeloid leukemia. J. Clin. Oncol. 2010;28:521–3.

[120]Rowe JM, Tallman MS. How I treat acute myeloid leukemia. Blood 2010;116:3147–56.

[121]Zuber J, Radtke I, Pardee TS, et al. Mouse models of human AML accurately predict chemotherapy response. Genes Dev. 2009;23:877–89.

[122]Abdul-Nabi AM, Yassin ER, Varghese N, Deshmukh H, Yaseen NR. In vitro transformation of primary human CD34 + cells by AML fusion oncogenes: early gene expression profiling reveals possible drug target in AML. PLoS One 2010;5:e12464.

[123]Camós M, Esteve J, Jares P, et al. Gene expression profiling of acute myeloid leukemia with translocation t(8;16) (p11;p13) and MYST3-CREBBP rearrangement reveals a distinctive signature with a specific pattern of HOX gene expression. Cancer Res. 2006;66:6947–54.

[124]Peterson LF, Boyapati A, Ahn EY, et al. Acute myeloid leukemia with the 8q22;21q22 translocation: secondary mutational events and alternative t(8;21) transcripts. Blood 2007;110:799–805.

[125]Abdul-Nabi AM, Yassin ER, Varghese N, Deshmukh H, Yaseen NR. In vitro transformation of primary human CD34 + cells by AML fusion oncogenes: early gene expression profiling reveals possible drug target in AML. PLoS One 2010;5:e12464.

[126]Abdul-Nabi AM, Yassin ER, Varghese N, Deshmukh H, Yaseen NR. In vitro transformation of primary human CD34 + cells by AML fusion oncogenes: early gene expression profiling reveals possible drug target in AML. PLoS One 2010;5:e12464.

[127]Miller BG, Stamatoyannopoulos JA. Integrative meta-analysis of differential gene expression in acute myeloid leukemia. PLoS One 2010;5:e9466.

CLINICAL TRIALS

In addition to chromosomal abnormalities, leukemic cells from AML patients show changes in gene expression. The term *gene expression* can refer to increases or decreases in the biosynthesis of mRNA, and it can also refer to changes in the rate of biosynthesis of the corresponding polypeptides. According to Miller and Stamatoyannopoulos (128), analysis of gene expression using microarrays revealed that poor prognosis in AML patients was associated with the up-regulation of several hundred different genes, such as *BCL11A, TBXAS1, HOXB5*, and *HOXA10*, while poor prognosis was associated with the down-regulation of several hundred different genes, including *EML4, C3AR1, SMG1*, and *SEMA3F*. Gene expression analysis can serve as a tool for predicting patient outcome, but it can also identify potential drug targets. The gene expression data were used as a basis for suggesting using *TBXAS1* and *SEMA3F* as drug targets (129).

AML is treated by two therapeutic steps (130). The first step is induction, which results in remission. The second step is postremission therapy, which prevents relapse. Drugs in use for treating AML include clofarabine (purine analog), laromustine (DNA alkylating agent), gemtuzumab ozogamicin (antibody), decitabine (inhibitor of DNA methyltransferase), and azacitidine (inhibitor of DNA methyltransferase) (131).

2. Acute Promyelocytic Leukemia

APL is a subset of AML, and comprises about 10% of adults with AML (132). APL manifests itself by spontaneous bleeding (133). The bleeding is potentially fatal, and it is recommended that treatment be started, after an emergency consultation with a hematologist, before the diagnosis is confirmed. Death can result from bleeding in the central nervous system, lungs, or gastrointestinal tract (134).

APL involves a chromosomal defect, where there is a translocation between chromosomes 15 and 17. This translocation generates the fusion gene involving the PML gene and retinoic acid receptor-alpha gene (RAR-alpha). PML stands for "promyelocyte." The resulting fusion gene and the expressed fusion protein are called PML-RAR-alpha. The fusion protein blocks the differentiation of the cells (135).

The disease is highly curable, where treatment involves all-trans-retinoic acid (a form of vitamin A) plus anthracycline. Patients also

[128]Miller BG, Stamatoyannopoulos JA. Integrative meta-analysis of differential gene expression in acute myeloid leukemia. PLoS One 2010;5:e9466.

[129]Miller BG, Stamatoyannopoulos JA. Integrative meta-analysis of differential gene expression in acute myeloid leukemia. PLoS One 2010;5:e9466.

[130]Rowe JM. Optimal induction and post-remission therapy for AML in first remission. Hematol. Am. Soc. Hematol. Educ. Program 2009;396−405.

[131]Schiller G. Current status of acute myeloid leukemia treatment in the elderly. Clin. Adv. Hematol. Oncol. 2009;7:580−2.

[132]Rowe JM. Optimal induction and post-remission therapy for AML in first remission. Hematol. Am. Soc. Hematol. Educ. Program 2009;396−405.

[133]Tallman MS, Altman JK. How I treat acute promyelocytic leukemia. Blood 2009;114:5126−35.

[134]Tallman MS, Abutalib SA, Altman JK. The double hazard of thrombophilia and bleeding in acute promyelocytic leukemia. Semin. Thromb. Hemost. 2007;33:330−8.

[135]de Thé H, Chen Z. Acute promyelocytic leukaemia: novel insights into the mechanisms of cure. Nat. Rev. Cancer 2010;10:775−83.

receive transfusions of platelets. APL can also be cured by administering all-trans-retinoic acid plus arsenic trioxide. Arsenic trioxide is As_2O_3. According to Nayak et al. (136), studies on APL patients have shown that all-trans-retinoic acid alone improves survival, arsenic trioxide alone improves survival, and the combination of both drugs further improves survival, that is, the effects are somewhat additive.

PML-RAR-alpha (fusion protein) retains both DNA-binding domains and ligand-binding domains of RAR-alpha (137). The fusion protein binds retinoic acid just as wild-type RAR-alpha binds retinoic acid. The fusion protein is thought to block cell differentiation by constitutively silencing retinoic-acid-responsive genes involved in the control of differentiation of hematopoietic precursor cells (138). The silencing of these genes, and the blocking of cell differentiation is reversed by administering retinoic acid (139). As reviewed by Nasr and de Thé (140), all-trans-retinoid acid induces the degradation of the PML-RAR-alpha fusion protein, and arsenic trioxide also provokes degradation of the PML-RAR-alpha fusion protein. Regarding the mechanism of action of arsenic trioxide, Goussetis et al. (141) find that it induces autophagy, a mechanism of cell death, while Shackelford et al. (142) find that arsenic trioxide induces apoptosis, another mechanism of cell death. Thus, when the combination of all-trans-retinoic acid and arsenic trioxide is used to treat PML, relief from cancer may result from killing of the cancer cells, but also by promoting the cancer cells to undergo cell differentiation to become non-transformed cells.

3. Methodology Tip—Platelets and Blood Clotting

Platelet transfusion is used in treating APL and the MDS. The relevance of platelets to blood clotting is as follows. The blood-clotting pathway is initiated when a wound releases tissue factor, and tissue factor is exposed to the bloodstream. Tissue factor resides in the walls of blood vessels (143,144). Following a rapid cascade of enzymatic events, prothrombin (catalytically inactive) is converted to

[136]Nayak S, Shen M, Bunaciu RP, Bloom SE, Varner JD, Yen A. Arsenic trioxide cooperates with all trans retinoic acid to enhance mitogen-activated protein kinase activation and differentiation in PML-RARalpha negative human myeloblastic leukemia cells. Leuk. Lymphoma 2010;51:1734−47.

[137]Segalla S, Rinaldi L, Kilstrup-Nielsen C, et al. Retinoic acid receptor alpha fusion to PML affects its transcriptional and chromatin-remodeling properties. Mol. Cell Biol. 2003;23:8795−808.

[138]Segalla S, Rinaldi L, Kilstrup-Nielsen C, et al. Retinoic acid receptor alpha fusion to PML affects its transcriptional and chromatin-remodeling properties. Mol. Cell Biol. 2003;23:8795−808.

[139]Minucci S, Monestiroli S, Giavara S, et al. PML-RAR induces promyelocytic leukemias with high efficiency following retroviral gene transfer into purified murine hematopoietic progenitors. Blood 2002;100:2989−95.

[140]Nasr R, de Thé H. Eradication of acute promyelocytic leukemia-initiating cells by PML/RARA-targeting. Int. J. Hematol. 2010;91:742−7.

[141]Goussetis DJ, Altman JK, Glaser H, McNeer JL, Tallman MS, Platanias LC. Autophagy is a critical mechanism for the induction of the antileukemic effects of arsenic trioxide. J. Biol. Chem. 2010;285:29989−97.

[142]Shackelford D, Kenific C, Blusztajn A, Waxman S, Ren R. Targeted degradation of the AML1/MDS1/EVI1 oncoprotein by arsenic trioxide. Cancer Res. 2006;66:11360−9.

[143]Mackman N, Taubman M. Tissue factor: past, present, and future. Arterioscler. Thromb. Vasc. Biol. 2009;29:1986−8.

[144]Mackman N. The many faces of tissue factor. J. Thromb. Haemost. 2009;7(Suppl. 1):136−9.

thrombin (catalytically active). Thrombin, in turn, catalyzes the activation of fibrinogen as well as the activation of platelets (145). In other words, thrombin activates two branches of the blood-clotting cascade (fibrinogen, platelets). The result is a blood clot, which takes the form of a network of crosslinked fibrin, where platelets are crosslinked to the fibrin.

4. Chronic Myeloid Leukemia

In the United States there are nearly 5000 new cases of CML per year (146). CML is a potentially fatal stem cell cancer that accounts for about 14% of all leukemias (147). More than 80% of patients complain of fatigue, regardless of the phase of CML. About 40% of these patients go to their primary care physicians for something unrelated, and in the process it is determined that their blood cell count is abnormally high. Jamieson et al. (148)

outlined the events leading to the immortalization of cancer cells in the myeloid leukemias, including CML.

Imatinib is used to treat newly diagnosed cases of CML. Where imatinib does not work, nilotinib or dasatinib, which are also tyrosine kinase inhibitors, can be used (149,150,151). As mentioned above, imatinib inhibits BCR-ABL tyrosine kinase.

The criteria for determining response to treatment include hematologic assessments and bone marrow cytogenetics (152), as well as time to treatment failure and PFS (153), Talpaz et al. (154) provide details on measuring hematologic and bone marrow cytogenetic responses during treatment of CML. Hughes and Branford (155) and Baccarani et al. (156) provide further information on using cytogenetics to measure response rates during treatment of CML.

[145]Brody T. Nutritional biochemistry. 2nd ed. San Diego, CA: Academic Press; 1999. pp. 524−39.

[146]National Cancer Institute. What you need to know about leukemia. NIH publication no.08-3775; 2008 (55 pp.).

[147]Sessions J. Chronic myeloid leukemia in 2007. J. Manage. Care Pharm. 2007;13(8 Suppl. A):4−7.

[148]Jamieson CH, Weissman IL, Passegué E. Chronic versus acute myelogenous leukemia: a question of self-renewal. Cancer Cell. 2004;6:531−3.

[149]Wei G, Rafiyath S, Liu D. First-line treatment for chronic myeloid leukemia: dasatinib, nilotinib, or imatinib. J. Hematol. Oncol. 2010;3:47.

[150]Terasawa T, Dahabreh I, Trikalinos TA. BCR-ABL mutation testing to predict response to tyrosine kinase inhibitors in patients with chronic myeloid leukemia. PLoS Curr. 2010;2:RRN1204.

[151]Baccarani M, Cortes J, Pane F, et al. Chronic myeloid leukemia: an update of concepts and management recommendations of European LeukemiaNet. J. Clin. Oncol. 2009;27:6041−51.

[152]Shah NP, Kantarjian HM, Kim DW, et al. Intermittent target inhibition with dasatinib 100 mg once daily preserves efficacy and improves tolerability in imatinib-resistant and -intolerant chronic-phase chronic myeloid leukemia. J. Clin. Oncol. 2008;26:3204−12.

[153]Kantarjian H, Pasquini R, Hamerschlak N, et al. Dasatinib or high-dose imatinib for chronic-phase chronic myeloid leukemia after failure of first-line imatinib: a randomized phase 2 trial. Blood 2007;109:5143−50.

[154]Talpaz M, Shah NP, Kantarjian H, et al. Dasatinib in imatinib-resistant Philadelphia chromosome-positive leukemias. New Engl. J. Med. 2006;354:2531−41.

[155]Hughes TP, Branford S. Monitoring disease response to tyrosine kinase inhibitor therapy in CML. Hematol. Am. Soc. Hematol. Educ. Program 2009:477−487.

[156]Baccarani M, Saglio G, Goldman J, et al. Evolving concepts in the management of chronic myeloid leukemia: recommendations from an expert panel on behalf of the European LeukemiaNet. Blood 2006;108:1809−20.

An organization in Europe, European Leukemia Net (157), recommends that response to treatments for CML include measuring cytology at various intervals, that is, at 3, 6, 12, and 18 months (158). Cytogenic response at the time point of 12 months has been used as a primary endpoint in clinical trials for CML (159). The term "housekeeping gene" refers to a gene used in the ordinary, day-to-day, metabolism of a typical or generic cell in the body, and that maintains constant expression, even when drugs are administered (160). Another endpoint used in CML clinical trials is genetic response, that is, the ratio of expression of BCR-ABL1 gene to the *ABL1* gene or to another housekeeping gene.

II. MYELODYSPLASTIC SYNDROMES

a. Introduction

Myelodysplastic syndromes (MDS) are a group of disorders involving anemia, neutropenia, and thrombocytopenia. The anemia results in chronic tiredness and shortness of breath, the neutropenia results in increased infections, and the thrombocytopenia (low platelets) results in increased bleeding and bruising. Hence, where a patient presents with anemia, infections, and bleeding, the physician might reasonably suspect MDS. The MDS are distinguished in that they can lead to another type of cancer, namely, AML (161). Even though MDS can occur at any age, most patients are older, and just over 70% of MDS patients are age 70 or older (162).

According to Bacher et al. (163), the diagnosis of MDS is not straightforward and may require a combination of techniques, such as cytochemistry using various stains, flow cytometry (a technique where cells are tagged with fluorescent antibodies), FISH, which involves hybridizing fluorescent nucleic acids to fixed cells, and molecular markers.

According to Barzi and Sekeres (164), higher-risk MDS patients survive only about 1.5 years, while lower-risk MDS patients survive about 3—7 years. The life-threatening aspects of MDS are hematopoietic insufficiency associated with severe anemia and fatal infections due to

---

[157] www.leukemia-net.org.

[158] Baccarani M, Cortes J, Pane F, et al. Chronic myeloid leukemia: an update of concepts and management recommendations of European LeukemiaNet. J. Clin. Oncol. 2009;27:6041—51.

[159] Tanimoto T, Hori A. To the editor. Second-generation BCR-ABL kinase inhibitors in CML. New Engl. J. Med. 2010;363:17 (1 p.).

[160] Wittwer C, Hahn M, Kaul K. Rapid cycle real-time PCR-methods and applications. New York: Springer; 2004. pp. 3—10.

[161] Barzi A, Sekeres MA. Myelodysplastic syndromes: a practical approach to diagnosis and treatment. Cleve. Clin. J. Med. 2010;77:37—44.

[162] Barzi A, Sekeres MA. Myelodysplastic syndromes: a practical approach to diagnosis and treatment. Cleve. Clin. J. Med. 2010;77:37—44.

[163] Bacher U, Haferlach T, Kern W, Weiss T, Schnittger S, Haferlach C. The impact of cytomorphology, cytogenetics, molecular genetics, and immunophenotyping in a comprehensive diagnostic workup of myelodysplastic syndromes. Cancer 2009;115:4524—32.

[164] Barzi A, Sekeres MA. Myelodysplastic syndromes: a practical approach to diagnosis and treatment. Cleve. Clin. J. Med. 2010;77:37—44.

neutropenia (low neutrophil count), plus the additional risk of leukemic transformation (165). Red blood cell transfusions may be used to treat the anemia, while platelet transfusions can be used to treat bleeding (166).

According to Orazi and Czader (167), exposure to benzene (168), diesel fuel, smoking, and immunosuppression, as well as chemotherapy or radiation therapy, are all risk factors for acquiring MDS. MDS has been associated with a number of chromosomal abnormalities, for example, those affecting chromosomes 5, 7, 8, 13, and 20, or the sex chromosomes. According to Komrokji and Bennett (169), a panel of diagnostic probes for the FISH technique is used for ensuring a proper diagnosis of MDS. These probes are specific for the 5q, 7q, 8q, and 20q chromosomal abnormalities. Malcovati and Nimer (170) provides a simple table for correlating each of these chromosomal abnormalities with each of seven different subtypes of MDS.

For most of these abnormalities, the relation between the abnormality and MDS is uncertain. In contrast, an association of a specific abnormality of chromosome 5 and MDS is well-established.

b. Classifying MDS and Assessing Prognosis

MDS is a collection of different diseases. The WHO classification system is used to identify the particular type of MDS. Each of these diseases can occur at a different severity. The International Prognostic Scoring System (IPSS), which in revised form is the IPSS-R, is available for scoring disease severity and prognosis (171). The IPSS-R has been validated (172). Ria et al. (173) and Steensma (174) provide side-by-side accounts of the WHO classification system and the IPSS. The IPSS score takes into account the fact that MDS can vary from being

[165]Greenberg PL, Young NS, Gattermann N. Myelodysplastic syndromes. Hematol. Am. Soc. Hematol. Educ. Program 2002:136−61.

[166]Latsko JM, Stone R, Shadduck RK, Breed C. MDS: Practical treatment approaches for physicians and nurses. Clin. Adv. Hematol. Oncol. 2005;3:1−7.

[167]Orazi A, Czader MB. Myelodysplastic syndromes. Am. J. Clin. Pathol. 2009;132:290−305.

[168]Galbraith D, Gross SA, Paustenbach D. Benzene and human health: a historical review and appraisal of associations with various diseases. Crit. Rev. Toxicol. 2010;40(Suppl. 2):1−46.

[169]Komrokji RS, Bennett JM. What is "WHO"?: myelodysplastic syndrome classification and prognosis. Am. Soc. Clin. Oncol. 2009;413−9.

[170]Malcovati L, Nimer SD. Myelodysplastic syndromes:diagnosis and staging. Cancer Control. 2008;15(No. 4, Suppl.):4−13.

[171]Bejar R, et al. Myelodysplastic syndromes: recent advancements in risk stratification and unmet therapeutic challenges. 2013 ASCO Educational Book; 2013. pp. e256−70.

[172]Voso MT, et al. Revised International Prognostic Scoring System (IPSS) predicts survival and leukemic evolution of myelodysplastic syndromes significantly better than IPSS and WHO Prognostic Scoring System: validation by the Gruppo Romano Mielodisplasie Italian Regional Database. J. Clin. Oncol. 2013;31:2671−7.

[173]Ria R, Moschetta M, Reale A, et al. Managing myelodysplastic symptoms in elderly patients. Clin. Interv. Aging 2009;4:413−23.

[174]Steensma DP. The changing classification of myelodysplastic syndromes: what's in a name? Hematol. Am. Soc. Hematol. Educ. Program 2009;645−55.

indolent to life-threatening (175). Indolent is a term of the art used to describe relatively benign lymphoproliferative diseases (176,177). The prognosis (risk) is used to guide treatment of MDS.

As reviewed by Orazi and Czader (178), the WHO system for classifying MDS provides these subtypes:

1. Refractory cytopenia with unilineage dysplasia with the subcategories of refractory anemia, refractory neutropenia, and refractory thrombocytopenia;
2. Refractory anemia with ring sideroblasts;
3. Refractory cytopenia with multilineage dysplasia;
4. Refractory anemia with excess of blasts (RAEB) with subcategories RAEB-1 and RAEB-2;
5. Unclassifiable MDS; and
6. MDS with isolated deletion (5q) chromosomal abnormality.

These MDS subtypes are based, in part, on the level or "depth" of anemia, neutropenia, or thrombocytopenia. The term *cytopenia* refers to the anemia, neutropenia, and thrombocytopenia (179).

While chromosomal abnormalities (dysplasias) are used for diagnosing MDS, these abnormalities also occur in deficiencies in folate or vitamin B12 (180). Hence a proper diagnosis requires exclusion of folate deficiency, exclusion of B12 deficiency, and may also require characterization of blood cells by flow cytometry (181,182). Flow cytometry in MDS mainly involves the analysis of white blood cells and immature red blood cells that still bear a nucleus. van de Loosdrecht et al. (183) provide a thorough review of the application of flow cytometry to MDS.

The IPSS score is a function of the percentage of blasts found in the bone marrow, the chromosomal abnormalities in bone marrow blood cells, and the blood cell counts, as indicated in Table 18.2 (184). What the IPSS score

[175]Ria R, Moschetta M, Reale A, et al. Managing myelodysplastic symptoms in elderly patients. Clin. Interv. Aging 2009;4:413–23.

[176]Cheson BD. The myelodysplastic syndromes. Oncologist 1997;2:28–39.

[177]Keating MJ. Leukemia: a model for drug development. Clin. Cancer Res. 1997;3:2598–604.

[178]Orazi A, Czader MB. Myelodysplastic syndromes. Am. J. Clin. Pathol. 2009;132:290–305.

[179]Kao JM, McMillan A, Greenberg PL. International MDS Risk Analysis Workshop (IMRAW)/IPSS reanalyzed: impact of cytopenias on clinical outcomes in myelodysplastic syndromes. Am. J. Hematol. 2008;83:765–70.

[180]Brody T. Nutritional biochemistry. 2nd ed. San Diego, CA: Academic Press; 1999. pp. 507, 512–4.

[181]van de Loosdrecht AA, Alhan C, Béné MC, et al. Standardization of flow cytometry in myelodysplastic syndromes: report from the first European LeukemiaNet working conference on flow cytometry in myelodysplastic syndromes. Haematologica 2009;94:1124–34.

[182]Ogata K, Della Porta MG, Malcovati L, et al. Diagnostic utility of flow cytometry in low-grade myelodysplastic syndromes: a prospective validation study. Haematologica 2009;94:1066–74.

[183]van de Loosdrecht AA, Alhan C, Béné MC, et al. Standardization of flow cytometry in myelodysplastic syndromes: report from the first European LeukemiaNet working conference on flow cytometry in myelodysplastic syndromes. Haematologica 2009;94:1124–34.

[184]Kouides PA, Bennett JM. Understanding myelodysplastic syndromes: a patient handbook. 2nd ed. Crosswicks, NJ: Myelodysplastic Syndromes Foundation; 2001.

TABLE 18.2 IPSS Score for MDS

Criterion	Score Value
BLASTS	
5% or less	0.0
5–10%	0.5
11–20%	1.5
21–30%	2.0
CYTOGENETICS	
Good[a]	0.0
Intermediate[a]	0.5
Poor[a]	1.0
BLOOD TEST FINDINGS	
0 or 1 of the findings	0.0
2 or 3 of the findings	0.5

[a]*Good: Normal set of 23 pairs of chromosomes, or a set having only partial loss of the long arm of chromosomes 5 or 20, or loss of the Y chromosome. Poor: Loss of one of the two (monosomy) 7 chromosomes, addition of a third (trisomy) 8 chromosome, or three or more total abnormalities. Intermediate is between "good" and "poor".*

measures is prognosis and risk (185). The IPSS is shown in Table 18.2. Blood test findings are defined as: neutrophils <1800 per μL; hematocrit <36% of red blood cells in total body volume; platelets <100,000 per μL).

c. Genetic Mutations in MDS for Use in Assessing Prognosis

IPSS-R is the primary criterion for assessing prognosis for MDS, and thus is the primary guide for determining treatment. Although gene mutations in MDS are not yet available for routine medical practice, mutations in genes such as *TP53*, *TUNX1*, *ASXL1*, *EZH2*, *RUNX1*, and *ETV6*, provide additional information on prognosis (186). Differences in survival of MDS patients with or without any of these mutations are clearly evident from Kaplan–Meier plots (187). Any given mutation can occur in all cancerous cells or, alternatively, the mutation can occur only in one subset of cancerous cell. The mutation profile can be used to guide treatment.

d. Treating MDS

Treatment of low-risk MDS patients depends on cytogenetics. For patients without del(5q), treatment is with agents that stimulate erythropoiesis such as erythropoietin (188), and for patients with del(5q), treatment is with lenalidomide (189,190,191). The term del(5q) refers to deletions of the long arm of

[185]Ria R, Moschetta M, Reale A, et al. Managing myelodysplastic symptoms in elderly patients. Clin. Interv. Aging 2009;4:413–23.

[186]Bejar R, et al. Clinical effect of point mutations in myelodysplastic syndromes. New Engl. J. Med. 2011;364:2496–506.

[187]Bejar R, et al. Myelodysplastic syndromes: recent advancements in risk stratification and unmet therapeutic challenges. 2013 ASCO Educational Book; 2013. pp. e256–70.

[188]Garcia-Manero G. Update on treatments for patients with myelodysplastic syndrome. Clin. Adv. Hematol. Oncol. 2010;8:407–9.

[189]Fenaux P, Ades L. How we treat lower-risk myelodysplastic syndromes. Blood 2013;121:4280–6.

[190]Ghosh N, et al. Expanding role of lenalidomide in hematologic malignancies. Cancer Manage. Res. 2015;7:105–19.

[191]Vozella F, Latagliata R, Carmosino I, et al. Lenalidomide for myelodysplastic syndromes with del(5q): how long should it last? Hematol. Oncol. 2015;33:48–51.

chromosome 5 (192,193). Breakpoints leading to deletions can vary, resulting in a variety different deletions in this chromosome. High-risk MDS patients may be treated with 5-azacytidine or with 5-aza-deoxycytidine (decitabine) (194). According to Atallah and Garcia-Manero (195), 5-azacytidine and 5-aza-deoxycytidine have comparable efficacies against MDS.

e. Transfusions in MDS

Many patients with MDS need transfusions of red blood cells at some point, while fewer patients need platelets (196). As detailed by Messa et al. (197), where a patient is treated with long-term tranfusions with red blood cells, the result may be toxicity due to iron overload. Transfusion dependency is a prognostic factor in MDS and portends worse prognosis (198).

Toxicity from long-term red blood cell transfusion is a potential side effect of chronic transfusions, but this is a risk only in patients with mild MDS (since patients with severe MDS die before iron toxicity occurs). Toxicity from free iron atoms results from the well-known Fenton reaction (199). To prevent iron toxicity, MDS patients are treated with iron chelator therapy.

In a nutshell, when assessing the prognostic factors for survival in MDS patients, the investigator needs separately to address the issue of whether anemia is severe enough to require transfusions (200), whether transfusions are prolonged enough to result in iron toxicity, and whether the potential for iron toxicity is so great as to require iron chelation therapy.

f. Chromosome 5 Abnormality and Lenalidomide for Treating MDS

According to List et al. (201), deletions involving the long arm of chromosome 5 are among the most common cytogenetic abnormalities found in patients with the MDS, with

[192]Westbrook CA, et al. Cytogenetic and molecular diagnosis of chromosome 5 deletions in myelodysplasia. Br. J. Haematol. 2000;110:847–55.

[193]Pedersen B, Jensen IM. Clinical and prognostic implications of chromosome 5q deletions: 96 high resolution studied patients. Leukemia 1991;5:566–73.

[194]Bernal T, Martinez-Camblor P, Sanchez-Garcia J, et al. Effectiveness of azacitidine in unselected high-risk myelodysplastic syndromes: results from the Spanish registry. Leukemia 2015. doi:10.1038/leu.2015.115.

[195]Atallah E, Garcia-Manero G. Use of hypomethylating agents in myelodysplastic syndromes. Clin. Adv. Hematol. Oncol. 2007;5:544–52.

[196]Barzi A, Sekeres MA. Myelodysplastic syndromes: a practical approach to diagnosis and treatment. Cleve. Clin. J. Med. 2010;77:37–44.

[197]Messa E, Cilloni D, Saglio G. Iron chelation therapy in myelodysplastic syndromes. Adv. Hematol. 2010;2010:756289 (8 pp.).

[198]Messa E, Cilloni D, Saglio G. Iron chelation therapy in myelodysplastic syndromes. Adv. Hematol. 2010;2010:756289 (8 pp.).

[199]Brody T. Nutritional biochemistry. 2nd ed. San Diego, CA: Academic Press; 1999. pp. 626–8, 903.

[200]Cazzola M, Malcovati L. Myelodysplastic syndromes—coping with ineffective hematopoiesis. New Engl. J. Med. 2005;352:536–8.

[201]List A, Dewald G, Bennett J, et al. Lenalidomide in the myelodysplastic syndrome with chromosome 5q deletion. New Engl. J. Med. 2006;355:1456–65.

frequencies from 16% to 28%. The MDS clinical trial of List et al. (202) demonstrated that lenalidomide is specifically toxic to cells containing a specific deletion in chromosome 5, namely, the 5q31 deletion. The inclusion criteria expressly required the 5q31 deletion in the affected cells of the study subjects. Therapy with lenalidomide resulted in remission in about half of the patients. The drug also restored production of red blood cells, apparently by its effect in suppressing the clone of myelodysplastic cells containing the 5q31 deletion. The investigators found that, "lenalidomide is selectively cytotoxic to 5q-deletion clones and restores red cell production in part by suppressing the myelodysplastic clone" (203).

g. Mechanism of Action of Lenalidomide

Studies of the mechanism of action of lenalidomide by Verhelle et al. (204) and Escoubet-Lozach et al. (205) revealed that the drug stimulates an increase in expression of the *p21WAF-1* gene, with the consequent halt in proliferation. In detail, $p21^{WAF-1}$, at increased levels, combines with various kinases, inhibits the kinases, where the result is reduced phosphorylation of pRB, and a consequent block of the cell cycle. In contrast, when lenalidomide

is added to normal cells (not cancer cells) the drug does not halt proliferation of the cells.

h. Mechanism of Action of 5-Aza-Deoxycytidine

5-Aza-deoxycytidine is a hypomethylating agent, that is, it reduces the amount of methyl groups that are naturally attached to deoxycytidine residues of the chromosomal DNA. As a consequence of this reduced methylation, genes are activated in the target cells, where the activation of genes that cause cell differentiation causes a cancerous cell to be noncancerous. The mechanism of action of 5-aza-deoxycytidine likely includes the following scenario (206). The drug is an analog of deoxycytidine, and is incorporated into the chromosome during DNA replication. Normally, specific residues of deoxycytidine in the mammalian chromosome are enzymatically methylated. Methylation is catalyzed by DNA methyltransferase. But when this enzyme attempts to catalyze the methylation of 5-aza-deoxycytidine, the enzyme becomes covalently bound to the DNA and is trapped. The consequence is a reduction of the amount of this enzyme in the cell, failure to methylate DNA, and the generation of under-methylated chromosomes.

[202]List A, Dewald G, Bennett J, et al. Lenalidomide in the myelodysplastic syndrome with chromosome 5q deletion. New Engl. J. Med. 2006;355:1456−65.

[203]List A, Dewald G, Bennett J, et al. Lenalidomide in the myelodysplastic syndrome with chromosome 5q deletion. New Engl. J. Med. 2006;355:1456−65.

[204]Verhelle D, Corral LG, Wong K, et al. Lenalidomide and CC-4047 inhibit the proliferation of malignant B cells while expanding normal CD34 + progenitor cells. Cancer Res. 2007;67:746−55.

[205]Escoubet-Lozach L, Lin IL, Jensen-Pergakes K, et al. Pomalidomide and lenalidomide induce p21 WAF-1 expression in both lymphoma and multiple myeloma through a LSD1-mediated epigenetic mechanism. Cancer Res. 2009;69:7347−56.

[206]Patel K, Dickson J, Din S, Macleod K, Jodrell D, Ramsahoye B. Targeting of 5-aza-2'-deoxycytidine residues by chromatin-associated DNMT1 induces proteasomal degradation of the free enzyme. Nucleic Acids Res. 2010;38:4313−24.

III. SUMMARY

Some of the topics relevant to solid tumors are also relevant to the hematological malignancies, for example, the endpoint of survival, prognostic factors regarding outcome for untreated patients, and predictive factors that predict the success of drugs. But the hematological malignancies are distinguished by the fact that the concept of metastasis is not applied, by the phenomenally high cure rate for some of the leukemias (HCL, APL), by the fact that the hematological neoplasms may be unusually difficult to distinguish from each other, and by the fact that the RECIST criteria are not used.

IV. CYTOGENETICS OF HEMATOLOGICAL CANCERS

a. Introduction

The human chromosomes are numbered 1–22, with two additional chromosomes called X and Y. Chromosomes 1–22 occur as two copies in every somatic cell. The X chromosome occurs as two copies in every female somatic cell, but only once in every male somatic cell. The Y chromosome occurs only once in every male somatic cell. Thus, the sex chromosomes in males are XY, and the sex chromosomes in females are XX. Altogether, human somatic cells have 46 chromosomes (207). During mitosis, the genome condenses to form chromosomes that can be seen using a light microscope. The appearance of these chromosomes is called the *karyotype*.

In a point in the cell cycle, that is, during metaphase, each of the chromosomes can be seen to have two arms, the p arm and the q arm. The letter p refers to the short arm, while q refers to the long arm. Within each arm, numbers are assigned to large areas called regions, and another set of numbers is used to refer to bands within the regions. Numbering starts from the centromere, and increases as one moves towards the tip of each arm (208).

To provide an example, the term "14q32" refers to the second band in the third region of the q arm of chromosome 14 (209). (It is not the case that the number 32 is read as thirty-two. Instead, it is read as three-two.) Another example is as follows. The breast cancer gene *BRCA1* is located at 17q21.31. This means that the gene is located on the q arm of chromosome 17, in region 2. Within region 2, the gene is located in band 1. Collectively, this may be called, "band two, one." Within band 21, the gene resides in sub-band 31. Regarding the number 31, the 3 refers to a sub-band, and the number 1 refers to a sub-band within sub-band 3 (210).

b. Cytogenetics for Diagnosis and Prediction—AML

The following cytogenetic markers are used for predicting outcome for AML (211). These markers predict favorable prognosis, intermediate prognosis, and poor prognosis, as indicated:

[207]Tijio JH, Levan A. The chromosome number in man. Hereditas 1956;42:1–6.

[208]Pasternak JJ. An introduction to human genetics. 2nd ed. Hoboken, NJ: John Wiley and Sons, Inc.; 2005. p. 27.

[209]Jorde LB, Carey JC, Bamshad MJ, White RL. Medical genetics. 3rd ed. St. Louis, MO: Mosby; 2003. p. 108.

[210]Pasternak JJ. An introduction to human genetics. 2nd ed. Hoboken, NJ: John Wiley and Sons, Inc.; 2005. pp. 27–8.

[211]Gregory TK, Wald D, Chen Y, Vermaat JM, Xiong Y, Tse W. Molecular prognostic markers for adult acute myeloid leukemia with normal cytogenetics. J. Hematol. Oncol. 2009;2:23.

- Favorable prognosis: inv(16); t(15;17); and t(8;21).
- Intermediate prognosis: no identifiable abnormal cytogenetics.
- Poor prognosis: monosomy 5; monosomy 7; and 11q23.

These cytogenetic markers result in the creation of a number of fusion genes, as indicated in the following table. AML patients with no identifiable abnormal cytogenetics (using the microscope) have been classified according to a number of specific genetic mutations, as determined by DNA sequencing, where these genetic mutations provide prognostic value. Table 18.3 discloses the prognostic value of these mutant genes.

c. Cytogenetics for Diagnosis and Prediction—ALL

Cytogenetic characteristics may be the most important prognostic factor for ALL, according to Cortes and Kantarjian (212). These abnormalities can take the form of changes in the number of chromosomes, or changes in the structure of the affected chromosomes, as shown in Table 18.4. All numbers (%) in the table are from Cortes and Kantarjian (213), unless specified otherwise.

This concerns some of the abnormalities listed in the table.

1. Numeric Abnormalities in ALL

Patients with hyperdiploid ALL, in particular those with more than 50 chromosomes, have the best prognosis. Hypodiploidy (less than 44 chromosomes), which is found in less than 2% of pediatric or adult cases, predicts a poor outcome. The rare cases with low hypodiploidy (33–39 chromosomes) and near-haploidy (23–29 chromosomes) have a particularly poor prognosis.

2. Structural Abnormality t(9;22) (Philadelphia Chromosome) in ALL

The outcome for ALL patients with blasts containing the Philadelphia chromosome is poor (214). The Philadelphia chromosome in ALL may be different from that found in CML. In ALL, this chromosome involves band 34 of the long arm of chromosome 9, splicing the proto-oncogene c-abl to band 11 of the long arm of chromosome 22 in the bcr gene. In 50–80% of cases of ALL, the breakpoint in 22q11 falls between exons b1 and b2 of the major breakpoint cluster region, as opposed to between b2 and b3 or b3 and b4 in CML. The difference is in the positions of the breakpoints occurring in the translocation, that is, breakpoints within the BCR gene. This difference in breakpoints results in a smaller polypeptide of 190 kDa (p190 BCR/ABL) in ALL, and a larger polypeptide in CML (210 kDa, p210 BCR/ABL) (215,216). Both polypeptides have increased tyrosine kinase activity.

---

[212]Cortes JE, Kantarjian HM. Acute lymphoblastic leukemia. A comprehensive review with emphasis on biology and therapy. Cancer 1995;76:2393–417.

[213]Cortes JE, Kantarjian HM. Acute lymphoblastic leukemia. A comprehensive review with emphasis on biology and therapy. Cancer 1995;76:2393–417.

[214]Cortes JE, Kantarjian HM. Acute lymphoblastic leukemia. A comprehensive review with emphasis on biology and therapy. Cancer 1995;76:2393–417.

[215]Score J, Calasanz MJ, Ottman O, et al. Analysis of genomic breakpoints in p190 and p210 BCR-ABL indicate distinct mechanisms of formation. Leukemia 2010;24:1742–50.

[216]Cortes JE, Kantarjian HM. Acute lymphoblastic leukemia. A comprehensive review with emphasis on biology and therapy. Cancer 1995;76:2393–417.

TABLE 18.3 Cytogenetics for Favorable, Intermediate, and Poor Prognosis for AML

FAVORABLE PROGNOSIS

Abnormal chromosome[a]	Commentary on the abnormal chromosome
inv(16)	The abnormal chromosome encodes the fusion gene, *CBFB/MYH11*[b]
t(15;17)	The abnormal chromosome encodes the fusion gene, PML/RAR-alpha[c,d]
t(8;21)	The abnormal chromosome encodes the fusion gene, *AML1/ETO*,[b,d,e] also called *RUNX1/MTG8*

INTERMEDIATE PROGNOSIS (NO IDENTIFIABLE CHROMOSOMAL ABNORMALITIES)

Abnormal gene[a]	Mutations or overexpression of the following genes indicate poor prognosis in patients not showing any chromosomal abnormalities
NPMI	Nucleophosmin. Nucleophosmin mutations occur in 50–60% of adult AML patients, where there are no chromosomal abnormalities
FLT3	Fms-like tyrosine kinase 3 gene
MLL	Mixed lineage leukemia gene
CEBP-alpha	CCAT/enhancer binding protein alpha
BAALC[f]	Brain and acute leukemia cytoplasmic
MN1	Meningioma 1
ERG[g]	ETS-related gene
AF1q	AF1q

POOR PROGNOSIS

Abnormal chromosome[a]	Commentary on the chromosomal abnormality
Monosomy 5	Monosomy 5 means loss of material from chromosome 5[h,i]
Monosomy 7	Monosomy 7 means loss of material from chromosome 7[j]
11q23	11q23 encompasses various chromosomal abnormalities.[k] Different AML patients show different fusion products, for example, t(9;11), t(11;19), t(6;11), where all of these indicate poor prognosis.[l] 11q23 encompasses an abnormality called MLL rearrangement, which involves the *MLL* gene. About 95% of patients with 11q23 abnormalities have the MLL rearrangement.[m] The MLL rearrangement occurs in two types of acute leukemias, AML and ALL. The term MLL refers to the mixed lineage leukemia gene, which encodes a transcription factor

[a]Gregory TK, Wald D, Chen Y, Vermaat JM, Xiong Y, Tse W. Molecular prognostic markers for adult acute myeloid leukemia with normal cytogenetics. J. Hematol. Oncol. 2009;2:23.

[b]Marcucci G, Mrózek K, Ruppert AS, et al. Prognostic factors and outcome of core binding factor acute myeloid leukemia patients with t(8;21) differ from those of patients with inv(16): a Cancer and Leukemia Group B study. J. Clin. Oncol. 2005;23:5705–17.

[c]Payton JE, Grieselhuber NR, Chang LW, et al. High throughput digital quantification of mRNA abundance in primary human acute myeloid leukemia samples. J. Clin. Invest. 2009;119:1714–26.

[d]Petrie K, Zelent A. AML1/ETO, a promiscuous fusion oncoprotein. Blood 2007;109:4109–10.

[e]Xiao Z, Greaves MF, Buffler P, et al. Molecular characterization of genomic AML1-ETO fusions in childhood leukemia. Leukemia 2001;15:1906–13.

[f]BAALC is located on chromosome 8 at 8q22.3. BAALC has GenBank Accession No. AF363578.

[g]ERG is located on chromosome 21, at 21q22.3. ERG has GenBank Accession No. NM_004449.

[h]Herry A, Douet-Guilbert N, Morel F, Le Bris MJ, De Braekeleer M. Redefining monosomy 5 by molecular cytogenetics in 23 patients with MDS/AML. Eur. J. Haematol. 2007;78:457–67.

[i]Bram S, Swolin B, Rödjer S, Stockelberg D, Ogärd I, Bäck H. Is monosomy 5 an uncommon aberration? Fluorescence in situ hybridization reveals translocations and deletions in myelodysplastic syndromes or acute myelocytic leukemia. Cancer Genet. Cytogenet. 2003;142:107–14.

[j]Hasle H, Alonzo TA, Auvrignon A, et al. Monosomy 7 and deletion 7q in children and adolescents with acute myeloid leukemia: an international retrospective study. Blood 2007;109:4641–7.

[k]Harrison CJ, Hills RK, Moorman AV, et al. Cytogenetics of childhood acute myeloid leukemia: United Kingdom Medical Research Council Treatment trials AML 10 and 12. J. Clin. Oncol. 2010;28:2674–81.

[l]Tamai H, Yamaguchi H, Hamaguchi H, et al. Clinical features of adult acute leukemia with 11q23 abnormalities in Japan: a co-operative multicenter study. Int. J. Hematol. 2008;87(2):195–202.

[m]Zangrando A, Dell'orto MC, Te Kronnie G, Basso G. MLL rearrangements in pediatric acute lymphoblastic and myeloblastic leukemias: MLL specific and lineage specific signatures. BMC Med. Genom. 2009;2:36 (12 pp.).

TABLE 18.4 Cytogenetic Abnormalities in ALL

Cytogenic Abnormality	Incidence in Children (%)	Incidence in Adults (%)
NUMERIC ABNORMALITIES		
Hyperdiploid	40–50	10–20
47–50 chromosomes	15–20	5–10
Over 50 chromosomes	25–30	5–10
Diploid	10–30	25–35
Hypodiploid	7–10, 5[a]	5–10, 5[a]; 18[b]
STRUCTURAL ABNORMALITIES		
Pseudodiploid	40–50	50–60; 69[b]
t(9;22)(q34;q11) "the Philadelphia chromosome"	3–5; 4[b]	15–25; 15[c]; 40[b]
t(8;14), t(8;2), and t(8;22)	3–5	5–10; 7[c]
t(4;11)(q21;q23)	5	5; 4[c]
t(1;19)(q23;p13.3)	5–7	Less than 5; 3[c]
4q11	Less than 5	5–10
7q35	Less than 5	Less than 5
t(12;21)(p13;q22)	25[d,e,f]	2–3[d,e,f]

[a]Harrison CJ, Moorman AV, Broadfield ZJ, et al. Three distinct subgroups of hypodiploidy in acute lymphoblastic leukaemia. Br. J. Haematol. 2004;125:552–9.

[b]De Braekeleer E, Douet-Guilbert N, Morel F, et al. Philadelphia chromosome-positive acute lymphoblastic leukemia: a cytogenetic study of 33 patients diagnosed between 1981 and 2008. Anticancer Res. 2010;30:569–73.

[c]Moorman AV, Chilton L, Wilkinson J, Ensor HM, Bown N, Proctor SJ. A population-based cytogenetic study of adults with acute lymphoblastic leukemia. Blood 2010;115:206–14.

[d]Brown P. TEL-AML1 in cord blood: 1% or 0.01%. Blood 2011;117:2–4.

[e]Frost BM, Forestier E, Gustafsson G, et al. Translocation t(12;21) is related to in vitro cellular drug sensitivity to doxorubicin and etoposide in childhood acute lymphoblastic leukemia. Blood 2004;104:2452–7.

[f]Garcia-Sanz R, Alaejos I, Orfao A, et al. Low frequency of the TEL/AML1 fusion gene in acute lymphoblastic leukemia in Spain. Br. J. Haematol. 1999;107:667–9.

3. Structural Abnormality t(1;19) in ALL

Translocation t(1;19) is the most common (5% of cases) translocation in children with ALL but is uncommon in adults. Patients with this abnormality typically exhibit other poor prognostic factors, such as high white blood cell counts and high lactate dehydrogenase levels, and have a poor prognosis (217).

4. Structural Abnormality t(12:21) in ALL

The following concerns the structural abnormality in ALL known as t(12;21). ALL commonly involves a chromosomal abnormality involving fusion of the *TEL* gene of chromosome 12 with

[217]Cortes JE, Kantarjian HM. Acute lymphoblastic leukemia. A comprehensive review with emphasis on biology and therapy. Cancer 1995;76:2393–417.

the *AML1* gene of chromosome 21, to produce a fusion gene. Expression of the fusion gene results in a fusion protein (218,219). The fusion product is named TEL-AML1 (also known as ETV6-RUNX1). TEL is also known as ETV6, while AML1 is also known as RUNX1. The chromosomal abnormality is named t(12;21), which refers to the fact that it is a translocation, and that the translocation involves chromosomes 12 and 21. The TEL-AML1 (ETV6/RUNX1) translocation appears to be a necessary, first step in the development of ALL, but this mutation alone is not sufficient to cause leukemia (220,221).

In B-cell precursor ALL, hyperdiploidy (more than 50 chromosomes) and TEL-AML1 fusion, which account for 25% and 23% of childhood cases but only 7% and 2% of adult cases, respectively, are associated with a favorable prognosis (222).

d. Cytogenetics for Diagnosis and Prediction—CML

Philadelphia chromosome encodes a mutant protein, that is, a fusion protein (*BCR/ABL1*), that is responsible for causing CML.

The BCR/ABL1 fusion protein is essential for initiation, maintenance, and progression of CML (223).

Where a patient's cells contain Philadelphia chromosome, the genotype is called Ph-positive.

However, in about 1% of patients with CML, the bone marrow cells appear to be Ph-negative, although the *BCR/ABL1* fusion gene still exists, where it may be located on chromosomes 22q11, 9q34, or even on a third chromosome (224). The failure to observe Philadelphia chromosome in Ph-negative CML patients has been explained by a scenario where a first translocation forms Philadelphia chromosome, resulting in generation of the *BCR/ABL1* fusion gene, followed by a second translocation that restores what appears to be of the original, normal chromosomes. Virgili et al. (225) have identified the locations of the *BCR/ABL1* fusion gene in a number of Ph-negative CML patients.

[218]Burmeister T, Gökbuget N, Schwartz S, et al. Clinical features and prognostic implications of TCF3-PBX1 and ETV6-RUNX1 in adult acute lymphoblastic leukemia. Haematologica 2010;95:241–6.

[219]Ford AM, Palmi C, Bueno C, et al. The TEL-AML1 leukemia fusion gene dysregulates the TGF-beta pathway in early B lineage progenitor cells. J. Clin. Invest. 2009;119:826–36.

[220]Wiemels JL, Hofmann J, Kang M, et al. Chromosome 12p deletions in TEL-AML1 childhood acute lymphoblastic leukemia are associated with retrotransposon elements and occur postnatally. Cancer Res. 2008;68:9935–44.

[221]Metzler M, Mann G, Monschein U, et al. Minimal residual disease analysis in children with t(12;21)-positive acute lymphoblastic leukemia: comparison of Ig/TCR rearrangements and the genomic fusion gene. Haematologica 2006;91:683–6.

[222]Pui C-H. Impact of molecular profiling and cytogenetics in acute lymphoblastic leukemia. Hematology 2005;10 (Suppl. 1):176–7.

[223]Nacheva EP, Brazma D, Virgili A, et al. Deletions of immunoglobulin heavy chain and T cell receptor gene regions are uniquely associated with lymphoid blast transformation of chronic myeloid leukemia. BMC Genom. 2010;11:41 (11 pp.).

[224]Virgili A, Brazma D, Reid AG, et al. FISH mapping of Philadelphia negative BCR/ABL1 positive CML. Mol. Cytogenet. 2008;1:14 (13 pp.).

[225]Virgili A, Brazma D, Reid AG, et al. FISH mapping of Philadelphia negative BCR/ABL1 positive CML. Mol. Cytogenet. 2008;1:14 (13 pp.).

In addition to t(9;22)(q34;q11) (Philadelphia chromosome), Brazma et al. (226) and Nacheva et al. (227) have identified a number of other chromosomal abnormalities in CML, where these abnormalities occur, for example, at 1p36, 5q21, 7p12, 8q24, 9p21, 9q34, 9q34, 14q11, 14q32, and 22q11. Moreover, a variety of gene mutations have been associated with CML, most notably, affecting *CDKN2A/2B*, *EVI-1*, *RB*, *MYC*, and *p53* genes (228). The possibility that these chromosomal abnormalities and genetic mutations contribute to the progression of CML, or can be used as a prognostic marker, is currently being explored. The following concerns the time point for conducting an analysis of chromosomal aberrations and gene mutations. Evidence suggests that the BCR/ABL1 fusion protein itself can induce the accumulation of additional genetic lesions, including point mutations, gene amplifications, genome loss and chromosome translocations, and that these mutations drive the malignant process (229).

e. Utility of Philadelphia Chromosome in Diagnosis, Drug Target, and for Assessing Response

Philadelphia chromosome, or its expressed mRNA and polypeptide, can be used as follows:

- Diagnosing leukemia;
- As a target of kinase inhibitors;
- To measure objective response to chemotherapy, for example, in the minimal residual disease (MRD) assay (230,231,232);
- In deciding to increase drug dose or to change to a second-line treatment (233).

Leukemias that are caused by a mutation called *Philadelphia chromosome* are CML and Philadelphia chromosome-positive ALL. The mutation is a translocation, identified as, t(9;22)(q34;q11). This abnormal chromosome contains a fusion gene, consisting of the *ABL* gene and the *BCR* gene, producing the *BCR-ABL* oncogene. This oncogene expresses an

[226]Brazma D, Grace C, Howard J, et al. Genomic profile of chronic myelogenous leukemia: imbalances associated with disease progression. Genes Chromosomes Cancer 2007;46:1039−50.

[227]Nacheva EP, Brazma D, Virgili A, et al. Deletions of immunoglobulin heavy chain and T cell receptor gene regions are uniquely associated with lymphoid blast transformation of chronic myeloid leukemia. BMC Genom. 2010;11:41 (11 pp.).

[228]Nacheva EP, Brazma D, Virgili A, et al. Deletions of immunoglobulin heavy chain and T cell receptor gene regions are uniquely associated with lymphoid blast transformation of chronic myeloid leukemia. BMC Genom. 2010;11:41 (11 pp.).

[229]Nacheva EP, Brazma D, Virgili A, et al. Deletions of immunoglobulin heavy chain and T cell receptor gene regions are uniquely associated with lymphoid blast transformation of chronic myeloid leukemia. BMC Genom. 2010;11:41 (11 pp.).

[230]Ottmann OG, Pfeifer H. Management of Philadelphia chromosome-positive acute lymphoblastic leukemia (Ph + ALL). Hematol. Am. Soc. Hematol. Educ. Program 2009:371−81.

[231]Bhojwani D, Howard SC, Pui CH. High-risk childhood acute lymphoblastic leukemia. Clin. Lymphoma Myeloma 2009;9(Suppl. 3):S222−30.

[232]Foroni L, Gerrard G, Nna E, et al. Technical aspects and clinical applications of measuring BCR-ABL1 transcripts number in chronic myeloid leukemia. Am. J. Hematol. 2009;84:517−22.

[233]Kantarjian HM, Shan J, Jones D, et al. Significance of increasing levels of minimal residual disease in patients with Philadelphia chromosome-positive chronic myelogenous leukemia in complete cytogenetic response. J. Clin. Oncol. 2009;27:3659−63.

enzyme that has a constitutive, abnormal tyrosine kinase activity. According to O'Brien et al. (234), the existence of this fusion gene is necessary and sufficient for the generation of leukemia.

The fusion proteins that are expressed in CML and in ALL are slightly different from each other, occurring as a p190 form and a p210 form. The p190 form of BCR-ABL causes ALL, while the p210 form of BCR-ABL is seen in the majority of patients with CML (235).

BCR-ABL is a target of tyrosine kinase inhibitor drugs, such as imatinib. Imatinib can provide dramatic results in patients with CML, as indicated by the endpoints of overall survival (86% overall survival at 7 years) and event-free survival (EFS) (81% EFS at 7 years) (236). In describing the influence of imatinib on BCR-ABL expression in a pivotal clinical trial, Druker et al. (237) reported that

after 1 year, levels of BCR-ABL transcripts had fallen by at least 1000-fold in 66 of 124 patients.

The studies of O'Brien et al. (238) and Druker et al. (239) established the utility of BCR-ABL expression as a prognostic marker. BCR-ABL mRNA levels indicate therapeutic response for patients with CML as well as for Philadelphia chromosome-positive ALL (240). Measurements of mRNA levels provide an accurate measure of the total leukemia cell mass and the degree to which the amount BCR-ABL mRNA is reduced by therapy (241). When reporting the expression of BCR-ABL in the clinical context, the amount of mRNA is stated using an international scale. The medical community has accepted the BCR-ABL assay as a prognostic tool, as shown by the clinical trial of Saglio et al. (242), where BCR-ABL expression was used as the primary endpoint in a study of CML. This study compared the efficacy of nilotinib (BCR-ABL inhibitor)

[234]O'Brien SG, Guilhot F, Larson RA, et al. Imatinib compared with interferon and low-dose cytarabine for newly diagnosed chronic-phase chronic myeloid leukemia. New Engl. J. Med. 2003;348:994−1004.

[235]Melo JV, Hewett DR. Wrapping BCR-ABL: it's in the bag. Blood 2010;116:3382−3.

[236]Hughes TP, Hochhaus A, Branford S, et al. Long-term prognostic significance of early molecular response to imatinib in newly diagnosed chronic myeloid leukemia: an analysis from the International Randomized Study of Interferon and STI571 (IRIS). Blood 2010;116:3758−65.

[237]Druker BJ, Guilhot F, O'Brien SG, et al. Five-year follow-up of patients receiving imatinib for chronic myeloid leukemia. New Engl. J. Med. 2006;355:2408−17.

[238]O'Brien SG, Guilhot F, Larson RA, et al. Imatinib compared with interferon and low-dose cytarabine for newly diagnosed chronic-phase chronic myeloid leukemia. New Engl. J. Med. 2003;348:994−1004.

[239]Druker BJ, Guilhot F, O'Brien SG, et al. Five-year follow-up of patients receiving imatinib for chronic myeloid leukemia. New Engl. J. Med. 2006;355:2408−17.

[240]White HE, Matejtschuk P, Rigsby P, et al. Establishment of the first World Health Organization International Genetic Reference Panel for quantitation of BCR-ABL mRNA. Blood 2010;116:e111−7.

[241]Hughes T, Deininger M, Hochhaus A, et al. Monitoring CML patients responding to treatment with tyrosine kinase inhibitors: review and recommendations for harmonizing current methodology for detecting BCR-ABL transcripts and kinase domain mutations and for expressing results. Blood 2006;108:28−37.

[242]Saglio G, Kim DW, Issaragrisil S, et al. Nilotinib versus imatinib for newly diagnosed chronic myeloid leukemia. New Engl. J. Med. 2010;362:2251−9.

with imatinib, and found nilotinib to be superior in efficacy. Jabbour et al. (243) described the uses and limitations of the BCR-ABL assay, as a prognostic tool.

f. Cytogenetics for Diagnosis and Prediction—CLL

In CLL, the most frequent aberrations are represented by 13q-, 11q-, +12, 6q-, 17p-, and 14q32/IGH translocations (244). Some of these forms of abnormal cytogenetics, as well as certain gene mutations, serve as prognostic markers in CLL. The 17p deletion (17p-), the 11q deletion (11q-), and the TP53 mutation, indicate a negative prognosis for CLL. Over 80% of CLL patients with the 17p deletion also carry a TP53 mutation. The 17p deletion and the TP53 can occur independently of each other, and both predict poor outcome (245). According to Badoux et al. (246), deletions of 17p or mutations of TP53 indicate a very poor prognosis, being predictive of a short time for disease progression, lack of response to therapy, and short overall survival.

In a study of 268 CLL patients, TP53 mutations occur in 3.7% of patients ($n = 10$), where 7/10 cases showed a concomitant 17p-deletion (247). Thus, there is a high prevalence of TP53 mutation in 17p-deleted patients. Only three (1.1%) of the newly diagnosed patients carried TP53 mutations without 17p-deletion.

A totally separate study of CLL found TP53 mutations in 8.5% of patients (28 of 328 patients), where TP53 mutations in the absence of 17p deletions were found in 4.5% of patients (248). The *TP53* gene is located on chromosome 17p13.1 (249). This gene encodes a transcription factor known as *p53*.

This introduces the biology of *p53*, and of *p53* mutations. The p53 protein is a tumor suppressor protein. This protein normally blocks tumor formation by triggering apoptosis (250). But various kinds of tumors encode a mutated *p53* that prevents *p53* from binding to DNA, prevents *p53* from regulating target genes, and allows tumor formation. Mutations in *p53* occur in a great variety of cancers, including cancer of the breast, head and neck, liver, bladder, brain, lung, colorectum, esophagus, ovary, and

[243]Jabbour E, Cortes JE, Kantarjian HM. Molecular monitoring in chronic myeloid leukemia: response to tyrosine kinase inhibitors and prognostic implications. Cancer 2008;112:2112−8.

[244]Cavazzini F, Ciccone M, Negrini M, Rigolin GM, Cuneo A. Clinicobiologic importance of cytogenetic lesions in chronic lymphocytic leukemia. Expert Rev. Hematol. 2009;2:305−14.

[245]Stilgenbauer S, Zenz T. Understanding and managing ultra high-risk chronic lymphocytic leukemia. Hematol. Am. Soc. Hematol. Educ. Program 2010;481−8.

[246]Badoux XC, Keating MJ, Wierda WG. What is the best frontline therapy for patients with CLL and 17p deletion? Curr. Hematol. Malig. Rep. 2011;6:36−46.

[247]Zainuddin N, Murray F, Kanduri M, et al. TP53 Mutations are infrequent in newly diagnosed chronic lymphocytic leukemia. Leuk. Res. 2011;35:272−4.

[248]Zenz T, Eichhorst B, Busch R, et al. TP53 mutation and survival in chronic lymphocytic leukemia. J. Clin. Oncol. 2010;28:4473−9.

[249]Chang H, Jiang AM, Qi CX. Aberrant nuclear p53 expression predicts hemizygous 17p (TP53) deletion in chronic lymphocytic leukemia. Am. J. Clin. Pathol. 2010;133:70−4.

[250]Wiman KG. Pharmacological reactivation of mutant p53: from protein structure to the cancer patient. Oncogene 2010;29:4245−52.

hematopoietic and lymphoid systems (251). Mutations in *p53* frequently occur at six discrete hotspot codons within the DNA-binding domain of the molecule, namely, at codons 175, 245, 248, 249, 273, and 282 (252). Where mutations occur, the strongest correlations between poor prognosis have been found mainly for breast cancer and CLL (253). But convincing correlations have not been found, for example, in the case of colorectal cancer.

g. Cytogenetics for Diagnosis and Prediction—MDS

Chromosomal abnormalities are detected in about 50% of patients with de novo MDS and in up to 80% of patients with MDS secondary to chemotherapy (254). Deletions of the long arm of chromosome 5 (del(5q)) are the most frequent chromosomal abnormality in de novo MDS.

The IPSS applies only to de novo MDS. This scoring system assigns a "risk category" for risk of death or transformation to AML. These risk categories reflect the percentage of bone marrow blasts, number of cytopenias, and presence or absence and type of chromosomal abnormalities. The chromosomal abnormalities, which are used to assign risk, are defined by the IPSS as good, poor, and intermediate. The chromosomal abnormalities associated

with good, poor, and intermediate prognosis are as follows (255):

- Good prognosis. Normal, isolated -Y, del (5q), and del(20q).
- Poor prognosis. Complex (≥3 abnormalities) and/or any chromosome 7 anomalies.
- Intermediate prognosis. All other abnormalities.

Because it is simple, the IPSS score is suitable for use as a gentle introduction to the cytogenetics of MDS. That said, the following serves as an introduction to the tremendous variability of MDS cytogenetics.

In a large study of MDS, Haase et al. (256) acquired cytogenetic data on 2072 MDS patients. Of these, 988 did not show chromosomal abnormalities, and 1084 had chromosomal abnormalities. Thus, about 50% showed abnormal cytogenetics. The variety of abnormalities was remarkable, as the abnormalities fell into 684 different categories. Many of the patients contained only one chromosomal abnormality (333 patients had only one abnormality). Some of the patients (83 patients) contained two abnormalities. A significant number of patients had three abnormalities (32 patients), four to six abnormalities (59 patients), or greater than six abnormalities (41 patients).

[251]Robles AI, Harris CC. Clinical outcomes and correlates of TP53 mutations and cancer. Cold Spring Harbor Perspect. Biol. 2010;2(15 pp.).

[252]Robles AI, Harris CC. Clinical outcomes and correlates of TP53 mutations and cancer. Cold Spring Harbor Perspect. Biol. 2010;2(15 pp.).

[253]Robles AI, Harris CC. Clinical outcomes and correlates of TP53 mutations and cancer. Cold Spring Harbor Perspect. Biol. 2010;2(15 pp.).

[254]Haase D, Germing U, Schanz J, et al. New insights into the prognostic impact of the karyotype in MDS and correlation with subtypes: evidence from a core dataset of 2124 patients. Blood 2007;110:4385–95.

[255]Haase D, Germing U, Schanz J, et al. New insights into the prognostic impact of the karyotype in MDS and correlation with subtypes: evidence from a core dataset of 2124 patients. Blood 2007;110:4385–95.

[256]Haase D, Germing U, Schanz J, et al. New insights into the prognostic impact of the karyotype in MDS and correlation with subtypes: evidence from a core dataset of 2124 patients. Blood 2007;110:4385–95.

The most frequent abnormalities were deletions of 5q, occurring in 30% of the patients presenting with chromosomal abnormalities (257). Another frequent anomaly was −7/del (7q), which occurred in 21% of the patients presenting with chromosomal abnormalities. Of the patients with abnormal cytogenetics, the best prognosis was found in patients with the del(5q) abnormality (with only this particular abnormality), with a mean survival time of 80 months. Poorer survival occurred with the −7/del(7q) abnormality, with a median survival time of 14 months. Very poor prognosis was with t(5q) (as the only abnormality), and here mean survival time was 4.4 months. MDS patients with normal cytogenetics had a mean survival time of 53 months (258). The following concerns patients with multiple abnormalities. In general, a sudden drop in survival time, for any given MDS patient, occurred when that patient's blasts contained three or more abnormalities. In publications relating to MDS, the term "complex" refers to three or more abnormalities.

The tremendous variability of MDS cytogenetics inspired Haase (259) to observe this contrast. At one end of the spectrum is CML, which is characterized by only one chromosomal abnormality (Philadelphia chromosome) while, at the other end of the spectrum, is MDS which has hundreds of different chromosomal abnormalities.

V. CHROMOSOMAL ABNORMALITIES IN SOLID TUMORS

Chromosomal abnormalities and cytogenetics are sometimes used in clinical trials on solid tumors, but at a frequency much less than that for hematological cancers. This reveals types of chromosomal analysis for solid tumors. In a study of colorectal cancer, Bardi et al. (260) found that structural changes in chromosome 8, structural changes in chromosome 16, and loss of chromosome 18, are correlated with shorter survival. In a manner somewhat reminiscent of the distinction of the various leukemias using cytogenetic analysis, the Bardi study also found that colon cancer and rectal cancer were distinguished by different patterns of abnormal cytogenetics. To provide another example, studies of breast cancer from Larson et al. (261) and from Heaphy et al. (262), identified certain chromosomal abnormalities that are correlated with poor prognosis for breast cancer patients. These

[257]Haase D, Germing U, Schanz J, et al. New insights into the prognostic impact of the karyotype in MDS and correlation with subtypes: evidence from a core dataset of 2124 patients. Blood 2007;110:4385−95.

[258]Haase D, Germing U, Schanz J, et al. New insights into the prognostic impact of the karyotype in MDS and correlation with subtypes: evidence from a core dataset of 2124 patients. Blood 2007;110:4385−95.

[259]Haase D. Cytogenetic features in myelodysplastic syndromes. Ann. Hematol. 2008;87:515−26.

[260]Bardi G, Fenger C, Johansson B, Mitelman F, Heim S. Tumor karyotype predicts clinical outcome in colorectal cancer patients. J. Clin. Oncol. 2004;22:2623−34.

[261]Larson PS, Schlechter BL, de las Morenas A, Garber JE, Cupples LA, Rosenberg CL. Allele imbalance, or loss of heterozygosity, in normal breast epithelium of sporadic breast cancer cases and BRCA1 gene mutation carriers is increased compared with reduction mammoplasty tissues. J. Clin. Oncol. 2005;23:8613−9.

[262]Heaphy CM, Bisoffi M, Joste NE, Baumgartner KB, Baumgartner RN, Griffith JK. Genomic instability demonstrates similarity between DCIS and invasive carcinomas. Breast Cancer Res. Treat. 2009;117:17−24.

abnormalities were allelic imbalances. Allelic imbalances are defined as a deviation from the normal 1:1 ratio of maternal and paternal alleles. Regarding chromosomal deletions, Ellsworth et al. (263) provided a diagram of all of the chromosomes, illustrating the most commonly deleted regions in breast cancers.

VI. ENDPOINTS IN HEMATOLOGICAL CANCERS

a. Introduction

Examples of a number of clinical endpoints, as well as data from several clinical trials, are shown below. Clinical endpoints used in clinical trials on hematological cancers include EFS, PFS, and overall survival. Earlier chapters in this textbook detailed the oncology endpoint of PFS, as well as other surrogate endpoints, and the gold standard endpoint of overall survival. This further develops the concept of surrogate endpoints, with a narrative on MRD.

b. Endpoint of Event-Free Survival

Event-free survival (EFS) is used in about 25% of all clinical trials on leukemia (264). This endpoint is used in about 7% of all oncology clinical trials, where it is used mainly for clinical trials in leukemia and lymphoma, but also sometimes for clinical trials in neuroblastoma, breast cancer, and lung cancer (265). This endpoint is rarely used in clinical trials in colorectal cancer, myelodysplastic disorder, prostate cancer, and melanoma.

Event-free survival may be the preferred endpoint, where the investigator wants the endpoint to reflect the primary treatment, and not subsequent treatments that are given where the study drug fails or subsequent treatments that are given if relapse occurs (266). Where the study drug fails, subsequent treatments are often not controlled by the investigator. In contrast to the endpoint of event-free survival, the endpoint of overall survival takes into account second-line treatments that are given where the study drug fails, or where the study drug is unacceptably toxic.

In some clinical trials, event-free survival may be the preferred endpoint, where the cancer in question can be reliably treated by existing drugs. In this situation, use of *overall survival* as the endpoint would not make much sense, as this particular endpoint would be triggered by so few study subjects. According to Basso et al. (267), recent advances for

---

[263]Ellsworth RE, Ellsworth DL, Lubert SM, Hooke J, Somiari RI, Shriver CD. High-throughput loss of heterozygosity mapping in 26 commonly deleted regions in breast cancer. Cancer Epidemiol. Biomark. Prev. 2003;12:915–9.

[264]Search in *Journal of Clinical Oncology* of all articles published from 1990 to 2011, with "leukemia" as search term in title/abstract, and "event-free survival" as search term in entire text. Search conducted March 9, 2011.

[265]A search in *Journal of Clinical Oncology*, conducted March 7, 2011, probed articles published from 1990 to 2011. Of 1145 articles containing the term "event-free survival" (anywhere in the article), some 531 articles contained the term "leukemia" or "lymphoma" in the title/abstract, 93 articles contained the term "breast," 89 contained "neuroblastoma," but only 19 contained "myelodysplastic," six contained "melanoma," three contained "prostate," and one contained "pancreatic" or "pancreas" in the title/abstract.

[266]Nachman JB. E-mail of March 10, 2011.

[267]Basso G, Veltroni M, Valsecchi MG, et al. Risk of relapse of childhood acute lymphoblastic leukemia is predicted by flow cytometric measurement of residual disease on day 15 bone marrow. J. Clin. Oncol. 2009;27:5168–74.

treating childhood ALL allow the "vast majority" of patients to achieve complete remission and then to be cured. In the words of another physician, "[i]n pediatric as opposed to adult oncology, event-free survival is the preferred end point for almost all of our trials. This is because of the generally high cure rates for our diseases" (268).

Event-free survival has been defined in a number of ways in clinical trials for the various leukemias, as documented in the following bullet points. The author's survey of oncology articles also revealed that a small proportion of articles failed to define event-free survival (269). Hence, the medical writer should be vigilant and ensure that this definition is included in any Clinical Study Protocols and manuscripts.

Event-free survival (EFS) was defined by:

- Creutzig et al. (270), in a study of AML, defined EFS as early death, resistant leukemia, relapse, secondary malignancy, or death resulting from any cause.
- Langebrake et al. (271), in a study of AML, defined EFS as failure to achieve remission, resistant leukemia, relapse, second malignancy, or death of any cause.
- Marcucci et al. (272), in a study of AML, defined EFS as failure to achieve CR, relapse, or death as a result of any cause. CR means complete remission (recovery of morphologically normal BM and blood counts (ie, neutrophils $\geq 1500/\mu L$ and platelets $\geq 100,000/\mu L$), and no circulating leukemic blasts or evidence of extramedullary leukemia).
- Rao et al. (273), in a study of AML, defined EFS as recurrence of AML or death.
- Basso et al. (274), in a clinical trial of ALL, defined EFS as death in induction, resistance, relapse, death in continuous CR, or secondary malignant neoplasm. CR means complete remission, defined as no physical signs of leukemia, bone marrow with active hematopoiesis, and fewer than 5% leukemic blast cells, normal CSF.
- Butturini et al. (275), in a clinical trial of ALL, defined EFS as death from any cause, failure to achieve remission after induction therapy, relapse in any site, and second malignancy.

[268]Nachman JB. E-mail of March 10, 2011.

[269]Survey of all 504 articles containing the term "event-free survival" published in *Journal of Clinical Oncology*, in the years 2005–11. This survey was conducted on March 7, 2011.

[270]Creutzig U, Zimmermann M, Lehrnbecher T, et al. Less toxicity by optimizing chemotherapy, but not by addition of granulocyte colony-stimulating factor in children and adolescents with acute myeloid leukemia: results of AML-BFM 98. J. Clin. Oncol. 2006;24:4499–506.

[271]Langebrake C, Creutzig U, Dworzak M, et al. Residual disease monitoring in childhood acute myeloid leukemia by multiparameter flow cytometry: the MRD-AML-BFM Study Group. J. Clin. Oncol. 2006;24:3686–92.

[272]Marcucci G, Maharry K, Whitman SP, et al. High expression levels of the ETS-related gene, ERG, predict adverse outcome and improve molecular risk-based classification of cytogenetically normal acute myeloid leukemia: a Cancer and Leukemia Group B study. J. Clin. Oncol. 2007;25:3337–43.

[273]Rao AV, Valk PJ, Metzeler KH, et al. Age-specific differences in oncogenic pathway dysregulation and anthracycline sensitivity in patients with acute myeloid leukemia. J. Clin. Oncol. 2009;27:5580–6.

[274]Basso G, Veltroni M, Valsecchi MG, et al. Risk of relapse of childhood acute lymphoblastic leukemia is predicted by flow cytometric measurement of residual disease on day 15 bone marrow. J. Clin. Oncol. 2009;27:5168–74.

[275]Butturini AM, Dorey FJ, Lange BJ, et al. Obesity and outcome in pediatric acute lymphoblastic leukemia. J. Clin. Oncol. 2007;25:2063–9.

- Nachman et al. (276), in a clinical trial of ALL, defined EFS as induction failure, induction death, relapse at any site, death in remission, or a second malignant neoplasm.
- Schultz et al. (277), in a clinical trial of ALL, defined EFS as induction failure, relapse at any site, secondary malignancy, or death.
- Cortes et al. (278), in a study of CML, defined EFS as death from any cause, loss of complete hematologic response, loss of complete cytogenetic response, discontinuation of therapy for toxicity or lack of efficacy, or progression to accelerated phase (AP) or blastic phase (BP).
- Caballero et al. (279), in a study of CLL, defined EFS as disease progression or death, and patients who did not reach disease response (complete or partial remission).
- Adès et al. (280), in a study of APL, defined EFS as treatment failure, death in first CR, and relapse. CR means complete remission, where there were separate definitions for hematologic CR and for molecular CR.

- Devine et al. (281), in a review of pediatric leukemias, defined EFS as occurrence of a major adverse clinical event such as failure to achieve remission, relapse, and death during remission.

Prof. Thomas Fleming provided comments regarding composite endpoints such as event-free survival (EFS) and progression-free survival (PFS) (282). PFS is a composite endpoint, because it is triggered by either the event of progression or the event of death. Prof. Fleming cautions against the use of broader composite endpoints, such as "discontinuation of treatment," instead of using narrower composite endpoints, such as EFS or PFS. The reason to avoid broader composite endpoints, is that it can result in meaningless information. Even the layperson can understand that the composite endpoint of "discontinuation of treatment" can be triggered by death of the subject, by the subject's withdrawal of his consent, or by a strike by bus drivers that prevents the subject from traveling to the clinic.

[276]Nachman JB, La MK, Hunger SP, et al. Young adults with acute lymphoblastic leukemia have an excellent outcome with chemotherapy alone and benefit from intensive postinduction treatment: a report from the children's oncology group. J. Clin. Oncol. 2009;27:5189–94.

[277]Schultz KR, Bowman WP, Aledo A, et al. Improved early event-free survival with imatinib in Philadelphia chromosome-positive acute lymphoblastic leukemia: a children's oncology group study. J. Clin. Oncol. 2009;27:5175–81.

[278]Cortes JE, Jones D, O'Brien S, et al. Results of dasatinib therapy in patients with early chronic-phase chronic myeloid leukemia. J. Clin. Oncol. 2010;28:398–404.

[279]Caballero D, García-Marco JA, Martino R, et al. Allogeneic transplant with reduced intensity conditioning regimens may overcome the poor prognosis of B-cell chronic lymphocytic leukemia with unmutated immunoglobulin variable heavy-chain gene and chromosomal abnormalities (11q- and 17p-). Clin. Cancer Res. 2005;11:7757–63.

[280]Adès L, Chevret S, Raffoux E, et al. Is cytarabine useful in the treatment of acute promyelocytic leukemia? Results of a randomized trial from the European Acute Promyelocytic Leukemia Group. J. Clin. Oncol. 2006;24:5703–10.

[281]Devine S, Dagher RN, Weiss KD, Santana VM. Good clinical practice and the conduct of clinical studies in pediatric oncology. Pediatr. Clin. North Am. 2008;55:187–209.

[282]Fleming TR. Addressing missing data in clinical trials. Ann. Intern. Med. 2011;154:113–7.

VII. CYTOGENETICS AS A PROGNOSTIC MARKER—THE GREVER STUDY OF CLL

The chromosomal abnormalities in CLL include:

- del(13q14.3),
- trisomy 12,
- del(17p13.1), and
- del(11q22.3).

The term "del" means chromosomal deletion. Of these, deletions of 17p13.1 and 11q22.3 are associated with poorer prognosis, while the 13q14.3 deletion is associated with better prognosis (283).

The following concerns a clinical trial on CLL, where one of the goals was to determine whether either of these two cytogenetic abnormalities, del(17p13.1), and del(11q22.3), might be correlated with poor survival, relative to survival of patients whose cells did not contain these particular abnormalities.

Grever et al. (284) conducted a clinical trial of CLL, where study subjects (235 subjects in total) were allocated to two arms. The two arms were:

- Arm A. Fludarabine alone.
- Arm B. Fludarabine plus cyclophosphamide.

TABLE 18.5 Response of CLL Patients to Fludarabine Alone or to Fludarabine Plus Cyclophosphamide

	Objective Response (Complete Response; CR) (%)	Progression-Free Survival (PFS)
Fludarabine alone	5.3	19.9 months
Fludarabine plus cyclophosphamide	24.6	33.5 months

Treatment was for six cycles, each cycle lasting 1 month, and all study subjects were monitored for about 50 months. The results are shown in Table 18.5. The results demonstrate that the combination of the two drugs worked better than fludarabine alone.

The following concerns the endpoint of CR. The Grever study used the endpoint of CR, where the definition was provided by another publication by the same researchers (285). The definition appears in footnote (286).

Now let us turn from data that distinguish Arm A treatment from Arm B treatment, to data that correlate cytogenetic abnormalities with PFS. This concerns methodology. The two types of chromosomal anomalies, del (17p13.1) and del(11q22.3), were determined by fluorescent probes. Peripheral blood mononuclear cells (PBMCs) were isolated at

---

[283]Woyach JA, Heerema NA, Zhao J, et al. Dic(17;18)(p11.2;p11.2) is a recurring abnormality in chronic lymphocytic leukaemia associated with aggressive disease. Br. J. Haematol. 2010;148:754–9.

[284]Grever MR, Lucas DM, Dewald GW, et al. Comprehensive assessment of genetic and molecular features predicting outcome in patients with chronic lymphocytic leukemia: results from the US Intergroup Phase III Trial E2997. J. Clin. Oncol. 2007;25:799–804.

[285]Blum KA, Young D, Broering S, et al. Computed tomography scans do not improve the predictive power of 1996 National Cancer Institute-Sponsored Working Group Chronic Lymphocytic Leukemia Response Criteria. J. Clin. Oncol. 2007;25:5624–9.

[286]Complete response was the absence of lymphadenopathy and organomegaly by physical examination, absolute lymphocyte count (ALC) no higher than 5000/μL, absolute neutrophil count (ANC) of at least 1,500/μL, platelets more than 100,000/μL, hemoglobin more than 11.0 g/dL, and bone marrow without lymphoid nodules and fewer than 30% lymphocytes.

baseline from each patient, that is, before administering any drugs. Two hundred cells (PBMCs) were evaluated using each fluorescent probe, and the results were expressed as the percentage of nuclei with an abnormal signal pattern for any probe and corresponding chromosomal anomaly. Cytogenetic analysis was by FISH, using methods suited for CLL (287).

For the purposes of cytogenetic analysis, survival data from all 235 subjects were pooled, and then separated into three different curves. The three curves appear in a Kaplan–Meier plot in the original journal article. The three curves did not correspond to different treatments but, instead, they corresponded to the cytogenetics of the leukemia. Thus, the three different curves corresponded to subjects where blood cells contained: (1) the del(17p13.1) chromosomal abnormality; (2) the del(11q22.3) chromosomal abnormality; and (3) other chromosomal abnormalities. The results were as follows. The median PFS was 10.8 months for patients with del(17p13.1) and 21.5 months for those with del(11q22.3). But median PFS was more favorable in the group of subjects not having either of these chromosomal abnormalities.

In comparing PFS of patients with these two chromosomal abnormalities with PFS of patients without these chromosomal abnormalities, the authors concluded that each of these two chromosomal abnormalities is prognostic of poor outcome. The authors went a step further, by using these results to recommend that alternative treatments should be pursued for patients with del(17p13.1) or del(11q22.3). These alternate treatments include use of alemtuzumab, flavopiridol, and stem cell transplantation.

This concerns semantics. In view of the heterogeneous nature of B-cell CLL, this disease has been classed according to cytogenetics, for example, whether the blasts have del(17p13.1) cyotogenetics or have del(11q22.3) cytogenetics. But sometimes, del(17p13.1) and del(11q22.3) are called biomarkers. The question of whether a given deletion is used to define a given type of CLL or is used to refer to a biomarker, is a matter of personal preference.

VIII. MINIMAL RESIDUAL DISEASE

Minimal residual disease (MRD) is a parameter used mainly in clinical trials of hematological cancers. The RECIST criteria, used as an endpoint in clinical trials on solid tumors, finds a counterpart in MRD. But unlike RECIST criteria, which is *not* often a reliable predictor of clinical response, MRD has been found to be an *excellent predictor* of clinical response in the hematological cancers (288).

MRD is a parameter used mainly in clinical trials in leukemia and lymphoma. This parameter is used in about 12% of all clinical trials of leukemia or lymphoma (289). MRD is also used in clinical trials in breast cancer, neuroblastoma, and ovarian cancer. But MRD is used only rarely in clinical trials in MDSs, melanoma, lung cancer, sarcoma, and colorectal cancer.

[287]Dewald GW, Brockman SR, Paternoster SF, et al. Chromosome anomalies detected by interphase fluorescence in situ hybridization: correlation with significant biological features of B-cell chronic lymphocytic leukaemia. Br. J. Haematol. 2003;121:287–95.

[288]Hedrick EE. Personal communication, March 2, 2011.

[289]Search of articles in *Journal of Clinical Oncology*, published between 1990 and 2011. The search was conducted on March 7, 2011.

The response to treatment in patients with leukemia has traditionally been assessed by counting blood cells using a microscope, and identifying residual leukemic blasts in samples from peripheral blood and from bone marrow. The task of identifying residual leukemic cells is difficult when leukemic calls are present in small numbers (290). Another problem with using the microscope is that, under some conditions, it might be impossible to distinguish between leukemic cells and normal cells (291).

Instead of using the microscope, residual leukemic cells can be measured by using techniques such as flow cytometry, or the polymerase chain reaction (PCR) method, to detect genes (markers) that are expressed in leukemic cells, but not expressed in normal cells. This approach refers to the detection of *submicroscopic levels of leukemic cells* (292). Gabert et al. (293), describe the various types of leukemias (ALL, CML, APL) that are frequently subjected to MRD analysis, and outline the specific fusion genes where gene expression is used to detect MRD.

When flow cytometry, PCR, or some other sensitive technique, is used to quantify residual leukemic cells, the term used to refer to the measured parameter is MRD.

In the context of leukemia, MRD refers to the detection of leukemic cells based on their expression of abnormal combinations of antigens that are not present on normal bone marrow cells (294). In commentary on ALL, Pui (295) finds that MRD levels on day 15 were a powerful prognostic factor.

In commentary on APL, Grimwade et al. (296) found that MRD monitoring successfully identified most patients subject to relapse and provided a powerful predictor of RFS. Thus, MRD is sometimes used as a surrogate endpoint in the hematological cancers, though the

[290]Campana D. Role of minimal residual disease monitoring in adult and pediatric acute lymphoblastic leukemia. Hematol. Oncol. Clin. North Am. 2009;23:1083—98.

[291]Campana D. Role of minimal residual disease monitoring in adult and pediatric acute lymphoblastic leukemia. Hematol. Oncol. Clin. North Am. 2009;23:1083—98.

[292]Basso G, Veltroni M, Valsecchi MG, et al. Risk of relapse of childhood acute lymphoblastic leukemia is predicted by flow cytometric measurement of residual disease on day 15 bone marrow. J. Clin. Oncol. 2009;27:5168—74.

[293]Gabert J, Beillard E, van der Velden VH, et al. Standardization and quality control studies of 'real-time' quantitative reverse transcriptase polymerase chain reaction of fusion gene transcripts for residual disease detection in leukemia—a Europe Against Cancer program. Leukemia 2003;17:2318—57.

[294]Borowitz MJ, Pullen DJ, Shuster JJ, et al. Minimal residual disease detection in childhood precursor-B-cell acute lymphoblastic leukemia: relation to other risk factors. A Children's Oncology Group study. Leukemia 2003;17:1566—72.

[295]Pui C-H. Toward a total cure for acute lymphoblastic leukemia. J. Clin. Oncol. 2009;27:5121—3.

[296]Grimwade D, Jovanovic JV, Hills RK, et al. Prospective minimal residual disease monitoring to predict relapse of acute promyelocytic leukemia and to direct pre-emptive arsenic trioxide therapy. J. Clin. Oncol. 2009;27:3650—8.

utility of MRD differs depending on the cancer (297,298,299).

MRD test results have the following utilities. Grimwade et al. (300) and Campana (301) find that MRD measurements can provide the risk of relapse, direct preemptive therapy, guide the selection of intensity and duration of treatment, and provide guidance for treatment of the leukemia with stem cell transplantation.

a. Example of Use of MRD and Relapse—The Scheuring Study of Philadelphia Chromosome-Positive ALL

In a study of ALL (Ph-positive ALL), Scheuring et al. (302) acquired samples of PBMCs and bone marrow immediately before chemotherapy, and after 2 weeks, after 4 weeks, and at monthly intervals thereafter. The authors determined the date of MRD. Because of the repeated samplings of PBMCs, they were able to determine the date when a significant increase in blasts in the PBMC sample occurred. This date was then compared to the date of relapse and graphed on the Kaplan—Meier plot. Relapse was defined as the reappearance of blasts in the PBMCs in a patient who had earlier achieved a

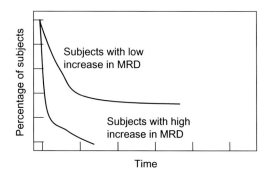

FIGURE 18.3 Schematic diagram of Kaplan—Meier plot of ALL. The plot shows the percentage of all subjects (*x* axis) versus time from date of significant increase in blasts until date of relapse. The *upper curve* corresponds to subjects with a low increase in MRD, while the *lower curve* corresponds to subjects with a high increase in MRD.

reduction in bone marrow blasts to less than 5%, with no detectable blasts in the PBMCs.

The schematic diagram of the Kaplan—Meier plot (Fig. 18.3) shows the proportion of patients, during the time course of the clinical trial, experiencing relapse. Two curves are shown in the Kaplan—Meier plot. The upper curve corresponds to subjects with a relatively low increase in MRD (when the increase was first detected), while the lower curve corresponds to subjects with a relatively high increase in MRD (when the increase was first detected). The authors

[297]Cazzaniga G, Gaipa G, Rossi V, Biondi A. Minimal residual disease as a surrogate marker for risk assignment to ALL patients. Rev. Clin. Exp. Hematol. 2003;7:292—323.

[298]Hallek M. The role of minimal residual disease elimination in the outcome of chronic lymphocytic leukemia. Hematol. Rep. 2005;1:30—2.

[299]Dreger P, Ritgen M, Böttcher S, Schmitz N, Kneba M. The prognostic impact of minimal residual disease assessment after stem cell transplantation for chronic lymphocytic leukemia: is achievement of molecular remission worthwhile? Leukemia 2005;19:1135—8.

[300]Grimwade D, Jovanovic JV, Hills RK, et al. Prospective minimal residual disease monitoring to predict relapse of acute promyelocytic leukemia and to direct pre-emptive arsenic trioxide therapy. J. Clin. Oncol. 2009;27:3650—8.

[301]Campana D. Minimal residual disease in acute lymphoblastic leukemia. Hematol. Am. Soc. Hematol. Educ. Program 2010;2010:7—12.

[302]Scheuring UJ, Pfeifer H, Wassmann B, et al. Serial minimal residual disease (MRD) analysis as a predictor of response duration in Philadelphia-positive acute lymphoblastic leukemia (Ph + ALL) during imatinib treatment. Leukemia 2003;17:1700—6.

discovered that, in assays of PBMC blasts, an increase that was under 5×10^{-4} was associated with a longer time to relapse, while an increase above 5×10^{-4} was associated with a shorter time to relapse (median 27 days to relapse) (Fig. 18.3).

The authors concluded that this assay method enabled detection of patients with poor prognosis, and in need of more aggressive therapy.

b. Example of Use of MRD and EFS— The Basso Study of Philadelphia Chromosome-Negative ALL

In a study of childhood ALL (Ph-negative ALL), Basso et al. (303) stratified patients according to MRD data that were collected from bone marrow samples on day 15 of the study. The MRD data were combined with established cytogenetics parameters, and this combination was used to define the following risk groups:

1. *High risk.* t(4;11)(q21;q23) or MLL/AF4, and testing positive for MRD, where blast counts were greater or equal to 10%. *MLL/AF4* refers to the fusion of *MLL* gene and *AF4* gene, a fusion product often found in infant ALL. The *MLL* gene is also known as *ALL1, HRX,* and *Hrx1*(304).
2. *Low risk.* Patients lacking the high-risk cytogenetics and testing negative for MRD, that is, where blast counts were under 0.1%.
3. *Intermediate risk.* Patients not meeting the criteria for high risk or for low risk.

All of the subjects were non-Philadelphia chromosome-positive. Chemotherapy was for

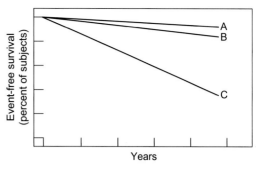

FIGURE 18.4 Schematic diagram of Kaplan−Meier plot of ALL. EFS is shown for patients stratified according to MRD. All patients received the same chemotherapy. At 15 days, bone marrow samples were withdrawn for use in MRD), where the results were used to define the three risk groups. The three strata were: (A) top line, under 0.1% blast cells; (B) middle line, between 0.1% and 10% blast cells; and (C) bottom line, greater or equal to 10% blast cells.

a 7-day period (days 1−7). The patients were followed for 5 years. The endpoint used in this clinical trial was EFS. EFS was a composite endpoint, that could be triggered by death, relapse, or by the appearance of a secondary malignant neoplasm. The Kaplan−Meier plot is schematically represented in Fig. 18.4.

The study found that where MRD was lowest (MRD under 0.1%), EFS data showed the most favorable outcome. The study also found that where MRD was greatest (MRD greater or equal to 10%), EFS data showed the worst outcome. The schematic diagram (Fig. 18.4) of the Kaplan−Meier plot discloses EFS for three different categories of patients.

EFS was used as an endpoint that was triggered by each individual patient, where results from individual patients are shown in the

[303]Basso G, Veltroni M, Valsecchi MG, et al. Risk of relapse of childhood acute lymphoblastic leukemia is predicted by flow cytometric measurement of residual disease on day 15 bone marrow. J. Clin. Oncol. 2009;27:5168−74.

[304]Cimino G, Cenfra N, Elia L, et al. The therapeutic response and clinical outcome of adults with ALL1(MLL)/AF4 fusion positive acute lymphoblastic leukemia according to the GIMEMA experience. Haematologica 2010;95:837−40.

Kaplan–Meier plot. But another endpoint, 5-year EFS was an endpoint corresponding to each of the three groups of patients. Five-year EFS refers to the percentage of subjects experiencing EFS at the 5-year time point. Please note that the term, "EFS," means *free of events*, and that it does not mean that *an event has occurred*. For the high-risk group, 5-year EFS was 46.1%. For the low-risk group, 5-year EFS was 89.9%. For the intermediate-risk group, 5-year EFS was 79.3%.

The authors concluded that patients with the lowest value for MRD, as determined by examination of bone marrow at 15 days, had an excellent outcome, as shown by the data which demonstrated that over 90% of these were relapse-free after 5 years. The authors found that the results will enable physicians to give more aggressive therapy to high-risk patients, and to give less aggressive and less toxic therapy to low-risk patients.

c. Methodology Tip—Flow Cytometry

In the clinical trial of Basso et al. (305), described above, flow cytometry was used for analyzing marrow cells and for generating data used for minimal residual disease analysis. In the analysis of blood cells by flow cytometry, the investigators tagged blood cells with antibodies specific for various markers, also called antigens, that are typically expressed on the surface of leukemic cells of the B-cell lineage and leukemic cells of the T-cell lineage. As detailed in another publication by Basso et al. (306), the CD19 marker is specific for B-cell ALL, and the CD7 marker is specific for T-cell ALL. As is the case with all applications of flow cytometry, the antibodies had been modified by covalent attachment of fluorescent dyes, to allow detection of tagged cells during passage through the flow cytometer. Details on the technique of flow cytometry, including guidance on choosing antibody tags, as it relates to the leukemias, are provided by Peters and Ansari (307), Uhrmacher et al. (308), and Al-Mawali et al. (309).

d. Using Cells Acquired After Chemotherapy (Not Before Chemotherapy) as a Prognostic Factor for Long-Term Relapse—The Cilloni Study

In a study of adult AML patients, Cilloni et al. (310) measured Wilms' tumor-1 gene (*WT1* gene) expression, as a reflection of MRD in patients with AML.

WT1 is not a fusion protein, but it is in a class of proteins that is conventionally known as *tumor antigens*. *WT1*, which stands for Wilms' tumor gene-1 (not written as Wilm's),

[305]Basso G, Veltroni M, Valsecchi MG, et al. Risk of relapse of childhood acute lymphoblastic leukemia is predicted by flow cytometric measurement of residual disease on day 15 bone marrow. J. Clin. Oncol. 2009;27:5168–74.

[306]Basso G, Buldini B, De Zen L, Orfao A. New methodologic approaches for immunophenotyping acute leukemias. Haematologica 2001;86:675–92.

[307]Peters JM, Ansari MQ. Multiparameter flow cytometry in the diagnosis and management of acute leukemia. Arch. Pathol. Lab. Med. 2011;135:44–54.

[308]Uhrmacher S, Erdfelder F, Kreuzer KA. Flow cytometry and polymerase chain reaction-based analyses of minimal residual disease in chronic lymphocytic leukemia. Adv. Hematol. 2010 (11 pp.).

[309]Al-Mawali A, Gillis D, Lewis I. The role of multiparameter flow cytometry for detection of minimal residual disease in acute myeloid leukemia. Am. J. Clin. Pathol. 2009;131:16–26.

[310]Cilloni D, Renneville A, Hermitte F, et al. Real-time quantitative polymerase chain reaction detection of minimal residual disease by standardized WT1 assay to enhance risk stratification in acute myeloid leukemia: a European LeukemiaNet study. J. Clin. Oncol. 2009;27:5195–201.

encodes a transcription factor. While this gene normally functions to regulate cell growth and differentiation, overexpression (311) or mutations (312) occur in a variety of leukemias, in MDS, and in most solid tumors. Hence, *WT1* has found utility as a marker for cancer cells, and as a drug target (313).

The following concerns the methodology of the Cilloni study. The authors assayed WT1 expression from a group of normal volunteers in order to arrive at a normal range. WT1 expression was notated as the ratio: [*WT1* gene mRNA]/[*Abelson* gene mRNA]. In other words, *Abelson* gene expression was used to normalize the value for *WT1* gene expression, using the technique of Beillard et al. (314). The normal expression range was 0–200 copies of *WT1* mRNA per 10,000 copies of *Abelson* gene mRNA, when testing bone marrow cells, and 0–50 copies of *WT1* mRNA per 10,000 copies of *Abelson* gene mRNA, when testing PBMCs.

Patients were treated with conventional chemotherapy, anthracycline plus cytarabine, where the pretreatment, baseline *WT1* gene expression levels exceeded 2×10^4 mRNA copies/10^4 *Abelson* gene mRNA copies.

Gene expression levels were measured in bone marrow cells taken at baseline, and again in bone marrow cells taken after the first cycle of chemotherapy. The first cycle was called "induction therapy." Thus, the series of the two bone marrow samples was called a paired pretreatment sample and a postinduction sample. Actually, in most of the patients, bone marrow samples were used for measuring gene expression, while in other patients, PBMCs were the source of cells.

Cilloni et al. (315) provide a Kaplan–Meier plot (not shown here) revealing the percent of patients relapsing versus length of complete remission. AML patients were treated with chemotherapy, followed by measuring the percentage of bone marrow cells that overexpressed Wilms' tumor gene, with normalization in terms of expression of the *Abelson* gene. The Kaplan–Meier plot shows two curves. The two curves corresponded to the subgroup of patients showing a great decrease in *WT1* gene expression, and to the subgroup of patients showing a small decrease in *WT1* gene expression, where *WT1* gene expression was compared before and after chemotherapy.

The authors discovered that a greater reduction in *WT1* gene expression after the first cycle of chemotherapy predicted a decreased risk of subsequent relapse (HR = 0.54; $P = 0.004$). The hazard ratio (HR) corresponds to the magnitude of the difference in the two curves, while the P value corresponds to the significance of this difference. The authors concluded that greater reduction in normalized

[311]Sugiyama H. WT1 (Wilms' tumor gene 1): biology and cancer immunotherapy. Jpn J. Clin. Oncol. 2010;40:377–87.

[312]Owen C, Fitzgibbon J, Paschka P. The clinical relevance of Wilms Tumour 1 (WT1) gene mutations in acute leukaemia. Hematol. Oncol. 2010;28:13–9.

[313]Oka Y, Tsuboi A, Oji Y, Kawase I, Sugiyama H. WT1 peptide vaccine for the treatment of cancer. Curr. Opin. Immunol. 2008;20:211–20.

[314]Beillard E, Pallisgaard N, van der Velden VH, et al. Evaluation of candidate control genes for diagnosis and residual disease detection in leukemic patients using 'real-time' quantitative reverse-transcriptase polymerase chain reaction (RQ-PCR)—a Europe against cancer program. Leukemia 2003;17:2474–86.

[315]Cilloni D, Renneville A, Hermitte F, et al. Real-time quantitative polymerase chain reaction detection of minimal residual disease by standardized WT1 assay to enhance risk stratification in acute myeloid leukemia: a European LeukemiaNet study. J. Clin. Oncol. 2009;27:5195–201.

WT1 transcript levels following anthracycline and cytarabine-based chemotherapy predicts a reduced risk of subsequent relapse.

e. Methodology Tip—Should Biomarkers be Measured Before or After Chemotherapy?

The Cilloni study (316) is distinguished from most other studies of oncology biomarkers, in that it found postchemotherapy measurements of a biomarker to have prognostic value. The Cilloni study directly addressed the possibility that prechemotherapy biomarker data might have prognostic value, and discovered they were not useful for this purpose. Penault-Llorca et al. (317) also studied the relative merits of measuring biomarkers before and after chemotherapy. In a study of breast cancer treated by chemotherapy, these authors found that HER2 negativity predicted better survival, and HER2 positivity predicted worse survival, in terms of the endpoint DFS. These authors also conducted their analysis with an endpoint other than DFS, namely, the endpoint of overall survival. Surprisingly, HER2 expression was found to predict overall survival only when HER2 expression was measured after chemotherapy. Where HER2 expression was measured before chemotherapy, there was no difference in overall survival in the HER2-negative patients and in the HER2-positive patients. None of the patients had received trastuzumab (the antibody that targets HER2). As a general proposition, researchers interested in prognostic markers prefer to use biopsies from chemotherapy-naive subjects, in order to avoid the potentially confounding effects of the therapy on the biomarker. However, the above studies reveal that taking biopsies before, as well as after, chemotherapy might be the most productive approach.

f. Example of Use of MRD—The Grimwade Study Using PML-RAR-Alpha Fusion Protein

Grimwade et al. (318) reveal the utility of collecting data on minimal residual disease during anticancer therapy. Minimal residual disease was measured by assays that detected expression of the mRNA encoding the fusion product, PML-RAR-alpha. Patients with APL were treated with standard chemotherapy, all-trans-retinoic acid. The patients experienced remission. Assays for fusion protein transcript were conducted on bone marrow samples at regular intervals following remission. Where levels of mRNA increased, after remission, and where the remission triggered a finding of minimal residual disease, patients were further treated with preemptive chemotherapy to prevent subsequent clinical remission. Evidence from this study suggested that use of minimal residual disease assays, coupled with preemptive therapy, can reduce subsequent relapse. The data indicated that this approach to treating APL can cut in half the rate of relapse.

[316]Cilloni D, Renneville A, Hermitte F, et al. Real-time quantitative polymerase chain reaction detection of minimal residual disease by standardized WT1 assay to enhance risk stratification in acute myeloid leukemia: a European LeukemiaNet study. J. Clin. Oncol. 2009;27:5195–201.

[317]Penault-Llorca F, Abrial C, Mouret-Reynier MA, et al. Achieving higher pathological complete response rates in HER-2-positive patients with induction chemotherapy without trastuzumab in operable breast cancer. Oncologist 2007;12:390–6.

[318]Grimwade D, Jovanovic JV, Hills RK, et al. Prospective minimal residual disease monitoring to predict relapse of acute promyelocytic leukemia and to direct pre-emptive arsenic trioxide therapy. J. Clin. Oncol. 2009;27:3650–58.

IX. CONFLUENCE OF CYTOGENETICS AND GENE EXPRESSION

Diagnostic, prognostic, and predictive information acquired from cytogenetics and from gene expression may or may not agree with each other. Fortunately, the confluence of these two fields, the ancient field of cytogenetics and the modern field of gene expression, has provided consistent results. This concerns pediatric acute lymphoblastic leukemia (ALL). ALL can be classified according to whether the leukemic cell is in the B-cell lineage (B-ALL) or the T-cell lineage (T-ALL) (319). Within these two classes, the ALL can be further classified according to cytogenetics, that is, abnormalities such as translocation, hyperploidy, and hypoploidy. Alternatively, or in addition, within these two classes of ALL, the disease can be classified according to gene expression. One goal of gene expression studies is to identify which genes are expressed in association with each chromosomal abnormality. Yeoh et al. (320) discovered that distinct groups of genes distinguish cases of leukemia that are B-cell lineage cases of ALL, such as, t(1;19)E2A-PBX1, t(9;22)BCR-ABL, and t(12;21)TEL-AML1, and MLL. The term "MLL" refers to the B-cell lineage ALL where there are rearrangements in the *MLL* gene on chromosome 11. To provide examples of these correlations, t(1;19)E2A-PBX1 leukemias were characterized by high expression of the *MERTK* gene, while MLL arrangement leukemias were characterized by high expression of the *HOXA9* gene and *MEIS1* gene.

Gene expression data have an advantage over cytogenetics, in that they can identify ALL patients where there are no chromosomal translocations. For example, only 30% of all cases of T-ALL have chromosomal translocations. Gene expression profiling of T-ALL provided an explanation for this, namely, that the oncogenes *HOX11*, *TAL1*, and *LYL1* that are involved in T-ALL translocations can also be overexpressed by other mechanisms, in patients where the leukemic cells lack translocations (321).

X. CONCLUDING REMARKS

When designing a clinical study on hematological malignancies, the investigator needs to identify methods of diagnosis, endpoints, prognostic markers that indicate risk for outcome of the disease, and predictive markers that mandate use of specific drugs. Methods of diagnosis include clinical methods, as well as blood counts, cytogenetics (chromosomal abnormalities), and genetic mutations. Prognostic aids include age of the patient, microscopic appearance of blood cells, cytogenetics, genetic mutations, and minimal residual disease. Endpoints include EFS, PFS, and overall survival.

Each of the above parameters can be separately evaluated where the patients are children versus adults, where the patients are treatment-naive versus patients having failed an earlier treatment, and where the patient has no coexisting genetic abnormalities

---

[319] Staudt LM. It's ALL in the diagnosis. Cancer Cell 2002;1:109–10.

[320] Yeoh EJ, Ross ME, Shurtleff SA, et al. Classification, subtype discovery, and prediction of outcome in pediatric acute lymphoblastic leukemia by gene expression profiling. Cancer Cell 2002;1:133–43.

[321] Staudt LM. It's ALL in the diagnosis. Cancer Cell 2002;1:109–10.

versus where there are coexisting genetic abnormalities.

Investigators need to be vigilant regarding the fact that some genes (and the corresponding fusion proteins) are identified by two or three different names, and not by just one name. Additionally, what must also be kept in mind is that the prevalence of some hematological disorders can vary markedly, depending on the geographic region of the world (322,323). Furthermore, investigators should be aware that diagnostic and prognostic methods can change dramatically as indicated, for example, by the fact that the t(12;21) (p13;q22) cytogenetic abnormality of ALL was not described until relatively recently, that is, in 1994 (324).

[322]Brown P. TEL-AML1 in cord blood: 1% or 0.01%. Blood 2011;117:2−4.

[323]Garcia-Sanz R, Alaejos I, Orfao A, et al. Low frequency of the TEL/AML1 fusion gene in acute lymphoblastic leukemia in Spain. Br. J. Haematol. 1999;107:667−9.

[324]Burmeister T, Gökbuget N, Schwartz S, et al. Clinical features and prognostic implications of TCF3-PBX1 and ETV6-RUNX1 in adult acute lymphoblastic leukemia. Haematologica 2010;95:241−6.

Biomarkers

I. INTRODUCTION

Biomarkers include proteins, peptides, cells, histological data, and genetic markers. Genetic markers encompass single genes, small collections of three or four genes, and large collections (arrays) of genes. Typically, when a gene is used a biomarker what is actually measured is the messenger RNA (mRNA) expressed by the gene. However, in the case of single nucleotide polymorphisms (SNPs), gene amplification, chromosomal abnormalities, what is measured is the gene itself. For genes that encode polypeptides, the term "gene" refers to the combination of regulatory sequences plus sequences encoding the polypeptide plus introns. Genetic markers include classical mRNA, as well as micro-RNA (miRNA) (1,2,3,4). Common biomarkers include low-density lipoprotein (LDL) cholesterol for assessing risk for atherosclerosis (5), prostate-specific antigen for assessing risk for prostate cancer (6,7), and human estrogen receptor-2 (*HER2*) to assess risk for breast cancer (8).

[1]Flamant S, Ritchie W, Guilhot J, et al. Micro-RNA response to imatinib mesylate in patients with chronic myeloid leukemia. Haematologica 2010;95:1325—33.

[2]Nonn L, Vaishnav A, Gallagher L, Gann PH. mRNA and micro-RNA expression analysis in laser-capture microdissected prostate biopsies: valuable tool for risk assessment and prevention trials. Exp. Mol. Pathol. 2010;88:45—51.

[3]Otaegui D, Baranzini SE, Armañanzas R, et al. Differential micro RNA expression in PBMC from multiple sclerosis patients. PLoS One 2009;4(7):e6309 (9 pp.).

[4]Nuovo GJ, Schmittgen TD. Benign metastasizing leiomyoma of the lung: clinicopathologic, immunohistochemical, and micro-RNA analyses. Diagn. Mol. Pathol. 2008;17:145—50.

[5]Brody T. Nutritional biochemistry. 2nd ed. San Diego, CA: Academic Press; 1999. pp. 311—76.

[6]Bratt O, Garmo H, Adolfsson J, et al. Effects of prostate-specific sntigen testing on familial prostate cancer risk estimates. J. Natl Cancer Inst. 2010 [Epub ahead of print].

[7]Chang SL, Harshman LC, Presti Jr JC. Impact of common medications on serum total prostate-specific antigen levels: analysis of the National Health and Nutrition Examination Survey. J. Clin. Oncol. 2010 [Epub ahead of print].

[8]Purdie CA, Baker L, Ashfield A, et al. Increased mortality in HER2 positive, oestrogen receptor positive invasive breast cancer: a population-based study. Br. J. Cancer 2010;103:475—81.

Clinical Trials.
DOI: http://dx.doi.org/10.1016/B978-0-12-804217-5.00019-9

Biomarkers are distinguished by their variety. They can take the form of membrane-bound proteins, serum antibodies, and serum chemokines, as shown by the following respective examples. PD-L1 expression by at least 50% of tumor cells in a tumor biopsy, is a biomarker for predicting efficacy of the anticancer drug, pembrolizumab (9). Peanut-specific serum IgE antibodies can be used for predicting risk for allergic reactions (10). Yet another biomarker is serum TARC for predicting risk for puritis in patients with atopic dermatitis (11). TARC, which is a chemokine, is a measure of Th2-type immune response, a type of immune response that characterizes atopic dermatitis.

Most laypersons have seen lists of biomarkers on printouts from their annual medical checkup. These printouts include biomarkers, as well as other parameters, such as blood cell counts and electrolytes. Blood cell counts and electrolytes are not considered biomarkers because they are clinically important in their own right, and are not used primarily to represent or predict any future-arising medical condition. In other words, an extremely low red blood cell count is, by definition, *anemia* (12). Moreover, a low red blood cell count has the following utility—it means that you have anemia right now; not that you are at increased risk for getting anemia some time in the next 5 years.

Biomarkers can take the form of an array or collection of genes. Because the device that contains this array is small, it is called a microarray. Any given microarray contains between 50 and 5000 genes or more. With use for any given patient, the number of genes that gives a positive signal, and the identities of the genes that give a positive signal, is likely to be unique, in a manner reminiscent of a fingerprint. Because of this fingerprint quality, the term *personalized medicine* is used to refer to the use of microarray data for guiding diagnosis and treatment. Microarrays have the utility of correlating the patient's fingerprint with a go/no go decision to treat the patient with a specific type of therapy. Researchers developing microarrays conduct research that is used to establish the correlation. Once the microarray is widely accepted or marketed, physicians can take advantage of the established correlation, and used the microarray to make go/no go decisions.

In clinical trials, biomarkers can be used to dictate subgroups used in the stratification of study subjects. Also, biomarkers can be used for purely exploratory purposes.

The utilities of biomarkers include:

- Identifying patients with a good prognosis versus poor prognosis (in absence of medical treatment).
- Identifying patients likely to respond to a given drug versus patients unlikely to respond to that drug.
- Identifying patients likely to experience adverse drug reactions to a given drug versus patients unlikely to experience adverse drug reactions.

[9]Garon EB, Rizvi NA, Hui R, et al. Pembrolizumab for the treatment of non-small-cell lung cancer. New Engl. J. Med. 2015. http://dx.doi.org/10.1056/NEJMoa1501824.

[10]Du Toit MB, Roberts G, Sayre PH, et al. Randomized trial of peanut consumption in infants at risk for peanut allergy. New Engl. J. Med. 2015;372:803–13.

[11]Beck LA, Thaci P, Hamilton JP, et al. Dupilumab treatment in adults with moderate-to severe atopic dermatitis. New Engl. J. Med. 2014;371:130–9.

[12]Brody T. Nutritional biochemistry. 2nd ed. San Diego, CA: Academic Press; 1999. p. 757.

a. Predictive Markers Versus Prognostic Markers

The most common uses for biomarkers are to determine the likely outcome of a disease in the absence of therapy, and to determine whether a given drug is likely to be effective against that disease. According to Mandrekar and Sargent [13], these two uses are referred to by the terms, *prognostic* marker and *predictive* marker, respectively. These concepts are illustrated below with data on breast cancer and colorectal cancer.

Overexpression of *HER2* by breast cancer cells increases invasiveness and tumorigenicity of breast cancer, where the oncogenic effects of *HER2* result from gene amplification rather than from mutations [14]. Trastuzumab (Herceptin®), an antibody that binds to *HER2*, generally mediates the killing only of tumors that overexpress *HER2* [15]. Tumors showing negative staining for *HER2* are not killed by *HER2*-targeted therapies. In fact, the package insert for Herceptin expressly states that this drug has been FDA-approved only for patients having tumors that overexpress *HER2*. The package insert reads, "Herceptin as a single agent is indicated for the treatment of patients with metastatic breast cancer whose tumors overexpress the HER2 protein and who have received one or more chemotherapy regimens for their metastatic disease" [16].

Breast cancer patients with *HER2* overexpression face bad news and good news. The bad news is that this overexpression is associated with a more aggressive cancer. But the good news is that this overexpression is associated with enhanced efficacy of Herceptin.

This concerns a different marker, *KRAS*. RAS is a protein that is part of a cell signaling pathway [17]. RAS actually represents a family of three different genes, namely, *KRAS*, *HRAS*, and *NRAS*. *KRAS*, also called Ki-RAS or Kirsten-RAS, was named after Werner Kirsten [18,19]. Oncogenic mutations in *KRAS* occur in about 40% of colorectal cancers. These mutations are associated with a somewhat poorer prognosis.

This concerns predicting responses of a patient to a drug. In summarizing the results from a clinical trial on colorectal cancer, Mandrekar and Sargent [20] state that *KRAS* status was assessed on 427 subjects, where 43% were found to have *KRAS* mutations. Subjects were then randomized to receive either anti-epidermal growth factor receptor (anti-EGFR) antibody (panitumumab) or placebo. The results demonstrated that the anti-EGFR antibody was more effective in subjects where tumors expressed wild-type *KRAS*, and less effective where tumors expressed mutated *KRAS*.

---

[13]Mandrekar SJ, Sargent DJ. Clinical trial designs for predictive biomarker validation: theoretical considerations and practical challenges. J. Clin. Oncol. 2009;27:4027−34.

[14]Purdie CA, Baker L, Ashfield A, et al. Increased mortality in HER2 positive, oestrogen receptor positive invasive breast cancer: a population-based study. Br. J. Cancer 2010;103:475−81.

[15]Gutierrez C, Schiff R. HER2: biology, detection, and clinical implications. Arch. Pathol. Lab. Med. 2011;135:55−62.

[16]Herceptin® trastuzumab. Package insert. Genentech, South San Francisco, CA; October 2003.

[17]Brody T. Nutritional biochemistry. 2nd ed. San Diego, CA: Academic Press; 1999. pp. 898−902.

[18]Russo A, Bazan V, Agnese V, Rodolico V, Gebbia N. Prognostic and predictive factors in colorectal cancer: Kirsten Ras in CRC (RASCAL) and TP53CRC collaborative studies. Ann. Oncol. 2005;16(Suppl. 4):iv 44−9.

[19]Kirsten WH, Schauf V, McCoy J. Properties of a murine sarcoma virus. Bibl. Haematol. 1970;36:246−9.

[20]Mandrekar SJ, Sargent DJ. Clinical trial designs for predictive biomarker validation: theoretical considerations and practical challenges. J. Clin. Oncol. 2009;27:4027−34.

The hazard ratio (HR) in comparing drug versus placebo was HR = 0.45 where the tumors had wild-type, nonmutated *KRAS*. The HR in comparing drug versus placebo was HR = 0.99, where tumors had mutated *KRAS*.

In view of results such as these, the American Society of Clinical Oncology (ASCO), recommended that only patients with wild-type *KRAS* be treated with anti-EGFR therapy, and that patients with mutated *KRAS* should not receive this treatment (21,22). In this chapter, mutated *KRAS* refers to mutations at codons 12 or 13.

To summarize, colorectal cancer patients with *KRAS* mutations face two types of bad news. The first bad news is that these mutations are prognostic for worse outcome. The second type of bad news is that anti-EGFR is not recommended, where the cancer expresses *KRAS* that is mutated at codons 12 or 13.

b. Including Biomarker Tests in the Study Design

Biomarker status can be an integral part of trial design, that is, for dictating the nature of the study schema. As indicated by three study schema, shown below, biomarker status can be used: (1) to serve as an inclusion or exclusion criterion (Fig. 19.1); (2) to stratify subjects (Fig. 19.2); and (3) to dictate the treatment, for example, drug A versus drug B (Fig. 19.3) (23).

c. Criteria for Surrogates

The following concerns surrogate markers, as well as markers that do not meet the stringent requirements for a marker to be considered a surrogate marker. According to the Prentice criteria (24,25), a valid surrogate is one that correlates with the true clinical outcome and fully captures the net effect of drug treatment. The term *surrogate* refers to a biological parameter, such as tumor shrinkage, cholesterol levels, blood pressure, bloodstream virus levels, or serum levels of a tumor antigen, where the measured value can replace the true clinical outcome, and contribute to convincing a regulatory agency to approve the study drug. Regarding these particular examples, tumor shrinkage can be a surrogate for

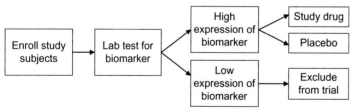

FIGURE 19.1 Biomarkers can be used when determining inclusion criteria or exclusion criteria.

[21]Bacolod MD, Barany F. Molecular profiling of colon tumors: the search for clinically relevant biomarkers of progression, prognosis, therapeutics, and predisposition. Ann. Surg. Oncol. 2011 (7 pp.).

[22]Allegra CJ, Jessup JM, Somerfield MR, et al. American Society of Clinical Oncology provisional clinical opinion: testing for KRAS gene mutations in patients with metastatic colorectal carcinoma to predict response to anti-epidermal growth factor receptor monoclonal antibody therapy. J. Clin. Oncol. 2009;27:2091−6.

[23]Freidlin B, McShane LM, Korn EL. Randomized clinical trials with biomarkers: design issues. J. Natl Cancer Inst. 2010;102:152−60.

[24]Fleming TR, DeMets DL. Surrogate end points in clinical trials: are we being misled? Ann. Intern. Med. 1996;125:605−13.

[25]Gill S, Sargent D. End points for adjuvant therapy trials: has the time come to accept disease-free survival as a surrogate end point for overall survival? Oncologist 2006;11:624−9.

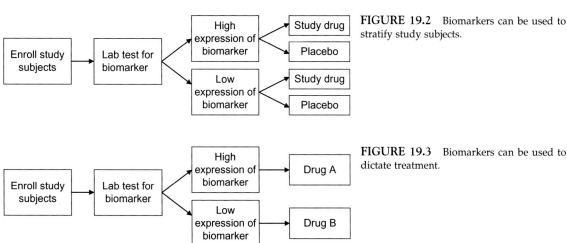

FIGURE 19.2 Biomarkers can be used to stratify study subjects.

FIGURE 19.3 Biomarkers can be used to dictate treatment.

total elimination of cancer, lowered cholesterol can be a surrogate for reduction in heart attack rate, lowered blood pressure can be a surrogate for reduced heart attack rate, reduced virus levels can be a surrogate for total cure from the virus, and reduced tumor antigen can be a surrogate for total cure from the cancer.

Fleming and DeMets (26) and Molenberghs et al. (27) warn that merely establishing a *correlation* between the proposed surrogate and the clinical endpoint is not sufficient to establish the parameter as an acceptable surrogate. What is also needed is that the proposed surrogate endpoint be validated, that is, experimentally tested using appropriate statistical methods. "From a regulatory perspective, a biomarker is not considered an acceptable surrogate endpoint for a determination of efficacy of a new drug unless it has been empirically shown to function as a valid indicator of clinical benefit" (28).

Fleming and DeMets (29) provided an insightful set of factors that may prevent a proposed surrogate, including proposed surrogates that are biomarkers, from being established as a valid surrogate. These factors are as follows:

1. The surrogate is not in the causal pathway of the disease process.
2. Of several causal pathways of disease, the study drug affects only the pathway mediated through the surrogate, and does not affect other pathways that can cause the disease.

[26] Fleming TR, DeMets DL. Surrogate end points in clinical trials: are we being misled? Ann. Intern. Med. 1996;125:605–13.

[27] Molenberghs G, Buyse M, Burzykowski T. The evaluation of surrogate endpoints. New York: Springer; 2005. p. 9.

[28] Molenberghs G, Buyse M, Burzykowski T. The evaluation of surrogate endpoints. New York: Springer; 2005. p. 7.

[29] Fleming TR, DeMets DL. Surrogate end points in clinical trials: are we being misled? Ann. Intern. Med. 1996;125:605–13.

3. The surrogate is not in the pathway of the drug's effect.
4. The study drug has mechanisms of action that are independent of the disease process.

d. Clinical Trials Focusing on Utility of a Biomarker

It is common practice, in clinical trials, to stratify subjects according to the grade or stage of the disease or pathological lesion, gender, and study site (city or nation). During the event of allocation and randomization, study personnel ensure that the number of subjects in each of these subgroups, for study drug subjects, is equal to the number of subjects in each corresponding subgroup, for control subjects.

But where the goal of a clinical trial is to assess the value of a biomarker, study subjects are also stratified into a first subgroup where biomarker is highly expressed, and into a subgroup where biomarker expression is low.

1. Biomarkers in Breast Cancer —The Stratton Study

Biomarkers relevant to breast cancer include *BRCA1* gene, *BRCA2* gene, human EGFR-2 (*HER2*), *estrogen receptor*, and *progesterone receptor*. Women with mutations in *BRCA1* or *BRCA2* are at increased risk for breast cancer (30). These women have a 50% chance of developing breast cancer. *BRCA1* mutations also result in an increased risk for ovarian cancer and, in men, prostate cancer. Women screening positive for these mutations have the choice of frequent cancer surveillance by magnetic resonance imaging, chemoprevention, or preemptive mastectomy (31). Table 19.1 lists the contribution of *BRCA1* mutations to ovarian cancer.

TABLE 19.1   Contribution of BRCA1 Mutations to Ovarian Cancer[a]

Patient	Mutation in *BRCA1* Gene
Breast cancer, age 50	Deletion of AA (adenine-adenine) at nucleotide 230
Ovarian cancer, age 38	Four base pair deletion at nucleotide 1942
Ovarian cancer, age 34	Four base pair deletion at nucleotide 3452
Breast cancer, age 38	Deletion of GT (guanine-thymine) at nucleotide 4287
Breast cancer, age 60	Conversion of C (cytosine) to T (thymidine) at nucleotide 4446, resulting in a stop codon
Breast cancer, age 44	Four base pair deletion at nucleotide 5149
Ovarian cancer, age 44	Insertion of C (cytosine) at nucleotide 5382
Ovarian cancer, age 40	Deletion of G (guanine) at nucleotide 5629

[a]*Stratton JF, Gayther SA, Russell P, et al. Contribution of BRCA1 mutations to ovarian cancer. New Engl. J. Med. 1997;336:1125–30.*

[30]Fong PC, Boss DS, Yap TA, et al. Inhibition of poly(ADP-ribose) polymerase in tumors from BRCA mutation carriers. New Engl. J. Med. 2009;361:123–34.

[31]Olopade OI, Grushko TA, Nanda R, Huo D. Advances in breast cancer: pathways to personalized medicine. Clin. Cancer Res. 2008;14:7988–99.

This provides the scientific background on BRCA1. BRCA1 is a 1863-amino-acid protein, thus requiring a nucleotide mRNA containing 5589 codons (one codon for each amino acid) (32). The amino acid sequence of wild-type human *BRCA1* can be found at GenBank Accession No. AAC37594.1. Some of the mutations in this gene that are associated with breast cancer and ovarian cancer are shown in Table 19.1 (33).

In conducting any kind of clinical trial, the investigator might want to test all subjects for expression of the genetic biomarker. The investigator might also want to go a step further by subjecting the genetic biomarker to tests that identify the exact structure of expected mutations. If the biomarker is a protein or peptide, the researcher should decide whether gene expression should be measured (hybridization-based assay), if protein expression should be measured (antibody-based immunoassay), or if both should be measured. The failure of a change in gene expression to result in a corresponding change in polypeptide expression has been thoroughly documented. See, for example, Hu et al. (34), Haynes et al. (35), Pennica et al. (36), and Oh et al. (37).

Drugs such as Herceptin and antiestrogen compounds cannot be fully understood, unless one is aware of breast cancers that cannot be treated with these particular drugs. Triple-negative breast cancer resists treatment by these particular agents (38). About 15% of all breast cancers show low expression of the following three genes: *HER2*, *estrogen receptor*, and *progesterone receptor*. Breast cancer tumors with this genetic profile are called *triple negative* (39,40,41). Generally, triple-negative breast cancers appear at a younger age, in particular in premenopausal African-American women, and have an especially poor prognosis. Triple-negative breast cancers are threefold more prevalent in premenopausal black women, than in other groups. Triple-negative breast cancers are diagnosed, not by gene expression, but by using immunohistology. Immunohistology, in this context, refers to using fluorescent antibodies that specifically

[32]Smith TM, Lee MK, Szabo CI, et al. Complete genomic sequence and analysis of 117 kb of human DNA containing the gene BRCA1. Genome Res. 1996;6:1029–49.

[33]Stratton JF, Gayther SA, Russell P, et al. Contribution of BRCA1 mutations to ovarian cancer. New Engl. J. Med. 1997;336:1125–30.

[34]Hu Y, Hines LM, Weng H, et al. Analysis of genomic and proteomic data using advanced literature mining. J. Proteome Res. 2003;2:405–12.

[35]Haynes PA, Gygi SP, Figeys D, Aebersold R. Proteome analysis: biological assay or data archive? Electrophoresis 1998;19:1862–71.

[36]Pennica D, Swanson TA, Welsh JW, et al. WISP genes are members of the connective tissue growth factor family that are up-regulated in wnt-1-transformed cells and aberrantly expressed in human colon tumors. Proc. Natl Acad. Sci. USA 1998;95:14717–22.

[37]Oh JM, Brichory F, Puravs E, et al. A database of protein expression in lung cancer. Proteomics 2001;1:1303–19.

[38]Hudis CA, Gianni L. Triple-negative breast cancer: an unmet medical need. Oncologist 2011;16(Suppl. 1):1–11.

[39]Berrada N, Delaloge S, André F. Treatment of triple-negative metastatic breast cancer: toward individualized targeted treatments or chemosensitization? Ann. Oncol. 2010;21(Suppl. 7):vii30–5.

[40]Anders C, Carey LA. Understanding and treating triple-negative breast cancer. Oncology (Williston Park) 2008;22:1233–9.

[41]Stead LA, Lash TL, Sobieraj JE, et al. Triple-negative breast cancers are increased in black women regardless of age or body mass index. Breast Cancer Res. 2009;11:R18.

bind to *HER2*, to *estrogen receptor*, or to *progesterone receptor*.

Triple-negative breast cancer cannot be treated with Herceptin or with antiestrogen drugs, since (by definition) the tumor cells do not contain the targets of these drugs (42). Hence, triple-negative breast cancer is treated with conventional small-molecule drugs. Triple-negative breast cancers overexpress human EGFR-1 (HER1). Although "HER1" has a name similar to "*HER2*," it is not the same protein. Because of this cancer's high expression of HER1, there has been some interest in treating triple-negative patients with cetuximab (Erbitux®), an antibody that binds to HER1 (43,44).

This introduces the function of *HER2*, and describes its relationship to other cell signaling proteins. HER2 is a membrane-bound protein that transmits signals, by way of a cell signaling pathway, to phosphatidylinositol-3,4,5-trisphosphate kinase (PI3K) (45,46). PI3K is in a class of enzymes called kinases. Kinases catalyze the phosphorylation of specific target molecules. Drugs that inhibit PI3 kinases are used for treating a variety of cancers (47). PI3 kinases, which catalyze the phosphorylation of certain lipids, regulate survival, proliferation, and apoptosis in normal cells as well as in cancer cells (48).

2. Biomarkers in Breast Cancer— The Vogel Study

Trastuzumab (Herceptin), an antibody that specifically binds to *HER2*, is used for treating breast cancer. In a study of 108 breast cancer patients, Vogel et al. (49) assessed the efficacy of trastuzumab, and attempted to find a correlation between expression of *HER2* in tumor biopsies with efficacy of the drug. Efficacy was measured by two endpoints, objective response and time to progression (TTP).

According to the endpoint of objective response, efficacy was found in 34% of patients who *overexpressed HER2*, but only in 7% in patients bearing tumors with *normal expression of HER2*. These measures of objective response represent the sum of data on complete response and partial response. Partial response was defined by a greater than 50% decrease in the sum of the products of the perpendicular diameters of all measurable lesions.

[42]Conlin AK, Seidman AD. Beyond cytotoxic chemotherapy for the first-line treatment of HER2-negative, hormone-insensitive metastatic breast cancer: current status and future opportunities. Clin. Breast Cancer 2008;8:215–23.

[43]Oliveras-Ferraros C, Vazquez-Martin A, López-Bonet E, et al. Growth and molecular interactions of the anti-EGFR antibody cetuximab and the DNA cross-linking agent cisplatin in gefitinib-resistant MDA-MB-468 cells: new prospects in the treatment of triple-negative/basal-like breast cancer. Int. J. Oncol. 2008;33:1165–76.

[44]Anders CK, Carey LA. Biology, metastatic patterns, and treatment of patients with triple-negative breast cancer. Clin. Breast Cancer 2009;9(Suppl. 2):S73–81.

[45]Fu X, et al. Biology and therapeutic potential of PI3K signaling in ER + /HER2-negative breast cancer. Breast 2013;22(Suppl. 2):S12–8.

[46]Yao E, Zhou W, Lee-Hoeflich ST, et al. Suppression of HER2/HER3-mediated growth of breast cancer cells with combinations of GDC-0941 PI3K inhibitor, trastuzumab, and pertuzumab. Clin. Cancer Res. 2009;15:4147–5416.

[47]Bunney TD, Katan M. Phosphoinositide signalling in cancer: beyond PI3K and PTEN. Nat. Rev. Cancer 2010;10:342–52.

[48]Chalhoub N, Baker SJ. PTEN and the PI3-kinase pathway in cancer. Annu. Rev. Pathol. 2009;4:127–50.

[49]Vogel CL, Cobleigh MA, Tripathy D, et al. Efficacy and safety of trastuzumab as a single agent in first-line treatment of HER2-overexpressing metastatic breast cancer. J. Clin. Oncol. 2002;20:719–26.

Thus, by the endpoint of objective response, patients bearing tumors that overexpressed *HER2* responded better to therapy than patients bearing tumors that did not overexpress *HER2*.

The authors also used the endpoint of TTP. Progression was defined as a 25% or greater increase in any measurable lesion or the appearance of a new lesion. Median TTP was calculated. Median TTP was 4.9 months in patients with *overexpressed HER2*, whereas median TTP was much shorter (1.7 months) in patients where tumors expressed *normal levels of HER2* ($P < 0.0001$). Thus, by the endpoint of median TTP, expression analysis showed that patients bearing tumors that overexpressed *HER2* responded better to therapy than patients bearing tumors that did not overexpress *HER2*.

An inclusion criterion for enrollment was that *HER2* be expressed at a level of 2 plus or 3 plus, as determined by an immunological technique, that is, antibody staining of tumor cells. But the correlation study between *HER2* expression and TTP used the fluorescence in situ hybridization (FISH) technique, not from antibody staining. In other words, the correlation between *HER2* expression and TTP was made by probing chromosomes using the FISH technique, a technique sensitive to changes in copy number of any given gene (gene amplification). In view of the results showing that median TTP was 4.9 months in patients with *overexpressed HER2*, whereas median TTP was only 1.7 months in patients where tumors

expressed *normal levels of HER2*, the authors concluded that the FISH technique can select patients likely to benefit from trastuzumab therapy. As a general proposition, any investigator interested in making use of correlations between gene expression and choices of treatment needs to take note if expression was measured by techniques sensitive to: (1) gene amplification; (2) expression of mRNA; or (3) expression of polypeptide.

A general question, relevant to all clinical trials involving trastuzumab, is whether overexpression of the *HER2 polypeptide* correlates with overexpression of the gene by the mechanism of *gene amplification*. The answer is no. Overexpression of *HER2* can result from gene amplification or, alternatively, it can result from changes in transcriptional regulation (50,51,52). An advantage of the FISH technique is that gene copy number cannot change during processing or storage of the tumor sample while, in contrast, *HER2* polypeptide can deteriorate during processing or storage. An advantage of immunological testing is that the antibody signal is relatively stable during storage while, in contrast, the hybridized complex of the FISH probe and genes is not particularly stable to storage (53). The take-home lesson is that clinicians faced with the decision of choosing between using the FISH technique and the antibody staining technique, need to know that the biology of gene expression is not the same as the biology of polypeptide expression, and the technical limitations of the FISH technique are not the same as the

[50]Magnifico A, Albano L, Campaner S, et al. Protein kinase Calpha determines HER2 fate in breast carcinoma cells with HER2 protein overexpression without gene amplification. Cancer Res. 2007;67:5308−17.

[51]Magnifico A, Albano L, Campaner S, et al. Tumor-initiating cells of HER2-positive carcinoma cell lines express the highest oncoprotein levels and are sensitive to trastuzumab. Clin. Cancer Res. 2009;15:2010−21.

[52]Gruver AM, Peerwani Z, Tubbs RR. Out of the darkness and into the light: bright field in situ hybridisation for delineation of ERBB2 (HER2) status in breast carcinoma. J. Clin. Pathol. 2010;63:210−9.

[53]Penault-Llorca F, Bilous M, Dowsett M, et al. Emerging technologies for assessing HER2 amplification. Am. J. Clin. Pathol. 2009;132:539−48.

technical limitations of the antibody staining technique.

3. Methodology Tip—FISH Technique

In situ hybridization was invented by Gall and Pardue (54). This technique can determine the location of a given gene on a chromosome, to identify the particular chromosome, and to measure the number of copies of that gene on the chromosome.

FISH means *fluorescence in situ hybridization*. This term appears on the Kaplan–Meier plot from the Vogel study (55), as described earlier in this chapter. FISH involves contacting a fluorescent-tagged nucleic acid with a permeabilized cell, and allowing the fluorescent nucleic acid to diffuse to the gene of interest and to hybridize with the gene of interest, thereby producing a fluorescent signal that is associated with the gene in a stable manner.

The signal is proportional to the number of copies of the gene in the cell. In an article discussing the reliability of the FISH technique for measuring HER2 expression in breast cancer tumors, Gunn et al. (56) compared the FISH technique, which measures the number of HER2 genes, with immunological techniques, which measures the amount of HER2 protein residing on the membrane of the cell.

This concerns gene amplification. Gene amplification can occur in mammals (57), bacteria (58), protozoans (59), and archaebacteria (60). Gall (61) has been credited with the discovery of gene amplification (62). Schimke and co-workers (63,64) conducted most of the early, detailed research on the mechanisms of gene amplification, in the context of studies explaining how cancer cells in patients treated with methotrexate became resistant to that drug.

[54]Gall JG, Pardue ML. Formation and detection of RNA–DNA hybrid molecules in cytological preparations. Proc. Natl Acad. Sci. USA 1969;63:378–83.

[55]Vogel CL, Cobleigh MA, Tripathy D, et al. Efficacy and safety of trastuzumab as a single agent in first-line treatment of HER2-overexpressing metastatic breast cancer. J. Clin. Oncol. 2002;20:719–26.

[56]Gunn S, Yeh IT, Lytvak I, et al. Clinical array-based karyotyping of breast cancer with equivocal HER2 status resolves gene copy number and reveals chromosome 17 complexity. BMC Cancer 2010;10:396–403.

[57]Schimke RT. Gene amplification, drug resistance, and cancer. Cancer Res. 1984;44:1735–42.

[58]Elliott KT, et al. Copy number change: evolving views on gene amplification. Future Microbiol. 2013;8:887–99.

[59]Chavchich M, Gerena L, Peters J, Chen N, Cheng Q, Kyle DE. Role of pfmdr1 amplification and expression in induction of resistance to artemisinin derivatives in *Plasmodium falciparum*. Antimicrob. Agents Chemother. 2010;54:2455–64.

[60]Lam WL, Doolittle WF. Mevinolin-resistant mutations identify a promoter and the gene for a eukaryote-like 3-hydroxy-3-methylglutaryl-coenzyme A reductase in the archaebacterium *Haloferax volcanii*. J. Biol. Chem. 1992;267:5829–34.

[61]Gall JG. Differential synthesis of the genes for ribosomal RNA during amphibian oögenesis. Proc. Natl Acad. Sci. USA 1968;60:553–60.

[62]Brown DD. E.B. Wilson Award Lecture, 1996. Differential gene action. Mol. Biol. Cell. 1997;8:547–53.

[63]Alt FW, Kellems RE, Schimke RT. Synthesis and degradation of folate reductase in sensitive and methotrexate-resistant lines of S-180 cells. J. Biol. Chem. 1976;251:3063–74.

[64]Schimke RT, Kaufman RJ, Alt FW, Kellems RF. Gene amplification and drug resistance in cultured murine cells. Science 1978;202:1051–5.

4. Circulating Tumor Cells as a Prognostic Biomarker for Colon Cancer—The Cohen Study

Circulating tumor cells (CTCs) can be used as a biomarker. In a study of colon cancer, Cohen et al. (65) stratified patients according to baseline levels of tumor cells circulating in the bloodstream. Prior to initiating chemotherapy, blood was withdrawn, tumor cells present in the bloodstream were analyzed, and patients were divided into two subgroups. The two subgroups were:

- *First subgroup.* Three or more tumor cells/ 7.5 mL whole blood.
- *Second subgroup.* Less than three tumor cells/7.5 mL whole blood.

Tumor cells were detected by an immunological method sensitive to cytokeratin. All of the patients were subsequently treated with one of the drugs, bevacizumab, irinotecan, or exaliplatin. There was no placebo group.

The median PFS was 4.5 months (high CTCs) and 7.9 months (low CTCs). The median overall survival was 9.4 months (high CTCs) and 18.5 months (low CTCs). The results demonstrated that lower baseline CTCs, as compared with higher baseline CTCs, are correlated with greater PFS ($P = 0.0002$) and also correlated with greater overall survival ($P < 0.0001$). The authors concluded that the biomarker of CTCs is a strong predictor for PFS and overall survival.

The CTC biomarker test has the following uses. First, it can serve as a stratification factor for clinical trials. Second, it can inform the physician if more aggressive chemotherapy is needed (high CTCs), or if less toxic chemotherapy is acceptable (low CTCs). Third, it can identify patients who can safely have prolonged treatment breaks in chemotherapy versus those who need to resume chemotherapy more quickly.

5. Methodology Tip—Circulating Tumor Cells as a Biomarker

Tumor cells circulating in the bloodstream can be used as a measure of solid tumors present in specific organs, and as a prognostic tool for survival to that solid tumor. It has been reported that all types of solid tumors give rise to CTCs, and that in all types of solid tumors, some of these find residence in the bone marrow (66). Once residing in the bone marrow, these cells may persist over many years and eventually disseminate into other organs. Hence, studies using tumor cells as a biomarker use peripheral blood mononuclear cells (PBMCs) as well as bone marrow as the source of cells. CTCs can be measured directly, using an immunoassay that employs antibodies and a microscope, or indirectly, using PBMCs with detection of tumor cells by a polymerase chain reaction (PCR)-based method (67). PBMCs, used as a source of unpurified lymphocytes by immunologists, also contain CTCs.

[65]Cohen SJ, Punt CJ, Iannotti N, Saidman BH, et al. Relationship of circulating tumor cells to tumor response, progression-free survival, and overall survival in patients with metastatic colorectal cancer. J. Clin. Oncol. 2008;26:3213–21.

[66]Riethdorf S, Wikman H, Pantel K. Review: biological relevance of disseminated tumor cells in cancer patients. Int. J. Cancer 2008;123:1991–2006.

[67]Vogelaar FJ, Mesker WE, Rijken AM, et al. Clinical impact of different detection methods for disseminated tumor cells in bone marrow of patients undergoing surgical resection of colorectal liver metastases: a prospective follow-up study. BMC Cancer 2010;10:153 (7 pp.).

A number of studies of colorectal cancer, for example, have used the PCR for measuring the number of tumor cells present in the bulk of unpurified PBMCs. Iinuma et al. (68) used PCR for quantifying tumor cells, where the target genes were carcinoembronic antigen and cytokeratin 20. In a careful methodological study, these authors found a statistical difference in CTC counts, when comparing normal control subjects with cancer patients, and found some overlap in count numbers between these two sets of subjects. Iinuma et al. (69), report a detection limit of one tumor cell in 3 million PBMCs.

6. Cytokeratin as a Soluble Protein Biomarker for Colon Cancer —The Koelink Study

This study concerned the tumor antigen, cytokeratin. The type of cytokeratin that was measured was CK18-Asp396, a degradation product of cytokeratin-18.

Koelink et al. (70) demonstrated that soluble cytokeratin is elevated in the blood plasma of patients with colon cancer and that it is correlated with outcome. Outcome was according to the endpoint of disease-free survival. In this study, patients were divided into two groups, namely, those with cytokeratin greater than the median plasma concentration (for the group of patients), and those with cytokeratin lower than the median concentration (for the group of patients). Scott et al. (71) reported similar findings on cytokeratin's use as a prognostic biomarker for colon cancer.

7. Tumor-Infiltrating T Cells as a Prognostic Biomarker for Colon Cancer—The Galon Study

The number and activation state of immune cells found to infiltrate a tumor can be prognostic of outcome, for example, prognostic of metastasis of the tumor (72). Figure 19.4, from a biopsy of a patient with colorectal cancer, illustrates the infiltration of tumor cells (blue in original article) with lymphocytes (T cells) (brown in original article) (73,74). The study found that the density of T cells near tumor cells was a better predictor of survival than traditional staging based on tumor size. The researchers divided their biopsy samples into two groups, depending on whether the concentrations of T cells were high or low. Patients whose tumors had an abundant

[68]Iinuma H, Okinaga K, Egami H, et al. Usefulness and clinical significance of quantitative real-time RT-PCR to detect isolated tumor cells in the peripheral blood and tumor drainage blood of patients with colorectal cancer. Int. J. Oncol. 2006;28:297–306.

[69]Iinuma H, Okinaga K, Egami H, et al. Usefulness and clinical significance of quantitative real-time RT-PCR to detect isolated tumor cells in the peripheral blood and tumor drainage blood of patients with colorectal cancer. Int. J. Oncol. 2006;28:297–306.

[70]Koelink PJ, Lamers CB, Hommes DW, Verspaget HW. Circulating cell death products predict clinical outcome of colorectal cancer patients. BMC Cancer 2009;9:88.

[71]Scott LC, Evans TR, Cassidy J, et al. Cytokeratin 18 in plasma of patients with gastrointestinal adenocarcinoma as a biomarker of tumour response. Br. J. Cancer 2009;101:410–7.

[72]Deschoolmeester V, Baay M, Specenier P, Lardon F, Vermorken JB. A review of the most promising biomarkers in colorectal cancer: one step closer to targeted therapy. Oncologist 2010;15:699–731.

[73]Galon J, Costes A, Sanchez-Cabo F, et al. Type, density, and location of immune cells within human colorectal tumors predict clinical outcome. Science 2006;313:1960–4.

[74]Couzin J. T Cells a boon for colon cancer prognosis. Science 2006;313:1868–9.

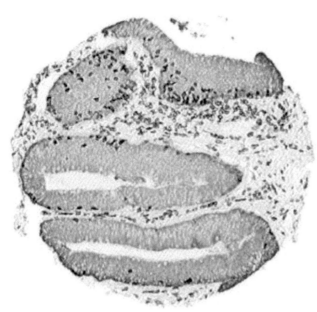

FIGURE 19.4 T cells (brown in original article) and tumor cells (blue in original article). The antibodies used for tagging T cells were antibodies that specifically bind CD3, CD8, CD45RO, and GZMB (granzyme B). The antibodies used for tagging tumor cells were antibodies against cytokeratin, and cytokeratin-8.

infiltrate of T cells had a 5-year survival rate of 73%, compared with 30% for patients with low densities of T cells around the tumor. Thus, the nature of a patient's immune response to a given tumor can be a good prognostic marker, where the prognostic value of this particular marker may be greater than that provided by traditional staging methods.

Immune cells have been used as biomarkers for predicting survival to colon cancer in studies by other investigators, for example, Pagès et al. (75), Pagès et al. (76), and Camus et al. (77).

8. Tumor-Infiltrating T Cells as a Prognostic Biomarker for Colon Cancer—The Morris Study

Morris et al. (78) evaluated the prognostic significance of lymphocytes, as markers, in colon cancer patients treated with surgery alone, or with surgery followed by 5-fluorouracil. Increased lymphocyte infiltration was associated with better survival in patients treated by *surgery plus 5-fluorouracil* (HR = 0.52). But increased lymphocyte infiltration was not associated with better (or worse) survival in patients treated by *surgery alone* (HR = 0.98). The study

[75]Pagès F, Kirilovsky A, Mlecnik B, et al. In situ cytotoxic and memory T cells predict outcome in patients with early-stage colorectal cancer. J. Clin. Oncol. 2009;27:5944–51.

[76]Pagès F, Berger A, Camus M, et al. Effector memory T cells, early metastasis, and survival in colorectal cancer. New Engl. J. Med. 2005;353:2654–66.

[77]Camus M, Tosolini M, Mlecnik B, et al. Coordination of intratumoral immune reaction and human colorectal cancer recurrence. Cancer Res. 2009;69:2685–93.

[78]Morris M, Platell C, Iacopetta B. Tumor-infiltrating lymphocytes and perforation in colon cancer predict positive response to 5-fluorouracil chemotherapy. Clin. Cancer Res. 2008;14:1413–7.

demonstrated that tumor-infiltrating lymphocytes is a parameter suitable for predicting efficacy of 5-fluorouracil. In this case, efficacy was measured according to the endpoint of overall survival.

The following concerns the hypothesis that chemotherapy creates a natural anticancer vaccine. The Morris study proposed that cytotoxic chemotherapy is a potent activator of antitumor immune responses, and referred to the hypothesis that chemotherapy creates a wave of dead or dying tumor cells that enter the antigen presentation pathway. To reiterate this scenario, antigen presentation involves uptake of antigen by dendritic cells, processing of antigen by DCs to peptides, presentation of the peptides by DCs to T cells, and activation of antigen-specific clones of T cells.

e. Lymphocytes Can Kill Cancer Cells, but Lymphocytes Can Also Cause Cancer

As described above, tumor-infiltrating lymphocytes can be associated with a favorable outcome, as documented above in the studies of Galon et al. (79) and Morris et al. (80) in patients with colorectal cancer. On the other hand, lymphocytes infiltrating the gut on a chronic basis can cause colorectal cancer. This untoward effect of lymphocytes has been extensively documented in diseases of chronic inflammation of the gut, such as Crohn's disease and ulcerative colitis (81,82). Inflammatory bowel disease (Crohn's disease; ulcerative colitis) must exist for at least 7 years before the risk of colorectal cancer increases. Toxic oxygen produced by infiltrating lymphocytes and neutrophils induces the mutations found in cells of the gut, where these mutations occur in oncogenes such as *p53*, *KRAS*, and *adenomatous polyposis coli* (83,84). The end-result of accumulated mutations in the relevant oncogenes is colorectal cancer (85).

It might also be pointed out that patients with Crohn's disease and ulcerative colitis have elevated C-reactive protein (CRP). About 75% of Crohn's disease patients have elevated CRP, while 30% of ulcerative colitis patients have increased CRP (86). CRP, which is detailed at the end of this chapter, finds use as a biomarker.

II. METHODOLOGY TIP—MICROARRAYS

Microarrays are a tool for measuring large numbers of different biomarkers, for example,

[79]Galon J, Costes A, Sanchez-Cabo F, et al. Type, density, and location of immune cells within human colorectal tumors predict clinical outcome. Science 2006;313:1960−4.

[80]Morris M, Platell C, Iacopetta B. Tumor-infiltrating lymphocytes and perforation in colon cancer predict positive response to 5-fluorouracil chemotherapy. Clin. Cancer Res. 2008;14:1413−7.

[81]Westbrook AM, Szakmary A, Schiestl RH. Mechanisms of intestinal inflammation and development of associated cancers: lessons learned from mouse models. Mutat. Res. 2010;705:40−59.

[82]Ullman TA, Itzkowitz SH. Intestinal inflammation and cancer. Gastroenterology 2011;140:1807−16.

[83]Itzkowitz SH, Yio X. Inflammation and cancer IV. Colorectal cancer in inflammatory bowel disease: the role of inflammation. Am. J. Physiol. Gastrointest. Liver Physiol. 2004;287:G7−17.

[84]Leedham SJ, Graham TA, Oukrif D, et al. Clonality, founder mutations, and field cancerization in human ulcerative colitis-associated neoplasia. Gastroenterology 2009;136:542−50.

[85]Brody T. Nutritional biochemistry. 2nd ed. San Diego, CA: Academic Press; 1999. pp. 879−917.

[86]Sidoroff M, Karikoski R, Raivio T, Savilahti E, Kolho KL. High-sensitivity C-reactive protein in paediatric inflammatory bowel disease. World J. Gastroenterol. 2010;16:2901−6.

50–5000 different genes, at the same time. In using a microarray, expression levels of genes can be measured by a technique that employ hybridization.

A DNA microarray takes the form of a solid support, such as a glass slide, silicon chip, or nylon membrane, on which single-stranded DNA (ssDNA) is attached (87). Typically, the slide or chip is divided into hundreds or thousands of different regions, where ssDNA, corresponding to a particular gene of interest, is attached to each individual region. The microarray can even contain ssDNA corresponding to every single gene in the human genome, about 50,000 genes. With a tissue biopsy, or with collected lymphocytes, the researchers first isolate the mRNA, and use standard techniques for generating single-stranded cDNA (complementary DNA). The cDNA is modified by attaching a fluorescent dye. This is followed by hybridizing the fluorescent cDNA to the DNA microarray, where the nucleotide sequence of the cDNA matches closely the sequence of one particular DNA that is attached to the slide. Where there is matching, hybridization occurs, and the signal from hybridization is processed to take the form of an array of squares that are colored green or red. Typically, a green square means that the expression of the gene is low, while a red square means that gene expression is high. Nonbinding fluorescent DNA needs to be washed away before measuring hybridized fluorescent DNA.

In published studies of clinical trials, it is typical for the study to be conducted in two parts. In the first part, the researcher uses a microarray containing a huge number of genes, perhaps 5000 genes, determines which genes show increased (or decreased) expression in patients who are helped by a drug, and determines which genes show increased (or decreased) expression in patients who are not helped by the drug. The researcher identifies which genes are most altered in the helped patients, versus in the nonhelped patients. There may be about 50 genes in this group. In the second two, the researcher manufactures a microarray containing these 50 genes, and then uses this microarray as a tool or device on a second group of patients. In short, tissue samples are taken from all patients before starting drug therapy, and the expression levels of the 50 genes are measured. Then, all subjects receive the same study drug. After treatment, the researcher determines whether the helped patients showed a gene expression profile that was predicted (or expected) from the predetermined gene profile. If the helped patients actually did show the expected gene expression profile, the researcher publishes the results.

According to FDA's Guidance for Industry on microarrays, where a microarray is used in a regulated clinical trial, the investigator should detail the set of data that was used to discover the genes in the microarray, as well as the set of data used to validate the microarray (88). When a microarray is used, FDA wants data on the clinical history, demographic of the human subjects used to generate both sets of data, as well as information on how the genes were chosen. Ioannidis (89) reviewed methods for validating gene arrays.

[87]Brennan DJ, O'Brien SL, Fagan A, et al. Application of DNA microarray technology in determining breast cancer prognosis and therapeutic response. Expert. Opin. Biol. Ther. 2005;5:1069–83.

[88]U.S. Department of Health and Human Services. Food and Drug Administration. Guidance for industry and FDA staff. Class II special controls guidance document: gene expression profiling test system for breast cancer prognosis; May 9, 2007.

[89]Ioannidis JP. Is molecular profiling ready for use in clinical decision making? Oncologist 2007;12:301–11.

a. Microarray Used in Ovarian Cancer—The Spentzos Study

In a study of ovarian cancer, Spentzos et al. (90) acquired tumor biopsies from 68 patients and analyzed the expression of a large number of genes. Treatment involved surgery followed by chemotherapy. In general, ovarian cancer is eradicated in 70% of cases, but the cancer usually returns, and when it returns it is unusually resistant to chemotherapy.

What is thus desired is a prognostic device to determine which patients will likely fail initial therapy. In the Spentzos study, ovarian tumor biopsies were collected at the time of surgery, but before chemotherapy. For their first study, seven samples from short-term survivors and seven samples from long-term survivors were analyzed. The result was a first list of genes, where changes in expression were associated with short-term survival, and a second list of genes where changes were associated with long-term survival. Then, after the surgery, patients received chemotherapy, and study personnel waited several years to determine which patients would be short-term survivors (death within 2 years), and which would be long-term survivors (over 5 years).

After collecting all survival data, the researchers sought a correlation between survival and gene expression, and arrived at a collection of 115 genes, which they named, "Ovarian Cancer Prognostic Profile."

With this profile in hand, the researchers applied it to a group of 68 patients, who were also treated with surgery, followed by tumor biopsy and gene analysis, and then chemotherapy. The authors drew a Kaplan–Meier plot. The first curve on the plot contained data points corresponding to all patients with a gene expression profile that, according to their diagnostic device, had a favorable prognosis. The second curve on the plot contained data points corresponding to all patients with a gene expression profile that, according to their diagnostic device, had a poor prognosis. The result was two well-separated curves on the Kaplan–Meier plot, where the degree of separation was measured by the hazard ratio (HR). The separation was statistically significant ($P = 0.004$). The authors concluded that patients showing an unfavorable prognosis would be appropriate candidates for maintenance therapy, or for treatment with new experimental drugs.

b. Microarray Used in Colon Cancer—The Wang Study

In a study of Dukes' B colon cancer, Wang et al. (91) acquired tumor biopsies from 74 patients, prepared cDNA from the biopsies, and analyzed the cDNA using a microarray that contained DNA corresponding to 22,000 different genes. (The term Dukes' is not a typo.) In the years following surgery, 31 patients had relapse within 3 years, whereas 43 patients remained cancer-free for over 3 years.

Eventually, the authors arrived at a 23-gene signature that served as a prognostic device.

With this device in hand, the authors studied a separate group of patients (36 patients). During surgery for the colon cancer, the researchers acquired tumor biopsies, analyzed each tumor sample with the 23-gene signature device, and allocated each patient into the good prognosis group or the poor prognosis group. Then, the researchers waited 6 years, and kept records of the survival time for each

[90]Spentzos D, Levine DA, Ramoni MF, et al. Gene expression signature with independent prognostic significance in epithelial ovarian cancer. J. Clin. Oncol. 2004;22:4700–10.

[91]Wang Y, Jatkoe T, Zhang Y, et al. Gene expression profiles and molecular markers to predict recurrence of Dukes' B colon cancer. J. Clin. Oncol. 2004;22:1564–71.

patient. The results were used to make a Kaplan–Meier plot containing two curves. The two curves were well-separated, where the separation was statistically significant ($P = 0.0001$). The issue was that Dukes' B colon cancer is treated with surgery, but that data on whether surgery should be followed by chemotherapy is conflicting, undecided, or controversial. The Wang study is expected to bring a decisive answer, by identifying patients likely to benefit from chemotherapy, prior to actually administering chemotherapy. In the authors' own words, "the prognosis signature would provide a powerful tool to select the patients who are at high risk and ensure that they receive adjuvant treatment."

Dukes' B colon cancer is not a specific type of colon cancer, but is part of a generic classification system for cancer of the large intestines (92). Dukes' A colon cancer involves invasion into but not through the bowel wall. Dukes' B involves invasion through the bowel wall, but not involving lymph nodes. Dukes' C involves invasion through the bowel wall, and also the lymph nodes, while Dukes' D involves all of the above, with widespread metastasis. This classification is similar to the more recently devised staging system, namely, Tumor (T), Node (N), Metastasis (M) staging (TNM staging) that is used for a variety of cancers.

c. Microarray Used in Liver Cancer—The Hoshida Study

In a study of hepatocelluar carcinoma (HCC), Hoshida et al. (93) acquired tumor biopsies from 307 patients, as well as biopsies from normal areas of the liver next to the tumor. In patients treated for HCC, what is desired is a diagnostic tool for predicting which patients are at greatest risk for recurrence. The researchers chose 6100 genes, and determined which of these genes were associated with long-term survival after surgery for HCC. In other words, the researchers determined whether there was a correlation between a change in expression (either an increase or decrease) for every single one of these 6100 genes, and long-term survival.

Gene expression data from *tumor samples* failed to show any correlation. To increase their chance of finding a useful result, the researchers also analyzed *normal liver samples* harvested from tissue adjacent to the liver tumor. This experiment worked. The authors arrived at a collection of 186 genes (a defined set of genes) useful for predicting risk for recurrence of HCC patients after "curative" surgery. The genes showing changes in expression, and that were most associated with poor prognosis, included *FSHB, SH3GL2, RBM34, NCAPH*, and *EGF*. The genes that showed changes in expression, and that were most associated with good prognosis, included *ALDH9A1, TTR, RLF, IPA1*, and *PFKFB1* (94). With the prognostic device in hand, the researchers then used it for testing liver samples from 234 other patients with HCC. The result was a success. The device predicted survival, and it predicted recurrence. The researchers concluded that their device can be used to identify patients in need of intensive follow-up after curative surgery.

---

[92]Shampo MA. Dukes and Broders, pathological classification of cancer of the rectum. J. Pelvic Surg. 2001;7:5–7.

[93]Hoshida Y, Villanueva A, Kobayashi M, et al. Gene expression in fixed tissues and outcome in hepatocellular carcinoma. New Engl. J. Med. 2008;359:1995–2004.

[94]Further information on these genes can be found at a web site of the US government, www.ncbi.nlm.nih.gov/pubmed.

III. C-REACTIVE PROTEIN

a. Introduction

The protein complex known as C-reactive protein (CRP) finds use as a biomarker for diseases having an immune component. CRP is an "acute phase protein," meaning that its levels in the blood increase dramatically, from under 0.003 mg/mL to about 1.0 mg/mL, within days of the start of inflammation. Interleukin-6 (IL-6) is the main inducer of CRP's acute-phase response. CRP has several biological functions, such as its ability to bind to phosphatidylcholine, including the phosphatidylcholine of infecting bacteria as well as the phosphatidylcholine that is exposed on dying human cells that are apoptotic or necrotic (95). CRP increases during autoimmune diseases, cancer, atherosclerosis, and heart attacks, as outlined:

• CRP is elevated in patients with chronic, pathological inflammation in the gut, as in Crohn's disease and ulcerative colitis. This inflammation increases the risk for colorectal cancer.
• Elevated CRP occurs in patients with colorectal cancer, nonsmall-cell lung cancer, prostate cancer, and breast cancer. CRP has been proposed to have prognostic value for these cancers, that is, to be a biomarker that predicts outcome of the disease.
• Where CRP levels in the bloodstream are slightly elevated (not markedly elevated) on a chronic basis, CRP serves as a prognostic factor for atherosclerosis.
• Acute changes in plasma CRP reflect tissue damage resulting from a heart attack. Acute, markedly elevated levels of CRP occur during a heart attack, where the CRP may contribute to the mechanism of tissue damage.

b. Biochemistry of C-Reactive Protein

C-reactive protein is a pattern-recognition molecule that mediates innate immune response. Because of CRP's role in innate immune response, CRP has a function analogous to other pattern-recognition molecules such as the toll-like receptors (TLRs) and nucleotide-binding oligomerization domain (NOD) proteins (96,97). Specifically, CRP binds to phosphocholine (PC) as a component of microbial capsular polysaccharide and mediates the innate immune response against microorganisms (98). Binding of CRP to the PC of bacteria promotes clearing of the bacteria from the bloodstream. CRP finds use in protecting against pneumococcal infections (99,100), *Salmonella*

[95]Pegues MA, et al. C-reactive protein exacerbates renal ischemia-reperfusion injury. Am. J. Physiol. Renal. Physiol. 2013;304:F1358−65.

[96]Lee MS, Kim YJ. Pattern-recognition receptor signaling initiated from extracellular, membrane, and cytoplasmic space. Mol. Cells 2007;23:1−10.

[97]Hartvigsen K, Chou MY, Hansen LF, et al. The role of innate immunity in atherogenesis. J. Lipid Res. 2009;50 (Suppl.):S388−93.

[98]Chang MK, Binder CJ, Torzewski M, Witztum JL. C-reactive protein binds to both oxidized LDL and apoptotic cells through recognition of a common ligand: phosphorylcholine of oxidized phospholipids. Proc. Natl Acad. Sci. USA 2002;99:13043−8.

[99]Kim JO, Romero-Steiner S, Sørensen UB, et al. Relationship between cell surface carbohydrates and intrastrain variation on opsonophagocytosis of *Streptococcus pneumoniae*. Infect. Immun. 1999;67:2327−33.

[100]Briles DE, Forman C, Horowitz JC, et al. Antipneumococcal effects of C-reactive protein and monoclonal antibodies to pneumococcal cell wall and capsular antigens. Infect. Immun. 1989;57:1457−64.

enterica (101), *Neisseria meningitis* (102), and malaria parasites (103).

CRP, TLRs, and NOD proteins are all used for pattern-recognition signaling (104). CRP consists of five identical proteins that are arranged around a central pore (105). The CRP polypeptide has the following sequence (106,107). The CRP polypeptide is 206 amino acids long. The polypeptide has a binding site for phosphatidylcholine, which comprises phenylalanine-66, threonine-76, and glutamate-81. The glutamate residue functions to bind the nitrogen atom of choline group of phosphatidylcholine (108). The amino acid sequence of human CRP is shown below (109):

```
MEKLLCFLVL   TSLSHAFGQT   DMSRKAFVFP
KESDTSYVSL   KAPLTKPLKA   FTVCLHFYTE
LSSTRGYSIF   SYATKRQDNE   ILIFWSKDIG
YSFTVGGSEI   LFEVPEVTVA   PVHICTSWES
ASGIVEFWVD   GKPRVRKSLK   KGYTVGAEAS
IILGQEQDSF   GGNFEGSQSL   VGDIGNVNMW
DFVLSPDEIN   TIYLGGPFSP   NVLNWRALKY
EVQGEVFTKP   QLWP
```

The following diagram outlines the pathway where IL-6 is expressed by leukocytes in an inflamed tissue, where the IL-6 travels through the bloodstream to the liver, and where the hepatocytes respond by expressing and secreting CRP. Injury to various parts of the body results in the expression of IL-6 as well as of other cytokines, which dramatically stimulate hepatocytes to release CRP (110). This increase is part of an event called the *acute-phase response*.

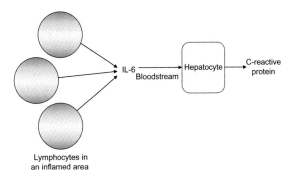

[101]Szalai AJ, VanCott JL, McGhee JR, Volanakis JE, Benjamin Jr WH. Human C-reactive protein is protective against fatal *Salmonella enterica* serovar typhimurium infection in transgenic mice. Infect. Immun. 2000;68:5652−6.

[102]Casey R, Newcombe J, McFadden J, Bodman-Smith KB. The acute-phase reactant C-reactive protein binds to phosphorylcholine-expressing *Neisseria meningitidis* and increases uptake by human phagocytes. Infect. Immun. 2008;76:1298−304.

[103]Pied S, Nussler A, Pontent M, et al. C-reactive protein protects against preerythrocytic stages of malaria. Infect Immun. 1989;57:278−82.

[104]Lee MS, Kim YJ. Pattern-recognition receptor signaling initiated from extracellular, membrane, and cytoplasmic space. Mol. Cells 2007;23:1−10.

[105]Black S, Kushner I, Samols D. C-reactive protein. J. Biol. Chem. 2004;279:48487−90.

[106]Tenchini ML, Marchetti L, Bossi E, Malcovati M. Lorenzetti R. Genbank accession no.: CAA39671.

[107]Oliveira EB, Gotschlich EC, Liu TY. Primary structure of human C-reactive protein. Proc. Natl Acad. Sci. USA 1977;74:3148−51.

[108]Gang TB, et al. The phosphatidyl-binding pocket on C-reactive protein is necessary for initial protection of mice against pneumococcal infection. J. Biol. Chem. 2012;287:43116−25.

[109]GenBank Accession No. M118880.

[110]Yue CC, Muller-Greven J, Dailey P, Lozanski G, Anderson V, Macintyre S. Identification of a C-reactive protein binding site in two hepatic carboxylesterases capable of retaining C-reactive protein within the endoplasmic reticulum. J. Biol. Chem. 1996;271:22245−50.

1. CRP as a Lung Cancer Biomarker —The Allin Study

C-reactive protein has found utility as a prognostic marker for a number of cancers, including liver cancer, lung cancer, and melanoma, as detailed below. Allin et al. (111) conducted an epidemiological study of 10,408 cancer-free Danish people. The authors acquired baseline plasma CRP levels, and followed the subjects for 16 years. Of all the subjects, 1624 developed cancer. The study excluded subjects who, at any time before or during the study, had cirrhosis of the liver. The authors divided baseline CRP into three groups, that is, low (under 1.0 mg/L), medium (1.0–3.0 mg/L), and high (over 3.0 mg/L). The authors discovered a significant association between elevated CRP (at baseline) with later development of lung cancer. Greater levels of baseline CRP were progressively associated with greater risk for lung cancer. The authors proposed that the association could be the result of undetected cancer (at baseline) where inflammation around the cancer caused expression of IL-6, where this IL-6 provoked hepatic expression of CRP. The authors also proposed that tumor cells could have been expressing the IL-6.

2. CRP as a Liver Cancer Biomarker —The Wong Study

This concerns surgery on the liver to remove metastatic tumors originating from colorectal cancer. Surgery is the standard treatment for this type of liver cancer. With surgery, liver cancer recurs in two-thirds of patients. Wong et al. (112) took plasma samples 1 day before liver surgery and measured plasma CRP. After surgery, patients were then followed for a prolonged period of time, where the median time of follow-up was 28 months. The authors found that elevated CRP was correlated with worse survival, and that normal CRP was correlated with better survival. Median survival of high CRP patients was 19 months, while median survival of normal-level CRP patients was 42.8 months ($P = 0.004$). The authors proposed that increased CRP was the result of greater nonspecific inflammation occurring in livers having a greater tumor burden.

The authors were careful to point out that there is an inverse relation between CRP and infiltration of tumors by lymphocytes. It should also be apparent, from the studies described in this chapter, that high CRP can mean poor prognosis, while high infiltration by lymphocytes of tumors can indicate favorable prognosis. The former parameter (CRP) reflects nonspecific immune response, while the latter parameter (infiltration) reflects antigen-specific immune response (113). In other words, a reader finding the opposite prognostic values of CRP and tumor infiltration to be contradictory, needs to realize that one reflects nonspecific immunity while the other reflects specific immunity.

3. CRP as a Melanoma Marker —The Findeisen Study

Melanoma, once metastasized, is an aggressive disease with a very poor prognosis.

[111]Allin KH, Bojesen SE, Nordestgaard BG. Baseline C-reactive protein is associated with incident cancer and survival in patients with cancer. J. Clin. Oncol. 2009;27:2217–24.

[112]Wong VK, Malik HZ, Hamady ZZ, et al. C-reactive protein as a predictor of prognosis following curative resection for colorectal liver metastases. Br. J. Cancer 2007;96:222–5.

[113]Canna K, McArdle PA, McMillan DC, et al. The relationship between tumour T-lymphocyte infiltration, the systemic inflammatory response and survival in patients undergoing curative resection for colorectal cancer. Br. J. Cancer 2005;92:651–4.

The melanoma study of Findeisen et al. (114) concerned early-stage melanoma, which has a relatively good prognosis. Staging of melanoma is according to the criteria set forth by the American Joint Committee on Cancer (AJCC) (115). The Findeisen study consisted of screening of serum proteins with the goal of discovering useful biomarkers. Screening involved the technique of mass spectroscopy, a technique that provided a unique fingerprint of peptides derived from each serum protein, where the fingerprint took the form of a number, that is, the mass/charge (m/z) ratio. This technique is outlined below. The Findeisen study reported the discovery of a protein identified as $m/z = 11.680$. This protein was later identified as *serum amyloid A*. The authors found that stage I melanoma patients expressing high levels of serum amyloid A had worse survival, compared to stage I melanoma patients with high serum amyloid A. Moreover, the authors also found that stage IV melanoma patients with high serum amyloid A had worse survival.

The following introduces CRP into this narrative. In view of the fact that serum amyloid A is an "acute phase protein," the researchers also sought correlations between other established acute-phase proteins, such as CRP, and survival to melanoma. The Findeisen study discovered that CRP expression was able to distinguish between poor-prognosis stage I melanoma patients and good-prognosis stage I melanoma patients. The authors concluded that the *combination of expression data on serum amyloid A and CRP* serves as an excellent prognostic biomarker for early-stage melanoma patients. Findeisen et al. (116) were also careful to note that serum lactic dehydrogenase, a traditional biomarker for advanced melanoma, failed to have any prognostic significance for early-stage melanoma. In another study, by Fang et al. (117), it was discovered that elevated CRP is associated with poorer survival to melanoma.

c. FDA's Decision-Making Process in Evaluating the Study Drug's Influence on CRP, for a Cancer Clinical Trial

FDA's *Medical Reviews, Pharmacological Reviews*, and *Statistical Reviews*, are published at the time that FDA publishes its *Approval Letter*. These reviews provide an intimate picture of the FDA's decision-making process.

This concerns a clinical trial on ruxolitib (Jakafi®), for treating myelofibrosis, a type of cancer. The information is from December 2014 of the FDA's website. The FDA reviewer observed that plasma levels of biomarkers associated with inflammation, such as *CRP, were elevated in myelofibrosis patients*, as compared to healthy persons. The reviewer also observed that *the study drug reduced CRP*, writing that, "[t]he levels of **C-reactive protein showed an 86% decrease** within 4 weeks of treatment with ruxolitinib." The study drug inhibits the enzyme, Janus kinase (JAK2).

The FDA reviewer described the connection between Janus kinase, a signaling protein

[114]Findeisen P, Zapatka M, Peccerella T, et al. Serum amyloid A as a prognostic marker in melanoma identified by proteomic profiling. J. Clin. Oncol. 2009;27:2199–208.

[115]Balch CM, Buzaid AC, Soong SJ, et al. Final version of the American Joint Committee on Cancer staging system for cutaneous melanoma. J. Clin. Oncol. 2001;19:3635–48.

[116]Findeisen P, Zapatka M, Peccerella T, et al. Serum amyloid A as a prognostic marker in melanoma identified by proteomic profiling. J. Clin. Oncol. 2009;27:2199–208.

[117]Fang S, Wang Y, Sui D, et al. C-reactive protein as a marker of melanoma progression. J. Clin. Oncoll. 2015;12:1389–96.

(STAT3), and plasma markers of inflammation, writing that the "data lends support to the widely held assumption that the JAK2 activating mutation and consequent activation of STAT3 leads to **increased inflammatory cytokines** in the plasma ... and that treatment with ruxolitinib reversed this." Focusing more on the drug's mechanism of action, the reviewer added that, "measurement of pSTAT3 activation is a surrogate for JAK2 [Janus kinase] activation, ... [t]his is a demonstration that ruxolitinib is inhibiting the enzymatic activity of JAK2 in vivo in patients on the ruxolitinib arm."

FDA's analysis of the study drug's influence on CRP is reflected in the *Pharmacodynamics* section of the package insert. Although the package insert did not mention CRP, it did mention part of the pathway (STAT3 activation) that provides inflammatory responses. The package insert for ruxolitinib (Jakafi) read:

> Ruxolitinib inhibits cytokine induced STAT3 phosphorylation in whole blood from healthy subjects and MF patients. Jakafi administration resulted in maximal inhibition of STAT3 phosphorylation 2 hours after dosing which returned to near baseline by 10 hours in both healthy subjects and myelofibrosis patients (118).

To conclude, the *Medical Review* illustrates how clinical trial data, which made use of the CRP biomarker, were included in the *Pharmacodynamics* section of the package insert.

d. C-Reactive Protein and Atherosclerosis

In addition to expression by hepatocytes, CRP is also expressed by cells in atherosclerotic lesions. CRP is found in the plasma, as well as in the extracellular matrix at the site of inflammation, such as atherosclerotic lesions (119). Expression of CRP by these lesions can result in local concentrations of CRP that are far in excess of plasma concentrations (120).

If CRP is eventually proven to contribute to the mechanism of atherosclerosis, it is likely that these high, local concentrations of CRP are a source of CRP's proinflammatory and proatherogenic effects (121). One possible mechanism of CRP, which is central to the established mechanism for atherosclerosis, is CRP's ability to mediate uptake of oxidized LDLs by macrophages (122). In atherosclerosis, it is a firmly established fact that chronic uptake of oxidized LDLs by macrophages results in the conversion of macrophages to foam cells, and eventually to formation of the atherosclerotic lesion (123,124). Singh et al.

---

[118]Package insert for JAKAFI™ (ruxolitinib) tablets, for oral use; November 2011 (23 pp.).

[119]Singh SK, et al. Exposing hidden functional sites of C-reactive protein by site-directed mutagenesis. J. Biol. Chem. 2012;287:3550–8.

[120]Wilson AM, Swan JD, Ding H, et al. Widespread vascular production of C-reactive protein (CRP) and a relationship between serum CRP, plaque CRP and intimal hypertrophy. Atherosclerosis 2007;191:175–81.

[121]Devaraj S, Singh U, Jialal I. The evolving role of C-reactive protein in atherothrombosis. Clin. Chem. 2009;55:229–38.

[122]Devaraj S, Singh U, Jialal I. The evolving role of C-reactive protein in atherothrombosis. Clin. Chem. 2009;55:229–38.

[123]Brody T. Nutritional biochemistry. 2nd ed. San Diego, CA: Academic Press; 1999. pp. 332–71.

[124]Galkina E, Ley K. Immune and inflammatory mechanisms of atherosclerosis. Annu. Rev. Immunol. 2009;27:165–97.

(125) provide straightforward evidence that CRP mediates uptake of oxidized LDLs by macrophages. CRP binds to PC that resides on oxidized lipoproteins (126).

The incidence of future cardiovascular disease events, that is, heart attacks and strokes, is increased among individuals with elevated baseline levels of CRP. Even modest elevations in stable baseline plasma CRP are correlated with an increased risk of future cardiovascular disease (127). CRP has an established utility in predicting risk for atherosclerosis. For this reason, use of CRP as a biomarker for atherosclerosis is outlined in this chapter. In brief, the risk of atherosclerosis (ischemic heart disease) was increased by a factor of 1.6 in persons who had CRP levels above 3 mg/L, as compared with persons who had CRP levels below 1 mg/L (128). In the chronic timeframe, high levels of plasma CRP are considered to be 3–10 mg/L (129).

While plasma CRP levels are dramatically correlated with the subsequent development of cardiovascular disease, it cannot be said that CRP satisfies the criteria set forth by Fleming and DeMets (130) for using CRP as a surrogate for cardiovascular disease. The reason that CRP fails is that the proposed surrogate (CRP) has not been conclusively demonstrated or proven to be in the causal pathway of atherosclerosis. Studies on humans using the methods of genetics have not supported the notion that CRP contributes to the mechanism of atherosclerosis (131,132).

Inflammation is part of the mechanism of atherosclerosis. LDLs are taken up by monocytes. The monocytes bind to endothelial cells of the coronary artery. The monocytes differentiate into macrophages, which accumulate in the artery, resulting in the "fatty streak," which later becomes an atherosclerotic lesion (133). The pathological accumulation of macrophages in the walls of blood vessels is one form of inflammation. CRP is expressed by arterial plaque and aortic endothelial cells. CRP contributes to

[125]Singh U, Dasu MR, Yancey PG, Afify A, Devaraj S, Jialal I. Human C-reactive protein promotes oxidized low density lipoprotein uptake and matrix metalloproteinase-9 release in Wistar rats. J. Lipid Res. 2008;49:1015–23.

[126]Hartvigsen K, Chou MY, Hansen LF, et al. The role of innate immunity in atherogenesis. J. Lipid Res. 2009;50 (Suppl.):S388–93.

[127]Teupser D, Weber O, Rao TN, Sass K, Thiery J, Fehling HJ. No reduction of atherosclerosis in C-reactive protein (CRP)-deficient mice. J. Biol. Chem. 2011;286:6272–9.

[128]Zacho J, Tybjaerg-Hansen A, Jensen JS, Grande P, Sillesen H, Nordestgaard BG. Genetically elevated C-reactive protein and ischemic vascular disease. New Engl. J. Med. 2008;359:1897–908.

[129]Hamer M, Chida Y, Stamatakis E. Association of very highly elevated C-reactive protein concentration with cardiovascular events and all-cause mortality. Clin. Chem. 2010;56:132–5.

[130]Fleming TR, DeMets DL. Surrogate end points in clinical trials: are we being misled? Ann. Intern. Med. 1996;125:605–13.

[131]C Reactive Protein Coronary Heart Disease Genetics Collaboration (CCGC), Wensley F, Gao P, et al. Association between C reactive protein and coronary heart disease: mendelian randomisation analysis based on individual participant data. Br. Med. J. 2011;342 (8 pp.).

[132]Elliott P, Chambers JC, Zhang W, et al. Genetic loci associated with C-reactive protein levels and risk of coronary heart disease. J. Am. Med. Assoc. 2009;302:37–48.

[133]Brody T. Nutritional biochemistry. 2nd ed. San Diego, CA: Academic Press; 1999. pp. 332–71.

atherosclerosis by promoting adhesion of plate-lets to the endothelial cells of the vasculature, thereby stimulating thrombus formation (134).

CRP is likely to be part of the mechanism for acute damage occurring during a heart attack (135). In this mechanism, CRP contri-butes to complement activation. During this acute timeframe, CRP levels in the blood-stream can reach 150–200 mg/L (136,137). The highest levels of plasma CRP occur at 2–4 days after myocardial infarction (138). These high values are much greater than CRP levels occurring in chronic timeframes. Ørn et al. (139) provide time-course data on plasma CRP in heart attack patients, and demonstrate that a peak (mean of 35 mg/L) occurs at 2 days.

IV. BIOMARKERS—SPECIALIZED TOPICS

a. Introduction

Individual biomarkers, as well as biomarker combinations, are typically used for these purposes.

- Diagnosing a disease,
- Assessing the prognosis of the disease,
- Predicting efficacy of a given drug,
- Predicting safety of a drug.

In using a panel of biomarkers, subgroups of study subjects are identified prior to initiat-ing treatment of subjects in a clinical trial, thus enabling the biomarker panel to identify sub-groups of particular interest.

b. Exploratory Biomarkers

Biomarkers that are used in clinical trials include those that are used as study endpoints, as well as those that are merely exploratory biomarkers. Exploratory biomarkers are used with the goal of arriving at a suitable panel that can subsequently be tested and validated, for use as an endpoint in future clinical trials. In an account of endpoints for clinical trials, Turk et al. (140) distinguished "exploratory endpoints" from biomarkers that are used to define a primary endpoint, multiple primary endpoints, secondary endpoints, and compos-ite endpoints. In using a composite endpoint, multiple endpoints are typically combined to produce a single variable, such as an index or score.

[134]Grad E, et al. Endothelial C-reactive protein increases platelet adhesion under flow conditions. Am. J. Physiol. Heart Circ. Physiol. 2011;301:H730–6.

[135]Casas JP, Shah T, Hingorani AD, Danesh J, Pepys MB. C-reactive protein and coronary heart disease: a critical review. J. Intern. Med. 2008;264:295–314.

[136]Pietilä KO, Harmoinen AP, Jokiniitty J, Pasternack AI. Serum C-reactive protein concentration in acute myocardial infarction and its relationship to mortality during 24 months of follow-up in patients under thrombolytic treatment. Eur. Heart J. 1996;17:1345–9.

[137]Griselli M, Herbert J, Hutchinson WL, et al. C-reactive protein and complement are important mediators of tissue damage in acute myocardial infarction. J. Exp. Med. 1999;190:1733–40.

[138]Pietilä KO, Harmoinen AP, Jokiniitty J, Pasternack AI. Serum C-reactive protein concentration in acute myocardial infarction and its relationship to mortality during 24 months of follow-up in patients under thrombolytic treatment. Eur. Heart J. 1996;17:1345–9.

[139]Ørn S, Manhenke C, Ueland T, et al. C-reactive protein, infarct size, microvascular obstruction, and left-ventricular remodelling following acute myocardial infarction. Eur. Heart J. 2009;30:1180–6.

[140]Turk DC, Dworkin RH, McDermott MP, et al. Analyzing multiple endpoints in clinical trials of pain treatments: IMMPACT recommendations. Pain 2008;139:485–93.

c. Endpoint That Is a Combination of a Biomarker and a Clinical Parameter

An endpoint can take the form of a composite that is the combination of a biomarker and a clinical parameter. Nolen and Lokshin (141) described the combination of a protein (carbohydrate antigen-125; CA125) and a clinical parameter (ultrasound). Where CA125 alone is used, this biomarker is sensitive to only half of early-stage ovarian cancers. A problem with using *ultrasound alone*, is a high rate of false positives (142). The composite endpoint provides the most reliable endpoint.

A panel of biomarkers, typically used with an algorithm to generate a score, is sometimes used in clinical trials. To this end, Pinsky and Zhu (143) stated that, "[a] widely held viewpoint in the field of predictive markers for disease holds that no single marker can provide high enough discrimination and that a panel of markers … will be needed." Although it might be intuitively obvious that a panel of markers is more accurate than using only one biomarker, attempts at discovering useful panels often fail. For example, one study which concerned CA125, an established biomarker for ovarian cancer, determined that a panel of eight biomarkers that included CA125 is no more predictive than CA125 alone (144). *False positives* occur with the CA125 biomarker, because CA125 can be elevated in benign conditions, such as endometriosis, pelvic inflammatory disease, pregnancy, and diverticulosis. Another problem with the CA125 biomarker, is *false negatives* in about half of early-stage ovarian cancers (145).

Another example of a combination of a biomarker with clinical parameters, is use of the CA125 biomarker and ultrasound and menopausal status clinical parameters. The algorithm takes the form (146):

Risk Malignancy Index

$$= [\text{serum concentration of } CA125]$$
$$\times [\text{ultrasound score}] \times [\text{menopausal status}]$$

The algorithm provides a score called the Risk Malignancy Index (RMI). The CA125 component of this score is the concentration of CA125 in serum (units/mL). The ultrasound component of this algorithm is itself the result of an algorithm. In other words, the ultrasound component is the result of the following sum. To arrive at this sum, one point is given for each of septations, solid areas, metastatic disease, ascites, and bilateral lesions, as determined by ultrasound. Regarding the menopausal component of this algorithm, one point is given if premenopausal, and three points is given if postmenopausal.

Jordan and Bristow (147) were careful to disclose that the risk malignancy index (RMI) has been periodically refined and updated

[141]Nolen BM, Lokshin AE. Biomarker testing for ovarian cancer: clinical utility of multiplex assays. Mol. Diagn. Ther. 2015;17:139–46.

[142]Yurkovetsky Z, Skates S, Lomakin A, et al. Development of a multimarker assay for early detection of ovarian cancer. J. Clin. Oncol. 2010;28:2159–66.

[143]Pinsky PF, Zhu CS. Building multi-marker algorithms for disease prediction—the role of correlations among markers. Biomarker Insights 2011;6:83–93.

[144]Pinsky PF, Zhu CS. Building multi-marker algorithms for disease prediction—the role of correlations among markers. Biomarker Insights 2011;6:83–93.

[145]Jordan SM, Bristow RE. Ovarian cancer biomarkers as diagnostic tests. Curr. Biomark. Findings 2013;3:35–42.

[146]Jordan SM, Bristow RE. Ovarian cancer biomarkers as diagnostic tests. Curr. Biomark. Findings 2013;3:35–42.

[147]Jordan SM, Bristow RE. Ovarian cancer biomarkers as diagnostic tests. Curr. Biomark. Findings 2013;3:35–42.

over the years. As a general proposition, medical writers need to be aware that the criteria for measuring the severity for various diseases are updated periodically. In oncology, for example, the RECIST criteria for measuring the size and number of solid tumors have been periodically updated, as indicated in the cited references (148,149,150,151).

This concerns an algorithm that generates a predictive score using only biomarker data, but no clinical parameters. The name of the algorithm is Risk of Ovarian Malignancy Algorithm (ROMA). According to one commentator, "ROMA is a reliable tool characterized by high accuracy and reproducibility to stratify patients into a high or a low ovarian cancer risk" (152). The ROMA algorithm makes use of simple arithmetic, and requires input of data from two biomarkers. The two biomarkers are CA125 and serum human epididymus protein (HE4) (153,154). Please note that, in addition to being expressed in ovarian cancers, HE4 is expressed in normal tissues of both males and females, where it is found in epithelial cells of the trachea, renal tubules, breast, and epididymus (155). The ROMA algorithm, which involves simple arithmetic, provides a score called "Predictive Index." The algorithm, which requires inputting the concentrations of both CA125 and HE4 is as follows (156):

$$\text{Predictive Index} = -1.25 + 2.38 \times \text{logarithm} \\ \times [HE4] + 0.0626 \\ \times \text{logarithm}[CA125]$$

This particular algorithm is used only for premenopausal women. A different, but equally simple algorithm, is used for postmenopausal women. To repeat, the Predictive Index stratifies patients into low and high risk of malignancy groups.

Yet another diagnostic test used in ovarian cancer, is the OVA-1 test. This test requires expression data from five biomarkers, CA125, prealbumin, apolipoprotein A-1, beta2-microglobulin, and transferrin. The OVA-1 score can be any number between 1 and 10 (157,158).

[148]Ronot M, Bouattour M, Wasserman J, et al. Alternative response criteria (Choi, European Association for the Study of the Liver, and Modified Response Evaluation Criteria in Solid Tumors [RECIST]) versus RECIST 1.1 in patients with advanced hepatocellular carcinoma treated with sorafenib. Oncologist 2014;19:394−402.

[149]Fournier L, et al. Imaging criteria for assessing tumour response: RECIST, mRECIST, Cheson. Diagn. Interv. Imaging 2014;95:689−703.

[150]Edeline J, et al. Comparison of tumor response by Response Evaluation Criteria in Solid Tumors (RECIST) and modified RECIST in patients treated with sorafenib for hepatocellular carcinoma. Cancer 2012;118:147−56.

[151]Lenioni R, Llovet JM. Modified RECIST (mRECIST) assessments for hepatocellular carcinoma. Semin. Liver Dis. 2010;30:52−60.

[152]Chudecka-Glaz AM. ROMA, an algorithm for ovarian cancer. Clin. Chim. Acta 2015;440C:143−51.

[153]Simmons AR, et al. The emerging role of HE4 in the evaluation of epithelial ovarian and endometrial carcinomas. Oncology (Williston Park) 2013;27:548−56.

[154]Jordan SM, Bristow RE. Ovarian cancer biomarkers as diagnostic tests. Curr. Biomark. Findings 2013;3:35−42.

[155]Simmons AR, et al. The emerging role of HE4 in the evaluation of epithelial ovarian and endometrial carcinomas. Oncology (Williston Park) 2013;27:548−56.

[156]Moore RG, McMeekin DS, Brown AK, et al. A novel multiple marker bioassay utilizing HE4 and CA125 for the prediction of ovarian cancer in patients with a pelvic mass. Gynecol. Oncol. 2009;112:40−6.

[157]Abraham J. OVA1 test for preoperative assessment of ovarian cancer. Commun. Oncol. 2010;7:249−51.

[158]Jordan SM, Bristow RE. Ovarian cancer biomarkers as diagnostic tests. Curr. Biomark. Findings 2013;3:35−42.

d. Summary

This bullet-point list outlines general concepts relating to biomarkers, including those described in the above examples:

- Diagnostic tests include those that are prognostic, that is, used for assessing the natural outcome of a disease, and those that are predictive, that is, for predicting a particular subject's response to a drug. Diagnostic tests can also predict toxicity of a drug in a particular subject.
- Separate biomarker tests have been designed for use prior to administration of the study drug, and for use after treatment with the study drug. In other words, a given biomarker test may take into account whether a patient is treatment-naive or is treatment-experienced.
- Tests that use biomarkers can take the form of a combination of a biomarker with one or more tests that assess clinical parameters.
- Biomarker tests can use one biomarker, or several biomarkers where each is used separately and where each gives an individual score, or alternatively, several biomarkers where data from all of the markers are processed by an algorithm to give a single score.
- Attempts to establish the utility of one biomarker, or a panel of biomarkers, for use with a given disease are likely to be complicated where the disease takes several forms. Jones and Libermann (159) warn that the quest to discover a biomarker panel can

be impaired, where the disease of interest takes various forms, as is the case with renal cancer. Renal cancer takes the forms of pRCC, chrRCC, and oncocytomas.

V. EXPLORING NEW TYPES OF BIOMARKERS

a. Introduction

A number of molecules, subcellular structures, and cells, have been established as part of the mechanisms of normal physiology, and of the physiology of disease, but have only begun to be explored for their suitability as biomarkers. These include miRNAs, circulating DNA, covalent modification of the chromosomes with methyl groups (epigenetics), exosomes, and CTCs. This outlines the use of miRNAs, circulating DNA, epigenetics, exosomes (a subcellular structure), and CTCs (160) as biomarkers.

b. Nucleic Acids in the Circulation

miRNAs are small single-stranded RNA molecules of 21−23 nucleotides in length. miRNAs are biosynthesized in cells, and a fraction are released from cells and found in the circulation. miRNAs are used in the regulation of about one-third of all genes. miRNAs are distinguished by their stability in tumors, in the circulatory system, and also during storage. Berger and Reiser (161) outlined the use

---

[159]Jones J, Libermann TA. Genomics of renal cell cancer: the biology behind and the therapy ahead. Clin. Cancer Res. 2007;13(2 Suppl.):685s−92s.

[160]Almufti R, et al. A critical review of the analytical approaches for circulating tumor biomarker kinetics during treatment. Ann. Oncol. 2014;25:41−56.

[161]Berger F, Reiser MF. Micro-RNAs as potential new molecular biomarkers in oncology: have they reached relevance for the clinical imaging sciences? Theranostics 2013;3:943−52.

of miRNAs as biomarkers for clinical trials in oncology. To provide a more specific example, Corcoran et al. (162) explored the use of a panel of miRNAs, as well as exosomes that contain miRNAs, for their potential to assess the clinical outcome in patients with prostate cancer.

In an example from lung adenocarcinoma, a panel of four miRNAs was found to be capable of distinguishing patients with lung adenocarcinoma from normal subjects (163). The four miRNAs were miR-21, miR-486, miR-375, and miR-200b. Please note that each of these names represents a different sequence of some 21–23 nucleotides. In detail, in patients with lung adenocarcinoma, the concentrations in sputum of miR-21, miR-200b, and miR-375 were higher than in normal subjects, while the concentration of miR-486 was lower. After investigating the panel of four biomarkers, the investigators successfully validated the panel, where this validation was conducted with 64 patients with lung adenocarcinoma.

The take-home lessons from this study are as follows. First, the study shows that a lung cancer biomarker can be provided by sputum (rather than from a lung biopsy). Secondly, the study demonstrates the utility of biomarkers with *increased expression* as well as the utility of biomarkers with *decreased expression*. And third, the study reveals that an exploratory

clinical trial and a validation clinical trial involve two separate study designs.

This concerns DNA circulating free in the bloodstream, that is, DNA that is free and not in any cells. In a study of 30 women, Dawson et al. (164) determined that circulating tumor DNA was detectable in nearly all of the women, while CTCs were detectable in 87% of the women. A goal of this study was to improve upon earlier findings that a biomarker protein (CA 15-3) had only moderate sensitivity in detecting breast cancer. Dawson et al. (165) and others (166) have used the term "liquid biopsy" to refer to the use of free DNA in the circulation, rather than tissue biopsies, for assessing tumor burden in patients. An advantage of a liquid biopsy is the ease of repeated sampling during the course of chemotherapy.

c. Exosomes

Regarding exosomes, most types of cells, including tumor cells, secrete small vesicles. These small vesicles have been called exosomes and microvesicles. Exosomes contain proteins, as well as various types of nucleic acids, including DNA, RNA, and miRNAs. Exosomes are found in blood plasma, ascites fluid, and urine. In the context of oncology, exosomes can be used as biomarkers for

---

[162]Corcoran C, et al. miR-34a is an intracellular and exosomal predictive biomarker for respose to docetaxel with clinical relevance to prostate cancer progression. The Prostate 2014;74:1320–34.

[163]Yu L, Todd NW, Xing L, et al. Early detection of lung adenocarcinoma in sputum by a panel of microRNA markers. Int. J. Cancer 2010;127:2870–8.

[164]Dawson SJ, Tsui DW, Murtaza M, et al. Analysis of circulating tumor DNA to monitor metastatic breast cancer. New Engl. J. Med. 2013;368:1199–209.

[165]Dawson SJ, Tsui DW, Murtaza M, et al. Analysis of circulating tumor DNA to monitor metastatic breast cancer. New Engl. J. Med. 2013;368:1199–209.

[166]Toss A, et al. CTC enumeration and characterization: moving towards personalized medicine. Ann. Transl. Med. 2014;2:108 (16 pp.).

assessing the progression of cancer in cancer patients, for assessing efficacy of a drug during treatment. When originating from tumor cells, exosomes contain DNA sequences corresponding to oncogenes, including oncogenes that bear mutations responsible for the cancer. Nucleic acids originating from oncogenes, and which are found in exosomes, and which are being explored for their utility as biomarkers, include *KRAS, TP53, MET,* and *HER2* (167).

d. Circulating Tumor Cells

This mainly concerns cancerous cells released from solid tumors. A definition that distinguishes between primary tumor cells, CTCs, and disseminated tumor cells (DTCs), is provided by the following statement. The statement is that, "the existence of circulating tumor cells (CTC) and the settlement of these cells in secondary organs, such as liver, bone, and lungs, as disseminated metastatic tumor cells (DTC), is generally accepted. These cells are believed to be rare members among the cellular population of primary tumor cells" (168).

Thus, it is the case that CTCs represent a transition point between the primary tumor and a location of settlement. Toss et al. (169)

commented on bone marrow as a location of settlement, referring to the "notion that bone marrow may be a 'perfect niche' in which tumor cells ... survive," where these settled cells are called DTCs.

For the analysis of CTCs, it is generally the case that a sample of peripheral blood is taken, leukocytes are removed, resulting in a population of cells expressing the epethelial cell protein, EpCAM. The cells are then tagged with fluorescent antibodies specific for cytokeratins expressed by epithelial cells (170).

In an example of a prognostic test based on CTCs, Wallwiener et al. (171) described the use of CTCs to monitor the progression of *metastatic breast cancer*. Using the cutoff point of five cells per 7.5 mL of blood, the authors found that a concentration of CTCs at levels of greater or equal to 5 cells/7.5 mL blood was associated with decreased survival to the breast cancer.

An advantage of CTCs, over DTCs, for use as a biomarker, is that CTCs are much easier to sample, especially where repeated sampling is desired. CTC counting has been characterized a "liquid biopsy," that is a non-invasive test for predicting and monitoring response to treatment in various cancers

[167]Carvalho J, Oliveira C. Extracellular vesicles-powerful markers of cancer evolution. Front. Immunol. 2015;5:1−2.

[168]Braun S, Naume B. Circulating and disseminated tumor cells. J. Clin. Oncol. 2005;23:1623−6.

[169]Toss A, et al. CTC enumeration and characterization: moving towards personalized medicine. Ann. Transl. Med. 2014;2:108 (16 pp.).

[170]Toss A, et al. CTC enumeration and characterization: moving towards personalized medicine. Ann. Transl. Med. 2014;2:108 (16 pp.).

[171]Wallwiener M, Riethdorf S, Hartkopf AD, et al. Serial enumeration of circulating tumor cells predicts treatment response and prognosis in metastatic breast cancer: a prospective study in 393 patients. BMC Cancer 2014;14:512 (12 pp.).

(172,173,174,175,176,177). When CTCs are measured, the nature and number of these cells represent those freshly released from the primary tumor, as well as those released from site of metastasis. Sites of metastasis can include the bone marrow. To this point, Cen et al. (178) state that, "[c]irculating tumor cells (CTCs) are tumor cells disseminated from primary and metastatic sites and can be isolated from peripheral blood."

Cen et al. (179) disclose another advantage of CTC over biopsies of the primary tumor, namely, the advantage that CTC sampling and analysis is more representative of the types of tumor cells in the patient's body. To this end, Cen et al. state that, "[t]raditional tumor biopsy sampling can only capture part of the tumor and is unable to represent the entire tumor cell population or identify changes that occur over time. Ongoing analysis of CTCs not only has the potential to represent all cells shed from primary pancreatic tumor and each metastatic site."

CTCs have been used in early-stage cancer, as well as in metastatic cancer (late-stage cancer). The following concerns the biology of CTCs in breast cancer. In short, cancerous cells from breast cancer tumors migrate to the bone marrow. The *breast cancer* cells that migrate to the bone and reside in the bone are called "disseminated tumor cells" (180). Once establishing residence in the bone marrow, the breast cancer cells represent "minimal residual disease," and can be detected directly by way of a bone marrow biopsy. When the cells representing minimal residual disease leave the bone marrow, they are called "circulating tumor cells," and can be detected without the need for a bone marrow biopsy.

Riethdorf and Pantel (181) disclose that *breast cancer* cells leave the primary tumor to become CTCs, and that these CTCs migrate to

[172]Toss A, et al. CTC enumeration and characterization: moving towards personalized medicine. Ann. Transl. Med. 2014;2:108 (16 pp.).

[173]Wallwiener M, Riethdorf S, Hartkopf AD, et al. Serial enumeration of circulating tumor cells predicts treatment response and prognosis in metastatic breast cancer: a prospective study in 393 patients. BMC Cancer 2014;14:512 (12 pp.).

[174]Grobe A, Blessman M, Hanken H, et al. Prognostic relevance of circulating tumor cells in blood and disseminated tumor cells in bone marrow of patients with squamous cell carcinoma of the oral cavity. Clin. Cancer Res. 2013;20:425-33.

[175]Broersen LH, et al. Clinical application of circulating tumor cells in breast cancer. Cell Oncol. (Dordr). 2014;37:9–15.

[176]Young R, Pailler E, Billiot F, et al. Circulating tumor cells in lung cancer. Acta Cytol. 2012;56:655–60.

[177]Liandou ES, Markou A. Circulating tumor cells in breast cancer: detection systems, molecular characterization, and future challenges. Clin. Chem. 2011;57:1242–55.

[178]Cen P, et al. Circulating tumor cells in the diagnosis and management of pancreatic cancer. Biochim. Biophys. Acta 2012;1826:350–6.

[179]Cen P, et al. Circulating tumor cells in the diagnosis and management of pancreatic cancer. Biochim. Biophys. Acta 2012;1826:350–6.

[180]Hartkopf AD, Wallwiener M, Hahn M, et al. Simultaneous detection of disseminated and circulating tumor cells in primary breast cancer patients. Cancer Res. Treatment 2012. http://dx.doi.org/10.4143/crt.2014.287.

[181]Riethdorf S, Pantel K. Disseminated tumor cells in bone marrow and circulating tumor cells in blood of breast cancer patients: current state of detection and characterization. Pathobiology 2008;75:140–8.

bone marrow, stating that the bone marrow "is a common homing and surviving organ not only for breast cancer cells but also for cancer cells from other organs. These cells are likely to escape from the host immune system in a dormant state until internal and/or external signals might enable them to move and grow out to overt metastases at different organs." In short, in cancers associated with various organs, individual cancer cells may migrate to the bone marrow and, after a period of residence, leave the bone marrow for the circulation and initiate new tumors.

A similar scenario, involving migration of CTCs to bone marrow, occurs in *head and neck squamous cell carcinoma* (HNSCC). According to Grobe et al. (182), "disseminated tumor cells (DTC) in bone marrow has been shown to be a ... prognostic indicator for patients with ... HNSCC ... studies on bone marrow samples from patients ... revealed a positive correlation of DTC detection to relapse and metastases. However, because repeated and sequential bone marrow analyses are only possible in selected patients during follow-up observations, analysis of peripheral blood has become a promising alternative to investigate tumor cell dissemination ... the presence of circulating tumor cells (CTC) in peripheral blood is associated with a worse prognosis."

Studies of CTCs and of DTCs are currently directed to the goal of establishing these cells as biomarkers for use in prognostic tests and predictive tests in cancer. The studies have addressed the correlation of CTCs with cancer and the correlation of DTCs with cancer. A number of studies have addressed the possible correlation of CTC measurements with DTC measurements (183,184,185,186,187). For example, Grobe et al. (188) state that there is a, "[l]ack of correlation between detection of CTCs and DTCs." Issues in the potential utility of CTCs as a biomarker include the need to capture more CTCs, in order to overcome the problem that the heterogeneity of CTCs prevents meaningful results from analysis of only a small number of these cells (189).

[182]Grobe A, Blessman M, Hanken H, et al. Prognostic relevance of circulating tumor cells in blood and disseminated tumor cells in bone marrow of patients with squamous cell carcinoma of the oral cavity. Clin. Cancer Res. 2013;20:425−33.

[183]Grobe A, Blessman M, Hanken, H, et al. Prognostic relevance of circulating tumor cells in blood and disseminated tumor cells in bone marrow of patients with squamous cell carcinoma of the oral cavity. Clin. Cancer Res. 2013;20:425−33.

[184]Hartkopf AD, Wallwiener M, Hahn M, et al. Simultaneous detection of disseminated and circulating tumor cells in primary breast cancer patients. Cancer Res. Treatment; 2015. http://dx.doi.org/10.4143/crt.2014.287.

[185]Riethdorf S, Pantel K. Disseminated tumor cells in bone marrow and circulating tumor cells in blood of breast cancer patients: current state of detection and characterization. Pathobiology 2008;75:140−8.

[186]Kruck S, et al. Disseminated and circulating tumor cells for monitoring chemotherapy in urological tumors. Anticancer Res. 2011;31:2053−8.

[187]Braun S, Naume B. Circulating and disseminated tumor cells. J. Clin. Oncol. 2005;23:1623−6.

[188]Grobe A, Blessman M, Hanken H, et al. Prognostic relevance of circulating tumor cells in blood and disseminated tumor cells in bone marrow of patients with squamous cell carcinoma of the oral cavity. Clin. Cancer Res. 2013;20:425−33.

[189]Andrews NA. Circulating and disseminated tumor cells: many challenges, and even more opportunities for the cancer and bone field. IBMS Bonekey. 2012; Article no. 12 (2012) Int. Bone and Mineral Society (IBMS) Nature Publishing.

As of 2012, CTC measurements and the relevant correlations have not yet been *validated* as a tool for making clinical decisions (190). For this reason, this author refrains from disclosing studies that have shown correlations that are merely promising.

e. Epigenetics

Current research is addressing the possible utility of epigenetics tests for the diagnosis of, for example, lung cancer (191), breast and ovarian cancer (192), hepatocellular carcinoma (193), and Alzheimer's disease (194). To provide an example, the analysis of methylation of about 40 genes has revealed that this methylation can be used as a biomarker for *renal cancer*. Increases and decreases in methylation of specific genes are both used to produce a score.

In a study of *multiple myeloma*, the degree of methylation of the *NFKB1* gene was found to be associated with response to treatment with a particular drug, where lower levels of NFKB1 methylation were associated with longer survival during chemotherapy (195). Epigenetic markers have also been proposed for use in autoimmune disease, such as multiple sclerosis and rheumatoid arthritis (196,197). In *rheumatoid arthritis*, loss of methylation (hypomethylation) has been observed in specific genes in T cells and in synovial fibroblasts in patients with rheumatoid arthritis. The methylation changes in T cells cause these cells to be autoreactive, while the methylation changes in synovial fibroblasts cause them to be more susceptible to autoimmune attack. To give an example of a specific gene, loss of methylation of the *MMP13* gene causes increased expression of this gene, leading to degradation of type II collagen in cartilage (198).

VI. SINGLE NUCLEOTIDE POLYMORPHISMS

a. Introduction

SNPs are variants in the genome occurring naturally in the human population. SNPs is often pronounced as "snips." Each individual inherits one allele copy from each parent, so that the individual genotype at an SNP site is *AA, BB,* or *AB.* The Human Genome Project, the SNP Consortium, and other groups, have

[190]Hayashi N, Yamauchi H. Role of circulating tumor cells and disseminated tumor cells in primary breast cancer. Breast Cancer 2012;19:110−7.

[191]Nikolaidis G, et al. DNA methylation biomarkers offer improved diagnostic efficiency in lung cancer. Cancer Res. 2012;72:5692−701.

[192]Wittenberger T, Sleigh S, Reisel D, et al. DNA methylation markers for early detection of women's cancer: promise and challenges. Epigenomics 2014;6:311−27.

[193]Villanueva A, Portela A, Sayols S, et al. DNA methylation-based prognosis and epidrivers in hepatocellular carcinoma. Hepatology; 2015. http://dx.doi.org/10.1002/hep.27732.

[194]De Jager PL, Srivastava G, Lunnon K, et al. Alzheimer's disease: early alterations in brain DNA methylation at ANK1, BIN1, RHBDF2 and other loci. Nat. Neurosci. 2014;17:1156−63.

[195]Fall DG, et al. Utilization of translational bioinformatics to identify novel biomarkers of bortezomib resistance in multiple myeloma. J. Cancer 2014;5:720−7.

[196]Gupta B, Hawkins RD. Epigenetics of autoimmune diseases. Immunol. Cell Biol. 2015;93:271−6.

[197]Van den Elsen P, et al. The epigenetics of multiple sclerosis and other related disorders. Multiple Sclerosis Relat. Disorders 2014;3:163−75.

[198]Gupta B, Hawkins RD. Epigenetics of autoimmune diseases. Immunol. Cell Biol. 2015;93:271−6.

identified about 15 million common DNA variants, mostly SNPs (199).

SNP is defined as a genomic locus where two or more alternative bases occur with appreciable frequency ($>1\%$). SNPs are the most frequent type of variation in the human genome, occurring once every several hundred base pairs throughout the genome (200). For any given SNP, the SNP can occur in a coding region but not result in a change in amino acid, it can occur in a coding region with an amino acid change, it can occur in a regulatory region where the result is a change in gene expression, or it can occur in a region between genes.

b. Examples of Lung Cancer, Colorectal Cancer, and Chronic Lymphocytic Leukemia

The practical utility of SNP analysis in the field of oncology is illustrated by the following. In brief, two SNPs within the *MMP-9* gene are associated with the risk of developing lung cancer with metastasis. To provide another example, SNPs within the UGT1A7 have been shown to predict the response of colorectal cancer patients to capecitabine (201).

This concerns chronic lymphocytic leukemia (CLL). CLL has a heterogeneous clinical course. This variability in clinical course has stimulated interest in discovering prognostic biomarkers.

One such biomarker is mRNA encoding lipoprotein lipase. High levels of mRNA expression are associated with very poor prognosis for this type of cancer. However, detection of mRNA expression is not the same as detecting SNPs. In a study of SNPs in the gene encoding lipoprotein lipase, among 248 patients with CLL, Rombout et al. (202) focused on the SNP that is known as **rs13702**. CLL patients with the wild-type genotype (T/T) had very poor prognosis, while CLL patients with C/C genotype or T/C genotype had better prognosis.

The SNP **rs13702** is located at position 19868772 on human chromosome 8 (203). After transcription of the gene encoding for lipoprotein lipase, SNP **rs13702** resides in the 3′-untranslated region of the mRNA encoding lipoprotein lipase. The change in nucleotide in this SNP disrupts a regulatory element that functions with a species of miRNA, namely, miRNA-410. To provide a bit of scientific background, microRNAs (miR) are small 20–24-nucleotide noncoding RNAs that act as posttranscriptional inhibitors of gene expression by binding to miR recognition elements within the 30 UTR of their target mRNAs (204).

In their exploration of various SNPs and their possible association with survival time in CLL patients, Rombout et al. (205) concluded that, of the three SNPs in the lipoprotein lipase gene, rs301, rs328, and rs13702, it is the case

[199]Iacobucci I, et al. Use of single nucleotide polymorphism array technology to improve the identification of chromosomal lesions in leukemia. Curr. Cancer Drug Targets 2013;13:791–810.

[200]Engle LJ, et al. Using high-throughput SNP technologies to study cancer. Oncogene 2006;25:1594–601.

[201]Engle LJ, et al. Using high-throughput SNP technologies to study cancer. Oncogene 2006;25:1594–601.

[202]Rombout A, et al. Lipoprotein lipase SNPs rs13702 and rs301 correlated with clinical outcome in chronic lymphocytic leukemia patients. PLoS One 2015;0121526 (15 pp.).

[203]Deo RC, et al. Genetic differences between the determinants of lipid profile phenotypes in African and European Americans: The Jackson Heart Study. PLoS Genetics 2009;e1000342 (11 pp.).

[204]Richardson K, Nettleton JA, Rotllan N, et al. Gain-of-function lipoprotein lipase variant rs13702 modulates lipid traits through disruption of a microRNA-410 Seed Site. Am. J. Hum. Genetics 2013;92:5–14.

[205]Rombout A, et al. Lipoprotein lipase SNPs rs13702 and rs301 correlated with clinical outcome in chronic lymphocytic leukemia patients. PLoS One 2015; (15 pp.).

that rs301 and **rs13702** correlated with survival time of the patients to their leukemia, whereas no association with survival time was observed for rs328.

c. FDA's Decision-Making Process in Utilizing SNP Biomarkers in the FDA's Approval of Sofosbuvir

At the time of drug approval, FDA publishes its *Approval Letter* along with its *Medical Review*, *Pharmacological Review*, *Statistical Review*, and other reviews. This is from FDA's approval of sofosbuvir for the indication of hepatitis C virus (HCV) infections. This is for NDA 204671, which can be found on Mar. 2015 on FDA's website. The SNP was located on the human chromosome near the gene encoding *IL-28B*. In the list of baseline characteristics of all study subjects, the Sponsor had disclosed the genotype for each subject, that is, whether the subject was CC, CT, or TT. This refers to the nucleotide of interest near the *IL-28B* gene.

The FDA reviewer stated that:

> [a] genetic polymorphism near the IL28B gene is a strong predictor of SVR [Sustained Virologic Reponse] in patients receiving therapy with peginterferon and ribavirin. Numerous studies have demonstrated that patients who carry the variant alleles (C/T and T/T genotypes) have lower SVR rates than individuals with the C/C genotype.

The FDA reviewer merely observed the predictive value of the polymorphism, and refrained from making any further comment. The term *Sustained Virologic Response* (SVR) is conventional for studies on HCV, and it refers to reduction of viral RNA in the bloodstream to levels below 25 IU/mL blood as measures at 12 weeks after study drug cessation. The FDA reviewer's identification of the polymorphism indicates that it is identical with SNP **rs12979860**. This polymorphism is detailed below.

d. SNP That Is Upstream of *IL-28B* Gene and HCV Infections

Scientific background information on SNPs associated with the gene encoding *IL-28B* is disclosed here. SNP **rs12979860** is located about 1000 bases upstream of the gene encoding *IL-28B*. The *IL-28B* gene resides on chromosome 19. More specifically the gene resides at position 19q13 on chromosome 19.

In various people, this SNP can occur in three genotypes, homozygous for C (C/C), heterozygous (C/T), and homozygous for T (T/T).

People who are homozygous for C are twice as likely to respond to anti-HCV therapy than people homozygous for T (T/T), where therapy is with peginterferon alpha and ribavirin. Also, spontaneous recovery from HCV occurs at a two-and-a-half-times greater rate. Regarding subgroups, the variant that predicts greater risk of infection (T) is more common among Africans than in Caucasians, where the prevalence is 50−70% in Kenyans and Nigerians (206,207,208). The fact that SNP **rs12979860** has been characterized for its prognostic value (disease outcome in absence of therapy) and predictive value (disease outcome with a specific drug) indicates that it is a biomarker that can reasonably be included as an exploratory endpoint in a clinical trial.

[206]Thio CL, Thomas DL. Interleukin-28b: a key piece of the hepatitis C virus recovery puzzle. Gastroenterology 2010;138:1240−3.

[207]Thomas DL, et al. Genetic variation in IL28B and spontaneous clearance of hepatitis C virus. Nature 2009;461:796−801.

[208]Howell CD, Gorden A, Ryan KA, et al. Single nucleotide polymorphism upstream of interleukin 28B associated with phase 1 and phase 2 of early viral kinetics in patients infected with HCV genotype 1. J. Hepatol. 2012;56. doi:10.1016/j.jhep.2011.10.004.

e. FDA's Decision-Making Process in Utilizing SNP Biomarkers in the FDA's Approval of Telaprevir

Background information on SNPs from one of FDA's *Medical Reviews*, and from the published literature, is disclosed above. What follows is actual data from a clinical trial that led to the approval of a drug for HCV.

The drug was telaprevir, in combination with two other drugs, ribavirin and pegylated interferon-alpha2a. The goal of the study was to assess use of the *IL-28B* genotype for predicting SVR. SVR is defined above.

The clinical trial is from NDA 201917, and the *Medical Review* is available from May 2011 of FDA's website. The FDA reviewer observed that, after the clinical trial was started, researchers discovered various SNPs occurring near the *IL-28B* gene in patients with chronic HCV. The genotypes, that is, mutations in the chromosomal DNA, took the following three forms: C/C, C/T, and T/T.

The FDA reviewer noted that the Sponsor wanted to stratify the subjects who were enrolled in the trial, but it was too late for a conventional stratification. As such, the Sponsor implemented a work-around, and by way of Consent Forms, obtained consent to identify the genotypes of the enrolled subjects. This illustrates the concepts of:

- Stratification by SNP genotype;
- Correlating SNP genotype with favorable response to the drug;
- Obtaining permission to conduct additional tests on study subjects, once the clinical trial is underway;
- Stratifying subjects according to being treatment-naive or treatment-experienced;
- Critique from the FDA reviewer.

The FDA reviewer wrote:

In 2009, numerous publications described a novel association between single nucleotide polymorphisms (SNPs) near the interleukin (IL) 28B gene locus and response to treatment in subjects with CHC [chronic hepatitis C] ... the investigators identified a particular SNP (rs12979860) strongly determined the outcome of HCV therapy. Three genotypes were identified: C/C, C/T and T/T. The discovery of the IL28B SNPs occurred after the Phase 3 trials had been fully enrolled and mostly completed. As such, it was not possible for the Applicant to stratify subjects at enrollment based on the IL28B genotype. Specific consent for genotyping for rs12979860 was obtained.

The FDA reviewer commented on the applicability of using SNPs in predicting outcome for treatment-naive subjects and treatment-specific subjects:

Treatment naïve C/C subjects appeared to respond favorably to PR [active control] alone, although SVR [sustained virologic response] rates were higher for all of the telaprevir-containing regimens in this subgroup. C/T carriers had lower response rates than C/C carriers in all treatment arms ... [i]n treatment experienced subjects, telaprevir appeared to benefit subjects of all genotypes by increasing SVR rates by 50–60% for each genotype compared to Pbo/PR [active control].

The reviewer's criticism was that, "[t]he above data must be interpreted with caution because ... the data were not collected and analyzed prospectively."

VII. VALIDATING BIOMARKERS

FDA's Guidance for Industry states that, "[f]or pivotal studies that require regulatory action for approval or labeling ... the bioanalytical methods should be fully validated" (209).

---

[209]U.S. Department of Health and Human Services. Food and Drug Administration. Guidance for industry. Bioanalytical method validation; 2013 (28 pp.).

Biomarker validation encompasses a number of activities (210). First, *analytical validity* refers to the accuracy, reliability, and reproducibility of the test that detects and quantifies a given biomarker. Second, *biologic validity* refers to establishing that expression of a biomarker is associated with a particular nonclinical endpoint, that is, an endpoint measured in studies with animals or by way of in vitro cell culture. Third, *clinical validity* refers to the demonstration that expression of a biomarker correlates with a clinical endpoint. McShane and Hayes (211) observed that establishing reliability and accuracy of a biomarker used in the prognosis of a disease, or for predicting efficacy of a drug, can be difficult in documenting that the drug has efficacy. FDA has issued a number of guidance documents that relate to biomarkers (as cited in 212,213,214). For example, FDA states that the Sponsor should include analytical assay validation reports, with information on, "strengths and limitations of the submitted data," "atypical parameters that define when and how the

biomarker should be used," and "if the biomarker is used to select or exclude study subjects, to optimize doses, to monitor drug safety" (215).

Regarding *clinical validity* of a biomarker, Scher et al. (216) state that a clinically qualified biomarker is one for which sufficient evidence has been generated for FDA acceptance for use in regulatory submissions, and that FDA has separate criteria for evaluating biomarkers that are prognostic biomarkers or predictive biomarkers. Scher et al. (217) also refer to validity of biomarkers that are measured in the timeframe *after* a drug is administered (rather than *before*), where the biomarker correlates with clinical efficacy.

Validation of an in vitro diagnostic test can involve tests on the reproducibility of test results, where data are acquired from the same test conducted at different study sites, different reagent lots, different operators, and for the same test repeated on different days. Validation studies of these types are typically required by the FDA, where a new type of

[210]McShane LM, Hayes DF. Publication of tumor research marker research results: the necessity for complete and transparent reporting. J. Clin. Oncol. 2012;34:4223–32.

[211]McShane LM, Hayes DF. Publication of tumor research marker research results: the necessity for complete and transparent reporting. J. Clin. Oncol. 2012;34:4223–32.

[212]U.S. Department of Health and Human Services. Food and Drug Administration. Guidance for industry. E16 biomarkers related to drug or biotechnology product development: context, structure, and format of qualification submissions; 2011 (12 pp.).

[213]U.S. Department of Health and Human Services. Food and Drug Administration. Guidance for industry and FDA staff. Qualification process for drug development tools; 2014 (32 pp.).

[214]U.S. Department of Health and Human Services. Food and Drug Administration. Guidance for industry. Use of histology in biomarker qualification studies; 2011 (12 pp.).

[215]U.S. Department of Health and Human Services. Food and Drug Administration. Guidance for industry. E16 biomarkers related to drug or biotechnology product development: context, structure, and format of qualification submissions; 2011 (12 pp.).

[216]Scher HI, et al. Validation and clinical utility of prostate cancer biomarkers. Nat. Rev. Clin. Oncol. 2013;10:225–34.

[217]Scher HI, et al. Validation and clinical utility of prostate cancer biomarkers. Nat. Rev. Clin. Oncol. 2013;10:225–34.

in vitro diagnostics test is submitted to the FDA by way of a submission known as the premarket approval (PMA) submission (218).

Validation tests that are typically included in a PMA submission are outlined below. Following this, is an account of the FDA's regulatory process for medical devices, such as medical devices that are in vitro diagnostic tests for biomarkers. The account of FDA's regulatory process for medical devices is not the same as that for FDA's regulatory process for a new drug (NDA; BLA). However, because FDA's approval for an in vitro diagnostic test may require a clinical trial for human subjects, it is the case that an account of medical device regulations fits into the scope of this textbook, and provides an interesting counterpoint for this textbook's account of FDA's drug-approval process.

VIII. BIOMARKER VALIDATION FROM FDA SUBMISSIONS FOR IN VITRO DIAGNOSTICS TESTS

a. Introduction

FDA's guidance for the validation of biomarkers that are to be used in clinical trials that are used in an NDA or BLA is somewhat sparse, as is evident in the cited Guidance for Industry documents (219,220). For this reason, detailed information on validation, as acquired

from 501(k) submissions and PMA submissions is revealed below.

Validation tests for in vitro diagnostics, are available from various FDA submissions. The examples are from *510(k) submissions* and from *PMA submissions*. The differences between 510(k) submissions and PMA submissions are outlined a later in this chapter. Information from these FDA submissions, as available on the FDA's website, provide guidance for validating many types of biomarkers that are to be used in a clinical trial. Information from the 510(k) submissions and PMA submissions is valuable for this purpose, in the situation where the Sponsor only intends to gain FDA approval of the drug, and also in the situation where the Sponsor wants FDA approval of the biomarker test.

b. Validation of Genomic DNA Diagnostic Reagent in a 510(k) Submission

This example is from FDA's approval of a medical device that takes the form of purified human DNA with a preservative (221). The DNA is genomic DNA isolated from B lymphocytes of human donors. Each human donor possesses genomic DNA with 1 of 10 different variations of the cytochrome P450 (2D6) gene. The purpose of this purified human DNA is for use as a control during routine tests of DNA from human patients, where the goal is to detect or identify 1 of the 10 variations.

---

[218]Derion T. Considerations for the planning and conduct of reproducibility studies of in vitro diagnostic tests for infective agents. Biotechnol. Annu. Rev. 2003;9:249–58.

[219]U.S. Department of Health and Human Services. Food and Drug Administration. Guidance for industry. E16 biomarkers related to drug or biotechnology product development: context, structure, and format of qualification submissions; 2011 (12 pp.).

[220]U.S. Department of Health and Human Services. Food and Drug Administration. Guidance for industry. Bioanalytical method validation; 2013 (28 pp.).

[221]510(k) Substantial Equivalence Determination Decision Summary for 510(k) no. K063224. Approval letter of Dec. 23, 2006. Approved by Jean M. Cooper, Office of In Vitro Diagnostic Device Evaluation and Safety, FDA. Documents accessed from FDA website on Mar. 1, 2015.

To repeat, the medical device that was the subject of the 510(k) submission was purified DNA.

Validation of the medical device (the genomic DNA) included the following tests. The tests measured integrity of the DNA, and stability under various storage conditions. Integrity of the DNA was measured by sequencing the DNA, and where validation took the form of assaying under different formats. As stated in the 510(k) Substantial Equivalence Determination Decision Summary, the FDA reviewer referred to these formats, writing that, "the correct genotype results were reproducible from lab-to-lab, lot-to-lot, and from run-to-run."

Referring to tests for integrity, the FDA reviewer wrote that "stability of three different lots of the … material were [sic] evaluated … by four methods … agarose gel, generation of PCR amplicon, bi-directional sequencing, and additional methodologies to evaluate specific alleles."

Moreover, stability of the genomic DNA was assessed under various storage conditions, that is, at 2−8°C, −30°C, at room temperature in a vial that was opened and closed at least 10 times, heated at 45°C for 5 days, and three freeze/thaw cycles.

To summarize, validation of the in vitro diagnostics reagent (the medical device) took three general approaches:

1. Testing in different laboratories, testing of different lots.
2. Testing using various assay methods to assess DNA integrity or structure, such as,

agarose gels, DNA sequencing, and the ability to amplify the sequence by PCR.
3. Stability testing using various storage conditions (222).

Although the medical device in question was relatively simple (just a reagent in a vial), this author points out that the same principles of validation are applicable to more complex reagents and procedures involving biomarkers, such as a device and method for conducting multiplex PCR analysis, or a device and method for detecting chromosomal mutations by FISH.

c. Validation PCR Reaction Diagnostic Test in a 519(k) Submission

To provide another example, the 510(k) no. k073014 submission concerned a medical device that comprised an array made of polyester film coated with spots, where each spot was designed to detect a specific sequence of DNA, a liquid reagent for conducting a PCR reaction, and a machine that comprises a microscope, where the machine conducts multiplex PCR reactions (223). This 510(k) submission assessed run-to-run variability, stability testing, the determination of the lowest level of detection, and the potential of chemicals found in blood to interfere with the test. These bullet points outline the approaches used for this 510(k) submission:

• Run-to-run variability, variability found with three different machines, site-to-site variability, variability with different operators.

---

[222]The author (Tom Brody) conducted the same type of quality control tests, on small-molecule biologicals, and instrumentation at Athena Neurosciences, South San Francisco, CA, in 1993−94. Hence, the author knows that the tests set forth by the FDA's 510(k) Substantial Equivalence Determination Decision Summary are generally applicable to reagents that are small molecules, biologicals, and machines or instrumentation.

[223]510(k) Substantial Equivalence Determination Decision Summary for 510(k) no. k073014. Approval letter of Jan. 28, 2008. Approved by Jean M. Cooper, Office of In Vitro Diagnostic Device Evaluation and Safety, FDA. Documents accessed from FDA website on Mar. 1, 2015.

- Stability testing with storage of the array and the liquid reagent for 180 days.
- Lowest concentration of DNA that can be detected per reaction mixture.
- Potential of compounds found in blood to interfere with the test. The compounds tested were bilirubin, cholesterol, and heparin.

To reiterate FDA's position on validation on biomarkers and other types of tests, FDA recommends that, "[f]or pivotal studies that require regulatory action for approval or labeling ... the bioanalytical methods should be fully validated" (224).

d. Validation PCR Reaction Diagnostic Test in a PMA Submission

The validation of a test for biomarkers taking the form of mutations in the *BRCA1* gene and *BRCA2* gene, are described. This example is from PMA no. P140020. The test is sensitive to mutations that are point mutations, deletions, and insertions. The goal of the diagnostic test is to aid in selecting ovarian cancer patients who are likely to be treatable with the drug, olaparib. The test includes a risk, in that a false positive will be treated with olaparib, and thus be susceptible to adverse drug reactions from olaparib. This risk compels the need to review this diagnostic test by way of a PMA submission.

According to the FDA reviewer "[a]ccuracy of the ... test was verified by comparison against a validated next generation sequencing ... assay ... [a]ll specimens were tested in a blinded manner. The specimens covered a range of variants, including single nucleotide variants, deletions ... and insertions." In this writing, the term variants is equivalent to the term, mutations. In granting approval to the application (225), the FDA reviewer concluded that the Sponsor's test was 100% accurate, writing that, "Percent Positive Agreement (PPA) = 100%."

The medical device under review took the form of a kit that included a blood collection tube and instructions, and information on using machines and reagents for analyzing variants in the genomic DNA of patients. The PMA submission required that the machines include a specific DNA-sequencing machine (Qiagen's QIAsymphony SP®) and a specific machine for imaging electrophoresis gels (Invitrogen's E-Gel Safe Imager®).

Validation of the blood samples, reagents, and machines, took these forms:

- Tests on metabolites found in blood (IgG, hemoglobin, albumin, bilirubin).
- Tests on additives used in blood processing (EDTA).
- Tests on chemicals used in handling the machines (ethanol, bleach). The goal was to determine how these added chemicals could interfere with the in vitro diagnostic test that was the subject of the PMA.

In performing the validation, IgG, hemoglobin, albumin, and bilirubin were intentionally added to (spiked) genomic DNA samples acquired from the blood cells of patients.

Regarding the results, the FDA reviewer wrote, "[t]reatment with each potentially interfering substance ... with the exception of IgG at 60 g/L, did not affect the performance of the test." Further commenting on the interfering properties of IgG, the reviewer wrote that, "[s]amples with IgG at 60 g/L yielded a no call rate of 33%, which failed to meet the

---

[224]U.S. Department of Health and Human Services. Food and Drug Administration. Guidance for industry. Bioanalytical method validation; 2013 (28 pp.).

[225]Premarket approval submission P140020 was approved on Dec. 19, 2014 by Alberto Gutierrez, Office of In Vitro Diagnostics and Radiological Health, FDA.

acceptance criteria … and demonstrated that IgG at … 60 g/L interferes with the assay." The term "no call" has been defined as, "inconclusive results" (226), "indeterminable" (227), and as "clear results cannot be obtained" (228).

Validation also included tests on *run-to-run* variation, involving three independent runs on the same set of 20 samples of genomic DNA, runs using three lots of reagent, and runs using three different operators. Other validation tests involved an intentional deviation from the instructions. Specifically, alternative temperatures for conducting the PCR reaction were tested, where the annealing temperatures were altered by 1°C, 2°C, and 3°C. This type of validation is sometimes called *guardbanding* (229,230). Moreover, validation also involved tests for *cross-contamination* between runs, where two sequential samples were evaluated for inter-run contamination. The FDA reviewer commented that, "carryover events leading to miscall results were not observed." Furthermore, *stability* tests were also conducted on whole blood specimens and on reagents. For example, stability of genomic DNA was tested by storing patients' blood at 4°C for 14, 30, and 37 days.

To summarize, validation in the PMA submission for the BRCA1 and BRCA2 tests involved:

- spiking of patient samples with contaminants;

- an account of conditions that result in "no call" results;
- run-to-run variation, lot-to-lot variation, operator-to-operator variation;
- guardbanding;
- cross-contamination;
- stability tests.

e. Summary

One of the main themes in this textbook is the use of biomarkers as endpoints in FDA-regulated clinical trials for drugs. Because FDA recommends that biomarkers be validated when used in these clinical trials, the present material provides concrete guidance on procedures for validating in vitro diagnostic tests, including reagents and machines that are used to detect various biomarkers. The most useful source of guidance on validating biomarkers comes from FDA's approval package of medical devices taking the form of an in vitro diagnostic test, in response to 510(k) submissions and PMA submissions.

f. Distinctions Between 510(k) Submission and PMA Submission, for Medical Devices

FDA's regulation of drugs and medical devices find an intersection where a clinical trial in support of drug approval makes use of in vitro biomarker tests. Depending on the

[226]Smith M, Visootsak J. Noninvasive screening tools for Down syndrome: a review. Int. J. Women's Health 2013;5:125–31.

[227]Smith M. A case of false negatives NIPT for Down syndrome—lessons learned. Case Reports Genetics 2014;2014:Article ID 823504 (3 pp.).

[228]Chang KC, et al. Development and validation of a clinical trial patient stratification assay that interrogates 27 mutation sites in MAPK pathway genes. PLoS One 2013;8:e72239 (17 pp.).

[229]Rozet E, et al. Methods for the validation of analytical methods involved in uniformity of dosage units tests. Anal. Chim. Acta 2013;760:46–52.

[230]Ermer J, Nethercote PW. Method validation in pharmaceutical analysis: a guide to best practice. 2nd ed. Weinhein: Wiley-VCH; 2014. pp. 43, 47–49, 56–57.

commercial needs of the sponsor, the goal of the clinical trial that uses in vitro biomarker tests may, or may not, be to gain FDA-approval for that particular test.

Medical devices, such as tongue depressors, in vitro biomarker tests, and X-ray machines, can be classified as either class I, class II, or class III. Class I medical devices pose a risk that is low to moderate, and are subjected to FDA regulations called "general controls." Class II medical devices pose a risk that is moderate to high, and are also subjected to general controls. Class I and class II medical devices require a submission called, "510(k)." The 510(k) is also known as *premarket notification* submission. Class III medical devices pose a high risk and require a *PMA* submission to FDA (231).

Class I and class II medical devices are usually evaluated on whether they are equivalent to devices that are already marketed, and it is only occasionally that these devices require data from clinical trials (232). Only a small percentage of 510(k) submissions require clinical data to support the application (233).

To provide an example of the decision-tree that determines whether 510(k) or PMA is to be used, an in vitro biomarker diagnostic test can be evaluated by the 510(k) regulatory path if it is equivalent to an existing marketed test. But if the in vitro biomarker diagnostic test is not equivalent to an existing test, and if it is used to make a critical medical decision on diagnosis or treatment, then PMA is the appropriate regulatory pathway (234). In other words, the 510(k) is a submission to FDA that demonstrates that the Sponsor's medical devices are at least as safe and effective as an existing legally marketed device that was not subjected to PMA (see, 21 CFR §807.92(a)(3)).

Also, if FDA has determined that general controls are not sufficient to evaluate safety and efficacy of class III medical devices these devices require a PMA application to obtain clearance for marketing (235). As is the case with clinical trials in support of drug approval, where a Sponsor submits a PMA application, the Sponsor must submit information on all applicable clinical trials to the ClinicalTrials.gov registry (236).

Classification as class I, II, or III, can depend on the *intended use* and on the *indications* for use. For an in vitro biomarker test, *intended use* can be the detection of a genetic mutation, while the *indication* describes why a patient would be tested for this mutation. In an *in vitro* biomarker test for measuring a new type of analyte, or for a new intended use of an existing analyte that has not yet been subjected to FDA review, the test (device) may automatically be placed in class III, and thus require a PMA application (237).

[231]U.S. Department of Health and Human Services. Food and Drug Administration. Guidance for industry. The 510(k) Program: evaluating substantial equivalence in premarket notifications [510(k)]; 2014 (39 pp.).

[232]Rising JP, Moscovitch B. Characteristics of pivotal trials and FDA review of innovative devices. PLoS One 2015;10:e0117235.

[233]Device advice: investigational device exemption (IDE). FDA website, accessed Mar. 1, 2015.

[234]Liotta LA, Petricoin EF. Regulatory approval pathways for molecular diagnostic technology. Methods Mol. Biol. 2012;823:409−20.

[235]U.S. Department of Health and Human Services. Food and Drug Administration. Guidance for industry and FDA staff. Premarket approval application filing review; 2003 (12 pp.).

[236]Form FDA-3674, ClinicalTrials.gov Data Bank. FDA website accessed Mar. 1, 2015.

[237]Mansfield E, et al. Food and Drug Administration regulation of in vitro diagnostic devices. J. Mol. Diagnost. 2005;7:2−7.

IX. CONCLUDING REMARKS

Biomarkers can be a basis for the stratification of study subjects. They can be used in a decision tree residing in the schema of a clinical trial. Or they can be used purely for exploratory purposes. Changes in expression of a biomarker, during the course of medical treatment, can be used to determine whether any given patient is a high-risk or low-risk patient. Biomarkers can also determine whether a particular drug will likely work for any given patient.

Regarding the studies described above, the Vogel study (238), showed that *HER2* can predict a drug's efficacy. The Cohen study (239) showed that CTCs can be used as a biomarker to predict survival time. The Koelink study (240) showed that a tumor protein found in the bloodstream, cytokeratin, can predict survival time. The Galon study (241,242) concerned a biomarker that took the form of immune cells clustering around a tumor, where the goal of using this biomarker was to predict survival. The Morris study (243) also involved immune cells, and here the goal was to predict whether a drug would be effective. This chapter also discloses use of gene arrays as a biomarker. Gene arrays are distinguished in that no single particular gene has a reliable prognostic value, but that a large collection of genes, having various unrelated functions (or even having unknown functions), can be used as a biomarker.

Although this textbook focuses mainly on oncology, CRP, which is mainly used as a biomarker for atherosclerosis, was also detailed above. CRP was detailed for a variety of reasons. First, there has been an increasing interest in using CRP as a biomarker for oncology. Second, the utility of CRP for oncology, as well as for atherosclerosis, provides an excellent teaching example regarding the principles set forth by Fleming and DeMets (244). It can be concluded that CRP is reasonable to use as an exploratory biomarker, suitable for use as an inclusion/exclusion criterion, reasonable to use as a basis for stratifying subjects into subgroups, and suitable for use in the clinic as a prognostic marker. However, in view of the lack of evidence that CRP plays a major role, or any role, in the mechanisms of cancer or

[238]Vogel CL, Cobleigh MA, Tripathy D, et al. Efficacy and safety of trastuzumab as a single agent in first-line treatment of HER2-overexpressing metastatic breast cancer. J. Clin. Oncol. 2002;20:719−26.

[239]Cohen SJ, Punt CJ, Iannotti N, et al. Relationship of circulating tumor cells to tumor response, progression-free survival, and overall survival in patients with metastatic colorectal cancer. J. Clin. Oncol. 2008;26:3213−21.

[240]Koelink PJ, Lamers CB, Hommes DW, Verspaget HW. Circulating cell death products predict clinical outcome of colorectal cancer patients. BMC Cancer 2009;9:88.

[241]Galon J, Costes A, Sanchez-Cabo F, et al. Type, density, and location of immune cells within human colorectal tumors predict clinical outcome. Science 2006;313:1960−4.

[242]Couzin J. T Cells a boon for colon cancer prognosis. Science 2006;313:1868−9.

[243]Morris M, Platell C, Iacopetta B. Tumor-infiltrating lymphocytes and perforation in colon cancer predict positive response to 5-fluorouracil chemotherapy. Clin. Cancer Res. 2008;14:1413−7.

[244]Fleming TR, DeMets DL. Surrogate end points in clinical trials: are we being misled? Ann. Intern. Med. 1996;125:605−13.

atherosclerosis, it cannot be concluded that CRP can serve as a surrogate marker for a clinical endpoint in regulated clinical trials. Any clinician interested in using CRP as a biomarker needs to take into account the fact that statin drugs, such as atorvastatin, can have a marked influence on CRP levels (245,246,247,248,249).

[245]Singh U, Devaraj S, Jialal I, Siegel D. Comparison effect of atorvastatin (10 versus 80 mg) on biomarkers of inflammation and oxidative stress in subjects with metabolic syndrome. Am. J. Cardiol. 2008;102:321−5.

[246]Deanfield JE, Sellier P, Thaulow E, et al. Potent anti-ischaemic effects of statins in chronic stable angina: incremental benefit beyond lipid lowering? Eur. Heart J. 2010;31:2650−9.

[247]Nissen SE, Tuzcu EM, Schoenhagen P, et al. Statin therapy, LDL cholesterol, C-reactive protein, and coronary artery disease. New Engl. J. Med. 2005;352:29−38.

[248]Gensini GF, Gori AM, Dilaghi B, et al. Effect of atorvastatin on circulating hsCRP concentrations: a sub-study of the achieve cholesterol targets fast with atorvastatin stratified titration (ACTFAST) study. Int. J. Cardiol. 2010;142:257−64.

[249]Ridker PM, Cannon CP, Morrow D, et al. C-reactive protein levels and outcomes after statin therapy. New Engl. J. Med. 2005;352:20−8.

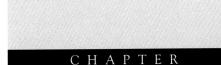

CHAPTER

20

Endpoints for Immune Diseases

I. INTRODUCTION

Immune diseases include multiple sclerosis, rheumatoid arthritis, psoriasis, ulcerative colitis, Crohn's disease, systemic lupus erythematosus (SLE), asthma, allergies, and chronic obstructive pulmonary disease (COPD). These are autoimmune diseases. Asthma, allergies, and COPD are diseases with an immune component, and these may be termed, inflammatory disorders. A common feature of these immune diseases is pathological behavior by white blood cells. Correspondingly, a common feature of the endpoints used in assessing these diseases is endpoints that assess tissue damage caused by white blood cells. This chapter details the endpoints used for clinical trials on multiple sclerosis.

II. SUBSETS OF MULTIPLE SCLEROSIS

Multiple sclerosis is a chronic autoimmune disease that involves attack by the immune system on the central nervous system. This disease tends to present in young adults, and it is twice as prevalent in women as in men. Common presenting symptoms include impaired vision with eye pain, paresthesias (numbness), weakness, and impaired coordination (1). A number of reviews on the clinical features, diagnosis, and treatment of multiple sclerosis are available (2,3,4). Endpoints and diagnostic tools for multiple sclerosis are provided by the *New England Journal of Medicine* from clinical trials on drugs such as, interferon beta-1a (5), glatiramer (6),

[1]Calabresi PA. Diagnosis and management of multiple sclerosis. Am. Fam. Physician 2004;70:1935−44.

[2]Feinstein A, et al. Treatment of progressive multiple sclerosis: what works, what does not, and what is needed. Lancet Neurol. 2015;14:194−207.

[3]Ontaneda D, et al. Clinical trials in progressive multiple sclerosis: lessons learned and future perspectives. Lancet Neurol. 2015;14:208−23.

[4]Filippi M, et al. Magnetic resonance outcome measures in multiple sclerosis trials: time to rethink? Curr. Opin. Neurol. 2014;27:290−9.

[5]Cohen JA, Barkhof F, Comi G, et al. Oral fingolimod or intramuscular interferon for relapsing multiple sclerosis. New Engl. J. Med. 2010;362:402−15.

[6]Fox RJ, Miller DH, Phillips JT, et al. Placebo-controlled phase 3 study of oral BG-12 or glatiramer in multiple sclerosis. New Engl. J. Med. 2012;367:1087−97.

Clinical Trials.
DOI: http://dx.doi.org/10.1016/B978-0-12-804217-5.00020-5

fingolimod (7), cladribine (8), natalizumab (9), and dimethyl fumarate (10,11).

The United States National Multiple Sclerosis Society has defined four types of MS:

- *Relapsing-remitting MS (RRMS).* Relapses, also known as "flares," occur followed by recovery periods. Frequency: about 65% (12). About 90% of untreated RRMS patients will transition to SPMS after 20 years (13).
- *Primary-progressive MS (PPMS).* The disease progresses steadily from the onset with no distinct relapse. Frequency: about 7.5% (14,15).
- *Secondary-progressive MS (SPMS).* Initially relapsing-remitting, the disease steadily worsens with or without flare-ups and with minor remissions. Frequency: in the absence of disease-modifying drugs, this form of the disease would occur at a frequency of about 20% (16).

- *Progressive-relapsing MS (PRMS).* The disease progresses steadily from the onset characterized by acute attacks, with or without recovery in between. Frequency: about 7.5% (17).

Drugs available for treating multiple sclerosis include:

- fingolimod,
- natalizumab,
- interferon-1-alpha,
- interferon-1-beta,
- cladribine,
- glatiramer acetate,
- dimethyl fumarate.

A disorder related to multiple sclerosis is *clinically isolated syndromes* (CIS). CIS includes optic neuritis, brainstem cord syndrome, and spinal cord syndrome. CIS is often a precursor to multiple sclerosis, and CIS patients

[7]Kappos L, Radue E, O'Connor P, et al. A placebo-controlled trial of oral fingolimod in relapsing multiple sclerosis. New Engl. J. Med. 2012;362:387–401.

[8]Giovannoni G, Comi G, Cook S, et al. A placebo-controlled trial of oral cladribine for relapsing multiple sclerosis. New Engl. J. Med. 2010;362:416–26.

[9]Polman CH, O'Connor PW, Havrdova E, et al. A randomized, placebo-controlled trial of natalizumab for relapsing multiple sclerosis. New Engl. J. Med. 2006;354:899–910.

[10]Fox RJ, Miller DH, Phillips JT, et al. Placebo-controlled phase 3 study of oral BG-12 or glatiramer in multiple sclerosis. New Engl. J. Med. 2012;367:1087–97.

[11]Gold R, Kappos L, Arnold DL, et al. Placebo-controlled phase 3 study of oral BG-12 for relapsing multiple sclerosis. New Engl. J. Med. 2012;367:1098–107.

[12]National Multiple Sclerosis Society. The multiple sclerosis trend report: perspectives from managed care, providers, and patients. Kikaku America Int.; 2007 (76 pp.).

[13]Gold R, Wolinsky JS, Amato MP, Comi G. Evolving expectations around early management of multiple sclerosis. Ther. Adv. Neurol. Disord. 2010;3:351–67.

[14]National Multiple Sclerosis Society. The multiple sclerosis trend report: perspectives from managed care, providers, and patients. Kikaku America Int.; 2007 (76 pp.).

[15]Thompson AJ, Polman CH, Miller DH, et al. Primary progressive multiple sclerosis. Brain 1997;120:1085–96.

[16]National Multiple Sclerosis Society. The multiple sclerosis trend report: perspectives from managed care, providers, and patients. Kikaku America Int.; 2007 (76 pp.).

[17]National Multiple Sclerosis Society. The multiple sclerosis trend report: perspectives from managed care, providers, and patients. Kikaku America Int.; 2007 (76 pp.).

frequently convert to multiple sclerosis (18). Gold et al. (19) state that certain drugs used for treating multiple sclerosis can delay conversion of CIS to multiple sclerosis.

a. Diagnosing Multiple Sclerosis

People must be diagnosed with a condition or disease in order to satisfy the inclusion criteria of any clinical trial. For many disorders, such as iron-deficiency anemia, the diagnostic criteria are straightforward, and can be found in standard manuals, such as *Henry's Clinical Diagnosis and Management by Laboratory Methods* (20). However, for many diseases, the diagnostic criteria are complex, require use of more than one type of technology, require dedicated experts, and are subject to revision from time to time. Such is the case with multiple sclerosis. There is no single clinical feature or diagnostic test that is sufficient to diagnose multiple sclerosis, and the diagnosis is mainly a clinical one (21).

The Poser criteria for diagnosing multiple sclerosis are an older diagnostic method, which have been replaced with the newer McDonald criteria (22,23). The Poser criteria (24) date from 1983, while the McDonald criteria (25) date from 2001. Moreover, the McDonald criteria have been replaced by the revised 2005 McDonald criteria (26,27).

When comparing the results of two different multiple sclerosis clinical trials, investigators need to be vigilant and determine whether the first trial used the Poser criteria and the second trial used the McDonald criteria. If both trials used the same set of criteria, then the results from both trials can reasonably be compared. But if the trials use different criteria, the comparison will likely result in spurious and

[18]Fisniku LK, Brex PA, Altmann DR, et al. Disability and T2 MRI lesions: a 20-year follow-up of patients with relapse onset of multiple sclerosis. Brain 2008;131:808−17.

[19]Gold R, Wolinsky JS, Amato MP, Comi G. Evolving expectations around early management of multiple sclerosis. Ther. Adv. Neurol. Disord. 2010;3:351−67.

[20]McPherson PA, Pincus MR. Henry's clinical diagnosis and management by laboratory methods. 22nd ed. Philadelphia, PA: Elsevier Saunders; 2011.

[21]Milo R, Miller A. Revised diagnostic criteria of multiple sclerosis. Autoimmun. Rev. 2014;13:518−24.

[22]Hawkes CH, Giovannoni G. The McDonald Criteria for Multiple Sclerosis: time for clarification. Mult. Scler. 2010;16:566−75.

[23]Fangerau T, Schimrigk S, Haupts M, et al. Diagnosis of multiple sclerosis: comparison of the Poser criteria and the new McDonald criteria. Acta Neurol. Scand. 2004;109:385−9.

[24]Poser CM, Paty DW, Scheinberg L, et al. New diagnostic criteria for multiple sclerosis: guidelines for research protocols. Ann. Neurol. 1983;13:227−31.

[25]McDonald WI, Compston A, Edan G, et al. Recommended diagnostic criteria for multiple sclerosis: guidelines from the International Panel on the diagnosis of multiple sclerosis. Ann. Neurol. 2001;50:121−7.

[26]Polman CH, Reingold SC, Edan G, et al. Diagnostic criteria for multiple sclerosis: 2005 revisions to the "McDonald Criteria". Ann. Neurol. 2005;58:840−6.

[27]McHugh JC, Galvin PL, Murphy RP. Retrospective comparison of the original and revised McDonald criteria in a general neurology practice in Ireland. Mult. Scler. 2008;14:81−5.

artifactual conclusions, as cautioned by Sormani et al. (28,29). In fact, Fraser et al. (30) warned "that the new McDonald criteria lead to more than double the number of patients with a diagnosis of MS at 1 year compared with the use of the Poser criteria." Some studies on multiple sclerosis have used both sets of criteria (31,32).

A question that arises, not just for multiple sclerosis, but for any disease, is what to do when a standard of criteria is changed after the study has been set in motion. In an appropriate response to a change in standards, Grasso et al. (33) reported, "[w]e enrolled 270 MS patients admitted … with definite MS, as diagnosed according to the Poser criteria. We revised all the diagnoses of the MS patients according to the new criteria recently formulated by McDonald."

b. Biomarkers and Surrogates for Diagnosing Multiple Sclerosis

This provides an account of exploratory biomarkers and of an objective measure of multiple sclerosis, prior to reviewing disability scales, such as the Kurtzke Expanded Disability Status Scale (EDSS) score, and prior to reviewing magnetic resonance imaging (MRI). MRI is a gross measure of pathology and MRI data are somewhat remote from the mechanism of action of the disease.

Neurofilament light chains (NFL) and neurofilament heavy chains (NFH), or peptide fragments thereof, are biomarkers that can be acquired from samples of cerebrospinal fluid (CSF) (34,35). CSF can be safely obtained by lumbar puncture, though this procedure is invasive (more so than blood samples, less than liver biopsy). Neurofilament is a cytoskeletal protein of axons, and its presence in CSF results from damage to axons. NFL levels may reflect acute damage to axons, and can be useful for diagnosing patients recently converting from CIS to multiple sclerosis, while NFH levels may reflect chronic irreversible damage (36). Kuhle et al. (37) determined that NFL levels in CSF correlate with EDSS score, and

[28]Sormani MP, Tintorè M, Rovaris M, et al. Will Rogers phenomenon in multiple sclerosis. Ann. Neurol. 2008;64:428–33.

[29]Sormani MP. The Will Rogers phenomenon: the effect of different diagnostic criteria. J. Neurol. Sci. 2009;287 (Suppl. 1):S46–9.

[30]Fraser C, Klistorner A, Graham S, Garrick R, Billson F, Grigg J. Multifocal visual evoked potential latency analysis: predicting progression to multiple sclerosis. Arch. Neurol. 2006;63:847–50.

[31]Korporal M, Haas J, Balint B, et al. Interferon beta-induced restoration of regulatory T-cell function in multiple sclerosis is prompted by an increase in newly generated naive regulatory T cells. Arch. Neurol. 2008;65:1434–9.

[32]Kuhle J, Pohl C, Mehling M, et al. Lack of association between antimyelin antibodies and progression to multiple sclerosis. New Engl. J. Med. 2007;356:371–8.

[33]Grasso MG, Pace L, Troisi E, Tonini A, Paolucci S. Prognostic factors in multiple sclerosis rehabilitation. Eur. J. Phys. Rehabil. Med. 2009;45:47–51.

[34]Gnanapavan S, et al. Guidelines for uniform reporting of body fluid biomarker studies in neurological disorders. Neurology 2014;83:1210–6.

[35]Friese MA, et al. Mechanisms of neurodegeneration and axonal dysfunction in multiple sclerosis. Nat. Rev. Neurol. 2014;10:225–38.

[36]Teunissen CE, Khalil M. Neurofilaments as biomarkers in multiple sclerosis. Mult. Scler. 2012;18:552–6.

[37]Kuhle J, Plattner K, Bestnick JP, et al. A comparative study of CSF neurofilament light and heavy chain protein in MS. Mult. Scler. 2013;19:1597–603.

proposed that NFL be a useful surrogate marker for testing efficacy of drugs for multiple sclerosis.

Eye pathology is a common initial finding in multiple sclerosis. About 20% of patients with multiple sclerosis have optical neuritis (38). Retinal nerve fiber layer (RNFL) thickness is an objective measure of optic neuritis. Optical coherence tomography (OCT) measures thickness of the RNFL (39). In patients with multiple sclerosis, annual thinning of the RNFL is about 2 μm/year, while in healthy controls, annual thinning is 0.2 μm/year (40). Data from OCT and from MRI provide complementary information about vision pathology in multiple sclerosis (41). Information on vision impairment in multiple sclerosis is also captured by the quality of life tool, the NEI-VFQ-25 questionnaire.

c. Endpoints for Multiple Sclerosis

Endpoints used in clinical trials for multiple sclerosis include:

- Percent of subjects with relapse at 96 weeks (relapse rate) (42);
- Percent of subjects experiencing relapse per year (relapse rate) (43,44);
- Proportion of subjects who are relapse-free at end of study (45,46);
- Change in EDSS score from baseline to end of study (47);
- Time to 3-month sustained change in EDSS score (defined as time to a sustained increase in EDSS score, of at least 1 point in EDSS score, or an increase of at least 1.5 points, if baseline EDSS score was zero, where sustained increase in EDSS score lasts for at least 3 months) (48,49), or where

[38]Balcer LJ, et al. Vision and vision-related outcome measures in multiple sclerosis. Brain 2015;138:11−7.

[39]Lee JY, et al. Axonal degeneration in multiple sclerosis: can we predict and prevent permanent disability. Acta Neuropathol. Commun. 2014;2:97 (16 pp.).

[40]Friese MA, et al. Mechanisms of neurodegeneration and axonal dysfunction in multiple sclerosis. Nat. Rev. Neurol. 2014;10:225−38.

[41]Balcer LJ, et al. Vision and vision-related outcome measures in multiple sclerosis. Brain 2015;138:11−7.

[42]Giovannoni G, Comi G, Cook S, et al. A placebo-controlled trial of oral cladribine for relapsing multiple sclerosis. New Engl. J. Med. 2010;362:416−26.

[43]Kappos L, Radue EW, O'Connor P, et al. A placebo-controlled trial of oral fingolimod in relapsing multiple sclerosis. New Engl. J. Med. 2010;362:387−401.

[44]Polman CH, O'Connor PW, Havrdova E, et al. A randomized, placebo-controlled trial of natalizumab for relapsing multiple sclerosis. New Engl. J. Med. 2006;354:899−910.

[45]Giovannoni G, Comi G, Cook S, et al. A placebo-controlled trial of oral cladribine for relapsing multiple sclerosis. New Engl. J. Med. 2010;362:416−26.

[46]Polman CH, O'Connor PW, Havrdova E, et al. A randomized, placebo-controlled trial of natalizumab for relapsing multiple sclerosis. New Engl. J. Med. 2006;354:899−910.

[47]Kappos L, Radue EW, O'Connor P, et al. A placebo-controlled trial of oral fingolimod in relapsing multiple sclerosis. New Engl. J. Med. 2010;362:387−401.

[48]Giovannoni G, Comi G, Cook S, et al. A placebo-controlled trial of oral cladribine for relapsing multiple sclerosis. New Engl. J. Med. 2010;362:416−26.

[49]Polman CH, O'Connor PW, Havrdova E, et al. A randomized, placebo-controlled trial of natalizumab for relapsing multiple sclerosis. New Engl. J. Med. 2006;354:899−910.

sustained increase in EDSS score lasts for at least 6 months (50);

- MRI imaging of gadolinium-enhancing T1-weighted brain lesions (number of lesions at end of study) (51,52,53);
- MRI imaging of T2-weighted brain lesions (number of new lesions; % change in lesion volume) (54,55,56).

Petkau et al. (57) and Rovira (58) address the concept that only certain endpoints used in multiple sclerosis clinical trials are accepted by the FDA for granting approval to a drug. These commentators also address the concept that a surrogate endpoint might be accepted as a primary endpoint, but only where the surrogate is firmly correlated with clinical response.

d. Timing for Measuring Endpoints

The study of Kappos et al. (59) provides an exemplary account of endpoints. Data on the various endpoints were captured at various times during the course of the clinical trial. Clinical assessments were performed at baseline, at 2 weeks, and at 1, 2, 3, 6, 9, 12, 15, 18, 21, and 24 months. Objective measurements were as follows. The EDSS (60) was determined every 3 months, and the Multiple Sclerosis Functional Composite (MSFC) score every 6 months. MRI scans were obtained at the screening visit and at 6, 12, and 24 months.

e. Primary Endpoint

The primary endpoint was the *annualized relapse rate*. The annualized relapse rate is defined as the number of confirmed relapses per year. The term "relapse" is defined by Dr J.A. Cohen, one of the investigators of two different clinical trials on fingolimod

[50]Jacobs LD, Cookfair DL, Rudick RA, et al. Intramuscular interferon beta-1a for disease progression in relapsing multiple sclerosis. The Multiple Sclerosis Collaborative Research Group (MSCRG). Ann. Neurol. 1996;39:285−94.

[51]Kappos L, Radue EW, O'Connor P, et al. A placebo-controlled trial of oral fingolimod in relapsing multiple sclerosis. New Engl. J. Med. 2010;362:387−401.

[52]Polman CH, O'Connor PW, Havrdova E, et al. A randomized, placebo-controlled trial of natalizumab for relapsing multiple sclerosis. New Engl. J. Med. 2006;354:899−910.

[53]Jacobs LD, Beck RW, Simon JH, et al. Intramuscular interferon beta-1a therapy initiated during a first demyelinating event in multiple sclerosis. CHAMPS Study Group. New Engl. J. Med. 2000;343:898−904.

[54]Kappos L, Radue EW, O'Connor P, et al. A placebo-controlled trial of oral fingolimod in relapsing multiple sclerosis. New Engl. J. Med. 2010;362:387−401.

[55]Polman CH, O'Connor PW, Havrdova E, et al. A randomized, placebo-controlled trial of natalizumab for relapsing multiple sclerosis. New Engl. J. Med. 2006;354:899−910.

[56]Jacobs LD, Beck RW, Simon JH, et al. Intramuscular interferon beta-1a therapy initiated during a first demyelinating event in multiple sclerosis. CHAMPS Study Group. New Engl. J. Med. 2000;343:898−904.

[57]Petkau J, Reingold SC, Held U, et al. Magnetic resonance imaging as a surrogate outcome for multiple sclerosis relapses. Mult. Scler. 2008;14:770−8.

[58]Rovira A. Tissue-specific MR imaging in multiple sclerosis. Am. J. Neuroradiol. 2009;30:1277−8.

[59]Kappos L, Radue EW, O'Connor P, et al. A placebo-controlled trial of oral fingolimod in relapsing multiple sclerosis. New Engl. J. Med. 2010;362:387−401.

[60]Kurtzke JF. Rating neurologic impairment in multiple sclerosis: an Expanded Disability Status Scale (EDSS). Neurology 1983;33:1444−52.

(61,62). According to Dr Cohen (63), "relapse" has two main components, one of which is subjective and the other objective. Relapse refers to the following composite:

1. *Subjective information.* Acute new or worsening symptoms consistent with neurologic symptoms caused by multiple sclerosis lasting at least 24 h. "Symptoms" is a subjective phenomenon experienced and reported by the patient. Spontaneous reports from a patient trigger the objective examination by the physician (64). Jacobs et al. (65), also disclosed that it is the patient that initiates the documentation of symptoms.

2. *Objective information.* A corresponding objective change in the neurologic exam performed by the neurologist, for example, the patient complains their leg became weaker 3 days ago and the exam today shows less strength than the previous study visit. The EDSS is a rating scale that summarizes and quantifies the findings on the neurologic exam. Most definitions in trials stipulate the amount of change on the EDSS that is required for the event to qualify as a relapse.

Moreover, according to Dr Cohen (66), to constitute a confirmed relapse, the symptoms must have been accompanied by an increase of at least half a point in the EDSS score, of one point in each of two EDSS functional-system scores, or of two points in one EDSS functional-system score (excluding scores for the bowel, bladder, or cerebral functional systems). Higher EDSS scores mean a more severe disability.

The EDSS scoring scheme appears in Table 20.1. As reviewed by John F. Kurtzke (67), the Kurtzke EDSS score has an origin in studies from the early 1950s (68).

f. Multiple Sclerosis Functional Composite Score

Another primary endpoint used in the Kappos et al. (69) study was the multiple sclerosis functional composite (MSFC) score, as set forth by a manual authored by Fischer et al. (70). This test includes a 25-foot walk, a nine-hole peg test, and a listening test. Regarding the 25-foot walk, for example, the manual states that the patient is instructed to walk 25 feet as quickly as possible. The task is immediately

[61]Cohen JA, Barkhof F, Comi G, et al. Oral fingolimod or intramuscular interferon for relapsing multiple sclerosis. New Engl. J. Med. 2010;362:402–15.

[62]Kappos L, Radue EW, O'Connor P, et al. A placebo-controlled trial of oral fingolimod in relapsing multiple sclerosis. New Engl. J. Med. 2010;362:387–401.

[63]Kind thanks to Dr J.A. Cohen, MD. E-mail of September 2, 2010.

[64]Cohen JA. E-mail of September 5, 2010.

[65]Jacobs LD, Beck RW, Simon JH, et al. Intramuscular interferon beta-1a therapy initiated during a first demyelinating event in multiple sclerosis. CHAMPS Study Group. New Engl. J. Med. 2000;343:898–904.

[66]Cohen JA. E-mail of September 2, 2010.

[67]Kurtzke JF. Historical and clinical perspectives of the expanded disability status scale. Neuroepidemiology 2008;31:1–9.

[68]Kurtzke JF. A new scale for evaluating disability in multiple sclerosis. Neurology 1955;5:580–3.

[69]Kappos L, Radue EW, O'Connor P, et al. A placebo-controlled trial of oral fingolimod in relapsing multiple sclerosis. New Engl. J. Med. 2010;362:387–401.

[70]Fischer JS, Jak AJ, Kniker JE, Rudick RA. Multiple Sclerosis Functional Composite (MSFC) Administration and Scoring Manual; 2001 (41 pp.).

TABLE 20.1 Kurtzke Expanded Disability Status Scale

0.0	Normal neurological examination
1.0	No disability, minimal signs in one functional systems (FS)
1.5	No disability, minimal signs in more than one FS
2.0	Minimal disability in one FS
2.5	Mild disability in one FS or minimal disability in two FS
3.0	Moderate disability in one FS, or mild disability in three or four FS. Fully ambulatory
3.5	Fully ambulatory but with moderate disability in one FS and more than minimal disability in several others
4.0	Fully ambulatory without aid, self-sufficient, up and about some 12 h a day despite relatively severe disability; able to walk without aid or rest some 500 m
4.5	Fully ambulatory without aid, up and about much of the day, able to work a full day, may otherwise have some limitation of full activity or require minimal assistance; characterized by relatively severe disability; able to walk without aid or rest some 300 m
5.0	Ambulatory without aid or rest for about 200 m; disability severe enough to impair full daily activities (work a full day without special provisions)
5.5	Ambulatory without aid or rest for about 100 m; disability severe enough to preclude full daily activities
6.0	Intermittent or unilateral constant assistance (cane, crutch, brace) required to walk about 100 m with or without resting
6.5	Constant bilateral assistance (canes, crutches, braces) required to walk about 20 m without resting
7.0	Unable to walk beyond approximately 5 m even with aid, essentially restricted to wheelchair; wheels self in standard wheelchair and transfers alone; up and about in wheelchair some 12 h a day
7.5	Unable to take more than a few steps; restricted to wheelchair; may need aid in transfer; wheels self but cannot carry on in standard wheelchair a full day; may require motorized wheelchair
8.0	Essentially restricted to bed or chair or perambulated in wheelchair, but may be out of bed itself much of the day; retains many self-care functions; generally has effective use of arms
8.5	Essentially restricted to bed much of day; has some effective use of arms; retains some self-care functions
9.0	Confined to bed; can still communicate and eat
9.5	Totally helpless bed patient; unable to communicate effectively or eat/swallow
10.5	Death due to MS

administered again by having the patient walk back the same distance. The instruction manual of Fischer et al. (71) also states that patients may use assisting devices when doing the walk, and that materials needed are a stopwatch, clipboard, *Timed 25-Foot Walk Record Form*, and a marked 25-foot distance in an unobstructed hallway.

g. Secondary Endpoints

The main secondary endpoint was the time to confirmed *disability progression*. Time to

[71]Fischer JS, Jak AJ, Kniker JE, Rudick RA. Multiple Sclerosis Functional Composite (MSFC) Administration and Scoring Manual; 2001 (41 pp.).

confirmed disability progression is defined as an increase of one point in the EDSS score, with an absence of relapse at the time of assessment and with all EDSS scores measured during that time meeting the criteria for disability progression.

Other secondary endpoints included the *time to a first relapse, time to disability progression* (confirmed after 6 months), changes in the EDSS score and MSFC between baseline and 24 months, and information from pictures of brain lesions. Brain lesions are viewed by the technique of MRI.

h. MRI and Detecting the Onset of Brain Lesions

Magnetic resonance imaging is used for diagnosing multiple sclerosis, and for monitoring the efficacy of drugs during clinical trials (72).

At the initial stage of multiple sclerosis, brain lesions are thin and long (Dawson's fingers), which is probably associated with the inflammatory changes around the medullary vein. These lesions create a dilated perivenular space (73). The perivascular inflammation plays a primary role in disrupting the blood—brain barrier, in myelin breakdown, and in the formation of new lesions (74). The following concerns this disruption. In multiple sclerosis, macrophages and cytotoxic T cells (CD8$^+$ T

cells), inflict damage on blood vessels, where the result is a breakdown of the blood—brain barrier, and where this breakdown permits an ever greater influx of immune cells from the circulatory system into the central nervous system (75).

The following concerns the correlation of MRI data with disability. What are introduced here are the terms, "T1 black holes," also known as "T1 hypointensities," and T2 hyperintensities. Chronic T1 black holes in multiple sclerosis are correlated with disability (76). This is explained by the fact where T1 hypointensities are a more restrictive and more destructive set of processes at the tissue level. T1-hypointense lesion load shows good correlation with disability (77). This contrasts with the situation with T2 hyperintensities. T2 hyperintensities are less correlated with disability. T2 hyperintensities represent several different pathologic changes including gliosis, demyelination, inflammation, and focal edema (78).

The following introduces the technique of administering gadolinium, in conjunction with MRI. An early event in multiple sclerosis lesions is inflammation, where this inflammation disrupts the blood—brain barrier. Disruption of the blood—brain barrier enables the entry of medical imaging agents, in particular gadolinium (79). Gadolinium is used, in conjunction with

[72]Wolbarst AB, et al. Medical imaging: essentials for physicians. Hoboken, NJ: Wiley-Blackwell; 2013.

[73]Ge Y. Multiple sclerosis: the role of MR imaging. Am. J. Neuroradiol. 2006;27:1165—76.

[74]Ge Y. Multiple sclerosis: the role of MR imaging. Am. J. Neuroradiol. 2006;27:1165—76.

[75]Lassmann H. Hypoxia-like tissue injury as a component of multiple sclerosis lesions. J. Neurol. Sci. 2003;206:187—91.

[76]Pirko I, Nolan TK, Holland SK, Johnson AJ. Multiple sclerosis: pathogenesis and MR imaging features of T1 hypointensities in a murine model. Radiology 2008;246:790—5.

[77]Pirko I, Nolan TK, Holland SK, Johnson AJ. Multiple sclerosis: pathogenesis and MR imaging features of T1 hypointensities in a murine model. Radiology 2008;246:790—5.

[78]Pirko I, Nolan TK, Holland SK, Johnson AJ. Multiple sclerosis: pathogenesis and MR imaging features of T1 hypointensities in a murine model. Radiology 2008;246:790—5.

[79]Tas MW, Barkhol F, van Walderveen MA, Polman CH, Hommes OR, Valk J. The effect of gadolinium on the sensitivity and specificity of MR in the initial diagnosis of multiple sclerosis. Am. J. Neuroradiol. 1995;16:259—64.

T1-weighted MRI, to produce what is called, "gadolinium-enhanced T1-weighted images" or, for brevity, "gadolinium-enhanced MRI" (80). Use of gadolinium in conjunction with T1-weighted MRI gives rise to a higher intensity of signal (81).

A standard dose of gadolinium is 0.1 mmol gadolinium per kilogram of body weight (82). A standard protocol for MRI takes the form of T1-weighted imaging and T2-weighted imaging, before the injection of contrast agent and T1-weighted imaging after the injection of contrast agent (83). Images may be acquired within the first 5–10 min after injection.

Newly arising lesions involve disruption of the blood–brain barrier (enhancing lesions), whereas older lesions may be inactive and not involve disruption of the blood–brain barrier (nonenhancing lesions) (84). According to Rice et al. (85), "[g]adolinium-enhanced T1 lesions represent areas of breakdown in the blood–

brain barrier and are generally believed to be sites of new inflammation that probably precede symptoms." Nonenhancing lesions are the result of earlier episodes of disease (86). In the words of Lövblad et al. (87), there are two patterns of enhancement that can appear when using gadolinium in conjunction with T1 MRI. These two patterns are uniform enhancement, reflecting the onset of a new lesion, and ring-like enhancement, indicating reactivation of an older lesion. Nonenhancing lesions are the result of earlier episodes of disease (88).

MRI is about 5–10-fold more sensitive to ongoing demyelination than clinical measures (89,90,91). This means that most lesions are clinically silent, and that most lesions, while detectable by MRI, do not impair the functions of the patient. By "functions of the patient," what is generally meant is functions measured by the EDSS scale.

[80]Tas MW, Barkhol F, van Walderveen MA, Polman CH, Hommes OR, Valk J. The effect of gadolinium on the sensitivity and specificity of MR in the initial diagnosis of multiple sclerosis. Am. J. Neuroradiol. 1995;16:259–64.

[81]Tas MW, Barkhol F, van Walderveen MA, Polman CH, Hommes OR, Valk J. The effect of gadolinium on the sensitivity and specificity of MR in the initial diagnosis of multiple sclerosis. Am. J. Neuroradiol. 1995;16:259–64.

[82]Maravilla KR, Maldjian JA, Schmalfuss IM, et al. Contrast enhancement of central nervous system lesions: multicenter intraindividual crossover comparative study of two MR contrast agents. Radiology 2006;240:389–400.

[83]Tas MW, Barkhol F, van Walderveen MA, Polman CH, Hommes OR, Valk J. The effect of gadolinium on the sensitivity and specificity of MR in the initial diagnosis of multiple sclerosis. Am. J. Neuroradiol. 1995;16:259–64.

[84]Tas MW, Barkhol F, van Walderveen MA, Polman CH, Hommes OR, Valk J. The effect of gadolinium on the sensitivity and specificity of MR in the initial diagnosis of multiple sclerosis. Am. J. Neuroradiol. 1995;16:259–64.

[85]Rice GP, Filippi M, Comi G. Cladribine and progressive MS: clinical and MRI outcomes of a multicenter controlled trial. Cladribine MRI Study Group. Neurology 2000;54:1145–55.

[86]Lövblad KO, Anzalone N, Dörfler A, et al. MR imaging in multiple sclerosis: review and recommendations for current practice. Am. J. Neuroradiol. 2010;31:983–9.

[87]Lövblad KO, Anzalone N, Dörfler A, et al. MR imaging in multiple sclerosis: review and recommendations for current practice. Am. J. Neuroradiol. 2010;31:983–9.

[88]Lövblad KO, Anzalone N, Dörfler A, et al. MR imaging in multiple sclerosis: review and recommendations for current practice. Am. J. Neuroradiol. 2010;31:983–9.

[89]Simon JH, Li D, Traboulsee A, Coyle PK, et al. Standardized MR imaging protocol for multiple sclerosis: Consortium of MS Centers consensus guidelines. Am. J. Neuroradiol. 2006;27:455–61.

[90]Ge Y. Multiple sclerosis: the role of MR imaging. Am. J. Neuroradiol. 2006;27:1165–76.

[91]Leist TP, Marks S. Magnetic resonance imaging and treatment effects of multiple sclerosis therapeutics. Neurology 2010;74(Suppl. 1):S54–61.

1. Example of MRI Photograph

With imaging by MRI, brain lesions in patients with multiple sclerosis can take the form of nodes, rings, and arcs (92). In a review article, Ge (93) provides a dramatic MRI picture of lesions from a 30-year-old woman (Fig. 20.1). The large lesions appear as nodes and rings. The arrows in the picture point to small lesions.

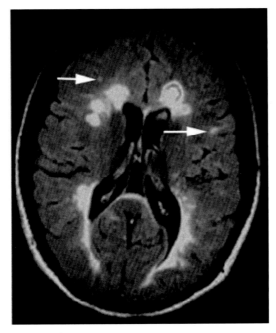

FIGURE 20.1 Magnetic resonance imaging. The photograph shows an MRI photograph of brain lesions of a patient with multiple sclerosis. The large lesions appear as nodes and rings. The arrows point to small lesions.

MRI images can be acquired under three conditions:

1. Noncontrast T1-weighted imaging;
2. Noncontrast T2-weighted imaging; and
3. Gadolinium-enhanced T1-weighted imaging.

The terms T1 and T2 are terms in physics, and refer to long relaxation time and to transverse relaxation time, respectfully.

2. T2-Weighted MRI

T2-weighted images are highly sensitive for the detection of MS lesions. (T2-weighted images are unenhanced, and do not involve administering gadolinium.) Such a sensitivity makes them very useful for diagnostics and for assessing the overall disease burden (by measuring the total hyperintense lesion volume on yearly scans) (94). T2-weighted MRI is considered the most sensitive diagnostic test for demonstrating disease dissemination, but with moderate specificity (95). Lesions detected with T2-weighted imaging are non-specific and T2 lesion load does not include the pathology. Therefore, although lesion load measures may not appear to adequately account for the patient's functional state, they provide important information in monitoring the natural history and treatment effects of the disease (96). Multiple sclerosis lesions detected by T2-weighted brain images appear as bright areas and are often referred to as T2-hyperintense lesions. Some of the T2-hyperintense lesions may resolve and wane

[92]He J, Grossman RI, Ge Y, Mannon LJ. Enhancing patterns in multiple sclerosis: evolution and persistence. Am. J. Neuroradiol. 2001;22:664−9.

[93]Ge Y. Multiple sclerosis: the role of MR imaging. Am. J. Neuroradiol. 2006;27:1165−76.

[94]Rovaris M, Rocca MA, Filippi M. Magnetic resonance-based techniques for the study and management of multiple sclerosis. Br. Med. Bull. 2003;65:133−44.

[95]Lövblad KO, Anzalone N, Dörfler A, et al. MR imaging in multiple sclerosis: review and recommendations for current practice. Am. J. Neuroradiol. 2010;31:983−9.

[96]Ge Y. Multiple sclerosis: the role of MR imaging. Am. J. Neuroradiol. 2006;27:1165−76.

over time (97). However, most newly formed T2 lesions chronically persist as "footprints" of damage. T2-hyperintense lesions in patients with multiple sclerosis are nonspecific for the underlying pathology, which may include varying degrees of inflammation, demyelination, gliosis, edema, ischemia, and axonal loss (98,99). In other words, T2-weighted MRI does not distinguish between these pathologic processes (100).

3. T1-Weighted MRI

T1-weighted images can take the form of T1 hypointensities (T1 black holes). With T1-weighted imaging, the acute lesions are often isointense (same intensity) to the normal white matter, but can be hypointense if chronic tissue injury or severe edema occurs. The accumulation of hypointense lesions may correlate with disease progression and disability (101). In the acute inflammatory phase, the lesion may disrupt the blood—brain barrier, leading to gadolinium enhancement of the T1-weighted image, and may last from days to weeks. T1-weighted scans, taken both before and after

administering gadolinium, allow discrimination between active and inactive MS lesions, since gadolinium enhancement occurs as a result of increased blood—brain barrier permeability and corresponds to areas with on-going inflammation (102). Lesions that are detected by gadolinium enhancement may vary in shape and size, and usually start as homogeneous enhancing nodules and subsequently progress to ring-like enhancements (103).

T1 hypointensities may be observed as a transient stage in the formation of a new lesion. However, about 30% of patients with multiple sclerosis also develop persistent T1 black holes. These black hole lesions are thought to represent severe tissue loss, including axonal damage (104). Hypointense lesions on a T1-weighted MRI scan are thought to represent irreversible axonal damage (105). The black holes that are detected in the brain by the T1 method relate to axon loss, matrix destruction, gliosis, and edema. In short, the T1 method picks up enlargements of the extracellular spaces in the brain (106). T1-hypointense lesions most commonly

[97]Neema M, Stankiewicz J, Arora A, Guss ZD, Bakshi R. MRI in multiple sclerosis: what's inside the toolbox? Neurotherapeutics 2007;4:602—17.

[98]Neema M, Stankiewicz J, Arora A, Guss ZD, Bakshi R. MRI in multiple sclerosis: what's inside the toolbox? Neurotherapeutics 2007;4:602—17.

[99]Leist TP, Marks S. Magnetic resonance imaging and treatment effects of multiple sclerosis therapeutics. Neurology 2010;74(Suppl. 1):S54—61.

[100]Leist TP, Marks S. Magnetic resonance imaging and treatment effects of multiple sclerosis therapeutics. Neurology 2010;74(Suppl. 1):S54—61.

[101]Ge Y. Multiple sclerosis: the role of MR imaging. Am. J. Neuroradiol. 2006;27:1165—76.

[102]Rovaris M, Rocca MA, Filippi M. Magnetic resonance-based techniques for the study and management of multiple sclerosis. Br. Med. Bull. 2003;65:133—44.

[103]Ge Y. Multiple sclerosis: the role of MR imaging. Am. J. Neuroradiol. 2006;27:1165—76.

[104]Pirko I, Nolan TK, Holland SK, Johnson AJ. Multiple sclerosis: pathogenesis and MR imaging features of T1 hypointensities in a murine model. Radiology 2008;246:790—5.

[105]Gold R, Wolinsky JS, Amato MP, Comi G. Evolving expectations around early management of multiple sclerosis. Ther. Adv. Neurol. Disord. 2010;3:351—67.

[106]Barkhof F, van Walderveen M. Characterization of tissue damage in multiple sclerosis by nuclear magnetic resonance. Philos. Trans. R. Soc. Lond. B Biol. Sci. 1999;35:1675—86.

develop initially as gadolinium-enhancing lesions and have about a 50% chance of being either transient, that is, lasting 6–12 months, or being permanent (107).

i. Results From the Gold Study

Gold et al. (108) conducted a clinical trial on subjects with relapsing-remitting multiple sclerosis. The study drug was dimethyl fumarate (Tecfidera®). The control arm received placebo. The drug had its origin in Germany during the 1950s, when it was thought (incorrectly) that psoriasis resulted from disruptions in the Krebs cycle (109) and because of the realization that the Krebs cycle includes fumarate as an intermediate (110). Psoriasis and multiple sclerosis are both autoimmune diseases.

The mechanism of action of dimethyl fumarate involves its influence on shifting lymphocytes in the body from expressing Th1-type cytokines to Th2-type cytokines. Also, dimethyl fumarate appears to stimulate a pathway that reduces the concentration of toxic oxygen, such as nitric oxide, hydrogen peroxide, and peroxynitrate. By stimulating the Nrf2 antioxidant response pathway, dimethyl fumarate reduces toxic oxygen, and thus reduces toxic oxygen's destruction of nerve tissue.

The Gold study enrolled 1237 subjects, and 952 subjects completed the trial. The researchers were careful to note that the rate of discontinuation was similar in the study drug arm (31%) and in the placebo arm (35%). The primary endpoint was:

- Percent of subjects having a relapse by 2 years into the study.

The secondary endpoints were:

- Number of new or enlarging lesions (mean number of lesions per subject). The Supplementary Appendix broke down the number of patients, in the study drug arm and the placebo arm, having zero lesions, one lesion, two lesions, three to four lesions, or five or more lesions.
- Total number of relapses divided by patient-years.
- The endpoint was the percent of patients that progressed to disability, according to the EDSS scale.

In greater detail, "relapse" was defined as new or recurrent neurological symptoms that lasted for at least 24 h, and that were accompanied by new objective neurological findings.

The Clinical Study Protocol (111) provided general information on the characteristics of a relapse, which is reproduced in the footnote (112). The Clinical Study Protocol is available on

---

[107]Neema M, Stankiewicz J, Arora A, Guss ZD, Bakshi R. MRI in multiple sclerosis: what's inside the toolbox? Neurotherapeutics 2007;4:602–17.

[108]Gold R, Kappos L, Arnold DL, et al. Placebo-controlled phase 3 study of oral BG-12 for relapsing multiple sclerosis. New Engl. J. Med. 2012;367:1098–107.

[109]Meissner M, et al. Dimethyl fumarate—only an anti-psoriatic medication? J. Dtsch. Dermatol. Ges. 2012;10:793–801.

[110]Krebs HA, Eggleston LV. The oxidation of pyruvate in pigeon breast muscle. Biochem. J. 1940;34:442–59.

[111]Clinical Study Protocol no. 109MS301 (ver. 6). Biogen IDEC (May 26, 2010).

[112]"Subjects with relapsing-remitting MS experience discrete episodes of neurologic dysfunction (referred to as relapses, exacerbations, or attacks), each lasting several days to several weeks, which occur intermittently over many years. Symptoms of such relapses include loss of vision or double vision, numbness or tingling sensation in the extremities, muscle weakness, slurred speech, difficulty with coordination, and bladder dysfunction. Early in the course of this phase of the disease, these symptoms tend to subside completely after each attack. Over time, recovery from attacks tends to be incomplete, leading to the accumulation of functional disability."

TABLE 20.2   Efficacy Data for the Endpoints in the Gold Study

PRIMARY ENDPOINT		
Percent of subjects having a relapse by 2 years	26–27% (study drug)	46% (placebo)
SECONDARY ENDPOINTS		
Number of new or enlarging lesions (mean number of lesions per subject)	2.6–4.4 (study drug)	17.0 (placebo)
Total number of relapses divided by patient-years in the study	0.17–0.19 (study drug)	0.36 (placebo)
Percent of patients that progressed to disability according to EDSS scale	16–18% (study drug)	27% (placebo)

the website of the *New England Journal of Medicine* (113).

Regarding new or enlarging lesions, these are the lesions as measured on T2-weighted images.

Regarding progression to disability, progression of multiple sclerosis in any given patient to a disability was defined as a 1.0-point increase in EDSS in patients with a baseline score of 1.0 or higher, or at least a 1.5-point increase in patients with a baseline score of zero. To trigger this endpoint, the increased score must be sustained for at least 12 weeks.

Table 20.2 discloses the efficacy data from the Gold study. The study drug was actually provided to subjects in two separate study drug arms, not just one arm. The efficacy results from these two arms were similar, and hence are disclosed as a range. As is readily evident, efficacy was dramatically greater in the study drug arm than in the placebo arm. The Gold study demonstrates the use of *clinical response*, which encompassed loss of vision, numbness or tingling sensations, muscle weakness, slurred speech, and *objective response*, which took the form of lesion size and number, as endpoints.

III. FDA'S DECISION-MAKING PROCESS IN EVALUATING ENDPOINTS FOR MULTIPLE SCLEROSIS

Fampridine (Ampyra®), which is also called 4-aminopyridine, improves the symptoms of multiple sclerosis, but does not influence the course of the disease itself. The drug improves conduction of action potentials in demyelinated nerve fibers and increases release of neurotransmitters in synapses and at neuromuscular junctions. Fampridine is fat-soluble and readily crosses the blood–brain barrier. According to articles on fampridine clinical trials, the drug increases in muscle strength and walking speed in a third of patients, as measured by *the endpoint of the 12-Item Walking Scale* (114,115).

[113]Gold R, Kappos L, Arnold DL, et al. Placebo-controlled phase 3 study of oral BG-12 for relapsing multiple sclerosis. New Engl. J. Med. 2012;367:1098–107.

[114]Lugaresi A. Pharmacology and clinical efficacy of dalfampridine for treating multiple sclerosis. Expert Opin. Drug Metab. Toxicol. 2015;11:295–306.

[115]Jensen HB, et al. 4-Aminopyridine for symptomatic treatment of multiple sclerosis: a systematic review. Ther. Adv. Neurol. Dis. 2014;7:97–113.

The FDA's decision-making process in the approval of fampridine is revealed by the facts that:

- During the timeline of drug approval process, the FDA complained that a particular endpoint was relatively meaningless, and require use of an additional endpoint.
- The FDA complained about the need to validate endpoints.
- The FDA agreed that where a Sponsor uses a nonvalidated endpoint, the FDA may accept this endpoint if additional supportive endpoints are also used to assess efficacy.

FDA's *Medical Review* and *Medical Summary*, which were published on FDA's website, along with the *Approval Letter*, included the following comments. Regarding meaningless endpoint, the FDA reviewer complained that the endpoint was such that it could be triggered by even a tiny increment of improvement, writing that:

> [t]he sponsor showed Timed Walk Responder rates were higher with fampridine treatment compared to placebo in both pivotal trials, yet the clinical meaningfulness of the benefit remains unclear. Though more patients on fampridine appear to walk faster, the magnitude of the improvement in walking speed suggests the improvement lacks clinical significance. The responder variable is limited by its ignoring the importance of the **extent of improvement** in walking speed. So, a small benefit in many patients given the treatment can result in a positive trial even in the **absence of a clinically meaningful benefit**.

Regarding validation of the endpoint, the reviewer wrote:

The Division questioned the clinical significance of results based on the analyses; it noted that the responder **criterion was neither validated** by that trial nor did it demonstrate maintenance of effect over time. The Division demanded **additional validation** of the sponsor's outcome measure of responder criterion. The agreements at that meeting were: to conduct a trial to demonstrate effect on two co-primary endpoints, walking speed and a global subjective measure, or have a sequential analysis to **validate** the clinical meaningfulness of the responder criterion and the maintenance of benefit.

The reviewer made a suggestion on how the endpoint could be validated, stating that, "[v]alidation … is from correlating results of timed 25-foot walk (T25FW) with scores on Guy's Neurological Disability Scale (GNDS) or EDSS."

Regarding the need for supportive endpoints, the reviewer wrote, "[s]upportive endpoints such as EDSS are potentially helpful, especially when MSWS-12 is not clearly validated by the Agency for MS trials. Only baseline EDSS was performed in the sponsor's trials."

The FDA complained that the Sponsor had only acquired baseline EDSS data. While baseline EDSS data are useful for proper stratification of study subjects, EDSS data can be used as an efficacy endpoint only if EDSS data are captured at the time of randomization and at a time point after the study drug was administered. Goldman et al. (116) and Pilutti et al. (117) provide guidance on validating the Timed 25-foot Walk (T25FW) scale for multiple sclerosis. Moore et al. (118) review the validation of tests for measuring health-related quality of life for multiple sclerosis patients.

[116]Goldman MD, et al. Clinically meaningful performance benchmarks in MS: timed 25-foot walk and the real world. Neurology 2013;81:1856−63.

[117]Pilutti LA, et al. Further validation of multiple sclerosis walking scale-12 scores based on spatiotemporal gait parameters. Arch. Phys. Med. Rehab. 2013;94:575−8.

[118]Moore F, et al. Two multiple sclerosis quality-of-life measures: comparison in a national sample. Can. J. Neurol. Sci. 2015;42:55−63.

IV. CONCLUDING REMARKS

A variety of endpoints are available for use in clinical trials on immune diseases. Some of these endpoints, which are observed and recorded by the clinician, relate to ability of the patient to function in ordinary daily activities, for example, "unable to take more than a few steps; restricted to wheelchair." Other endpoints require special equipment and extensive training, for example, MRI. An ongoing theme in this book is criteria for diagnosing a disease, as well criteria for assessing the stage of the disease after it is properly diagnosed. As emphasized in this book, these criteria may be revised once every few years with publication of the new standards in a medical journal. As is the case with the endpoint of objective response in clinical trials for solid tumors (RECIST criteria), data from MRI are used in nearly all clinical trials on multiple sclerosis. Another similarity, is that data on objective response in clinical trials on solid tumors and data from MRI imaging in multiple sclerosis, are usually relegated to be secondary endpoints in clinical trials (and are not often primary endpoints).

21

Endpoints for Infections

I. INTRODUCTION

Infections include bacterial infections, protozoal infections, and viral infections. Endpoints used in clinical trials for infections can include direct measurements of the infecting agent, measurements of physiological functions that are impaired by the infecting agent, and measurements of immune responses against the infecting agent.

Infections are not necessarily fatal. For example, regarding Chagas' disease, which is caused by infections with *Trypanosoma cruzi*, "the disease enters the chronic phase, which usually involves a clinically latent period ... lasting 10–30 years, although it may be lifelong" (1). Thus, endpoints that track survival, such as overall survival or progression-free survival, may be irrelevant in clinical trials on infections. Another issue in determining drug efficacy is that there may not exist any test to determine a cure. In the words of Molina et al.

(2) "[o]ne of the limitations of clinical trials ... in chronic Chagas' disease is that there is no definite test to determine cure." For these reasons, surrogate endpoints may be the only available endpoint available for clinical trials on infectious diseases.

This chapter establishes a context for understanding endpoints for clinical trials on infectious diseases by detailing the physiology of hepatitis C virus (HCV) infections, and endpoints used for clinical trials on HCV. HCV infections are often chronic and fatal.

II. CLINICAL AND IMMUNOLOGICAL FEATURES OF HCV INFECTIONS

Hepatitis C virus (HCV) was identified in 1989 (3). About 170 million people worldwide are infected with HCV, with about 4 million of

---

[1]Pérez-Molina JA, Pérez-Ayala A, Moreno S, et al. Use of benznidazole to treat chronic Chagas' disease: a systematic review with a meta-analysis. J. Antimicrob. Chemother. 2009;64:1139–47.

[2]Molina I, Prat J, Salvador F, et al. Randomized trial of posaconazole and benznidazloe for chronic Chagas' disease. New Engl. J. Med. 2014;370:1899–908.

[3]Rehermann B. Hepatitis C virus versus innate and adaptive immune responses: a tale of coevolution and coexistence. J. Clin. Invest. 2009;119:1745–54.

these in the United States (4). About 20% of patients with chronic HCV will have cirrhosis within 20 years, and 1–4% of cirrhotic HCV patients will develop hepatocellular carcinoma (HCC) per year. HCV is the most common reason for liver transplantation. Almost 5000 liver transplants were performed in the United States in 2000, where about 40% of the recipients had chronic HCV.

HCV infections are typically not diagnosed until alanine aminotransferase (ALT) levels rise, which occurs at 8–12 weeks after initial infection. At this time, HCV-specific antibodies and T cells become detectable (5,6).

HCV infections have the following adverse consequences (7):

- Chronic hepatitis;
- Increased risk for liver cirrhosis;
- Increased risk for liver cancer (HCC);
- Failure of drug treatment. For example, therapy with interferon and ribavirin does not work in about half of treated patients (8,9);
- Requirement for a liver transplant.

From 60% to 80% of HCV-infected people develop chronic hepatitis, that is, pathological inflammation of the liver (10). The frequencies of liver cirrhosis and HCC are documented by Prasad et al. (11). In a study of 2452 patients with HCV infections, 339 patients (14%) were found to have cirrhosis, while 54 had HCC (about 2%). Patients with cirrhosis secondary to chronic infection with HCV are at particular risk for HCC, though in patients with chronic HCV without cirrhosis, HCC is rare (12).

III. ACUTE HCV VERSUS CHRONIC HCV

HCV infections are classed as acute infections (newly acquired infections) and as chronic infections. In acute infections, many patients are asymptomatic or develop only unspecific symptoms such as fatigue, low-grade fever, myalgia, or nausea. Jaundice only occurs in 20–30% of cases. When detected and treated, most cases of acute HCV infection can

[4]Gordon FD, Kwo P, Vargas HE. Treatment of hepatitis C in liver transplant recipients. Liver Transpl. 2009;15:126–35.

[5]Rehermann B. Hepatitis C virus versus innate and adaptive immune responses: a tale of coevolution and coexistence. J. Clin. Invest. 2009;119:1745–54.

[6]Wiegand J, Deterding K, Cornberg M, Wedemeyer H. Treatment of acute hepatitis C: the success of monotherapy with (pegylated) interferon alpha. J. Antimicrob. Chemother. 2008;62:860–5.

[7]Shin EC, Capone S, Cortese R, et al. The kinetics of hepatitis C virus-specific CD8 T-cell responses in the blood mirror those in the liver in acute hepatitis C virus infection. J. Virol. 2008;82:9782–8.

[8]Rehermann B. Hepatitis C virus versus innate and adaptive immune responses: a tale of coevolution and coexistence. J. Clin. Invest. 2009;119:1745–54.

[9]Taylor MW, Tsukahara T, Brodsky L, et al. Changes in gene expression during pegylated interferon and ribavirin therapy of chronic hepatitis C virus distinguish responders from nonresponders to antiviral therapy. J. Virol. 2007;81:3391–401.

[10]Rehermann B. Hepatitis C virus versus innate and adaptive immune responses: a tale of coevolution and coexistence. J. Clin. Invest. 2009;119:1745–54.

[11]Prasad L, Spicher VM, Zwahlen M, et al. Cohort profile: the Swiss Hepatitis C Cohort Study (SCCS). Int. J. Epidemiol. 2007;36:731–7.

[12]Nash KL, Woodall T, Brown AS, Davies SE, Alexander GJ. Hepatocellular carcinoma in patients with chronic hepatitis C virus infection without cirrhosis. World J. Gastroenterol. 2010;16:4061–5.

be cured (13). Most HCV infections persist, but some spontaneously resolve during the first year of infection. In about 80% of infected people, the virus is able to avoid clearance by the immune system, and the result is chronic HCV infection (14,15). In a study of 251 HCV patients, Huang et al. (16) reported that 34% spontaneously cleared the HCV infection, while 66% had a chronic HCV infection. The Huang study implicated differences in the human genome as responsible for the patient's ability to clear the infection, or to suffer from a chronic infection. This difference took the form of a polymorphism in the DNA sequence of the human interferon (IFN)-gamma gene. This polymorphism occurred in one of the promoters of this gene. Patients resolving the infection, and patients with chronic infection, had different DNA sequences in this promoter.

The fact that some people infected with HCV spontaneously recover, while others progress and suffer from chronic HCV, has further bases in the immune system. Most people infected with HCV mount CD8$^+$ T-cell responses. However, what distinguishes people who recover from acute HCV and those who progress to chronic HCV, is that those who quickly recover also mount an effective CD4$^+$ T-cell response (in addition to the CD8$^+$ T-cell response), while those who progress to chronic HCV mount only CD8$^+$ T-cell

responses, but fail to mount a CD4$^+$ T-cell response (17). In other words, although increased numbers of viral antigen-specific CD8$^+$ T cells are present in most patients, these cells are not maximally activated, where inadequate inactivation occurs because of lack of CD4$^+$ T-cell response. CD4$^+$ T cells serve as Mother Nature's adjuvant.

Smyk-Pearson et al. (18) characterized CD8$^+$ T cells that specifically recognize and kill HCV infections, but that have not been helped by CD4$^+$ T cells. These CD8$^+$ T cells are helpless, impaired in the ability to generate a secondary response upon rechallenge, where the unhelped memory cytotoxic T lymphocytes divided less and were unable to provide complete protection against HCV.

IV. DRUGS AGAINST HCV

Traditionally, the most commonly used anti-HCV drugs are IFN-alfa2 and ribavirin. Ribavirin, which is a guanosine analog, is effective against a variety of viruses, that is, viruses with a DNA genome and viruses with a ribonucleic acid (RNA) genome. With HCV, ribavirin's effect is transient, but when combined with IFN-alpha, the combination can permanently eradicate that particular HCV

[13]Weigand K, Stremmel W, Encke J. Treatment of hepatitis C virus infection. World J. Gastroenterol. 2007;13:1897—905.

[14]Wölfl M, Rutebemberwa A, Mosbruger T, et al. Hepatitis C virus immune escape via exploitation of a hole in the T cell repertoire. J. Immunol. 2008;181:6435—46.

[15]Blackard JT, Shata MT, Shire NJ, Sherman KE. Acute hepatitis C virus infection: a chronic problem. Hepatology 2008;47:321—31.

[16]Huang Y, Yang H, Borg BB, et al. A functional SNP of interferon-gamma gene is important for interferon-alpha-induced and spontaneous recovery from hepatitis C virus infection. Proc. Natl Acad. Sci. USA 2007;104:985—90.

[17]Smyk-Pearson S, Tester IA, Klarquist J, et al. Spontaneous recovery in acute human hepatitis C virus infection: functional T-cell thresholds and relative importance of CD4 help. J. Virol. 2008;82:1827—37.

[18]Smyk-Pearson S, Tester IA, Klarquist J, et al. Spontaneous recovery in acute human hepatitis C virus infection: functional T-cell thresholds and relative importance of CD4 help. J. Virol. 2008;82:1827—37.

infection (19). Interferon-alpha is abbreviated as both IFN-alpha and IFN-alfa. Proposed mechanisms of ribavirin are:

- Ribavirin promotes signaling by interferon, thereby enhancing interferon's effects against HCV (20,21). Microarray analyses demonstrated that ribavirin increases induction of interferon-stimulated genes.
- Ribavirin inhibits the enzyme, inosine monophosphate dehydrogenase (22). This is a key enzyme in the biosynthesis of nucleotides (23). This inhibition results in depletion of intracellular guanosine pools (pools needed for viral replication).
- Ribavirin may provoke mutations in the viral genome, where the result of the mutations is termination of the viral lifecycle. A study of human subjects treated for 1 year with ribivirin plus interferon showed an increase in mutations in the HCV genome, for example, C→U and G→A mutations (24). But in a 24-week study of human subjects with chronic HCV infection, Chevaliez et al. (25), determined that ribavirin monotherapy (or ribavirin plus IFN-alpha) did not influence HCV's mutation rate.

Although treatment of HCV involves ribavirin in combination with one or more other drugs such as pegylated IFN-alfa-2, an effort has been to eliminate both of these drugs because of their adverse effects. IFN-alfa-2 is a naturally occurring cytokine, but when used as a drug, it is chemically modified by attaching polyethylene glycol (PEG). PEG is an inert polymer that, when covalently attached to the interferon, increases its half-life in the bloodstream. Thus, the drug is called, "pegylated IFN-alfa-2."

The majority of acute HCV infections become chronic. Until the year 2011, the only approved therapies for chronic HCV were those that included IFN-alfa-2. The success rates of these IFN-alfa-2-based therapies ranged from 40% to 90% depending on the genotype of the infecting virus (26). In 2011, two small-molecule drugs, boceprevir and telaprevir, which act directly on HCV-encoded proteins, were approved by the FDA.

Drugs against HCV also include boceprevir, telaprevir, and simeprevir. These drugs inhibit an enzyme that is encoded by the genome of this virus, namely, *NS3/4A protease*. Anti-HCV drugs also include ledipasvir, daclatasvir, and

[19]Thomas E, Feld JJ, Li Q, Hu Z, Fried MW, Liang TJ. Ribavirin potentiates interferon action by augmenting interferon-stimulated gene induction in hepatitis C virus cell culture models. Hepatology 2011;53:32—41.

[20]Feld JJ, Lutchman GA, Heller T, et al. Ribavirin improves early responses to peginterferon through improved interferon signaling. Gastroenterology 2010;139:154—62.

[21]Thomas E, Feld JJ, Li Q, Hu Z, Fried MW, Liang TJ. Ribavirin potentiates interferon action by augmenting interferon-stimulated gene induction in hepatitis C virus cell culture models. Hepatology 2011;53:32—41.

[22]Mori K, Ikeda M, Ariumi Y, Dansako H, Wakita T, Kato N. Mechanism of action of ribavirin in a novel hepatitis C virus replication cell system. Virus Res. 2011;157:61—70.

[23]Pal S, Bera B, Nair V. Inhibition of inosine monophosphate dehydrogenase (IMPDH) by the antiviral compound, 2-vinylinosine monophosphate. Bioorg. Med. Chem. 2002;10:3615—8.

[24]Cuevas JM, González-Candelas F, Moya A, Sanjuán R. Effect of ribavirin on the mutation rate and spectrum of hepatitis C virus in vivo. J. Virol. 2009;83:5760—4.

[25]Chevaliez S, Brillet R, Lázaro E, Hézode C, Pawlotsky JM. Analysis of ribavirin mutagenicity in human hepatitis C virus infection. J. Virol. 2007;81:7732—41.

[26]Abdel-Hakeem MS, Bedard N, Badr G, et al. Comparison of immune restoration in early versus late alpha interferon therapy against hepatitis C virus. J. Virol. 2010;84:10429—35.

samatasvir, and these drugs target one of the nonstructural proteins of HCV, that is, **NS5A**. The drug sofosbuvir targets the nonstructural protein **NS5B** (27,28). The term "nonstructural" means that the protein is not part of the infective viral particle and that, instead, it is used to mediate maturation or assembly of the viral particle inside of the host cell.

A variety of drugs have been used in clinical trials on HCV, as indicated:

- peginterferon-alfa-2 (29,30,31,32),
- sofosbuvir (33,34,35,36),
- ledipasvir (37,38),
- boceprevir (39,40),
- telaprevir (41),

[27]Liu D, et al. Fast HCV RNA elimination and NS5A redistribution by NS5A inhibitors studied by a multiplex assay approach. Antimicrob. Agents Chemother. 2015;2015:pii: AAC.00223-15.

[28]Kirby BJ, et al. Pharmacokinetic, pharmacodynamic, and drug-interaction profile of the hepatitis C virus NS5B polymerase inhibitor sofosbuvir. Clin. Pharmacokinet. 2015;Mar 31 [Epub ahead of print].

[29]Lawitz E, Mangia A, Wyles D, et al. Sofosbuvir for previously untreated chronic hepatitis C infection. New Engl. J. Med. 369:1878—87.

[30]Lok AS, Gardiner, DF, Lawitz E, et al. Preliminary study of two antiviral agents for hepatitis C genotype 1. New Engl. J. Med. 2012;366:216—24.

[31]Bacon BR, Gordon SC, Lawitz E, et al. Boceprevir for previously treated chronic HCV genotype 1 infection. New Engl. J. Med. 2011;364:1207—17.

[32]Poordad F, McCone J, Bacon BR, et al. Boceprevir for untreated chronic HCV genotype 1 infection. New Engl. J. Med. 2011;364:1195—206.

[33]Lawitz E, Mangia A, Wyles D, et al. Sofosbuvir for previously untreated chronic hepatitis C infection. New Engl. J. Med. 369:1878—87.

[34]Kowdley KV, Gordon SC, Reddy KR, et al. Ledipasvir and sofosbuvir for 8 or 12 weeks for chronic HCV without cirrhosis. New Engl. J. Med. 2014;370:1879—88.

[35]Gane EJ, et al. Nucleotide polymerase inhibitor sofosbuvir plus ribavirin for hepatitis C. New Engl. J. Med. 2013;368:34—44.

[36]Afdhal N, Zeuzem S, Kwo P, et al. Ledipasvir and sofosbuvir for untreated HCV genotype 1 infection. New Engl. J. Med. 2014;370:1889—98.

[37]Kowdley KV, Gordon SC, Reddy KR, et al. Ledipasvir and sofosbuvir for 8 or 12 weeks for chronic HCV without cirrhosis. New Engl. J. Med. 2014;370:1879—88.

[38]Afdhal N, Zeuzem S, Kwo P, et al. Ledipasvir and sofosbuvir for untreated HCV genotype 1 infection. New Engl. J. Med. 2014;370:1889—98.

[39]Bacon BR, Gordon SC, Lawitz E, et al. Boceprevir for previously treated chronic HCV genotype 1 infection. New Engl. J. Med. 2011;364:1207—17.

[40]Poordad F, McCone J, Bacon BR, et al. Boceprevir for untreated chronic HCV genotype 1 infection. New Engl. J. Med. 2011;364:1195—206.

[41]Jacobson IM, McHutchison JG, Dusheiko G, et al. Telaprevir for previously untreated chronic hepatitis C virus infection. New Engl. J. Med. 2011;364:2405—16.

- daclatasvir (42),
- dasabuvir (43),
- ombitasvir (44,45),
- ABT-333 (46),
- asunaprevir (47),
- ritonavir (48,49).

All of the cited clinical trials used the indicated drug in combination with one or more anti-HCV drugs, where this other drug typically included ribavirin. FDA's Guidance for Industry provides a background for conducting clinical trials on HCV (50).

In the scientific literature, various spellings are used for interferon-alpha, including "interferon-alpha," "alpha-interferon," "interferon-alfa," and names that use the Greek letter alpha. This textbook uses the name that best corresponds to that from the published study being described.

V. IMMUNE RESPONSES AGAINST HCV

Immune response, in particular, response by cytotoxic T cells (CD8[+] T cells), plays a major role in combating HCV infections. CD8[+] T cells destroy HCV by killing liver cells that contain the virus. CD8[+] T cells use a second, independent mechanism for combating HCV, namely, expression of IFN-gamma. IFN-gamma released by CD8[+] T cells has a direct, negative effect on the virus, that is, it inhibits viral replication (51). IFN-gamma is also called "gamma-interferon."

HCV-specific CD8[+] T cells can be detected by way of biopsies of the liver, and more conveniently, in blood samples (52). Hence, the immune system's response against HCV infections can be easily be determined by acquiring blood samples, and by characterizing the

---

[42]Lok AS, Gardiner, DF, Lawitz E, et al. Preliminary study of two antiviral agents for hepatitis C genotype 1. New Engl. J. Med. 2012;366:216−24.

[43]Ferenci P, Bernstein D, Lalezari J, et al. ABT-450/r-ombitasvir and dasabuvir with or without ribavirin for HCV. New Engl. J. Med. 2014;370:1983−92.

[44]Poordad F, Hezode C, Trinh R, et al. ABT-450/r-ombitasvir and dasabuvir with ribavirin for hepatitis C with cirrhosis. New Engl. J. Med. 2014;370:1973−82.

[45]Ferenci P, Bernstein D, Lalezari J, et al. ABT-450/r-ombitasvir and dasabuvir with or without ribavirin for HCV. New Engl. J. Med. 370:1983−92.

[46]Kowdley KV, Lawitz E, Poordad F, et al. Phase 2b trial of interferon-free therapy for hepatitis C virus genotype 1. New Engl. J. Med. 2014;370:222−32.

[47]Lok AS, Gardiner, DF, Lawitz E, et al. Preliminary study of two antiviral agents for hepatitis C genotype 1. New Engl. J. Med. 2012;366:216−24.

[48]Kowdley KV, Lawitz E, Poordad F, et al. Phase 2b trial of interferon-free therapy for hepatitis C virus genotype 1. New Engl. J. Med. 2014;370:222−32.

[49]Ferenci P, Bernstein D, Lalezari J, et al. ABT-450/r-ombitasvir and dasabuvir with or without ribavirin for HCV. New Engl. J. Med. 2014:370:1983−92.

[50]U.S. Department of Health and Human Services. Food and Drug Administration. Guidance for industry. Chronic hepatitis C virus infection: developing direct-acting antiviral drugs for treatment; 2013 (39 pp.).

[51]Huang Y, Yang H, Borg BB, et al. A functional SNP of interferon-gamma gene is important for interferon-alpha-induced and spontaneous recovery from hepatitis C virus infection. Proc. Natl Acad. Sci. USA 2007;104:985−90.

[52]Shin EC, Capone S, Cortese R, et al. The kinetics of hepatitis C virus-specific CD8 T-cell responses in the blood mirror those in the liver in acute hepatitis C virus infection. J. Virol. 2008;82:9782−8.

number and antigen-specificity of the T cells in the blood sample. Responses by helper T cells (CD4$^+$ T cells) are essential for an effective response by the cytotoxic T cells. CD4$^+$ T cells contribute to the immune response to HCV in two ways, namely, by expressing cytokines and by directly contacting CD8$^+$ T cells (53). This direct contact involves CD40 ligand of the helper T cell to CD40 receptor of the cytotoxic T cell. The result is the CD40L/CD40R complex.

VI. KINETICS OF HCV INFECTIONS

The following narrative describes the studies in the bulletpoint list. These are all time-course studies:

- untreated acute HCV infections;
- untreated fluctuating or intermittent acute HCV infections;
- untreated chronic HCV infections;
- biphasic response to IFN-alpha;
- sustained responders versus nonsustained responders, with IFN-alpha treatment.

HCV infections follow one of two different natural courses. These are:

1. acute infections that spontaneously resolve and
2. chronic infections that do not resolve spontaneously (54).

After exposure to HCV, there is a lag time of 1−3 weeks before serum HCV-RNA can be detected. The appearance of anti-HCV antibodies, which is called seroconversion, occurs at 4−10 weeks after exposure to HCV (55).

Acute HCV infections, which occur in about 20% of HCV infections, mean HCV infections where the patient spontaneously recovers within about 6 months. During the acute phase, serum HCV-RNA levels can fluctuate widely and may even be transiently undetectable. Levels of HCV in the bloodstream are usually determined by measuring the viral genome, which consists of RNA, and where measurement is by the polymerase chain reaction (56).

Loomba et al. (57) provides serum HCV-RNA data from three patients who showed the fluctuating pattern (Fig. 21.1). Meyer et al. (58) also shows data on the fluctuating nature of HCV-RNA that sometimes occurs with acute HCV. Where spontaneous clearance does

[53]Semmo N, Klenerman P. CD4 + T cell responses in hepatitis C virus infection. World J. Gastroenterol. 2007;13:4831−8.

[54]Scott JD, Gretch DR. Molecular diagnostics of hepatitis C virus infection: a systematic review. J. Am. Med. Assoc. 2007;297:724−32.

[55]Santantonio T, Wiegand J, Gerlach JT. Acute hepatitis C: current status and remaining challenges. J. Hepatol. 2008;49:625−33.

[56]Elkady A, Tanaka Y, Kurbanov F, et al. Performance of two real-time RT-PCR assays for quantitation of hepatitis C virus RNA: evaluation on HCV genotypes 1−4. J. Med. Virol. 2010;82:1878−88.

[57]Loomba R, Rivera MM, McBurney R, et al. The natural history of acute hepatitis C: clinical presentation, laboratory findings and treatment outcomes. Aliment. Pharmacol. Ther. 2011;33:559−65.

[58]Meyer MF, Lehmann M, Cornberg M, et al. Clearance of low levels of HCV viremia in the absence of a strong adaptive immune response. Virol. J. 2007;4:58 (11 pp.).

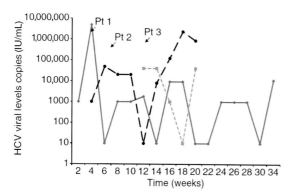

FIGURE 21.1 Serum levels of HCV-RNA. What is shown is the fluctuating pattern of HCV-RNA from three different, untreated HCV patients.

occur, the time for spontaneous clearance of acute HCV varies between 1 and 12 months (59). Figure 21.2, which is from Gordon et al. (60), provides serum levels of HCV-RNA from patients with chronic HCV infections. Depending on the particular patient, the HCV-RNA levels increased, decreased, or were stable, over the course of time. The patients were not treated with drugs for HCV. Also shown are serum levels of ALT. Serum ALT is an enzyme that is used to monitor liver damage, for example, from HCV infections.

The kinetics of serum HCV-RNA, over the course of time, is illustrated. The example is with therapy using IFN-alpha. Typically, IFN-alpha therapy results in a biphasic decrease in serum HCV-RNA. Zeuzem and Herrmann (61)

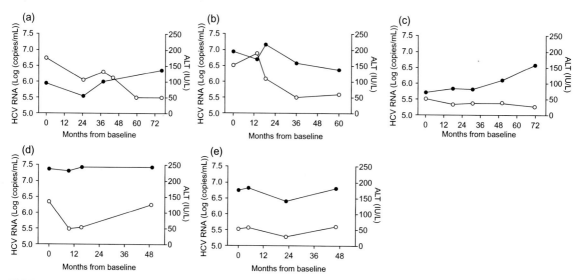

FIGURE 21.2 Chronic HCV infection. Data on HCV-RNA (*black dots*) as well as on serum ALT (*open circles*), are shown over the course of 48–72 months. Data from five different untreated HCV patients are shown.

[59]Wang CC, Krantz E, Klarquist J, et al. Acute hepatitis C in a contemporary US cohort: modes of acquisition and factors influencing viral clearance. J. Infect. Dis. 2007;196:1474–82.

[60]Gordon SC, Dailey PJ, Silverman AL, Khan BA, Kodali VP, Wilber JC. Sequential serum hepatitis C viral RNA levels longitudinally assessed by branched DNA signal amplification. Hepatology 1998;28:1702–6.

[61]Zeuzem S, Herrmann E. Dynamics of hepatitis C virus infection. Ann. Hepatol. 2002;1:56–63.

reports that, after starting IFN-alpha therapy, there is an initial delay of about 9 h where HCV-RNA does not change, followed typically by a rapid decrease and then by a gradual decrease in HCV-RNA. Variations on this theme occur, for example, where there is a rapid decline, followed by a prolonged plateau in serum HCV-RNA, or a rapid decline followed by a rebound in HCV-RNA. Almost all patients treated with IFN-alpha show the initial rapid phase (62). Neumann et al. (63) and Medeiros-Filho et al. (64) provides excellent data showing the biphasic response to IFN-alpha treatment.

The following time-course study distinguishes responders from nonresponders. In a study patients with chronic hepatitis Calleja et al. (65) administered the combination of ribavirin plus IFN-alpha. The patients had not yet been treated for HCV, and were therefore treatment-naive. Serum HCV-RNA (black dots) was followed over the course of time, as indicated in the following figures. Serum ALT was also measured. After conducting the study, the researchers categorized patient data into those who were responders (Fig. 21.3) and those who were nonresponders (Fig. 21.4). Patients who fail to respond to therapy with ribavirin plus IFN-alpha, that is, "nonresponders," represent an overwhelming public health problem, as disclosed in further detail below.

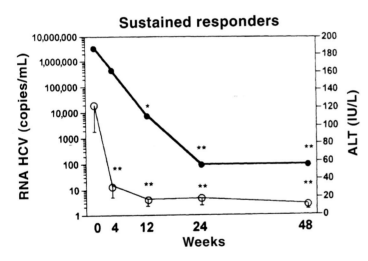

FIGURE 21.3 Time course of serum HCV-RNA during treatment with IFN-alpha2b plus ribavirin therapy, in responders. The HCV-RNA assay detection limit was somewhat less than 100 copies per mL. *Black dots* indicate HCV-RNA. *Open circles* represent serum ALT.

[62]Zeuzem S. Hepatitis C virus: kinetics and quasispecies evolution during anti-viral therapy. Forum (Genova) 2000;10:32−42.

[63]Neumann AU, Lam NP, Dahari H, et al. Hepatitis C viral dynamics in vivo and the antiviral efficacy of interferon-alpha therapy. Science 1998;282:103−7.

[64]Medeiros-Filho JE, de Carvalho Mello IM, Pinho JR, et al. Differences in viral kinetics between genotypes 1 and 3 of hepatitis C virus and between cirrhotic and non-cirrhotic patients during antiviral therapy. World J. Gastroenterol. 2006;12:7271−7.

[65]Calleja JL, Albillos A, Rossi I, et al. Time course of serum hepatitis C virus-RNA during chronic hepatitis C treatment accurately predicts the type of response. Aliment. Pharmacol. Ther. 2001;15:241−9.

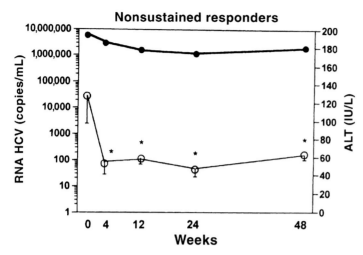

FIGURE 21.4 Time course of serum HCV-RNA during treatment with IFN-alpha2b plus ribavirin therapy, in nonresponders. The HCV-RNA assay detection limit was <100 copies per mL. *Black dots* indicate HCV-RNA. *Open circles* represent serum ALT.

VII. RESPONDERS VERSUS NONRESPONDERS

About half of people with chronic HCV fail to respond to therapy with ribavirin plus IFN-alpha. The problem of nonresponsiveness is more prevalent with African-Americans than with Caucasian-Americans. Studies addressing the mechanism of these failures have taken the following approach. Researchers have taken samples of white blood cells from responders and nonresponders undergoing treatment with the standard of care. With the white blood cells in hand, the researchers analyzed the expression of hundreds of genes, where the goal was to measure increases in expression (and decreases in expression), and where interest focused on genes associated with effective antiviral immune responses.

IFN-alpha binds to interferon receptors on the cell surface membrane, where this binding may influence the rate of transcription of about 1000 genes. The term "expression," in the context of genetic expression studies, refers to changes in the amount of messenger RNA (mRNA) as well as to changes in the amount of the relevant polypeptide. In performing this type of experiment, Taylor et al. (66) found that, in nonresponders, gene expression is subdued, relative to gene expression in responders. Expression in nonresponders was relatively low, for example, for the following four genes. These genes are known to be relevant to immune response against HCV:

- *2'5'-oligoadenylate synthetase,*
- *MX1,*
- *IRF-7,*
- *Toll-like receptor-7 (TLR7).*

TLR7 is a protein of the immune system that mediates immune activity in response to viral nucleic acids, specifically, in response to viral RNA. When a viral nucleic acid binds to TLR7 the result is a general enhancement of immune response, including responses to specific antigens, such as HCV antigens.

In another study addressing the genes responsible for nonresponse to therapy,

[66]Taylor MW, Tsukahara T, Brodsky L, et al. Changes in gene expression during pegylated interferon and ribavirin therapy of chronic hepatitis C virus distinguish responders from nonresponders to antiviral therapy. J. Virol. 2007;81:3391−401.

Golden-Mason et al. (67) discovered that one culprit is a gene called *programmed death-1 (PD-1)*. PD-1 is a protein of immune cells that, when expressed at elevated levels, impairs activity of the immune cell. In healthy people, PD-1 is typically expressed at low levels on immune cells, for example, on CD4$^+$ T cells, CD8$^+$ T cells, and NK cells. But in patients with chronic HCV who fail to respond to the standard of care, PD-1 expression is elevated. This effect is especially pronounced in African-Americans. In this situation, PD-1 is not indiscriminately elevated in all immune cells. PD-1 is specifically and dramatically elevated in CD8$^+$ T cells that are specific for HCV antigens.

To view the big picture, a goal of HCV researchers is to identify genes responsible for failure to mount an immune response to acute HCV infections, as these are the genes that permit acute HCV infections to become chronic HCV infections. It is also a goal to identify genes that prevent effective treatment with the standard of care. One reason for these goals is to develop screening programs for patients who are likely or not likely to respond to any give anti-HCV drug. Screening programs of this type are in a field of endeavor called, *personalized medicine*.

VIII. ENDPOINTS IN CLINICAL TRIALS AGAINST HCV

Endpoints used in clinical trials against hepatitis C include those that directly measure the virus, such as plasma *HCV-RNA levels* (68), *sustained virologic response* (SVR) (69), and relapse rate, endpoints that indirectly indicate liver damage, such as serum aminotransferases, endpoints that directly measure liver damage, such as histology scores, and endpoints that detect disorders that result from chronic HCV infections, such as liver fibrosis (70), hepatic decompensation, and hepatocellular carcinoma (HCC).

Guidance for assessing *liver fibrosis* with HCV infections is available (71,72). Regarding *hepatic decompensation*, once is cirrhosis is established, patients have a 3−6% annual risk of hepatic decompensation (variceal hemorrhage, ascites, encephalopathy). Following an episode of decompensation the risk of death in the following year is 15−20% (73). Regarding HCC, HCV

[67]Golden-Mason L, Klarquist J, Wahed AS, Rosen HR. Cutting edge: programmed death-1 expression is increased on immunocytes in chronic hepatitis C virus and predicts failure of response to antiviral therapy: race-dependent differences. J. Immunol. 2008;180:3637−41.

[68]Pyne MT, et al. HCV RNA measurement in samples with diverse genotypes using versions 1 and 2 of the Roche COBAS® AmpliPrep/ COBAS® TaqMan® HCV test. J. Clin. Virol. 2015;65:54v57.

[69]Smith-Palmer J, et al. Achieving sustained virologic response in hepatitis C: a systematic review of the clinical, economic and quality of life benefits. BMC Infect. Dis. 15:19. http://dx.doi.org/10.1186/s12879-015-0748-8.

[70]Hoefs JC, et al. Rate of progression of hepatic fibrosis in patients with chronic hepatitis C: results from the HALT-C Trial. Gastroenterology 2011;141:900−8.

[71]Leroy V, Sturm N, Faure P, et al. Prospective evaluation of FibroTest®, FibroMeter®, and HepaScore® for staging liver fibrosis in chronic hepatitis B: comparison with hepatitis C. J. Hepatol. 2014;61:28−34.

[72]Degos F, Perez P, Roche B, et al. Diagnostic accuracy of FibroScan and comparison to liver fibrosis biomarkers in chronic viral hepatitis: a multicenter prospective study (the FIBROSTIC study). J. Hepatol. 2010;53:1013−21.

[73]Westbrook RH, Dusheiko G. Natural history of hepatitis C. J. Hepatol. 2014;61(1 Suppl.):S5−68.

infects about 170 million people worldwide. Chronic HCV can progress to HCC, with a total of 195,000 cases worldwide (74).

This concerns mechanisms of liver damage in HCV infections and potential biomarkers. Colman et al. (75) studied genetic expression in short-term HCV infections, as determined with cultured liver cells. Smalling et al. (76) characterized genetic expression in the development and progression of chronic HCV. Ueda et al. (77) have published mRNA expression profiles of tumor lesions in patients with HCV-induced HCC. Bolen et al. (78) assessed the response of patients to chronic HCV infections by assaying gene expression in white blood cells. This type of assay is more convenient and less invasive than liver biopsies. The researchers identified a distinct gene expression for chronic HCV, where the expressed genes included those related to inflammation. The set of induced genes was validated in a second cohort of patients. While the goal is to determine "an HCV signature," issues to overcome include the notion that HCV might not be expected to influence gene expression in white blood cells, contradictory reports on whether HCV infects white blood cells, and the issue of whether HCV-induced changes in white blood cell gene expression are similar to HCV-induced changes in liver cell gene expression.

a. Endpoints of the McHutchison Study

In a study of chronic HCV, McHutchison et al. (79) treated subjects according to these three study arms:

- *Arm A*. Ribavirin plus pegylated IFN-alpha2a.
- *Arm B*. Ribavirin plus standard-dose pegylated IFN-alpha2b.
- *Arm C*. Ribavirin plus low-dose pegylated IFN-alpha2b.

The subjects were not previously treated for HCV infection, that is, they were treatment-naive. The primary endpoint was undetectable HCV-RNA levels 24 weeks after the completion of therapy. The parameter of "undetectable" was a function of the assay method, and for the assay method used, the lower limit of detection was 27 international units (IU) of HCV-RNA per mL. HCV-RNA was measured in samples of blood plasma.

Secondary endpoints included the rates of response during the treatment phase and relapse. Relapse was defined as *undetectable* HCV-RNA level at the end of the treatment phase (48 weeks), where there was a subsequent *detectable* HCV-RNA level during the follow-up period. The follow-up period was the 24-week period following the 48-week treatment period.

---

[74]Lee MH, Yang HI, Lu SN, et al. Hepatitis C virus seromarkers and subsequent risk of hepatocellular carcinoma: long-term predictors from a community-based cohort study. J. Clin. Oncol. 2010;28:4587–93.

[75]Colman H, et al. Genome-wide analysis of host mRNA translation during hepatitis C virus infection. J. Virol. 2013;87:6668–77.

[76]Smalling RL, Delker DA, Zhang Y, et al. Genome-wide transcriptome analysis identifies novel gene signatures implicated in human chronic liver disease. Am. J. Physiol. Gastrointest. Liver Physiol. 2013;305:G364–74.

[77]Ueda T, et al. Gene expression profiling of hepatitis B- and hepatitis C-related hepatocellular carcinoma using graphical Gaussian modeling. Genomics 2013:101:238–48.

[78]Bolen CR, et al. The blood transcriptional signature of chronic hepatitis C virus is consistent with an ongoing interferon-mediated antiviral response. J. Interferon Cytokine Res. 2013;33:15–23.

[79]McHutchison JG, Lawitz EJ, Shiffman ML, et al. Peginterferon alfa-2b or alfa-2a with ribavirin for treatment of hepatitis C infection. New Engl. J. Med. 2009;361:580–93.

To ensure that the characteristics of subjects in each of the three study arms were similar, subjects were stratified as follows:

- *First stratum*. Plasma levels of HCV-RNA (less than or equal to 600,000 IU/mL vs greater than 600,000 IU/mL) and
- *Second stratum*. Race (African-American vs non-African-American).

The results were as follows. The values for SVR were about the same for all three arms, that is, about 40%. In the words of the authors, "the rates of sustained virologic response were similar among the three groups."

The values for relapse rate were more favorable to the patients receiving IFN-alpha-2b (about 22% relapse rate), and less favorable for patients receiving IFN-alpha-2a (31.5% relapse rate). According to the authors, "patients treated with peginterferon-alfa-2a were more likely to have a response while receiving therapy, followed by relapse after the completion of therapy."

b. Endpoints of the Di Bisceglie Study

The clinical trial of chronic HCV by Di Bisceglie et al. (80) had two study arms, as indicated:

- *Arm A*. Pegylated IFN-alpha-2a.
- *Arm B*. Placebo (no drugs).

All of the subjects had chronic hepatitis C and advanced fibrosis. All of the subjects had been previously treated with pegylated interferon and ribavirin, but had not responded. As mentioned earlier in this chapter, it is the case

that SVR occurs in only half of patients treated with the standard of care. Subjects were stratified in order to ensure that the characteristics of subjects allocated to Arm A and Arm B were similar. Stratification was according to stage of liver fibrosis (noncirrhotic fibrosis vs cirrhotic fibrosis).

Regarding ethics, it should be noted that where potential study subjects had earlier failed to respond to treatment by the standard of care, administering placebo in a subsequent clinical trial is ethical. According to Daugherty et al. (81) and Amdur and Biddle (82), placebo controls are increasingly being used when the standard of care is ineffective.

The Di Bisceglie study addressed the possibility that long-term "maintenance" therapy with interferon might be effective in controlling the disease.

The primary endpoint was progression of liver disease. Progression of liver disease encompasses all of these events:

- death,
- hepatocellular carcinoma,
- hepatic decompensation, for example, variceal hemorrhage,
- increase in fibrosis score, as determined with liver biopsies.

The secondary endpoints were:

- serum aminotransferase,
- serum HCV-RNA,
- histologic necroinflammatory scores (determined with liver biopsies at baseline, at 1.5 years, and 3.5 years).

The study drug did not improve the primary endpoint. The response rate, as

---

[80]Di Bisceglie AM, Shiffman ML, Everson GT, et al. Prolonged therapy of advanced chronic hepatitis C with low-dose peginterferon. New Engl. J. Med. 2008;359:2429–41.

[81]Daugherty CK, Ratain MJ, Emanuel EJ, Farrell AT, Schilsky RL. Ethical, scientific, and regulatory perspectives regarding the use of placebos in cancer clinical trials. J. Clin. Oncol. 2008;26:1371–8.

[82]Amdur RJ, Biddle CJ. An algorithm for evaluating the ethics of a placebo-controlled trial. Int. J. Cancer 2001;96:261–9.

measured with the unit of percent, was 34.1% in the treatment group and 33.8% in the placebo group (HR = 1.01; $P = 0.90$).

Regarding the secondary endpoints, serum aminotransferase, serum HCV-RNA, and histologic necroinflammatory scores, all decreased significantly ($P < 0.001$) with treatment. A SVR occurred in 18 treated subjects (3.5%) but in only one placebo subject.

The authors concluded that the long-term maintenance therapy is associated with decreases in serum HCV-RNA levels, serum ALT levels, and histologic necroinflammatory scores. Unfortunately, therapy was not associated with a reduction in clinical outcomes or in the progression of fibrosis.

IX. CONCLUDING REMARKS

A variety of endpoints can be used for assessing infection severity and for determining drug efficacy. The best account of endpoints for HCV infections is in the cited studies published in *New England Journal of Medicine*, and the Clinical Study Protocols that are published with these articles and that are available on the *Journal*'s website. For HCV, these endpoints include indirect assessment of liver damage by way of serum aminotransferases (83), direct assessment of liver damage using liver biopsies, and the measurement of viral nucleic acids in the bloodstream.

[83]McPherson PA, Pincus MR. Henry's clinical diagnosis and management by laboratory methods. 22nd ed. Philadelphia, PA: Elsevier Saunders; 2011.

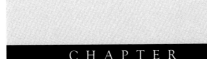

CHAPTER

22

Health-Related Quality of Life Tools—Oncology

I. INTRODUCTION

This chapter concerns health-related quality of life (HRQoL) tools in general, as well as HRQoL tools for oncology, while the next two chapters concern HRQoL tools for immune diseases and infections. The terms HRQoL tools, HRQoL instruments, and HRQoL questionnaires, all mean the same thing.

HRQoL tools are filled out by study subjects, and are used to capture information on mental state and physical functions. Alternatively, the HRQoL tool can be filled out by a healthcare worker while interviewing the patient. HRQoL tools directly capture the patient's perceived response to treatment, and may be more reliable than observer-reported measures, because they are not influenced by differences in judgment of different interviewers. On the other hand, reporting by a patient may be unreliable, for example, where the questionnaire is not easily understood or is not completed by one or more patients (1).

According to FDA's Guidance for Industry, HRQoL tools involve domains, as indicated by the following excerpt (2).

> HRQL is a **multidomain** concept that represents the patient's general perception of the effect of illness and treatment on physical, psychological, and social aspects of life. Claiming a ... meaningful improvement in HRQL implies: (1) that all HRQL domains that are important to interpreting change in how the clinical trial's population feels or functions as a result of the targeted disease and its treatment were measured; (2) that a general improvement was demonstrated; and (3) that no decrement was demonstrated in any **domain**.

This Guidance for Industry further states that each domain consists of items, for example, two items or four items, and that two or more domains are combined by way of an algorithm to generate a general concept score. The SF-36, an instrument commonly used for assessing

[1]Ralston J. Comments on: guidance for industry patient reported outcome measures: use in medical product development to support labeling claims. Northbrook, IL: ClinPhone, Inc.; 2006. 8 pp.

[2]U.S. Department of Health and Human Services. Food and Drug Administration. Guidance for industry. Patient-reported outcome measures: use in medical product development to support labeling claims; 2009 (43 pp.).

HRQoL in cancer (3), multiple sclerosis (4), hepatitis C virus infections (5), and other diseases, provides examples of items and domains.

SF-36 questions fall into eight domains: physical function, physical role limitations, vitality, general health perceptions, pain, social function, emotional role limitations, and mental health. The domain of physical function has 10 items (10 questions), that capture, for example, ability to carry groceries, walk, climb stairs, and dressing. The domain of pain has two items, which are concerned with the amount of pain experienced in the previous 4 weeks, and the extent to which pain interferes with normal work activities. The domain of mental health has five items, which concern anxiety and depression. The domain scores are then used to calculate summary scores. The SF-36 tool has two summary scores, physical summary score and mental summary score. In a description that ties together items, domains, and scores, Schroeder et al. (6), stated that, "HRQOL was assessed with the SF-36 ... [t]his self-administered ... [instrument] consists of 36 items and assesses eight dimensions [domains] (physical functioning, role limitations due to physical health, bodily pain, general health perception, vitality, social function, role limitations due to emotional health, and mental health), which are aggregated to product physical and mental summary ... scores."

According to Patrick et al. (7), improvement in HRQoL is a highly sought-after claim by pharmaceutical companies, though regulatory bodies may not readily accept HRQoL data as a component for regulatory approval (8). Another term, quality of life (QOL), is sometimes used interchangeably with HRQoL, but they are not exactly the same thing. QOL encompasses more things than HRQoL. According to Patrick et al. (9), "QOL is affected not only by health status but also by ... safe environment, adequate housing, guaranteed income and freedom."

When used for clinical trials, it has been recommended that HRQoL tools be administered on at least three occasions, that is, before

[3]Schroeder PR, Haugen BR, Pacini F, et al. A comparison of short-term changes in health-related quality of life in thyroid carcinoma patients undergoing diagnostic evaluation with recombinant human thyrotropin compared with thyroid hormone withdrawal. J. Clin. Endocrinol. Metabl. 2006;91:878–84.

[4]Pittock SJ, et al. Quality of life is favorable for most patients with multiple sclerosis. Arch. Neurol. 2004;61:679–86.

[5]Bernstein D, et al. Relationship of health-related quality of life to treatment adherence and sustained response in chronic hepatitis C patients. Hepatology 2002;35:704–8.

[6]Schroeder PR, Haugen BR, Pacini F, et al. A comparison of short-term changes in health-related quality of life in thyroid carcinoma patients undergoing diagnostic evaluation with recombinant human thyrotropin compared with thyroid hormone withdrawal. J. Clin. Endocrinol. Metabl. 2006;91:878–84.

[7]Patrick DL, Burke LB, Powers JH, et al. Patient-reported outcomes to support medical product labeling claims: FDA perspective. Value Health 2007;10(Suppl. 2):S125–37.

[8]Bottomley A, Jones D, Claassens L. Patient-reported outcomes: assessment and current perspectives of the guidelines of the Food and Drug Administration and the reflection paper of the European Medicines Agency. Eur. J. Cancer 2009;45:347–53.

[9]Patrick DL, Burke LB, Powers JH, et al. Patient-reported outcomes to support medical product labeling claims: FDA perspective. Value Health 2007;10(Suppl. 2):S125–37.

treatment begins, and on two different occasions during treatment (10). Regarding baseline HRQoL data, "[b]aseline QOL information is highly prognostic in advanced disease (of many sorts), and several have called for such assessment at baseline to stratify or determine eligibility, but it has never taken hold" (11).

Data on HRQoL are typically collected at baseline and during the course of the trial, for arriving at conclusions relating to safety and efficacy of the study drug. Baseline data on HRQoL can be used in the stratification of study subjects, or merely for collecting data on subgroups.

Poor compliance by the study subjects, that is, failure or inability of study subjects to fill out the questionnaires, may be a problem. Michael and Tannock (12) and Olschewski et al. (13) discuss various issues relating to compliance in filling out HRQoL questionnaires.

One desirable characteristic of HRQoL questionnaires is that they are drafted to be at the reading level of a 10-year-old (14). In this respect, HRQoL questionnaires are somewhat similar to consent forms used in clinical trials. The need to keep the reading level of consent forms at the level of a 10−12-year-old child is well established (15,16,17,18,19).

II. SUMMARY

When HRQoL tools are used in clinical trials, the following is desired:

- HRQoL questionnaires should be administered at baseline, as well as during the treatment phase of the trial.
- The HRQoL instrument should be validated before use in the trial.
- During the clinical trial, the investigator should make efforts to ensure high compliance with filling out the HRQoL questionnaires. It is preferred that the rates

[10]Kopec JA, Yothers G, Ganz PA, et al. Quality of life in operable colon cancer patients receiving oral compared with intravenous chemotherapy: results from National Surgical Adjuvant Breast and Bowel Project Trial C-06. J. Clin. Oncol. 2007;25:424−30.

[11]Cella D. E-mail of September 8, 2010.

[12]Michael M, Tannock IF. Measuring health-related quality of life in clinical trials that evaluate the role of chemotherapy in cancer treatment. Can. Med. Assoc. J. 1998;158:1727−34.

[13]Olschewski M, Schulgen G, Schumacher M, Altman DG. Quality of life assessment in clinical cancer research. Br. J. Cancer 1994;70:1−5.

[14]Webster K, Cella D, Yost K. The Functional Assessment of Chronic Illness Therapy (FACIT) Measurement System: properties, applications, and interpretation. Health Qual. Life Outcomes 2003;1:79.

[15]Coyne CA, Xu R, Raich P, et al. Randomized, controlled trial of an easy-to-read informed consent statement for clinical trial participation: a study of the Eastern Cooperative Oncology Group. J. Clin. Oncol. 2003;21:836−42.

[16]Sudore RL, Landefeld CS, Williams BA, Barnes DE, Lindquist K, Schillinger D. Use of a modified informed consent process among vulnerable patients: a descriptive study. J. Gen. Intern. Med. 2006;21:867−73.

[17]Sudore RL, Landefeld CS, Barnes DE, et al. An advance directive redesigned to meet the literacy level of most adults: a randomized trial. Patient Educ. Couns. 2007;69:165−95.

[18]Flory J, Emanuel E. Interventions to improve research participants' understanding in informed consent for research: a systematic review. J. Am. Med. Assoc. 2004;292:1593−601.

[19]Davis TC, Holcombe RF, Berkel HJ, Pramanik S, Divers SG. Informed consent for clinical trials: a comparative study of standard versus simplified forms. J. Natl Cancer Inst. 1998;90:668−74.

of compliance be equivalent in both study arms (20).

- When randomizing subjects into two study arms, it is desired that the average HRQoL scores for both study arms be roughly the same. The investigator should decide whether results from HRQoL tools, taken at baseline, are to be used in stratifying study subjects. This decision necessarily must occur prior to administering the study drug or control treatment.
- HRQoL questionnaires should be written at a reasonably low reading level.

III. HRQoL TOOLS TAKE ON INCREASED IMPORTANCE WHEN CAPTURING DATA ON ADVERSE EVENTS, OR IN TRIALS ON PALLIATIVE TREATMENTS

The European Organisation for Research and Treatment of Cancer (EORTC), an oncology organization, provides the following advice on HRQoL tools (21). Typically, HRQoL measurements are not taken in phase I and phase II trials, because the primary aim of these studies is to determine safety and efficacy, and because patient numbers are usually small. HRQoL measurements take on greater importance, in the context of clinical trials that compare two different palliative treatments, and in clinical trials where the study drug and an active control drug are not expected to differ in terms of efficacy. HRQoL tools also take on increased relevance in clinical trials where toxicity in one of the study arms is a major issue, for example, when comparing high-dose chemotherapy versus low-dose chemotherapy.

HRQoL tools are used in two types of clinical trials, *disease treatment trials* and *symptom management trials*. Joly et al. (22) found that in disease treatment trials, HRQoL results are typically used as a secondary endpoint, but rarely as a primary endpoint. In symptom management trials, HRQoL results are usually used as a secondary endpoint, and are sometimes used as a primary endpoint. Hauser and Walsh (23) describe various categories of HRQoL scales.

The importance of HRQoL endpoints can increase where the study drug does not much influence endpoints involving survival. In other words, if the study drug and the active control drug show no significant difference in terms of halting tumor growth, in reducing the rate of metastasis, or in enhancing survival, data from HRQoL tools can be a deciding factor in gaining regulatory approval for the study drug.

[20]Bottomley A, Biganzoli L, Cufer T, et al. Randomized, controlled trial investigating short-term health-related quality of life with doxorubicin and paclitaxel versus doxorubicin and cyclophosphamide as first-line chemotherapy in patients with metastatic breast cancer: European Organization for Research and Treatment of Cancer Breast Cancer Group, Investigational Drug Branch for Breast Cancer and the New Drug Development Group Study. J. Clin. Oncol. 2004;22:2576–86.

[21]EORTC Quality of Life Group. Guidelines for assessing quality of life in EORTC clinical trials. Brussels: EORTC; 2002 (32 pp.).

[22]Joly F, Vardy J, Pintilie M, Tannock IF. Quality of life and/or symptom control in randomized clinical trials for patients with advanced cancer. Ann. Oncol. 2007;18:1935–42.

[23]Hauser K, Walsh D. Visual analogue scales and assessment of quality of life in cancer. J. Support Oncol. 2008;6:277–82.

Di Maio and Perrone (24), as well as Frost and Sloan (25), find that HRQoL data are particularly helpful when two treatments result in similar survival outcomes but exhibit differences in QOL outcomes. In other words, where the clinical efficacy of two drugs is found to be equivalent, there is little question that a prospective patient would like to know whether one of the two drugs is more associated with favorable outcomes that are measured by the parameters of depression, anxiety, self-esteem, or hopefulness.

IV. SCHEDULING THE ADMINISTRATION OF HRQoL TOOLS

HRQoL tools can be administered a set number of days or weeks after randomization (independently of treatment schedules), or they can be administered to coincide with treatment cycles (26). In chemotherapy involving several courses of treatment (rounds of treatment), assessments are usually scheduled to take place immediately before the next course of treatment. Coupling the time of the HRQoL with treatment time, rather than a set calendar time, is useful. If the HRQoL tool is required to be administered shortly before each round of chemotherapy, the investigator can be assured that the HRQoL tool will only capture data relating to chronic conditions of the patient, but if the HRQoL tool is tied to specific calendar dates, and where dates of chemotherapy for some patients need to be rescheduled, the result is that the HRQoL tool

will capture chronic characteristics for some patients, and acute characteristics of other patients. In other words, if the investigator prefers that HRQoL data be acquired shortly prior to a round of chemotherapy, but where chemotherapy for a given patient needs to be rescheduled a few days earlier, a calendar-based HRQoL tool will inadvertently capture the acute effects of the chemotherapy.

Consider this hypothetical involving study drug and active control drug, where the study drug has the property of provoking immediate toxicity, and the control drug has the property of delayed (but severe) toxicity. Adverse events that influence the patient's quality of life materialize shortly after administering the study drug, but in the case of the control drug, have a delayed effect (27). Hence, in this hypothetical, administering the HRQoL tool shortly after chemotherapy will show poor outcome for the study drug, but will show favorable outcome for the active control drug. This favorable outcome for the control drug is an artifact, and can result in false conclusions in the study.

V. HRQoL TOOLS IN ONCOLOGY

a. Introduction

This provides examples of HRQoL tools from clinical trials on colorectal cancer, melanoma, non-small-cell lung cancer (NSCLC), and breast cancer. The lessons from these trials may be applicable to HRQoL tools for drugs used for treating a variety of other diseases,

[24]Di Maio M, Perrone F. Quality of life in elderly patients with cancer. Health Qual. Life Outcomes 2003;1:44.

[25]Frost MH, Sloan JA. Quality of life measurements: a soft outcome-or is it? Am. J. Manag. Care 2002;8:S574−9.

[26]EORTC Quality of Life Group. Guidelines for assessing quality of life in EORTC clinical trials. Brussels: EORTC; 2002 (32 pp.).

[27]EORTC Quality of Life Group. Guidelines for assessing quality of life in EORTC clinical trials. Brussels: EORTC; 2002 (32 pp.).

including other cancers, chronic immune disorders, and chronic infections.

Data from HRQoL tools are often used as endpoints in oncology clinical trials. Buchanan et al. (28) identified about 20 different instruments for measuring HRQoL for cancer patients enrolled in clinical trials. Wilson et al. (29) compared the discriminatory abilities, and the degrees of overlap in questions, of these questionnaires. HRQoL tools for various chronic disorders, including cancer, include:

- *SF-36®* [RAND 36-Item Health Survey (SF-36)];
- *EORTC* (European Organisation for Research and Treatment of Cancer Quality of Life Questionnaire);
- *FACT* (Functional Assessment of Cancer Treatment);
- *FLIC* (Functional Living Index: Cancer), also known as the Manitoba Functional Living Cancer Questionnaire;
- *GWB* (Rand General Well-Being Scale);
- *SQLI* (Spitzer Quality of Life Index); and
- *V-RQOL* (Voice-Related Quality of Life), for use in clinical trials on laryngeal cancer (30).

The EORTC provides over 15 questionnaires or *modules*. The core module is the QLQ-C30 Core questionnaire. Specialty modules are also available, but when these are administered, the core module must also be used. The specialty modules include: Lung, Breast, Head and Neck, Ovarian, Esophageal, Gastric, Cervix, Multiple Myeloma, Oesophago-Gastric, Prostate, Colorectal Liver Metastases, Colorectal, and Brain Modules.

FACIT.org (31) provides a large number of questionnaires on chronic diseases, including cancer in general (FACT-G), specific types of cancer, such as FACT-B for breast cancer, FACT-Br for brain cancer, and FACT-C for colorectal cancer, as well as for multiple sclerosis, and human immunodeficiency virus. FACIT means, Functional Assessment of Chronic Illness Therapy. The FACIT.org website provides literature references that document the use and validation of some of these questionnaires. FACIT questionnaires can be administered by self-report or interview (face-to-face or telephone) (32).

b. Symptoms and Functioning

Within the endpoint of HRQoL, one finds the two groups, namely, symptoms and functioning.

1. Symptoms

Buchanan et al. (33) defined symptoms as subjective evidence of disease and how the

---

[28]Buchanan DR, O'Mara AM, Kelaghan JW, Minasian LM. Quality-of-life assessment in the symptom management trials of the National Cancer Institute-supported Community Clinical Oncology Program. J. Clin. Oncol. 2005;23:591–8.

[29]Wilson RW, Hutson LM, Vanstry D. Comparison of 2 quality-of-life questionnaires in women treated for breast cancer: the RAND 36-Item Health Survey and the Functional Living Index-Cancer. Phys. Ther. 2005;85:851–60.

[30]Fung K, Lyden TH, Lee J, et al. Voice and swallowing outcomes of an organ-preservation trial for advanced laryngeal cancer. Int. J. Radiat. Oncol. Biol. Phys. 2005;63:1395–9.

[31]FACT.org, 381 South Cottage Hill Ave., Elmhurst, IL.

[32]Webster K, Cella D, Yost K. The Functional Assessment of Chronic Illness Therapy (FACIT) Measurement system: properties, applications, and interpretation. Health Qual. Life Outcomes 2003;1:79.

[33]Buchanan DR, O'Mara AM, Kelaghan JW, Sgambati M, McCaskill-Stevens W, Minasian L. Challenges and recommendations for advancing the state-of-the-science of quality of life assessment in symptom management trials. Cancer 2007;110:1621–8.

patient feels, for example, pain, fatigue, nausea, or depression. Symptoms can be classed as physical or mental. Symptoms are not the same thing as signs. Signs, such as temperature, blood pressure, or tumor size and number, are objective. Hofman et al. (34) report that fatigue is one of the most common symptoms of cancer, that it can result from the cancer, where it may occur in nearly half of patients at the time of diagnosis, and that it can result from the anticancer therapy. Moreover, these authors reported that fatigue can have downstream consequences on emotional symptoms, for example, a loss of emotional control, feelings of isolation and solitude, and feelings of dejection. According to Ryan et al. (35), cancer-related fatigue is frequently reported as the most distressing symptom associated with cancer and its treatment, even more so than pain, nausea, or vomiting.

2. Functioning

Functioning refers to the patient's ability to perform various actions, such as the ability to climb stairs. Symptoms, such as severe pain, can prevent functions, such as the ability to climb stairs. Also, functional impairments, such as inability to climb stairs or to dress oneself, can have increase symptoms, such as depression. Hofman et al. (36) report that fatigue can have the downstream consequences of impaired ability on functions, for example, cooking, housecleaning, and carrying things.

c. Formats for Disclosing HRQoL Results

Results from HRQoL tools can be disclosed by way of text, table, or histogram. In a study of NSCLC, Ramlau et al. (37) administered the Lung Cancer Symptom Scale (LCSS) questionnaire, a HRQoL tool covering nine parameters. These authors disclosed the results in the form of a forest plot, a type of histogram that more clearly displays information than with a typical histogram. Typically, forest plots include the confidence interval. The clinical trial contained two arms (Arm A: toptecan; Arm B: docetaxel). What is shown below is not the forest plot, but a more simple table. The confidence intervals do not appear in this table. The HRQoL results (Table 22.1) show changes in each parameter over a 3-month interval. During the course of treatment, HRQoL scores for each parameter declined, in the case of both drugs. The decline, over a period of 3 months, for every single parameter was more severe with topotecan. The most dramatic difference, when comparing the two study arms, was in the parameter of appetite. In an analysis of the LCSS quality-of-life questionnaire, Hollen et al. (38), found that optimal data could be acquired by administering the questionnaire at intervals of once every 3 weeks, while the data were less reliable when administered every 4 weeks.

[34]Hofman M, Ryan JL, Figueroa-Moseley CD, Jean-Pierre P, Morrow GR. Cancer-related fatigue: the scale of the problem. Oncologist 2007;12(Suppl. 1):4−10.

[35]Ryan JL, Carroll JK, Ryan EP, Mustian KM, Fiscella K, Morrow GR. Mechanisms of cancer-related fatigue. Oncologist 2007;12(Suppl. 1):22−34.

[36]Hofman M, Ryan JL, Figueroa-Moseley CD, Jean-Pierre P, Morrow GR. Cancer-related fatigue: the scale of the problem. Oncologist 2007;12(Suppl. 1):4−10.

[37]Ramlau R, Gervais R, Krzakowski M, et al. Phase III study comparing oral topotecan to intravenous docetaxel in patients with pretreated advanced non-small-cell lung cancer. J. Clin. Oncol. 2006;24:2800−7.

[38]Hollen PJ, Gralla RJ, Rittenberg CN. Quality of life as a clinical trial endpoint: determining the appropriate interval for repeated assessments in patients with advanced lung cancer. Support Care Cancer 2004;12:767−73.

TABLE 22.1 HRQoL Changes Using the Lung Cancer Symptom Scale (LCSS)

	Parameter	Change Over 3 Months	
		Topotecan	Docetaxel
1	Appetite	− 12.6	− 3.13
2	Fatigue	− 9.26	− 7.23
3	Coughing	− 4.53	− 1.07
4	Shortness of breath	− 13.6	− 7.89
5	Blood in sputum	− 1.68	− 1.13
6	Pain	− 6.25	− 4.23
7	Symptoms from lung cancer	− 9.84	− 4.26
8	Normal activities	− 8.99	− 5.88
9	Global quality of life	− 13.2	− 8.45

d. Colorectal Cancer

HRQoL data from a representative number of clinical trials on colorectal cancer are shown in Table 22.2 (39). On occasion, clinical trials may administer HRQoL tools during the course of the trial, but fail to acquire baseline HRQoL information. Moreover, on occasion, publications on clinical trials may disclose that HRQoL data were captured, but may fail to identify the HRQoL instrument that was used (40).

Let us first review results from the clinical trials of two groups of investigators, the Sobrero group and the Giacchetti group. Sobrero et al. (41) provide an unusually thorough analysis of the various parameters detected by the HRQoL tool. Moreover, these authors clearly articulated how HRQoL results can be used, in conjunction with survival results. The authors found that the HRQoL results supported the survival benefit. Physical, emotional, cognitive functioning, and global health status were significantly better with cetuximab and irinotecan.

Now, let us turn to the Giacchetti study. In the methods section of the publication, Giacchetti et al. (42) state that, "[s]econdary end points were PFS, objective response rate, safety, and quality of life." However, the tool used for assessing QoL, the times of administration of the questionnaire, and HRQoL data, are not revealed.

On the other hand, 2 years after this publication, the HRQoL data from this same study were revealed in a separate paper. The separate paper was by Efficace et al. (43). HRQoL was determined using EORTC QLQ-C30, but

[39]The author used the search tool of Journal of Clinical Oncology to search for the previous 10 years (2000 to 2011), using the search terms "HRQOL" or "quality of life." The author conducted the same search with New England Journal of Medicine. Most of the articles acquired from this search are reported in this table.

[40]Hurwitz H, Fehrenbacher L, Novotny W, et al. Bevacizumab plus irinotecan, fluorouracil, and leucovorin for metastatic colorectal cancer. New Engl. J. Med. 2004;350:2335−42.

[41]Sobrero AF, Maurel J, Fehrenbacher L, et al. EPIC: phase III trial of cetuximab plus irinotecan after fluoropyrimidine and oxaliplatin failure in patients with metastatic colorectal cancer. J. Clin. Oncol. 2008;26:2311−9.

[42]Giacchetti S, Bjarnason G, Garufi C, et al. Phase III trial comparing 4-day chronomodulated therapy versus 2-day conventional delivery of fluorouracil, leucovorin, and oxaliplatin as first-line chemotherapy of metastatic colorectal cancer: the European Organisation for Research and Treatment of Cancer Chronotherapy Group. J. Clin. Oncol. 2006;24:3562−9.

[43]Efficace F, Innominato PF, Bjarnason G, et al. Validation of patient's self-reported social functioning as an independent prognostic factor for survival in metastatic colorectal cancer patients: results of an international study by the Chronotherapy Group of the European Organisation for Research and Treatment of Cancer. J. Clin. Oncol. 2008;26:2020−6.

TABLE 22.2 HRQoL in Clinical Studies of Colorectal Cancer

Colorectal Cancer	Instrument	Was HRQoL Captured at Baseline?	HRQoL Used as Endpoint
Au et al.[a]	EORTC QLQ-30	Yes	Taken at 4, 8, 16, 24 weeks
Falcone et al.[b]	EORTC QLQ-30	Yes	Taken at beginning of each cycle
Giacchetti et al.[c] and Efficace et al.[d]	EORTC QLQ-30	Yes	No. HRQoL was determined only at baseline
	The study reported that secondary endpoints were progression-free survival, the response rate, the duration of the response, safety, and the quality of life, however the paper failed to provide any information on the HRQoL instrument, or on the HRQoL results		
Jayne et al.[e]	EORTC QLC-30 and QLQ-CR38	Yes	2 weeks, 3, 6, 18, and 36 months. No significant correlation between clinical endpoints and HRQoL
Jonker et al.[f]	EORTC QLC-30	Yes	Taken at 4, 8, 16, and 24 weeks
	Conclusion: As compared with supportive care alone, cetuximab (study drug) treatment was associated with less deterioration in physical function at 8 weeks ($P < 0.05$) and 16 weeks ($P = 0.03$). Further information on HRQoL data from the same study is found in Karapetis et al.[g]		
Kemeny et al.[h]	Four instruments: Rand 36-Item Health Status Profile; the Memorial Symptom Assessment Scale; the Medical Outcomes Study Social Support Questionnaire; and the Medical Outcomes Study Sexual Functioning Scale	Yes	HRQoL data captured every 3 months
	Conclusion: HRQoL analysis showed a correlation between study drug and physical functioning, but not in social functioning, role functioning-emotional, or general health perceptions		
Kozuch et al.[i]	Two instruments: EORTC QLC-30 and CRC-specific Quality of Life Questionnaire module	Not stated	The authors found there was insufficient data to draw a conclusion
Saltz et al.[j]	EORTC QLC-30	Yes	Every 4 weeks
	Conclusion: The triple-drug group had a smaller decrease in function than the two-drug group ($P < 0.05$)		
Sobrero et al.[k]	EORTC QLC-30	Yes	At 3 weeks, then every 6 weeks
	Conclusion: The study drug group was significantly more effective in maintaining HRQoL. Advantages were seen with fatigue ($P = 0.005$), nausea or vomiting ($P < 0.001$), insomnia ($P = 0.04$), pain ($P < 0.001$), diarrhea ($P = 0.02$), global health status ($P = 0.047$), physical functioning ($P = 0.002$), role functioning ($P = 0.003$), emotional functioning ($P = 0.002$), and cognitive functioning ($P < 0.001$), and no differences were seen in the social functioning ($P = 0.774$)		

(Continued)

TABLE 22.2 (Continued)

Colorectal Cancer	Instrument	Was HRQoL Captured at Baseline?	HRQoL Used as Endpoint
Tol et al.[l]	EORTC QLC-30	Yes	Every 9 weeks
	Conclusion: Overall quality of life and global health status were similar in the two groups at baseline while after treatment both measures improved significantly more in the CB group (two drugs) (P = 0.007) than in the CBC group (three drugs) (P = 0.03)		
Twelves et al.[m]	EORTC QLC-30, used as primary endpoint	Yes	At about 8, 16, and 25 weeks
	Conclusion: At week 25 of treatment, scores for global health status in the two groups showed similar small increases from baseline (<5% in raw scores), indicating improvement in the quality of life		

[a] Au HJ, Karapetis CS, O'Callaghan CJ, et al. Health-related quality of life in patients with advanced colorectal cancer treated with cetuximab: overall and KRAS-specific results of the NCIC CTG and AGITG CO.17 Trial. J. Clin. Oncol. 2009;27:1822–8.

[b] Falcone A, Ricci S, Brunetti I, et al. Phase III trial of infusional fluorouracil, leucovorin, oxaliplatin, and irinotecan (FOLFOXIRI) compared with infusional fluorouracil, leucovorin, and irinotecan (FOLFIRI) as first-line treatment for metastatic colorectal cancer: the Gruppo Oncologico Nord Ovest. J. Clin. Oncol. 2007;25:1670–6.

[c] Giacchetti S, Bjarnason G, Garufi C, et al. Phase III trial comparing 4-day chronomodulated therapy versus 2-day conventional delivery of fluorouracil, leucovorin, and oxaliplatin as first-line chemotherapy of metastatic colorectal cancer: the European Organisation for Research and Treatment of Cancer Chronotherapy Group. J. Clin. Oncol. 2006;24:3562–9.

[d] Efficace F, Innominato PF, Bjarnason G, et al. Validation of patient's self-reported social functioning as an independent prognostic factor for survival in metastatic colorectal cancer patients: results of an international study by the Chronotherapy Group of the European Organisation for Research and Treatment of Cancer. J. Clin. Oncol. 2008;26:2020–6.

[e] Jayne DG, Guillou PJ, Thorpe H, et al. Randomized trial of laparoscopic-assisted resection of colorectal carcinoma: 3-year results of the UK MRC CLASICC Trial Group. J. Clin. Oncol. 2007;25:3061–8.

[f] Jonker DJ, O'Callaghan CJ, Karapetis CS, et al. Cetuximab for the treatment of colorectal cancer. New Engl. J. Med. 2007;357:2040–8.

[g] Karapetis CS, Khambata-Ford S, Jonker DJ, et al. K-ras mutations and benefit from cetuximab in advanced colorectal cancer. New Engl. J. Med. 2008;359:1757–65.

[h] Kemeny NE, Niedzwiecki D, Hollis DR, et al. Hepatic arterial infusion versus systemic therapy for hepatic metastases from colorectal cancer: a randomized trial of efficacy, quality of life, and molecular markers (CALGB 9481). J. Clin. Oncol. 2006;24:1395–403.

[i] Kozuch PS, Rocha-Lima CM, Dragovich T, et al. Bortezomib with or without irinotecan in relapsed or refractory colorectal cancer: results from a randomized phase II study. J. Clin. Oncol. 2008;26:2320–6.

[j] Saltz LB, Cox JV, Blanke C, et al. Irinotecan plus fluorouracil and leucovorin for metastatic colorectal cancer. Irinotecan Study Group. New Engl. J. Med. 2000;343:905–14.

[k] Sobrero AF, Maurel J, Fehrenbacher L, et al. EPIC: phase III trial of cetuximab plus irinotecan after fluoropyrimidine and oxaliplatin failure in patients with metastatic colorectal cancer. J. Clin. Oncol. 2008;26:2311–9.

[l] Tol J, Koopman M, Cats A, et al. Chemotherapy, bevacizumab, and cetuximab in metastatic colorectal cancer. New Engl. J. Med. 2009;360:563–72.

[m] Twelves C, Wong A, Nowacki MP, et al. Capecitabine as adjuvant treatment for stage III colon cancer. New Engl. J. Med. 2005;352:2696–704.

only at baseline. The results demonstrated a 2-year survival rate of 22% for patients scoring in the lower third of the social functioning scale, and 2-year survivals rates of 42–43% for patients scoring in the middle third and upper third of the social functioning scale.

e. Melanoma

HRQoL results from melanoma clinical trials are shown in Table 22.3. Let us dwell briefly on the Bottomley study. Bottomley et al. (44) included interferon-alpha in one of the study arms. Interferon-alpha resulted in deterioration in HRQoL, where the deterioration was so great, that it rendered inconsequential any benefit found in the study arm that had included the interferon-alpha.

In comments on this particular study, Janku and Kurzrock (45) remarked that the Bottomley group "are to be congratulated" for their study of HRQoL in melanoma, and that this study showed "remarkable deterioration" in global HLRQoL using the EORTC Quality-of-Life Questionnaire C30. In other words, the benefit of the Bottomley study is that it provided clear-cut and decisive evidence that interferon-alpha should not be used.

Another interesting nuance regarding the collection of HRQoL data, is the paper of Mohr et al. (46), complaining about the fact that one particular clinical trial on melanoma failed to report on HRQoL.

f. Non-small-Cell Lung Cancer

This concerns the Shepherd clinical trial, the Bezjak clinical trial, and the Bonomi clinical trial, as outlined below.

1. The Shepard Study

Shepherd et al. (47) provided a detailed account of HRQoL results, as shown in Table 22.4. HRQoL were separated into data regarding pain, dyspnea, cough, fatigue, and emotional.

The authors included a discussion of the HRQoL results, along with the survival results, finding that, "[m]ore patients in the erlotinib group than in the placebo group had reductions in dyspnea, pain, and cough ... [t]he analysis of the quality of life showed that symptom improvement was also associated with significantly improved physical function."

In addition to the detailed account of several categories of the HRQoL tool, what is unique about the Shepherd study is that it expressly stated that, for study centers in non-English-speaking countries, only validated HRQoL tools were used. The validation of HRQoL tools is an on-going concern, including the need to validate HRQoL tools that are in various languages,

[44]Bottomley A, Coens C, Suciu S, et al. Adjuvant therapy with pegylated interferon alfa-2b versus observation in resected stage III melanoma: a phase III randomized controlled trial of health-related quality of life and symptoms by the European Organisation for Research and Treatment of Cancer Melanoma Group. Clin. Oncol. 2009;27:2916–23.

[45]Janku F, Kurzrock R. Adjuvant interferon in high-risk melanoma: end of the era? J. Clin. Oncol. 2010;28:e15–6.

[46]Mohr P, Hauschild A, Trefzer U, Weichenthal M. Quality of life in patients receiving high-dose interferon alfa-2b after resected high-risk melanoma. J. Clin. Oncol. 2009;27:e70.

[47]Shepherd FA, Rodrigues Pereira J, Ciuleanu T, et al. Erlotinib in previously treated non-small-cell lung cancer. New Engl. J. Med. 2005;353:123–312.

TABLE 22.3 Health-Related Quality of Life in Clinical Studies of Melanoma

Melanoma	Instrument	HRQoL at Baseline	HRQoL Used as Endpoint
Avril et al.[a]	EORTC QLQ-C30	Yes	At end of the induction (neoadjuvant) cycle, at each maintenance cycle, then at the end of the study in the fotemustine arm and at each cycle and end of study in the dacarbazine (DTIC) arm
			Conclusion: No significant differences in HRQoL were found between treatment groups
Bottomley et al.[b]	EORTC QLQ-C30	Yes	Months 3, 12, 24, 36, 48, and 60
			Conclusion: Patients receiving study drug (interferon) had a significant lowering of global HRQoL levels as compared with patients in the observation arm (P less or equal to 0.0004), at all the points following chemotherapy. In other words, HRQoL was worse in the study drug arm. Social functioning, fatigue, and appetite loss were key factors that could account for the lower HRQOL
Hillner et al.[c]	EORTC QLQ-C30	Yes	Yes, but times of data collection were not disclosed
			Conclusion: Although available data showed that TEM (study drug) patients compared with DTIC (active control) patients were more likely to maintain or improve their quality-of-life score at 12 and 24 weeks, the number of patients responding was small, and this was not a primary endpoint. Therefore, a quality-adjusted survival analysis was not performed
Kaufmann et al.[d]	None		The authors expressly stated that HRQoL data were not collected
Middleton et al.[e]	EORTC QLQ-C30	Yes	HRQoL questionnaire was administered on day 1 of cycle 1 and after completion of each subsequent treatment cycle
			Conclusion: Improvement in HRQoL scores from baseline to 12 weeks indicated a significant advantage in the physical and cognitive functioning domains for the temozolomide-treated (study drug) group compared with the DTIC-treated (active control) group. Both arms showed similar results in terms of the endpoint of survival. Thus, the superior results, for temozolomide, in terms of HRQoL, served as a basis for recommending this drug over DTIC
Pectasides et al.[f]	None	None	None
			Conclusion: Although Pectasides et al. stated that their goals included improving patient quality of life, the study did not include any HRQoL instrument. In a letter to the editor, Mohr et al.[g] complained that the study of Pectasides et al. had failed to disclose information on HRQoL. In particular, Mohr et al. were disappointed to see that information on fatigue was not presented
Richtig et al.[h]	Visual analog scale	Yes	6 months and 2 years
			Conclusion: There were only marginal differences in HRQoL between treatment groups

[a]Avril MF, Aamdal S, Grob JJ, et al. Fotemustine compared with dacarbazine in patients with disseminated malignant melanoma: a phase III study. J. Clin. Oncol. 2004;22:1118–25.

[b]Bottomley A, Coens C, Suciu S, et al. Adjuvant therapy with pegylated interferon alfa-2b versus observation in resected stage III melanoma: a phase III randomized controlled trial of health-related quality of life and symptoms by the European Organisation for Research and Treatment of Cancer Melanoma Group. J. Clin. Oncol. 2009;27:2916–23.

[c]Hillner BE, Agarwala S, Middleton MR. Post hoc economic analysis of temozolomide versus dacarbazine in the treatment of advanced metastatic melanoma. J. Clin. Oncol. 2000;18:1474–80.

[d]Kaufmann R, Spieth K, Leiter U, et al. Temozolomide in combination with interferon-alfa versus temozolomide alone in patients with advanced metastatic melanoma: a randomized, phase III, multicenter study from the Dermatologic Cooperative Oncology Group. J. Clin. Oncol. 2005;23:9001–7.

[e]Middleton MR, Grob JJ, Aaronson N, et al. Randomized phase III study of temozolomide versus dacarbazine in the treatment of patients with advanced metastatic malignant melanoma. J. Clin. Oncol. 2000;18:158–66.

[f]Pectasides D, Dafni U, Bafaloukos D, et al. Randomized phase III study of 1 month versus 1 year of adjuvant high-dose interferon alfa-2b in patients with resected high-risk melanoma. J. Clin. Oncol. 2009;27:939–44.

[g]Mohr P, Hauschild A, Trefzer U, Weichenthal M. Quality of life in patients receiving high-dose interferon alfa-2b after resected high-risk melanoma. J. Clin. Oncol. 2009;27:e70.

[h]Richtig E, Soyer HP, Posch M, et al. Prospective, randomized, multicenter, double-blind placebo-controlled trial comparing adjuvant interferon alfa and isotretinoin with interferon alfa alone in stage IIA and IIB melanoma: European Cooperative Adjuvant Melanoma Treatment Study Group. J. Clin. Oncol. 2005;23:8655–63.

TABLE 22.4 HRQoL Results From the Shepherd Study

	Erlotinib (Study Drug)			Placebo			P Value (Significance of Difference Between Study Drug and Placebo)
	Improved	Stable	Worsen	Improve	Stable	Worsen	
Pain	42	15	43	28	20	51	0.01
Dyspnea	34	27	40	23	33	44	0.03
Cough	44	24	32	27	31	41	0.00
Fatigue	45	4	51	36	8	55	0.06
Emotional	39	24	37	30	36	35	0.01

for example, Portuguese (48), Chinese (49), German (50), and Italian (51).

2. The Bezjak Study

Bezjak et al. (52) reported one particularly useful aspect of HRQoL, namely, that the adverse influence of study drug on HRQoL was only temporary. Hence, this result might influence the decisions of the physicians and patients to request this chemotherapy. In the author's words, "[f]unctional impairment is not unusual for individuals who are taking chemotherapy ... however, by 9 months, when most of the acute adverse effects of chemotherapy have resolved, there is a return to normal function. The only persistent symptom scale score differences, specifically peripheral neuropathy and ototoxicity."

The Bezjak study provides an excellent demonstration of good methodology. If the investigator wishes to capture HRQoL data, it is poor methodology to administer the HRQoL tool only at one time, and good methodology to administer the HRQoL tools at two or three different time points during the course of the clinical trial.

3. The Bonomi Study

The Bonomi clinical trial reveals a problem that might arise, where the HRQoL tool is administered at several different times during the course of the study. In a clinical trial of lung cancer, Bonomi et al. (53) collected information on HRQoL. These authors documented the problem that, as the clinical study progressed, compliance with filling out the

[48]Pais-Ribeiro J, Pinto C, Santo C. Validation study of the Portuguese version of the QLC-C30-V.3. Psicologia, Saude & Doencas 2008;9:89−102.

[49]Wan C, Meng Q, Yang Z, et al. Validation of the simplified Chinese version of EORTC QLQ-C30 from the measurements of five types of inpatients with cancer. Ann. Oncol. 2008;19:2053−60.

[50]Bestmann B, Rohde V, Siebmann JU, Galalae R, Weidner W, Küchler T. Validation of the German prostate-specific module. World J. Urol. 2006;24:94−100.

[51]Zotti P, Lugli D, Vaccher E, Vidotto G, Franchin G, Barzan L. The EORTC quality of life questionnaire-head and neck 35 in Italian laryngectomized patients. European organization for research and treatment of cancer. Qual. Life Res. 2000;9:1147−53.

[52]Bezjak A, Lee CW, Ding K, et al. Quality-of-life outcomes for adjuvant chemotherapy in early-stage non-small-cell lung cancer: results from a randomized trial, JBR.10. J Clin Oncol. 2008;26:5052−9.

[53]Bonomi P, Kim K, Fairclough D, et al. Comparison of survival and quality of life in advanced non-small-cell lung cancer patients treated with two dose levels of paclitaxel combined with cisplatin versus etoposide with cisplatin: results of an Eastern Cooperative Oncology Group trial. J. Clin. Oncol. 2000;18:623−31.

questionnaire decreased, and that there was some evidence that growing noncompliance introduced bias into the results.

4. Representative List of Clinical Trials

Now that the take-home lessons from the Shepherd study, the Bezjak study, and the Bonomi study, have been reviewed, the following provides study design information regarding HRQoL from these clinical trials, as well as from one additional clinical trial (Table 22.5).

g. HRQoL in Breast Cancer

Perry et al. (54) summarized the HRQoL tools, about 20 in all, that have been used in clinical trials on breast cancer. The following narrative focuses on only two trials, the Watanabe study and the Muss study.

h. HRQoL in Chronic Lymphocytic Leukemia

The Clinical Study Protocol for a trial for a leukemia drug provides an exemplary account of the use of an HRQoL tool. The HRQoL tool was the FACT-Leu questionnaire, which is configured for use with leukemia patients (55). HRQoL data were used as one of the secondary endpoints. The Protocol provided the following guidance on how the HRQoL data should be interpreted (56):

> Change in HRQL domain and symptom scores based on ... FACT-Leu ... defined as the change from baseline and the time to definitive increments or decrements of 10%, 20%, and 40% from baseline; **time to definitive increment** (better than baseline by the specified amount) is the interval from randomization to the first timepoint when the HRQL measure is consistently better than at baseline ... and **time to definitive HRQL decrement** (worse than baseline by the specified amount) is the interval from randomization to the earliest death or the first timepoint when the HRQL measure is consistently worse than at baseline.

The FACT-Leu questionnaire took the form of rows of checkboxes requesting choice of severity, for questions such as:

- I have lack of energy;
- I have nausea;
- I am forced to spend time in bed;
- I feel close to my friends;
- I get emotional support from my friends;
- My family has accepted my illness;
- I feel sad;
- I feel nervous;
- I worry about dying.

The Clinical Study Protocol also included background information on the evaluation of HRQoL in leukemia clinical trials, which is excerpted below (57). Although it might be

---

[54]Perry S, Kowalski TL, Chang CH. Quality of life assessment in women with breast cancer: benefits, acceptability and utilization. Health Qual. Life Outcomes 2007;5:24—37.

[55]Cella D, et al. Measuring health-related quality of life in leukemia: the Functional Assessment of Cancer Therapy-Leukemia (FACT-Leu) questionnaire. Value Health 2012;15:1051—8.

[56]A phase 3, randomized, double-blind, placebo-controlled study evaluating the efficacy and safety of GS-1101 (CAL-101) in combination with rituximab for previously treated chronic lymphocytic leukemia. Protocol GS-US-312-0116. November 18, 2011.

[57]A phase 3, randomized, double-blind, placebo-controlled study evaluating the efficacy and safety of GS-1101 (CAL-101) in combination with rituximab for previously treated chronic lymphocytic leukemia. Protocol GS-US-312-0116. November 18, 2011.

TABLE 22.5 Health-Related Quality of Life in Clinical Studies of Nonsmall-Cell Lung Cancer (NSCLC)

	Instrument	HRQoL at Baseline	HRQoL Used as Endpoint
Bezjak et al.[a]	Two instruments were used: EORTC QLQ-C30, and a lung-cancer-specific questionnaire QLQ-LC13	Yes	After 5 weeks, 9 weeks, and 3, 6, 9, and 12 months
	Conclusion: The study compared surgery only, with surgery followed by chemotherapy. Patients in the chemotherapy arm had better scores in symptom items of nausea ($P = 0.001$) and fever ($P = 0.1$), but worse scores for numbness ($P < 0.001$), pins, and needles ($P = 0.02$), and loss of hearing ($P = 0.03$)		
Bonomi et al.[b]	Functional Assessment of Cancer-Lung (FACT-L)	Yes	Taken 6, 12, and 26 weeks after the first course of chemotherapy
	Conclusion: All three regimens demonstrated significant decreases in the scores over 6 months, but there were no significant differences between the regimens ($P = 0.59$ for the total FACT scores)		
Shepherd et al.[c]	Two instruments: EORTC QLQ-C30 (cancer in general) and EORTC QLQ-LC13 (for lung cancer)	Yes	Every 4 weeks
	Conclusion: Analyses of the quality of life found that more patients receiving erlotinib had improvement in cough, pain, and dyspnea and in the domain of overall physical function		
Mok et al.[d]	Functional Assessment of Cancer Therapy Lung (FACT-L)	Yes	At week 1, and at 3-week intervals until day 127, and once every 6 weeks until disease progression, and when study drug was discontinued
	Conclusion: Significantly more patients in the gefitinib group than in the carboplatin-paclitaxel group had improvement in quality of life ($P = 0.01$)		

[a]Bezjak A, Lee CW, Ding K, et al. Quality-of-life outcomes for adjuvant chemotherapy in early-stage non-small-cell lung cancer: results from a randomized trial, JBR.10. J. Clin. Oncol. 2008;26:5052−9.
[b]Bonomi P, Kim K, Fairclough D, et al. Comparison of survival and quality of life in advanced non-small-cell lung cancer patients treated with two dose levels of paclitaxel combined with cisplatin versus etoposide with cisplatin: results of an Eastern Cooperative Oncology Group trial. J. Clin. Oncol. 2000;18:623−31.
[c]Shepherd FA, Rodrigues Pereira J, Ciuleanu T, et al. Erlotinib in previously treated non-small-cell lung cancer. New Engl. J. Med. 2005;353:123−312.
[d]Mok TS, Wu YL, Thongprasert S, et al. Gefitinib or carboplatin-paclitaxel in pulmonary adenocarcinoma. New Engl. J. Med. 2009;361:947−57.

suggested that this background information is excessive to include in a Clinical Study Protocol, the fact that the information is from a Sponsor of a chronic lymphocytic leukemia (CLL) trial establishes the reliability of the information:

Health-Related Quality of Life. Direct patient reporting of outcomes using standardized methods has become an increasingly important component of therapeutic assessment. Evaluation of patient-reported outcomes (PROs) is particularly relevant in patients who cannot be cured of disease ... PRO questionnaires have been previously used in CLL to understand how patients differ from the general population in terms of health concerns ... to understand differences in perceptions of well-being in younger vs older patients ... to determine how treatment affects HRQL ... [p]atients with CLL have overtly impaired well-being relative to comparable controls ... [f]atigue is cited as a common complaint, being present in the substantial majority of patients ... [f]actors associated with lower overall HRQL have included older age, greater fatigue, severity of comorbid health conditions, advanced stage, and ongoing treatment for CLL ... [y]ounger patients appear to have worse emotional and social well-being but older patients experience worse physical HRQL.

1. Where Survival Data Are Identical in Both Study Arms, HRQoL Data Turn the Tide—The Watanabe Study

Watanabe et al. (58) provide an elegant narrative regarding HRQoL data, for a clinical study of women, after surgery, who received either uracil plus tegafur (UFT) (group 1), or cyclophosphamide, methotrexate, and 5-fluorouracil (CMF) (group 2). The study shows graphs of various measures of QoL, for the two groups, over a 2-year period. For example, one graph disclosing the parameter of "upset by hair loss," shows that the CMF group peaked at 1−4 months, and then returned towards baseline while, in contrast, the UFT group remained at baseline.

Data on survival for the UFT group and the CMF group were essentially identical. In view of these identical results, the authors turned to the HRQoL data for guidance. In finding the quality-of-life data to be better in the UFT group, the authors recommended UFT, over CMF, as the proper treatment for breast cancer. Thus data on HRQoL played a role in concluding that one of the study arm treatments was better than the other.

This concerns prognostic factors. There has been some interest in using HRQoL data, for example, on fatigue and emotional states, acquired before drug treatment is initiated, as a prognostic factor for later-arising parameters of efficacy (59,60).

2. HRQoL Data Demonstrate That Long-Term Treatment Is Well Tolerated—The Muss Clinical Trial

HRQoL data were evaluated for a drug that was intended for chronic administration, and used to prevent recurrence of breast cancer. Muss et al. (61) studied breast cancer survivors, who had earlier been treated with surgery and chemotherapy, and were subsequently randomized into two groups. Group 1 received letrozole, and group 2 received placebo, both on a chronic basis. The issue to be decided was whether women who were treated for breast cancer, and were cancer-free, are likely to make the decision to take letrozole on a chronic basis, with the expectation that there would be a small percentage reduction in the chance of relapse.

The authors found that HRQoL assessment in older patients showed only a modest decrease in HRQoL with letrozole treatment, compared with placebo. The authors found that letrozole was well tolerated by older women, and recommended the drug should be considered for subsequent extended adjuvant endocrine therapy with letrozole for healthy older patients who have completed 5 years of tamoxifen.

[58]Watanabe T, Sano M, Takashima S, et al. Oral uracil and tegafur compared with classic cyclophosphamide, methotrexate, fluorouracil as postoperative chemotherapy in patients with node-negative, high-risk breast cancer: National Surgical Adjuvant Study for Breast Cancer 01. Trial. J. Clin. Oncol. 2009;27:1368−74.

[59]Goodwin PJ, Ennis M, Bordeleau LJ, et al. Health-related quality of life and psychosocial status in breast cancer prognosis: analysis of multiple variables. J. Clin. Oncol. 2004;22:4184−92.

[60]Bottomley A, Biganzoli L, Cufer T, et al. Randomized, controlled trial investigating short-term health-related quality of life with doxorubicin and paclitaxel versus doxorubicin and cyclophosphamide as first-line chemotherapy in patients with metastatic breast cancer: European Organization for Research and Treatment of Cancer Breast Cancer Group, Investigational Drug Branch for Breast Cancer and the New Drug Development Group Study. J. Clin. Oncol. 2004;22:2576−86.

[61]Muss HB, Tu D, Ingle JN, et al. Efficacy, toxicity, and quality of life in older women with early-stage breast cancer treated with letrozole or placebo after 5 years of tamoxifen: NCIC CTG intergroup trial MA.17. J. Clin. Oncol. 2008;26:1956−64.

VI. DECISIONS ON COUNSELING; DECISIONS ON CHEMOTHERAPY VERSUS SURGERY

This further concerns HRQoL tools in oncology. Data on HRQoL can provide guidance, where the clinician needs to decide if counseling is needed, or where the clinician needs to decide between two courses of therapy. For example, where a cancer patient faces surgery, and where data from the SF-36 form shows poor social functioning, the clinician may decide to provide the patient with counseling, in order to improve outcome to the surgery (62). Moreover, where SF-36 data reveal that the patient has cramps and decreased appetite, these results can guide the physician to make an informed choice between two treatment options, for example, chemotherapy versus surgery (63).

VII. CONCLUDING REMARKS

Variables and issues in HRQoL methodology include:

- HRQoL tools were administered, but only at baseline. See, for example, Efficace et al. (64).
- HRQoL tools administered at various intervals during the course of the clinical trial.
- HRQoL scores were determined to be similar, at baseline, in the study drug group and control group. See, for example, Tol et al. (65).
- HRQoL tools administered at various intervals during the course of a clinical trial, but compliance was poor, or dwindled over time. See, for example, Bonomi et al. (66), Michael and Tannock (67), and Olschewski et al. (68).

[62]Anthony T, Hynan LS, Rosen D, et al. The association of pretreatment health-related quality of life with surgical complications for patients undergoing open surgical resection for colorectal cancer. Ann. Surg. 2003;238:690−6.

[63]Anthony T, Hynan LS, Rosen D, et al. The association of pretreatment health-related quality of life with surgical complications for patients undergoing open surgical resection for colorectal cancer. Ann. Surg. 2003;238:690−6.

[64]Efficace F, Innominato PF, Bjarnason G, et al. Validation of patient's self-reported social functioning as an independent prognostic factor for survival in metastatic colorectal cancer patients: results of an international study by the Chronotherapy Group of the European Organisation for Research and Treatment of Cancer. J. Clin. Oncol. 2008;26:2020−6.

[65]Tol J, Koopman M, Cats A, et al. Chemotherapy, bevacizumab, and cetuximab in metastatic colorectal cancer. New Engl. J. Med. 2009;360:563−72.

[66]Bonomi P, Kim K, Fairclough D, et al. Comparison of survival and quality of life in advanced non-small-cell lung cancer patients treated with two dose levels of paclitaxel combined with cisplatin versus etoposide with cisplatin: results of an Eastern Cooperative Oncology Group trial. J. Clin. Oncol. 2000;18:623−31.

[67]Michael M, Tannock IF. Measuring health-related quality of life in clinical trials that evaluate the role of chemotherapy in cancer treatment. Can. Med. Assoc. J. 1998;158:1727−34.

[68]Olschewski M, Schulgen G, Schumacher M, Altman DG. Quality of life assessment in clinical cancer research. Br. J. Cancer 1994;70:1−5.

- In some clinical trials on cancer, HRQoL tools were not at all used. See, for example, Pectasides et al. (69).

Issues in efficacy and safety are summarized by the bullet points:

- HRQoL for study drug was found superior to HRQoL from control treatment, where study drug also resulted in superior survival. See, for example, Sobrero et al. (70).
- HRQoL for study drug was superior to HRQoL from control treatment, in the context where study drug did not provide superior survival over survival with control treatment. See, for example, Middleton et al. (71).
- Where the overall HRQoL score fails to indicate any advantage of the study drug over control treatment, separate analysis of the separate components of the HRQoL tool may enable a conclusion. See, for example, Kemeny et al. (72). Shepherd et al. (73), also provide a breakdown showing the various parameters that were captured by the HRQoL tool.

[69]Pectasides D, Dafni U, Bafaloukos D, et al. Randomized phase III study of 1 month versus 1 year of adjuvant high-dose interferon alfa-2b in patients with resected high-risk melanoma. J. Clin. Oncol. 2009;27:939—44.

[70]Sobrero AF, Maurel J, Fehrenbacher L, et al. EPIC: phase III trial of cetuximab plus irinotecan after fluoropyrimidine and oxaliplatin failure in patients with metastatic colorectal cancer. J. Clin. Oncol. 2008;26:2311—9.

[71]Middleton MR, Grob JJ, Aaronson N, et al. Randomized phase III study of temozolomide versus dacarbazine in the treatment of patients with advanced metastatic malignant melanoma. J. Clin. Oncol. 2000;18:158—66.

[72]Kemeny NE, Niedzwiecki D, Hollis DR, et al. Hepatic arterial infusion versus systemic therapy for hepatic metastases from colorectal cancer: a randomized trial of efficacy, quality of life, and molecular markers (CALGB 9481). J. Clin. Oncol. 2006;24:1395—403.

[73]Shepherd FA, Rodrigues Pereira J, Ciuleanu T, et al. Erlotinib in previously treated non-small-cell lung cancer. New Engl. J. Med. 2005;353:123—312.

23

Health-Related Quality-of-Life Tools—Immune Disorders

I. INTRODUCTION

Chapter 22's account of health-related quality-of-life (HRQoL) tools for cancer is extended here to another class of chronic disorders, the autoimmune disorders. This chapter contains a reproduction of a HRQoL questionnaire, outlines its use for a variety of autoimmune diseases, and focuses on multiple sclerosis.

HRQoL tools express, in numbers, the influence of a patient's disease and treatment on self-reported well-being (1). The questions may address physical well-being, social well-being, and emotional well-being. In a study of multiple sclerosis patients, Moore et al. (2) compared two separate HRQoL instruments, the MUSiQoL questionnaire and the MSQOL-54 questionnaire. The researchers found that one

of these instruments was easier to understand and answer, while the other was more relevant to the quality of life of the multiple sclerosis patient.

This discloses the SF-36® HRQoL questionnaire, which is used for a variety of diseases. The SF-36 form contains 36 questions, which reside in eight different categories. "SF" means short form.

II. SHORT FORM SF-36 QUESTIONNAIRE

The SF-36 questionnaire (SF-36) contains 36 items that assess patients' health status and its impact on their lives (Table 23.1). SF-36 is a structured, self-report questionnaire that a patient can complete with little or no counseling

---

[1]Anthony T, Hynan LS, Rosen D, et al. The association of pretreatment health-related quality of life with surgical complications for patients undergoing open surgical resection for colorectal cancer. Ann. Surg. 2003;238:690−6.

[2]Moore F, et al. Two multiple sclerosis quality of life measures: comparison in a national sample. Can. J. Neurol. Sci. 2015;42:55−63.

Clinical Trials.
DOI: http://dx.doi.org/10.1016/B978-0-12-804217-5.00023-0

TABLE 23.1   Short Form SF-36 Questionnaire.[a,b,c]

1. In general, would you say your health is: (1) Excellent; (2) Very good; (3) Good; (4) Fair; (5) Poor.

For each statement please circle the one number that indicates how TRUE or FALSE that statement is for you.

	Definitely true	Mostly true	Not sure	Mostly false	Definitely false
2. I seem to get sick a little easier than other people	1	2	3	4	5
3. I am as healthy as anybody I know	1	2	3	4	5
4. I expect my health to get worse	1	2	3	4	5
5. My health is excellent	1	2	3	4	5

6. Compared to 1 year ago, how would you rate your health in general now? (circle one):

(1) Much better

(2) Somewhat better

(3) Same

(4) Somewhat worse

(5) Much worse

Now think about the activities you might do during a typical day. Does your health limit you in these activities? If so, how much? Please circle 1, 2, or 3 on each item to indicate how much your health limits you.

	Yes, limited a lot	Yes, limited a little	No, not limited at all
7. Vigorous activities, such as running, lifting heavy objects, participating in strenuous sports	1	2	3
8. Moderate activities, such as moving a table, pushing a vacuum cleaner, bowling, or playing golf	1	2	3
9. Lifting or carrying groceries	1	2	3
10. Climbing several flights of stairs	1	2	3
11. Climbing one flight of stairs	1	2	3
12. Bending, kneeling, or stooping	1	2	3
13. Walking more than 1 mile	1	2	3
14. Walking several blocks	1	2	3
15. Walking one block	1	2	3
16. Bathing and dressing yourself	1	2	3

During the past 4 weeks, have you had any of the following problems with your work or other regular daily activities as a result of your physical health? Please circle "1" (Yes) or "2" (No) for each item.

	Yes	No
17. Cut down on the amount of time you could spend on work or other activities	1	2
18. Accomplished less than you would like	1	2

19. Were limited in the kind of work or other activities   1   2

20. Had difficulty performing the work or other activities (eg, it took extra effort)   1   2

21. How much bodily pain have you had during the past 4 weeks? (circle one): (1) None; (2) Very mild; (3) Mild; (4) Moderate; (5) Severe; (6) Very severe.

22. During the past 4 weeks, how much did pain interfere with your normal work (including work both outside the home and housework)? (circle one): (1) Not at all; (2) A little bit; (3) Moderately; (4) Quite a bit; (5) Extremely.

During the past 4 weeks, have you had any of the following problems with your work or other regular daily activities, as a result of any emotional problems, such as feeling depressed or anxious? Please circle "1" (Yes) or "2" (No) for each item.

	Yes	No
23. Cut down on the amount of time you could spend on work or other activities	1	2
24. Accomplished less than you would like	1	2
25. Did do work or other activities less carefully than usual	1	2

26. During the past 4 weeks, to what extent have your physical health or emotional problems interfered with your normal social activities with family, friends, neighbors, or groups? (circle one number): (1) Not at all; (2) Slightly; (3) Moderately; (4) Quite a bit; (5) Extremely.

The next set of questions is about how you feel and how things have been with you during the past 4 weeks. For each question, please circle the one number for the answer that comes closest to the way you have been feeling. How much time during the past 4 weeks:

	All of the time	Most of the time	A good bit of the time	A little of the time	None of the time
27. Did you feel full of pep?	1	2	3	4	5
28. Have you been a very nervous person?	1	2	3	4	5
29. Have you felt so down in the dumps that nothing could cheer you up?	1	2	3	4	5
30. Have you felt calm and peaceful?	1	2	3	4	5
31. Did you have a lot of energy?	1	2	3	4	5
32. Have you felt downhearted and blue?	1	2	3	4	5
33. Did you feel worn out?	1	2	3	4	5
34. Have you been a happy person?	1	2	3	4	5
35. Did you feel tired?	1	2	3	4	5
36. Finally, during the past 4 weeks, how much of the time has your physical health or emotional problems interfered with your social activities (like visiting with friends, relatives, etc.)?	1	2	3	4	5

[a]Ware JE, Kosinski M, Bjorner JB, et al. SF-36v2® Health Survey: administrative guide for clinical trial investigators. Lincoln, RI: QualityMetric, Inc.
[b]SF-36®, SF36v2®, SF-12®, and SF-12v2® are trademarks of the Medical Outcomes Trust and are used under license. The SF-8™, SF-10™, ACTTM, and PIQ-6™ are copyrighted by QualityMetric Incorporated.
[c]Ritvo PG, Fischer JS, Miller DM, Andrews H, Paty DW, LaRocca NG. Multiple sclerosis quality of life inventory: a user's manual. New York: National Multiple Sclerosis Society; 1997.

from an interviewer. SF-36, as provided by Ware et al. (3) by and Ritvo et al. (4), is reproduced below. SF-36 occurs in various revised forms.

SF-36 is composed of eight multi-item scales (Physical Functioning, Role-Physical, Bodily Pain, General Health, Vitality, Social Functioning, Role-Emotional, Mental Health), with scores for each of these scales (or dimensions) ranging from 0 to 100. Higher scores indicate higher HRQoL. SF-36 scores range from 0 (worst) to 100 (best) (5).

This instrument addresses health concepts from the patient's perspective. There is no single overall score for the SF-36. The SF-36 form generates eight subscales and two summary scores. The eight subscales are: physical functioning, role limitations due to physical problems, bodily pain, general health perceptions, vitality, social functioning, role limitations due to emotional problems, and mental health. The two summary scores are the Physical Component Summary (PCS) score and the Mental Component Summary (MCS) score (6). PCS and MCS are derived by aggregating individual scores. The PCS and MCS scores for the general population in the United States are each 50 (7).

Shown below are short accounts on the use of SF-36 for various immune disorders, followed by a more detailed analysis of the use of SF-36 for multiple sclerosis.

a. Arthritis

In a study of arthritis, the SF-36 form showed that administering infliximab followed by sulfasalazine gives better outcome than drugs given in the reverse order, sulfasalazine followed by infliximab (8).

b. Psoriasis

When the SF-36 form was used by subjects in a clinical trial on psoriasis, data from SF-36 demonstrated that the *placebo* had little or no effect on HRQoL, whereas the *study drug* (infliximab) resulted in dramatic improvements in response to questions relating to general feelings of accomplishments at work, or to general feelings about doing work carefully (9).

[3]Ware JE, Kosinski M, Bjorner JB, et al. SF-36v2® Health Survey: administrative guide for clinical trial investigators. Lincoln, RI: QualityMetric, Inc.

[4]Ritvo PG, Fischer JS, Miller DM, Andrews H, Paty DW, LaRocca NG. Multiple sclerosis quality of life inventory: a user's manual. New York: National Multiple Sclerosis Society; 1997.

[5]van der Kooij SM, de Vries-Bouwstra JK, Goekoop-Ruiterman YP, et al. Patient-reported outcomes in a randomized trial comparing four different treatment strategies in recent-onset rheumatoid arthritis. Arthritis Rheum. 2009;61:4−12.

[6]Rudick RA, Miller D, Hass S, et al. Health-related quality of life in multiple sclerosis: effects of natalizumab. Ann. Neurol. 2007;62:335−46.

[7]Reich K, Nestle FO, Wu Y, et al. Infliximab treatment improves productivity among patients with moderate-to-severe psoriasis. Eur. J. Dermatol. 2007;17:381−6.

[8]van der Kooij SM, de Vries-Bouwstra JK, Goekoop-Ruiterman YP, et al. Patient-reported outcomes in a randomized trial comparing four different treatment strategies in recent-onset rheumatoid arthritis. Arthritis Rheum. 2009;61:4−12.

[9]Reich K, Nestle FO, Wu Y, et al. Infliximab treatment improves productivity among patients with moderate-to-severe psoriasis. Eur. J. Dermatol. 2007;17:381−6.

c. Crohn's Disease

When the SF-36 form was used with patients suffering from Crohn's disease, Cadahia et al. (10) found that the study drug (infliximab) resulted in improvements in the physical role (PR) scale, but no change in the physical function (PF) scale. The PR scale of SF-36 is determined by questions about time required to complete tasks, difficulties in completing tasks, and ability to accomplish things. In contrast, the PF scale reflects questions on bending, walking, climbing, and lifting.

d. Chronic Obstructive Pulmonary Disease

When the SF-36 form was used by subjects in a clinical trial on chronic obstructive pulmonary disease (COPD), Eaton et al. (11) found that administering oxygen gas resulted in an improvement in HRQoL, for example, in reduction of anxiety. In this study, the experimental group received oxygen from a tank of compressed gas, while the placebo group received air from a tank of compressed gas. The authors were careful to point out that the requirement of both groups of subjects to carry a heavy tank of compressed gas might have reduced quality of life. The authors concluded that their study was one of the first to provide justification to the widespread belief that COPD patients can benefit from oxygen.

e. Multiple Sclerosis

HRQoL questionnaires are used for clinical studies, as well as in ordinary medical practice, for patients diagnosed with multiple sclerosis. These questionnaires are used for a number of reasons. Multiple sclerosis produces a deterioration in HRQoL. Thus, use of the HRQoL instruments can be used to measure drug efficacy in clinical trials on multiple sclerosis (12). Additionally, some of the factors measured by HRQoL forms, such as fatigue, pain, bladder or bowel control, and physical functioning, cannot be readily measured by laboratory tests (13). Moreover, according to Mowry et al. (14), data from HRQoL questionnaires may be used as a surrogate for clinical outcomes.

III. HRQoL INSTRUMENTS SPECIFIC FOR MULTIPLE SCLEROSIS

The SF-36 form is a generic form, suitable for use with many disorders, including multiple sclerosis. Depending on needs and resources, an investigator may wish to use an HRQoL instrument that is specific for multiple sclerosis. These specific instruments include the Multiple Sclerosis Quality of Life Inventory (MSQLI), and others. MSQLI includes the questions found on SF-36 plus

[10]Cadahia V, García-Carbonero A, Vivas S, et al. Infliximab improves quality of life in the short-term in patients with fistulizing Crohn's disease in clinical practice. Rev. Esp. Enferm. Dig. 2004;96:369−74.

[11]Eaton T, Garrett JE, Young P, et al. Ambulatory oxygen improves quality of life of COPD patients: a randomised controlled study. Eur. Respir. J. 2002;20:306−12.

[12]Rudick RA, Miller D, Hass S, et al. Health-related quality of life in multiple sclerosis: effects of natalizumab. Ann. Neurol. 2007;62:335−46.

[13]Robinson Jr D, Zhao N, Gathany T, Kim LL, Cella D, Revicki D. Health perceptions and clinical characteristics of relapsing-remitting multiple sclerosis patients: baseline data from an international clinical trial. Curr. Med. Res. Opin. 2009;25:1121−30.

[14]Mowry EM, Beheshtian A, Waubant E, et al. Quality of life in multiple sclerosis is associated with lesion burden and brain volume measures. Neurology 2009;72:1760−5.

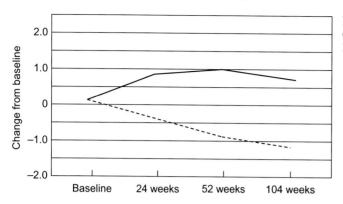

FIGURE 23.1 PCS in the Rudick study. Change in PCS scale with administration of natalizumab (solid line) or placebo (dashes).

additional questions. Other multiple-sclerosis-specific questionnaires include MS Quality of Life-54 (QOL-54) (15), Functional Assessment of Multiple Sclerosis, the Fatigue Impact Scale (16), and visual analog scales (17).

a. The Rudick Study

The Rudick study on multiple sclerosis compared outcome, where subjects were administered an antibody (natalizumab; Tysabri®) or a placebo. Rudick et al. (18) evaluated the relationship between HRQoL scores and clinical measures of multiple sclerosis. Subjects received either natalizumab (627 subjects) or placebo (315 subjects). All subjects had a form of the disease known as, relapsing-remitting multiple sclerosis.

SF-36 was used to calculate the PCS (Fig. 23.1) and the MCS (Fig. 23.2). When

comparing the study drug with placebo, improvements were found with the study drug, where the improvements were sustained over the entire 104-week duration of the clinical study.

Of practical use to future patients is that these results justify counseling patients that they may expect improvements in HRQoL by 24 weeks of therapy with the antibody. In other words, because of the Rudick study, physicians may be justified in stating, "You should expect to feel somewhat better by or before 24 weeks of treatment."

In the Rudick study, clinical endpoints were measured by the EDSS score and also the volume of brain lesions, where brain lesions were measured by magnetic resonance imaging (MRI). The authors found that subjects who experienced sustained worsening of EDSS score also had worsened PCS scores and MCS scores. Moreover, subjects with a greater

[15]Fischer JS, LaRocca NG, Miller DM, Ritvo PG, Andrews H, Paty D. Recent developments in the assessment of quality of life in multiple sclerosis (MS). Mult. Scler. 1999;5:251—9.

[16]Melanson M, Grossberndt A, Klowak M, et al. Fatigue and cognition in patients with relapsing multiple sclerosis treated with interferon beta. Int. J. Neurosci. 2010;120:631—40.

[17]Kos D, Nagels G, D'Hooghe MB, Duportail M, Kerckhofs E. A rapid screening tool for fatigue impact in multiple sclerosis. BMC Neurol. 2006;6:27.

[18]Rudick RA, Miller D, Hass S, et al. Health-related quality of life in multiple sclerosis: effects of natalizumab. Ann. Neurol. 2007;62:335—46.

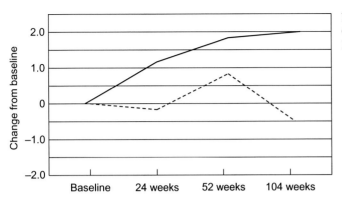

FIGURE 23.2 MCS scale in the Rudick study. Change in MCS scale with administration of natalizumab (solid line) or placebo (dashes).

relapse rate correlated with worse HRQoL scores. Additionally, the study found that subjects with more serious lesions, according to MRI also had worse HRQoL scores. Twork et al. (19) compared the EDSS instrument with the HRQoL instrument, as described below.

b. EDSS Score Versus HRQoL Score

The EDSS scale is described in Chapter 20. Please note that although the EDSS score is acquired by way of a questionnaire, it does not assess HRQoL. Twork et al. (20) conducted a side-by-side comparison of the goals of a HRQoL instrument specific for multiple sclerosis (MSQOL-54) and the EDSS questionnaire. The EDSS instrument is a questionnaire used for multiple sclerosis, but it is not an HRQoL instrument. These authors found that there was some overlap between these two types of instruments, and that there is a moderate correlation between results from use of the first instrument and the second instrument.

c. Interferon-Alfa-2a —The Nortvedt Study

In a clinical trial of 97 multiple sclerosis subjects, Nortvedt et al. (21) administered low-dose interferon-alfa-2a, high-dose interferon-alfa-2a, or placebo. Study drugs and placebo were administered for 6 months, followed by a 6-month follow-up period. The investigators were careful to administer SF-36 at baseline, 3 months, 6 months, and 12 months.

The study drug prevented the development of new lesions, as measured by MRI. This effect was quite dramatic. However, the study drug did not result in any significant improvement of HRQoL, as assessed by the SF-36 form.

[19]Twork S, Wiesmeth S, Spindler M, et al. Disability status and quality of life in multiple sclerosis: non-linearity of the Expanded Disability Status Scale (EDSS). Health Qual. Life Outcomes 2010;8:55.

[20]Twork S, Wiesmeth S, Spindler M, et al. Disability status and quality of life in multiple sclerosis: non-linearity of the Expanded Disability Status Scale (EDSS). Health Qual. Life Outcomes 2010;8:55.

[21]Nortvedt MW, Riise T, Myhr KM, Nyland HI, Hanestad BR. Type I interferons and the quality of life of multiple sclerosis patients. Results from a clinical trial on interferon alfa-2a. Mult. Scler. 1999;5:317–22.

d. Interferon-Beta-1a
—The Jongen Study

In a clinical trial of 284 multiple sclerosis patients, Jongen et al. (22) treated all patients with interferon-beta-1a (Avonex®). The response was assessed by tests for physical outcome, that is, the Multiple Sclerosis Functional Composite (MSFC), which includes a timed 25-foot walk. Response was also assessed by a HRQoL instrument, that is, the MS54QoL questionnaire. Data from the physical tests and HRQoL tests were captured at baseline and at 3, 6, 12, 18, and 24 months.

The MSFC scores did not change significantly.

In contrast, HRQoL scores did improve. The physical score component of the HRQoL instrument improved somewhat, while the mental score component of the HRQoL instrument improved only slightly. The researchers examined the subgroups of the study population, and in reviewing data from the subgroups, the authors concluded that, "after 2 years of treatment, HRQoL was increased, especially in younger patients with low disability."

e. Glatiramer Acetate
—The Zwibel Study

Zwibel (23) conducted a clinical trial on multiple sclerosis patients. All patients received daily injections of glatiramer acetate. The study involved 805 patients, some of whom had already been treated with interferon-beta-1b, while the rest were treatment-naive. Glatiramer acetate is a synthetic random polypeptide, containing L-alanine, L-glutamate, L-lysine, and L-tyrosine. The drug inhibits Th1-type immune response and promotes Th2-type immune response (24,25).

This was a single-arm study, that is, all patients received the study drug. Efficacy was assessed by the EDSS scale every 6 months, while safety was assessed every 3 months, for a period of up to 3.5 years.

Results from the HRQoL data were published separately (26). The results demonstrated that improvements in HRQoL were found in only treatment-naive patients ($P < 0.001$). In patients having previously received interferon-beta-1b for multiple sclerosis, there was no significant improvement in HRQoL during the glatiramer acetate trial ($P = 0.13$). The study enables the clinician to predict that, for any given treatment-naive patient, there is a 40% chance that glitiramer acetate therapy will improve HRQoL, and that this improvement will be found at 6 months and will be maintained until at least 12 months, with continued glitiramer acetate therapy.

---

[22]Jongen PJ, Sindic C, Carton H, et al. Improvement of health-related quality of life in relapsing remitting multiple sclerosis patients after 2 years of treatment with intramuscular interferon-beta-1a. J. Neurol. 2010;257:584—9.

[23]Zwibel HL. Copolymer-1 treatment study principal investigators. Glatiramer acetate in treatment-naïve and prior interferon-beta-1b-treated multiple sclerosis patients. Acta Neurol. Scand. 2006;113:378—86.

[24]Jasny E, Eisenblatter M, Matz-Rensing K, et al. IL-12-impaired and IL-12-secreting dendritic cells produce IL-23 upon CD154 restimulation. J. Immunol. 2008;180:6629—39.

[25]Vieira PL, Heystek HC, Wormmeester J, Wierenga EA, Kapsenberg ML. Glatiramer acetate (copolymer-1, copaxone) promotes Th2 cell development and increased IL-10 production through modulation of dendritic cells. J. Immunol. 2003;170:4483—8.

[26]Jongen PJ, Lehnick D, Sanders E, et al. Health-related quality of life in relapsing remitting multiple sclerosis patients during treatment with glatiramer acetate: a prospective, observational, international, multi-centre study. Health Qual Life Outcomes 2010;8:133.

f. Meditation Training —The Grossman Study

Grossman et al. (27,28) conducted a clinical trial with 150 multiple sclerosis patients. Half of the subjects participated in an 8-week trial of meditation, while the other half did not receive mediation training. Training involved eight weekly 2.5-h classes of exercises while lying or sitting, and included yoga posturing.

Two different HRQoL instruments were used, namely, the Profile of Health-Related Quality of Life in Chronic Disorders (PQOLC scale) and the Hamburg Quality of Life Questionnaire in Multiple Sclerosis (HAQUAMS) scale.

HRQoL in the meditation group was significantly improved, as determined immediately after the trial, and as determined at 6 months after the trial's conclusion (6-month follow-up). Immediately after the trial, improvement by PQOLC was significant, and improvement by HAQUAMS was also significant. The authors observed that earlier trials have shown that HRQoL is often independent of the extent of the disease, and that drugs used to treat multiple sclerosis tend not to result in corresponding improvements in HRQoL. In view of these findings, and in view of the improvements found in the Grossman trial, meditation-training can be a reasonable additional treatment for patients receiving drugs such as fingolimod or natalizumab. According to one commentator, "generally speaking, patients with all forms of MS should be able to benefit from meditation" (29).

IV. CONCLUDING REMARKS

HRQoL tools assess the effects of immune diseases on the patient's life, and assess the efficacy of drugs on the disease. Drugs against immune disorders, in particular the interferons, can result in depression and thus reduce HRQoL. HRQoL tools are of increased importance when drugs with the adverse effect of depression are used.

Clinical trials testing drugs for multiple sclerosis have generally not assessed HRQoL, possibly because previously conducted studies have shown that these drugs do not improve HRQoL (30). However, it is still the case that HRQoL is a day-to-day concern for victims of multiple sclerosis. HRQoL tools have had particular utility in revealing the beneficial influence of meditation and yoga for multiple sclerosis patients. It might be noted that, at the time of this writing, there were about 100 FDA-approved clinical trials where the intervention was yoga. Some of these trials are identified in the footnote (31).

[27]Grossman P, Kappos L, Gensicke H, et al. MS quality of life, depression, and fatigue improve after mindfulness training: a randomized trial. Neurology 2010;75:1141–9.

[28]Tavee J, Stone L. Healing the mind. Meditation and multiple sclerosis. Neurology 2010;75:1130–1.

[29]Tavee J. E-mail of December 21, 2010.

[30]Barten LJ, Allington DR, Procacci KA, Rivey MP. New approaches in the management of multiple sclerosis. Drug Des. Devel. Ther. 2010;4:343–66.

[31]Yoga Study in Breast Cancer Patients NCT00476203; Yoga for the Management of HIV-Metabolic Syndromes NCT00627380; Yoga Therapy in Treating Patients With Malignant Brain Tumors NCT01234805; Development and Evaluation of Modified Yoga in Systemic Lupus Erythematosus NCT01176643; Yoga to Reduce Cancer Fatigue NCT00583739; Yoga for Arthritis NCT00349869.

24

Health-Related Quality-of-Life Tools—Infections

I. INTRODUCTION

When assessing infections that are chronic and debilitating, health-related quality-of-life (HRQoL) questionnaires are used in clinical trials, epidemiological surveys, and in everyday clinical practice. This chapter focuses on HRQoL tools for an exemplary infection, hepatitis C virus (HCV). HRQoL tools used for chronic HCV infections include SF-36® form (1), Beck Depression Inventory (2), Liver Disease Symptom Index (3), Mishel Uncertainty in Illness Scale (4), Functional Assessment of Chronic Illness Therapy-Fatigue (FACIT-F) (5), Chronic Liver Disease Questionnaire-HCV (CLDQ-HCV) (6), and Work Productivity and Activity Index: Specific Health Problem (WPAI:SHP) (7).

HRQoL tools include many items (individual questions), which fall into a smaller

[1]Conversano C, et al. Interferon alpha therapy in patients with chronic hepatitis C infection: quality of life and depression. Hematol. Rep. 2015;7:5632. http://dx.doi.org/10.4081/ hr.2015.5632.

[2]Sherman KE, Sherman SN, Chenier T, Tsevat J. Health values of patients with chronic hepatitis C infection. Arch. Intern. Med. 2004;164:2377–82.

[3]Gutteling JJ, de Man RA, van der Plas SM, Schalm SW, Busschbach JJ, Darlington AS. Determinants of quality of life in chronic liver patients. Aliment Pharmacol. Ther. 2006;23:1629–35.

[4]Bailey Jr DE, Landerman L, Barroso J, et al. Uncertainty, symptoms, and quality of life in persons with chronic hepatitis C. Psychosomatics 2009;50:138–46.

[5]Younossi ZM, et al. Improvement of health-related quality of life and work productivity in chronic hepatitis C patients with early and advanced fibrosis treated with ledipasvir and sofosbuvir. J. Hepatol. 2015;pii:S0168-8278 (15)00192-0. http://dx.doi.org/10.1016/j.jhep.2015.03.014.

[6]Younossi ZM, et al. Improvement of health-related quality of life and work productivity in chronic hepatitis C patients with early and advanced fibrosis treated with ledipasvir and sofosbuvir. J. Hepatol. 2015;pii:S0168-8278 (15)00192-0. http://dx.doi.org/10.1016/j.jhep.2015.03.014.

[7]Younossi ZM, et al. Improvement of health-related quality of life and work productivity in chronic hepatitis C patients with early and advanced fibrosis treated with ledipasvir and sofosbuvir. J. Hepatol. 2015;pii:S0168-8278 (15)00192-0. http://dx.doi.org/10.1016/j.jhep.2015.03.014.

number of domains, where the domains are used to generate a score. It is interesting to point out that the analysis of clinical trial results can involve, not just a final score, but also contemplation of the various domains. For example, in an analysis of HRQoL results for HCV infections, Conversano et al. (8) commented on the data on the various domains, writing that, "[c]onsidering the whole sample of our study, during IFN-alpha treatment most of the SF-36 **domains** decreased, with the exception of general and mental health scores."

Dramatic shifts in drugs available for treating HCV infections resulted in improvements of HRQoL for patients. The standard of care for chronic HCV, until the year 2013, was the combination of *interferon-alfa-2* and *ribavirin*. In 2013, the combination of *sofosbuvir* and *ledipasvir* was approved for treating HCV. The approved drug combination did not include interferon-alfa-2 or ribavirin. An advantage of the new therapy was absence of the side effects of depression and anemia.

The package label for interferon-alfa-2b (9) provides warnings against depression and anemia, in its writings about "depression and suicidal behavior" and "suppresses bone marrow function and may result in severe ... anemia." In contrast, a view of the package insert for the sofosbuvir/ledipasvir combination reveals the absence of any warnings about depression or anemia (10). In an account of differences in HRQoL that are found with interferon versus drugs such as sofosbuvir, one commentator observed that, the HRQoL, "of the new IFN-free regimens as compared to the IFN-containing are very favorable ... these results ... indicate better tolerability of these new regimens, which could ... lead to better compliance to treatment with very low drop-out rates due to side effects" (11).

In the scientific literature, various spellings are used for interferon-alpha, including "interferon-alpha," "alpha-interferon," "interferon-alfa," and names that use the Greek letter alpha. This textbook uses the name that best corresponds to that from the published study being described in this book.

II. HRQoL TOOLS WITH CHRONIC HCV

Chronic HCV infections are typically silent (12). But signs and symptoms can occur with advanced chronic HCV. In some patients, symptoms do not develop until onset of advanced cirrhosis of the liver or of hepatocellular carcinoma (HCC). Thus, while HRQoL instruments may not reliably reflect HCV-induced hepatitis, HRQoL data most definitely can capture the symptoms of advanced cirrhosis and liver cancer.

In the era prior to the introduction of sofosbuvir and ledipasvir, the standard of care for chronic HCV was ribavirin plus interferon-alpha-2a or ribavirin plus interferon-alpha-2b

---

[8]Conversano C, et al. Interferon alpha therapy in patients with chronic hepatitis C infection: quality of life and depression. Hematol. Rep. 2015;7:5632. http://dx.doi.org/10.4081/ hr.2015.5632.

[9]Package insert for INTRON® A. Interferon alfa-2b, recombinant for injection; October 2014 (39 pp.).

[10]Package insert for HARVONI® (ledipasvir and sofosbuvir) tablets, for oral use; March 2015 (32 pp.).

[11]Younossi Z, Henry L. The impact of the new antiviral regimens on patient reported outcomes and health economics of patients with chronic hepatitis C. Dig. Liver Dis. 2014;46:S186—96.

[12]Bonkovsky HL, Snow KK, Malet PF, et al. Health-related quality of life in patients with chronic hepatitis C and advanced fibrosis. J. Hepatol. 2007;46:420—31.

(13,14). In each case, the pegylated derivative of interferon is used. In about 60% of chronic HCV patients, this treatment with ribavirin plus IFN-alpha eradicates the virus. But IFN-alpha has the established adverse drug reactions of depression, anxiety, and irritability. These effects are separate from the disease-induced adverse events of fatigue and weakness (15). The success rate of this standard of care ranges from 45% to 95%, where success is defined as sustained eradication of HCV (16).

Eradication of HCV requires adherence to the drug treatment schedule. Interferon-induced depression is a major source of failure to take anti-HCV drugs. Interferon-alpha can also cause depression when used for other indications, that is, hepatitis B virus and melanoma. From 15% to 60% of patients receiving interferon-alpha get psychiatric side effects, such as depression (17).

The relationship between interferon-alpha and depression has produced the following irony. Loftis et al. (18) observed that the cure rate was better on chronic HCV patients who developed depression, and that the cure rate was lower in chronic HCV patients who did not develop depression. In other words, the cure rate was better in patients who developed depression, apparently because these patients allowed themselves to be treated to the extent

that the drug caused recovery from the virus, as well as the adverse drug reaction of depression.

a. Example of Hepatitis C Virus HRQoL—The Mathew Study

Mathew et al. (19) conducted a study on patients with chronic HCV. All patients received ribavirin plus IFN-alpha-2b. HRQoL questionnaires (SF-36®) were administered at 0 weeks (baseline), 24 weeks, 48 weeks, and at 72 weeks after end of treatment. Drugs were administered from baseline until 48 weeks. The HRQoL data collected at 72 weeks constitutes follow-up data.

The study involved 152 patients. The result of this study was that 25 patients out of the 152 patients achieved sustained virological response, meaning that the drug worked.

Some of the results are shown in Table 24.1. For assembling this table, scores at baseline were set at zero. What is shown is data at 24 weeks, which was at the half-way point in the treatment scheme, and data at 72 weeks, which was long after completion of the study. The results demonstrate that, for the patients destined to be responders, the HRQoL scores tended to plummet during treatment, but then after treatment, were much better than the

[13]Toniutto P, Fabris C, Bitetto D, Fornasiere E, Rapetti R. Updates on antiviral therapy for chronic hepatitis C. Discov. Med. 2007;7:27−32.

[14]Shimakami T, Lanford RE, Lemon SM. Hepatitis C: recent successes and continuing challenges in the development of improved treatment modalities. Curr. Opin. Pharmacol. 2009;9:537−44.

[15]Fontana RJ, Schwartz SM, Gebremariam A, Lok AS, Moyer CA. Emotional distress during interferon-alpha-2B and ribavirin treatment of chronic hepatitis C. Psychosomatics 2002;43:378−85.

[16]Horsmans Y. Interferon-induced depression in chronic hepatitis C. J. Antimicrob. Chemother. 2006;58:711−3.

[17]Horsmans Y. Interferon-induced depression in chronic hepatitis C. J. Antimicrob. Chemother. 2006;58:711−3.

[18]Loftis JM, Socherman RE, Howell CD, et al. Association of interferon-alpha-induced depression and improved treatment response in patients with hepatitis C. Neurosci. Lett. 2004;365:87−91.

[19]Mathew A, Peiffer LP, Rhoades K, McGarrity TJ. Improvement in quality of life measures in patients with refractory hepatitis C, responding to re-treatment with Pegylated interferon alpha-2b and ribavirin. Health Qual. Life Outcomes 2006;4:30−8.

TABLE 24.1 HRQoL Results From the Mathew Study

S-36 Scores	$t = 24$ Weeks	$t = 72$ Weeks (Follow-Up)
RESPONDERS		
Vitality score	− 8.28	+ 5.69
Bodily pain score	− 3.31	+ 1.96
Role emotional score	− 4.98	+ 5.50
NONRESPONDERS		
Vitality score	− 3.47	+ 2.05
Bodily pain score	− 3.73	+ 1.32
Role emotional score	− 1.20	− 0.63

scores found at baseline. In contrast, for the patients destined to be nonresponders, the scores decreased slightly (got a little worse), and then after treatment rose slightly. Hence, these particular scores might justify providing HCV patients with this advice. Generally, patients who feel the worst during treatment end up responding favorably to the treatment, and end up feeling the best once treatment has been completed.

b. Concluding Remarks

The clinical trial of Mathew et al. (20) provides a detailed account of the various reporting categories on the SF-36® form. This study is distinguished in that SF-36 data were collected repeatedly during dosing, as well as during the follow-up period. While this study failed to state how the results could be used to gain regulatory approval for the drug, the study did seem to provide a basis for giving patients advice on what to expect, in terms of quality of life, during and after anti-HCV treatment.

HRQoL tools are not often used in most clinical trials on chronic HCV (21). Instead, HRQoL tools for HCV are more used in ordinary clinical practice, when treating chronic HCV. HRQoL is a particular concern because interferon-alpha has the established adverse drug reaction of causing depression, and also because depression can arise from the HCV viral infection itself. HCV-induced depression arising from the infection itself was demonstrated by the fatigue-induced depression found in untreated HCV patients (22).

This concerns liver transplants. Chronic HCV-induced end-stage liver disease and chronic HCV-induced HCC are major reasons for liver transplants (23). Thus, HRQoL questionnaires have also been used in this context for liver transplants, that is, with HCV patients before and after a liver transplant (24).

[20]Mathew A, Peiffer LP, Rhoades K, McGarrity TJ. Improvement in quality of life measures in patients with refractory hepatitis C, responding to re-treatment with Pegylated interferon alpha-2b and ribavirin. Health Qual. Life Outcomes 2006;4:30−8.

[21]Bonkovsky HL, Snow KK, Malet PF, et al. Health-related quality of life in patients with chronic hepatitis C and advanced fibrosis. J. Hepatol. 2007;46:420−31.

[22]Castera L, Constant A, Bernard PH, de Ledinghen V, Couzigou P. Psychological impact of chronic hepatitis C: comparison with other stressful life events and chronic diseases. World J. Gastroenterol. 2006;12:1545−50.

[23]Kim WR, Terrault NA, Pedersen RA, et al. Trends in waiting list registration for liver transplantation for viral hepatitis in the United States. Gastroenterology 2009;137:1680−6.

[24]Russell RT, Feurer ID, Wisawatapnimit P, Lillie ES, Castaldo ET, Pinson CW. Profile of health-related quality of life outcomes after liver transplantation: univariate effects and multivariate models. HPB (Oxford) 2008;10:30−7.

25

Drug Safety

I. INTRODUCTION

The term *pharmacovigilance* refers to the process of identifying and responding to drug safety issues, where this process occurs during clinical trials as well as after regulatory approval (1). Drug safety data are collected or "captured" during the course of clinical trials intended for regulatory approval, as well as after approval (2).

The goals of phase I clinical trials include determining drug safety, characterizing the drug's pharmacokinetic (PK) and pharmacodynamic (PD) properties, and acquiring information useful for arriving at the most optimal dose for phase II and phase III clinical trials. Information on optimal dose encompasses the amount of drug to be administered, route of administration, and timing of doses. The main goals of phase II and III clinical trials are to acquire information on both safety and efficacy.

Safety is determined by capturing adverse events (AEs), and then determining which AEs result from the disease, which AEs likely arise from the drug, and which AEs are irrelevant to the disease or to the drug. Adverse events encompass all unfavorable events, including those caused by the drug, those caused by the disease being treated, and those resulting from causes that appear irrelevant to the drug or disease, such as automobile accidents. The subset of AEs that is caused by any given drug is called *adverse drug reactions* (ADRs).

Adverse events may be observed and captured by the clinician or, alternatively, by the study subject. Adverse events, and other information on the disease and drug that are captured by the study subject, are called patient-reported outcomes (PROs) (3).

Generally, regulatory approval is a function of both efficacy and safety. But extra emphasis may be placed on safety in a type of trial design called a noninferiority clinical trial.

[1]Talbot JC, Nilsson BS. Pharmacovigilance in the pharmaceutical industry. Br. J. Clin. Pharmacol. 1998;45:427–31.

[2]Scharf O, Colevas AD. Adverse event reporting in publications compared with sponsor database for cancer clinical trials. J. Clin. Oncol. 2006;24:3933–8.

[3]U.S. Department of Health and Human Services. Food and Drug Administration. Guidance for industry. Patient-reported outcome measures: use in medical product development to support labeling claims; December 2009 (43 pp.).

In this type of trial, the basis of approval can be more a function of improved safety, and less a function (or not at all a function) of improved efficacy. According to the European Medicines Agency (EMA), "a noninferiority trial aims to demonstrate that the test product is not worse than the comparator by more than a pre-specified, small amount" (4). In comments on noninferiority trials, Pocock (5) observed that the main motivation of the sponsor may be to demonstrate that, "[t]he new treatment has less side-effects," or that "[t]he new treatment is less invasive." According to the FDA's Guidance for Industry (6), noninferiority trials find a basis in the Code of Federal Regulations (CFR) (21 CFR §314.126 (a)(2)(iv)).

Castle and Kelly (7) caution that details for reporting adverse events to regulatory agencies can differ in the United States and in Europe. These differences include whether all adverse events are to be reported, or if only AEs with a likely causal relation should be reported. In Europe, safety reports submitted by the CIOMS form are restricted to ADRs, that is, adverse events where the physician has judged it a reasonable possibility that the observed clinical occurrence was caused by the drug (8). Another difference is whether the AE is reported as arising from a specific drug, or from a class of drugs. Yet another difference is whether the AE is reported as arising from the drug, with reference to the chemical name, or with reference to the drug's brand name.

The above list of differences between US and European requirements is likely to change, over the course of time. But the take-home lesson is that investigators need to be vigilant regarding differences in safety reporting that might exist between US and European regulatory agencies.

a. Overview of Drug Safety

The topics of this chapter appear in the order shown by the bullet points:

- *Examples of adverse events.* Safety data from a publication devoted to adverse events arising from interferon-treatment.
- *Planning for adverse events in the design of clinical studies.* In designing a clinical trial, and writing the Clinical Study Protocol, the investigator might need to include special instructions regarding AEs that are expected, that is, expected from the disease or treatment. These special instructions include techniques for monitoring AEs and for modifying doses in response to AEs.
- *Dose modification.* One type of special instruction is *dose modification.* Examples from actual Clinical Study Protocols are included in this chapter.
- *Safety definitions.* The relevant safety definitions are those provided by regulatory agencies (not definitions from medical textbooks or journal articles). Accurate interpretations of data from any clinical trial, and accurate review by regulatory agencies, hinges on the investigator's awareness of and conformity to these safety definitions.

---

[4]European Medicines Agency. Guideline on the choice of the non-inferiority margin; 2005 (11 pp.).

[5]Pocock SJ. The pros and cons of noninferiority trials. Fundam. Clin. Pharmacol. 2003;17:483–90.

[6]U.S. Department of Health and Human Services. Food and Drug Administration. Guidance for industry. Non-inferiority clinical trials; March 2010.

[7]Castle GH, Kelly B. Global harmonization is not all that global: divergent approaches in drug safety. Food Drug Law J. 2008;63:601.

[8]Mann RD, Andrews EB. Pharmacovigilance. 2nd ed. New York: Wiley; 2007. p. 289.

- *Classification of adverse events as induced by disease versus induced by the study drug.* Proper alignment of any given AE with the safety definitions might require an awareness of whether the AE was induced by the disease, induced by the study drug, produced by the simultaneous presence of both disease and study drug, or produced by the study drug in combination with lingering biochemical or physiological effects from a previously administered drug.

- *Classification of adverse events by considerations used by statisticians.* This further develops the topics of intent-to-treat (ITT) analysis and per protocol (PP) analysis.

- *Classification of adverse events as anticipated versus unanticipated.* An awareness of this classification can influence how AEs are reported to regulatory agencies.

- *Using adverse event data to acquire cause-and-effect information on ADRs.* An awareness of this issue can also influence how AEs are reported to regulatory agencies. This introduces the Naranjo algorithm.

- *Paradoxical ADRs.* The paradoxical nature of some AEs may impair an investigator's ability to anticipate these AEs before embarking on a clinical trial, and may impact the way the paradoxical AEs are reported to regulatory agencies.

- *Monitoring and evaluating adverse events.* This material constitutes a shift in the chapter from issues that are medical and scientific, to issues relating to the processes of managing drug safety reporting. This introduces the job of the data manager, and a form called the Case Report Form (CRF).

- *Adverse events—capturing, transmitting, and evaluating data on adverse events.* This introduces the topic of transmitting and routing of reports of AEs, from any given clinical trial.

- *Forms for reporting of adverse events.* This reveals special forms for capturing AEs from individual patients, for use in clinical trials, or for use by the general public outside of any clinical trial.

- *Risk minimization tools.* This focuses mainly on *Dear Healthcare Professional* letters. Candid, unbiased accounts of risk minimization tools, such as *Dear Healthcare Professional* letters, consent forms, and package inserts, are available from published courtroom cases. Information about the content of these letters can also be found on the FDA's website at the location, "Approved Risk Evaluation and Mitigation Strategies (REMS)." The most comprehensive and reliable source of information on REMS is that which is published on the FDA's website, for any given drug, at the same time that the FDA publishes its *Approval Letter.*

- *Patient-reported outcomes.* PROs encompass both safety and efficacy reporting.

- *Data and Safety Monitoring Committee.* This Committee plays a major role in regulated clinical trials. The Committee meets at regular intervals, reviews data on safety and efficacy, has the authority to unblind data, and recommends (but does not mandate) changes in the clinical trial. A typical recommendation is that of halting the clinical trial.

b. Examples of Adverse Events

The example of interferon-alpha-2b (IFN-alpha-2b) provides a concrete example of various adverse events. This drug is mainly used for treating melanoma (9), leukemias and

[9]Hauschild A, Gogas H, Tarhini A, et al. Practical guidelines for the management of interferon-alpha-2b side effects in patients receiving adjuvant treatment for melanoma: expert opinion. Cancer 2008;112:982−94.

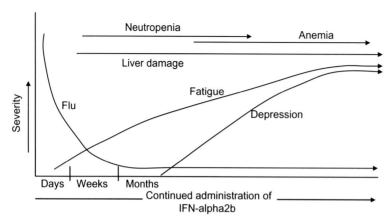

FIGURE 25.1 Adverse events occurring with administration of IFN-alpha-2b. The adverse events include hematological parameters, that is, neutrophil counts and red blood cell counts, as well as PROs, fatigue and depression.

lymphomas (10,11,12), and infections by hepatitis B virus and hepatitis C virus (13,14), IFN-alpha-2b, as well as all other interferons, are in a class of proteins called cytokines. Hauschild et al. (15), provides a review of the adverse events produced by IFN-alpha-2b.

Figure 25.1 (16) describes the adverse events in this bulletpoint list:

- flu,
- neutropenia,
- hepatic damage,
- anemia,
- fatigue,
- depression.

The figure shows the time course of AEs, with continued drug administration, over the course of days, weeks, and months. The listed AEs are those that were specifically caused by the drug.

Neutropenia refers to low neutrophil counts. Neutrophils, which represent the first line of defense against invading bacteria, are part of the innate immunity component of the immune system. Anemia refers to low red blood cell counts. Liver damage is routinely determined

[10]Smith SM, Johnson J, Cheson BD, et al. Recombinant interferon-alpha2b added to oral cyclophosphamide either as induction or maintenance in treatment-naive follicular lymphoma: final analysis of CALGB 8691. Leuk. Lymphoma 2009;50:1606–17.

[11]Baccarani M, Martinelli G, Rosti G, et al. Imatinib and pegylated human recombinant interferon-alpha2b in early chronic-phase chronic myeloid leukemia. Blood 2004;104:4245–51.

[12]Sirohi B, Powles R, Lawrence D, et al. An open, randomized, controlled, phase II, single centre, two-period crossover study to compare the quality of life and toxicity experienced on PEG interferon with interferon-alpha2b in patients with multiple myeloma maintained on a steady dose of interferon-alpha2b. Ann. Oncol. 2007;18:1388–94.

[13]Lee S, Kim IH, Kim SH, et al. Efficacy and tolerability of pegylated interferon-alpha2a plus ribavirin versus pegylated interferon-alpha2b plus ribavirin in treatment-naive chronic hepatitis C patients. Intervirology 2010;53:146–153.

[14]Shamliyan TA, MacDonald R, Shaukat A, et al. Antiviral therapy for adults with chronic hepatitis B: a systematic review for a National Institutes of Health Consensus Development Conference. Ann. Intern. Med. 2009;150:111–24.

[15]Hauschild A, Gogas H, Tarhini A, et al. Practical guidelines for the management of interferon-alpha-2b side effects in patients receiving adjuvant treatment for melanoma: expert opinion. Cancer 2008;112:982–94.

[16]Hauschild A, Gogas H, Tarhini A, et al. Practical guidelines for the management of interferon-alpha-2b side effects in patients receiving adjuvant treatment for melanoma: expert opinion. Cancer 2008;112:982–94.

by laboratory tests for the serum levels of the enzyme, alanine aminotransferase (ALT). This enzyme was formerly known as glutamate pyruvate transaminase (SGPT).

The presentation of the ADR of flu-like symptoms declined with continued administration of the drug. In other words, the patient develops tolerance. This phenomenon of tolerance is called *tachyphylaxis*. The flu-like symptoms are fever, chills, headache, myalgia, nausea, and vomiting. Fatigue increases in intensity as therapy continues and it can be very debilitating. Levels of hepatic enzymes, as measured in serum samples, are assayed on a weekly basis in order to monitor drug-induced liver toxicity. Where liver toxicity presents, the physician may respond by lowering the dose, or delaying dosing, of the IFN-alpha2b. In the context of a clinical trial, this response is called *dose modification*.

c. Anticipating Adverse Events in the Design of Clinical Studies

Planning the study design includes planning which types of adverse events should be monitored. According to the ICH Guidelines (17):

> [a] hierarchy of organ systems can be developed according to their importance with respect to life-supporting functions. Vital organs or systems, the functions of which are acutely critical for life, such as the cardiovascular, respiratory and central nervous systems, are considered to be the most important ones to assess in safety pharmacology studies. Other organ systems, such as the renal or gastrointestinal system, the functions of which can be transiently disrupted by adverse pharmacodynamic effects without

causing irreversible harm, are of less immediate investigative concern.

The ICH Guidelines specifically focus on adverse events involving the immune system, and where these adverse events reside in two categories, namely, where a study drug impairs the immune system, and where the study drug induces immune-system-mediated harm to various tissues of the body (18):

> Toxicity to the immune system encompasses a variety of adverse effects. These include suppression or enhancement of the immune response. Suppression of the immune response can lead to decreased host resistance to infectious agents or tumor cells. Enhancing the immune response can exaggerate autoimmune diseases or hypersensitivity. Drug or drug--protein adducts might also be recognized as foreign and stimulate an anti-drug response. Subsequent exposures to the drug can lead to hypersensitivity (allergic) reactions.

d. Dose Modification as Part of the Clinical Study Protocol

The Clinical Study Protocol optionally includes instructions for dose modification. Dose modifications can include changing dose levels, delaying doses, changing the frequency of dosing, permanent discontinuation, and so on. Where dose modification is not appropriate, then the Clinical Study Protocol should state that dose modification is not allowed. An example of this prohibition appears, for example, in a Clinical Study Protocol for a cystic fibrosis drug. The Protocol reads "**Dose Modification for Toxicity.** No change in dosing of lumacaftor or ivacaftor is permitted" (19).

[17]ICH Harmonised Tripartite Guideline. Safety pharmacology studies for human pharmaceuticals S7A. Step 4 version; November 2000. 9 pp.

[18]ICH Harmonised Tripartite Guideline. Immunotoxicity studies for human pharmaceuticals S8. Step 4 version; September 2005. 14 pp.

[19]Clinical Study Protocol A Phase 3, randomized, double-blind, placebo-controlled, parallel-group study to evaluate the efficacy and safety of lumacaftor in combination with ivacaftor in subjects aged 12 years and older with cystic fibrosis, homozygous for the f508del-CFTR mutation vertex study number: VX12-809-103 Lumacaftor IND No: 79,521 Ivacaftor IND No: 74,633 EUDRACT No: 2012-003989-40.

Clinical trials can include dose modifications that *reduce dosing*, as detailed below, but also dose modifications that *increase dosing*. Increased dosing was used, for example, in the following clinical trial on leukemia. Where a starting dose of 400 mg imatinib per day was found to produce only partial response, the dose was increased to two 400 mg imatinib doses per day (20). *Dose escalations* have also been used, for example (21), in clinical trials of nonsmall-cell lung cancer (NSCLC) (22), breast cancer (23), and colorectal cancer (24), with the goal of improving drug efficacy against the cancer. Where an unanticipated need arises to increase dosing, and if the Protocol provides no guidance for increased dosing, the Protocol will likely need to be amended to allow for the increased dose. Bander et al. (25) provide an example of a dose-increasing amendment. Amending the Clinical Study Protocol requires approval by the Institutional Review Board (IRB) and the FDA.

Dose reduction is the more common type of dose modification. Dose modification encompasses dose reduction and delays in administering doses subsequent to an intolerable adverse event. In clinical trials involving cytotoxic drugs,

it is useful to include instructions in the Clinical Study Protocol for reducing or delaying the dose, in the event that a drug-related adverse event occurs. Where drug-related adverse events are detected in the course of a clinical trial, the presence of a dose-reduction scheme in the Protocol enables the investigator to lower the dose and retain the subject in the clinical trial. But absence of any dose reduction or dose-delaying instructions may necessitate discontinuing the subject from the clinical trial, or a time-consuming amendment to the Protocol.

Guidance for writing dose modification instructions comes from the medical literature, as revealed by these representative examples. This is an example of a dose modification scheme from a Clinical Study Protocol on leukemia, where the study drugs were *imatinib* and *nilotinib*. As is evident, the safety parameter of interest is blood platelets. As can be seen, dose modification includes withholding the drug until recovery occurs, as well as dose reduction (26,27):

If platelets $\leq 100 \times 10^9$/L, withhold treatment with study drug until recovery to at least $>100 \times 10^9$/L and resume treatment at same dose.

[20]O'Brien SG, Guilhot F, Larson RA, et al. Imatinib compared with interferon and low-dose cytarabine for newly diagnosed chronic-phase chronic myeloid leukemia. New Engl. J. Med. 2003;348:994−1004.

[21]These examples were found by inputting the search term "could be escalated."

[22]Schiller JH, Larson T, Ou SH, et al. Efficacy and safety of axitinib in patients with advanced non-small-cell lung cancer: results from a phase II study. J. Clin. Oncol. 2009;27:3836−41.

[23]O'Shaughnessy J, Miles D, Vukelja S, et al. Superior survival with capecitabine plus docetaxel combination therapy in anthracycline-pretreated patients with advanced breast cancer: phase III trial results. J. Clin. Oncol. 2002;20:2812−23.

[24]Van Cutsem E, Twelves C, Cassidy J, et al. Oral capecitabine compared with intravenous fluorouracil plus leucovorin in patients with metastatic colorectal cancer: results of a large phase III study. J. Clin. Oncol. 2001;19:4097−106.

[25]Bander NH, Milowsky MI, Nanus DM, et al. Phase I trial of 177lutetium-labeled J591, a monoclonal antibody to prostate-specific membrane antigen, in patients with androgen-independent prostate cancer. J. Clin. Oncol. 2005;23:4591−601.

[26]Clinical Study Protocol for Saglio G, Kim D-W, Issaragrisil S, et al. Nilotinib versus imatinib for newly diagnosed chronic myeloid leukemia. New Engl. J. Med. 2010;362:2251−9.

[27]Quote reproduced by permission of Dr G. Saglio. E-mail of April 25, 2011.

If recurrence of platelets $\leq 100 \times 10^9$/L, then withhold treatment until recovery to at least $>100 \times 10^9$/L and resume treatment at 50% of the dose to a minimum dose of 300 mg/day for imatinib. The nilotinib dose may be reduced to a minimum of 400 mg/day. If the platelet count remains below 100×10^9/L, then imatinib or nilotinib should be ceased or management with anticoagulation therapy re-evaluated at the discretion of the Investigator.

In an oncology clinical trial with *sorafenib*, Zhao et al. (28) mandated that unacceptable toxicity must trigger a dose modification scheme consisting of delaying the next dose until the toxicity subsided. Zhao et al. (29) mandated an alternate dose modification scheme, where dose must be reduced by one level, that is, from two doses per day (b.i.d.) to one dose per day, or a reduction of one dose per day (q.d.) to one dose every other day (q.o.d.). Moreover, the dose modification scheme also mandated that subjects requiring over two dose modifications must be dropped from the study.

In an oncology clinical trial with *temozolomide*, Siena et al. (30) set forth a dose modification scheme that included both dose delay and dose reduction. The authors observed that thrombocytopenia was the adverse event that most frequently necessitated dose reduction or treatment discontinuation. In the following dose modification scheme, ANC means *absolute neutrophil count*: "The dose was reduced to 125 mg/m^2/day if ANC was <500 cells/μl for 5 days, if ANC was <500 cells/μl with fever and/or platelet count $<25\,000$/μl." (31).

Hauschild et al. (32) provide comprehensive instructions for dose modification, with separate instructions correlated with the type of adverse event, where the adverse events include psoriasis, granulocytopenia, depression, fatigue, and hepatotoxicity. The drug in question is *IFN-alpha-2b*, a drug specifically noted for the ADRs of depression and fatigue.

Li et al. (33) describe a common situation, namely, the administration of two concurrent drugs. In this case, the two drugs were *tipifarnib* and *fulvestrant*. The dose modification scheme mandated that, in the situation where tipifarnib was held for toxicity, the dosing of the other drug (fulvestrant) should not be modified.

[28]Zhao JD, Liu J, Ren ZG, et al. Maintenance of Sorafenib following combined therapy of three-dimensional conformal radiation therapy/intensity-modulated radiation therapy and transcatheter arterial chemoembolization in patients with locally advanced hepatocellular carcinoma: a phase I/II study. Radiat. Oncol. 2010;5:12 (7 pp.).

[29]Zhao JD, Liu J, Ren ZG, et al. Maintenance of Sorafenib following combined therapy of three-dimensional conformal radiation therapy/intensity-modulated radiation therapy and transcatheter arterial chemoembolization in patients with locally advanced hepatocellular carcinoma: a phase I/II study. Radiat. Oncol. 2010;5:12 (7 pp.).

[30]Siena S, Crinò L, Danova M, et al. Dose-dense temozolomide regimen for the treatment of brain metastases from melanoma, breast cancer, or lung cancer not amenable to surgery or radiosurgery: a multicenter phase II study. Ann. Oncol. 2010;21:655−61.

[31]Siena S, Crinò L, Danova M, et al. Dose-dense temozolomide regimen for the treatment of brain metastases from melanoma, breast cancer, or lung cancer not amenable to surgery or radiosurgery: a multicenter phase II study. Ann. Oncol. 2010;21:655−61.

[32]Hauschild A, Gogas H, Tarhini A, et al. Practical guidelines for the management of interferon-alpha-2b side effects in patients receiving adjuvant treatment for melanoma: expert opinion. Cancer 2008;112:982−94.

[33]Li T, Christos PJ, Sparano JA, et al. Phase II trial of the farnesyltransferase inhibitor tipifarnib plus fulvestrant in hormone receptor-positive metastatic breast cancer: New York Cancer Consortium Trial P6205. Ann. Oncol. 2009;20:642−7.

Dose modification may take the form of interrupting treatment, and later resuming treatment (34). Where a dose interruption scheme is included in the Clinical Study Protocol, data from subjects with interrupted doses do not have to be excluded from the ITT analysis.

Dose modification schemes for a variety of other anticancer drugs have been published, for example, for oxaliplatin (35), sunitinib plus bevacizumab combination (36), dasatinib (37), and bortexomib (38).

Other examples of dose modification schemes can be found in Clinical Study Protocols from studies on human immunodeficiency virus (HIV) (39), on colorectal cancer (40), on adrenocortical carcinoma (41), on NSCLC (42), and on cancer of the head and neck (43), as cited.

An adverse event need not be life-threatening in order to mandate dose modification. In a description of skin reactions from sorafenib and sunitinib, Lacouture et al. (44) detail the hand and foot skin reactions occurring with use of these drugs, and schemes for dose reduction. The hand and foot skin reactions include blisters, necrosis, pain, reduction in mobility, and loss of weight-bearing ability of feet. The recommended dose reduction is a 50% reduction in drug dose for at least 7 days, while the recommended drug delay is discontinuing the drug for at least 7 days. These recommendations are keyed to, or coupled with, a standard grading scale for skin reaction severity.

Abnormal laboratory values can trigger the requirement for withholding or discontinuing the study drug, placebo, or active control.

[34]Llovet JM, Ricci S, Mazzaferro V, et al. Sorafenib in advanced hepatocellular carcinoma. New Engl. J. Med. 2008;359:378–90.

[35]Saif MW, Reardon J. Management of oxaliplatin-induced peripheral neuropathy. Ther. Clin. Risk Manag. 2005;1:249–58.

[36]Rini BI, Garcia JA, Cooney MM, et al. A phase I study of sunitinib plus bevacizumab in advanced solid tumors. Clin. Cancer Res. 2009;15:6277–83.

[37]Cortes J, Rousselot P, Kim DW, et al. Dasatinib induces complete hematologic and cytogenetic responses in patients with imatinib-resistant or -intolerant chronic myeloid leukemia in blast crisis. Blood 2007;109:3207–13.

[38]Argyriou AA, Iconomou G, Kalofonos HP. Bortezomib-induced peripheral neuropathy in multiple myeloma: a comprehensive review of the literature. Blood 2008;112:1593–9.

[39]Sax PE, Tierney C, Collier AC, et al. Abacavir–lamivudine versus tenofovir–emtricitabine for initial HIV-1 therapy. New Engl. J. Med. 2009;361:2230–40.

[40]STUDY ID (ML 19033) EUDRACT no: 2006-002295-18 Avastin and Chemotherapy followed by Avastin alone or in combination with Tarceva for the treatment of metastatic colorectal cancer.

[41]First International Randomized Trial in Locally Advanced and Metastatic Adrenocortical Carcinoma Treatment (FIRM-ACT) Etoposide, Doxorubicin, Cisplatin and Mitotane vs. Streptozotocin and Mitotane. Collaborative Group for Adrenocortical Carcinoma Therapy-COACT-CLINICAL STUDY PROTOCOL; April 12, 2004.

[42]A Phase III Randomized Trial of Adjuvant Chemotherapy With or Without Bevacizumab for Patients With Completely Resected Stage IB (>4 cm)—IIIA Non-Small Cell Lung Cancer (NSCLC). E1501. Revised April 2008.

[43]A Randomized Phase II Trial of Concurrent Radiation and Chemotherapy for Advanced Squamous Cell Carcinomas of the Head and Neck. RTOG 97-03; September 8, 1998.

[44]Lacouture ME, Wu S, Robert C, et al. Evolving strategies for the management of hand-foot skin reaction associated with the multitargeted kinase inhibitors sorafenib and sunitinib. Oncologist 2008;13:1001–11.

TABLE 25.1 Laboratory Criteria Requiring Withholding or Permanent Discontinuation of Blinded Study Treatment With BG00012/Placebo

Laboratory Parameter	Laboratory Result	Required Action
AST (SGOT) or ALT (SGPT)	$>3 \times$ ULN	The Investigator should repeat the test as soon as possible. If retest value confirms AST or ALT $>3 \times$ ULN, the study treatment must be withheld. If the value remains $>3 \times$ ULN for greater or equal to 4 weeks after discontinuation of study treatment, then the subject **must *permanently* discontinue study treatment**
Creatinine	$>1.2 \times$ ULN	The Investigator should repeat the test as soon as possible. If retest value confirms that creatinine $>1.2 \times$ ULN, the study treatment must be withheld. If the value remains $>1.2 \times$ ULN for ≥ 4 weeks after discontinuation of study treatment, then the subject **must *permanently* discontinue study treatment**
White blood cell (WBC)	$<2000/mm^3$	The Investigator should repeat the test as soon as possible. If retest value confirms that WBC $<2000/mm^3$, the study treatment must be withheld. If the value remains $<2000/mm^3$ for greater or equal to 4 weeks after discontinuation of study treatment, then the subject **must *permanently* discontinue study treatment**
Urine cytology	Positive	Urine cytology must be performed on any subject who has hematuria of unknown etiology on two consecutive visits. If urine cytology is positive, then the subject **must *permanently* discontinue study treatment**

An exemplary account of instructions for dose withholding or permanent discontinuation, in response to abnormal laboratory values, is provided in a Clinical Study Protocol used in a clinical trial on multiple sclerosis (45,46). The Protocol provided brief instructions and a table (see Table 25.1). The instructions read, "Dosing Interruption for Abnormal Laboratory Values ... treatment with [study drug or] placebo must be temporarily withheld when any of the following laboratory values meet the threshold limits defined in Table 11.2-1." This table is reproduced here, as Table 25.1.

Table 25.1 provides instructions for dose withholding and also for permanent discontinuation. The emphasis (bold) is in the original table. The term "ULN" means, upper limit of normal. The terms AST (SGOT) and ALT (SGPT) refer to enzymes (aminotransferases) that are released by the liver into the serum, where elevated serum levels indicate liver damage. In the table, the term "BG00012" is the study drug, which is also known as dimethyl fumarate.

e. FDA's Warning Letter on Dose Modification

On occasion, the FDA issues Warning Letters to the Sponsor when there are repeated and uncorrected violations of instructions in the Clinical Study Protocol, or of other

[45]A Randomized, Multicenter, Placebo-Controlled and Active Reference (Glatiramer Acetate) Comparison Study to Evaluate the Efficacy and Safety of BG00012 in Subjects With Relapsing-Remitting Multiple Sclerosis. EUDRA CT NO: 2006-003697-10. DATE: 09 January 2008. Protocol No. 109MS302. Version 4.

[46]The Clinical Study Protocol is a supplement to, Fox RJ, Miller DH, Phillips JT, et al. Placebo-controlled phase 3 study of oral BG-12 or glatiramer in multiple sclerosis. New Engl. J. Med. 2012;367:1087−97.

requirements set forth by Title 21 of the CFR. This provides an example of a Warning Letter that complained about the Sponsor's failure to comply with the dose modification scheme. The Warning Letter reiterated the dose modification scheme, and then complained about failure of the Sponsor to comply with this scheme. The Warning Letter stated that (47):

> From our review of the FDA establishment inspection report … and your … written response, we conclude that you did not adhere to the applicable … FDA regulations governing the conduct of clinical investigations … [t]he … Protocol required that you … hold or adjust the dose of the investigational drug in managing specific drug-related adverse events … Protocol requires that you stop dosing … in subjects with an increase of 0.5 mg/dL from a normal baseline creatinine that is greater than the institutional upper limit of normal (IULN) … until serum creatinine returns to within 10% of baseline. Subject 222626, who was randomized to Treatment Arm 2 (clodronate), met this protocol criterion for stopping the dosing of clodronate, and yet the subject continued to receive clodronate for more than one year after meeting the criterion … [f]or Subject 222626, you failed to stop dosing of clodronate until January 24, 2012, more than one year after you should have done so.

The Warning Letter concluded with the warning that "[w]ithin fifteen (15) working days of your receipt of this letter, you should notify this office of the actions you have taken to prevent similar violations in the future. Failure to address the violations … may result in regulatory action without further notice."

II. SAFETY DEFINITIONS

a. Definitions From US and European Regulatory Agencies

FDA's Guidance for Industry provides the following definitions for safety terms (48). The EMA also provides safety definitions, but these definitions may differ somewhat from those of the FDA (49). Investigators and medical writers need to compare safety definitions in these three sources: CFR, ICH Guidelines, and the FDA's Guidance for Industry.

Definitions for adverse events find a basis in the CFR. For example, 21 CFR 310.305(b) provides that adverse events include (50):

> Any adverse event associated with the use of a drug in humans, whether or not considered drug related, including the following: An adverse event occurring in the course of the use of a drug product in professional practice; an adverse event occurring from drug overdose whether accidental or intentional; an adverse event occurring from drug abuse; an adverse event occurring from drug withdrawal; and any failure of expected pharmacological action.

This part of the CFR also defines a serious adverse drug experience, as follows (51):

> Any adverse drug experience occurring at any dose that results in any of the following outcomes: Death, a life-threatening adverse drug experience, inpatient hospitalization or prolongation of existing hospitalization, a persistent or significant disability/incapacity, or a congenital anomaly/birth defect.

---

[47]FDA Warning Letter Ref: 14-HFD-45-04-0, dated April 28, 2014, issued by Dr Sean Y. Kassim, Ph.D. Acting Director, CDER, FDA.

[48]U.S. Department of Health and Human Services. Food and Drug Administration. Guidance for industry. E6 good clinical practice:consolidated guidance; April 1996.

[49]ICH Topic E 2 A Clinical Safety Data Management: Definitions and Standards for Expedited Reporting; June 1995.

[50]21 CFR 310.305(b) (April 1, 2010 version).

[51]21 CFR 310.305(b) (April 1, 2010 version).

Important medical events that may not result in death, be life-threatening, or require hospitalization may be considered a serious adverse drug experience when, based upon appropriate medical judgment, they may jeopardize the patient or subject and may require medical or surgical intervention to prevent one of the outcomes listed in this definition. Examples of such medical events include allergic bronchospasm requiring intensive treatment in an emergency room or at home, blood dyscrasias or convulsions that do not result in inpatient hospitalization, or the development of drug dependency or drug abuse.

The investigator and medical writer may want to review the *Federal Register*, from time to time, to learn of proposed definitions relating to drug safety and efficacy. In the *Federal Register*, when there is an actual change in the law, it is called a "Final Rule."

1. Adverse Events

FDA's Guidance for Industry provides the following definition of adverse events (AEs) (52):

> An AE is any untoward medical occurrence in a patient or clinical investigation subject administered a pharmaceutical product and that does not necessarily have a causal relationship with this treatment. An AE can therefore be any unfavorable and unintended sign (including an abnormal laboratory finding), symptom, or disease temporally associated with the use of a medicinal (investigational) product, whether or not related to the medicinal (investigational) product.

2. Serious Adverse Event

FDA's Guidance for Industry provides the following definition of serious adverse events (SAEs) (53):

> Any untoward medical occurrence that at any dose:
>
> - Results in death,
> - Is life-threatening,
> - Requires inpatient hospitalization or prolongation of existing hospitalization,
> - Results in persistent or significant disability/incapacity, or
> - Is a congenital anomaly/birth defect.

3. Abnormal Laboratory Values can be Adverse Events, and They can Also be SAEs

FDA's Guidance for Industry (54) teaches that abnormal laboratory values can be considered to be adverse events, and can also be considered to be SAEs and therefore subject to the applicable reporting requirements. Regarding abnormal laboratory values of liver-related laboratory values (aminotransferases; bilirubin), highly abnormal liver-related laboratory values (55), "should be handled as a serious unexpected adverse event associated with the use of the drug and reported to the FDA promptly (i.e., even before all other possible causes of liver injury have been excluded). It should be promptly reported to the FDA before fully working up the patient to rule out other

[52]U.S. Department of Health and Human Services. Food and Drug Administration. Guidance for industry. E6 good clinical practice: consolidated guidance; April 1996.

[53]U.S. Department of Health and Human Services. Food and Drug Administration. Guidance for industry. E6 good clinical practice:consolidated guidance; April 1996.

[54]U.S. Department of Health and Human Services. Food and Drug Administration. Guidance for industry. Drug-induced liver injury: premarketing clinical evaluation; July 2009 (25 pp.).

[55]U.S. Department of Health and Human Services. Food and Drug Administration. Guidance for industry. Drug-induced liver injury: premarketing clinical evaluation; July 2009 (25 pp.).

etiologies." Abnormal liver transaminase levels, that is, as measured in the serum, are distinguished in that they are often the result of factors other than the study drug, such as hepatitis C virus and nonalcoholic steatohepatitis (56). An excerpt from a Clinical Study Protocol on a drug for hepatitis C virus establishes that the medical writer has the option of including instructions (in the Protocol) for reporting laboratory values. The excerpt reads (57), "laboratory abnormalities (e.g. clinical chemistry, hematology, urinalysis) independent of the underlying medical condition that require medical or surgical intervention or lead to investigational medicinal product interruption or discontinuation must be recorded as an AE, as well as an SAE, if applicable."

4. Adverse Drug Reaction

FDA's Guidance for Industry provides the following definition of ADRs (58):

In the pre-approval clinical experience with a new medicinal product or its new usages, particularly as the therapeutic dose(s) may not be established, all noxious and unintended responses to a medicinal product related to any dose should be considered adverse drug reactions. The phrase "responses to a medicinal product" means that a causal relationship between a medicinal product and an adverse event is at least a reasonable possibility, i.e., the relationship cannot be ruled out. Regarding marketed medicinal products: A response to a drug

that is noxious and unintended and that occurs at doses normally used in man for prophylaxis, diagnosis, or therapy of diseases or for modification of physiological function.

5. Unexpected Adverse Drug Reactions

FDA's Guidance for Industry provides the following definition of unexpected drug reactions (59):

An "unexpected adverse drug reaction" is an adverse reaction, the nature or severity of which is not consistent with the applicable product information (e.g., Investigator's Brochure for an unapproved investigational product or package insert/summary of product characteristics for an approved product).

This provides an example where a Clinical Study Protocol expressly stated that a given drug-related adverse event was expected. The narrative based expectedness on the mechanism of action. This is from a clinical trial on leukemia. The Protocol read (60):

Treatment-related lymphocytosis, for the purposes of this protocol, is defined as an elevation in blood lymphocyte count of >50% compared to baseline that occurs in the setting of ... improvement in at least one other disease-related parameter including lymph node size, spleen size, hematologic parameters (Hgb or platelet count), or disease-related symptoms. Given the **known mechanism of action** of BCR-inhibiting agents including ibrutinib,

[56] U.S. Department of Health and Human Services. Food and Drug Administration. Guidance for industry. Drug-induced liver injury: premarketing clinical evaluation; July 2009 (25 pp.).

[57] The Clinical Study Protocol was included as a supplement to, Jacobson IM, Gordon SC, Kowdley KV, et al. Sofosbuvir for hepatitis C genotype 2 or 3 in patients without treatment options. New Engl. J. Med. 2013;368:1867–77.

[58] U.S. Department of Health and Human Services. Food and Drug Administration. Guidance for industry. E6 good clinical practice:consolidated guidance; April 1996.

[59] U.S. Department of Health and Human Services. Food and Drug Administration. Guidance for industry. E6 good clinical practice: consolidated guidance; April 1996.

[60] A randomized, multicenter, open-label, phase 3 study of the Bruton's tyrosine kinase (BTK) inhibitor ibrutinib versus ofatumumab in patients with relapsed or refractory chronic lymphocytic leukemia/small lymphocytic lymphoma. NCT01578707; Phase 3. ORIGINAL PROTOCOL PCYC-1112-CA.

treatment-related lymphocytosis is an **expected and frequent pharmacodynamic phenomenon** observed with initiation (or re-initiation) of ibrutinib. Ibrutinib associated treatment-related lymphocytosis generally occurs within the first few weeks of therapy, peaks within the first few months, and resolves slowly.

6. Potential Confusion in Defining Adverse Events

Defining terms used to characterize drug safety is not a trivial issue. Ioannidis et al. (61) find that some publications use the terms *side effects* and *adverse effects* to mean the same thing, thus creating confusion. Regarding this inappropriate use of terms, Ioannidis et al. (62) complain that, some authors use the term *adverse events* synonymously with *side effects.* What is inappropriate is that the term *side effects* implies that the drug causes the side effect while, in contrast, the term adverse effects does not imply causality.

Moreover, ICH Guidelines (63) expressly recommend not using the term, side effect, writing that, "[t]he old term 'side effect' has been used in various ways in the past, usually to describe negative (unfavourable) effects, but also positive (favourable) effects. It is recommended that this term no longer be used and particularly should not be regarded as synonymous with adverse event or adverse reaction."

The CFR distinguishes between adverse events that are "expected" and that are "anticipated." To quote from 21 CFR §312.32(a),

> Unexpected adverse drug experience: Any adverse drug experience, the specificity or severity of

which is not consistent with the current investigator brochure ... [u]nexpected, as used in this definition, refers to an adverse drug experience that has not been previously observed (e.g., included in the investigator brochure) rather than from the perspective of such experience not being anticipated from the pharmacological properties of the pharmaceutical product.

To repeat, "expected" is not synonymous with "anticipated."

b. Classification of Adverse Events as Induced by Disease Versus Induced by the Study Drug

This distinguishes between AEs due to the disease and drug-induced AEs. This particular example is from the Council for International Organizations of Medical Sciences (CIOMS). The example provided by CIOMS concerns the AE of skin eruptions (64):

> In diagnosing a cutaneous eruption that may be an adverse drug reaction it is important to decide whether the eruption is due to the disease, primarily due to the drug, or due possibly to an interaction between the disease and the drug. Cutaneous reactions frequently occur when patients are receiving a number of drugs, and thus etiological relationship may be difficult to assess. When patients take drugs for a febrile disorder [increased body temperature] that ultimately proves to be an infection, an eruption may be due to the underlying disorder or the prescribed drug.

This concerns AEs that are accidents, such as accidents occurring when using machinery. Where a subject enrolled in a clinical study is

[61]Ioannidis JP, Evans SJ, Gøtzsche PC, et al. Better reporting of harms in randomized trials: an extension of the CONSORT statement. Ann. Intern. Med. 2004;141:781–8.

[62]Ioannidis JP, Evans SJ, Gøtzsche PC, et al. Better reporting of harms in randomized trials: an extension of the CONSORT statement. Ann. Intern. Med. 2004;141:781–8.

[63]ICH Topic E 2 A Clinical Safety Data Management: Definitions and Standards for Expedited Reporting; June 1995.

[64]Bankowski Z, Bruppacher R, Crusius I, Gallagher J, Kremer G, Venulet J. Reporting adverse drug reactions. Geneva: Council for International Organizations of Medical Sciences; 1999. 146 pp.

injured by an automobile accident, for example, on the way to the clinic, this injury is classified as an AE (65,66,67,68,69,70,71). Although some publications may state that injuries from accidents are not AEs (72), it is actually improper to exclude accidents from AEs. The layperson can readily appreciate the fact that drugs can cause drowsiness, or result in impaired vision (73), where the result is an accident that produces injury.

c. Classification of Adverse Events by Considerations Used by Statisticians

Adverse events can also be classified according to how a statistician would approach the data. These approaches include the following reporting (74):

- AEs by ITT analysis;
- AEs by PP analysis;

- Use of a severity threshold, that is, reporting of AEs only above a certain severity grade;
- Use of a prevalence threshold, that is, reporting of AEs occurring only above a certain percentage of patients;
- Outcomes of AEs, such as treatment discontinuations, dose reductions, and withdrawals from the study.

Although these types of adverse events generally fall under the umbrella of the biostatistician serving a clinical study, a typical medical writer will be familiar with all of these concepts.

d. ITT Analysis Versus PP Analysis for Assessing Safety

Clinical trials in regulated settings require collection of data on safety and efficacy. The FDA grants marketing approval for drug

[65]Soni MG, Carabin IG, Griffiths JC, Burdock GA. Safety of ephedra: lessons learned. Toxicol. Lett. 2004;150:97–110.

[66]Dienstag JL, Cianciara J, Karayalcin S, et al. Durability of serologic response after lamivudine treatment of chronic hepatitis B. Hepatology 2003;37:748–55.

[67]Douglas Jr JS, Holmes Jr DR, Kereiakes DJ, et al. Coronary stent restenosis in patients treated with cilostazol. Circulation 2005;112:2826–32.

[68]Garber A, Henry R, Ratner R, et al. Liraglutide versus glimepiride monotherapy for type 2 diabetes (LEAD-3 Mono): a randomised, 52-week, phase III, double-blind, parallel-treatment trial. Lancet 2009;373:473–81.

[69]Ramulu P. Glaucoma and disability: which tasks are affected, and at what stage of disease? Curr. Opin. Ophthalmol. 2009;20:92–8.

[70]Leung N, Peng CY, Hann HW, et al. Early hepatitis B virus DNA reduction in hepatitis B e antigen-positive patients with chronic hepatitis B: a randomized international study of entecavir versus adefovir. Hepatology 2009;49:72–9.

[71]Ennever JF. A user's guide to the RASCAL IRB module. Ver. 2.1. Columbia University Medical Center; 2006. 117 pp.

[72]NIMH Multisite HIV Prevention Trial. Definition of adverse reactions in clinical trials of a behavioral intervention. AIDS 1997;11:S55–7.

[73]Ramulu P. Glaucoma and disability: which tasks are affected, and at what stage of disease? Curr. Opin. Ophthalmol. 2009;20:92–8.

[74]Chowers MY, Gottesman BS, Leibovici L, Pielmeier U, Andreassen S, Paul M. Reporting of adverse events in randomized controlled trials of highly active antiretroviral therapy: systematic review. J. Antimicrob. Chemother. 2009;64:239–50.

products based on a review of safety and efficacy data (75). The EMA also requires that clinical trials provide data on safety and efficacy (76).

Safety data may be analyzed in ways that are different than for efficacy data. ITT analysis, modified ITT analysis, and PP analysis, have been applied differently for safety data and efficacy data. Where safety analysis is presented from a clinical trial, it is typically presented by way of ITT analysis, as the FDA requires all subjects exposed to the drug to be reported in the safety analysis (77).

Efficacy can be assessed by ITT analysis, but also by methods that apply to more restricted and smaller groups of study subjects. It is often the case that safety is assessed only by ITT analysis, or a slight variant thereof, while efficacy is assessed by ITT analysis and also by modified ITT analysis.

For example, adverse events from chemotherapy can be assessed within hours of administering the study drug. In the case of chemotherapy with cisplatin, the time to emesis is about 19 h (78). In the case of chemotherapy with cyclophosphamide, time to emesis is about 9 h (79). In the case of antibody therapy for multiple sclerosis, the time to an adverse allergic reaction is 2 h (80). In contrast, data on efficacy of drugs for chronic diseases may not reasonably be captured within the first few days after beginning therapy. Hence, it is intuitively obvious that ITT analysis is appropriate for analyzing data on safety, while smaller patient groups, that exclude certain study subjects, may be just as appropriate for assessing data on efficacy.

The following scenario refers to chronic diseases that require prolonged treatment to show efficacy, but may require only 1 day of treatment to show drug-related adverse events. Chronic diseases include, for example, cancer, multiple sclerosis, and hepatitis C.

ITT analysis may be reasonable for capturing safety data, because it includes subjects who present with adverse effects even with one dose. But modified ITT analysis, which can exclude subjects who, within the first week of the beginning the study, are found not to have satisfied the inclusion criteria or exclusion criteria, is a reasonable approach for assessing efficacy data.

In a study of antibiotics for peritonitis, Dupont et al. (81) assessed safety by ITT analysis, and assessed efficacy by modified ITT analysis.

[75]McKee A, Farrell AT, Pazdur R, Woodcock J. The role of the U.S. Food and Drug Administration review process: clinical trial endpoints in oncology. The Oncologist 2010;15(Suppl. 1):13–8.

[76]European Medicines Agency. ICH Topic E6. Notes for guidance on good clinical practice; July 2002.

[77]Weigelt JA. E-mail of August 15, 2010.

[78]Kris MG, Pendergrass KB, Navari RM, et al. Prevention of acute emesis in cancer patients following high-dose cisplatin with the combination of oral dolasetron and dexamethasone. J. Clin. Oncol. 1997;15:2135–8.

[79]Crucitt MA, Hyman W, Grote T, et al. Efficacy and tolerability of oral ondansetron versus prochlorperazine in the prevention of emesis associated with cyclophosphamide-based chemotherapy and maintenance of health-related quality of life. Clin. Ther. 1996;18:778–88.

[80]Krumbholz M, Pellkofer H, Gold R, Hoffmann LA, Hohlfeld R, Kümpfel T. Delayed allergic reaction to natalizumab associated with early formation of neutralizing antibodies. Arch. Neurol. 2007;64:1331–3.

[81]Dupont H, Carbon C, Carlet J. Monotherapy with a broad-spectrum beta-lactam is as effective as its combination with an aminoglycoside in treatment of severe generalized peritonitis: a multicenter randomized controlled trial. Antimicrobial Agents Chemother. 2000;44:2028–33.

In a study of intravenous iron given to anemic cancer patients, Auerbach et al. (82) defined the analyses for the safety group and for the efficacy group in different ways. The group used for assessing safety was by ITT analysis, defined as all subjects receiving at least one dose of study drug. The group used for assessing efficacy was by modified ITT analysis, defined as all subjects who were randomly assigned and having at least one postbaseline observation.

In a study of ovarian cancer by Berek et al. (83), the group of subjects evaluated for safety was the same as the group evaluated for efficacy. In both cases, modified ITT analysis was used. The study had enrolled 147 subjects, but two subjects withdrew before treatment; hence the modified ITT group consisted of 145 subjects.

In a study of antibiotic treatment of tuberculosis, Conde et al. (84) used ITT analysis (170 patients) for safety analysis, and modified ITT analysis (146 patients) for efficacy analysis. Patients found to have negative cultures, contaminated cultures, or contained drug-resistant tuberculosis, were excluded from the efficacy analysis.

In a study of treating anemia with erythropoietin, Waltzman et al. (85) assessed safety using ITT analysis and efficacy using modified ITT analysis. Patients (358 in total) were enrolled and randomized, and received at least one dose of study drug. Safety analysis was conducted on these 358 patients. The modified ITT group (352 patients) consisted of all patients who had received at least one dose of study drug, and had at least one postbaseline hemoglobin value, or a transfusion.

This provides a study design uniquely configured for the possibility that safety data can be gathered, but where drug efficacy data cannot be logically gathered. The study drug was an antiemetic, that is, a drug that prevents vomiting in response to chemotherapy. This possibility that drug efficacy data could not be gathered materialized where the study drug (antiemetic) is administered, but where *chemotherapy is not administered*. In a study of an antiemetic used for treating nausea during chemotherapy, Warr et al. (86) used different-sized groups for safety analysis and efficacy analysis. Safety analysis was conducted on all 866 patients who were enrolled and randomized. The antiemetic study drug was given to 438 patients, while a control antiemetic was given to 428 patients. From these, a smaller group of 857 subjects was used, in a modified ITT group, for efficacy analysis. The modified ITT group was defined as, "a patient *must have received chemotherapy*, been administered a dose of the study drug, and have at least one post-treatment assessment on day 1 (required for

[82]Auerbach M, Ballard H, Trout JR, et al. Intravenous iron optimizes the response to recombinant human erythropoietin in cancer patients with chemotherapy-related anemia: a multicenter, open-label, randomized trial. J. Clin. Oncol. 2004;22:1301−7.

[83]Berek JS, Taylor PT, Gordon A, et al. Randomized, placebo-controlled study of oregovomab for consolidation of clinical remission in patients with advanced ovarian cancer. J. Clin. Oncol. 22:3507−16.

[84]Conde MB, Efron A, Loredo, et al. Moxifloxacin in the initial therapy of tuberculosis: a randomized, phase 2 trial. Lancet 2009;373:1183−9.

[85]Waltzman R, Croot C, Justice GR, Fesen MR, Charu V, Williams D. Randomized comparison of Epoetin Alfa (40,000 U weekly) and Darbepoetin Alfa (200 μg every 2 weeks) in anemic patients with cancer receiving chemotherapy. The Oncologist 2005;10:642−50.

[86]Warr DG, Hesketh PJ, Gralla RJ, et al. Efficacy and tolerability of aprepitant for the prevention of chemotherapy-induced nausea and vomiting in patients with breast cancer after moderately emetogenic chemotherapy. J. Clin. Oncol. 2005;23:2822−30.

acute phase) and day 2 (required for both delayed phase and overall analyses)." This study is distinguished by the fact that useful *safety data* can be obtained where the patient had received an antiemetic and chemotherapy, that useful safety data can also be obtained where a patient receives antiemetic but no chemotherapy, but that useful *efficacy data* cannot be obtained where the patient receives antiemetic but no nausea-inducing chemotherapy.

In a study of fungal infections, Walsh et al. (87) used the modified ITT group for assessing both safety and efficacy.

In a study of breast cancer, Krainick-Strobel et al. (88) assessed safety on a group of 32 subjects, defined as, "all patients treated with at least one dose of study medication." In contrast, efficacy was assessed on smaller groups of subjects, that is, the ITT group and the PP group. The ITT group excluded both untreated patients and those who took study medication for less than 4 months (<105 days). The PP group was defined as the group which excluded, from the ITT subset, all patients with major protocol violations. The major protocol violations included an interval of more than 30 days between the last dose of study

drug and breast surgery; the patient's refusal to undergo surgery; deviations from clinically relevant selection criteria; and any treatment with prohibited medication.

In a study of pancreatic cancer, Chauffert et al. (89) assessed safety by ITT analysis, and efficacy by both ITT analysis and PP analysis.

In a study of antibiotics for treating fungal infections, Vazquez et al. (90) used ITT analysis for assessing safety and modified ITT analysis for assessing efficacy.

In a study of bacterial infections treated with antibiotics by Pichichero et al. (91), safety was assessed only by ITT analysis, while efficacy was assessed by both ITT analysis and modified ITT analysis.

Patients with bacterial infections are typically treated immediately with antibacterials, because there is no time to conduct laboratory tests to provide a solid diagnosis. As a consequence, at least in the context of clinical trials for antibacterial drugs, PP analysis and ITT analysis are both conducted. In this situation, the FDA may not evaluate efficacy data collected on patients in the ITT group, who were later excluded from the PP group. However, in this situation, the FDA will still require safety

[87]Walsh TJ, Goodman JL, Pappas P, et al. Safety, tolerance, and pharmacokinetics of high-dose liposomal amphotericin B (AmBisome) in patients infected with *Aspergillus* species and other filamentous fungi: maximum tolerated dose study. Antimicrobial Agents Chemother. 2001;45:3487−96.

[88]Krainick-Strobel UE, Lichtenegger W, Wallwiener D, et al. Neoadjuvant letrozole in postmenopausal estrogen and/or progesterone receptor positive breast cancer: a phase IIb/III trial to investigate optimal duration of preoperative endocrine therapy. BMC Cancer 2008;8:62−72.

[89]Chauffert B, Mornex F, Bonnetain F. Phase III trial comparing intensive induction chemoradiotherapy (60 Gy, infusional 5-FU and intermittent cisplatin) followed by maintenance gemcitabine with gemcitabine alone for locally advanced unresectable pancreatic cancer. Definitive results of the 2000−01 FFCD/SFRO study. Ann. Oncol. 2008;19:1592−9.

[90]Vazquez JA, Skiest DJ, Tissot-Dupont H, Lennox JL, Boparai MS, Isaacs R. Safety and efficacy of posaconazole in the long-term treatment of azole-refractory oropharyngeal and esophageal candidiasis in patients with HIV infection. HIV Clin. Trials 2007;8:86−97.

[91]Pichichero ME, Casey JR, Block SL, et al. Pharmacodynamic analysis and clinical trial of amoxicillin sprinkle administered once daily for 7 days compared to penicillin V potassium administered four times daily for 10 days in the treatment of tonsillopharyngitis due to *Streptococcus pyogenes* in children. Antimicrobial Agents Chemother. 2008;52:2512−20.

data. In other words, even if the patient was found not to be suffering from the infection that was required by the Clinical Study Protocol, the safety data will still be valid. The FDA requires (92):

> that safety be reported for all patients who received the drug, irrespective of whether a pathogen was identified or not. For purposes of efficacy, the population of interest varies by indication. While for some, the primary analysis is only in patients who had identified micro-organisms, for others it may be patients with a well-defined clinical entity, even if culture results are not positive.

To summarize, investigators may be inclined to analyze efficacy data by ITT analysis, modified ITT analysis, or PP analysis, and may decide to analyze safety data by ITT analysis, modified ITT analysis, or by PP analysis. These decisions are influenced by the following factors.

First, FDA requires all safety data, that is, data from the ITT population, not just from the PP population. Hence, while an investigator may analyze efficacy by way of PP analysis (thereby excluding study subjects who missed a few doses), missing a drug-taking schedule will not influence the validity of the existing safety data.

Safety data on any drug may be obtained within an hour of administering the drug. If a patient vomits or has a change in blood pressure within an hour or so of receiving the drug, the investigator can easily capture these adverse events. In contrast, efficacy can usually not be determined within an hour of receiving the drug, in particular, for diseases such as cancer and infections. In this way,

safety data may have a different character than efficacy data.

If a study subject drops out of the study at a time point that is, for example, 1 week into a 2-year clinical study, any person would be able to understand that any safety data acquired in that 2-week period will be valuable. In contrast, any person can understand that efficacy data, acquired on the patient who drops out 2 weeks into the study, could be of questionable use.

e. Anticipated Versus Unanticipated Adverse Events

Investigators may need to distinguish between anticipated AEs and unanticipated AEs. This distinction informs the investigator whether or not any given AE needs to be reported to outside reviewers, such as the Data Monitoring Committee (DMC) or IRB. According to FDA's Guidance for Industry, unanticipated AEs are classified as follows (93):

- Unanticipated AEs include AEs that are uncommon and that are typically associated with drugs. A single occurrence of a serious, unexpected event that is uncommon but that is strongly associated with drug exposure, may include angioedema, agranulocytosis, hepatic injury, or Stevens—Johnson syndrome (SJS). SJS is a severe rash that occurs in response to various types of drug (94).
- Unanticipated AEs include AEs that are uncommon and not typically associated with drugs. A single occurrence, or more

---

[92]Drug Information RL, Division of Drug Information, Center for Drug Evaluation and Research, Food and Drug Administration. E-mail of October 15, 2010 from FDA.

[93]U.S. Department of Health and Human Services. Food and Drug Administration. Guidance for clinical investigators, sponsors, and IRBs. Adverse event reporting to IRBs—improving human subject protection; January 2009.

[94]Iannini P, Mandell L, Felmingham J, Patou G, Tillotson GS. Adverse cutaneous reactions and drugs: a focus on antimicrobials. J. Chemother. 2006;18:127—39.

often a small number of occurrences, of a serious, unexpected event that is not commonly associated with drug exposure, but uncommon in the study population, for example, tendon rupture or progressive multifocal leukoencephalopathy (PML). PML is caused by a virus called John Cunningham virus (JC virus), and is associated with a drug used for multiple sclerosis (natalizumab).

- Unanticipated AEs include AEs that are not uncommon, but that occur in the study at a greater rate than usual, for example, at a rate above the baseline rate.
- Unanticipated AEs also include any safety findings, including findings based on animal data or epidemiological data, that would cause the Sponsor to modify the investigator's brochure, Clinical Study Protocol, or consent form. (The term adverse event is not used in the context of animal studies. Instead, the term "toxicity" is used for animal data.)

In the context of preapproval reporting, the Office of Human Research Protections (OHRP) has stated that an unexpected (or unanticipated) adverse event includes any adverse event occurring in one or more subjects participating in a research protocol, the nature, severity, or frequency of which is not consistent with either, "the known or foreseeable risk of adverse events associated with the procedures involved in the research that are described in … the protocol-related documents, such as the **IRB-approved research protocol**, any applicable **investigator brochure**, and the current IRB-approved **informed consent document**" (95).

The fact that the Investigator's Brochure can be used to distinguish between an adverse event that is anticipated and unanticipated, is revealed by one of FDA's Warning Letters. The Warning Letter states that (96,97), "We disagree that a hospitalization for somatic transformation was an anticipated event, because this type of reaction was not described in the **Investigator's Brochure**."

Please note that according to the OHRP, the term "unanticipated" encompasses "unexpected," as is evident from the following excerpt. Also, please note that the term "unanticipated" encompasses other adverse events, in addition to those that are "unexpected." The excerpt reads (98):

> What are *unanticipated problems*? … OHRP considers *unanticipated problems*, in general, to include any incident, experience, or outcome that meets all of the following criteria: unexpected (in terms of nature, severity, or frequency).

The classification of ADRs into anticipated versus unanticipated was based on a scheme

---

[95]Office for Human Research Protections (OHRP) Department of Health and Human Services (HHS). Guidance on reviewing and reporting unanticipated problems involving risks to subjects or others and adverse events; January 15, 2007.

[96]Warning Letter to Emord and Associates, P.C. (the letter has no Warning Letter No.) (March 16, 2007) from Mary Malarkey, Office of Compliance and Biologics Quality, CBER, U.S. Food and Drug Administration. The letter sent to Emord and Associates is an attachment to Warning Letter No. CBER-07-06 (February 1, 2007), as available on FDA's website.

[97]Warning Letter No. CBER-07-06 (February 1, 2007) from Mary A. Malarkey, Office of Compliance and Biologics Quality, CDER, U.S. Food and Drug Administration.

[98]Office for Human Research Protections (OHRP) Department of Health and Human Services (HHS). Guidance on reviewing and reporting unanticipated problems involving risks to subjects or others and adverse events, January 15, 2007.

originally proposed by Hurwitz and Wade (99). Wilke et al. (100) provided a well-organized description of anticipated drug reactions and unanticipated ADRs. Anticipated ADRs include those that are extensions of the drug's intended therapeutic effect.

In contrast, examples of unanticipated ADRs that seem not to be related to lowering cholesterol include the effect of statins (cholesterol-lowering drug) in causing myalgia (muscle pain). Unanticipated ADRs also encompass those resulting in a response to the drug, by patients having specific genetic mutations.

Wilke et al. (101) identified a number of mutations, in human patients, that can give rise to unanticipated ADRs. These mutations include the CYP2C9 and VKORC1 mutations, which increase risk for bleeding during warfarin treatment (102), mutations in glucose-6-phosphate dehydrogenase can give rise to hemolytic anemia during treatment with sulfonylurea drugs, as is the case with glipizide, a drug that stimulates the pancreas to secrete insulin in diabetics (103), and mutations in

UDP-glucuronosyl transferase 1A1 (UGT1A1) can give rise to neutropenia, with administration of the anticancer drug irinotecan (104). The package inserts for these drugs identify these mutations, and warn of the ADRs, as indicated in the footnoted package inserts.

III. QT INTERVAL PROLONGATION

a. Introduction

Cardiac drug safety information is captured on a routine basis in various types of clinical trials, for example, in clinical trials for oncology drugs and antibiotics (105,106,107). Cardiac adverse event information is provided by electrocardiograms (ECG) and, in particular, by a pattern on the ECG called the "QT interval." Instructions for monitoring the QT interval and other parameters of cardiac physiology are sometimes included in the Clinical

[99]Hurwitz N, Wade OL. Intensive hospital monitoring of adverse reactions to drugs. Br. Med. J. 1969;1:531–6.

[100]Wilke RA, Lin DW, Roden DM, et al. Identifying genetic risk factors for serious adverse drug reactions: current progress and challenges. Nat. Rev. Drug Discov. 2007;6:904–16.

[101]Wilke RA, Lin DW, Roden DM, et al. Identifying genetic risk factors for serious adverse drug reactions: current progress and challenges. Nat. Rev. Drug Discov. 2007;6:904–16.

[102]Roth M. The warfarin revised package insert: is the information in the label "too thin"? Hous. J. Health L. Policy 2009;9:279–308.

[103]Package insert. Glipizide (Glucotrol®) Pfizer, New York, NY; August 2010.

[104]Package insert. Irenotecan (Camptosar®) Sun Pharmaceuticals, India; June 2009.

[105]Shah RR, Morganroth J. Update on cardiovascular safety of tyrosine kinase inhibitors: with a special focus on QT interval, left ventricular dysfunction and overall risk/benefit. Drug Saf. 2015;38:693–710.

[106]Wernicke J, et al. An evaluation of the cardiovascular safety profile of duloxetine: findings from 42 placebo-controlled studies. Drug Saf. 2007;30:437–55.

[107]Morganroth J. A definitive or thorough phase 1 QT ECG trial as a requirement for drug safety assessment. J. Electrocardiol. 2004;37:25–9.

Study Protocol, either as part of the inclusion/exclusion criteria, or as part of the instructions for safety monitoring (108,109,110,111,112).

b. Electrophysiology of the QT Interval

The QT interval is the part of the ECG measurement that describes the period between the onset of ventricular depolarization and the end of the repolarization process (113). Regarding repolarization, FDA's Guidance for Industry provides tests for determining the influence of any drug on the heart and on the influence of the drug to delay cardiac repolarization (114).

A drug's influence on cardiac repolarization is assessed by detecting prolongation of the QT interval. The QT interval represents the duration of ventricular depolarization and subsequent repolarization. This duration resides between the beginning of the QRS complex to the end of the T wave. The pathological consequence of this delay (the prolongation) is the development of cardiac arrythmias, such as the type of arrhythmia called, torsade de pointes.

[108]Clinical Research Protocol. PREVAIL: a multinational phase 3, randomized, double-blind, placebo-controlled efficacy and safety study of oral MDV3100 in chemotherapy-naïve patients with progressive metastatic prostate cancer who have failed androgen deprivation therapy. Protocol Number: MDV3100-03. This Protocol was a supplement to: Beer TM, Armstrong AJ, Rathkopf DE, et al. Enzalutamide in metastatic prostate cancer before chemotherapy. New Engl. J. Med. 2014;371:424–33.

[109]Protocol: GED-301-01-11. EUDRACT No. 2011-002640-27. A phase II multicenter, randomized, double-blind, controlled vs placebo, dosefinding study on the efficacy and safety of GED-0301, in patients with active Crohn's disease (Ileo-Colitis). This Protocol was a supplement to: Monteleone G, Neurath MF, Ardizzone S, et al. Mongersen, an oral *SMAD7* antisense oligonucleotide, and Crohn's disease. New Engl. J. Med. 2015;372:1104–13.

[110]Protocol No. 109MS302. A randomized, multicenter, placebo-controlled and active reference (glatiramer acetate) comparison study to evaluate the efficacy and safety of BG00012 in subjects with relapsing-remitting multiple sclerosis. EUDRA CT No: 2006-003697-10. Date: 09 January 2008. Version 4. This Protocol was a supplement to: Fox RJ, Miller DH, Phillips JT, et al. Placebo-controlled phase 3 study of oral BG-12 or glatiramer in multiple sclerosis. New Engl. J. Med. 2012;367:1087–97.

[111]Clinical Study Protocol M13-099. A randomized, open-label study to evaluate the safety and efficacy of ABT-450/Ritonavir/ABT-267 (ABT-450/r/ABT-267) and ABT-333 coadministered with ribavirin (RBV) in adults with genotype 1 chronic hepatitis C virus (HCV) infection and cirrhosis (TURQUOISE-II). Date: 21 August 2012. EudraCT No: 2012-003088-23. This Protocol was a supplement to: Poordad F, Hezode C, Trinh R, et al. ABT-450/r–ombitasvir and dasabuvir with ribavirin for hepatitis C with cirrhosis. New Engl. J. Med. 2014;370:1973–82.

[112]Clinical Study Protocol. A phase 3, randomized, double-blind, placebo-controlled, parallel-group study to evaluate the efficacy and safety of lumacaftor in combination with ivacaftor in subjects aged 12 years and older with cystic fibrosis, homozygous for the *F508del-CFTR* mutation. Vertex Study Number: VX12-809-103. Lumacaftor IND Number: 79,521. Ivacaftor IND Number: 74,633. EUDRACT No: 2012-003989-40. Date: 05 February 2014 (Version 3.0). This Protocol was a supplement to: Wainwright CE, Elborn JS, Ramsey BW, et al. Lumacaftor–ivacaftor in patients with cystic fibrosis homozygous for Phe508del *CFTR*. New. Engl. J. Med. 2011;365:1663–72.

[113]Ball A. Quinalone-induced QT interval prolongation: a not-so-unexpected class effect. J. Antimicrob. Chemother. 2000;45:557–9.

[114]U.S. Department of Health and Human Services. Food and Drug Administration. Guidance for industry. E14. Clinical evaluation of QT/QTc interval prolongation potential for non-antiarrhythmic drugs; October 2005 (16 pp.).

Torsade de pointes can lead to sudden death. QT prolongation is a biomarker for a drug's risk of causing arrhythmias. FDA's Guidance for Industry recommends that the Clinical Study Protocol includes instructions that the study drug be discontinued if there is a marked prolongation of the QT/QTc interval, especially if the measurement is reproduced in repeated ECG (115). FDA's Guidance states that the threshold for discontinuing the drug is an increase of greater than 500 ms, or of greater than 60 ms over the baseline reading.

This concerns the QTc interval, in contrast to the QT interval. The lower case letter "c" in the term "QTc" refers to a corrected value of the QT interval. As stated by FDA's Guidance, "[b]ecause of its inverse relationship to heart rate, the measured QT interval is routinely corrected by means of various formulae to a less heart rate dependent value known as the QTc interval" (116). While FDA recommends that corrections be made using either Bazette's formula or Fridericia's formula, FDA also recommends reporting both corrected and uncorrected QT interval data. Referring to this correction, Humland Turner (117) teach that, "[p]recise categorization of the normal QT interval for a given individual is impractical since it changes with every heartbeat ... [s]ince the QT interval is impacted by heart rate, tending to be shorter as heart rate increases, it is typically corrected for heart rate by ... mathematical formulae, resulting in QTc data." The normal QTc for the healthy adult male is 350–460 ms, and for the healthy adult female is 360–470 ms. The finding of a prolonged QT interval represents the prolongation of action potential of at least some cells in the ventricular myocardium (118).

For drug safety studies with animals and cultured cells, FDA provides a concise Guidance for Industry (119), with background information teaching that ventricular polarization is the net result of the activities of many membrane ion channels and transporters, including transporters that are sodium, potassium, and calcium channels. FDA's Guidance recommends that the investigator use in vitro tests that measure action potential duration and ion currents, and that these tests can use single cells (cardiomyocytes) or multicellular structures, such as a Purkinje fibers, or other cells of the heart such as epicardial cells, midmyocardial cells, and endocardial cells (120). Regarding ion channels, the ion channels most associated with drug-induced QT prolongation

[115]U.S. Department of Health and Human Services. Food and Drug Administration. Guidance for industry. E14. Clinical evaluation of QT/QTc interval prolongation potential for non-antiarrhythmic drugs; October 2005 (16 pp.).

[116]U.S. Department of Health and Human Services. Food and Drug Administration. Guidance for industry. E14. Clinical evaluation of QT/QTc interval prolongation potential for non-antiarrhythmic drugs; October 2005 (16 pp.).

[117]Huml RA, Turner JR. The current regulatory landscape for cardiac and cardiovascular safety assessments: part I. Regulatory Focus; January 2011:43–8.

[118]Roden DM. Drug-induced prolongation of the QT interval. New Engl. J. Med. 2004;350:1013–22.

[119]U.S. Department of Health and Human Services. Food and Drug Administration. Guidance for industry. S7B. Nonclinical evaluation of the potential for delayed ventricular repolarization (QT interval prolongation) by human pharmaceuticals; October 2005 (10 pp.).

[120]Roden DM. Drug-induced prolongation of the QT interval. New Engl. J. Med. 2004;350:1013–22.

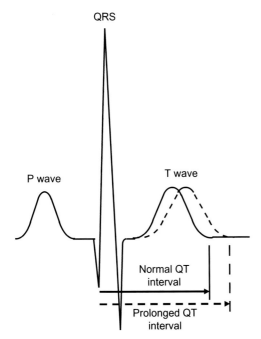

FIGURE 25.2 Drug-induced QT interval prolongation. Redrawn from Introduction to Antiarrhythmic Agents, by Dr Munther K. Homoud, M.D., Tufts-New England Medical Center, Spring 2008. *Permission to reproduce image granted by Dr Munther K. Homoud, M.D., Co-Director, New England Cardiac Arrhythmia Center, Tufts University School of Medicine, Medford, MA (e-mail of Jul. 22, 2015).*

Figure 25.2 reproduces a typical textbook example of the QT interval and QT interval prolongation (122). The X-axis has the unit of milliseconds and the Y-axis has the unit of millivolts. The letter "P" refers to the P wave. P wave represents atrial depolarization. The term "QRS" refers to QRS complex. QRS complex involves ventricular depolarization. QRS complex is produced by the upstroke of the action potential. The letter "T" is T wave. Finlayson et al. (123) provide a rudimentary introduction to the ECG readout, "the P wave represents the combined electrical activity of action potential depolarisation in the atria ... [t]he QRS complex of the ECG corresponds to the action potential depolarisation as it occurs in the ventricles ... while the T wave is associated with ventricular repolarisation." Finlayson et al. continue, "[t]hus the QT interval of an ECG represents the duration of the ventricular action potential, plus the time associated with transmission across the myocardium ... [i]t therefore follows that a prolongation of the QT interval corresponds to a prolongation of the ventricular action potential."

c. Torsade De Pointes and Further Details on the QT Interval

The term, "torsade de pointes" was devised in 1966 to describe a peculiar appearance of ventricular tachycardia occurring in an elderly woman (124,125). Most drugs that cause TdP

are I_{Kr}, I_{Ks}, and the sodium channel. I_{Kr} refers to inward potassium rectifier channel, and I_{Ks} refers to slowly activating delayed rectified potassium channel (121).

[121]Nachimuthu S, et al. Drug-induced QT interval prolongation: mechanisms and clinical management. Therapeutic Adv. Drug Safety 2012;3:241−53.

[122]Redrawn from, Introduction to Antiarrhythmic Agents, by Dr Munther K. Homoud, M.D., Tufts-New England Medical Center, Spring 2008. Permission to reproduce image granted by Dr Munther K. Homoud, M.D., Co-Director, New England Cardiac Arrhythmia Center, Tufts University School of Medicine, Medford, MA (e-mail of July 22, 2015).

[123]Finlayson K, et al. Acquired QT interval prolongation and HERG: implications for drug discovery and development. Eur. P. Pharmacol. 2004;500:129−42.

[124]Roden DM. Drug-induced prolongation of the QT interval. New Engl. J. Med. 2004;350:1013−22.

[125]Dessertenne F. La tachycardie ventriculaire à deux foyers opposés variables. Arch. Mal. Coeur 1966;59:263−72.

prolong the QT interval by blocking cardiac potassium ion channels, more specifically, the potassium channel responsible for the rapid repolarizing current I_{Kr} (126). The "mouth" of this channel is unusually wide for a potassium ion-selective channel, permitting access to many drugs. The channel is composed of proteins encoded for by two genes. The human ether-related a-go-go (HERG) gene encodes for the pore-forming HERG protein and the KCNE2 gene encodes for the accessory protein, MinK-related peptide 1 (127). In addition to acting directly at the mouth of the HERG protein, other mechanisms for drug-induced QTc prolongation include blockade of both I_{Kr} and I_{Ks}, as occurs with azimilidine, and inhibition of HERG trafficking to the cell membrane, as occurs with pentamidine and arsenic trioxide (128). The term, trafficking to the cell membrane, refers to the process where newly biosynthesized polypeptides, which are destined to be membrane-bound proteins, are inserted into the plasma membrane. Fluoxetine, which is an antidepressant, prolongs the QTc interval by two

mechanisms, direct block of the HERG channel and disruption of HERG trafficking to the cardiac cell membrane (129).

According to various commentators (130,131), the relation between QT prolongation and the risk of TdP is complex and unpredictable. Assessment of risk for TdP versus the health benefit of any drug, may be finely balanced, thus impairing clear-cut individual clinical judgments. The resulting problem for drug safety monitoring is as follows. Torsades de pointes and sudden death are unpredictable and rare. The detection of these adverse events requires large sample sizes that are achieved only after a drug is on the market (132). Regarding this point, another commentator stated that, "[e]ven in the presence of QT prolongation, however TdP may occur as rarely as once in every 10,000 patient-years of exposure to a compound ... clinical TdP is notoriously difficult to assess during the pharmaceutical development process" (133).

The mechanism by which QT prolongation leads to torsades de pointes is outlined in an excellent review by Nachimuthu et al. (134).

[126]Ritter JM. Cardiac safety, drug-induced QT prolongation and torsade de pointes (TdP). Br. J. Pharmacol. 2012;73:331−4.

[127]Sides GD. QT interval prolongation as a biomarker for torsades de pointes and sudden death in drug development. Disease Markers 2002;18:57−62.

[128]Heist EK, Ruskin JN. Drug-induced arrhythmias. Circulation 2010;122:1426−35.

[129]Heist EK, Ruskin JN. Drug-induced arrhythmias. Circulation 2010;122:1426−35.

[130]Ritter JM. Cardiac safety, drug-induced QT prolongation and torsade de pointes (TdP). Br. J. Pharmacol. 2012;73:331−4 Heist EK, Ruskin JN. Drug-induced arrhythmias. Circulation 2010;122:1426−35. Ritter JM. Cardiac safety, drug-induced QT prolongation and torsade de pointes (TdP). Br. J. Pharmacol. 2012;73:331−4.

[131]Heist EK, Ruskin JN. Drug-induced arrhythmias. Circulation 2010;122:1426−35.

[132]Sides GD. QT interval prolongation as a biomarker for torsades de pointes and sudden death in drug development. Disease Markers 2002;18:57−62.

[133]Miram S, et al. Application of cardiac electrophysiology simulations to pro-arrhythmic safety testing. Br. J. Pharmacol. 2012;167:932−45.

[134]Nachimuthu S, et al. Drug-induced QT interval prolongation: mechanisms and clinical management. Therapeutic Adv. Drug Safety 2012;3:241−53.

This mechanism begins with the event where, "[p]rolongation of ventricular repolarization often leads to oscillation in the membrane potential called early after depolarization (EAD)" (135).

d. Drugs That Increase Risk for QT Interval Prolongation

During the 1960s, it began to be recognized that certain drugs induced heart arrhythmias and with an increased QT interval. The first drug associated with QT prolongations was quinidine, an antimalarial (136). In the early 1920s, it was reported that about 1% of patients treated with quinidine experienced sudden death. Symptoms that likely took the form of torsades de pointes were also observed, as illustrated by the following example. Shortly after the patient was treated with quinidine, they developed abrupt loss of consciousness and seizure-like activity (137). Arrhythmias related to noncardiac medications, including antihistamines and antipsychotics, were also reported in the 1960s and 1970s, but they were also poorly understood by clinicians.

Regarding quinidine, the Centers for Disease Control and Prevention (CDC) provides a warning about QT prolongation in its Guidelines (138):

> quinidine gluconate is cardiotoxic and so a baseline EKG should be obtained before initiating therapy ... [a]t the dosages required for the treatment of falciparum malaria, quinidine gluconate may cause ventricular arrhythmia, hypotension, hypoglycemia, and prolongation of the QTc interval. The quinidine gluconate infusion should be slowed or stopped for an increase in the QRS complex by >50%, a QTc interval >0.6 seconds, a QTc interval that is prolonged by more than 25% of the baseline value

Wroblewski et al. (139) provides an exemplary account of several malaria patients treated with quinidine, revealing that this drug resulted in an increase in the QT interval to 531, 543, 704, and 550 ms, in various patients.

This further concerns drugs that increase the risk for QT interval prolongation. Please note that the drugs described in the present narrative are not intended for cardiac uses. In addition to quinidine, drugs that pose an increased risk for QT prolongation include (140,141,142):

- Terfenadine (antihistamine for treating allergies) (143);

[135]Nachimuthu S, et al. Drug-induced QT interval prolongation: mechanisms and clinical management. Therapeutic Adv. Drug Safety 2012;3:241−53.

[136]Kannankeril P, et al. Drug-induced long QT syndrome. Pharm. Revs. 2010;62:760−81.

[137]Kannankeril P, et al. Drug-induced long QT syndrome. Pharm. Revs. 2010;62:760−81.

[138]Centers for Disease Control and Prevention. Treatment of malaria (guidelines for clinicians); July 2013 (8 pp.).

[139]Wroblewski HA, et al. High risk of QT interval prolongation and torsades de pointes associated with intravenous quinidine used for treatment of resistant malaria or babesiosis. Antimicrobial Agents Chemother. 2012;56:4495−9.

[140]Roden DM. Drug-induced prolongation of the QT interval. New Engl. J. Med. 2004;350:1013−22.

[141]Thomas SH, et al. Concentration dependent cardiotoxicity of terodiline in patients treated for urinary incontinence. Br. Heart J. 1995;74:53−6.

[142]Morganroth J. Cardiac repolarization and the safety of new drugs by electrocardiography. Clin. Pharmacol. Therapeutics 2007;81:108−13.

[143]Roden DM. Drug-induced prolongation of the QT interval. New Engl. J. Med. 2004;350:1013−22.

- Grepafloxacin (antibiotic) (144);
- Terodiline (for urinary incontinence) (145);
- Cisapride (promotes peristalsis during swallowing) (146);
- Erythromycin (antibiotic) (147);
- Thioridazine (antipsychotic) (148).

e. Terfenadine and the Issue of Drug–Drug Interactions

This concerns drug–drug interactions. A dramatic example of a drug–drug interaction is provided by the fact that drugs that inhibit cytochrome CYP3A also prevent CYP3A from engaging in its usual catabolism of xenobiotics, including drugs. This concerns the drug, terfenadine. The consequence of co-administering terfenadine in combination with a drug that inhibits CYP3A, such as erythromycin or ketoconazole, is an increase in levels of terfenadine, dramatically potentiating the ability of terfenadine to prolong the QT interval, with the consequences of torsades de pointes and death (149).

Terfenadine administered alone results in only a small prolongation of QT interval (only 6 ms) when this drug is administered at recommended doses (150). Remarking on the same minimal effect of terfenadein, another commentator stated that, "at standard clinical doses, terfenadine is associated with relatively minor QTc prolongation and low proarrhythmic risk when used as monotherapy, QTc prolongation, 18 milliseconds at peak plasma concentrations" (151).

A study of nine human subjects by Honig et al. (152), reveals that administered erythromycin provokes increases in blood levels of terfenadine, and of levels of the active form of terenadine (acid metabolite), resulting in increases in QT interval. In addition to potentiating terfenadine's ability to cause QT interval prolongation, Hancox et al. (153) point out that erythromycin alone can increase the QT interval.

In 1997, FDA required that terfenadine be withdrawn from the market. The following provides an interesting take-home lesson about pro-drugs. A pro-drug is a drug that requires metabolism in the patient's body in order to have a pharmacological effect. Terfenadine is a

[144]Ball A. Quinalone-induced QT interval prolongation: a not-so-unexpected class effect. J. Antimicrobial Chemother. 2000;45:557–9.

[145]Roden DM. Drug-induced prolongation of the QT interval. New Engl. J. Med. 2004;350:1013–22.

[146]Yap YG, Camm AJ. Drug induced QT prolongation and torsades de pointes. Heart 2003;89:1363–72.

[147]Ray WA, Murray KT, Meredith S, et al. Oral erythromycin and the risk of sudden death from cardiac causes. New Engl. J. Med. 2004;351:1089–96.

[148]Kannankeril P, et al. Drug-induced long QT syndrome. Pharm. Revs. 2010;62:760–81.

[149]Roden DM. Drug-induced prolongation of the QT interval. New Engl. J. Med. 2004;350:1013–22.

[150]Roden DM. Drug-induced prolongation of the QT interval. New Engl. J. Med. 2004;350:1013–22.

[151]Heist EK, Ruskin JN. Drug-induced arrhythmias. Circulation 2010;122:1426–35.

[152]Honig PK, et al. Changes in the pharmacokinetics and electrocardiographic pharmacodynamics of terfenadine with concomitant administration of erythromycin. Clin. Pharmacol. Therapeutics 1992;52:231–8.

[153]Hancox JC, et al. Erythromycin, QTc interval prolongation, and torsade de pointes: case reports, major risk factors and illness severity. Ther. Adv. Infect. Dis. 2014;2:47–59.

pro-drug that needs to be metabolized to another compound, fexofenadine, in order to have its antihistamine effect. At the same time that FDA withdrew terfenadine, they approved the active metabolite, fexofenadine (154). The withdrawn product was known by the tradename, Seldane®, while the active metabolite is known as Allegra-D®. Fexofenadine does not result in a statistically significant increase in risk of QT prolongation or in torsades de pointes. It has been reported that, "[a]nalysis of trial evidence from all phases of fexofenadine's clinical development in over 6,000 patients ... showed no statistically significant increases in mean QTc or serious cardiac arrhythmias, including torsades de pointes" (155).

f. Cisapride and Its Regulatory History

This concerns part of the regulatory history of cisapride. Cisapride is a gastrointestinal promotility agent used for gastroesophageal reflux disease and delayed gastric emptying time. The drug blocks both the I_{Kr} channel and the I_{Ks} channel (156).

Cisapride was marketed from 1993 to 1999, and was withdrawn from the market in 2000.

During the marketing period, FDA received adverse event reports from 341 patients. These patients included 117 who developed QT prolongation, 107 with torsades de pointes, 18 with ventricular fibrillation, 27 with ventricular tachycardia, 25 with cardiac arrest, and 15 with sudden death (157). The deaths were directly or indirectly associated with an arrhythmic event. In Jun. 1998, FDA informed practitioners of adverse cardiac events through additions to the boxed warning in the label and by requiring "Dear Health Care Professional" letters sent by the drug's manufacturer (158). The boxed warning and the letters did not concern all uses of cisapride, but addressed increased risk in patients taking concurrent medications that interfere with cisapride metabolism, that prolong the QT interval, or that have other diseases that predispose to such arrhythmias. Eventually, the manufacturer voluntarily withdrew the drug from the market. In the words of Smalley et al. (159), "[i]n March 2000, prior to when an FDA advisory committee was scheduled to review cisapride's benefits and risks for the approved indication, the manufacturer terminated marketing of cisapride in the United States effective as of July 2000."

[154]Anonymous. New FDA approvals. The Nurse Practitioner. 1998;23:116.

[155]Craig-McFeely PM, et al. Evaluation of the safety of fexofenadine from experience gained in general practice use in England in 1997. Eur. J. Clin. Pharmacol. 2001;57:313–20.

[156]Nachimuthu S, et al. Drug-induced QT interval prolongation: mechanisms and clinical management. Therapeutic Adv. Drug Safety 2012;3:241–53.

[157]Wysowski DK, et al. Postmarketing reports of QT prolongation and ventricular arrhythmia in association with cisapride and Food and Drug Administration regulatory actions. Am. J. Gastroenterol. 2001;96:1698–703.

[158]Smalley W, et al. Contraindicated use of cisapride: impact of food and drug administration regulatory action. J. Am. Med. Assoc. 2000;284:3036–9.

[159]Smalley W, et al. Contraindicated use of cisapride: impact of food and drug administration regulatory action. J. Am. Med. Assoc. 2000;284:3036–9.

g. Erythromycin—Data From Recombinant HERG, Purkinje Fibers, and Patients

1. Introduction

Erythromycin, clarithromycin (160), and azithromycin (161) are macrolide antibiotics. The macrolide antibiotics are polyketides. Polyketides are biosynthesized by way of polyketide synthase (162). These antibiotics can impair the I_{Kr} potassium channel and result in QT interval prolongation, with the consequence of cardiac arrhythmias such as torsades de pointes, ventricular tachycardia, and ventricular fibrillation (163).

2. Data From Recombinant Cells

Although the best in vitro model for drug safety testing on cardiac function is cardiac tissue taken from healthy humans, this tissue is not readily available. Another reasonable model is a permanent line of human cultured cells. One line of human cells, human embryonic kidney cells (HEK-293), has low levels of membrane-bound inward (rapid activating delayed) rectifier potassium channel (I_{Kr}). I_{Kr} is the product of the human ether-a-go-go-related gene (hERG). Elkins et al. (164) modified

HIK-293 cells by transfecting with the hERG gene, thereby resulting in the potassium channel being expressed by the cells, and then incorporated in the plasma membrane of the cells. In creating this transfected cell, the goal of the authors was for drug screening, that is, for "the removal of candidate compounds in the preclinical stages that are likely to have poor pharmacokinetic and toxicity profiles."

Crumb (165) used the above hERG gene-transfected cells for testing the influence of erythromycin on the electrophysiology of the cells. The researcher exposed cells to a variety of concentrations of erythromycin, from 0.001 mM up to 0.10 mM. The result was a progressively severe block of ion currents mediated by the potassium channel (I_{Kr}). The researcher also provided evidence that erythromycin binds to an extracellular portion of this potassium channel, whereas two other drugs, thioridazine and terfenadine, bind to an intracellular portion of this potassium channel. Thioridazine has been established to increase QT interval and also to increase risk for torsade de pointes (166).

3. Data From Purkinje Fibers

Purkinje fibers isolated from a dog were used for electrophysiology experiments (167).

---

[160]Vieweg WV, et al. Clarithromycin, QTc interval prolongation and torsades de pointes: the need to study case reports. Ther. Adv. Infect. Dis. 2013;1:121–38.

[161]Hancox JC, et al. Azithromycin, cardiovascular risks, QTc interval prolongation, torsade de pointes, and regulatory issues: a narrative review based on the study of case reports. Ther. Adv. Infect. Dis. 2013;1:155–65.

[162]Park SR, et al. Genetic engineering of macrolide biosynthesis: past advances, current state, and future prospects. Appl. Microbiol. Biotechnol. 2010;85:1227–39.

[163]Albert RK, et al. Macrolide antibiotics and the risk of cardiac arrhythmias. Am. J. Respir. Crit. Care Med. 2014;189:1173–80.

[164]Elkins S, et al. Three-dimensional quantitative structure–activity relationship for inhibition of human ether-a-go-go-related gene potassium channel. J. Pharmacol. Exp. Ther. 2002;301:427–34.

[165]Crumb WJ. Allosteric effects of erythromycin pretreatment on thioridazine block of hERG potassium channels. Br. J. Pharmacol. 2014;171:1668–75.

[166]Kannankeril P, et al. Drug-induced long QT syndrome. Pharm. Revs. 2010;62:760–81.

[167]Rubart M, et al. Electrophysiolical mechanisms in a canine model of erythromycin-associated long QT syndrome. Circulation 1993;88:1832–44.

An excerpt from the method for isolating the Purkinje fibers reads, "Purkinje cells were isolated by connective tissue into approximately circular and elliptical bundles composed of 5 to 24 ... cells juxtaposed in a bundle" (168). The method for taking electrophysiology data reads, in part, "[t]he proximal recording electrode was positioned greater than 1 Purkinje bundle diameter ... from the site of current injection to avoid problems with three-dimensional flow of current near the current electrode tip ... [t]he distal recording electrode was positioned a mean of 1221 micrometers from the current site" (169). Action potentials were recorded with microelectrodes, and were measured before and at various times (60, 90, and 120 min) after adding erythromycin to the solution bathing the Purkinje fibers (170). Erythromycin was added at 20 mg/L and at higher levels up to 200 mg/L. The results demonstrated that erythromycin increased the duration of the action potential, where this increase occurred in the plateau region of the action potential. Without erythromycin, the action potential was about 400 ms, while adding erythromycin, at progressively increasing concentrations resulted in a corresponding increase in action potential duration.

The authors were careful to point out that the concentrations found to provoke an increase in action potential duration with the in vitro experiments with Purkinje fibers overlapped the peak serum concentration (30 mg/L) found in human subjects dosed with erythromycin. Thus, the nature of this study supports the use of Purkinje fiber experiments, not merely for acquiring information on mechanisms, but also to predict safety in human subjects. This author has documented the difference between experiments suitable only to determine mechanisms, from those suitable for assessing efficacy and safety in humans (171).

4. Data From Patients

In an analysis of publicly available data on 1476 cases of sudden death from cardiac causes, Ray et al. (172) assessed the risk of death associated with erythromycin. Included in the analysis was assessing the risk of sudden death associated with erythromycin, where patients were not taking other antibiotics. The results of the analysis demonstrated that the rate of sudden death from cardiac causes was *twice as high* among users of erythromycin, as compared to patients not taking erythromycin. In an analysis of patients taking erythromycin in combination with a drug that inhibited CYP3A, the results demonstrated that the rate of sudden death from cardiac causes was *five times as high*, as compared to patients taking neither erythromycin nor CYP3A inhibitors. The CYP3A inhibitors that were used for this analysis were diltiazem, verapamil, and troleandomycin. Ray et al. concluded that the combination of erythromycin and CYP3A inhibitors should be avoided.

[168]Pressler ML, et al. Effects of extracellular calcium ions, verapamil, and lanthanum on active and passive properties of canine cardiac purkinje fibers. Circ. Res. 1982;51:637−51.

[169]Pressler ML, et al. Effects of extracellular calcium ions, verapamil, and lanthanum on active and passive properties of canine cardiac purkinje fibers. Circ. Res. 1982;51:637−51.

[170]Rubart M, et al. Electrophysiolical mechanisms in a canine model of erythromycin-associated long QT syndrome. Circulation 1993;88:1832−44.

[171]Brody T. Enabling claims under 35 USC §112 to methods of medical treatment or diagnosis, based on *in vitro* cell culture models and animal models. J. Patent Trademark Off. Soc. 2015;97:328−411.

[172]Ray WA, Murray KT, Meredith S, et al. Oral erythromycin and the risk of sudden death from cardiac causes. New Engl. J. Med. 2004;351:1089−96.

It is interesting to note that a package insert for erythromycin includes information on QT interval prolongation in the Warnings section (173):

> **WARNINGS.**... *QT Prolongation.* **Erythromycin** has been associated with prolongation of the QT interval and infrequent cases of arrhythmia. Cases of torsades de pointes have been spontaneously reported during postmarketing surveillance in patients receiving erythromycin. Fatalities have been reported. Erythromycin should be avoided in patients with known prolongation of the QT interval, patients with ongoing proarrhythmic conditions such as uncorrected hypokalemia or hypomagnesemia, clinically significant bradycardia, and in patients receiving Class IA (quinidine, procainamide) or Class III (dofetilide, amiodarone, sotalol) antiarrhythmic agents. Elderly patients may be more susceptible to drug-associated effects on the QT interval.

h. FDA's Decision-Making Process in Evaluating QT Intervals

FDA provides Sponsors with the opportunity to consult with the FDA's *QT Interdisciplinary Review Team* (QT-IRT). This *Review Team* was established in 2006 to provide expert review advice to sponsors, and to help assess whether there is any relation between drug concentrations and change in QT interval. FDA's *Manual of Policies and Procedures* (174) states that the *Review Team* may be available for consulting about serious ventricular arrhythmias, and that the *Review Team* will meet with a sponsor about specific product development issues only if requested to do so by a review division. FDA's review division prepares statements of development or regulatory questions to be answered by the *Review Team*.

This concerns an FDA-submission for *ivacaftor*, a drug for treating cystic fibrosis.

The FDA-submission was evaluated by the QT-IRT (175). The evaluation was published on FDA's website at Jan. 2012, for NDA 202188. The *Review Team* decided that the highest dose used with human volunteers resulted in QT interval changes that were well within the safe limit. The *Review Team* wrote:

> QT-IRT recommends the following label language. Our recommendations are suggestions only. We defer final decisions regarding labeling to the review division. The effect of multiple doses of **iva-caftor** 150 mg and 450 mg twice daily on QTc interval was evaluated in a randomized, placebo- and active-controlled (moxifloxacin 400 mg) ... QT study in 72 healthy subjects. In a study with demonstrated ability to detect small effects, the ... QTc ... was below 10 ms, the threshold for regulatory concern. The dose of 450 mg twice daily ivacaftor is adequate to represent the high exposure clinical scenario.

A separate document, the *Medical Review*, referred to two different safety studies, the first involving increasing doses of the study drug, and the second involving multiple doses of a constant amount of study drug. Please note that the *Medical Review* refers to the use of Fridericia's formula, not to Bazett's formula. The *Medical Review*, concluded that the study drug (ivacaftor; VX-770) did not show any significant toxicities:

> A thorough QT study was conducted for this program, and reviewed by the QT study interdisciplinary review team. The study consisted of 2 parts: **Part A** in which 8 subjects were enrolled to evaluate the safety and tolerability of increasing doses of VX-770 up to 450 mg every 12 hours (q12h), followed by **Part B** to determine if therapeutic or supratherapeutic systemic exposure to **multiple doses** of VX-770 up to 450 mg q12h prolongs the mean Fridericia-corrected QT (QTcF) interval by more than 5 milliseconds. No significant toxicities were identified in **Part A**.

---

[173]Package insert for ERY-TAB (Erythromycin delayed-release tablets, USP) Enteric-coated. Arbor Pharmaceuticals, LLC; July 2013.

[174]Manual of Policies and Procedures. Center for Drug Evaluation and Research. Interdisciplinary review team for QT studies; February 3, 2012 (10 pp.).

[175]Interdisciplinary Review Team for QT Studies Consultation: Thorough QT Study Review.

The actual effect of **multiple doses of VX-770 150 mg and 450 mg on QTc was evaluated in Part B**; a double-blind, randomized, placebo- and active-controlled … study in which 72 subjects received VX-770 150 mg q 12h, VX-770 450 mg q 12h, placebo, and moxifloxacin 400 mg (the active comparator). The … supra-therapeutic dose of 450 mg q 12h produced mean Cmax approximately 4 times higher than the mean Cmax for the therapeutic dose of 150 mg q 12h. No significant QTc prolongation effect of VX-770 at the doses tested was detected.

i. Clinical Study Protocol's Instructions for QT Interval Testing for a Clinical Trial on Cystic Fibrosis

The Clinical Study Protocol used for a study on *ivacaftor*, a drug for treating cystic fibrosis, provides instructions relating to QT interval (176,177). This Protocol is related to the NDA that is described in the preceding paragraphs. The relationship between the NDA and this Protocol is demonstrated by the timeline outlined in footnote (178).

Excerpts from this Protocol illustrated the drug discontinuation instructions:

> If the QTc value remains above the threshold value (greater than 45 msec from the average of the 3 predose values on Day 1 or greater than 500 msec) on repeated measurement or is noted on greater than 2 occasions with no identified alternative etiology for the increased QTc study drug, then discontinuation from study drug treatment may be

required after discussion with the medical monitor. Subjects in whom treatment is discontinued for increased QTc should have their QTc monitored closely until it normalizes or returns to baseline.

The Protocol also discloses Fridericia's correction as well as Bazett's correction, for use in the analysis of the ECG data:

> A cardiologist … will review each ECG to confirm if intervals were calculated correctly and to provide an interpretation, including a suggested clinical significance, as applicable … [t]he values reported by the central ECG diagnostic service will be used for data analysis. The PR, QT, and QTc for HR intervals (including **Fridericia's correction** $[QTcF = QT/RR^{1/3}]$ and **Bazett's correction** $[QTcB = QT/RR^{0.50}]$), QRS duration, and HR will be captured in the ECG database.

j. The Electrocardiogram

The electrocardiogram (ECG) is used for diagnosing intraventricular conduction disturbances and arrhythmias. ECG readings are used for detecting electrolyte abnormalities, particularly of serum potassium and calcium, for detecting genetic cardiac abnormalities, and for monitoring patients treated with antiarrhythmic drugs and noncardiac drugs. The American Heart Association has issued a series of six guidelines for conducting and interpreting ECGs for different patient groups (179). ECG measurements are

[176]Clinical Study Protocol. A phase 3, randomized, double-blind, placebo-controlled, parallel-group study to evaluate the efficacy and safety of lumacaftor in combination with ivacaftor in subjects aged 12 years and older with cystic fibrosis, homozygous for the *F508del-CFTR* Mutation. Vertex Study Number: VX12-809-103. Lumacaftor IND Number: 79,521. Ivacaftor IND Number: 74,633. EUDRACT Number: 2012-003989-40. Date of Protocol: 05 February 2014 (Version 3.0) Replaces Version 2.0, dated 25 July 2013.

[177]The Clinical Study Protocol was provided as a supplement to Wainwright CE, Elborn JS, Ramsey BW, et al. Lumacaftor—ivacaftor in patients with cystic fibrosis homozygous for Phe508del *CFTR*. New. Engl. J. Med. 2011;365:1663—72.

[178]First, the Sponsor submitted an Investigational New Drug (IND) application (IND No. 74,633). The Clinical Study Protocol, that is, Protocol No. VX12-809-103, was part of this submitted IND. FDA's review of this IND referred to VX12-809-103.

[179]Kligfield P, Gettes GS, Bailey JJ, et al. Recommendations for the standardization and interpretation of the electrocardiogram. Part I: The electrocardiogram and its technology. Circulation 115:1306—24.

acquired by pairs of electrodes placed at various parts of the patient's body, where these electrode pairs and the tracings that result are called "leads" (180).

The fourth in this series of six guidelines concerns the QT interval, as well as other features of the ECG (181). An excerpt from this fourth paper provides guidance for which leads should be used for measuring the QT interval, "[w]hen the QT interval is measured in individual leads, the lead showing the longest QT should be used ... [t]his is usually V2 or V3. However, if this measurement differs by more than 40 ms from that in other leads, the measurement may be in error, and measurements from adjacent leads should be considered." Sheppard et al. (182) provide excellent diagrams of the positioning of ECG leads on a patient, according to standard placement procedure, as well as by a modified procedure.

k. Summary of QT Interval

Animal toxicology studies and clinical safety studies include tests on the study drug's influence on heart electrophysiology. These tests take the form of measurements on isolated Purkinje fibers (animal studies) and ECG measurements (human studies). The ECG measurements establish whether or not the drug increases the QT interval. The medical literature provides a wealth of caution, regarding the potential consequences of drug-induced QT interval prolongation, and the consequences of drug–drug interactions that prolong the QT interval.

IV. STEVENS–JOHNSON SYNDROME

Stevens-Johnson syndrome (SJS) is a recurring issue in clinical trials, as well as for some marketed drugs. FDA's Guidance for Industry (183) on reporting adverse drug reactions states that SJS is an unanticipated problem encountered in clinical trials. Tohkin et al. (184) provides an account of adverse drug reaction reporting of SJS, and reveals that at least 100 different drugs have been found to cause SJS and a related skin disorder, toxic epidermal necrosis (TEN).

SJS (185) and TEN are rare disorders that can be caused by allopurinol,

[180]Sheppard HP, Barker TA, Ransinghe AM, et al. Does modifying electrode placement of the 12 lead ECG matter in healthy subjects? Int. J. Cardiol. 2011;152:184–91.

[181]Rautaharju PM, Surawicz B, Gettes LS, et al. AHA/ACCF/HRS recommendations for the standardization and interpretation of the electrocardiogram: part IV: the ST segment, T and U waves, and the QT interval: a scientific statement from the American Heart Association Electrocardiography and Arrhythmias Committee, Council on Clinical Cardiology; the American College of Cardiology Foundation; and the Heart Rhythm Society. Endorsed by the International Society for Computerized Electrocardiology. J. Am. Coll. Cardiol. 2009;53:982–92.

[182]Sheppard HP, Barker TA, Ransinghe AM, et al. Does modifying electrode placement of the 12 lead ECG matter in healthy subjects? Int. J. Cardiol. 2011;152:184–91.

[183]U.S. Department of Health and Human Services. Food and Drug Administration. Guidance for industry. Guidance for clinical investigators, sponsors, and IRBs. Adverse event reporting to IRBs. Improving human subject protection; January 2009 (9 pp.).

[184]Tohkin M, Ishiguro A, Kaniwa N, Saito Y, Kurose K, Hasegawa R. Prediction of severe adverse drug reactions using pharmacogenetic biomarkers. Drug Metab Pharmacokinet. 2010;25:122–33.

[185]Stevens AM, Johnson FC. A new eruptive fever associated with stomatitis and ophthalmia. Am. J. Dis. Child 1922;24:526–33.

trimethoprim-sulfamethaxole, sulfonamide drugs in general, aminopenicillins, cephalosporins, quinolones, carbamazepine, phenytoin, phenobarbitol, and nonsteroidal antiinflammatory drugs (NSAIDs) of the oxicam type (meloxicam, prioxicam, tenoxicam) (186,187,188).

SJS has a mortality of 1–5% and involves detachment of up to 10% of the epidermis (total body skin area) (189,190,191). TEN has a mortality of 25–30% and involves detachment of greater than 30% of the epidermis. A transitional SJS/TEN has been defined as an epidermal detachment between 10% and 30% (192). These two syndromes involve blisters, sloughing off of sheets of skin (193) full-thickness epidermal necrolysis, and extensive apoptosis of keratinocytes (194).

The drug reactions of SJS and TEN are self-limiting, where treatment involves stopping the drug, correcting electrolyte imbalances, and preventing sepsis. SJS (when severe) and TEN can have consequences similar to those of severe burns, that is, massive fluid losses, electrolyte imbalances, and infections (195). Eye involvement is frequent and can include conjunctivitis, erosion of the cornea, and blindness.

Photographs of skin lesions of SJS have been published, where the lesions were caused by lamotrigine (196), tetrazepam (197), penicillin (198), trimethoprim and sulfamethoxazole (199),

[186]Harr T, French LE. Toxic epidermal necrolysis and Stevens–Johnson syndrome. Orphanet J. Rare Dis. 2010;5:39.

[187]Ghislain PD, Roujeau JC. Treatment of severe drug reactions: Stevens–Johnson syndrome, toxic epidermal necrolysis and hypersensitivity syndrome. Dermatol. Online J. 2002;8:5.

[188]Mockenhaupt M, Viboud C, Dunant A, et al. Stevens–Johnson syndrome and toxic epidermal necrolysis: assessment of medication risks with emphasis on recently marketed drugs. The EuroSCAR-study. J. Invest. Dermatol. 2008;128:35–44.

[189]Harr T, French LE. Toxic epidermal necrolysis and Stevens–Johnson syndrome. Orphanet J. Rare Dis. 2010;5:39.

[190]Ghislain PD, Roujeau JC. Treatment of severe drug reactions: Stevens–Johnson syndrome, toxic epidermal necrolysis and hypersensitivity syndrome. Dermatol. Online J. 2002;8:5.

[191]Mockenhaupt M, Viboud C, Dunant A, et al. Stevens–Johnson syndrome and toxic epidermal necrolysis: assessment of medication risks with emphasis on recently marketed drugs. The EuroSCAR-study. J. Invest. Dermatol. 2008;128:35–44.

[192]Ghislain PD, Roujeau JC. Treatment of severe drug reactions: Stevens–Johnson syndrome, toxic epidermal necrolysis and hypersensitivity syndrome. Dermatol. Online J. 2002;8:5.

[193]De Rojas MV, Dart JK, Saw VP. The natural history of Stevens–Johnson syndrome: patterns of chronic ocular disease and the role of systemic immunosuppressive therapy. Br. J. Ophthalmol. 2007;91:1048–53.

[194]Harr T, French LE. Toxic epidermal necrolysis and Stevens–Johnson syndrome. Orphanet. J. Rare Dis. 2010;5:39.

[195]Harr T, French LE. Toxic epidermal necrolysis and Stevens–Johnson syndrome. Orphanet. J. Rare Dis. 2010;5:39.

[196]Wetter DA, Camilleri MJ. Clinical, etiologic, and histopathologic features of Stevens–Johnson syndrome during an 8-year period at Mayo Clinic. Mayo Clin Proc. 2010;85:131–8.

[197]Torres MJ, Mayorga C, Blanca M. Nonimmediate allergic reactions induced by drugs: pathogenesis and diagnostic tests. J. Investig. Allergol. Clin. Immunol. 2009;19:80–90.

[198]Cram DL. Life-threatening dermatoses. Calif. Med. 1973;118:5–12.

[199]Assaad D, From L, Ricciatti D, Shapero H. Toxic epidermal necrolysis in Stevens–Johnson syndrome. Can. Med. Assoc. J. 1978;118:154–6.

vaccines (200), and by recombinant antibodies (201,202,203). Corneal damage is the most severe long-term complication of SJS and TEN (204). Tsubota et al. (205) and De Rojas et al. (206) provide photographs of eye damage in SJS. FDA's Guidance for Industry documents relating to smallpox vaccines (207) and lamotrigine (208) also specifically warn against SJS.

V. IDIOSYNCRATIC DRUG REACTIONS

Stevens-Johnson syndrome is the most well-defined of the idiosyncratic drug reactions, and thus was described above. Idiosyncratic drug reactions generally take the form of an indistinct and variably defined group of disorders. Uetrecht and Naisbitt (209) defined an idiosyncratic drug reaction as, "an adverse reaction that does not occur in most patients treated with a drug and does not involve the therapeutic effect of the drug ... they are unpredictable and often life threatening."

The major locations of idiosyncratic drug reactions in humans are:

- skin,
- liver,
- bone marrow, resulting in hematological disorders.

Regarding the amount of drug that provokes the reaction, these reactions usually occur at a dose level below the level required for therapeutic efficacy, as well as at therapeutic levels (210). Gruchalla (211) pointed out that idiosyncratic drug reactions are those that are "neither predictable nor common," and that the reaction is not dose-dependent.

[200]Chopra A, Drage LA, Hanson EM, Touchet NL. Stevens—Johnson syndrome after immunization with smallpox, anthrax, and tetanus vaccines. Mayo Clin Proc. 2004;79:1193—6.

[201]Brown BA, Torabi M. Incidence of infusion-associated reactions with rituximab for treating multiple sclerosis: a retrospective analysis of patients treated at a US centre. Drug Saf. 2011;34:117—23.

[202]Scheinfeld N. A review of rituximab in cutaneous medicine. Dermatol. Online J. 2006;12:3.

[203]Salama M, Lawrance IC. Stevens—Johnson syndrome complicating adalimumab therapy in Crohn's disease. World J. Gastroenterol. 2009;15:4449—52.

[204]De Rojas MV, Dart JK, Saw VP. The natural history of Stevens Johnson syndrome: patterns of chronic ocular disease and the role of systemic immunosuppressive therapy. Br. J. Ophthalmol. 2007;91:1048—53.

[205]Tsubota K, Satake Y, Kaido M, et al. Treatment of severe ocular-surface disorders with corneal epithelial stem-cell transplantation. N. Engl. J. Med. 1999;340:1697—703.

[206]De Rojas MV, Dart JK, Saw VP. The natural history of Stevens Johnson syndrome: patterns of chronic ocular disease and the role of systemic immunosuppressive therapy. Br. J. Ophthalmol. 2007;91:1048—53.

[207]U.S. Department of Health and Human Services. Food and Drug Administration. Guidance for industry. Vaccinia virus developing drugs to mitigate complications from smallpox vaccination; March 2004 (40 pp.).

[208]U.S. Department of Health and Human Services. Food and Drug Administration. Guidance for industry. Nonclinical safety evaluation of pediatric drug products; February 2003 (22 pp.).

[209]Uetrecht J, Naisbitt DJ. Idiosyncratic adverse drug reactions: current concepts. Pharmacol. Revs. 2013;65:779—808.

[210]Uetrecht J, Naisbitt DJ. Idiosyncratic adverse drug reactions: current concepts. Pharmacol. Revs. 2013;65:779—808.

[211]Gruchalla RS. Drug metabolism, danger signals, and drug-induced hypersensitivity. Curr. Revs. Allergy Clin. Immunol. 2011;108:475—88.

An additional mode for classifying idiosyncratic drug reactions is by the delay before the reaction presents (212). Classification by delay is:

- Almost immediate, such as urticaria, angioedema, rhinoconjunctivitis, or anaphylaxis (213,214);
- 1−2 weeks, such as simple rashes (215);
- 2−3 weeks, such as generalized hypersensitivity;
- 1−2 months, such as hepatotoxicity and agranulocytosis;
- 1 year or more, such as autoimmune reactions.

Idiosyncratic drug reactions can proceed by way of a pathway that does *not involve an immune response*, or by way of a pathway that *does involve an immune response*. The immune response can involve direct, spontaneous reaction of the drug with a protein, with the creation of a protein that bears a hapten group. Alternatively, the immune response can involve enzymatic activation of the drug, followed by condensation of the activated drug with a protein, with the creation of a hapten. Hepten-mediated immune reactions have been reviewed (216).

The spontaneous formation of haptens occurs with drugs such as penicillins and cephalosporins, which have a beta-lactam ring that can spontaneously react proteins to generate the hapten. Enzymatic activation of drugs can be mediated, for example, by cytochrome P450 or peroxidase (217). Enzymatic activation of drugs can result in the conversion of drug into a reactive epoxy compound.

Idiosyncratic drug reactions are a frequent cause of acute liver failure (218). In fact, idiosyncratic drug-induced liver injury is a common reason for not receiving FDA-approval, or for the FDA's withdrawal of a drug from marketing. Idiosyncratic drug reactions to the liver tend to arise from antibacterials and NSAIDs. Serious reactions of this type usually occur at doses greater than 10 mg/day.

The anticonvulsants carbamazepine and phenytoin are associated with idiosyncratic drug reactions, where these reactions include fever, neutropenia, and skin rash (including Stevens-Johnson syndrome) (219).

A number of animal models have been developed for use in studying idiosyncratic drug reactions. To be a valid model, the drug-induced

---

[212]Ng W, Lobach AR, Zhu X, et al. Animal models of idiopathic drug reactions. Adv. Pharmacol. 2012;63:81−135.

[213]Sanchez-Borges M, et al. Hypersensitivity reactions to non beta-lactam antimicrobial agents, a statement of the WAO special committee on drug allergy. World Allergy Org. J. 2013;6:18 (23 pp.).

[214]Andrade RJ, Tulkens PM. Hepatic safety of antibiotics used in primary care. J. Antimicrob. Chemother. 2011;66:1431−46.

[215]Ng W, Lobach AR, Zhu X, et al. Animal models of idiopathic drug reactions. Adv. Pharmacol. 2012;63:81−135.

[216]Erkes DA, Selvan SR. Hapten-induced contact hypersensitivity, autoimmune reactions, and tumor regression: plausibility of mediating antitumor immunity. J. Immunol. Res. 2014;2014:175265 (28 pp.).

[217]Lu W, Uetrecht JP. Peroxidase-mediated bioactivation of hydroxylated metabolites of carbamazepine and phenytoin. Drug Metabol. Disposition 2008;36:1624−36.

[218]Lammert C, et al. Relationship between daily dose of oral medications and idiosyncratic drug-induced liver injury: search for signals. Hepatology 2008;47:2003−9.

[219]Lu W, Uetrecht JP. Peroxidase-mediated bioactivation of hydroxylated metabolites of carbamazepine and phenytoin. Drug Metabol. Disposition 2008;36:1624−36.

reaction in animals must resemble that occurring in humans (220,221). Animal models for idiosyncratic drug reactions include the "nevirapine-induced skin rash" test in rats (222). Please note that, in humans, nevirapine can result in SJS and liver toxicity. The acetaminophen-induced liver injury test in mice is a model for liver toxicity. The halothane-induced liver injury test in guinea pigs is another model. The clozapine-induced hematological toxicity test in rats has been used to study the idiosyncratic drug reaction taking the form of agranulocytosis (223).

Sulfamethoxazole-induced hypersensitivy in dogs and the penicillamine-induced reaction in rats are additional animal models (224). This example provides a context for all types of animal models that are intended for use in FDA-regulated drug development. According to Adamo et al. (225) basic exploratory studies do not have to following FDA's regulations on Good Laboratory Practice (GLP), but GLP regulations "do apply to subsequent safety and toxicology studies" that are intended for FDA-submission. Further information on GLP is cited (226,227).

VI. FDA'S DECISION-MAKING PROCESS IN EVALUATING ADVERSE EVENTS

a. FDA's Decision-Making Process in Evaluating Ipilimumab, and Stevens-Johnson Syndrome

This is from FDA's approval of *ipilimumab*, for the indication of melanoma. This example is from biologics license application (BLA) 125377, at Mar. 2015 of FDA's website. The FDA reviewer commented on the adverse event of SJS, writing that:

> [s]evere, life-threatening or fatal immune-mediated dermatitis (eg, Stevens–Johnson syndrome ... occurred in 13 (2.5%) YERVOY-treated patients ... [o]ne ... patient died as a result of toxic epidermal necrolysis and one additional patient required hospitalization for severe dermatitis.

As a consequence of this adverse reaction, the Sponsor wrote and submitted a REMS to the FDA, and agreed to transmit this REMS to all physicians who are members of several

---

[220]Shenton JM, et al. Animal models of idiosyncratic drug reactions. Chem.-Biol. Interactions 2004;150:53–70.

[221]Brody T. Enabling claims under 35 USC §112 to methods of medical treatment or diagnosis, based on in vitro cell culture models and animal models. Journal Patent Trademark Office Society; 2015 (in press).

[222]Ng W, Lobach AR, Zhu X, et al. Animal models of idiopathic drug reactions. Adv. Pharmacol. 2012;63:81–135.

[223]Ng W, Lobach AR, Zhu X, et al. Animal models of idiopathic drug reactions. Adv. Pharmacol. 2012;63:81–135.

[224]Shenton JM, et al. Animal models of idiosyncratic drug reactions. Chem.-Biol. Interactions 2004;150:53–70.

[225]Adamo JE, Bauer G, Berro M, et al. A roadmap for academic health centers to establish Good Laboratory Practice–compliant infrastructure. Acad. Med. 2012;87:279–84.

[226]The Code of Federal Regulations includes a section on Good Laboratory Practice (GLP), namely, 21 CFR §58. For example, 21 CFR 58.120 requires that, "[e]ach study shall have an approved written protocol that ... shall contain ... [a] description ... of the diet in the study ... each dosage level, expressed in milligrams per kilogram of body weight."

[227]Lee CS, Lee JY. Good Laboratory Practice (GLP) regulations: interpretation techniques and review of selected compliance issues. Drug Infor. J. 2006;40:33–8.

medical organizations, including the American Society of Clinical Oncology (ASCO). The REMS took the form of listed documents, each of which was required by the FDA:

- A Dear Healthcare Provider Letter informing healthcare providers about the incidence, type, severity and management of immune-mediated adverse reactions caused by YERVOY;
- The Immune-Mediated Adverse Reaction Management Guide;
- The Patient Wallet Card;
- The Nursing Immune-Mediated Adverse Reaction Symptom Checklist;

The Management Guide, which took the form of a booklet, included the writing:

> ipilimumab ... can result in severe and fatal inflammation of the skin, including Stevens– Johnson syndrome (SJS) and toxic epidermal necrolysis (TEN) ... Advise patients to report skin-related changes ... Monitor patients for the most common manifestations of immune-mediated dermatitis, such as rash and pruritus ... Withhold YERVOY dosing in patients with moderate to severe signs and symptoms.

b. FDA's Decision-Making Process in Evaluating Vemurafenib, and Stevens-Johnson Syndrome

This is from FDA's review of *vemurafenib* (Zelboraf®), for treating melanoma. The information is from FDA's evaluation of NDA 202429, as available at July 2013 on FDA's website. The FDA reviewer stated that, "[r]ash and pruritis were common adverse events with vemurafenib ... **the patient with Stevens–Johnson syndrome** that appeared 17 days after initiation of treatment ... demonstrate that vemurafenib has the potential to cause severe hypersensitivity reactions. The labeling includes severe hypersensitivity reactions under Warnings & Precautions."

A view of the package insert reveals that, in the *Warnings and Precautions* section, it reads, "[s]evere dermatological reactions, including **Stevens–Johnson syndrome** and toxic epidermal necrolysis. Discontinue ZELBORAF for severe dermatological reactions" (228). Also, the *Adverse Reactions* section reads, "[m]ost common adverse reactions ... are arthralgia, rash, alopecia."

The Sponsor did not propose to use any REMS, and the FDA did not require any REMS. Regarding the risks, including skin rash, the FDA reviewer wrote that, "[t]hese risks include cutaneous squamous cell carcinoma (cuSCC), QT-prolongation ... rash ... and fatigue. The sponsor believes that all the risks can be managed with appropriate labeling and routine pharmacovigilance." To conclude, although the adverse event of SJS did occur, it was apparently not prevalent enough to require any more than a warning in the *Warnings and Precautions* section of the package insert.

VII. DRUG-INDUCED LIVER INJURY

a. Introduction

Drug-induced liver injury has been defined by a set of criteria known as "Hy's law." Hy's law originated in an observation by Dr Hyman Zimmerman regarding elevated liver enzyme levels and drug-induced jaundice, where the drug caused hepatocellular injury and death in 10–50% of cases. Zimmerman's observation took the form of two biomarkers that were predictive of hepatocellular injury. FDA characterizes drug-induced liver injury as an idiosyncratic drug reaction, and considers Hy's law to be a biomarker-based algorithm for liver injury, where this algorithm is a surrogate for histological examination on a liver

[228]Package insert for ZELBORAF® (vemurafenib) tablet, oral; November 2014 (15 pp.).

biopsy (229). A biography of Dr Zimmerman and of Dr Robert Temple's invention of Hy's law is available (230).

b. Hy's Law

Hy's law is used during drug development to assess a drug's potential to cause severe drug-induced liver injury. FDA has standardized Hy's law to four components:

1. Serum ALT or aspartate aminotransferase (AST) elevation of greater than $3\times$ upper limit of normal.
2. Total bilirubin elevation greater than $2\times$ upper limit of normal.
3. Absence of initial findings of cholestasis. Absence of cholestasis is assessed by absence of elevation of serum alkaline phosphatase to geater than $2\times$ upper limit of normal.
4. No other reason can be found to explain the increased enzyme levels and increased bilirubin levels, aside from the administered drug.

FDA's Guidance for Industry (231) points out that drug-induced liver injury (DILI) is a type of adverse event that occurs only rarely, in its writing that, "a typical NDA or biologics license application (BLA) database usually will not show any cases of severe DILI, even for a drug that can cause such injury, because the rate of severe injury is usually relatively low (1/10,000 or less)."

According to the FDA, "[f]inding one Hy's law case in a clinical trial … is worrisome, finding two is … highly predictive that the drug has the potential to cause severe DILI when given to a large population" (232).

To provide background information, drug-induced liver injury can result from liver injury that is of the hepatocellular or cholestatic type. The cholestatic Drug-induced liver injury, if diagnosed early, is typically reversible upon drug discontinuation, and less commonly progresses to a severe outcome (233). In a study of human subjects, Kleiner et al. (234) distinguished between drug-induced liver injury that is hepatocellular injury and drug-induced liver injury that is cholestatic injury. The former involves inflammation, necrosis, apoptosis, and hemorrhage, while the latter involves bile plugs and duct paucity. This study involved liver histology. Please note that, in contrast, Hy's law involves use of serum enzyme data.

FDA's Guidance provides examples of drug-induced liver injury analysis for the drugs bromfenac, troglitazone, and ximelagatran. This provides the example of Hy's law analysis for another drug, rivaroxaban. In a study of 42 cases of liver injury associated with rivaroxaban, Liakoni et al. (235) found that 13 of the patients fulfilled the criteria of Hy's law.

[229]U.S. Department of Health and Human Services. Food and Drug Administration. Guidance for industry. Drug-induced liver injury: premarketing clinical evaluation; July 2009 (25 pp.).

[230]Reuben A. Hy's law. Hepatology 2004;39:574–8.

[231]U.S. Department of Health and Human Services. Food and Drug Administration. Guidance for industry. Drug-induced liver injury: premarketing clinical evaluation; July 2009 (25 pp.).

[232]U.S. Department of Health and Human Services. Food and Drug Administration. Guidance for industry. Drug-induced liver injury: premarketing clinical evaluation; July 2009 (25 pp.).

[233]Regev A. Drug-induced liver injury: morbidity, mortality, and Hy's law. Gastroenterology 2014;147:20–4.

[234]Kleiner DE, Chalasani NP, Lee WM, et al. Hepatic histological findings in suspected drug-induced liver injury: systematic evaluation and clinical associations. Hepatology 2014;59:661–70.

[235]Liakoni E, et al. Symptomatic hepatocellular liver injury with hyperbilirubinemia in two patients treated with rivaroxaban. Intern. Med. 2014;174:1683–6.

Researchers have explored the possibility of devising an animal model that is equivalent to Hy's law (236). ALT levels were found to be correlated with hepatocellular necrosis, while total bilirubin correlated with bile duct injury.

c. Application of Hy's Law in the FDA's Approval of Pazopanib

Hy's law is frequently mentioned in FDA's *Medical Review*s for various drugs. This example is from NDA 22465 (Apr. 2015 on the FDA website) for *pazopanib*, for the indication of renal cell carcinoma. The writing is generally applicable to all drugs, not just to pazopanib.

The review wrote that, "Hy's Law serves as an ominous indicator of the potential for a drug to cause serious and severe hepatic injury. In non-oncologic settings, if 2 or more patients in 1000 meet the criteria for Hy's Law, hepatic failure or death is likely to be seen in at least 2 patients in 10,000 ... such estimation has been observed with ... troglitazone, bromfenac, ximelagatran, and dilevalol."

Referring to the Sponsor's drug (pazopanib), the reviewer wrote that, "[t]he estimated rate of Hy's Law cases in the pazopanib ... population is about 4 patients per 1000." The reviewer was careful to mention sources with the potential to confound the Hy's law analysis, writing that, "[t]he above estimated rates of Hy's Law cases may be underestimated since several ... patients were eliminated due to the presence of a confounding factor such as ... elevated alkaline phosphatase, ... cholecystitis, ... or use of acetaminophen or herbs. Such cases ... illustrate the difficulty in identifying Hy's Law cases. It is critical to point out that a confounding factor does not necessarily act as an excluding factor."

d. Application of Hy's Law in the FDA's Approval of Pertuzumab, Where the Issue Was Liver Damage in the Placebo Arm

This example illustrates FDA's analysis of a Hy's law case that occurs in the placebo arm. This example is from BLA 125409 for *pertuzumab*, an antibody used for the indication of breast cancer. The *Medical Review* is from Mar. 2015 of FDA's website. The reviewer wrote that, "[a] single patient ... was found to meet criteria for Hy's law ... [h]owever, this patient ... was in the placebo treatment arm and did not receive pertuzumab." The reviewer was careful to point out that the study drug arm was with pertuzumab and docetaxel, while the placebo arm was with placebo plus docetaxel. But the reviewer refrained from commenting on the possible association of docetaxel with liver damage.

e. Application of Hy's Law in the FDA's Approval of Pramipexole, Where the Issue Was Ambiguous Causality

This example illustrates how the FDA confronts ambiguous data. This is from the FDA's approval of *pramipexole*, for the indication of Parkinson's disease. The review is available from NDA 022421, from Mar. 2015 on the FDA's website. The FDA reviewer wrote:

> The patient ... describes ... four painful event [sic] thought to be related to his gallbladder ... [t]he Sponsor concluded that this event is not related to drug. While the reviewer agrees that there is **insufficient data to attribute this to drug** [sic], there remains some question. It is possible that this subject has some tendency to susceptibility to drug induced hepatic dysfunction. There is no post-marketing data to suggest drug related liver dysfunction.

---

[236]Tonomura Y, et al. Diagnostic and predictive performance and standardized threshold of traditional biomarkers for drug-induced liver injury in rats. J. Appl. Toxicol. 2015;35:165–72.

These comments illustrate a recurring theme that occurs for all FDA-regulated clinical trials. This theme is that, where causation cannot be established by the clinical trial, information on causality is expected to materialize once the drug is marketed in the general population.

VIII. ASSESSING CAUSALITY

a. Using Raw Data on Adverse Events to Acquire Cause-and-Effect Data on ADRs

The Naranjo questionnaire consists of 10 questions that capture information regarding any given adverse event (237,238,239,240). These questions are shown below:

1. Are there previous conclusive reports on this reaction?
2. Did the adverse event appear after the suspected drug was administered?
3. Did the adverse reaction improve when the drug was discontinued or a specific antagonist was administered?
4. Did the adverse reaction reappear when the drug was readministered?
5. Are there alternative causes (other than the drug) that could on their own have caused the reaction?
6. Did the reaction reappear when a placebo was given?
7. Was the drug detected in the blood (or other fluids) in concentrations known to be toxic?
8. Was the reaction more severe when the dose was increased or less severe when the dose was decreased?
9. Did the patient have a similar reaction to the same or similar drugs in any previous exposure?
10. Was the adverse event confirmed by any objective evidence?

The questionnaire includes factors such as prior adverse reports, the timing of the adverse reaction, whether the adverse reaction stopped when the drug was discontinued and whether it reappeared when the drug was resumed, dosage levels, and alternative causes of the AE (241). The questionnaire uses a point system, with assigned points being added or subtracted to the overall score depending on the questionnaire responses to the questionnaire. These calculations yield a total score, that informs the drug safety scientist whether the cause was "highly probable," "probable," "possible," or "doubtful." In detail, Naranjo scores of 9 or 10 indicate that an event was "definitely" an ADR; scores of 5–8 rate the likelihood as "probable"; scores of 1–4 are "possible"; and scores of less than 1 are "doubtful" (242). To summarize, the Naranjo algorithm, or a similar decision-making process, bridges the gap between raw data taking

---

[237]Naranjo CA, Busto U, Sellers EM, et al. A method for estimating the probability of adverse drug reactions. Clin. Pharmacol. Ther. 1981;30:239–45.

[238]van Jaarsveld CH, Jahangier ZN, Jacobs JW, et al. Toxicity of anti-rheumatic drugs in a randomized clinical trial of early rheumatoid arthritis. Rheumatology (Oxford) 2000;39:1374–82.

[239]Papastavros T, Dolovich LR, Holbrook A, Whitehead L, Loeb M. Adverse events associated with pyrazinamide and levofloxacin in the treatment of latent multidrug-resistant tuberculosis. Can. Med. Assoc. J. 2002;167:131–6.

[240]Oberg KC. Adverse drug reactions. Am. J. Pharmaceut. Educat. 1999;63:199–204.

[241]Kami S, Kendall v. Hoffman-La Roche, Inc., et al., No. A-2633-08T3, N. J. Super. App.

[242]Kelly WN. How can I recognize an adverse drug event. Medscape CME Pharmacists; February 12, 2008.

the form of a documented AE, and data that are classified as an ADR. An additional scale, that is, a scale that is an alternative to the Naranjo scale, is the RUCAM scale (243).

Bright (244) reveals issues that can impair discovery of a cause, that is, of a connection between the drug and the AE, as follows. Recognition of a relationship between a drug and an AE can be impaired where the AE is a common condition in the population of study subjects, where there is a time delay between drug use and the AE, and where the AE occurred in a different organ in the body than the organ that was being treated by the drug.

The fact that gray areas need to be navigated when assessing causality is revealed by the following excerpt from Clinical Study Protocol on a study of leukemia (245). The fact that gray areas are involved is evident from the terms, "reasonable possibility," "[a]nother cause ... is more plausible," and "current knowledge ... indicates." The excerpt from the Protocol reads:

> Causality. The Investigator is to assess the causal relation (i.e., whether there is a reasonable possibility that the study drug caused the event) using the following definitions:
> Not Related: Another cause of the AE is more plausible; a temporal sequence cannot be established

with the onset of the AE and administration of the investigational product; or, a causal relationship is considered biologically implausible.
> Unlikely: The current knowledge or information about the AE indicates that a relationship to the investigational product is unlikely.
> Possibly Related: There is a clinically plausible time sequence between onset of the AE and administration of the investigational product, but the AE could also be attributed to concurrent or underlying disease, or the use of other drugs or procedures. Possibly related should be used when the investigational product is one of several biologically plausible AE causes.
> Related: The AE is clearly related to use of the investigational product.

Another example of a Clinical Study Protocol that reiterates part of the Naranjo criteria is cited (246,247). This Protocol concerned a study of prostate cancer.

b. Where Adverse Events Caused by the Disease Are of the Same Type as Adverse Events Caused by the Study Drug

One of the issues that arises with adverse event reporting, is how to capture and report a drug-related adverse event that is also associated with the disease alone (without drug). An answer is to monitor the frequency of the

[243]Miljkovic MM, Dobric S, Dragojevic-Simic V. Consistency between causality assessments obtained with two scales and their agreement with clinical judgments in hepatotoxicity. Pharmacoepidemiol. Drug Saf. 2011;20:272–85.

[244]Bright RA. Strategy for surveillance of adverse drug events. Food Drug Law J. 2007;62:605–15.

[245]A randomized, multicenter, open-label, phase 3 study of the bruton's tyrosine kinase (BTK) inhibitor ibrutinib versus ofatumumab in patients with relapsed or refractory chronic lymphocytic leukemia/small lymphocytic lymphoma. NCT01578707; Phase 3. ORIGINAL PROTOCOL PCYC-1112-CA.

[246]Clinical Research Protocol. Study title: PREVAIL: a multinational phase 3, randomized, double-blind, placebo-controlled efficacy and safety study of oral MDV3100 in chemotherapy-naïve patients with progressive metastatic prostate cancer who have failed androgen deprivation therapy protocol no: MDV3100-03.

[247]Clinical Study Protocol available as supplement to, Beer TM, Armstrong AJ, Rathkopf DE, et al. Enzalutamide in metastatic prostate cancer before chemotherapy. New Engl. J. Med. 2014;371:424–33.

adverse event, and to compare frequency in the untreated disease with frequency with drug treatment. Guidance is provided by a Protocol from a leukemia clinical trial (248). The Protocol contained the following instructions, followed by a list of adverse events associated with the disease alone.

> **Protocol-specified Serious Adverse Events.** FDA guidance also directs Sponsors to specify AEs that may be common in the study population and as such may not meet the guidance criteria for expedited reporting. Per the guidance, a limited number of occurrences of an AE, in a study population in which occurrences of the event are anticipated independent of drug exposure; do not constitute an adequate basis to conclude that the event is a "suspected adverse reaction." An individual occurrence of one of these SAEs is uninformative as a single case, and therefore it will not be considered as a "suspected adverse reaction." The SAEs outlined below are anticipated to occur in the population under study independent of drug exposure. The occurrence of these SAEs will be monitored by [the Sponsor] and an expedited report will be submitted if an aggregate analysis indicates that the events are occurring more frequently in the drug-treatment group than in a concurrent or historical control group.

The list in its entirety was (249): "Pneumonia, Fatigue, Asthenia, Thrombocytopenia, Anemia, Neutropenia, Febrile neutropenia, Leukopenia, Urinary tract infection, Upper respiratory infection, Fever/pyrexia, Abdominal pain, Back pain, Sepsis/bacteremia, Cellulitis."

c. Including Examples of Judgments by Clinical Trial Personnel of Causality in the Clinical Study Protocol

This describes a novel approach for helping study personnel assess causality of adverse events. The Clinical Study Protocol for a phase III clinical trial included, in the Appendix, case histories of patients from an earlier-completed clinical trial. The study drug was antisense nucleic acid, for treating Crohn's disease. The case histories were short, and focused on causality of an adverse event. The Appendix included a half-dozen case histories. One of these is reproduced below (250). ULN means upper limit of normal. The adverse events in question was high serum bilirubin, and an allergy:

> Patient # 102, a 39 year old male, was enrolled on 17/05/2010. Start/end date of study drug administration: 18/05/2010–24/05/2010. The patient medical history was: Crohn's disease (CD) since 1992, appendicectomy on 1991, peach allergy with bronchospams. On day 1, before the first dose, the patient had total bilirubin increased (1.72 mg/dl). The value decreased to Not Clinically Significant ... values on **investigator's judgement**, on day 8. On day 3 (May the 20th), the patient showed direct bilirubin increased (0.51 mg/dl; UNL: 0.30 mg/dl). The parameter value decreased to 0.42 mg/dl at day 8. On day 28, the event was considered resolved, when the direct bilirubin was within the normal range. The event, mild in intensity, was **judged unlikely related by the investigator** and did not require specific

---

[248] A randomized, multicenter, open-label, phase 3 study of the Bruton's tyrosine kinase (BTK) inhibitor ibrutinib versus ofatumumab in patients with relapsed or refractory chronic lymphocytic leukemia/small lymphocytic lymphoma. NCT01578707; Phase 3. ORIGINAL PROTOCOL PCYC-1112-CA.

[249] A randomized, multicenter, open-label, phase 3 study of the Bruton's tyrosine kinase (BTK) inhibitor ibrutinib versus ofatumumab in patients with relapsed or refractory chronic lymphocytic leukemia/small lymphocytic lymphoma. NCT01578707; Phase 3. ORIGINAL PROTOCOL PCYC-1112-CA.

[250] A phase II multicenter, randomized, double-blind, controlled vs placebo, dosefinding study on the efficacy and safety of GED-0301, in patients with active Crohn's disease (Ileo-Colitis). Protocol: GED-301-01-11. EUDRACT NUMBER 2011-002640-27.

treatment. At day 84, both the direct and total bilirubin were within the normal range. Between day visits 8 and 28 (11th June), the patient suffered from seasonal allergy of the upper airways. On July 2010, the event resolved (between day 28 and day 84), was mild in intensity, and was **judged unlikely related to study treatment**. The event was treated with antihistamines.

d. FDA's Decision-Making Process in Assessing Causality

This concerns *fingolimod*, for treating multiple sclerosis. The information is from the *Medical Review* for IND 022527, available from Jul. 2011 on FDA's website. The *Medical Review* stated that, "[o]n Day 3 of study therapy the patient developed generalized edema with symptoms of feeling bad, dyspnea … and increase in bilateral pitting edema … in the face, eyelids, hands, and feet."

As is evident, the FDA reviewer applied elements from the Naranjo questionnaire in assessing causality. The FDA reviewer assessed whether the adverse event of generalized edema was related to the study drug, writing that (emphasis added), "[t]he events appear to be **drug related, because it started 3 days into treatment and improved after drug discontinuation**, however, the cause of the edema remains unknown."

The FDA reviewer recommended that, in future and ongoing studies, attention should be focused on edema. To this point, the review wrote, "[f]our patients presented fluid retention/edema leading to study drug discontinuation during fingolimod treatment. … [w]eight should be measured and 24 hour protein should be collected in patients who develop edema in future and ongoing studies." However, it was not the case that any warning against fluid retention and generalized edema materialized in the package insert.

IX. PARADOXICAL ADVERSE DRUG REACTIONS

a. Introduction

An interesting aspect of adverse drug reactions is that they can take the form of a paradox. For example, a drug for preventing nausea may cause nausea, an antidepressant can increase depression, drugs used to treat bronchial spasms can induce bronchial spasms, and an anticancer drug can cause a new type of cancer.

Regarding nausea, drugs that are used to prevent nausea and vomiting may also cause nausea and vomiting. For example, aprepitant (Emend®) is used to prevent chemotherapy-induced nausea and vomiting. Although detailed information is not available on this matter, one source expressly states that this drug may induce vomiting (251), while another source clearly states that it may induce nausea (252). The existence of paradoxical adverse drug reactions can influence the clinician's decision to classify the adverse event as either expected or as unexpected.

b. Paradox With Chemotherapy for Cancer

The phenomenon where therapy for a first type of cancer has the downstream consequence

---

[251]Package insert. Aprepitant. Cigna Pharmacy Coverage Policy; December 15, 2009.

[252]Package insert. Emend. Merck; March 2010.

of causing a second type of cancer has been thoroughly documented (253,254,255,256,257, 258,259,260,261).

Radiation and chemotherapy can inflict damage on the chromosome. Damage to DNA includes strand breaks, apurinic sites, apyrimidinic sites, intrastrand crosslinks, interstrand crosslinks, and the incorporation of incorrect bases. Cisplatin, for example, crosslinks DNA. Methotrexate and 5-fluorouracil result in the incorporation of an incorrect base, namely, uracil. The mechanism of action of radiation and of chemotherapy, in cancer therapy, is to cause mutations, that is, mutations that are so extensive and severe that the tumor cell cannot survive.

On the other hand, radiation or chemotherapy can also inflict damage to the DNA of normal cells, and in the case where damage is slight, and the normal cell survives, and where the damage resulted in a mutation in a gene used for cell signaling, cell cycle control, or cell growth, the normal cell may be converted to a cancer cell.

This scenario has been documented in the case of breast cancer. Leukemia following chemotherapy for breast cancer was studied among patients diagnosed during 1973—85. Among 13,734 women given initial chemotherapy, 24 women developed acute nonlymphocytic leukemia, compared to only two women, as expected based on general population rates (262).

The fact that any type of chemotherapy that results in DNA damage may cause cancer (even if such cancer has not been observed) has prompted a warning in the package insert for methotrexate.

[253]Carneiro BA, Kaminer L, Eldibany M, Sreekantaiah C, Kaul K, Locker GY. Oxaliplatin-related acute myelogenous leukemia. Oncologist 2006;11:261—2.

[254]Barzi A, Sekeres MA. Myelodysplastic syndromes: a practical approach to diagnosis and treatment. Cleve. Clin. J. Med. 2010;77:37—44.

[255]Flaig TW, Tangen CM, Hussain MH, et al. Randomization reveals unexpected acute leukemias in Southwest Oncology Group prostate cancer trial. J. Clin. Oncol. 2008;26:1532—6.

[256]Le Deley MC, Suzan F, Cutuli B, et al. Anthracyclines, mitoxantrone, radiotherapy, and granulocyte colony-stimulating factor: risk factors for leukemia and myelodysplastic syndrome after breast cancer. J. Clin. Oncol. 2007;25:292—300.

[257]Beaumont M, Sanz M, Carli PM, et al. Therapy-related acute promyelocytic leukemia. J. Clin. Oncol. 2003;21:2123—37.

[258]Praga C, Bergh J, Bliss J, et al. Risk of acute myeloid leukemia and myelodysplastic syndrome in trials of adjuvant epirubicin for early breast cancer: correlation with doses of epirubicin and cyclophosphamide. J. Clin. Oncol. 2005;23:4179—91.

[259]Crump M, Tu D, Shepherd L, et al. Risk of acute leukemia following epirubicin-based adjuvant chemotherapy: a report from the National Cancer Institute of Canada Clinical Trials Group. J. Clin. Oncol. 2003;21:3066—71.

[260]Chaplain G, Milan C, Sgro C, Carli PM, Bonithon-Kopp C. Increased risk of acute leukemia after adjuvant chemotherapy for breast cancer: a population-based study. J. Clin. Oncol. 2000;18:2836—42.

[261]Patt DA, Duan Z, Fang S, Hortobagyi GN, Giordano SH. Acute myeloid leukemia after adjuvant breast cancer therapy in older women: understanding risk. J. Clin. Oncol. 2007;25:3871—6.

[262]Curtis RE, Boice JD, Moloney WC, Ries LG, Flannery JT. Leukemia following chemotherapy for breast cancer. Cancer Res. 50:2741—6.

The package insert for low-dose *methotrexate* mentions cancer (neoplasms), but does not expressly assert that cancer is a risk (263):

> No controlled human data exist regarding the risk of neoplasia with methotrexate. Methotrexate has been evaluated in a number of animal studies for carcinogenic potential with inconclusive results. Although there is evidence that methotrexate causes chromosomal damage to animal somatic cells and human bone marrow cells, the clinical significance remains uncertain. Non-Hodgkin's lymphoma and other tumors have been reported in patients receiving low-dose oral methotrexate.

Please also note that *etoposide*, which is used to treat various cancers, such as ovarian cancer, can cause leukemia (264).

c. FDA's Decision-Making Process in Evaluating Hematological Cancers Induced by an Anticancer Drug

This information is from FDA's *Medical Review* of *olaparib* (Lynparza®) for ovarian cancer (265). The FDA reviewer observed that hematological cancers materialized during treatment for ovarian cancer. The hematological cancers were myelodysplastic syndromes (MDS) and acute myeloid leukemia (AML). The FDA reviewer wrote that:

> In Study 19, three patients on olaparib treatment (2.2%) have been diagnosed with or had laboratory abnormalities suggestive of MDS or AML … [t]he

sponsor estimates that 2,618 patients have been treated with olaparib to date. There have been 21 total cases of MDS and/or AML reported among these patients (0.8%), not including the additional suspected case from Study 19. Of these 21 patients, 16 have died, with 12 deaths due to MDS/AML.

The FDA reviewer added that, "[t]he reported incidence in the olaparib database is higher than the expected incidence in the general population or in an ovarian cancer population treated with platinum-based therapy."

The comments in the *Medical Review* are mirrored on the package insert, in the *Warnings and Precautions* section, which warns that, "Myelodysplastic syndrome/Acute Myeloid Leukemia … occurred in patients exposed to Lynparza, and in some cases were fatal. Monitor patients for hematological toxicity at baseline and monthy thereafter. Discontinue if MDA/AML is confirmed" (266).

d. Paradox With Growth Factors for Cancer

A paradox can occur where a growth factor is administered as part of anticancer therapy.

Women receiving chemotherapy for breast cancer have received a small-molecule drug in combination with a growth factor. Growth factors administered to cancer patients include granulocyte colony-stimulating factor (G-CSF) and granulocyte-macrophage colony-stimulating factor (GM-CSF) (267).

[263]Bedford Laboratories, Bedford, OH. Package Insert. Methotrexate injection USP; April 2005.

[264]Dunton CJ. Management of treatment-related toxicity in advanced ovarian cancer. The Oncologist 2002;7(Suppl. 5):11–9.

[265]Medical Review for olaparib (Lynparza®) for NDA 206162, from December 2014 on FDA's website.

[266]Package insert for LYNPARZA™ (olaparib) capsules, for oral use; December 2014 (4 pp.).

[267]Hershman D, Neugut AI, Jacobson JS, et al. Acute myeloid leukemia or myelodysplastic syndrome following use of granulocyte colony-stimulating factors during breast cancer adjuvant chemotherapy. J. Natl Cancer Inst. 2007;99:196–205.

The desired effect of the administered growth factor is prevention of neutropenia (268). The prophylactic administration of the growth factor reduces the need for chemotherapy dose reductions and delays that may limit chemotherapy dose intensity. By reducing the need for dose reductions, the administered growth factor increases the potential for prolonged disease-free and overall survival in the curative setting (269).

Neutropenia is the primary dose-limiting toxicity in patients treated with chemotherapy that suppresses the formation of white blood cells (myelosuppressive chemotherapy), leading to morbidity and mortality, and disrupting treatment with curative regimens. The use of granulocyte G-CSFs, as primary prophylaxis starting in the first cycle of chemotherapy, can reduce the rates of febrile neutropenia and neutropenia-related hospitalization.

However, the undesired effect of the growth factor is that the antiapoptotic effect of G-CSF or GM-CSF saves cancer cells from chemotherapy-induced killing, thereby permitting the cancer cells to develop into a myeloid cancer.

Administration of these growth factors has been associated with increased risks for cancer as well as dysplasia. Dysplasia refers to aborm-alities of chromosomal structure that can be precursors to cancer. The use of G-CSF was associated with a doubling in the risk of subsequent AML or MDS among the population that we studied, although the absolute risk remained low. Growth factors have also been administered to enhance immune response against an anticancer vaccine (270). In any situation where the data suggest that a growth factor can be used as a drug against cancer, researchers and the FDA have been unusually cautious.

e. Paradox With Antidepressants and Depression

Antidepressants can have the effect of increasing depression and inducing suicide (271). This adverse drug reaction can occur when initiating therapy with the antidepressant. For example, fluoxetine (Prozac®) can result in increased depression and increased suicide risk in children and adolescents (272,273). This effect, which has been extensively documented, is distinguished by the following time line:

• May 2003: Manufacturer of notifies FDA of clinical trial data indicating an increased risk of suicidal thoughts and actions in children and adolescents.
• Oct. 2003: FDA issues a public health advisory on possible safety risks related to use of antidepressants.

---

[268]Rader M. Granulocyte colony-stimulating factor use in patients with chemotherapy-induced neutropenia: clinical and economic benefits. Oncology (Williston Park) 2006;20(5 Suppl. 4):16–21.

[269]Lyman GH. Guidelines of the National Comprehensive Cancer Network on the use of myeloid growth factors with cancer chemotherapy: a review of the evidence. J. Natl Compr. Canc. Netw. 2005;3:557–71.

[270]Parmiani G, Castelli C, Pilla L, Santinami M, Colombo MP, Rivoltini L. Opposite immune functions of GM-CSF administered as vaccine adjuvant in cancer patients. Ann. Oncol. 2007;18:226–32.

[271]Friedman RA, Leon AC. Expanding the black box-depression, antidepressants, and the risk of suicide. New Engl. J. Med. 2007;356:2343–6.

[272]Busch SH, Barry CL. Pediatric antidepressant use after the black-box warning. Health Aff. (Millwood) 2009;28:724–33.

[273]Leon AC. The revised warning for antidepressants and suicidality: unveiling the black box of statistical analyses. Am. J. Psychiatry 2007;164:1786–9.

- Sep. 2004: FDA advisory committees vote in favor of recommending the FDA issue a black box warning on the antidepressant product labels.
- Jan. 2005: Manufacturers are required to begin including a black box warning on antidepressant product labels.

f. Paradoxes With Drugs for Treating Bronchial Constriction

Isoproterenol, a drug used for treating asthma, can cause symptoms of asthma, when administered in excessive doses. In an article on various issues relating to package inserts, Goyan (274) wrote that:

> the first patient package insert was required by FDA in 1968, when it was recognized, at least implicitly, that some drugs could not be used properly unless certain information was conveyed to patients as well as to prescribers or dispensers. Thus, in June 1968, FDA required that each isoproterenol inhalation drug dispensed to a patient bear a two-sentence warning on the container advising of an association between repeated and excessive use and severe paradoxical bronchoconstriction. FDA required the warning because inappropriate use by patients was actually causing the condition the drug was intended to treat.

This particular adverse drug reaction may have been due, in part, to the fact that the drug contains sulfite. Sulfite has the well-known effect, at least in asthmatics, of causing allergic-type symptoms, including anaphylaxis (275). The package insert for isoproterenol includes "sulfite sensitivitiy is seen more frequently in asthmatic than in nonasthmatic people" (276). Moreover, the package insert explicitly warns of an additional paradox with this drug, "isoproterenol hydrochloride injection has paradoxically been reported to worsen heart block" (277). Still another drug for treating bronchial constriction or spasms, albuterol, has also documented to have the paradoxical adverse drug reaction of causing bronchial spasms (278). Yet another bronchodilator, ipratropium, has also been found to have the "paradoxical" effect of causing bronchial spasms. According to the package insert, "[i]nhaled medicines, including ATROVENT HFA Inhalation Aerosol, may cause paradoxical bronchospasm" (279).

X. CAPTURING ADVERSE EVENTS

a. Introduction

In clinical trials, AEs need to be monitored and captured, transmitted to various personnel stored in a database, and evaluated. Some AE data are captured on a scheduled and orderly basis, such as data from the laboratory analysis of blood and urine. But other AEs, such as vomiting, seizures, or death, need to be captured as soon as they occur. For any given clinical trial, at least in the context of oncology,

[274]Goyan J. Fourteen fallacies about patient package inserts. Western J. Med. 1981;134:463−8.

[275]Brody T. Nutritional biochemistry. San Diego, CA: Academic Press; 1999. pp. 821−2.

[276]Package insert. Isoproterenol. Isuprel®. Hospira, Inc., Lake Forest, IL; 2004.

[277]Package insert. Isoproterenol. Isuprel®. Hospira, Inc., Lake Forest, IL; 2004.

[278]Spooner LM, Olin JL. Paradoxical bronchoconstriction with albuterol administered by metered-dose inhaler and nebulizer solution. Ann. Pharmacother. 2005;39:1924−7.

[279]Package insert. Ipratropium. Atrovent®. Boehringer Ingelheim, Ridgefield, CT; July 2010.

about 50 AEs occur per study subject, with about 2000–3000 AEs in all during the lifetime of the clinical trial (280).

Personnel involved in recording, routing, and evaluating AEs include the study chair (a physician), data monitors, statisticians, as well as the IRB, Data and Safety Monitoring Committee (DSMC), and federal regulatory officials. To reveal one fine-grained detail of the process of AE reporting, this process may involve, "each night, an automated computer program e-mails the study chair, study statistician, and data monitor to notify them of any event that was reported the previous day and to report a cumulative summary of all events observed on that study" (281). Regarding the IRB, some clinical studies may require all AEs that are serious and unanticipated be reported to the IRB within 48 h of the event (282).

The "point man" in this scenario is the clinical research associate (CRA). The CRA (283,284) manages patient recruitment strategies to ensure target patient numbers are met, ensures that SAEs are reported according to standard operating procedures (SOPs), for any amendments to the Clinical Study Protocol, arranges monitoring visits at appropriate time intervals and writes monitoring reports, including deviations and deficiencies, and prepares follow-up letters to investigators, and

tracks completed case report forms sent to data management, track issued and resolved data queries. In filling out the case report forms, the CRA records the name of the AE, for example, a seizure, vomiting, or anemia, when it occurred, when it was reported to the investigator, whether the AE was on-going, the severity of the AE, whether the AE can be attributed to the study drug or medical device, whether the AE resulted in hospitalization, or if the AE was reported to the Sponsor or to any regulatory agency (FDA, EMA), or if that particular AE was in the Consent Form (285).

b. The Data Manager's Tasks Include Documenting Missing Data

The data manager is an expert in computer systems, in capturing remote data, and in quality control. The data manager reports missing data and discrepancies to the principal investigator.

Data management also includes making certain that the names of adverse events, and the names of various medications, found on forms provided by various study sites, are consistent with standard names found in appropriate dictionaries. These dictionaries take the form of the MedDRA dictionary, which may be used

---

[280]Mahoney MR, Sargent DJ, O'Connell MJ, Goldberg RM, Schaefer P, Buckner JC. Dealing with a deluge of data: an assessment of adverse event data on North Central Cancer Treatment Group trials. J. Clin. Oncol. 2005;23:9275–81.

[281]Goldberg RM, Sargent DJ, Morton RF, Mahoney MR, Krook JE, O'Connell MJ. Early detection of toxicity and adjustment of ongoing clinical trials: the history and performance of the North Central Cancer Treatment Group's real-time toxicity monitoring program. J. Clin. Oncol. 2002;20:4591–6.

[282]Columbia University and Columbia University Medical Center IRB Policy; April 13, 2004.

[283]American College of Radiology Imaging Network (ACRIN). Template for clinical study protocol.

[284]Young RC. Data and safety monitoring plan. Ensuring patient safety and the integrity of clinical research (ver. 1.61). Fox Chase Cancer Center, Philadelphia, PA.

[285]London JW, Smalley KJ, Conner K, Smith JB. The automation of clinical trial serious adverse event reporting workflow. Clin. Trials 2009;6:446–54.

TABLE 25.2 Example of a Definition of an Adverse Event

Adverse Event	Grade 1	Grade 2	Grade 3	Grade 4	Grade 5
Seizure	Brief partial seizure, no loss of consciousness	Brief generalized seizure	Multiple seizures despite medical intervention	Life-threatening; prolonged repetitive seizures	Death

for all types of clinical trials, and the CTCAE dictionary, which is used for oncology clinical trials, for adverse events. Medical Dictionary for Regulatory Activities (MedDRA) is a dictionary of adverse events, developed by the International Conference on Harmonization (ICH). The MedDRA dictionary contains over 80,000 terms. In cancer treatment trials, a standard dictionary for use in reporting adverse event data is Common Terminology Criteria for Adverse Events (CTCAE) (286,287). CTCAE was developed by the National Cancer Institute (NCI). The CTCAE (ver. 3) dictionary contains 1059 terms. The clinician acquires information about the AE, consults the CTCAE, and then transmits the AE using the appropriate term to the data manager (288).

The terms in CTCAE allow for severity grading. For each term, the physician can choose between one of four grades, mild, moderate, severe, or life-threatening (289). The

MedDRA system does not allow severity grading. An example of one of CTCAE's definitions is shown in Table 25.2. It is evident that, even though CTCAE is intended for use in oncology clinical trials, the following adverse event is not an adverse event specifically associated with cancer or with anticancer drugs (290):

MedDRA is used for regulatory reporting, while CTCAE is used for publications in oncology journals. Both dictionaries (MedDRA and CTCAE) may be used concurrently for an oncology study that is funded by the NCI, thereby requiring use of CTCAE, and that is used for regulatory approval, where there is the preferred use of MedDRA (291). According to FDA's Guidance for Industry, the FDA does not impose any particular dictionary, but does prefer that the MedDRA dictionary be used, writing "the FDA prefers that applicants use the Medical Dictionary for Regulatory Activities (MedDRA)" (292). Moreover, the

[286]Edgerly M, Fojo T. Is there room for improvement in adverse event reporting in the era of targeted therapies? J. Natl Cancer Inst. 2008;100:240−2.

[287]Trotti A, Colevas AD, Setser A, et al. CTCAE v3.0: development of a comprehensive grading system for the adverse effects of cancer treatment. Semin. Radiat. Oncol. 2003;13:176−81.

[288]Basch E, Jia X, Heller G, et al. Adverse symptom event reporting by patients vs clinicians: relationships with clinical outcomes. J. Natl Cancer Inst. 2009;101:1624−32.

[289]Trotti A, Colevas AD, Setser A, Basch E. Patient-reported outcomes and the evolution of adverse event reporting in oncology. J. Clin. Oncol. 2007;25:5121−7.

[290]Common Terminology Criteria for Adverse Events (CTCAE) Ver. 4.0. May 28, 2009 (v4.03: June 14, 2010).

[291]Trotti A, Colevas AD, Setser A, Basch E. Patient-reported outcomes and the evolution of adverse event reporting in oncology. J. Clin. Oncol. 2007;25:5121−7.

[292]U.S. Department of Health and Human Services. Food and Drug Administration. Guidance for industry. Providing regulatory submissions in electronic format—postmarketing expedited safety report; May 2001.

FDA prefers that only one dictionary be used (293). But note, that the FDA does not require the use of MedDRA for reporting of adverse events in any study or for spontaneous reporting of adverse events (294).

While CTCAE was designed for use in oncology clinical trials it has, on occasion, been used for trials on other diseases, such as HIV and hypertension (295).

The CTCAE dictionary fits into the MedDRA dictionary. Where a clinical trial is funded by NCI, the investigator is always required to send adverse event reports to NCI, using CTCAE, for example, CTCAE version 4.0 (296). All of the CTCAE version 4.0 terms are MedDRA terms, that is, CTCAE version 4.0 is a subset of MedDRA. For clinical trials used for gaining FDA-approval, the FDA will likely accept data on adverse events that use only CTCAE terminology (297).

c. Examples of Missing Data in Documents Submitted to the FDA

Missing information can prevent or delay regulatory approval of any drug. This provides an example where missing data was an issue. The example is from the approval process for *cetuximab* (Erbitux®), an antibody used for treating cancer. At an earlier part of the approval process, the FDA complained that, "[t]he review team identified several major clinical and scientific deficiencies including ... missing data ... the totality of the deficiencies rendered the application unacceptable for filing and a Refuse to File letter was issued on December 28, 2001" (298,299). But at a later part of the approval process, the FDA wrote that, "[m]inor protocol deviations as per applicant (5.3.5.1.1) are as follow [sic] ... patient did not provide 2 consents" (300,301). Thus, a fair amount of missing data, during an early part of the approval process, delayed the approval process for the drug. But when the drug was finally approved, the fact that two consent forms were missing did not prevent the FDA from approving the drug.

d. Writing Style in Case Report Forms

The case report form (CRF) is the instrument used for reporting adverse events in

---

[293]U.S. Department of Health and Human Services. Food and Drug Administration. Guidance for industry. Premarketing risk assessment; March 2005.

[294]Mozzicato P. E-mail of April 4, 2011.

[295]National Cancer Institute. CTCAE FAQ. (<https://cabig-kc.nci.nih.gov/Vocab/KC/index.php/ CTCAE_FAQ#> What is the rationale and purpose of CTCAE.3F) [accessed 25.11.10].

[296]Till B. Investigational Drug Branch, Cancer Therapy Evaluation Program Technical Resources International, Inc. E-mail of November 30, 2010.

[297]Till B. Investigational Drug Branch, Cancer Therapy Evaluation Program Technical Resources International, Inc. E-mail of November 30, 2010.

[298]Keegan P. Memorandum of February 12, 2004 in administrative and correspondence documents (35 pp. total).

[299]United States Food and Drug Administration. Center for Drug Evaluation and Research (CDER). Application No. STN/BLA 125084; ERBITUX (Cetuximab). All of the correspondence documents are incorporated by reference in an approval letter dated February 12, 2004.

[300]Clinical Review Section of Application No. STN/BLA 125084 (p. 51 of 149 pp. total, no date provided).

[301]United States Food and Drug Administration. Center for Drug Evaluation and Research (CDER). Application No. STN/BLA 125084; ERBITUX (Cetuximab). All of the correspondence documents are incorporated by reference in an approval letter dated February 12, 2004.

TABLE 25.3 Example of Questions for Patients With Poorly Written Questions (Left) and Adequately Written Questions (Right)

	Poor Writing	Better Writing
Avoid double negatives	Is the patient currently not taking asthma medication? ☐Y ☐N	Is the patient currently taking asthma medication? ☐Y ☐N
Specify time points	How would you rate your pain? ☐severe ☐mild	How would you rate your pain since your last visit? ☐severe ☐mild
Avoid two questions in one sentence	Were answers 28–32 reviewed by the nutritionist and was the patient eligible? ☐Y ☐N	Were answers 28–32 reviewed by the nutritionists? ☐Y ☐N

clinical trials. Moon (302) details the content and appearance of a typical CRF used for clinical trials. Some CRFs may capture only AEs occurring at a given point in time, while other CRFs may be designed to capture cumulative information on AEs. An example of a poor CRF may contain fields for inputting WBC counts, where the field looks like this:

Neutrophils _____; Lymphocytes _____.
  In contrast, a high-quality CRF will include the unit, and the field will look like this:
Neutrophils (cells/mL blood) _____;
Lymphocytes (cells/mL blood) _____.

CRFs should avoid double negatives, and should specify time points where appropriate, and should avoid lumping more than one question in a single sentence. This advice for a bad CRF and a good CRF is shown below (Table 25.3) (303).

Ene-Iordache et al. (304) describe issues relating to electronic CRFs, such as the requirement for the data-entry person to add an electronic signature, and the issue of the audit trail. Moreover, Headlee (305) teaches that CRFs may be designed in parallel with the writing of the Clinical Study Protocol, and that the form should include check boxes to capture AEs expected from the drug of interest, such as neurological AEs. Also, this author recommends using check boxes instead of spaces for writing, where appropriate, to increase the efficiency of filling, and the legibility, of the forms.

e. Adverse Events—Capturing, Transmitting, and Evaluating Data on Adverse Events

The following diagrams illustrate the overall processes used for capturing, evaluating, and

[302]Moon KK. Techniques for designing case report forms in clinical trials. ScianNews 2006;9:1 (7 pp.).

[303]NHMRC Clinical Trials Centre, University of Sydney. Outreach. An Australian initiative to support clinical trials; September 2009. 2 pp.

[304]Ene-Iordache B, Carminati S, Antiga L, et al. Developing regulatory-compliant electronic case report forms for clinical trials: experience with the demand trial. J. Am. Med. Inform. Assoc. 2009;16:404–8.

[305]Headlee D. The paper trail: CRFs, source documents and data collection tools. SoCRA Source; May 2004;30 (4 pp.).

performing quality control of SAEs. The processes used for AEs are somewhat different than for SAEs, in view of the fact that typical AEs are not submitted to regulatory agencies while, in contrast, SAEs may be submitted.

Thus, the big picture is revealed by the following small pictures. The arrows begin at the party that initiates the process of capturing events. The investigational site is the initiating party, in the first diagram, because this site is where the study subject experiences the AE, for example, vomiting, fatigue, anorexia, or a seizure. In contrast, for the next diagram, follow-up is initiated by the sponsor's safety group, for example, by the director of drug safety. The first two diagrams show the process, where a contract research organization (CRO) is not involved, while the next two diagrams show the sponsor had hired a CRO to perform capture, store, and perform quality control work, on adverse event data.

Title 21 of the CFR dictates the time line of some of the reporting procedures (306):

> The sponsor shall notify FDA and all participating investigators ... of ... [a]ny adverse experience associated with the use of the drug that is both serious and unexpected; or [a]ny finding from tests in laboratory animals that suggest a significant risk for human subjects including reports of mutagenicity, teratogenicity, or carcinogenicity. Each notification shall be made as soon as possible and in no event later than 15 calendar days after the sponsor's initial receipt of the information. Each written notification may be submitted on FDA Form 3500A or in a narrative format ... [t]he sponsor shall also notify FDA by telephone or by facsimile transmission of any unexpected fatal or life-threatening

experience associated with the use of drug as soon as possible but in no event later than 7 calendar days after the sponsor's initial receipt of the information.

The CFR also dictates the requirement for following up reports of adverse events. In short, if an adverse event was found initially not to be serious enough to report, but upon follow-up was determined to be serious enough to report, then the investigator must report it (307):

> The sponsor shall promptly investigate all safety information received by it ... [f]ollow up information to a safety report shall be submitted as soon as the relevant information is available.

These bullet points summarize the above information:

- The investigator can use a special form (MedWatch Form 3500A) to submit the report. A similar form, MedWatch Form 3500 is reproduced below.
- The FDA is only interested in receiving information about AEs that are serious and unexpected.
- The FDA must be provided with relevant data from animal testing.
- The sponsor must transmit the information to FDA, and also to participating investigators.
- What is provided is a 7-day deadline for SAEs that are unexpected fatal or life-threatening experiences.

Figures 25.3–25.6 outline the flow of information in adverse event reporting.

---

[306]21 CFR §312.32 (c) (April 1, 2006).

[307]21 CFR §312.32 (d) (April 1, 2006).

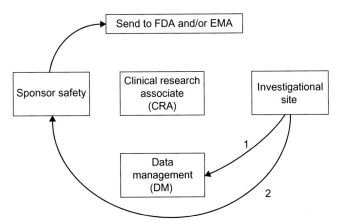

FIGURE 25.3 Initial report of SAE (situation where there is no CRO). One paper trail for processing adverse events starts at the investigational site, then continues to data management. Another paper trail begins at the investigational site, and proceeds to the sponsor's drug safety group, and then to regulatory agencies.

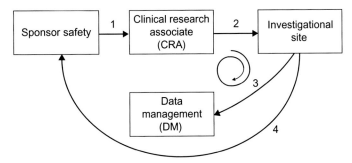

FIGURE 25.4 Follow-up to report of SAE (situation where there is no CRO). Follow-up of an SAE involves getting missing data, rationale according to the investigator's assessment, and information on resolution of the SAE. After the sponsor initiates follow-up, the next few subsequent steps are shown above. Following these steps, what occurs is a reiterative process, involving three parties, the CRA, the investigational site, and data management personnel, until the CRF is completely filled in. The reiterative process is indicated by the spiral.

XI. FDA'S WARNING LETTERS ABOUT FAILURE TO REPORT SAES

a. Failure to Report Adverse Events to the IRB

As stated above, the Sponsor needs to report certain adverse events to the IRB. The following Warning Letter concerns the issue of reporting requirements to the IRB. This reveals a paper trail that began with the FDA's inspection of the Sponsor's facility, which was followed by an exchange of letters between the Sponsor and the FDA, and ultimately the FDA's issuance of a Warning Letter. The Warning Letter (308) complained that the Sponsor had failed to report a SAE to the IRB. This Warning Letter was based on 21 CFR §312.66, which requires that, "[t[he investigator

[308]Warning Letter Ref. #: 09-HFD-45-01-02, dated February 2, 2009, to Family Practice Associates from Dr T. Purohit-Sheth, MD, Branch Chief, CDER, FDA.

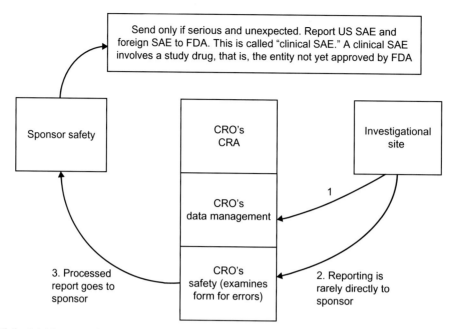

FIGURE 25.5   Initial report of SAE (situation where there is a CRO).

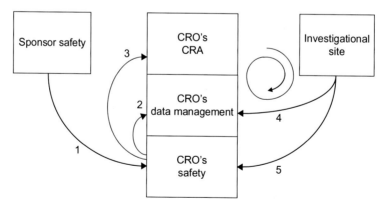

FIGURE 25.6   Follow-up report of SAE (situation where there is a CRO). Follow-up of an AE involves tracking down any missing data. The Sponsor's safety director initiates this follow-up, but is not involved in subsequent steps. After the initial few steps, shown above, what occurs is a reiterative process involving three parties, where the CRO's CRA and the CRO's data management personnel, contact the investigational site to make certain that all information for the CRF is filled out. The reiterative process is shown by the spiral.

shall … promptly report to the IRB all … unanticipated problems involving risk to human subjects." After citing this section of the CFR, the Warning Letter complained that:

> You failed to promptly report to the IRB all unanticipated problems involving risk to human subjects or others … your site was informed on December 12, 2006 that Subject … had been admitted to the hospital for a bilateral pulmonary embolism … and had remained in the intensive care unit for one week. You failed to notify the IRB per IRB requirements within three business days of becoming aware of this serious adverse event, and you reported this event to the IRB on February 12, 2007 as a protocol deviation rather than an adverse event.
>
> In your Undated Letter, you noted in response that Ms. [redacted] was the primary study coordinator for this protocol. This response is inadequate, because your site became aware of this event after Ms. [redacted] employment termination from your site … [i]t is your responsibility to ensure adherence to each requirement of the law and relevant FDA regulations. You must address these deficiencies and establish procedures to ensure that any ongoing or future studies will be in compliance with FDA regulations … [f]ailure to adequately and promptly explain the violations noted above may result in regulatory action without further notice.

b. Failure to Report Adverse Events to the FDA

The Sponsor has a duty to report adverse events to the FDA, including adverse events that occur after FDA-approval and during the marketing timeframe. Section 314.80 provides the applicable rule, which states that (21 CFR §314.80):

> Each applicant having an approved application … shall promptly review all adverse drug experience information obtained … from any source, foreign or domestic, including information derived from … postmarketing clinical investigations, postmarketing epidemiological/surveillance studies, reports in the scientific literature … applicant shall report each adverse drug experience that is both serious and unexpected, whether foreign or domestic, as soon as possible but in no case later than 15 calendar days of initial receipt of the information by the applicant.

In a Warning Letter to the Sponsor, FDA complained that the Sponsor had failed to comply with the requirement to transmit adverse event reports to the FDA, on a timely basis, in the timeframe after drug approval, that is, in the postmarketing timeframe. The Warning Letter complained that (309):

> The first postmarketing adverse drug experience (ADE) reporting compliance inspection of [redacted] Therapeutics was conducted in 2006. Observations from the 2006 inspection included late submission of 15-day Alert reports … [a]dditionally, during the 2009 inspection, the FDA Investigator noted that your firm did not complete corrective actions until 2007, even though your response to FDA, dated January 19, 2006, stated that all corrections had been made.
>
> Specific violations observed during the August 15, 2011 through September 9, 2011, inspection include … [f]ailure to submit all adverse drug experiences (ADEs) that are both serious and unexpected to FDA within 15 calendar days of initial receipt of the information as required by 21 CFR 314.80 … [f]rom January 22, 2010 through August 15, 2011, you submitted … late ADE reports to the Agency. These … reports contained both serious and unexpected adverse drug experiences, including but not limited to, deaths, irregular heartbeats, arrhythmia, acute fulminant hepatitis, hypersensitivity, and memory impairment that should have been submitted to the New Drug Application (NDA) within 15 days of initial receipt of the information … [f]or example, report [redacted] which described a patient who expired, was due to the Agency on August 28, 2010, but not received until January 10, 2011, approximately 136 days late.

---

[309]Warning Letter NYK-2012-18, dated May 10, 2012, issued by Ronald M. Pace, District Director, New York District, FDA.

The Warning Letter acknowledged that the Sponsor (application holder) had used a CRO to do its adverse event reporting, but stated that this did not relieve the Sponsor of its responsibility to comply with the applicable regulations. To this point, the Warning Letter stated:

> As part of your firm's corrective action plan for late reporting ... your firm voluntarily terminated its relationship with the contractor processing individual case safety reports ... and entered into an agreement with a different contractor for adverse event report processing. However, of the ... late reports noted above, [more late reports] occurred after you implemented your corrective action plan ... [a]s the holder of approved applications, [the Sponsor] has the obligation to report serious and unexpected adverse drug experiences to FDA within 15 calendar days of initial receipt of the information ... [i]f the application holder elects to out-source drug safety, [the application holder] retains the responsibility to ensure that it is done in a manner consistent with FDA regulations.

XII. DRUGS THAT CREATE RISK FOR INFECTIONS

a. Drugs That Inhibit the Immune System

Drugs that inhibit the immune system are used for treating autoimmune diseases, such as multiple sclerosis, rheumatoid arthritis, psoriasis, and inflammatory bowel disease. Autoimmune diseases result from pathological behaviors of T cells and other immune cells.

But it is self-evident that any drug that suppresses the immune system might increase the risk for infections. In the words of one commentator, a safety problem with therapies that inhibit the immune system and reduce pathological inflammation is that, "as flip side of the coin, treatment ... leaves the patient more susceptible to infection by inducing a certain extent of immunosuppression" (310).

b. Drugs That Inhibit Tumor Necrosis Factor-Alpha

Drugs that inhibit tumor necrosis factor-alpha (TNF-alpha) inhibit immune response and are used to treat rheumatoid arthritis. TNF-alpha is a cytokine. These inhibitory drugs, which include, *etanercept, infliximab,* and *adalimumab,* have all been associated with increased risk for infections, such as tuberculosis, hepatitis B virus (311), and fungal infections. For example, immunosuppressive therapy with anti-TNF-alpha antibodies increases the risk for *Pneumocystis* fungus (312).

In fact, the package label for *etanercept* (Enbrel®) includes a black box warning regarding infections (313). Although the drug is for treating an autoimmune disease (psoriatic arthritis), the drug also increases the risk for infections. The black box warning reads:

> SERIOUS INFECTIONS. Increased risk of serious infections leading to hospitalization or death, including tuberculosis (TB), bacterial sepsis, invasive fungal infections (such as histoplasmosis), and infections due to other opportunistic pathogens.

---

[310]De Keyser F. Choice of biologic therapy for patients with rheumatoid arthritis: the infection perspective. Curr. Rheumatol. Revs. 2011;7:77–87.

[311]De Keyser F. Choice of biologic therapy for patients with rheumatoid arthritis: the infection perspective. Curr. Rheumatol. Revs. 2011;7:77–87.

[312]Bello-Irizarry SN, et al. MyD88 signaling regulates both host defense and immunopathogenesis during Pneumocystis infection. J. Immunol. 2014;192:282–92.

[313]Package label for Enbrel® (etanercept) solution for subcutaneous use; March 2015.

The *Warnings and Precautions* section of the package insert cautions against fungal infections:

> WARNINGS AND PRECAUTIONS. Do not start Enbrel during an active infection. If an infection develops, monitor carefully and stop Enbrel if infection becomes serious. Consider empiric anti-fungal therapy for patients at risk for invasive fungal infections who develop a severe systemic illness on Enbrel (those who reside or travel to regions where mycoses are endemic).

The mechanism of TNF-alpha, in combating infections, has been reviewed (314). In short, bacteria, which possess molecules that stimulate toll-like receptors (TLRs), contact macrophages during the course of infection, and stimulate the TLRs of the macrophage, with the consequent expression of TNF-alpha.

c. Drugs That Inhibit Migration of T Cells to the Central Nervous System

Natalizumab (Tysabri®) is another immunosuppressive drug that is used to treat an autoimmune disease, that is, multiple sclerosis. The drug impairs the passage of T cells into the central nervous system, thus preventing pathological inflammation of the central nervous system. Unfortunately, a rare consequence is infections by JC virus in the central nervous system, resulting in a disorder called progressive multifocal leukoencephalopathy (315,316). The package label for natalizumab includes a black box warning regarding this disorder (317):

> WARNING: PROGRESSIVE MULTIFOCAL LEUKOENCEPHALOPATHY. TYSABRI increases the risk of progressive multifocal leukoencephalopathy (PML), an opportunistic viral infection of the brain that usually leads to death or severe disability.

d. Antibody Drugs That Inhibit Epidermal Growth Factor Receptor

Recombinant antibodies that bind to epidermal growth factor receptor (EGFR) are used for treating solid tumors. These antibodies include *cetuximab* and *panitumumab*, which are used for treating colorectal cancer. However, clinical trials using these drugs for treating colorectal cancer demonstrated an increased risk for infections.

Altan and Burtness documented the fact that the association between the anticancer drug and infections was not suspected, writing that, "[u]ntil recently, the infections observed during treatment with EGFR ... directed antibodies have not been attributed to ... the antibodies themselves ... [t]he mechanism of action for this effect has not been established" (318). Please note that, it was eventually discovered that EGF (ligand)

---

[314] Parameswaran N, Patial S. Tumor necrosis factor-alpha signaling in macrophages. Crit. Rev. Eukaryot. Gene Expr. 2010;20:87–103.

[315] van Rossum JA, et al. Safety, anxiety and natalizumab continuation in JC virus-seropositive MS patients. Multiple Sclerosis J. 2014;20:108–11.

[316] Tavazzi E, et al. Progressive multifocal leukoencephalopathy: an unexpected complication of modern therapeutic monoclonal antibody therapies. Clin. Microbiol. Infect. 2011;17:1776–80.

[317] Package insert for TYSABRI (natalizumab) injection for intravenous use; December 2013 (29 pp.).

[318] Altan M, Burtness B. EGFR-directed antibodies increase the risk of severe infection in cancer patients. BMC Med. 2015;13:37 (3 pp.).

and EGFR (receptor), and associated signaling pathways, are used to mediate innate immune response against infections (319,320). The behavior of FDA reviewers in documenting associations between *cetuximab* and infections is revealed below. The *Medical Review* is dated Oct. 2, 2007, long before concrete information was available on the association, or on the relevant mechanisms, of EGFR-mediated signaling and infections.

e. FDA's Decision-Making Process in Evaluating the Association of Cetuximab With Infections

This concerns FDA's review of the anti-EGFR antibody *cetuximab* for treating colorectal cancer. The information is from BLA 125084 from Mar. 2015 of FDA's website. The *Medical Review* is dated from a much earlier year, 2007, a time when it was not suspected that EGFR-mediated signaling was relevant to infections. The FDA reviewer's comments reveal how the FDA handles an adverse event, where causality is not suspected.

The FDA reviewer wrote, "Infectious events are noted to be more common in the cetuximab/arm of this and other controlled studies. **A causal link** between this patient's Gram negative sepsis [bacterial infection] and cetuximab **cannot be excluded**."

Further comments from the FDA reviewer revealed that the FDA did not suspect that EGFR-mediated pathways were used for innate immunity against infections. The FDA reviewer wrote, "[a]dministration of cetuximab causes or predisposes toward infections, possibly due to catheter use, increased number of medical procedures . . . other iatrogenic events."

The reviewer's comments about catheter use being a cause of infections was reasonable, in view of the fact that chronic catheter use does result in infections (321,322).

The take-home lesson is that the Sponsor should ensure documentation of all adverse events, even if a causal connection between the study drug and adverse event is unknown.

The package insert for *cetuximab* provides information about infections in the *Warnings and Precautions* section, the *Adverse Reactions* section, and in the *Clinical Trials Experience* section. The *Clinical Trials Experience* section reads "Infections: The incidence of infection was variable across studies, ranging from 13–35%. Sepsis occurred in 1–4% of patients" (323). (There was a black box warning, but it did not mention infections.)

f. Package Insert for a Drug That is a Potentialy Immunosuppressive Drug (Glatiramer)

Because, as a class of compounds, immunosuppressive drugs increase the risk for infections, it is interesting to point out that the package label for one drug that influences

---

[319]Feng Z, et al. Epithelial innate immune response to Acinetobacter baumannii challenge. Infect. Immunity 2014;82:4458–65.

[320]Yamashita M, et al. EGFR is essential for TLR3 signaling. Sci. Signal. 2012;5(233):ra50. http://dx.doi.org/10.1126/scisignal.2002581.

[321]Giare-Patel, K, et al. WO2013/070951. Novel enhanced formulations for coating medical devices. Int. Publication Date, 16 May 2013.

[322]This patent application (WO2013/070951) was drafted and submitted by Tom Brody.

[323]Package insert for ERBITUX® (cetuximab) Injection, for Intravenous Infusion; April 2015 (14 pp.).

the immune system, *glatiramer* (Copaxone®), expressly states that *increased infections have not been found*. The *Warnings and Precautions* section for the package insert reads (324):

> Because COPAXONE can modify immune response, it may interfere with immune functions … in a way that would undermine the body's … defenses against infection. There is no evidence that COPAXONE does this.

Dr Masha Hareli also commented on the fact that glatiramer has not been found to increase the risk for infections, explaining that, "[i]nterestingly, Copaxone does not cause immunosuppression, as you would presume, due to its short half-life" (325).

XIII. FDA'S DECISION-MAKING PROCESS ON ADVERSE EVENTS THAT APPEAR IRRELEVANT TO THE STUDY DRUG

a. Introduction

This provides examples of comments by FDA reviewers, for evaluating adverse events that seem unrelated to the study drug. Despite the apparently unrelated nature, the adverse event was recorded in the drug safety database and not ignored. In all cases, the FDA reviewer referred to reasoning or judgment on whether the adverse event was related to the drug. The take-home lesson is that study investigators and medical writers should not ignore adverse events, even when appearing to be extremely remote from the mechanism of action of the study drug.

b. Dimethyl Fumarate for Multiple Sclerosis

The example of *dimethyl fumarate* is from NDA 204063, which is available at Mar. 2013 on FDA's website. Dimethyl fumarate is metabolized in the body to fumaric acid which is a naturally occurring component of most foods and hence, at first glance, might not be expected to present any life-threatening safety issues. However, the clinical trial was for multiple sclerosis, which can be fatal. The *Medical Review* noted that the causes of death included, "traumatic brain injury following bicycle accident, motor vehicle accident, complications from MS (multiple sclerosis) relapse." The Review noted that the subject, "experienced a traumatic brain injury resulting from a bicycle accident … as the subject attempted to avoid a collision with a driver who was under the influence of alcohol." The reasoned conclusion in the *Medical Review* was that, "there does not appear to be a meaningful difference in mortality between" the study drug and placebo.

c. Irbesartan for Hypertension

The example of *irbesartan* is from NDA 20758, at Jan. 2015 on FDA's website. The adverse event was an automobile accident. According to the *Medical Review*, the "subject … was a 55 year old male with a 32-year history of hypertension. After 20 months on … irbesartan … he died in a motor vehicle accident. Relationship to study drug was considered unlikely, but no description appears to rule out sudden incapacitation of the subject prior to the accident." Although the conclusion contained no details, the FDA

---

[324] Package insert for COPAXONE (glatiramer acetate injection) for subcutaneous use; January 2014 (8 pp.).

[325] Kind response from Dr Masha Hareli, Ph.D., in e-mail of May 1, 2015.

reviewer's comments were reasonable in that they left open the possibility of "sudden incapacitation" related to the study drug.

d. Everolimus for Preventing Rejection of Kidney Transplants

This is from a clinical trial for *everolimus*, a drug for preventing rejection of kidney transplants. The information is from NDA 21560, from Jan. 2015 on FDA's website. A male study subject died as a result of a motor vehicle accident where, according to the FDA reviewer, the "real cause of death … is the motor vehicle accident." The reviewer states that the subject remained alive for 13 days following the accident, and that, "the final event causing the death … might have been pulmonary emboli occurring 13 days after" the accident. The take-home lesson is that, where an accident is the initiating event that results in death, safety reporting should include the final event most closely associated with the death.

e. Tavaborole for Fungal Infections

The example of *tavaborole* is from NDA 204427, at Jan. 2015 on the FDA's website. The study drug, tavaborole, took the form of a topical solution for applying directly to toenails infected with fungus. Please note the remote nature of a drug that is applied topically, and to possible causes of falling down. The *Medical Review* described one death, writing that, "[t]he subject was 61 years old female … [s]he was treated with tavaborole … from July 26, 2006 until November 6, 2006 … she fell down and, according to the death certificate, died of head trauma." Although reasons were not expressly stated, the FDA reviewer stated that the trauma "was not considered by investigators

as related to the treatment … I agree with the investigator's assessment that event was not likely related to the drug."

XIV. POSTMARKETING REPORTING OF ADVERSE EVENTS

a. Introduction

After regulatory approval of a drug, there is continued surveillance of drug safety. Healthcare professionals, as well as the general public, can submit drug safety reports to the FDA by way of a MedWatch form. There are two different versions of the MedWatch form, one of which is used by pharmaceutical companies, and the other by consumers in the postmarketing context.

The MedWatch form provides a rapid way to communicate SAEs to the FDA. This form is used for any SAE, especially those that might not be listed on the package insert, including fatalities, hospitalization, and other medically significant events. The FDA welcomes the use of MedWatch forms to report therapeutic failures, for example, if a patient needed to switch to another brand of the same drug, to report errors in the dosing instructions, and to report suspected counterfeit drugs or contaminated drugs. In the context of postapproval reporting, Nebeker et al. (326), stated that, "the FDA is interested in receiving reports on serious, unexpected adverse drug reactions (not adverse drug events) from marketed drugs. Unexpected reactions are those whose nature or severity is not consistent with the product label."

The MedWatch form finds use by physicians who treat members of the general public (not clinical trial subjects), as demonstrated by this example. Injuries to patients resulted from

[326]Nebeker JR, Barach P, Samore MH. Clarifying adverse drug events: a clinician's guide to terminology, documentation, and reporting. Ann. Intern. Med. 2004;140:795–801.

confusion with Lanoxin® (heart medicine) and Levoxine® (thyroid medicine) (327,328). Patients were receiving Lanoxin, when they should have been receiving Levoxine. The confusion was accentuated by the fact that the dosages were the same (0.125 mg). The medication errors and injuries were reported to the FDA using MedWatch forms and, as a result, the name of Levoxine was changed to Levoxyl® (329).

b. The MedWatch Form and the CIOMS I Form

A reproduction of the MedWatch form is shown below. The form can be mailed to the FDA or transmitted by way of the internet. The reproduced form is a slightly simplified version of the real form. The following discloses the time-line of how MedWatch forms influence the regulatory process. The FDA receives reports of adverse drug events primarily from physicians and pharmacists who submit them on MedWatch forms, as well as from information supplied by pharmaceutical companies.

After a sufficient number of reports, including reports published in medical journals, have accumulated implicating the drug, the division of the FDA that had initially reviewed and approved the drug examines the newly acquired data on AEs (330). If the FDA reviewers agree that the data are compelling enough to require regulatory action, the FDA notifies the manufacturer and requests the action. This action may take the form of a change in the package insert, a *Dear Healthcare Professional* letter, or withdrawal of the drug from the market. In Great Britain, the equivalent of the MedWatch form is the Yellow Card (331). The Yellow Card is administered by the Medicines and Healthcare products Regulatory Agency (MHRA) (332), located in London, UK. The MHRA is the British equivalent of the US FDA (333). The Yellow Card is not used in clinical trials, but by the public and healthcare professionals in the postmarketing context (334,335). In Great Britain, the CIOMS I form is used for reporting by manufacturers of suspected ADRs to regulatory authorities, but it is not used by healthcare professionals or patients. The FDA allows receipt of CIOMS forms in lieu of MedWatch forms (336).

[327]Pourmatobbed G. The naming of drugs is a difficult matter. New Engl. J. Med. 1994;311:1163.

[328]http://video.google.com/videoplay?docid = 7028108578849636582#

[329]FDA Advise-ERR:Medication errors associated with levothyroxine products. ISMP Medication Safety Alert!; September 6, 2000.

[330]Wysowski DK, Swartz L. Adverse drug event surveillance and drug withdrawals in the United States, 1969−2002: the importance of reporting suspected reactions. Arch. Intern. Med. 2005;165:1363−9.

[331]McLernon DJ, Bond CM, Hannaford PC, et al. Adverse drug reaction reporting in the UK: a retrospective observational comparison of yellow card reports submitted by patients and healthcare professionals. Drug Saf. 2010;33:775−88.

[332]http://www.mhra.gov.uk/index.htm

[333]Arnold BDC. E-mail of March 27, 2011.

[334]Stevenson D. E-mail of March 25, 2011.

[335]Heffer S. E-mail of April 1, 2011.

[336]Klepper M. E-mail of April 6, 2011.

c. CIOMS

CIOMS is an international, nongovernmental, organization established jointly by WHO and the United Nations Educational, Scientific and Cultural Organization (UNESCO) in 1949. It provides a range of guidance on issues ranging from bioethics, health policy, drug development and use, and international nomenclature of diseases, as well as on assessing and monitoring adverse events (337).

d. The CIOMS I Form

This concerns adverse events that occur outside the United States. For reporting these AEs to the FDA, drug companies can use either an international form (CIOMS I form) or FDA Form 3500A (338). However, for adverse events that occur within the United States, drug companies must use FDA Form 3500A, and must not use the CIOMS I Form. The CIOMS I form is available in electronic format (339).

There is only the CIOMS I form (there do not exist CIOMS II or CIOMS III forms). The CIOMS I form is used for both pre- and post-marketing reporting. Reporting is mandatory only for the Marketing Authorization Holder, but voluntary for consumers and physicians

(340). In Great Britain, the MHRA will accept information filled out on a CIOMS I form by a member of the public or healthcare professional, as long as it has the four minimum reporting requirements: a patient identifier, suspect drug, suspect reaction, and reporter details, however in practice, this route for reporting safety issues in Great Britain is rarely used (341).

Investigators need to be aware of different reporting requirements in the United States and in Europe. According to one commentator, in Europe, it is the case regulators accept the ICH concept that manufacturers should report only those events that the reporting physician or the manufacturer believe have a causal relationship with a drug (342). However, the United States has been slow to adopt these standards, and prefers companies to report all adverse experiences, irrespective of the likelihood of a causal relationship (Fig. 25.7).

e. Postmarketing Surveillance

Postmarketing safety reporting to the FDA can use a format mandated by the FDA (Periodic Adverse Drug Experience Report; PADER) or, with permission, can utilize the Periodic Safety Update Report (PSUR) format (343). The PSUR provides an update of

[337]Castle GH, Kelly B. Harmonization is not all that global: divergent approaches in drug safety. Food Drug Law J. 2008;63:601–22.

[338]U.S. Department of Health and Human Services. Food and Drug Administration. Guidance for industry. Postmarketing safety reporting for human drug and biological products including vaccines; March 2001.

[339]Drug safety reporting duties in Switzerland. Swissmedic, Hallerstrasse 7, CH-300 Bern 9 (document dated May 13, 2009).

[340]Andrews EB. E-mail of April 1, 2011.

[341]Heffer S. E-mail of April 1, 2011.

[342]Castle GH, Kelly B. Global harmonization is not all that global:divergent approaches in drug safety. Food Drug Law J. 2008;63:601.

[343]U.S. Department of Health and Human Services. Food and Drug Administration. Guidance for industry. Providing regulatory submissions in electronic format—postmarketing periodic adverse drug experience reports; June 2003 (16 pp.).

U.S. Department of Health and Human Services
Food and Drug Administration

Form Approved: OMB No. 09010-0291

MEDWATCH

The FDA Safety Information and Adverse Event Reporting Program

A. PATIENT INFORMATION

1. Patient Identifier	2. Age at Time of Event or Date of Birth:	3. Sex	4. Weight
In confidence		☐ Female ☐ Male	___ lbs or ___kgs.

B. ADVERSE EVENT, PRODUCT PROBLEM OR ERROR
Check all that apply:
1. ☐ Adverse Event ☐ Product Problem (e.g., defects/malfunctions)
☐ Product Use Error ☐ Problem with Different Manufacturer of Same Medicine

2. Outcomes Attributed to Adverse Event
(Check all that apply)
☐ Death (mm/dd/yyyy) ☐ Disability or Permanent Damage
☐ Life-threatening ☐ Congenital Anomaly/Birth Defect
☐ Hospitalization ☐ Other Serious (Important Medical Events)
☐ Required Intervention to Prevent Permanent Impairment/Damage (Devices

3. Date of Event (mm/dd/yyyy)

4. Date of This Report (mm/dd/yyyy)

5. Describe Event or Problem or Produce Use Error

6. Relevant Tests/Laboratory Data, Including Dates

7. Other Relevant History, Including Preexisting Medical Conditions (e.g., allergies, race, pregnancy, smoking and alcohol use, hepatic/renal problems, etc.)

C. PRODUCT AVAILABILITY
Product Available for Evaluation?
☐ Yes ☐ No ☐ Returned to Manufacturer on: (mm/dd/yyyy)

D. SUSPECT PRODUCT(S)
1. Name, Strength, Manufacturer (from product label)
2. Dose or Amount Frequency Route
3. Dates of Use (If unknown, give duration) from/to (or best estimate).
4. Diagnosis or Reason for Use (Indication)
5. Event Abated After Use Stopped or Dose Reduced?
☐ Yes ☐ No ☐ Doesn't Apply
6. Lot #
7. Expiration Date
8. Event Reappeared After Reintroduction?
☐ Yes ☐ No ☐ Doesn't Apply
9. NDC# or Unique ID

E. OTHER (CONCOMITANT) MEDICAL PRODUCTS
Product names and therapy dates (exclude treatment of event)

F. REPORTER (See confidentiality section on back)
1. Name and Address
Name
Address
City State Zip

Phone #	E-mail
2. Health Professional? ☐ Yes ☐ No	3. Occupation

FORM FDA 3500 (1/09) Submission of a report does not constitute an admission that medical personnel or the product contributed to the event.

FIGURE 25.7 MedWatch form. The MedWatch form is provided by the US Food and Drug Administration for reporting adverse events.

worldwide safety experiences of drugs. With the PSUR submission, the sponsor summarizes newly obtained information and evaluates the risk—benefit profile of the drug (344). PSURs present the worldwide safety experience of a medicinal product at defined times postauthorization, in order to report new safety information and relate the data to patient exposure, summarize market authorization status in different countries, and indicate whether changes should be made to safety information supplied with the product (345). Ordinarily, all dosage forms and formulations as well as indications for a given pharmacologically active substance should be covered in one PSUR. Separate presentations of data for different dosage forms, indications, or populations, for example, children versus adults, may be used. The PSUR may contain safety information acquired from a number of sources, including spontaneous notifications from healthcare professionals, spontaneous notifications from consumers, sponsored clinical studies, the published medical literature, and from ADR reporting systems used by regulatory agencies (346).

The following compares safety reporting by way of two different formats, the PSUR and the individual case safety report (ICSR). According to Michael Klepper (347), the majority of ICSRs, are based on single subjects and is used for expedited reporting (IND reports during premarketing and 15-day alert reports during postmarketing), whereas the PSUR is an aggregate report of both expedited and nonexpedited ICSRs (as well as other information) that was received by the sponsor, primarily on the marketed drug. Therefore Periodic Reports (PSUR) are bigger and more inclusive than ICSRs (348).

Once a drug is approved the sponsor has to send in a PADER (21 CFR §314.80) quarterly for the first 3 years after drug approval, then annually thereafter. The PSUR is used in Europe and elsewhere and may eventually replace the PADER. The FDA will accept the PSUR in lieu of the PADER upon request, but the PSUR must also be submitted quarterly for the first 3 years, then annually (349).

XV. RISK MINIMIZATION TOOLS

Risk minimization tools are proposed by the Sponsor and evaluated by FDA reviewers during the drug-submission and approval process. Risk minimization tools include REMS in the United States, and the *Risk Management Plans* (RMP) in the European Union, as well as common features such as the *Medication Guide, Dear Healthcare Professional Letter*, and black box warnings on the package insert.

---

[344]Pfizer. What are cumulative reports of safety? Version 1, August 2008 (4 pp.).

[345]U.S. Department of Health and Human Services. Food and Drug Administration. Guidance for industry. E2C. Clinical safety data management: periodic safety update reports for marketed drugs; November 1996 (21 pp.).

[346]U.S. Department of Health and Human Services. Food and Drug Administration. Guidance for industry. E2C. Clinical safety data management: periodic safety update reports for marketed drugs; November 1996 (21 pp.).

[347]Klepper M. E-mail of April 6, 2011.

[348]Klepper M. E-mail of April 6, 2011.

[349]Klepper M. E-mail of April 6, 2011.

a. Introduction to Risk Evaluation and Mitigation Strategies

The US FDA Amendments Act of 2007 granted the FDA new powers to enhance drug safety by requiring the pharmaceutical industry to develop Risk Evaluation and Mitigation Strategies (REMS) (350).

As part of the drug approval process, the FDA may require a Sponsor to submit a REMS. In submitting the REMS, the Sponsor explains how "the benefits of a drug outweigh the risks of the drug" (351). The Sponsor may voluntarily submit the REMS without having been required to do so by the FDA. Any submitted REMS is actually only a proposed REMS, because the FDA determines which parts of the REMS are necessary, that is, necessary during the course of the FDA-regulated clinical trial or necessary during marketing of the approved drug. REMS has a basis in Title 21 of the United States Code (21 USC §355), which states that the FDA considers these factors in evaluating a submitted REMS:

1. Size of the population likely to use the drug;
2. Seriousness of the disease or condition that is to be treated by the drug;
3. Expected benefit of the drug, with respect to the disease or condition;
4. Expected duration of treatment with the drug;
5. Seriousness of known or potential adverse events related to the drug;
6. Whether the drug is a new type of molecule.

Risk Evaluation and Mitigation Strategies find a basis in the CFR, which concerns "use of investigational new drugs and approved drugs where availability is limited by a ... REMS" (21 CFR §312.302). Section 312.302 requires that the FDA determine if "patients to be treated have a serious or immediately life-threatening disease or condition, and there is no comparable ... alternative therapy." Section 312.302 also requires that, "the potential patient benefit justifies the potential risks." When submitted, the REMS must be submitted to the FDA using Form FDA 1571. Form FDA 1571 is detailed in Chapter 33, in the material on the timeline of the FDA-approval process.

Along with the REMS, the Sponsor may submit these optional documents (352):

- *Medication Guide* (21 CFR §208);
- Patient Package Insert;
- Communication plan to healthcare providers, where this plan supports supplementation of some part of the REMS. This communication plan often takes the form of a "Dear Health Care Professional" letter plus internet-based information.

If the Sponsor submits a *Medication Guide*, the Sponsor must ensure that it "is available for distribution to patients who are dispensed the drug" (353). The content of the *Medication Guide* and Patient Package Insert are somewhat redundant, as is evident from the FDA's

[350]Nicholson SC, et al. Risk evaluation and mitigation strategies (REMS): educating the prescriber. Drug Saf. 2012;35:91–104.

[351]U.S. Department of Health and Human Services. Food and Drug Administration. Guidance for industry. Format and content of proposed risk evaluation and mitigation strategies (REMS), REMS assessments, and proposed REMS modifications; September 2009 (36 pp.).

[352]U.S. Department of Health and Human Services. Food and Drug Administration. Guidance for industry. Format and content of proposed risk evaluation and mitigation strategies (REMS), REMS assessments, and proposed REMS modifications; September 2009 (36 pp.).

[353]U.S. Department of Health and Human Services. Food and Drug Administration. Guidance for industry. Format and content of proposed risk evaluation and mitigation strategies (REMS), REMS assessments, and proposed REMS modifications; September 2009 (36 pp.).

statement that, "[h]aving both a required patient package insert and a *Medication Guide* for the same drug is not expected to occur frequently."

FDA's Guidance for Industry also suggests these optional elements to include in the REMS. The REMS may require that the physician have a particular type of training or certification, that the staff at pharmacies read the educational materials before dispensing the drug, that the drug be disposed to patients only in a hospital pharmacy, that patients receive counseling, and that all patients be enrolled in a registry.

b. Registries

As mentioned above, REMS may include a requirement that all patients taking the drug in question be enrolled in a registry. FDA-approved versions of any REMS that accompanies the approval of any drug can be accessed from the FDA's website by the procedure described in footnote (354).

- **Registry for lenalidomide**
  This REMS was part of the drug approval process for *lenalidomide* (Revlimid®). This is from NDA 021880, available on Dec. 2005 on the FDA's website. This REMS states that:

    > Upon receiving a report of pregnancy … Celgene [Sponsor] will enroll the female patient into the REVLIMID Pregnancy Exposure Registry. The objectives of the **registry are to monitor pregnancy** outcomes … and to understand why … REVLIMID … was unsuccessful," for the pregnancy case in question.

- **Registry for fingolimod**
  The REMS for another drug, *fingolimod*. The information is from NDA 22527, at Sep. 2010 on FDA's website. This REMS also refers to a registry. Fingolimod (Gilenya) is for the indication of multiple sclerosis. The REMS states that:

    > [s]ince there are no adequate and well-controlled studies of GILENYA in pregnant women, a **pregnancy registry** has been established … [p]rescribers with eligible patients, or patients themselves, can contact the Pregnancy Exposure Registry by … sending an email to grr@outcom.

- **Registry for ustekinumab**
  This REMS is for *ustekinumab* (Stelara®) for psoriasis. The information is from BLA 125261 from Sep. 2009 of the FDA's website. The REMS stated that the registry:

    > is a voluntary, disease specific **registry** … that collects information from psoriasis patients and their treating physicians. Since this registry will continue for 10 years, it will help us better understand the risk of long-latency serious events, such as malignancies.

- **Registry for teduglutide**

  This concerns *teduglutide*, a 33-amino-acid oligopeptide for treating short bowel syndrome. The information is from NDA 203441, from Jan. 2015 of FDA's website. In addition to requiring an REMS, the FDA required that the Sponsor create a registry. According to FDA's *Medical Review*, "[p]anel members expressed the need for a **registry** for colorectal and other cancers that follows patients for at least 10 years, in addition to the REMS."

---

[354]On FDA website, click on DRUG tab, click on Search Drug Approvals by Month Using Drugs@FDA, then choose the month and year, then choose the drug, and finally click on "Approval History, Letters, Reviews, and related documents."

The FDA recommended a registry, because even though the drug was for treating short bowel syndrome (which is not particularly relevant to cancer), it was the case that the drug (teduglutide) is a *growth factor*, and that some evidence suggests that administering growth factors may increase the risk for cancer (355,356). The FDA reviewer provided the following decision tree, which was recommended for including in the package label. In short, the package label should state that the drug should not be used in patients with gastrointestinal cancer, and that for patients with other types of cancer, the drug should be used only after a risk–benefit analysis.

c. *Dear Healthcare Professional* Letters

Dear Healthcare Professional letters are one form of risk minimization tool. These letters are issued in the postmarketing context.

The *Dear Healthcare Professional* letter fits into a broader context, namely that of risk minimization tools. These tools include: (1) Patient package insert; (2) Medication guide; (3) Dear Healthcare Professional letter; (4) Prescription sticker attached to the prescription; (5) Patient information leaflet; (6) Consent forms; and (7) Limiting number of pills in each bottle (357,358).

The medication guide must conform to the CFR (21 CFR §208), must be provided by the pharmacist to the patient with every new prescription and with every refill (359), and must be written in nontechnical language (360). Patient package inserts are also mandated by the FDA, at least for oral contraceptives (21 CFR §310.501) and for estrogens (21 CFR §310.515). The patient information leaflet is generally written by a party other than the drug manufacturer. Consent forms are described in Chapter 30. Prescription stickers, which are written by the manufacturer in collaboration with the FDA (361), have been issued for isotretinoin, fentanyl, clozapine, thalidomide, alosetron, mifepristone, dofetlide, bosentan, and oxybate (362).

[355]DiVall SA, Radovick S. Growth hormone and treatment controversy; long term safety of rGH. Curr. Pediatr. Rep. 2013;1:128–32.

[356]Ibrahim YH, Yee D. Insulin-like growth factor-I and cancer risk. Growth Horm. IGF Res. 2004;14:261–9.

[357]U.S. Department of Health and Human Services. Food and Drug Administration. Guidance for industry. Development and use of risk management action plans; March 2005 (27 pp.).

[358]Lee LY, Kortepeter CM, Willy ME, Nourjah P. Drug-risk communication to pharmacists: assessing the impact of risk-minimization strategies on the practice of pharmacy. J. Am. Pharm. Assoc. 2008;48:494–500.

[359]Lee LY, Kortepeter CM, Willy ME, Nourjah P. Drug-risk communication to pharmacists: assessing the impact of risk-minimization strategies on the practice of pharmacy. J. Am. Pharm. Assoc. 2008;48:494–500.

[360]U.S. Department of Health and Human Services. Food and Drug Administration. Guidance for industry. Drug safety information—FDA's communication to the public; March 2007 (17 pp.).

[361]Food and Drug Administration. CDER 2002 report to the nation: improving public health through human drugs. Rockville, MD: Food and Drug Administration.

[362]Lee LY, Kortepeter CM, Willy ME, Nourjah P. Drug-risk communication to pharmacists: assessing the impact of risk-minimization strategies on the practice of pharmacy. J. Am. Pharm. Assoc. 2008;48:494–500.

In a survey of *Dear Healthcare Professional* letters by Mazor et al. (363), the warnings were found to fall into the following categories:

- Change involves black box warning, addition, or revision.
- Revised to be consistent with another product.
- Change involves drug interaction.
- Change involves actions to be taken or avoided, for example, laboratory tests.
- Change gives information about specific patient group.
- Change defined by clinical condition.
- Change gives information about who should not get drug or about who is at increased risk.
- Change includes reference to fatal adverse events.

The following provides an example of a real *Dear Healthcare Professional Letter*. Within 6 months of marketing linezolid, also known as Zyvox®, MedWatch reports were sent to the FDA reporting myelosuppression. As a result, the FDA required the Zyvox package insert to include a warning regarding this drug-related adverse event.

And, as a further result of the reporting by MedWatch, the manufacture sent a *Dear Healthcare Professional* letter to the medical community, reproduced in part below. The *Dear Healthcare Professional* letter is a standard mechanism, used by the FDA, for warning physicians of AEs after marketing a new drug. Typically, these letters are sent within 1 year to up to 5 years after approval of any given drug (364). Drug withdrawals are extremely rare, compared to the frequency of *Dear Healthcare Professional* letters. Information on drug withdrawals, for safety reasons, can be found in the *Federal Register* and on the website of the FDA (365).

According to Giezen et al. (366), most *Dear Healthcare Professional* letters concern safety issues regarding hepatobiliary disorders, blood and lymphatic system disorders, cardiac disorders, and nervous system disorders. In a survey of about 2000 pharmacists who had received the *Dear Healthcare Professional* letters, Lee et al. (367), discovered that about 40% always read the letter, and that one-third often read it, and that 6% rarely read it. *Dear Healthcare Professional* letters are generally sent at the request of the FDA, though the

[363]Mazor KM, Andrade SE, Auger J, Fish L, Gurwitz JH. Communicating safety information to physicians: an examination of dear doctor letters. Pharmacoepidemiol. Drug Saf. 2005;14:869–75.

[364]Giezen TJ, Mantel-Teeuwisse AK, Straus SM, Schellekens H, Leufkens HG, Egberts AC. Safety-related regulatory actions for biologicals approved in the United States and the European Union. J. Am. Med. Assoc. 2008;300:1887–96.

[365]Lasser KE, Allen PD, Woolhandler SJ, Himmelstein DU, Wolfe SM, Bor DH. Timing of new black box warnings and withdrawals for prescription medications. J. Am. Med. Assoc. 2002;287:2215–20.

[366]Giezen TJ, Mantel-Teeuwisse AK, Straus SM, Schellekens H, Leufkens HG, Egberts AC. Safety-related regulatory actions for biologicals approved in the United States and the European Union. J. Am. Med. Assoc. 2008;300:1887–96.

[367]Lee LY, Kortepeter CM, Willy ME, Nourjah P. Drug-risk communication to pharmacists: assessing the impact of risk-minimization strategies on the practice of pharmacy. J. Am. Pharm. Assoc. 2008;48:494–500.

administrative law does not provide authority to require such communications (368). Shatin et al. (369) report that compliance with recommendations is low, as measured by the continued co-prescribing and co-dispensing of contraindicated drug combinations or completing recommended testing following label changes and mailed warnings.

The *Dear Healthcare Professional* letter reproduced below refers to the MedWatch reporting system (370). The letter provides a crystal-clear example of the responsible and ethical activities of the consumer, manufacturer, and the regulatory agency, in monitoring, reporting, and responding to adverse events of marketed drugs.

Dear Health Care Professional:

This letter is to advise you of important, new, safety information that has been added to the prescribing information for ZYVOX™ (linezolid injection, tablets and for oral suspension), a synthetic antibacterial agent of the oxazolidinone class. ZYVOX is indicated for the treatment of adult patients with the following infections caused by susceptible strains of designated microorganisms: vancomycin-resistant *Enterococcus faecium*, including cases with concurrent bacteremia; nosocomial pneumonia; complicated and uncomplicated skin and skin structure infections; and community-acquired pneumonia, including cases with concurrent bacteremia.

Pharmacia and the U. S. Food and Drug Administration (FDA) have received reports from the spontaneous reporting system of myelosuppression in patients receiving ZYVOX.

To communicate this important safety information, the following has been added to the WARNINGS section of the labeling:

Myelosuppression (including anemia, leukopenia, pancytopenia, and thrombocytopenia) has been

reported in patients receiving linezolid. In cases where the outcome is known, when linezolid was discontinued, the affected hematologic parameters have risen toward pretreatment levels. Complete blood counts should be monitored weekly in patients who receive linezolid, particularly in those who receive linezolid for longer than two weeks, those with pre-existing myelosuppression, those receiving concomitant drugs that produce bone marrow suppression, or those with a chronic infection who have received previous or concomitant antibiotic therapy. Discontinuation of therapy with linezolid should be considered in patients who develop or have worsening myelosuppression.

Changes consistent with the added warning have been made to the ADVERSE REACTIONS section and are as follows:

Postmarketing Experience. Myelosuppression (including anemia, leukopenia, pancytopenia, and thrombocytopenia) has been reported during postmarketing use of ZYVOX (see WARNINGS). These events have been chosen for inclusion due to either their seriousness, frequency of reporting, possible causal connection to ZYVOX, or a combination of these factors. Because they are reported voluntarily from a population of unknown size, estimates of frequency cannot be made and a causal relationship cannot be precisely established.

Our primary concern is the safety and well-being of patients who receive ZYVOX. If you become aware of any case(s) of the events described above, in patients treated with ZYVOX, please report the event promptly.

You may contact Pharmacia at 1-800-253-8600 extension 38244, or the FDA MedWatch program, by phone at 1-800-FDA-1088 ... Sincerely, ...

A medical journal characterized the collaboration between the FDA and the manufacturer in favorable terms (371). According to this journal, the manufacturer and the FDA worked together to change the labeling so that the

[368]Shatin D, Gardner JS, Stergachis A, Blough D, Graham D. Impact of mailed warning to prescribers on the co-prescription of tramadol and antidepressants. Pharmacoepidemiol. Drug Saf. 2005;14:149−54.

[369]Shatin D, Gardner JS, Stergachis A, Blough D, Graham D. Impact of mailed warning to prescribers on the co-prescription of tramadol and antidepressants. Pharmacoepidemiol. Drug Saf. 2005;14:149−54.

[370]Dear Health Care Professional letter. Peapack, NJ: Pharmacia Corp.; March 2001.

[371]FDA MedWatch Program Update: managing risk of use of medical products—the Zyvox example. Action Report Medical Board of California 2002;80:11.

warning of possible mylosuppression was added. The journal characterized the change as a success story, in that a product came on market with promise of significant efficacy, but rare adverse events materialized after marketing in the general population. The problem was found within the first year of marketing and the manufacturer was able to transmit the new safety information to the medical community.

d. *Dear Healthcare Professional* Letter Regarding Birth Control Pills

The issue of *Dear Healthcare Professional* arises, on occasion, during litigation between patients and pharmaceutical companies (372). *Dear Healthcare Professional* letters are part of a larger warning system, that includes the sum of package inserts, Physician's Desk Reference (PDR), and visits to doctors by the sales force (detailmen). Issues relating to a manufacturer's duty to warn, specifically relevant to the sales force, are the frequency of visits of the doctor, and training of the sales force regarding the warning in question. *Mahr v. G.D. Searle* (373) illustrates the concept that the sum of all of the above methods is part of the big picture for transmitting warnings to doctors, and that the sum of all of the above methods can determine whether a company is liable for insufficiently transmitting warnings to physicians. This particular case concerned pulmonary embolisms caused by birth control pills. *Mahr v. G.D. Searle* also illustrates the utility of *Dear Health Care Professional* letters in transmitting warnings where a gray area is thought to exist, that is, where there is no compelling reason to

believe that a drug caused the ADR in question. Thus, this courtroom opinion reveals the situation where the *Dear Healthcare Professional* letter "indicated that no causal connection between oral contraceptives and thromboembolic disorders had been demonstrated," but also "requested physicians to report to the company all instances of thrombophlebitic disease" (374).

The goal of this narrative is solely to illustrate some general principles that might be learned from the courtroom case, showing how the *Dear Healthcare Professional* letter fits into the various methods for warning physicians and patients.

e. *Dear Healthcare Professional* Letter Regarding Acne Medicine

Snyder v. Hoffman-LaRoche (375) further demonstrates that providing warnings to physicians (and patients) is the sum of a variety of tools, including the Dear Healthcare Professional letter, consent forms, a Medication Guide for pharmacists to distribute with the drug prescriptions, and oral counseling by the physician to the patient. In this context, the consent form is administered in the course of ordinary medical practice, not as part of a clinical trial. This courtroom opinion concerned an acne drug (13-cis-retinoic acid, Accutane®) that may have the ADR of inducing depression.

The time line is as follows. In Feb. 1998, the manufacturer amended the package insert to include the warning, "WARNINGS: Psychiatric Disorders: Accutane may cause depression, psychosis, and, rarely, suicidal ideation, suicide

---

[372]Search on LEXIS NEXIS® conducted on March 23, 2011, using search terms, "dear healthcare" and "dear health care," where the documents searched were all U.S. state and U.S. federal courts from the years 2000 to 2011. The result was about 40 relevant cases.

[373]Mahr v. G.D. Searle. 72 Ill. App. 3d 540; 390 N.E.2d 1214; 1979 Ill. App. LEXIS 2655.

[374]Mahr v. G.D. Searle. 72 Ill. App. 3d 540; 390 N.E.2d 1214; 1979 Ill. App. LEXIS 2655.

[375]Snyder v. Hoffman-Laroche. Middle District Florida, 2008 U.S. Dist. LEXIS 92017.

attempts, and suicide. Discontinuation of Accutane therapy may be insufficient; further evaluation may be necessary." The manufacturer provided additional warnings in the form of a "Dear Doctor" letter to physicians from Feb. 1998, the 1999 issue of the PDR, an information brochure to physicians entitled "Important Information Concerning Your Treatment with Accutane." In Jan. 2001, the manufacturer disseminated an Informed Consent Agreement for physcians to administer to all patients. The Informed Consent (to be read by patients) included the language, "I understand that some patients, while taking Accutane or soon after stopping Accutane, have become depressed or developed other serious mental problems. Signs of these problems include feelings of sadness, irritability, unusual tiredness, trouble concentrating, and loss of appetite." The Informed Consent also read, "Once I start taking Accutane, I agree to stop using Accutane and tell my provider right away if any of the following happen. I start to feel sad or have crying spells, lose interest in my usual activities,..."

On or about Feb. 2000, the physician first prescribed the drug to Mr Snyder for treating acne. Treatment was continued until Sep. 2003. But in Feb. 2005, the patient (Mr Snyder) committed suicide.

The goal of this narrative is solely to reveal general principles that can be learned from the courtroom case, regarding how the *Dear Healthcare Professional* letter fits into the various methods for warning physicians and patients.

f. *Dear Healthcare Professional* Letter Regarding Appetite Suppressants

In re Brisco et al. (376) provides one more illustration of a *Dear Healthcare Professional*

letter, this time, where the goal is to inform physicians that a drug was withdrawn from the market. As in the above examples, the *Dear Healthcare Professional* letter was used in combination with other methods for warning physicians and patients. To quote from this courtroom opinion, "The publicity began on September 15, 1997. At 5:00 p.m., the Houston CBS news affiliate started the broadcast with a report that ... diet drugs had been pulled from the market, announcing that the Food and Drug Administration is urging millions of dieters to stop taking them as they have been linked to serious heart problems. Similar newscasts kicked off the five o'clock news for both the ABC and NBC affiliate station in the Houston area ... furthermore, [the manufacturer] sent a *Dear Health Care Provider Letter* to approximately 450,000 physicians and pharmacists in which it informed them of the withdrawal of the drugs from the market and of the potential association between use of the drugs and instances of valvular heart disease" (377).

The purpose of this narrative is solely to reveal general principles that can be learned regarding how *Dear Healthcare Professional* letters fit into the array of available methods for warning physicians and patients.

XVI. FDA'S DECISION-MAKING PROCESS IN EVALUATING RISK MINIMIZATION TOOLS

a. Introduction

The comments from FDA reviewers provide concrete guidance to all Sponsors regarding the content of their draft REMS, and whether they should submit any REMS with their NDA or BLA.

[376]In re Brisco, et al. 448 F.3d 201, U.S. Court of Appeals, 3rd Circuit, 2006 U.S. App. LEXIS 11990.

[377]In re Brisco, et al. 448 F.3d 201, U.S. Court of Appeals, 3rd Circuit, 2006 U.S. App. LEXIS 11990.

One theme in the following commentary is the relationship between the *Medication Guide* and the package insert. The take-home lesson is that the medical writer needs to ensure that the warnings in the *Medication Guide* are consistent with warnings on the package insert in the *Warnings and Precautions* section of the package insert, and with the warnings in the *Drug–Drug Interactions* section of the package insert.

b. Recommendation Against Any REMS, Because Oncologists Are Highly Experienced With the Risks, and Because of the Restricted Distribution

This concerns *vismodegib* for basal cell carcinoma. The information is from NDA 203388, on FDA's website at Dec. 2013. In FDA's *Medical Review*, the reviewer wrote:

> [t]his reviewer finds that despite the serious nature of the teratogenic risk of vismodegib, a **REMS should not be required** for the following reasons: the standard of medical care in oncology ... provides adequate safeguards through the familiarity with the risk ... and patient monitoring. In the treatment of cancer, oncologist [sic] have a long history with ... highly toxic and teratogenic drugs dating back to the 1940's ... [o]ncology drugs have ... limited distribution ... restricted distribution to oncologists and specialty pharmacies.

The take-home lesson is that, if the relevant physicians are highly trained in the relevant specialty, and if the distribution of the drug is limited, a REMS might not be needed.

c. Requirement for a REMS Because of Danger of QT Prolongation

The FDA required a REMS with its approval of *vandetanib* for thyroid cancer. This drug also concerns cancer and, and it also concerns a small number of patients. Thus, it is interesting to point out that for two drugs, *vismodegib* and

vandetanib, each of which was for cancer, and each of which was for marketing to a small number of patients, the FDA required an REMS for one of the drugs, but did not require an REMS for the other drug.

This is from the FDA's approval of *vandetanib*. This is from NDA 22405 from Jul. 2013 on the FDA's website. In the *Medical Review*, the FDA reviewer stated that:

> [o]n January 21, 2011, FDA formally informed Astra-Zeneca [the Sponsor] that a **REMS is necessary** to ensure that the benefits of **vandetanib** outweigh the risks of QT prolongation and torsades de pointe ... [t]he goal of the REMS is to educate prescribers about ... management of QT prolongation and to help minimize the occurrence of torsades de pointe and sudden death and to inform patients about the serious risks associated with vandetanib.

The FDA reviewer further outlined the components of the *required REMS*, that is, a slide set and a telephone interview of physicians.

d. Recommendation Against Any REMS, Because Data on the Mechanism of the Drug Safety Issue Are Not Yet Available

This is from FDA's *Medical Review* of *ibrutinib*, for mantle cell lymphoma. The information is from NDA 205552, available from the FDA's website at Nov. 2013. The safety issue was bleeding events that occurred during clinical trials on ibrutinib.

The Sponsor did not propose any REMS for ibrutinib. In agreement with this, the FDA's reviewer recommended against any REMS, writing that:

> [u]sing a REMS to prevent patients at higher risk of bleeding from receiving ibrutinib **would *not* be helpful because we cannot identify the important risk factors** at this time ... [i]mplementing a REMS for ibrutinib without a better understanding of factors that may contribute to the risk of bleeding may restrict therapy without evidence establishing who

is at risk for bleeding events, and may create a barrier that prevents patients who could benefit from the drug from receiving it. It would not be appropriate to exclude all patients with risk factors from bleeding from receiving ibrutinib until additional data are available to better understand the bleeding safety signal.

In using the term "bleeding safety signal," the FDA reviewer was likely referring to the need for biomarkers that had the potential to correlate ibrutinib dosage with the adverse event of hemorrhage.

Instead of requiring that the Sponsor submit an REMS, FDA stated that:

> an in vitro study will be required to examine the effect of ibrutinib on platelet aggregation." In addition to requiring this experiment to test mechanisms of ibrutinib's apparent interference with blood clotting, FDA referred to its requirement for "enhanced pharmacovigilance to obtain information about bleeding events that occur in patients receiving ibrutinib. Information from the … pharmacovigilance program will … identify risk factors for bleeding with ibrutinib.

As a consequence, the *Warnings and Precautions* section of the package insert of ibrutinib included a warning about the association of ibrutinib with bleeding, and also included a statement that the mechanism for this association was not understood (378):

> Fatal bleeding events have occurred in patients treated with IMBRUVICA. Grade 3 or higher bleeding events (subdural hematoma, gastrointestinal bleeding, hematuria and post procedural hemorrhage) have occurred in up to 6% of patients. Bleeding events of any grade, including bruising and petechiae, occurred in approximately half of patients treated with IMBRUVICA. The mechanism for the bleeding events is not well understood.

The take-home lesson is that, where the mechanism of action is not known, FDA may refrain from requiring a REMS, and instead require a warning about the poorly understood risks, in the *Warnings and Precautions* section of the package insert.

e. Requirement for a *Medication Guide* With Vandetanib

With the approval of *vandetanib* (Caprelsa) (NDA 22405), FDA's website provides a five-page *Medication Guide*. The REMS stated that a *Medication Guide* will be dispensed to patients with each prescription, in accordance with 21 CFR §208.24. The *Medication Guide*, which is for patients to read, states, "Read this *Medication Guide* before you start taking CAPRELSA and each time you get a refill … [t]his *Medication Guide* does not take the place of talking to your healthcare provider."

The Guide also provides the warning that:

> CAPRELSA can cause a change in the electrical activity of your heart called QT prolongation, which can cause irregular heartbeats and that may lead to death … [y]our healthcare provider should perform tests to check the levels of your blood potassium, calcium, magnesium, and thyroid-stimulating hormone … [b]efore starting CAPRELSA … [r]egularly during CAPRELSA treatment: 2 to 4 weeks after starting CAPRELSA, 8 to 12 weeks after starting CAPRESLA.

As is evident, the *Medication Guide* attempts to lift the patient's awareness level towards the physician's awareness level, thus promoting a more effective partnership between the patient and physician in being vigilant of expected risks.

f. Requirement for a *Dear Healthcare Provider* Letter and a *Medication Guide*, for Telavancin

This provides a "poster-boy" of an REMS. In this author's opinion, the REMS is a poster-boy because the REMS required a large number of instruments for managing risks.

---

[378]Package insert for, IMBRUVICA® (ibrutinib) capsules, for oral use; January 2015 (26 pp.).

This concerns *telavancin* (Vibativ®), an antibiotic for Gram-positive bacterial infections. The information is from NDA 22110, from Dec. 2013 of the FDA's website. In the *Summary Review*, which was published with the Approval Letter, the FDA reviewer stated that, "[t]he need for a REMS was based on the findings of teratogenicity in animal species." The reviewer further stated that the REMS needs to include a *Medication Guide*, a *Dear Healthcare Provider* letter, and a registry for patients exposed to the drug during pregnancy. Furthermore, the REMS required surveys of women of child-bearing potential that are repeated annually, in order "to assess their understanding of the potential risk of fetal development toxicity if they are exposed to telavancin while pregnant."

The *Dear Healthcare Provider* letter describes the fetal effects of the study drug on animals, how to prevent pregnancy, and information on the registry. The REMS required that a "*Dear Healthcare Provider* (DHCP) Letter will be sent within 60 days, and again at 6 months, 1 and 2 years." The REMS required that the Sponsor send the letters to 18 different medical organizations, such as the American Thoracic Society and the American Medical Association, and that these organizations distribute the letters to all its members.

g. Warnings in the *Medication Guide* That Correspond to the *Warnings and Precautions* Section of the Package Label

This further concerns the REMS for *telavancin*. The *Medication Guide* instructed the patient to "[r]ead this *Medication Guide* before you receive VIBATIV." The *Guide* stated that the drug increases the risk of death in patients with kidney problems, and instructed patients to be vigilant in getting blood tests to assess kidney functions. Finally, the *Guide* warned the patient taking the Sponsor's drug (*telavancin*) and taking NSAIDs, ACE inhibitors, diuretics, anticoagulants, and antiarrhythmics.

The *Medication Guide* available on the manufacturer's website (www.vibative.com) includes the following warnings:

> **Tell your healthcare provider about all the medicines you take**, including prescription and non-prescription medicines, vitamins, and herbal supplements. VIBATIV and other medicines can affect each other causing side effects. Especially tell your healthcare provider if you take:
>
> - a Non-Steroidal Anti-Inflammatory Drug (NSAID)
> - certain blood pressure medicines called ACE Inhibitors or ARBs
> - water pills (diuretics)
> - a blood thinner, medicine to control your heart rate or rhythm (antiarrhythmics)
>
> Ask your healthcare provider or pharmacist for a list of these medicines, if you are not sure.

Please note that these warnings in the *Medication Guide* are not the same as warnings about drug–drug interactions (379). The package insert for telavancin does not include any warning about drug–drug interactions. The closest that the package insert gets to a *drug–drug interactions* warning is warnings about *drug–test interactions* (380). In short, a

---

[379]"The medication guide provides information to the patient—specifically to warn their HCP [healthcare provider] about any other medications they are taking. This is not due to any drug–drug interactions with Telavancin, but due to the potential for increasing adverse event rates with the medications listed in the Med Guide (i.e. NSAIDs, loop diuretics, ACEIs, ARBs, and antiarrhythmics)." Kind advice from Dr Christine Slover, PharmD, Theravance Biopharma Antibiotics of South San Francisco, CA, in e-mail dated April 7, 2015.

[380]Package insert for, VIBATIV® (telavancin) for injection, for intravenous use; December 2014 (37 pp.). The package insert was acquired from www.vibativ.com on April 7, 2015.

problem with televancin is that it interferes with certain blood coagulation tests and with a urine dipstick protein test.

The *Medication Guide*'s warnings about NSAID drugs, ACE inhibitors, water pills, and blood thinners, find a counterpart in the *Warnings and Precautions* section of the package insert. The *Warnings and Precautions* warns that "renal adverse event rates were also higher in patients who received concomitant medications known to affect kidney function (e.g., non-steroidal anti-inflammatory drugs, ACE inhibitors, and loop diuretics)" (381).

h. Warnings in the *Medication Guide* That Correspond to the *Warnings and Precautions* Section of the Package Label

This illustrates how warnings in the *Medication Guide* may be mirrored in the *Warnings and Precautions* section of the package label. This information is from NDA 22465, available on FDA's website at Apr. 2011.

FDA's approval was for *pazopanib* (Votrient®), for the indication of renal cell carcinoma. The FDA reviewer noted that, "the applicant has already specified all the important risks as warnings and precautions in the proposed package label for pazopanib," and further recommended a REMS that included the implementation of a *Medication Guide* and performing postmarketing pharmacoviligance to monitor liver toxicity. FDA stated that the goal of the *Medication Guide* was to, "convey

the risks of life-threatening hepatotoxicity, especially the occurrence of severe and fatal hepatotoxicity." In setting forth the requirements for the proposed REMS, FDA stated that the Sponsor:

> will ensure that a Medication Guide is available for distribution to patients with each ... pazopanib ... prescription in accordance with 21 CFR 208.24 ... [and] will include a statement, "Dispense the Medication Guide" ... to each patient ... on the label of each container ... of ... pazopanib.

XVII. EUROPEAN UNION'S RISK MANAGEMENT TOOLS

FDA's REMS finds a counterpart in the RMP of the European Union. The European Union includes various agencies, including *Germany's Federal Institute for Drugs and Medical Devices* (BfArM) and France's *Agence Nationale de Security du Medicament et des Produits de Sante* (ANSM) (382). In the European Union, pharmaceutical companies must submit a *Risk Evaluation and Mitigation Strategy* at the time of application for a marketing authorization. In 2005, EMA introduced the RMP for planning pharmacovigilance and risk management for new drugs. At an earlier time, regulatory authorities had mainly relied on spontaneous reports and industry or investigator-initiated studies (383). In a study of drugs approved by FDA and approved by EMA, Lis et al. (384)

---

[381]Package insert for, VIBATIV® (telavancin) for injection, for intravenous use; December 2014 (37 pp.). The package insert was acquired from www.vibativ.com on April 7, 2015.

[382]Dowlat HA. The importance and impact of the EU RMP and US REMS to risk—benefit Assessments. Biopractice. Feb. 2011;8 (5 pp.).

[383]Vermeer NS, Duijnhoven RG, Straus SM, et al. Risk management plans as a tool for proactive pharmacovigilance: a cohort study of newly approved drugs in Europe. Clin. Pharmacol. Ther. 2014;96:723–31.

[384]Lis et al. Comparisons of Food and Drug Administration and European Medicines Agency risk management implementation for recent pharmaceutical approvals: report of the International Society for Pharmacoeconomics and outcomes research risk benefit management working group. Value Health 2012;15:1108–18.

compared elements of the relevant REMS and *RMP*, respectively, and tabulated the frequency of use of a *Medication Guide*. The general conclusion was that the REMS and *RMP*, "[b]oth allow flexibility in product-specific actions, recognizing adverse effects of potential concern."

Motivation for using a *RMP* is evident from the warning in the EMA's Guidelines that, "not all actual or potential risks will have been identified at the time when an initial authorisation is sought and many of the risks ... will only be discovered ... post-authorisation" (385).

The EMA's Guidelines also state that risk management includes pharmacovigilance activities and "implementation of risk minimisation and mitigation." Correspondence between the EMA's Guidelines and the FDA's REMS is evident from the statement that, "it may be appropriate to have a risk minimisation plan ... there could be diverse educational needs for different specialists ... [f]or example an active substance which causes ... QT prolongation ... might need educational material if intended for use in general practice or orthopedic surgery" (386). In this writing, the EMA's Guidelines point out that education on QT prolongation is likely to be needed by doctors in general practice or by orthopedic surgeons, but not by doctors who are cardiologists. The EMA's Guidelines further state that, "[r]isk minimisation may consist of ... Direct Healthcare Professional communications" and that "[a]ny educational material should be non-promotional."

XVIII. SUMMARY

Risk Evaluation and Mitigation Strategies in the United States, and *RMP* in the European Union, include the common features of the *Medication Guide, Dear Healthcare Professional* letters, and requirements for enhanced pharmacovigilance once the drug is marketed. FDA's *Medical Review*s that published with FDA's *Approval Letters* reveal FDA's decision-making process that leads to the requirement for an REMS, or from refraining from requiring any REMS. FDA's *Medical Review*s also disclose how certain elements of the *Medication Guide* and *Package Insert* can track each other.

XIX. PATIENT-REPORTED OUTCOME

a. Introduction

Patient-Reported Outcome (PRO) is a tool for capturing data on safety and efficacy. Data from patients may be classed as those that are detectable *only by clinicians* and data detectable *only by patients*, as exemplified by the following:

- Data detectable only by clinicians: tachycardia; neutropenia.
- Data detectable only by patients: fatigue; depression; light-headedness; nausea, pain; headaches.

Clinicians can interview study subjects on data that is only patient-reportable. Special

---

[385]European Medicines Agency. Guideline on good pharmacovigilance practices (GVP) module V-risk management systems (Rev. 1); April 2014 (60 pp.).

[386]European Medicines Agency. Guideline on good pharmacovigilance practices (GVP) module V-risk management systems (Rev. 1); April 2014 (60 pp.).

instruments (questionnaires) are available for capturing patient-reported data. For example, the NCI provides the Patient-Reported Outcomes version of the Common Terminology Criteria for Adverse Events (PRO-CTCAE) (387). Where a clinician interviews a patient, and where the patient responds, the clinician needs to find counterparts of terms, used by the patient, in the MedDRA dictionary (388).

HRQoL questionnaires also capture patient-reported data. According to FDA's Guidance for Industry (389):

> [a] PRO is any report of the status of a patient's health condition that comes directly from the patient, without interpretation of the patient's response by a clinician or anyone else. The outcome can be measured in absolute terms (e.g., severity of a symptom, sign, or state of a disease) or as a change from a previous measure.

According to Scoggins and Patrick (390), information captured by PROs include data captured by HRQoL questionnaires. PROs constitute a broader category than parameters relating to HRQoL. An example of a PRO that does not fit into the categories of questions found in HRQoL instruments is menopausal hot flashes. In a clinical trial on a drug used for treating hot flashes, data on efficacy were captured by "questionnaires on the frequency and severity of their hot flashes using an electronic diary" (391).

b. PROs—Example of Head and Neck Cancer

Patrick et al. (392) provide a hypothetical example of an instrument for capturing patient-reported outcomes, where the goal of the instrument is to capture information for justifying certain claims on a package insert. This example is for a drug for head and neck cancer. The PRO instrument of the hypothetical of Patrick et al. (393), included these questions:

1. How often do you need to spit?
2. How much difficulty do you have swallowing your saliva?
3. How much difficulty do you have swallowing liquids?
4. How much difficulty do you have swallowing soft foods?
5. How much difficulty do you have swallowing solid foods?

---

[387]U.S. Department of Health and Human Services, National Institutes of Health, Division of Cancer Control and Population Sciences. Patient-reported outcomes version of the common terminology criteria for adverse events (PRO-CTCAE); July 2010 (2 pp.).

[388]Trotti AM. E-mail of November 22, 2010.

[389]U.S. Department of Health and Human Services. Food and Drug Administration. Guidance for industry. Patient-reported outcome measures: use in medical product development to support labeling claims; December 2009.

[390]Scoggins JF, Patrick DL. The use of patient-reported outcomes instruments in registered clinical trials: evidence from ClinicalTrials.gov. Comtemp. Clin. Trials 2009;30:289—92.

[391]Breeze3:Study of Gabapentin Extended Release in the Treatment of Vasomotor Symptoms (Hot Flashes) in Postmenopausal Women. Sponsored by Depomed, Inc. www.clinicaltrials.gov [accessed 22.12.10].

[392]Patrick DL, Burke LB, Powers JH, et al. Patient-reported outcomes to support medical product labeling claims: FDA perspective. Value Health 2007;10(Suppl. 2):S125—37.

[393]Patrick DL, Burke LB, Powers JH, et al. Patient-reported outcomes to support medical product labeling claims: FDA perspective. Value Health 2007;10(Suppl. 2):S125—37.

The example of Patrick et al. (394) was used to justify the following claim on the package insert, "improves swallowing in patients being treated for head and neck cancer."

A real-life example of a drug that improves swallowing in patients being treated for head and neck cancer is palifermin. In a clinical trial for palifermin, clinicians used a standard instrument for assessing the ability to swallow. This instrument (395), which was provided by the World Health Organization (WHO), provides a list of severities in impaired swallowing, and enables the choice between:

1. "Patient is able to eat a normal diet";
2. "Patient experiences extreme difficulty swallowing solid food and requires a liquid diet"; and
3. "Patient is unable to swallow and must receive nutrition ... via surgically implanted feeding tube."

As a result of using this list during the clinical trial, the package insert for palifermin disclosed the following benefit, "[p]atients reported significant decreases in mouth and throat soreness and swallowing limitation" (396).

Thus, the hypothetical example of Patrick et al. (397), which concerned PROs, finds a real-world counterpart in the package insert for palifermin. Paliformin is used to reduce injury to the mouth, during chemotherapy or radiotherapy for head and neck cancer. While the clinical trial on palifermin did not use a PRO instrument, the palifermin example does

concern subjective patient responses, where maximal capture of the relevant information requires either an interview between the clinician and patient, or a PRO instrument. It was the case with the palifermin package insert that a standard grading scale (398) was used in conjunction with interviews between the clinician and patient.

XX. SUMMARY OF REPORTING SYSTEMS

To view the big picture, adverse event data can be reported by the following four systems:

- As adverse events, using the MedDRA dictionary, where data are collected by the clinician.
- As adverse events, using the CTCAE dictionary, where data from oncology clinical trials are collected by the clinician.
- As PROs, where data are collected by an instrument filled out by the patient.
- As HRQoL instruments, where data are also collected by an instrument filled out by the patient. HRQoL instruments are detailed in a separate chapter in this book.

An investigator would not indiscriminately use all of these methods for capturing safety data, in view of the burden and expense involved (399). The instruments that are chosen will be a function of whether the study drug has any relevance to the patient's

---

[394]Patrick DL, Burke LB, Powers JH, et al. Patient-reported outcomes to support medical product labeling claims: FDA perspective. Value Health 2007;10(Suppl. 2):S125−37.

[395]WHO Scale for Grading the Severity of Oral Mucositis.

[396]Cigna Health Care Coverage Position. Palifermin (Kepivance®) October 15, 2005.

[397]Patrick DL, Burke LB, Powers JH, et al. Patient-reported outcomes to support medical product labeling claims: FDA perspective. Value Health 2007;10(Suppl. 2):S125−37.

[398]WHO Scale for Grading the Severity of Oral Mucositis.

[399]Trotti A, Colevas AD, Setser A, Basch E. Patient-reported outcomes and the evolution of adverse event reporting in oncology. J. Clin. Oncol. 2007;25:5121−7.

subjective responses, such as pain, fatigue, nausea, or depression.

XXI. DATA AND SAFETY MONITORING COMMITTEE

a. Introduction

The Data and Safety Monitoring Committee (DSMC), also known as a Data Monitoring Committee (DMC), is a group of about six people, appointed by the sponsor or investigator, that serves as an independent monitor of the clinical trial, as it progresses. DMCs are not used in all clinical trials, but are strongly recommended for trials where one of the endpoints is death, trials for life-threatening diseases, and trials with huge numbers of study subjects (400). Use of DMCs in clinical trials had an origin in the Greenberg Report (401).

What is monitored is data on safety, data on efficacy, and adherence to the terms in the Clinical Study Protocol, as the clinical study unfolds and progresses. Members of the DMC include an expert in the disease being studied, an expert in the design of clinical trials, a statistician, and an expert in medical ethics. The members of the DMC must not be affiliated with the sponsor, investigator, for example, a pharmaceutical company, or with a competing pharmaceutical company. The primary goal of the DMC is to protect the safety of the study subjects, in the context of a clinical trial on an experimental drug (402). The DMC has the power to unblind the study subjects, and determine whether any given data point is from a subject receiving placebo or study drug. Two reports are often prepared by the DMC, one for the open session and one for the closed session (403). The open session report may be a subset of the closed session report or entirely separate.

The DMC meets at regular intervals, for example, every 6 months, to review the available data. This analysis is called "interim analysis," whereas analysis performed at the conclusion of the clinical trial is called "final analysis" (404,405). Once the clinical trial is underway, the DMC can recommend stopping the trial because of benefit (406,407), safety, or futility (408). The meaning of these three

[400]Grant AM, Altman, DG, Babiker AB, et al. Issues in data monitoring and interim analysis of trials. Health Technol. Assessment 2005;9 (246 pp.).

[401]Halperin M, DeMets DL, Ware JH. Early methodological developments for clinical trials at the National Heart, Lung and Blood Institute. Stat. Med. 1990;9:881−92.

[402]Cuzick J, Howell A, Forbes J. Early stopping of clinical trials. Breast Cancer Res. 2005;7:181−3.

[403]Grant AM, Altman, DG, Babiker AB, et al. Issues in data monitoring and interim analysis of trials. Health Technol. Assessment 2005;9(7) (246 pp.).

[404]Trotta F, Apolone G, Garattini S, Tafuri G. Stopping a trial early in oncology: for patients or for industry? Ann. Oncol. 2008;19:1347−53.

[405]Fernandes RM, van der Lee JH, Offringa M. A systematic review of the reporting of Data Monitoring Committees' roles, interim analysis and early termination in pediatric clinical trials. BMC Pediatr. 2009;9:77.

[406]Montori VM, Devereaux PJ, Adhikari NK, et al. Randomized trials stopped early for benefit: a systematic review. J. Am. Med. Assoc. 2005;294:2203−9.

[407]Mueller PS, Montori VM, Bassler D, Koenig BA, Guyatt GH. Ethical issues in stopping randomized trials early because of apparent benefit. Ann. Intern. Med. 2007;146:878−81.

[408]Schoenfeld DA. Pro/con clinical debate: it is acceptable to stop large multicentre randomized controlled trials at interim analysis for futility. Pro: futility stopping can speed up the development of effective treatments. Crit. Care 2005;9:34−6.

concepts, as far as the present clinical trial is concerned, is that the data available to date convincingly show that the drug works, that the toxicity of the drug is overwhelmingly unacceptable, and that there is little hope that the drug can ever be shown to work, respectively. To repeat, the DMC cannot mandate that the trial be stopped, or that the Clinical Study Protocol be amended. The DMC can only make recommendations to the Sponsor or investigator.

For any clinical trial, all study subjects must read, understand, and sign a consent form. But where unforeseen adverse events occur, the DMC may suggest that a new consent form be drafted, that is, a "re-consent form," and that study subjects read and sign the reconsent form. In addition, where unforeseen adverse events occur, the DMC may suggest that the Clinical Study Protocol be amended to identify the newly emerging adverse events.

Where adverse events seem to affect only one of the subgroups of the clinical study, the DMC may suggest that subjects in this particular subgroup be dropped from the study, and that potential subjects falling in this subgroup be excluded, during the on-going process of enrollment. This function of the DMC clearly shows the wisdom and advantage of defining subgroups in the Clinical Study Protocol. Hence, in configuring the subgroups in the study population, the investigator or medical writer should divide subjects into those with high, moderate, and low risk, for any foreseeable ADRs. It is much better to exclude one particular subgroup from the clinical trial than to terminate the entire clinical trial.

Along similar lines, the DMC may recommend increased surveillance of specific adverse events, where the DMC suspects that a certain type of adverse event is not being adequately detected (409).

The FDA's Establishment and Operation of Clinical Trial Data Monitoring Committees provides a brief introduction to the DMC's structure and functions (410). DeMets et al. (411) have written an indispensable account of the activities ofDSMCs.

b. The DMC Charter

The responsibilities of the DSMC are formally set forth in a DMC Charter (or DSMC Charter). The DMC Charter, which can be written by a medical writer, is tailored to the needs of the clinical trial. The Charter can provide a schedule of meetings used for interim analysis. The meetings may be scheduled according to calendar dates, or in a manner that tracks the number of patients being enrolled as the trial unfolds. If the clinical trial has stopping rules, the Charter provides the statistical bases for stopping for benefit, stopping for safety, and stopping for futility. The following is a draft of a DMC Charter, based on a composite of the author's own work, in combination with a published DMC Charter (412). The name of the company, *PharmaDrug, Inc.*, is fictional.

[409]Grant AM, Altman DG, Babiker AB, et al. Issues in data monitoring and interim analysis of trials. Health Technol. Assessment 2005;9(7) (246 pp.).

[410]U.S. Department of Health and Human Services. Food and Drug Administration. Guidance for clinical trial sponsors. Establishment and Operation of Clinical Trial Data Monitoring Committees; March 2006.

[411]DeMets DL, Furberg CD, Friedman LM. Data monitoring in clinical trials.New York: Springer; 2006.

[412]Data Monitoring Committee (DMC) Charter for the Eurother3235 Trial (version 1.0 27/04/2009).

DATA SAFETY MONITORING BOARD CHARTER

Clinical Study Protocol No.: _____

_____ _____ _____
MD   Signature   Date

_____
(DMC chairperson)

_____ _____ _____
MD, MPH   Signature   Date

_____
(DMC member)

_____ _____ _____
PhD   Signature   Date

_____
(DMC biostatistician)

INTRODUCTION

This DMC Charter is for protocol no. _____ of *PharmaDrug, Inc.* (*PharmaDrug*). This Charter describes the roles and responsibilities of the Board and outlines the plan for communicating study data to the sponsor. The study Synopsis of the clinical trial is provided in Appendix A.

ROLE OF THE BOARD

The DMC will evaluate the safety parameters of the ongoing study of the study drug in combination with cisplatin for treating NSCLC, following the treatment and posttreatment period of each arm of the study. The sponsor can require that the DMC examine the safety data more frequently. The DMC will examine safety issues, and issues relating to the design and administration of, and compliance with, the study. The frequency of DMC meetings may be increased, for example, where safety issues arise. Efficacy will also be addressed.

The goals of the DMC will include:

- Protecting patient welfare.
- Monitoring interim safety data.
- Identifying safety issues and suggesting solutions regarding study design and conduct.
- Evaluating the nature and frequency of AEs reported from each treatment arm, including clinical assessments of all AEs and SAEs that could lead to discontinuation of the study drug.
- Advise sponsor on the need for modifying the study design or conduct, based on safety data.
- Provide interim review of adverse events (AEs) observed in each study arm.
- Based on safety data, advise sponsor regarding the need for modifying the study design or conduct.
- Based on safety data, advise sponsor on proposals for dose escalation, dose modification, dose continuation, or termination of the study.

The DMC is not responsible for reviewing the final study results, although such results may be made available to the Board, where found appropriate.

BOARD MEMBERSHIP

The DMC is an independent body of experts that serves in an advisory capacity to *PharmaDrug* to ensure that clinical trial participants are not exposed to unreasonable or unnecessary risks of the study drug in combination with cisplatin.

The DMC will consist of three voting members: two clinicians with expertise in oncology, one of which will be the DMC Chairperson (Chair), and a biostatistician. Each member's curriculum vitae will be kept in the files at *PharmaDrug*. Current Board membership is disclosed on the title page of this DMC Charter. In the event that a DMC member withdraws from the Board, *PharmaDrug* may appoint a replacement.

TERM

The duration of membership for the DMC will encompass the analysis of safety data from Clinical Study Protocol no. _____. The DMC may be asked to review the final safety study results.

CONFLICT OF INTEREST AND FINANCIAL DISCLOSURE

DMC members will be completely independent of study investigators and must have no financial, scientific, or other conflict of interest with the sponsor of the clinical trial. The DMC must not actively conduct any of the studies under the Board's review, and may not have any significant financial interest in the study's conduct or outcome.

Additionally, DMC members must disclose any potential conflict of interest involving, for example, pharmaceutical companies, manufacturers or distributors, CROs, and the like. Conflict of interest may be determined by assessing any financial arrangement, consultancy agreement (either directly or through a third party), research support, or other relationship that could be construed as introducing bias.

Members must advise the sponsor and the other members of the DMC of any existing or arising conflict of interest, including financial interests. If this conflict is considered by the sponsor to be significant and likely to impact objectivity, sponsor will find a replacement member. If this conflict is considered significant and likely to materially impact objectivity, the sponsor may ask the member to resign from the DMC. Where the DMC member resigns, the sponsor will identify a replacement and decide whether to approve the candidate.

The sponsor is free to appoint replacement DMC members.

COMPENSATION

A contract specifying fees to be paid to DMC members for each meeting, or for each data review, will be provided by *PharmaDrug* to DMC members. In addition to the payment of fees, the sponsor will reimburse all travel and other reasonable expenses incurred while attending DMC meetings.

BOARD MEETINGS AND REPORTS

DMC meetings will be held via teleconferences or in person. *PharmaDrug* or its designee will be responsible for arranging all meetings.

ORGANIZATIONAL MEETING

The first DMC meeting will be an organizational meeting, and will allow members to discuss logistic issues relating to future DMC meetings, for example, frequency of data reviews, content of data reviews, and the meeting format. The DMC Charter will also be reviewed and finalized at this meeting, with input from the Sponsor. Conflicts of interest will also be addressed. In addition to DMC members, representatives from *PharmaDrug* including the medical monitor, data managers, project managers, statisticians, and pharmacovigilance staff, may also participate in the organizational meeting.

INTERIM REVIEW MEETINGS

Regularly scheduled safety review meetings will be conducted after approximately ____ subjects, and after approximately ____ subjects have completed at least ____ cycles of treatment. The frequency of interim review meetings may be changed, as desired, by the DMC or by the sponsor.

FORMAT

Interim review meetings will be conducted in three consecutive sessions:

- An Open Session for reviewing administrative aspects of the study and the safety data.
- A Closed Session for discussing blinded safety data (if still blinded) and unblinded safety data (if unblinded), and for arriving at recommendations for the Sponsor.
- A Wrap-Up Session for communications between the DMC and the sponsor.

PARTICIPANTS

The Open Session and Wrap-Up session will be open to DMC members and to *PharmaDrug*. Other individuals identified by *PharmaDrug* may also participate in the Open and Wrap-Up sessions. The closed meeting will be for voting members only, optionally with a nonvoting Independent Reporting Statistician. It is recognized that including further nonvoting members may introduce bias.

REVIEW MATERIALS

Before each scheduled DMC meeting, *PharmaDrug* will prepare a packet of summary materials for the Board's review. These review materials will be sent to DMC members at least 1 week before each scheduled meeting. The DMC will keep an accurate minute of their discussions. Separate sections will be required for the open and closed sessions. The DMC Chair will sign off any minutes or notes. A sealed copy will be sent to the independent statistician.

The following concerns closed sessions. All DMC members should meet face-to-face in order for the DMC to make any formal recommendations regarding stopping or modifying the study. In the event that a timely face-to-face meeting cannot be held, members of the committee may confer by teleconference. Closed session participants will review information that includes, but is not limited to, the following. In closed DMC sessions consider data summarized by treatment arm (treatment arms coded as A and B), or unblinded data if needed. The following topics may be discussed:

- Safety-related data, including adverse events (AEs) and SAEs.
- Number of deaths and life-threatening events.
- Adverse events, or possible indications of drug toxicity, presenting as hematological values, serum chemistry, urinalysis, and the like.
- Events leading to discontinuation or withdrawal.

Open session materials will summarize results within the study. The following information will be summarized:

- Enrollment, including enrollment exceptions, subject accrual and drop-out rates, and deviations from the Clinical Study Protocol.
- Subject demographics, including demographics of subgroups in the subject population, and baseline characteristics.
- Study drug dosing information.
- Safety data, including adverse events or lab abnormalities that may represent dose-limiting toxicities.
- Missing data, including identification of specific study sites that are lagging in providing data, and the frequency of nonreported safety data.

At open sessions, the above material should be discussed in aggregate, not separately by study arms.

PERIODIC REPORTS TO THE DMC

Summaries of SAE data will be provided to the DMC members on a monthly basis. Blinded SAE listings will be distributed to the DMC at the first day of each month. DMC members will acknowledge the receipt of, and their review of, these listings, by way of e-mail to the Independent Reporting Statistician and DMC project administrator. If any safety concerns arise, the DMC Chair may request the DMC to schedule an ad hoc teleconference as soon as possible. Serious, unexpected AEs will be distributed immediately to all DMC members with summaries and narratives. The Chair may communicate with other members of the DMC, and vice versa, should any safety concerns that may arise.

UNSCHEDULED MEETINGS

PharmaDrug, Inc., reserves the right to request unscheduled meetings of the DMC, for example, in the event of notification of SAEs. Any such request will be made in writing to the DMC Chair. The DMC may request additional meetings with *PharmaDrug* and these requests must be made in writing by the DMC Chair directly to *PharmaDrug*. If the DMC decides to hold an unscheduled meeting, it must notify *PharmaDrug* immediately after the DMC has made the decision to hold this meeting.

DMC RECOMMENDATIONS

At each DMC meeting, the DMC will evaluate the nature and frequency of adverse events, decide on unblinding of safety data, and (if unblinded) evaluate whether there are significant differences in drug safety between the various study arms. The DMC will also evaluate safety issues in individual subjects

and determine whether adverse events or laboratory abnormalities represent dose-limiting toxicity.

The DMC may make a recommendation regarding any aspect of the conduct or design of the study, including early termination for safety reasons, dose reduction, dose escalation, change in number of subjects in the trial, termination of a subgroup, or any other modification of the Study Protocol. The DMC Chair will communicate recommendations to sponsor within _____ days of the DMC meeting.

Final decision-making authority regarding the study belongs to the sponsor. If the DMC recommends stopping or modifying the trial, the Sponsor may, at its discretion, meet immediately with the DMC to review the available data and recommendations. The Sponsor may also seek advice from regulatory bodies or from external experts. The Sponsor will make a decision to accept or reject the DMC's recommendation, to accept or reject recommendations from outside experts or regulatory bodies, and will relay its decision to the DMC and to relevant regulatory bodies.

In the event that the Sponsor decides to stop, extend, or otherwise modify the trial, it will inform all investigators and the relevant regulatory bodies. The DMC will not make any information public without prior approval from the Sponsor.

OUTSIDE EXPERTS

Where an issue cannot be resolved by way of a teleconference, the DMC should convene by way of a face-to-face meeting. The DMC is free to consult outside experts in the event of an impasse, after acquiring written permission from the sponsor. The sponsor is free to evaluate the technical expertise and conflict of interest of the outside experts, before the outside experts are admitted to participate.

ACCESS TO INTERIM RESULTS

To maintain the integrity of the study, all study information and interim results must be strictly controlled. DMC review materials may not be given to anyone other than members of the Closed Sessions. Copies of these review materials must not be made.

STOPPING RULES

The DMC will not use a formal statistical stopping rule for decision-making based on the safety reviews.

The study may be stopped early or design modifications may be recommended in case of safety needs or possible optimization based on the DSMC review of the safety data. Possible recommendations include no action needed and trial continues as planned; early stopping due, for example, to clear benefit or harm of a treatment, futility, or external evidence, or stopping recruitment within a subgroup. Other possible recommendations include stopping the trial on the basis of futility of recruitment, extending recruitment, or extending follow-up time, and sanctioning or proposing changes to the Clinical Study Protocol.

Three futility analyses will be performed, the first when 300 adverse events of death have been noted, the second when 450 adverse events of death have been recorded, and the third when 600 adverse events of death have been recorded. The last futility analysis will coincide with the formal interim analysis of overall survival for superiority. Following such an analysis, the DMC may recommend terminating the study for futility. At this time, the sponsor, after reviewing the summarized data, may decide to terminate the study.

If the interim overall survival results show that the study drug confers a significant benefit, then this could form the basis of a submission for an approval, and the study would be terminated at that time. If the interim overall survival results are not statistically significant, and the study is not terminated following a futility assessment, then the study would continue to enroll subjects and accumulate data until 900 adverse events of deaths have been recorded. At this time, the study will be terminated and a final analysis of the overall survival data will be conducted.

COMMUNICATIONS

Meeting Minutes

Minutes of the Open Session and Wrap-Up Session will be prepared by *PharmaDrug* and will be distributed to appropriate members of DMC and *PharmaDrug*. Minutes of the Closed Session will be prepared by the DMC. Under 21 CFR §312.58, the FDA may request copies of the meeting minutes.

OTHER COMMUNICATIONS

PharmaDrug, Inc., urges that any communication between the DMC and *PharmaDrug* outside the meeting format, be directed through the DMC Chair and *PharmaDrug*'s Drug Safety group, respectively. These pathways of communication will ensure the DMC's role as an objective and independent entity.

SPONSOR'S DECISIONS AND ANNOUNCEMENTS

In the event that any significant development results from DMC recommendations, *PharmaDrug, Inc.*, will be responsible for notifying investigators, regulatory agencies, ethics committees, and IRBs. The DMC will not make any public announcements without prior written permission from *PharmaDrug, Inc.*

TIMETABLE

Organizational Meeting _____ (date)
First DMC Meeting _____ (date)
Second DMC Meeting _____ (date)

CONTACT INFORMATION

_____

_____

DMC chairperson

_____

_____

DMC member

_____

_____

DMC biostatistician

_____

_____

PharmaDrug, Inc., Chief Medical Officer

_____

_____

PharmaDrug, Inc., Director of Drug Safety
  APPENDIX A (Synopsis of Clinical Study
Protocol)

XXII. CONCLUDING REMARKS

The issue of drug safety can be divided into a handful of topics. The topic of medical manifestations of adverse events is readily appreciated by any layperson, as these often include nausea, vomiting, and low blood cell counts. The topic of definitions is more subtle, as these definitions reflect definitions set forth by regulatory agencies. In addition to definitions, adverse events can fall into other categories, such as classifications created by statisticians, for example, ITT analysis versus PP analysis of adverse events, categories requiring clinical judgment, and categories requiring a knowledge of pharmacology and biochemistry. The above-mentioned topics are a prerequisite for understanding the following topics, that is, the topics of data management and process in clinical trials, as it applies to drug safety. Data management and process encompasses use of various tools for capturing drug safety data, such as case report forms, MedWatch forms, Yellow Card forms, and CIOMS I forms. Data management and process also encompasses tools for transmitting safety data to regulatory agencies, and to nonregulatory agencies, such as the Sponsor and to the DSMC. FDA's Guidance for Industry document on good pharmacovigilance practices provides an indispensable overview, and recommendations, on many of the above topics (413).

---

[413]Department of Health and Human Services. Food and Drug Administration. Guidance for industry. Good pharmacovigilance practices and pharmacoepidemiologic assessment; March 2005 (20 pp.).

26

Mechanism of Action of Diseases and Drugs—Part I

I. INTRODUCTION

Mechanism of action (MOA), as it applies to a disease, refers to the summation of changes in the normal physiology that contribute to the pathology of a disease. This include changes that are genetic, biochemical, related to cell biology, and physiological changes. Genetic changes include changes in the structures of genes, including germline mutations and somatic mutations. Germline mutations are mutations that are inherited from a parent, while somatic mutations occur after birth. Somatic mutations can be acquired, for example, from ultraviolet light or from cigarette smoking. Genetic changes also encompass those of epigenetics, such as gene methylation. Biochemical changes include changes in protein structure, such as the change in hemoglobin structure in sickle cell anemia. Changes in cell biology include alterations in cell maturation, activation, degranulation, and chemotaxis. Physiological changes include fibrosis,

neovascularization, and hypertension. Where a disease involves an infecting agent, the mechanism of action includes interactions of the infecting agent with the human host.

Drugs can influence the following targets:

- *Genes and RNA.* The term "gene" refers to the combination of the coding regions, introns, and regulatory elements. Drugs with a specific action at the genome include vectors used for gene therapy (1). Some drugs, such as cisplatin, have a nonspecific influence on the chromosome and do not target any particular gene. Drugs that target RNA include antisense RNA and micro-RNA (2).
- *Soluble proteins.* Drugs can interact with soluble proteins, such as drugs that inhibit (or activate) enzymes, transcription factors, and cytokines.
- *Membrane-bound proteins.* Drugs that interact with membrane-bound proteins, such as ion channels in nerves, hormone receptors, and cytokine receptors.

[1]Kotterman MA, Schaffer DV. Engineering adeno-associated viruses for clinical gene therapy. Nat. Rev. Genet. 2014;15:445−51.

[2]Kaboli PJ, et al. MicroRNA-based therapy and breast cancer: a comprehensive review of novel therapeutic strategies from diagnosis to treatment. Pharmacol. Res. 2015;pii:S1043-6618(15)00083-3. http://dx.doi.org/10.1016/j.phrs.2015.04.015.

- *Macromolecular structures.* Drugs that target macromolecular structures, such as the cytoskeleton and the extracellular matrix.
- *Metabolites.* Drugs that interact directly with metabolites, such as the drug, asparaginase (3).
- *Drugs requiring in vivo processing.* Drugs that require in vivo procession prior to acting on any target, include vaccines, as well as pro-drugs such as dimethyl fumarate (4) or isoniazid (5). This processing should be included as part of the MOA.

The terms "specific" and "nonspecific" are used in describing the MOA of some drugs. Iron is a drug for treating iron-deficiency anemia (6). However, iron (in the form of heme) binds to many proteins in the body, most of which have little or no relevance to anemia (7). The binding of iron, in the form of heme, is likely to be of similar strength, with binding to many different kinds of iron-requiring proteins. Hence, the researcher interested in describing the MOA of this drug would need to determine the target that is most relevant to the disease. In contrast, antibodies bind specifically to only one target. This statement refers to binding of the variable region of the antibody to its target antigen. Although antibodies do bind nonspecifically to countless other proteins, this binding is dramatically weaker than the binding to the target antigen.

Certain characteristics of drugs, such as the binding of a drug to a nutrient transport protein, typically albumin, the identity of transporters that allow the drug to enter cells, the identity of transporters that extrude the drug from cells, and pathways of drug degradation, are more properly classified as pharmacokinetic properties, not MOA properties.

A knowledge of the MOA of drugs is useful for a variety of reasons, as indicated by the following bullet points:

- *Regulatory approval for conducting a clinical trial.* Information on the MOA can play a vital role, along with information on safety and efficacy, in the decision to move forward to sponsor a clinical trial (8).
- *Package inserts.* Disclosures of MOA are required in documents for submitting to regulatory agencies, and may be required in the package insert.
- *Justifying a surrogate endpoint.* MOA can help justify use of a surrogate endpoint. The MOA helps establish the connection between the surrogate endpoint and the clinical endpoint.
- *Justifying exploratory endpoints.* The MOA can justify the proposal that there is a connection between an exploratory endpoint and a clinical endpoint. The goals of exploratory endpoints are to identify

[3]Chen SH. Asparaginase therapy in pediatric acute lymphoblastic leukemia: a focus on the mode of drug resistance. Pediatr. Neonatol. 2014;S1875−S9572.

[4]Linker RA, Gold R. Dimethyl fumarate for treatment of multiple sclerosis: mechanism of action, effectiveness, and side effects. Curr. Neurol. Neurosci. Rep. 2013;13:394. http://dx.doi.org/10.1007/s11910-013-0394-8.

[5]Kamachi S, et al. Crystal structure of the catalase-peroxidase KatG W78F mutant from *Synechococcus elongatus* PCC7942 in complex with the antitubercular pro-drug isoniazid. FEBS Lett. 2015;589:131−7.

[6]Plummer ES, et al. Intravenous low molecular weight iron dextran in children with iron deficiency anemia unresponsive to oral iron. Pediatr. Blood Cancer 2013;60:1747−53.

[7]Tsiftsoglou AS, et al. Heme as key regulator of major mammalian cellular functions: molecular, cellular, and pharmacological aspects. Pharmacol. Ther. 2006;111:327−45.

[8]Roberts TG, Lynch TJ, Chabner BA. The phase III trial in the era of targeted therapy: unraveling the "go or no go" decision. J. Clin. Oncol. 2003;21:3683−95.

candidates for useful surrogate endpoints, and to identify tools for distinguishing subgroups in the patient population.

- *Designing schedule of drug administration.* The MOA can provide guidance for clinical trial design, in the case of clinical trials that involve administering a combination of drugs, for example, drugs that have a synergistic effect, or drugs that have a cumulative toxic effect.
- *Designing and interpreting safety studies.* According to the ICH Guidelines, "the mechanism of action may suggest specific adverse effects, e.g., proarrhythmia is a common feature of antiarrhythmic agents" (9). This means that a clinical trial on an antiarrhythmic agent should include safety tests that are specific for measuring proarrhythmia. The proarrhythmia that may be caused by antiarrhythmic drugs is well documented (10,11). Moreover, according to the ICH Guidelines, "[m]echanistic studies are often useful for the interpretation of tumor findings in a carcinogenicity study and can provide a perspective on their relevance to human risk assessment" (12). In the context of carcinogenesis studies, "[m]echanistic studies in recent years have permitted the distinction between effects that are specific to the rodent model and those that are likely to have relevance for humans" (13).

FDA-submissions, from the Investigator's Brochure to the Package Insert, include information on the MOA of the study drug. Knowledge of the MOA can play a part in persuading regulatory agencies that a new drug should be effective for a given indication, or that an old drug should be effective for a new indication.

II. MOA AND THE PACKAGE INSERT

Information on the MOA is required in the package insert. According to FDA's Guidance for Industry, the package insert must contain information on the MOA, and "should be discussed at various levels, including the cellular, receptor, or membrane level … , the physiologic system level (target organ), and the whole body level, depending on what is known. Only reasonably well-characterized mechanisms should be described, and care must be taken to avoid speculative and undocumented suggestions of therapeutic advantages (21 CFR §201.56 (a)(2))" (14).

III. MOA AND SURROGATE ENDPOINTS

Where a surrogate endpoint is to be used as part of the basis for regulatory approval, the

[9]ICH Harmonised Tripartite Guideline. Safety pharmacology studies for human pharmaceuticals S7A. Step 4 version; November 2000, 9 pp.

[10]Carlsson L, Duker G, Jacobson I. New pharmacological targets and treatments for atrial fibrillation. Trends Pharmacol. Sci. 2010;31:364–71.

[11]Dobrev D, Nattel S. New antiarrhythmic drugs for treatment of atrial fibrillation. Lancet 2010;375:1212–23.

[12]ICH Harmonised Tripartite Guideline. Testing for carcinogenicity of pharmaceuticals S1B. Step 4 version; July 1997. 7 pp.

[13]ICH Harmonised Tripartite Guideline. Testing for carcinogenicity of pharmaceuticals S1B. Step 4 version; July 1997. 7 pp.

[14]Department of Health and Human Services. Food and Drug Administration. Guidance for industry. Clinical pharmacology section of labeling for human prescription drug and biological products-content and format; February 2009.

investigator will likely need to provide evidence that the surrogate is related to the clinical endpoint. If the surrogate endpoint is low-density lipoprotein cholesterol (LDL-cholesterol) and if the clinical endpoint is heart attack, the principal investigator or medical writer will need to draft arguments that rely on the mechanisms of action, to argue that drugs that reduce LDL-cholesterol are likely also to reduce the incidence of heart attacks.

Clinical endpoints can include markers that are surrogate endpoints, or that are merely proposed surrogate endpoints. In this situation, the investigator provides the biochemical or physiological mechanisms that connect the surrogate endpoint with the clinical endpoint. The Prentice criteria (15,16) set forth criteria for determining whether a proposed surrogate endpoint is relevant to a clinical endpoint. The Prentice criteria are discussed in Chapter 19. The fact that the FDA accepts data on surrogate endpoints as part of the basis for regulatory approval is established by the relevant statutes, for example, 21 USC §356 (17), and by the relative administrative law, for example, 21 CFR §314.510.

IV. MOA AND EXPECTED ADVERSE DRUG REACTIONS

Knowledge of the MOA can provide insight into the expected adverse drug reactions (18).

For example, if it is established that Drug A, which inhibits Biochemical Pathway A, results in a certain type of adverse drug reaction, and if the study drug also inhibits Biochemical Pathway A, then it might be useful for the package insert for the study drug to disclose these expected adverse drug reactions. The package inserts that come with marketed drugs may include a warning regarding a *class of drugs* with a common MOA. According to the FDA's Guidance for Industry (19) on drug labeling, the package insert should disclose expected adverse drug reactions, where these are based only on expectations (not on actual observations). This warning should be included in the package insert, providing that the expected adverse drug reaction is serious or clinically significant. The expected adverse drug reaction can be based on what is known about the pharmacology, chemistry, or *class of the drug*.

V. FDA'S WARNING LETTER REGARDING ASSESSING SAFETY OF THE STUDY DRUG, ACCORDING TO ITS MEMBERSHIP IN A PARTICULAR CLASS OF DRUGS

Many of the FDA's Warning Letters concern failures of the Sponsor to follow instructions in the Clinical Study Protocol and issues

[15]Fleming TR, DeMets DL. Surrogate end points in clinical trials: are we being misled? Ann. Intern. Med. 1996;125:605—13.

[16]Gill S, Sargent D. End points for adjuvant therapy trials: has the time come to accept disease-free survival as a surrogate end point for overall survival? Oncologist 2006;11:624—9.

[17]21 USC 356, in effect as of January 24, 2002.

[18]Wilke RA, Lin DW, Roden DM, et al. Identifying genetic risk factors for serious adverse drug reactions: current progress and challenges. Nat. Rev. Drug Discov. 2007;6:904—16.

[19]U.S. Department of Health and Human Services. Food and Drug Administration. Guidance for industry warnings and precautions, contraindications, and boxed warning sections of labeling for human prescription drug and biological products-content and format; January 2006. 11 pp.

relating to the Investigational Review Board (IRB). The following letter concerns the IRB and, more specifically, the need for the Sponsor and the IRB to take into account adverse events associated with the class of drugs. This refers to the class of drugs of which the study drug is a member. The letter referred to the study drug and to its membership in a class of drugs associated with serious cardiovascular events. The letter complained that (20), "[w]ith this drug class, there is a well established association with the potential for increased risk of serious cardiovascular events. However, there is no evidence in the IRB meeting minutes … to indicate that the IRB considered this risk in determining whether risks to subject were minimized … it is incumbent upon the IRB to conduct a thorough, independent, systematic, non-arbitrary analysis of risks and benefits."

VI. MOA AND DRUG COMBINATIONS

Once the mechanisms of action of various drugs are known, this knowledge can guide the design of therapies, for example, therapeutic approaches that include combinations of drugs. One particular approach is to administer two drugs, where the two drugs have different mechanisms of action, and where these two mechanisms are related in a way that would be expected to result in synergy between the two drugs.

a. Drug Combinations That Are Complementary or Synergistic

Ifosfamide in combination with *etoposide* is used in anticancer therapy. As reviewed by Grier et al. (21), ifosfamide has the effect of alkylating chromosomal DNA, while etoposide has the effect of uncoiling chromosomal DNA. When ifosfamide is administered, the result is increased alkylation of the DNA, where this is followed by the action of DNA repair enzymes, where the DNA repair enzymes cleave the tumor cell's chromosome, thereby killing the tumor cell. When etoposide is administered, the result is increased uncoiling of the DNA of the tumor's chromosome, which is expected to enhance the enzyme-mediated cleavage, and enhance killing of the tumor cell. The end-result of administering both drugs together is a synergistic increase in tumor killing. Miles et al. (22) describe the combination of *capecitabine* plus *docetaxel*. These two drugs have distinctly separate mechanisms of action, and their effects are synergistic. Moreover, they are both toxic, but their toxicities do not overlap. The MOA of any drug encompasses its toxicity. Piccart et al. (23) describe another example of drugs with complementary mechanisms, namely, *cisplatin* plus *gemcitabine*.

b. Drug Combinations That Avoid Inducing Cross-Resistance

Drug-resistance is a common problem in oncology, bacterial infections, and viral infections. In oncology, drug resistance can arise

[20]Warning Letter No. 10-HFD-45-04-03 (April 26, 2010) from Dr Leslie K. Ball, MD, Office of Compliance, CDER, U.S. Food and Drug Administration.

[21]Grier HE, Krailo MD, Tarbell NJ, et al. Addition of ifosfamide and etoposide to standard chemotherapy for Ewing's sarcoma and primitive neuroectodermal tumor of bone. New Engl. J. Med. 2003;348:694−701.

[22]Miles D, von Minckwitz G, Seidman AD. Combination versus sequential single-agent therapy in metastatic breast cancer. Oncologist 2002;7(Suppl. 6):13−9.

[23]Piccart MJ, Lamb H, Vermorken JB. Current and future potential roles of the platinum drugs in the treatment of ovarian cancer. Ann. Oncol. 2001;12:1195−203.

where a tumor increases the activity of a pump that forces drugs out of the tumor cell, or where the target of the drug acquires a mutation that enables the target to avoid the inhibiting action of the drug. Cross-resistance is the phenomenon where a patient is being treated with one drug, and where the tumor acquires a type of drug resistance that enables it to avoid being killed by a variety of drugs. Puhalla et al. (24) describe drug combinations, in the context of treatment regimens, where a first drug is administered for several weeks, and where this is followed by a second drug, also administered for several weeks. These authors have warned that if one of these drugs is known to induce cross-resistance, then this particular drug should not be the first that is administered, but instead should be the second.

VII. MOA OF DISEASES WITH AN IMMUNE COMPONENT

a. Introduction

Disorders with an immune component include:

- autoimmune diseases,
- inflammatory disorders,
- cancer,
- infections.

Cancer includes solid tumors and hematological cancers, such as leukemia and myelodysplastic syndromes. Infections include those from bacteria, viruses, and fungi. Autoimmune diseases include multiple sclerosis, rheumatoid arthritis, ulcerative colitis, Crohn's disease, psoriasis, and systemic lupus erythematosus. Inflammatory disorders include asthma, allergies such as allergic rhinitis, atopic dermatitis, and chronic obstructive pulmonary disease (COPD).

One approach for treating infections and cancer is to stimulate immune response. Another approach is to use drugs that are directly toxic against the infecting agent or the cancer cell. Conversely, the goal in treating autoimmune diseases and inflammatory disorders, is to administer drugs that dampen immune response.

An introduction to the mechanism of cancer is provided, followed by an introduction to the inflammatory disorders, as exemplified by asthma. Subsequent chapters provide more details on cancer, infections as exemplified by hepatitis C virus (HCV), and autoimmune diseases, as illustrated by multiple sclerosis. The mechanisms of all immune disorders share a number of components in common, and are thus likely to have a shared relevance.

An understanding of immunology may be enhanced by the organization provided by the following immunology pie chart.

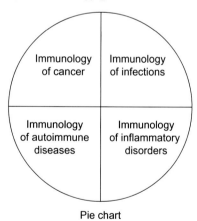

Pie chart

Cancer is distinguished by direct attack against cancer cells by CD8$^+$ T cells and by

---

[24]Puhalla S, Mrozek E, Young D, et al. Randomized phase II adjuvant trial of dose-dense docetaxel before or after doxorubicin plus cyclophosphamide in axillary node-positive breast cancer. J. Clin. Oncol. 2008;26:1691–7.

natural killer cells (NK cells), where the result is killed cancer cells. On the other hand, cancer is also distinguished by an impaired immune response against cancer cells, where this impairment results from the fact that tumor antigens are derived from self-antigens and are not usually recognized as foreign antigens, from the fact that cancer does not express immune adjuvants (unlike the case with infections), and because cancer cells mount an antiinflammatory response. The immune adjuvants expressed by viruses and bacteria, and the corresponding receptors in the human host, take the form of:

- Flagellin, muramyl-dipeptide, bacterial lipopolysaccharide, peptidoglycan, and double-stranded RNA. These are sometimes called toll-like receptor (TLR)-agonists, and they are recognized by the TLRs (25).
- Muramyl-dipeptide and daminopimelate-containing GlcNAc-tripeptide. These are recognized by the NOD-like receptors (26).
- Cyclic dinucleotides. These are recognized by the STING pathway (27).

b. Lymphocytes Infiltrate Tumors

When tumors grow in the body, various lymphocytes infiltrate the tumor. Mechanisms of immune response against cancer, for example of melanoma, were shown by Azimi et al. (28) who demonstrated various phases of interactions between tumor-infiltrating lymphocytes (TILs) and the tumor. At first, lymphocytes are in direct contact with tumor cells, where the lymphocytes disrupt "tumor nests" and later, the melanoma cells are destroyed. Pages et al. (29) provide a comprehensive identification of the various types of immune cells that infiltrate colorectal cancer tumors. Histological data for breast carcinoma were published, demonstrating the visualization of TILs in the tumors, and comparison with tumor tissue lacking in TILs (30). The lymphocytes were stained with hematoxylin and eosin. The degree of infiltration may provide a biomarker that is prognostic for survival of the patient, that is, the more TILs the better the prognosis.

Use of TILs as a biomarker depends on one or more variables, such as the location of the lymphocytes at the site of the tumor (31).

[25]Kawasaki T, Kawai T. Toll-like receptor signaling pathways. Front. Immunol. 2014;5:461. http://dx.doi.org/10.3389/fimmu.2014.00461.

[26]Corridoni D, et al. The dual role of nod-like receptors in mucosal innate immunity and chronic intestinal inflammation. Front. Immunol. 2014;5:317. http://dx.doi.org/10.3389/fimmu.2014.00317. eCollection

[27]Dubensky TW, et al. Rationale, progress and development of vaccines utilizing STING-activating cyclic dinucleotide adjuvants. Ther. Adv. Vaccines 2013;1:131−43.

[28]Azimi F, Scolyer RA, Rumcheva P, et al. Tumor-infiltrating lymphocyte grade is an independent predictor of sentinel lymph node status and survival in patients with cutaneous melanoma. J. Clin. Oncol. 2012;30:2678−83.

[29]Pages F, Berger A, Camus M, et al. Effector memory T cells, early metastasis, and survival in colorectal cancer. New Engl. J. Med. 2005;535:2654−66.

[30]Denkert C, von Minckwitz G, Brase JC, et al. Tumor-infiltrating lymphocytes and response to neoadjuvant chemotherapy with or without carboplatin in human epidermal growth factor receptor 2-positive and triple-negative primary breast cancers. J. Clin. Oncol. 2015;33:983−91.

[31]Ocana A, Diez-Gonzalez L, Adrover E, et al. Tumor-infiltrating lymphocytes in breast cancer: ready for prime time? J. Clin. Oncol. 2015;33:1298−9.

c. T Cells and NK Cells Kill Cancer Cells

Most T cells reside in tissues, such as lymphoid tissues, intestines, lungs, and skin, while a small percentage resides in the bloodstream. At birth, all T cells are naive, and memory T cells arise and develop in response to exposure to antigens. By the second decade of life, in humans, about 35% of the T cells in the bloodstream are memory T cells (32).

Upon interaction with dendritic cells (DCs), naive $CD4^+$ T cells and naive $CD8^+$ T cells differentiate into antigen-specific T cells, where CD4 + T cells become Th1 cells, Th2 cells, or Th17 cells, and $CD8^+$ T cells become effector cytotoxic T cells (cytotoxic T lymphocytes, CTLs) (33).

Immune response against cancer cells by effector cytotoxic T cells is by way of adaptive immunity, while immune response against cancer cells by NK cells, also called "natural killer cells," is by way of innate immunity. NK cells received their name because of their ability for spontaneous "natural" cytotoxicity against cancer cells and virus-infected cells. The name also invokes the fact that NK cells can kill their targets without need for any adaptive immune response (34).

Cytotoxic T cells and NK cells each independently can kill cancer cells by direct contact, where an immune synapse is formed.

Where the cells contact each other, the target cell can be killed by way of degranulation, where fusion of an intracellular vesicle (the granule) with the plasma membrane results in release of perforin and granzyme (35,36). Perforin creates momentary pores in the target cell, allowing granzyme to enter, and once inside the target cell, granzyme activates apoptosis and the target cell is killed. The pores, which are only 10 nanometers in diameter, are rapidly repaired. The immune system uses this method for killing cancer cells, and also for killing cells that are infected with viruses.

Cytotoxic T cells and NK cells also kill target cells, with direct contact, by way of another mechanism, namely by way of the ligands, FasL and TRAIL (37). These ligands transmit signals to the corresponding receptors on the target cell, and the target cell is killed. Swann and Smyth (38) provided an elegant colored drawing showing cytotoxic T cells, NK cells, and other immune cells, busily attacking a tumor.

d. Immune Evasion With Tumor-Associated Macrophages

Immune response against tumors is also mediated by another type of white blood cell, the macrophage. Macrophages occur as two subsets, M1 macrophages and M2

[32]Farber DL, et al. Human memory T cells: generation, compartmentalization and homeostasis. Nat. Rev. Immunol. 2014;14:24—35.

[33]Palucka K, Banchereau J. Cancer immunotherapy via dendritic cells. Nat. Rev. Cancer. 2012;12:265—77.

[34]Campbell KS, Hasegawa J. NK cell biology: an update and future directions. J. Allergy Clin. Immunol. 2013;132:536—44.

[35]Lopez JA, Susanto O, Jenkins MR, et al. Perforin forms transient pores on the target cell plasma membrane to facilitate rapid access to granzymes during killer cell attack. Blood 2013;121:2659—68.

[36]Molyguine AM, et al. ELISPOT assay for monitoring cytotoxic T lymphocytes (CTL) activity in cancer vaccine clinical trials. Cells 2012;1:111—26.

[37]Galli F, et al. NK cell imaging by in vitro and in vivo labeling approaches. Q. J. Nucl. Med. Mol. Imaging 2014;58:276—83.

[38]Swann JB, Smyth MJ. Immune surveillance of tumors. J. Clin. Inv. 2007;117:1137—46.

macrophages. M1 macrophages are activated by the Th1-type cytokine, interferon-gamma (IFN-gamma). M1 macrophages express proinflammatory cytokines, interleukin-12 (IL-12) and IL-23. M2 macrophages are activated by Th2-type cytokines (IL-4, IL-10, and IL-13). M2 macrophages are involved in scavenging cellular debris and in tissue repair.

M2 macrophages can also be immunosuppressive, that is, they can inhibit immune attack against cancer cells (39). Cancer cells express various chemokines, such as **CCL2**, which attracts and recruits M2 macrophages. The recruited M2 macrophages differentiate into immunosuppressive macrophages and, when physically associated with tumors, they are called "tumor-associated macrophages" (TAMs). TAMs resemble M2 macrophages.

The following dwells on the topic of TAMs, and also discloses other techniques that are used by the tumor to evade immune response. Solid tumors are characterized by hypoxia (low-oxygen environment), and energy metabolism in tumors uses anaerobic glycolysis to a greater extent, and oxidative phosphorylation to a lesser extent. Tumor hypoxia was discovered by Otto Warburg (40,41). The hypoxia induces the tumor cells to express various proteins, including **CCL2**, **VEGF**, **EMAPII**, which attract macrophages to the vicinity of the tumor (42). And once attracted the TAMs secrete high amounts of **VEGF** (which stimulates vascularization of the tumors), and also secrete IL-10, an antiinflammatory cytokine (43).

e. Immune Evasion Caused by Activity of T Regulatory Cells

This introduces the topic of T regulatory cells (Tregs). "Tregs" is pronounced, "tee-regs." Tumor-associated macrophages secrete chemokines, such as CCL17, which recruit Tregs to the tumor. Tregs, formerly called suppressor T cells, function to dampen immune response.

Tregs are CD4$^+$ T cells, and they occur in various subsets, including CD4$^+$ CD25$^+$ FOXP3 Tregs, and IL-10-producing Tregs (Tr1 cells) (44,45,46). CD25 and FOXP3 are used as biomarkers for identifying Tregs, and for distinguishing them from other types of lymphocytes. Tregs are beneficial to human health, in that they prevent inappropriate immune response against normal cells in the body, and prevent massive autoimmunity.

This utility of Tregs was dramatically shown by a naturally occurring mutant mouse,

[39]Colvin EK. Tumor-associated macrophages contribute to tumor progression in ovarian cancer. Front. Oncol. 2014;Article 137 (6 pp.).

[40]Warburg O. Uber den Stoffwechsel der tumoren. Berlin: Springer; 1926.

[41]Garber K. Energy boost: the Warburg effect returns in a new theory of cancer. J. Natl Cancer Inst. 2004;96:1805−6.

[42]Stockman C, et al. The impact of the immune system on tumor: angiogenesis and vascular remodeling. Front. Oncol. 2014;Article 69.

[43]Ostuni R, et al. Macrophages and men: from mechanisms to therapeutic implications. Trends Immunol. 2015;36:229−39.

[44]Shevach EM, Thornton AM. tTregs, pTregs and iTregs: similarities and differences. Immunol. Rev. 2014;259:88−102.

[45]Kleinewietfeld M, Hafler DA. Regulatory T cells in autoimmune neuroinflammation. Immunol. Rev. 2014;259:231−44.

[46]Mougiakakos D, et al. Naturally occurring regulatory T cells show reduced sensitivity toward oxidative stress-induced cell death. Blood 2009;113:3542−5.

the "scurfy mouse." Scurfy mouse has a genetic defect in the *FOXP3* gene. These mice lack Tregs, and their T cells proliferate indefinitely, leading to massive inflammation, overwhelming autoimmunity, and death (47).

But the Tregs that are associated with tumors only help the tumor evade immune attack. Tregs exert their immunosuppressive influences by killing $CD8^+$ T cells by way of the death receptor (CD95) and by secreting immunosuppressive cytokines, IL-10 and TGF-beta (48,49). Regarding TGF-beta, this cytokine is expressed by a wide variety of tumors. TGF-beta occurs at high levels in the plasma of cancer patients. The immunosuppressive effects of TGF-beta take the form of inhibiting cytotoxic lymphocytes, that is, inhibiting their expression of granzyme and of IFN-gamma (50).

f. Immune Evasion With PD-1 Signaling

PD-L1 (ligand) is a membrane-bound protein that is expressed by various tumor cells. PD-L1 is not just expressed by tumor cells, but it may also be expressed by the lymphocytes that infiltrate tumors (51).

PD-1 is the corresponding receptor. PD-1 is expressed by most kinds of lymphocytes that may infiltrate into the tumor. PD-1 is expressed by T cells, B cells, monocytes, natural killer T cells (NK cells), and macrophages (52,53).

Where the tumor cell's PD-L1 engages PD-1 of a T cell, the result is that the tumor can inhibit attack by the T cell (54). In the words of Garon et al. (55), "[o]ne hallmark of cancer is immune evasion, in which the immune system does not mount an effective antitumor response ... PD-1 is a negative costimulatory receptor expressed ... on the surface of activated T cells. The binding of PD-1 to ... PD-L1 ... can inhibit a cytotoxic T-cell response. Tumors can co-opt this pathway to escape T-cell-induced antitumor activity."

This binding of PD-L1 to PD-1, which is a part of immune evasion, is vividly illustrated by the fact that blocking antibodies against either the ligand (PD-L1) or the receptor (PD-1) can dramatically increase survival against cancer. In other words, the antibody prevents the tumor from engaging in this tactic of immune evasion.

[47]Eghtesad S, et al. The companions: regulatory T cells and gene therapy. Immunology 2009;27:68−73.

[48]Kleinewietfeld M, Hafler DA. Regulatory T cells in autoimmune neuroinflammation. Immunol. Rev. 2014;259:231−44.

[49]Brunkow ME, Jeffery EW, Hjerrild KA, et al. Disruption of a new forkhead/winged-helix protein, scurfin, results in fetal lymphoproliferative disorder of the scurfy mouse. Nat. Genet. 2001;27:68−73.

[50]Lin R, Chen L, Chen G, et al. Targeting miR-23a in CD8 + cytotoxic T lymphocytes prevents tumor-dependent immunosuppression. J. Clin. Invest. 2014;124:5352−67.

[51]Herbst RS, Soria JC, Kowanetz M, et al. Predictive correlates of response to the anti-PD-L1 antibody MPDL3280A in cancer patients. Nature 2014;515:563−7.

[52]McDermott DG, Atkins MB. PD-1 is a potential target in cancer therapy. Cancer Med. 2013;2:662−73.

[53]Huang X, Venet F, Wang YL, et al. PD-1 expression by macrophages plays a pathologic role in altering microbial clearance and the innate inflammatory response to sepsis. Proc. Natl Acad. Sci. 2009;106:6303−8.

[54]Pardoll D, Drake C. Immunotherapy earns its spot in the ranks of cancer therapy. J. Exp. Med. 2012;209:201−9.

[55]Garon EB, Rizvi NA, Hua R, et al. Pembrolizumab for the treatment of non-small-cell lung cancer. New Engl. J. Med. 2015. http://dx.doi.org/10.1056/NEJMoa1501824.

Pembrolizumab (anti-PD-1 antibody) improves survival against nonsmall-cell lung cancer (NSCLC) (56) as well as against melanoma (57). Another anti-PD-1 antibody, *nivolumab* improves survival against Hodgkin's lymphoma (58). Nivolumab also improves survival against NSCLC (59). Moreover, nivolumab improves survival against melanoma (60) and renal cell carcinoma (61). An antibody against the corresponding ligand, that is, anti-PD-L1 antibody, can improve survival against NSCLC, melanoma, and renal cell cancer (62,63).

VIII. IMMUNE SYSTEM PATHOLOGY IN INFLAMMATORY DISORDERS

Inflammatory disorders include asthma, COPD, allergies, and atopic dermatitis. Inflammatory disorders are characterized by the infiltration and activation of mast cells, eosinophils, and basophils.

The following provides an exemplary mechanism for asthma. Only one mechanistic feature of asthma is described, namely, a pathway leading from IL-4 and IL-13, to bronchial smooth muscle cells, to spasms. In a nutshell, the fact that an antibody that blocks the binding of IL-4 and IL-13 to its receptor relieves the symptoms of asthma, establishes that this receptor is part of the disease mechanism.

A clinical trial on *dupilumab* for treating asthma demonstrates that signaling via IL-4 receptor is part of the mechanism of asthma (64). The antibody binds to the alpha subunit of the receptor, and hence the antibody is an anti-IL4Ra antibody. Asthma is characterized by Th2-type immune response and by eosinophil infiltration. IL-4 and IL-13 occur at increased levels in the airways during asthma. IL-4 is expressed by T cells, while IL-13 is expressed by T cells, mast cells, eosinophils, and basophils. Both of these cytokines bind to the same receptor, IL-4R.

[56]Garon EB, Rizvi NA, Hua R, et al. Pembrolizumab for the treatment of non-small-cell lung cancer. New Engl. J. Med. 2015. http://dx.doi.org/10.1056/NEJMoa1501824.

[57]Robert C, Schachter J, Long GV, et al. Pembrolizumab versus Ipilimumab in Advanced Melanoma. New Engl. J. Med. 2015; Apr 19 [Epub ahead of print].

[58]Ansell SM, Lesokhin AM, Borrello I, et al. PD-1 blockade with nivolumab in relapsed or refractory Hodgkin's lymphoma. New Engl. J. Med. 2015;372:311−9.

[59]Gettinger SN, Horn L, Gandhi L, et al. Overall survival and long-term safety of nivolumab (anti-programmed death 1 antibody, BMS-936558, ONO-4538) in patients with previously treated advanced non-small-cell lung cancer. J. Clin. Oncol. 2015;pii:JCO.2014.58.3708.

[60]Robert C, Long GV, Dutriaux C, et al. Nivolumab in previously untreated melanoma without BRAF mutation. New Engl. J. Med. 2015;372:320−30.

[61]McDermott DF, Drake CG, Sznol M, et al. Survival, durable response, and long-term safety in patients with previously treated advanced renal cell carcinoma receiving nivolumab. J. Clin. Oncol. 2015;pii:JCO.2014.58.1041.

[62]Brahmer JR, Tykodi SS, Chow LQ, et al. Safety and activity of anti-PD-L1 antibody in patients with advanced cancer. New Engl. J. Med. 2012;366:2455−65.

[63]Herbst RS, Soria JC, Kowanetz M, et al. Predictive correlates of response to the anti-PD-L1 antibody MPDL3280A in cancer patients. Nature 2014;515:563−7.

[64]Wenzel S, Ford L, Pearlman D, et al. Dupilumab in persistent asthma with elevated eosinophil levels. New Engl. J. Med. 2013;368:2455−66.

According to Wenzel et al. (65), half of asthma patients have increased Th2-type inflammation, where there is increased expression of IL-4 and IL-13. Most asthma patients can be successfully treated with the combination of inhaled glucocorticoids plus long-acting beta-agonists, but about 20% of asthma patients do not respond to this therapy. In a study of patients with asthma that was not controllable by the combination of these two kinds of drugs, it was found that administered *dupilumab* was dramatically effective. Efficacy was measured by a test for lung function (forced respiratory volume in 1 s test; FEV_1 test), and by questionnaires filled out by the study subjects (SNOT-22 score; ACQ5 questionnaire).

Efficacy of *dupilumab* was also shown by plasma-level assays for two chemokines, TARC and eotaxin-3. TARC is also known as CCL17, and eotaxin-3 is also called CCL26. TARC is the ligand for CCR4, a receptor that occurs on T cells (66). TARC is thymus and activation-regulated chemokine. According to Wenzel et al. "[l]evels of TARC, eotaxin-3, and IgE ... remained unchanged with placebo. In contrast, with dupilumab, TARC and eotaxin-3 levels were decreased at week 1 and remained lower than baseline values through week 12. With dupilumab, the IgE level was also lower than the baseline value at week 4."

The literature establishes a mechanism of action that connects increased plasma levels of the cytokines IL-4 and IL-13, as a cause of constriction of smooth muscle of the airways. Asthma is a pulmonary disorder that is characterized by increased susceptibility to bronchospasms. Direct activation of smooth muscle by IL-4 or IL-13 is sufficient to induce airway hyper-responsiveness (AHR). In the words of Perkins et al. (67), "[t]hese observations demonstrated that AHR can be induced through direct, in vivo effects of IL-4R signaling on smooth muscle and were consistent with previous in vitro evidence that IL-4R signaling can increase smooth muscle contractility."

Airway smooth muscle cells express receptors for IL-4 and IL-13. These cytokines act on the smooth muscle cells to induce contractile and relaxant responses, proliferation, and the ability of smooth muscle cells to generate chemokines such as eotaxin and TARC (68). TARC acts on the chemokine receptor CCR4, which is expressed on T cells (69). TARC attracts T cells into the asthmatic airways. Plasma and bronchial fluids, in asthma patients, have elevated levels of TARC.

The following narrative helps establish a role for TARC, as expressed by airway smooth muscle cells, in the mechanism of airway smooth muscle contraction in asthma.

[65]Wenzel S, Ford L, Pearlman D, et al. Dupilumab in persistent asthma with elevated eosinophil levels. New Engl. J. Med. 2013;368:2455−66.

[66]Ying S, O'Connor B, Ratoff J, et al. Expression and cellular provenance of thymic stromal lymphopoietin and chemokines in patients with severe asthma and chronic obstructive pulmonary disease. J. Immunol. 2008;181:2790−8.

[67]Perkins C, et al. Selective stimulation of IL-4 receptor on smooth muscle induces airway hyperresponsiveness in mice. J. Exp. Med. 2011;208:853−67.

[68]Shore SA. Direct effects of Th2 cytokines on airway smooth muscle. Curr. Opin. Pharmacol. 2004;4:235−40.

[69]Leung TF, et al. Plasma TARC concentration may be a useful marker for asthmatic exacerbation in children. Eur. Respir. J. 2003;21:616−20.

According to Faffe et al. (70), "[b]ecause IL-4 or IL-13 is required for TARC release and since TARC is a chemotactic factor for the Th2 cells that express IL-4 and IL-13, these results suggest that airway smooth muscle participates in a **positive feedback loop** that promotes the recruitment of Th2 cells to the airways."

As stated above, Wenzel et al. (71) disclose that the study drug reduced plasma *eotaxin-3* levels. Eotaxin-3 is a chemokine that is also known as CCL26. The following incorporates eotaxin-3, as part of the narrative on the MOA of asthma. According to Provost et al. (72):

> [e]osinophils play a significant role in asthma pathogenesis. During asthma exacerbations ... eosinophils infiltrate the bronchial mucosa and lumen of asthmatics. This recruitment of eosinophils occurs in response to chemoattractants. The CC chemokines eotaxin-1/CCL11, eotaxin-2/CCL24, and **eotaxin-3/CCL26** are potent chemoattractants for eosinophils ... [l]ung-derived eotaxins can induce eosinophil mobilization from the bone marrow to the bronchial mucosa and locally stimulate the release of **ROS and cationic proteins**, resulting in the typical epithelial cell damage observed in asthma.

The utility of eosinophils in killing infections, and the pathology of eosinophils in asthma, are summarized by Felton et al. (73):

> [e]osinophils, granulocytic cells of the innate immune system, are primarily involved in defense against parasitic infections ... [u]nregulated or prolonged inflammatory responses in the lungs can lead to tissue damage, disrupting normal tissue architecture ... [f]ailure to resolve inflammation underlies the development ... of inflammatory lung diseases including asthma.

The utility in killing infections, and the pathological features of asthma, are further described by Felton et al. (74):

> eosinophil degranulation contributes to both the removal of the inflammatory stimuli and also the propagation of inflammation. Eosinophil-derived granules contain ... major basic protein, **eosinophil cationic protein**, eosinophil peroxidase, and eosinophil-derived neurotoxin, which are known to be cytotoxic to airway epithelial cells.

Damage to tissues from reactive oxygen, as occurs in asthma, can be detected by oxidative products of proteins, lipids, and nucleic acids (75). One form of reactive oxygen species is *peroxynitrite*. Peroxynitrite is generated by reaction of nitric oxide (NO) with superoxide. Nitric oxide is produced, at increased levels, by eosinophils in patients with asthma

[70]Faffe DS, et al. IL-13 and IL-4 promote TARC release in human airway smooth muscle cells: role of IL-4 receptor genotype. Am. J. Physiol. Lung Cell Mol. Physiol. 2003;285:L907—14.

[71]Wenzel S, Ford L, Pearlman D, et al. Dupilumab in persistent asthma with elevated eosinophil levels. New Engl. J. Med. 2013;368:2455—66.

[72]Provost V, et al. CCL26/eotaxin-3 is more effective to induce the migration of eosinophils of asthmatics than CCL11/eotaxin-1 and CCL24/eotaxin-2. J. Leukoc. Biol. 2013;94:213—22.

[73]Felton JM, et al. Eosinophils in the lung—modulating apoptosis and efferocytosis in airway inflammation. Front. Immunol. 2014;5:302. http://dx.doi.org/10.3389/fimmu.2014.00302

[74]Felton JM, et al. Eosinophils in the lung—modulating apoptosis and efferocytosis in airway inflammation. Front. Immunol. 2014;5:302. http://dx.doi.org/10.3389/fimmu.2014.00302

[75]Fujisawa T. Role of oxygen radicals on bronchial asthma. Curr. Drug Targets Inflamm. Allergy 2005;4:505—9.

(76,77,78,79). Kanazawa et al. (80) report that *peroxynitrite* is increased in airway epithelial cells and eosinophils in asthmatic patients compared with normal control subjects. To conclude, the above discloses the MOA of an inflammatory disorder. Chapter 27 describes the MOAs of various autoimmune diseases.

IX. CELLS OF THE IMMUNE SYSTEM

Cells of the immune system include DCs, T cells, B cells, NK cells, macrophages, Kupffer cells, microglia, and neutrophils. Kupffer cells (81) are resident macrophages that are part of the liver and do not circulate in the bloodstream, while microglia (82) are macrophages of the central nervous system. The term antigen-presenting cell (APC) refers to cells that can form an immune synapse with a T cell, where the APC presents an antigen once the immune synapse is formed, and where the antigen is presented by way of the major histocompatibility complex (MHC) class I or MHC class II of the APC, to the T cell. The consequence of antigen presentation is activation of the T cell. APCs include DCs, macrophages, and B cells.

In diagrams, all of these cells may be represented as a circle. Usually though, DCs are drawn in the shape of a starfish, because of the fact that DCs have dendrites or branches (83,84). There are two lineages of DCs, the myeloid DCs and plasmacytoid DCs (pDCs). The former type of DC resembles a starfish, while the latter is round (85). The long dendrites of DCs are believed to contribute to the remarkable efficiency by which DCs take up, process, and present antigen to T cells (86).

Immune response, as it applies to infections, cancer, inflammatory disorders, and autoimmune diseases, involves the following chain of events. DCs take up antigens, and present the

[76]Hebestreit H, et al. Disruption of Fas receptor signaling by nitric oxide in eosinophils. J. Exp. Med. 1998;187:415–25.

[77]Smith AD, et al. Use of exhaled nitric oxide measurements to guide treatment in chronic asthma. New Engl. J. Med. 2005;352:2163–73.

[78]van Vliet D, et al. Prediction of asthma exacerbations in children by innovative exhaled inflammatory markers: results of a longitudinal study. PLoS One 2015;10:e0119434. http://dx.doi.org/10.1371/journal.pone.0119434.

[79]Wenzel S, Ford L, Pearlman D, et al. Dupilumab in persistent asthma with elevated eosinophil levels. New Engl. J. Med. 2013;368:2455–66.

[80]Kanazawa H, et al. Decreased peroxynitrite inhibitory activity in induced sputum in patients with bronchial asthma. Thorax 2002;57:509–12.

[81]Tomita M, Yamamoto K, Kobashi H, Ohmoto M, Tsuji T. Immunohistochemical phenotyping of liver macrophages in normal and diseased human liver. Hepatology 1994;20:317–25.

[82]Rock RB, Gekker G, Hu S, et al. Role of microglia in central nervous system infections. Clin. Microbiol. Rev. 2004;17:942–64.

[83]Blanco P, Palucka AK, Pascual V, Banchereau J. Dendritic cells and cytokines in human inflammatory and autoimmune diseases. Cytokine Growth Factor Rev. 2008;19:41–52.

[84]Randolph GJ, Ochando J, Partida-Sánchez S. Migration of dendritic cell subsets and their precursors. Annu. Rev. Immunol. 2008;26:293–316.

[85]Wu L, Dakic A. Development of dendritic cell system. Cell Mol. Immunol. 2004;1:112–8.

[86]Swetman CA, Leverrier Y, Garg R, et al. Extension, retraction and contraction in the formation of a dendritic cell dendrite: distinct roles for Rho GTPases. Eur. J. Immunol. 2002;32:2074–83.

antigens to T cells, where the result is an activated T cell. In turn, the activated T cell proliferates, resulting in an increased population of T cells specific for that antigen, and where the activated T cell can respond extremely quickly the next time it encounters the antigen. Once stimulated with antigen, T cells can kill human cells that are infected with viruses or bacteria, thereby removing the infection, or the T cells can kill tumor cells. Regarding inflammatory disorders and autoimmune diseases, once stimulated with antigen, T cells can attack human cells, causing damage to human tissue.

A simple version of this scenario appears below (Fig. 26.1). In step 1, the DC takes up antigens. In step 2, the antigens are processed and mounted on a protein complex called MHC, where the processed antigens are bound to the outside surface of the DC. In step 3, which involves the immune synapse, the DC presents the antigen to a T cell. The T cell can be either a CD4$^+$ T cell or a CD8$^+$ T cell. In step 4, as a consequence of events taking place at the immune synapse, the T cell becomes activated, and it proliferates. In step 5, the T cell after proliferation contacts a tumor cell or an infected cell. In step 6, the activated T cell encounters a cell that contains the same antigen on its surface, and the T cell kills the cell (indicated by the bolt of lighting). In a variation of this scenario, taking place during an autoimmune disease, the T cell inflicts damage on a healthy human cell. In a separate pathway, occurring at the same time, the DC presents processed

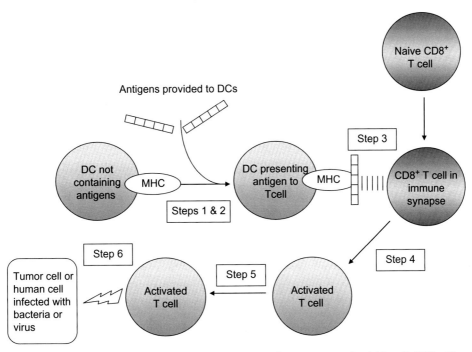

FIGURE 26.1 The immune response involves the introduction of antigens to a dendritic cell (DC), either by uptake from the environment or via biosynthesis by a bacterium or virus inside of the DC. The DC then processes the antigen to short peptides, and presents the peptides to waiting CD4$^+$ T cells or CD8$^+$ T cells. This results in the activation of the T cell. In the case of activated CD8$^+$ T cells, the T cell is then able to kill human cells where those human cells bear the same antigen on their outside surface.

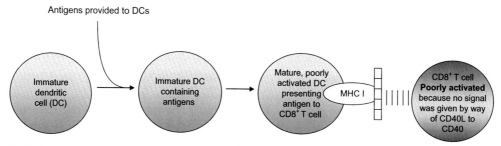

FIGURE 26.2 Dendritic cell (DC) acquires antigen, processes the antigen, and presents the processed antigen to a CD8⁺ T cell. Antigen processing and presentation by a DC that is poorly activated. The DC shown in this figure can present antigen to T cells, resulting in an activated T cell, but activation is not optimal, and the T cell cannot mount an effective and vigorous immune response.

antigens to the other type of T cell, namely, CD4⁺ T cells, resulting in the activation and proliferation of these CD4⁺ T cells.

The following diagrams illustrate further details of the immune system, showing the activation of DCs, where the consequence of this activation is that the DC more effectively activates the T cell. The first picture shows a nonactivated DC, where formation of the immune synapse results in a *poorly activated T cell*. The second picture shows the activation of a DC by an immune adjuvant, where this particular immune adjuvant is a TLR-agonist, and where the consequence is a *highly activated T cell*. The third picture shows the activation of a DC by a CD4⁺ T cell, where the consequence is a *highly activated T cell*. A property of a poorly activated CD8⁺ T cell is that it may be stimulated to proliferate, but it will function poorly in killing target cells. A property of a highly activated CD8⁺ T cell is that it is stimulated to proliferate, and that it can also function effectively in killing target cells. CD4⁺ T cells are also called helper T cells. CD8⁺ T cells function to kill other cells and for this reason are also called CTLs. The little arrays of lines represent the binding interaction between two proteins. This binding involves the formation of hydrogen bonds. It is conventional, in organic chemistry, to use an array of parallel lines to represent a hydrogen bond. The

segmented ribbon represents a peptide, that is, an oligomer of about 10 amino acids (Figures 26.2–26.4).

This concerns NK cells and antibodies. NK cells kill cells by way of antibody-dependent cell cytotoxicity (ADCC). In ADCC, an antibody binds to the surface of a human cell that is infected with a virus or bacteria, to form a complex. This complex mediates the binding of the NK cell to the infected cell, where the result is that the NK cell kills the infected human cell, thereby curing the infection. NK cells can kill tumor cells by the same mechanism, that is, where a tumor-specific antibody binds to the tumor cell. ADCC involves a sandwich of two cells, where the antibody resides inside the sandwich. B cells produce antibodies.

X. DRUGS THAT MODULATE THE IMMUNE SYSTEM

a. Introduction

In autoimmune diseases and inflammatory disorders, the relevant drugs are intended to inhibit the immune system, whereas in cancer and chronic infections, the drugs are intended to stimulate the immune system. Drugs that modulate the immune system are indicated by

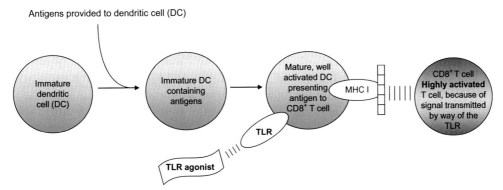

FIGURE 26.3 Antigen processing and presentation by a DC that is highly activated. DCs can be activated by a number of naturally occurring agents, such as a TLR agonist. TLR agonists are components of viruses and bacteria. The result is a highly activated CD8[+] T cell.

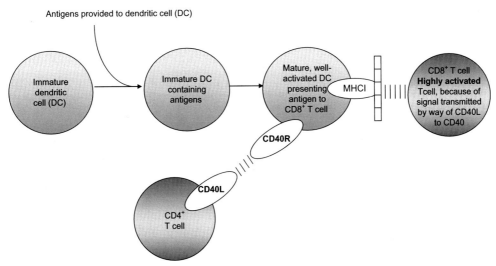

FIGURE 26.4 Antigen processing and presentation by a DC that is highly activated. DCs can be activated by a number of naturally occurring agents, such as a CD40 ligand. The DC is activated by a CD4[+] T cell, where this activation involves contact of CD40 ligand of the CD4[+] T cell with CD40 receptor of the DC. The end-result, after formation of the immune synapse, is a highly activated CD8[+] T cell.

the following bullet points. A few token examples are then disclosed.

- Vaccines,
- Cytokines,
- TLR agonists,
- Inhibitors of Tregs.

b. Vaccines

Vaccines have the longest history of use of all of the immune-modulating drugs (87). Edward Jenner is the scientist most associated with the invention of vaccination. Jenner's vaccination of

[87]Plotkin SA, editor. History of vaccine development. New York: Springer, Inc.; 2011.

a boy, James Phipps, involved the removal of fluid from a cowpox lesion on the hand of Sarah Nelmes. The fluid was inserted into two incisions in the skin of Phipps' arm. After 7 days the boy became slightly unwell, but soon recovered (88). Vaccination had a basis in the earlier practice of variolation, which had been practiced in China as early as the Sung Dynasty (AD 960–1280) (89).

c. Cytokines

The cytokines encompass three categories of molecules, namely, cytokines, chemokines, and certain growth factors (90). Interferon was the first cytokine to be described, as documented in a paper from 1957 (91). Cytokines function as autocrine signals (secretion and stimulation of the same cell), paracrine and juxtacrine signals (stimulation of nearby cells), or endocrine signals (circulating in the peripheral blood to act on cells remote to the source of production). A small proportion of cytokines have been used as drugs. For example, IL-12 (92), IFN-gamma (93), and IFN-alpha (94), have been tested, or are in actual use, for treating various cancers and immune disorders. The cytokine, granulocyte-macrophage colony-stimulating factor, has shown promising results for treating melanoma (95), lymphoma (96), and breast cancer (97). Interferon, in combination with a small molecule (ribavirin), was formerly the gold standard for treating HCV infections (98).

[88]Morgan AJ, Parker S. Translational mini-review series on vaccines: the Edward Jenner Museum and the history of vaccination. Clin. Exp. Immunol. 2007;147:389–94.

[89]Oldstone MBA. Viruses, plagues, and history: past, present and future. New York: Oxford University Press; 2009. p. 74.

[90]Tarrant JM. Blood cytokines as biomarkers of in vivo toxicity in preclinical safety assessment: considerations for their use. Toxicol. Sci. 2010;117:4–16.

[91]Isaacs A, Lindenmann J. Virus interference. I. The interferon. Proc. R. Soc. Lond. B Biol. Sci. 1957;147:258–67.

[92]Alatrash G, Hutson TE, Molto L, et al. Clinical and immunologic effects of subcutaneously administered interleukin-12 and interferon alfa-2b: phase I trial of patients with metastatic renal cell carcinoma or malignant melanoma. J. Clin. Oncol. 2004;22:2891–900.

[93]Miller CH, Maher SG, Young HA. Clinical use of interferon-gamma. Ann. N. Y. Acad. Sci. 2009;1182:69–79.

[94]Bottomley A, Coens C, Suciu S, et al. Adjuvant therapy with pegylated interferon alfa-2b versus observation in resected stage III melanoma: a phase III randomized controlled trial of health-related quality of life and symptoms by the European Organisation for Research and Treatment of Cancer Melanoma Group. J. Clin. Oncol. 2009;27:2916–23.

[95]Sato T, Eschelman DJ, Gonsalves CF, et al. Immunoembolization of malignant liver tumors, including uveal melanoma, using granulocyte-macrophage colony-stimulating factor. J. Clin. Oncol. 2008;26:5436–42.

[96]Cartron G, Zhao-Yang L, Baudard M, et al. Granulocyte-macrophage colony-stimulating factor potentiates rituximab in patients with relapsed follicular lymphoma: results of a phase II study. J. Clin. Oncol. 2008;26:2725–31.

[97]Emens LA, Asquith JM, Leatherman JM, et al. Timed sequential treatment with cyclophosphamide, doxorubicin, and an allogeneic granulocyte-macrophage colony-stimulating factor-secreting breast tumor vaccine: a chemotherapy dose-ranging factorial study of safety and immune activation. J. Clin. Oncol. 2009;27:5911–8.

[98]Lee S, Kim IH, Kim SH, et al. Efficacy and tolerability of pegylated interferon-alpha2a plus ribavirin versus pegylated interferon-alpha2b plus ribavirin in treatment-naive chronic hepatitis C patients. Intervirology 2010;53:146–53.

d. Toll-Like Receptor Agonists

The term toll-like receptor (TLR) agonist refers to a chemical that stimulates a TLR. The cited references in the following narrative identify oncology clinical trials using TLR agonists.

The TLRs consist of a class of 10 proteins. Each of the TLRs responds to a different agonist or ligand. For example, CpG-oligodeoxynucleotides stimulate TLR9 (99,100). TLR9 recognizes unmethylated CpG sequences in DNA molecules. CpG sites are relatively rare on vertebrate genomes in comparison to bacterial genomes or viral DNA. Synthetic CpG-oligodeoxynucleotides are analogs of naturally occurring viral and bacterial DNA. Coban et al. (101) provide a diagram showing the cell signaling pathway induced by administered CpG-oligodeoxynucleotides.

The immune system responds effectively to most viral and bacterial infections, for two reasons. The first is that viruses and bacteria contain foreign antigens, while the second is that viruses and bacteria provide naturally occurring TLR agonists. In contrast to the situation with infections, the immune system generally fails to respond effectively to tumors. This failure results from the fact tumor antigens are self-antigens (or closely resemble self-antigens), and also from the fact that tumors do not express TLR agonists. For this reason, TLR agonists have been used as drugs, and administered to cancer patients, in conjunction with chemotherapy, as in the clinical study of Manegold et al. (102). The actual CPG molecule that was used was identified as PF-3512676, also known as CPG7909. The safety and efficacy of CPG7909 have been assessed in many studies of cancer (103,104,105).

Polyinosinic:polycytidylic acid is another immune adjuvant that specifically binds to TLR3 (106,107). Glucopyranosyl lipid A (GLA)

[99]Lou Y, Liu C, Lizée G, et al. Antitumor activity mediated by CpG: the route of administration is critical. J. Immunother. 2011;34:279−88.

[100]Holtick U, Scheulen ME, von Bergwelt-Baildon MS, Weihrauch MR. Toll-like receptor 9 agonists as cancer therapeutics. Expert Opin. Investig. Drugs 2011;20:361−72.

[101]Coban C, Koyama S, Takeshita F, Akira S, Ishii KJ. Molecular and cellular mechanisms of DNA vaccines. Hum. Vaccin. 2008;4:453−6.

[102]Manegold C, Gravenor D, Woytowitz D, et al. Randomized phase II trial of a toll-like receptor 9 agonist oligodeoxynucleotide, PF-3512676, in combination with first-line taxane plus platinum chemotherapy for advanced-stage non-small-cell lung cancer. J. Clin. Oncol. 2008;26:3979−86.

[103]Yamada K, Nakao M, Fukuyama C, et al. Phase I study of TLR9 agonist PF-3512676 in combination with carboplatin and paclitaxel in patients with advanced non-small-cell lung cancer. Cancer Sci. 2010;101:188−95.

[104]Iwahashi M, Katsuda M, Nakamori M, et al. Vaccination with peptides derived from cancer-testis antigens in combination with CpG-7909 elicits strong specific CD8 + T cell response in patients with metastatic esophageal squamous cell carcinoma. Cancer Sci. 2010;101:2510−7.

[105]Brody JD, Ai WZ, Czerwinski DK, et al. In situ vaccination with a TLR9 agonist induces systemic lymphoma regression: a phase I/II study. J. Clin. Oncol. 2010;28:4324−32.

[106]Amos SM, Pegram HJ, Westwood JA, et al. Adoptive immunotherapy combined with intratumoral TLR agonist delivery eradicates established melanoma in mice. Cancer Immunol. Immunother. 2011; February 16 [Epub ahead of print].

[107]Okada H, Kalinski P, Ueda R, et al. Induction of CD8 + T-cell responses against novel glioma-associated antigen peptides and clinical activity by vaccinations with {alpha}-type 1 polarized dendritic cells and polyinosinic-polycytidylic acid stabilized by lysine and carboxymethylcellulose in patients with recurrent malignant glioma. J. Clin. Oncol. 2011;29:330−6.

is a TLR4 agonist being tested for efficacy in treating cancer (108). Imiquimod, a TLR7 agonist, is being used to treat cancer (109,110,111). *Listeria monocytogenes* (112) is a bacterium that naturally expresses three TLR agonists, namely, peptidoglycan, bacterial DNA, and flagellin. Peptidoglycan of *Listeria* is an agonist of TLR2 (113). Flagellin of *Listeria* is an agonist of TLR5 (114). Bacterial nucleic acids are an agonist of TLR9 (115).

e. Methodology Tip—Fine-Tuning of Immune Adjuvants When Treating Cancer

As is the case with many clinical trials, a number of clinical trials using CPG-oligodeoxynucleotides (CPGs) as an immune adjuvant have failed to show efficacy. But fine-tuning of the treatment schedule may overcome this problem. One issue is whether an immune adjuvant administered concurrently with chemotherapy, or at a different time, can each influence efficacy. In the case of CPG, Nierkens et al. (116) have shown that, where disruption of the tumor and where CPG administration occur concurrently, the CPG be an effective antitumor agent, but where CPG is administered a day or so before (or after) tumor disruption, the CPG is not effective. In general, tumor disruption can be accomplished by cytotoxic drugs, radiation, or cryoablation. The issue of the route of administration also needs to be addressed, in clinical trials that use drugs. In the case of CPG, Lou et al. (117) have shown that the route of administration can influence efficacy, where intratumor injection improves efficacy over intravenous injection.

f. Inhibitors of Tregs

Tregs, formerly called suppressor T cells, function to reduce the inflammatory response. Although Tregs are useful for preventing

[108]Fox CB, Friede M, Reed SG, Ireton GC. Synthetic natural TLR4 agonists as safe and effective vaccine adjuvants. In: Endotoxins: structure, function, and regulation, vol. 53, Subcellular biochemistry. New York: Springer; 2010. pp. 303–21.

[109]van Seters M, van Beurden M, ten Kate FJ, et al. Treatment of vulvar intraepithelial neoplasia with topical imiquimod. New Engl. J. Med. 2008;358:1465–73.

[110]Lu H, Wagner WM, Gad E, et al. Treatment failure of a TLR-7 agonist occurs due to self-regulation of acute inflammation and can be overcome by IL-10 blockade. J. Immunol. 2010;184:5360–7.

[111]Valins W, Amini S, Berman B. The expression of toll-like receptors in dermatological diseases and the therapeutic effect of current and newer topical toll-like receptor modulators. Clin. Aesthet. Dermatol. 2010;3:20–9.

[112]Skoberne M, Yewdall A, Bahjat KS, et al. KBMA *Listeria monocytogenes* is an effective vector for DC-mediated induction of antitumor immunity. J. Clin. Invest. 2008;118:3990–4001.

[113]Way SS, Thompson LJ, Lopes JE, et al. Characterization of flagellin expression and its role in *Listeria monocytogenes* infection and immunity. Cell Microbiol. 2004;6:235–42.

[114]Way SS, Thompson LJ, Lopes JE, et al. Characterization of flagellin expression and its role in *Listeria monocytogenes* infection and immunity. Cell Microbiol. 2004;6:235–42.

[115]Plitas G, Chaudhry UI, Kingham TP, Raab JR, DeMatteo RP. NK dendritic cells are innate immune responders to *Listeria monocytogenes* infection. J. Immunol. 2007;178:4411–6.

[116]Nierkens S, den Brok MH, Sutmuller RP, et al. In vivo colocalization of antigen and CpG within dendritic cells is associated with the efficacy of cancer immunotherapy. Cancer Res. 2008;68:5390–6.

[117]Lou Y, Liu C, Lizée G, et al. Antitumor activity mediated by CpG: the route of administration is critical. J. Immunother. 2011;34:279–88.

pathological inflammation, and for preventing massive autoimmunity, Tregs sometimes prevent the body from mounting an effective immune response against cancer or chronic infections. The antibody, anti-GITR antibody, is a drug that inhibits Tregs. GITR stands for *Glucocorticoid-Induced TNF receptor-Related* protein. GITR is a membrane-bound protein that transmits signals to the cell. GITR is activated when GITR ligand (GITRL) binds to GITR, forming the GITRL/GITR complex. GITRL and GITR are each membrane-bound proteins. GITRL is expressed by parencymal tissue cells, while GITR is expressed by Tregs (118). Anti-GITR antibody is being tested with the goal of increasing the immune response against cancer (119). In order to reduce the activity of Tregs, the anti-GITR antibody needs to be an agonistic antibody (it must not be a blocking antibody). Agonistic anti-GITR antibody has proven effective in various animal models of cancer (120). In addition to cancer, another vexing problem is chronic infections, such as parasitic infections. Agonistic anti-GITR antibody has also been shown to be effective against parasitic infections (121,122).

Cyclophosphamide, a drug commonly used against cancer, inhibits Tregs (123). Tregs act as a brake against the immune system, reducing immune response against self-antigens. Hence, Tregs are important for preventing indiscriminate, pathological inflammation of all organs of the body. Tregs also may reduce immune response against tumor antigens and infecting agents and, in this context, Treg activity may be undesired.

The mechanisms of cyclophosphamide include eliminating Tregs, enhancing expansion of antigen-specific T cells, inducing survival factors for T cells (type I interferon; IL-7; IL-15), and activating DCs (124). The structure of cyclophosphamide is shown below.

[118]Azuma M. Role of the glucocorticoid-induced TNFR-related protein (GITR)-GITR ligand pathway in innate and adaptive immunity. Crit. Rev. Immunol. 2010;30:547−57.

[119]Boczkowski D, Lee J, Pruitt S, Nair S. Dendritic cells engineered to secrete anti-GITR antibodies are effective adjuvants to dendritic cell-based immunotherapy. Cancer Gene Ther. 2009;16:900−11.

[120]Kamimura Y, Iwai H, Piao J, Hashiguchi M, Azuma M. The glucocorticoid-induced TNF receptor-related protein (GITR)-GITR ligand pathway acts as a mediator of cutaneous dendritic cell migration and promotes T cell-mediated acquired immunity. J. Immunol. 2009;182:2708−16.

[121]Haque A, Stanley AC, Amante FH, et al. Therapeutic glucocorticoid-induced TNF receptor-mediated amplification of CD4 + T cell responses enhances antiparasitic immunity. J. Immunol. 2010;184:2583−92.

[122]D'Elia R, Behnke JM, Bradley JE, Else KJ. Regulatory T cells: a role in the control of helminth-driven intestinal pathology and worm survival. J. Immunol. 2009;182:2340−8.

[123]Loeffler M, Krüger JA, Reisfeld RA. Immunostimulatory effects of low-dose cyclophosphamide are controlled by inducible nitric oxide synthase. Cancer Res. 2005;65:5027−30.

[124]Salem ML, Al-Khami AA, El-Naggar SA, et al. Cyclophosphamide induces dynamic alterations in the host microenvironments resulting in a Flt3 ligand-dependent expansion of dendritic cells. J. Immunol. 2010;184:1737−47.

XI. IMMUNOLOGY CAN BE ORGANIZED AS PAIRS OF CONCEPTS

a. Introduction

Although immunology is one of the least predictable of all the sciences, this situation is mitigated by the fact that many of the concepts in cellular immunology occur as pairs.

For example, many immune cells, such as DCs and T cells, can assume two different cytokine expression patterns, that is, they can express Th1-type cytokines or Th2-type cytokines. Also, T cells occur as two types, $CD4^+$ T cells and $CD8^+$ T cells, and once stimulated by a presented antigen, the T cells can undergo two consecutive responses, naive immune response followed at a later time by memory immune response. Such an abundance of pairs is rarely found in any other field of science, except, perhaps for physics. High school students are familiar with the wave/particle duality of light, with positive and negative electric fields, and with matter and antimatter.

b. Th1-Type Response and Th2-Type Response

By secreting cytokines, DCs can stimulate subsequent Th1-type immune response, or Th2-type immune response. For example, *Salmonella* bacteria can infect DCs, and once inside, provoke the activation of the DCs, and stimulate the DC to express IL-12 (125). This IL-12, in turn, stimulates downstream Th1-type immune responses that include expression of IFN-gamma (126). IL-12 is a master controller, as it stimulates Th1-type response and inhibits Th2-type response (127). Th1-type response is identified most with expression of IFN-gamma.

To provide another example, certain allergens, and helminths such as *Schistosoma mansoni* (128) and *Nippostrongylus brasiliensis*, stimulate DCs to express Th2-type cytokines (129,130). The separation of immune response into Th1-type and Th2-type is a simplification, in view of the fact that an additional type of response by T cells is Th17-type immune response. Th17 response occurs in the pathology of certain autoimmune disorders, such as multiple sclerosis and ulcerative colitis.

The designation Th, which occurs in the terms Th1 and Th2, refers to T helper cells. T helper cells are $CD4^+$ T cells. A similar division occurs with $CD8^+$ T cells, and here the corresponding responses by the $CD8^+$ T cells, are sometimes called Tc1-response and Tc2-response (131).

[125]Brzoza KL, Rockel AB, Hiltbold EM. Cytoplasmic entry of *Listeria monocytogenes* enhances dendritic cell maturation and T Cell differentiation and function. J. Immunol. 2004;173:2641—51.

[126]Lucey DR, Clerici M, Shearer GM. Type 1 and type 2 cytokine dysregulation in human infectious, neoplastic, and inflammatory diseases. Clin. Microbiol. Rev. 1996;9:532—62.

[127]Romani L, Puccetti P, Bistoni F. Interleukin-12 in infectious diseases. Clin. Microbiol. Rev. 1997;10:611—36.

[128]de Jong EC, Vieira PL, Pawel Kalinski P, et al. Microbial compounds selectively induce Th1 cell-promoting or Th2 cell-promoting dendritic cells in vitro with diverse Th cell-polarizing signals. J. Immunol. 2002;168:1704—9.

[129]MacDonald AS, Maizels RM. Alarming dendritic cells for Th2 induction. J. Exp. Med. 2008;205:13—7.

[130]Ishiwata K, Watanabe N, Guo M, et al. Costimulator B7-DC attenuates strong Th2 responses induced by *Nippostrongylus brasiliensis*. J. Immunol. 2010;184:2086—94.

[131]O'Donnell H, McSorley SJ. Salmonella as a model for non-cognate Th1 cell stimulation. Front. Immunol. 2014;5: Article 621 (13 pp.).

c. CD4$^+$ T Cells and CD8$^+$ T Cells

The term "CD" means *cluster of differentiation* (132,133). Proteins that are numbered with cluster of differentiation numbers are among the hundreds of membrane-bound proteins residing on the surface of lymphocytes. CD4 is a membrane-bound protein, identified by GenBank Accession No. NM_000616. CD8 is also a membrane-bound protein, identified by GenBank Accession No. NM_001145873.

d. Myeloid DCs and Plasmacytoid DCs

DCs are classified as myeloid DCs and plasmacytoid DCs (134,135).

Myeloid DCs and pDCs have different functions. Myeloid DCs are responsible for presenting antigens to T cells. In contrast to myeloid DCs, pDCs are a rare subset of DCs. pDCs contribute to antiviral immunity through their ability to produce high levels of IFN-alpha upon activation. pDCs are early responders during systemic viral infections and, in some cases, are the sole producers of IFN-alpha. IFN-alpha expression is crucial for viral clearance during primary viral infections (136). Also, pDCs are found in the microenvironment in tumors (137). IFN-alpha, along with IFN-beta, IFN-omega, IFN-epsilon, IFN-kappa, and IFN-tau, are classified as type I interferons (138,139).

This distinguishes type I interferons from type II interferon. In contrast to the situation with type I interferons, there exists only one type II interferon, namely, IFN-gamma (140,141,142,143). The classification of interferons into type I and type II interferon is not the same as, and is not directly relevant to, the concept of Th1-type and Th2-type response.

[132]Zola H, Swart B. The human leucocyte differentiation antigens (HLDA) workshops: the evolving role of antibodies in research, diagnosis and therapy. Cell Res. 2005;15:691−4.

[133]Lai L, Alaverdi N, Maltais L, Morse HC. Mouse cell surface antigens: nomenclature and immunophenotyping. J. Immunol. 1998;160:3861−8.

[134]Shortman K, et al. Plasmacytoid dendritic cell development. Adv. Immunol. 2013;120:105−26.

[135]Sathe P, et al. Convergent differentiation: myeloid and lymphoid pathways to murine plasmacytoid dendritic cells. Blood 2013;121:11−9.

[136]Flores M, et al. FcγRIIB prevents inflammatory Type I IFN production from plasmacytoid dendritic cells during a viral memory response. J. Immunol. 2015;194:4240−50.

[137]Conrad C, et al. Plasmacytoid dendritic cells promote immunosuppression in ovarian cancer via ICOS costimulation of Foxp3þ T-regulatory cells. Cancer Res. 2012;72:5240−90.

[138]Davidson S, et al. Disease-promoting effects of type I interferons in viral, bacterial, and coinfections. J. Interferon Cytokine Res. 2015;35:252−64.

[139]Wijesundara D, et al. Unraveling the convoluted biological roles of type I interferons in infection and immunity: a way forward for therapeutics and vaccine design. Front. Immunol. 2014;5:Article 412 (7 pp.).

[140]Platanias LC, Fish EN. Signaling pathways activated by interferons. Exp. Hematol. 1999;27:1583−92.

[141]Beiting DP. Protozoan parasites and type I interferons: a cold case reopened. Trends Parasitol. 2014;30:491−8.

[142]Gao B, et al. A 59 extended IFN-stimulating response element is crucial for IFN-g-induced tripartite motif 22 expression via interaction with IFN regulatory factor-1. J. Immunol. 2010;185:2314−23.

[143]Obeid D, Bauvois B. Interferons: mechanisms, biological activities and survey of their use in human disease. Curr. Bioactive Compounds 2006;2 (14 pp.).

e. Externally Acquired Antigens Versus Internally Acquired Antigens

DCs can present internally acquired antigens, that is, antigens newly biosynthesized in the DC, and these are presented by MHC class I (144,145). DCs can present externally acquired antigens, and these are presented by MHC class II.

f. Polypeptide Antigens can Contain Both MHC Class I and MHC Class II Epitopes

During processing of a polypeptide antigen by a DC, the polypeptide is cleaved into dozens of distinct oligopeptides. For any given polypeptide, some of these oligopeptides are presented by way of MHC class I, while others are presented by way of MHC class II. Where a polypeptide contains only regions that are eventually presented by way of MHC class I, the result is formation of an immune synapse with CD8[+] T cells. Where a polypeptide contains only regions that are eventually presented by way of MHC class II, the result is formation of an immune synapse with CD4[+] T cells. Using MHC class I, DCs present antigens to CD8[+] T cells (146). Using MHC class II, DCs present antigens to CD4[+] T cells.

g. Two Different Mechanisms of CTL Response (Fas-Dependent and Perforin-Dependent)

CD8[+] T cells kill target cell either by a Fas-dependent mechanism or a perforin-dependent mechanism (147).

h. Naive Response and Memory Response

The response of T cells takes the form of either naive immune response or memory immune response (148,149). Naive immune response occurs where the T cell is, for the first time, presented with a given antigen. Memory immune response occurs where the same T cell is presented, on a second later occasion, with the same antigen.

i. Innate Immunity and Specific Immunity

Immune response takes two forms, namely, innate immunity and specific immunity.

[144]Qian SB, Reits E, Neefjes J, Deslich JM, Bennink JR, Yewdell JW. Tight linkage between translation and MHC class I peptide ligand generation implies specialized antigen processing for defective ribosomal products. J. Immunol. 2006;177:227−33.

[145]Boes M, Stoppelenburg AJ, Sillé FC. Endosomal processing for antigen presentation mediated by CD1 and Class I major histocompatibility complex: roads to display or destruction. Immunology 2009;127:163−70.

[146]Lauvau G, Glaichenhaus N. Mini-review: presentation of pathogen-derived antigens in vivo. Eur. J. Immunol. 2004;34:913−20.

[147]Harty JT, Tvinnereim AR, White DW. CD8[+] T cell effector mechanisms in resistance to infection. Annu. Rev. Immunol. 2000;18:275−308.

[148]Griffin JP, Orme IM. Evolution of CD4 T-cell subsets following infection of naive and memory immune mice with *Mycobacterium tuberculosis*. Infect. Immun. 1994;62:1683−90.

[149]Serbina NV, Flynn JL. CD8[+] T Cells participate in the memory immune response to *Mycobacterium tuberculosis*. Infect. Immun. 2001;69:4320−8.

Specific immunity is mounted against certain specific antigens, such as protein expressed by the tuberculosis bacterium (150), in the case of immune response against tuberculosis infections, against a tumor antigen, such as mesothelin (151), in the case of immune response against pancreatic cancer, or against myelin proteins, in the case of multiple sclerosis (152). In contrast, innate immunity is stimulated by certain molecules, or more accurately classes of molecules, that are shared by many bacteria or shared by many viruses. These molecules include bacterial lipopolysaccharide, bacterial peptidoglycan, and viral nucleic acids. Each of these molecules, or more accurately classes of molecules, binds to a toll-like receptor (153). TLRs are expressed by DCs, neutrophils, and other cells of the immune system.

The importance of specific immunity is self-evident to any person familiar with vaccines. However, what is less well-known to the layperson, is that an efficient specific immune response often requires simultaneous stimulation of the innate immune system. In the case of bacterial infections, where a vaccine is administered, the bacterial infection generates its own innate immune response (there is no need for the physician to administer a drug that stimulates the innate immune response). But in the case of vaccines against cancer the physician needs to administer a drug that stimulates innate immunity. These types of drugs, which may be administered with chemotherapy or a vaccine, against infections or cancer, are called *immune adjuvants*. Immune adjuvants include CpG-oligonucleotides, imiquimod, and bacillus Calmette-Guerin (BCG). BCG is used for treating bladder cancer (154).

j. Expression of a Given Receptor Protein by NK Cells and Expression of the Same Receptor by Tregs

This provides a specialized type of paired concepts. This is the situation where a receptor that occurs on one type of immune cell can trigger an immune response that is opposite that where the same receptor is expressed on a different type of immune cell. In this example, the receptor protein is CD25. CD25 is part of the IL-2 receptor. In this example, the two types of immune cells are NK cells and Tregs.

Certain signaling molecules may be expressed on the plasma membrane of NK cells, a type of immune cell that kills other cells, and also on Tregs, a type of immune cell that is immunosuppressive. CD25 is part of the IL-2 receptor, that is, it is an IL-2 receptor alpha chain. The fact that CD25 is expressed by NK cells and also by Tregs suggests that CD25-mediated signaling may have different downstream results, depending on the cell in question, because of the fact that NK cells are cytotoxic, while Tregs are immunosuppressive. The immunosuppressive activity of Tregs

[150]Caccamo N, Guggino G, Meraviglia S, et al. Analysis of Mycobacterium tuberculosis-specific CD8 T-cells in patients with active tuberculosis and in individuals with latent infection. PLoS One 2009;4:e5528.

[151]Hassan R, Ho M. Mesothelin targeted cancer immunotherapy. Eur. J. Cancer 2008;44:46−53.

[152]Forooghian F, Cheung RK, Smith WC, O'Connor P, Dosch HM. Enolase and arrestin are novel nonmyelin autoantigens in multiple sclerosis. J. Clin. Immunol. 2007;27:388−96.

[153]Parker LC, Whyte MK, Dower SK, Sabroe I. The expression and roles of Toll-like receptors in the biology of the human neutrophil. J. Leukoc. Biol. 2005;77:886−92.

[154]Alexandroff AB, Nicholson S, Patel PM, Jackson AM. Recent advances in bacillus Calmette-Guerin immunotherapy in bladder cancer. Immunotherapy 2010;2:551−60.

includes its action in attenuating CD8$^+$ T cells and preventing CD8$^+$ T cells from causing pathological inflammation. In the words of Hodi and Dranoff (155), "regulatory T cells (Tregs) inhibit tumor-specific CD8$^+$ T-cell killing and restrict the effector functions of NK cells."

The fact that the same signaling molecule is expressed by NK cells and by Tregs is dramatically illustrated by the MOA of the anti-CD25 antibody, daclizumab (156). Daclizumab is used to treat multiple sclerosis, because of its ability to stimulate NK cells, where the stimulated NK cells kill the CD8$^+$ T cells responsible for the pathology of multiple sclerosis. Specifically it is the case that daclizumab stimulates a subset of NK cells called CD56^{bright} NK cells (157).

Regarding the ability of these NK cells to kill certain CD8$^+$ T cells, Bielekova (158) explained that:

> [b]ecause daclizumab expanded numbers of CD56^{bright} NK cells in the peripheral blood to up to 500% ... daclizumab-treated MS patients provided a unique opportunity to study the immunoregulatory functions of these cells in detail ... we observed that ... when NK cells were present during T-cell activation, survival of activated T cells was severely limited. Subsequent mechanistic studies demonstrated that this phenomenon was due to NK-cell mediated cytotoxicity toward activated autologous T cells.

In contrast, daclizumab may also be used to treat cancer (159,160), by way of its ability to inhibit the activity of Tregs. The story of the anti-CD25 antibody daclizumab provides a dramatic example of how the field of immunology can be organized as pairs of concepts.

XII. CONCLUDING REMARKS

Most drugs have a relatively simple mechanism of action. For example, warfarin prevents formation of mature blood-clotting proteins. Aspirin inhibits cyclooxygenase. Furosemide inhibits an ion transporter. Cisplatin crosslinks the DNA of the chromosome. All of these mechanisms of action can be demonstrated by in vitro techniques using cultured cells or by an experiment taking the form of a reaction in a test tube.

In contrast, drugs that work on the immune system influence what is called the *immune network*. The immune network comprises about a dozen different types of immune cells, each of which occurs in various subsets, various states of maturation, and various states of activation. Also, the immune network includes at least 100 different proteins that comprise the cytokines and cytokine receptors. In contrast to the mechanisms of action of warfarin, aspirin, furosomide, and cisplatin, the mechanisms of action of drugs that modulate the immune system cannot be adequately represented by experiments with a test tube or cell culture dish.

[155]Hodi FS, Dranoff G. The biological importance of tumor-infiltrating lymphocytes. J. Cutan. Pathol. 2011;37:48−53.

[156]Bielekova B. Daclizumab therapy for multiple sclerosis. Neurotherapeutics 2013;10:55−67.

[157]Bielekova B, et al. How implementation of systems biology into clinical trials accelerates understanding of diseases. Front. Neurol. 2014;5:Article 102 (9 pp.).

[158]Bielekova, B. Daclizumab therapy for multiple sclerosis. Neurotherapeutics 2013;10:55−67.

[159]Tse BW, et al. Antibody-based immunotherapy for ovarian cancer? Ann. Oncol. 2014;25:322−31.

[160]Barbi J, et al. Treg functional stability and its responsiveness to the microenvironment. Immunol. Rev. 2014;259:115−39.

Mechanism of Action—Part II (Cancer)

I. INTRODUCTION

Drugs against cancer include small-molecule drugs, such as methotrexate and cisplatin, as well as biologicals, such as cytokines, antibodies, and vaccines.

Small-molecule anticancer drugs include drugs that cause damage to the genome, such as methotrexate, 5-fluorouracil, and cisplatin. Fluorouracil, for example, is widely used for the treatment of colorectal, pancreatic, breast, head and neck, gastric, and ovarian cancers (1). DNA damage arises in different ways, depending on the drug. Damage can be caused by incorporation of the drug as part of the polynucleotide chain, by covalent damage directly to the double-stranded helix (other than by incorporation into the chain), or by provoking imbalances in the normal pools of deoxynucleotides, resulting in abnormal incorporation of a naturally occurring deoxynucleotide, for example, dUTP, into the chromosome.

For the above drugs, it is possible to provide a generic mechanism of action (MOA). As shown in the following diagram, drugs that act on the genome often have the following mechanism. First, the drug is incorporated, resulting in DNA damage, second apoptosis is activated, and third, apoptosis kills the cancer cell. This mechanism is responsible, at least in part, for the cytotoxic effects of methotrexate (2), 5-fluorouracil (3), cladribine (4),

---

[1]Rose MG, Farrell MP, Schmitz JC. Thymidylate synthase: a critical target for cancer chemotherapy. Clin. Colorectal Cancer 2002;1:220−9.

[2]Huschtscha LI, Bartier WA, Ross CE, Tattersall MH. Characteristics of cancer cell death after exposure to cytotoxic drugs in vitro. Br. J. Cancer 1996;73:54−60.

[3]Huschtscha LI, Bartier WA, Ross CE, Tattersall MH. Characteristics of cancer cell death after exposure to cytotoxic drugs in vitro. Br. J. Cancer 1996;73:54−60.

[4]Ceruti S, Beltrami E, Matarrese P, et al. A key role for caspase-2 and caspase-3 in the apoptosis induced by 2-chloro-2′-deoxy-adenosine (cladribine) and 2-chloro-adenosine in human astrocytoma cells. Mol. Pharmacol. 2003;63:1437−47.

gemcitabine (5,6), and cisplatin (7). Cladribine, which selectively kills lymphocytes, has the unique distinction of being used to treat two very different diseases. Cladribine is used to cure leukemia (hairy cell leukemia (8)) and to treat multiple sclerosis, two diseases with a pathology involving lymphocytes.

evidence suggests that damage to tumor cells, as caused by these drugs, causes the release of tumor antigens, facilitating capture of the antigens by immune cells. The capture of tumor antigens by immune cells is the first step in the immune response against cancer.

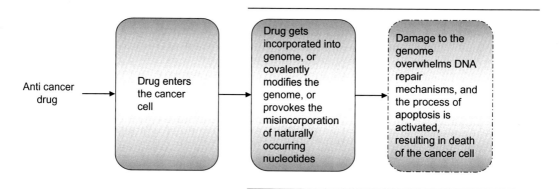

Small-molecule anticancer drugs include drugs that disrupt the cytoskeleton, such as the taxanes. The taxanes include paclitaxel and docetaxel, which are used for treating breast cancer, ovarian cancer, non-small cell lung cancer (NSCLC), and prostate cancer (9).

Drugs that directly kill tumor cells do so in a manner independent of the immune system. However, as indicated below,

But it is usually the case that, where there is tumor, the immune system fails to mount an effective response against the tumor.

Most tumors are not efficiently rejected, even when tumor antigens are recognized by $CD4^+$ T cells and $CD8^+$ T cells (10). In vitro experiments show that these T cells can recognize tumor cells and kill them, but in vivo, these T cells are prevented from gaining access to the tumors. According to Preynat-Seauve

[5]Pauwels B, Vermorken JB, Wouters A, et al. The role of apoptotic cell death in the radiosensitising effect of gemcitabine. Br. J. Cancer 2009;101:628—36.

[6]Plunkett W, Huang P, Gandhi V. Preclinical characteristics of gemcitabine. Anticancer Drugs 1995;6(Suppl. 6):7—13.

[7]Basu A, Krishnamurthy S. Cellular responses to cisplatin-induced DNA damage. J. Nucleic Acids 2010;2010. pii: 201367.

[8]Wanko SO, de Castro C. Hairy cell leukemia: an elusive but treatable disease. Oncologist 2006;11:780—9.

[9]Hennenfent KL, Govindan R. Novel formulations of taxanes: a review. Old wine in a new bottle? Ann. Oncol. 2006;17:735—49.

[10]Chaput N, Darrasse-Jèze G, Bergot AS, et al. Regulatory T cells prevent CD8 T cell maturation by inhibiting CD4 Th cells at tumor sites. J. Immunol. 2007;179:4969—78.

et al. (11), tumors grow in an immunoprivileged site, that is, they reside in an environment that cannot be scrutinized by the immune system. However, anticancer therapy can disrupt this immunoprivileged condition.

a. Mechanisms of Immune Response Against Tumors

Chemotherapy or radiation can kill cancer cells, where the mechanism of cell death is apoptosis or necrosis of the cancer cells, and where cell death results in the release of tumor antigens into interstitial fluids. Fragments of killed tumor cells, and released tumor antigens, can be taken up by dendritic cells (DCs) (12).

Although tumor cells and tumor antigens may be taken up by DCs, this does not necessarily mean that the DCs will subsequently present tumor antigens to T cells in an effective manner, that is, in a manner that will stimulate the T cells to kill tumor cells.

In the absence of an activating environment, the DC that takes up tumor antigens may cause tolerance to the tumor. In studies of tumors in animals, den Brok et al. (13) and Van Oosten and Griffith (14) inflicted physical damage on tumors. The damage was inflicted in the presence and absence of a TLR-agonist. The TLR-agonist was CpG-oligonucleotide. While tumor debris in the animal was an effective antigen depot for DCs, an effective immune response requires an immune adjuvant, such as a TLR-agonist. According to Cuenca et al. (15), where DCs capture tumor antigens but without stimulation, the DCs will travel to the lymph nodes and communicate with T cells, but instead of causing the T cells to be active against tumors, the T cells will be caused to be tolerogenic T cells. Human cancers often contain $CD8^+$ T cells, that is, tumor-infiltrating $CD8^+$ T cells, that are antigen-specific but do not lyse tumor cells (16).

Immune adjuvants useful for treating cancer can take the form of a TLR-agonist such as CpG-oligonucleotide, polyinosinic:polycytidylic acid, an adjuvant that binds to TLR3 (17,18), imiquimod, bacillus Calmette-Guerin

[11]Preynat-Seauve O, Contassot E, Schuler P, Piguet V, French LE, Huard B. Extralymphatic tumors prepare draining lymph nodes to invasion via a T-cell cross-tolerance process. Cancer Res. 2007;67:5009−16.

[12]van der Most RG, Currie A, Robinson BW, Lake RA. Cranking the immunologic engine with chemotherapy: using context to drive tumor antigen cross-presentation towards useful antitumor immunity. Cancer Res. 2006;66:601−4.

[13]den Brok MH, Sutmuller RP, Nierkens S, et al. Synergy between in situ cryoablation and TLR9 stimulation results in a highly effective in vivo dendritic cell vaccine. Cancer Res. 2006;66:7285−92.

[14]Van Oosten RL, Griffith TS. Activation of tumor-specific CD8 + T Cells after intratumoral Ad5-TRAIL/CpG oligodeoxynucleotide combination therapy. Cancer Res. 2007;67:11980−90.

[15]Cuenca A, Cheng F, Wang H, et al. Extra-lymphatic solid tumor growth is not immunologically ignored and results in early induction of antigen-specific T-cell anergy: dominant role of cross-tolerance to tumor antigens. Cancer Res. 2003;63:9007−15.

[16]Koneru M, Schaer D, Monu N, Ayala A, Frey AB. Defective proximal TCR signaling inhibits CD8 + tumor-infiltrating lymphocyte lytic function. J. Immunol. 2005;174:1830−40.

[17]Amos SM, Pegram HJ, Westwood JA, et al. Adoptive immunotherapy combined with intratumoral TLR agonist delivery eradicates established melanoma in mice. Cancer Immunol. Immunother. 2011; Feb 16 [Epub ahead of print].

[18]Okada H, Kalinski P, Ueda R, et al. Induction of CD8 + T-cell responses against novel glioma-associated antigen peptides and clinical activity by vaccinations with {alpha}-type 1 polarized dendritic cells and polyinosinic-polycytidylic acid stabilized by lysine and carboxymethylcellulose in patients with recurrent malignant glioma. J. Clin. Oncol. 2011;29:330−6.

(19), and *Listeria monocytogenes* (expressing recombinant tumor antigens) (20,21,22). In the case of bacterial adjuvants, the bacterium as a whole may be called an immune adjuvant. But the bacterium as a whole is not required for stimulating a toll-like receptor. What stimulates the toll-like receptor is the various components of the bacterium, such as flagellin, peptidoglycan, and bacterial DNA.

Immune adjuvants can take the form of a reagent that activates CD4$^+$ T cells. Knutson et al. (23) and Disis et al. (24) describe the use of reagents that activate CD4$^+$ T cells, in the treatment of breast cancer. Where CD4$^+$ T cells are stimulated, either by infecting bacteria or viruses or by an administered drug, the CD4$^+$ T cells serve as Mother Nature's immune adjuvant. The activated CD4$^+$ T cells are Mother Nature's immune adjuvant because, without them, CD8$^+$ T cells are not able to reach their

full potential for mediating an attack against infections.

Manegold et al. (25) provides an excellent diagram showing a DC that is activating a CD8$^+$ T cell, and showing the activated CCD8$^+$ T cell attacking a tumor cell.

After activation by DCs, CD8$^+$ T cells leave the lymph nodes and enter the circulatory system, where they may encounter tumors. When the CD8$^+$ T cells encounter tumors, they may find that chemotherapy or irradiation has enhanced the ability to kill the tumor cell (by mechanisms in addition to activation of the DC).

For example, chemotherapy or irradiation can enhance immune response against tumors by stimulating the living tumor cells to express Fas-receptor (26). Fas-receptor is targeted by CD8$^+$ T cells (which bear Fas-ligand), when the CD8$^+$ T cells kill tumor cells. Moreover, chemotherapy (27), radiation (28), or

[19]Alexandroff AB, Nicholson S, Patel PM, Jackson AM. Recent advances in bacillus Calmette-Guerin immunotherapy in bladder cancer. Immunotherapy 2010;2:551–60.

[20]Brockstedt DG, Bahjat KS, Giedlin MA, et al. Killed but metabolically active microbes: a new vaccine paradigm for eliciting effector T-cell responses and protective immunity. Nat. Med. 2005;11:853–60.

[21]Brockstedt DG, Giedlin MA, Leong ML, et al. *Listeria*-based cancer vaccines that segregate immunogenicity from toxicity. Proc. Natl Acad. Sci. USA 2004;101:13832–7.

[22]Leong ML, Hampl J, Liu W, et al. Impact of preexisting vector-specific immunity on vaccine potency: characterization of *Listeria monocytogenes*-specific humoral and cellular immunity in humans and modeling studies using recombinant vaccines in mice. Infect. Immun. 2009;77:3958–68.

[23]Knutson KL, Schiffman K, Disis ML. Immunization with a HER-2/neu helper peptide vaccine generates HER-2/neu CD8 T-cell immunity in cancer patients. J. Clin. Invest. 2001;107:477–84.

[24]Disis ML, Wallace DR, Gooley TA, et al. Concurrent trastuzumab and HER2/neu-specific vaccination in patients with metastatic breast cancer. J. Clin. Oncol. 2009;27:4685–92.

[25]Manegold C, Gravenor D, Woytowitz D, et al. Randomized phase II trial of a toll-like receptor 9 agonist oligodeoxynucleotide, PF-3512676, in combination with first-line taxane plus platinum chemotherapy for advanced-stage non-small-cell lung cancer. J. Clin. Oncol. 2008;26:3979–86.

[26]Chakraborty M, Abrams SI, Camphausen K. Irradiation of tumor cells up-regulates Fas and enhances CTL lytic activity and CTL adoptive immunotherapy. J. Immunol. 2003;170:6338–47.

[27]Alagkiozidis I, Facciabene A, Carpenito C, et al. Increased immunogenicity of surviving tumor cells enables cooperation between liposomal doxorubicin and IL-18. J. Transl. Med. 2009;7:104.

[28]Ciernik IF, Romero P, Berzofsky JA, Carbone DP. Ionizing radiation enhances immunogenicity of cells expressing a tumor-specific T-cell epitope. Int. J. Radiat. Oncol. Biol. Phys. 1999;45:735–41.

interferon-gamma (29), can enhance the tumor cell's behavior in expressing certain tumor antigens, that is, expression by major histocompatibility complex (MHC) class I by the tumor cell. Interferon-gamma, which is a Th1-type cytokine, is produced by immune cells, or it can be administered as a drug, for the treatment of cancer or infections.

The following concerns CD4$^+$ T cells, also known as helper T cells. CD4$^+$ T cells contribute to immune response against tumors in a number of ways. According to Chaput et al. (30), several mechanisms are possible. CD4$^+$ T cells contribute directly to CD8$^+$ T-cell function by increasing their survival, by improving division and effector function, and by modifying the trafficking of CD8$^+$ T cells into tumor sites.

Colorectal cancers are commonly infiltrated by immune cells. The most frequent among these are T cells and B cells, though natural killer cells (NK cells), DCs, macrophages, and neutrophils also infiltrate tumors. According to Morris et al (31), increased number of tumor-infiltrating lymphocytes are correlated with increased survival of the patient.

b. NK Cells and ADCC

NK cells can kill cancer cells by way of antibody-dependent cell cytotoxicity (ADCC). Although NK cells are classified as part of the innate immune response pathway it is the case that ADCC depends on the presence of antibodies, either antibodies that are naturally acquired by way of adaptive immune response,

or administered antibodies. When the antibody is present, it serves as a bridge between the NK cell and the tumor. Manegold et al. (32) provide a diagram showing the expression of antibodies by a B cell, the binding of these antibodies to a tumor cell resulting in a "decorated tumor cell," and the subsequent attack by NK cells against the antibody-decorated tumor cell.

As disclosed in Chapter 1, antibodies contain four polypeptide chains, two heavy chains and two light chains (see in-text diagram). The four chains are covalently attached to each other by way of disulfide bonds (bonds not shown). When fully assembled, the antibody contains a constant region and a variable region. The constant region contains regions that can bind tightly to Fc receptors, for example, Fc receptors on the surface of NK cells. The variable region, which recognizes a specific antigen, binds tightly to the antigen. In drawings of antibodies, the antibody takes the form of tweezers, where the Fc receptor-binding region is the handle of the tweezers, and the variable region is the tweezer prongs.

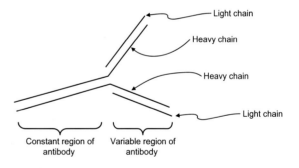

[29]Weidanz JA, Nguyen T, Woodburn T, et al. Levels of specific peptide-HLA class I complex predicts tumor cell susceptibility to CTL killing. J Immunol. 2006;177:5088−97.

[30]Chaput N, Darrasse-Jèze G, Bergot AS, et al. Regulatory T cells prevent CD8 T cell maturation by inhibiting CD4 Th cells at tumor sites. J. Immunol. 2007;179:4969−78.

[31]Morris M, Platell C, Iacopetta B. Tumor-infiltrating lymphocytes and perforation in colon cancer predict positive response to 5-fluorouracil chemotherapy. Clin. Cancer Res. 2008;14:1413−7.

[32]Manegold C, Gravenor D, Woytowitz D, et al. Randomized phase II trial of a toll-like receptor 9 agonist oligodeoxynucleotide, PF-3512676, in combination with first-line taxane plus platinum chemotherapy for advanced-stage non-small-cell lung cancer. J. Clin. Oncol. 2008;26:3979−86.

When antibodies mediate tumor killing by NK cells, the antibody bridges the Fc receptor of the NK cell and the target antigen of the tumor cell. The antigen residing on the surface of the tumor cell can be a typical membrane-bound protein, or it can take the form of a peptide that is being presented by MHC class I of the tumor cell (33). Either way, the combination of the NK cell and antibody can induce the NK cell to kill the tumor cell. The formation of the bridge is shown in Figure 27.1.

The mechanism of killing is as follows. When the NK cell contacts the tumor cell, vesicles (granules) inside the NK cell discharge their contents (degranulation) next to the tumor cell, where the discharged contents cause the tumor cell to be lysed and killed. The contents of the granules include perforin and granzyme (34). NK cells are not antigen-specific, in contrast to the situation of CD8$^+$ T cells. CD8$^+$ T cells also kill their target cells by releasing perforin and granzyme. "Opsonization" is a term from classical immunology. The function of the antibody is to opsonize the tumor cell (35).

Some pharmaceutical antibodies kill cancer cells by way of ADCC. Trastuzumab (Herceptin®), which binds to HER2 that is

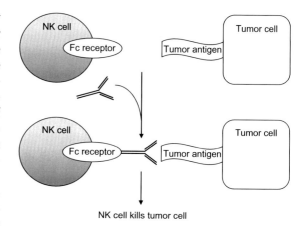

FIGURE 27.1 Antibody-dependent cell cytotoxicity. NK cells mediate ADCC. ADCC involves a sandwich of an NK cell and a target cell, where an antibody resides inside the sandwich. In order for the NK cell to kill the target cell, what is also required is the expression of specific pairs of activating/inhibiting ligands and receptors, which reside on both the NK cell and the target cell. These pairs are not shown in the diagram.

expressed on the surface of the cancer cell, mediates killing of breast cancer cells by way of ADCC (36,37,38). HER2 is human epidermal growth factor receptor-2. Cetuximab (Erbitux®), which binds to HER1 on the surface of the cancer cell, mediates ADCC (39). Cetuximab is

[33]Wittman VP, Woodburn D, Nguyen T, et al. Antibody targeting to a class I MHC-peptide epitope promotes tumor cell death. J. Immunol. 2006;177:4187−95.

[34]Moretta A, Bottino C, Vitale M, et al. Activating receptors and coreceptors involved in human natural killer cell-mediated cytolysis. Annu. Rev. Immunol. 2001;19:197−223.

[35]Zamai L, Ponti C, Mirandola P, et al. NK cells and cancer. J. Immunol. 2007;178:4011−6.

[36]Petricevic B, et al. Trastuzumab mediates antibody-dependent cell-mediated cytotoxicity and phagocytosis to the same extent in both adjuvant and metastatic HER2/neu breast cancer patients. J. Transl. Med. 2013;11:307 (11 pp.).

[37]Varchetta S, Gibelli N, Oliviero B, et al. Elements related to heterogeneity of antibody-dependent cell cytotoxicity in patients under trastuzumab therapy for primary operable breast cancer overexpressing Her2. Cancer Res. 2007;67:11991−9.

[38]Arnould L, Gelly M, Penault-Llorca F, et al. Trastuzumab-based treatment of HER2-positive breast cancer: an antibody-dependent cellular cytotoxicity mechanism? Br. J. Cancer 2006;94:259−67.

[39]Vincenzi B, Zoccoli A, Pantano F, Venditti O, Galluzzo S. Cetuximab: from bench to bedside. Curr. Cancer Drug Targets 2010;10:80−95.

used to treat colorectal cancer. HER1 is human epidermal growth factor-1 (40). The MOA of ADCC is made more interesting by the fact that activating CD137 of the NK cell can increase the NK cell's ability to kill its target. CD137, also known as 4-1BB, is a membrane-bound protein of the NK cell. Triggering CD137 by artificial means using an anti-CD137 antibody (41), or by natural means by way of the CD137 ligand that is expressed by one type of T cell (gammadelta T cells) (42), enhances the ability of the T cell to kill its target.

c. Regulatory T Cells

Anticancer drugs also include drugs that block normally occurring mechanisms that set upper limits to immune response. Upper limits to immune response are imposed by a class of T cells called T-regulatory cells (Tregs). If Tregs did not exist, it is likely that every human being would suffer from various auto-immune disorders, and would die from mas-sive inflammation (43). In fact, a component of the MOA of some autoimmune diseases is naturally occurring mutations that impair function of the Tregs (44). Consistent with this mechanism in autoimmune diseases is the fact that an antibody that inhibits Treg activity (anti-CD25 antibody; daclizumab), may be effective in treating cancer (45,46). In short, the fact that Treg activity can protect tumors from being attacked by $CD8^+$ T cells, serves as the rationale for impairing Treg activity, in the treatment of cancer.

Various types of Treg exist, but the most physiologically relevant type of Treg is $CD4^+CD25^+$ T cells. These Tregs are distin-guished by their expression of the transcrip-tion factor, Foxp3 (47). The gene and the protein are called Foxp3, while the encoded protein is sometimes called "scurfin." Foxp3 means, "forkhead box protein-3." The $CD4^+CD25^+$ Tregs account for about 10% of all the $CD4^+$ T cells in the body.

Tregs guard against autoimmunity, but in the context of a cancer patient, what is desir-able is to inhibit Tregs (48). Cancer patients may have increased levels of Tregs and, in par-ticular, an increase in Tregs infiltrating their

[40]Assenat E, Azria D, Mollevi C, et al. Dual targeting of HER1/EGFR and HER2 with cetuximab and trastuzumab in patients with metastatic pancreatic cancer after gemcitabine failure: results of the "THERAPY" phase 1-2 trial. Oncotarget 2015;6:12796−808.

[41]Kohrt HE, Colevas AD, Houot R, et al. Targeting CD137 enhances efficacy of cetuximab. J. Clin. Invest. 2014;124:2668−82.

[42]Maniar A, et al. Human gammadelta T lymphocytes induce robust NK cell-mediated antitumor cytotoxicity through CD137 engagement. Blood 2010;116:1726−33.

[43]Kim JM, et al. Regulatory T cells prevent catastrophic autoimmunity throughout the lifespan of mice. Nat. Immunol. 2006;8:191−7.

[44]Barbi J, et al. Treg functional stability and its responsiveness to the microenvironment. Immunol. Rev. 2014;259:115−39.

[45]Tse BW, et al. Antibody-based immunotherapy for ovarian cancer? Ann. Oncol. 2014;25:322−31.

[46]Barbi J, et al. Treg functional stability and its responsiveness to the microenvironment. Immunol. Rev. 2014;259:115−39.

[47]Barbi J, et al. Treg functional stability and its responsiveness to the microenvironment. Immunol. Rev. 2014;259:115−39.

[48]Siddiqui SA, Frigola X, Bonne-Annee S, et al. Tumor-infiltrating Foxp3-CD4 + CD25 + T cells predict poor survival in renal cell carcinoma. Clin. Cancer Res. 2007;13:2075−81.

tumors (49,50). In fact, the presence of Tregs in a tumor (tumor-infiltrating Tregs) serves as a prognostic factor for the survival of the patient (51). Where the tumor mass is infiltrated with a great number of Tregs, this means that the patient has a poorer chance of survival.

Cyclophosphamide is a common oncology drug that inhibits Tregs (52). By inhibiting Tregs, this drug releases normal physiological braking mechanisms that set upper limits on the immune system, thereby enabling a more vigorous immune response against tumors. Fluorouracil may also inhibit Tregs (53). Moreover, an anti-GITR antibody targets Tregs and blocks the immunosuppressive activity of Tregs (54,55). GITR, which may be pronounced as *guitar*, stands for glucocorticoid-induced tumor necrosis factor receptor. Anti-GITR antibodies, such as MK-4166 and TRX518, are being tested for treating cancer (56). "MK" and "TRX" stand for the pharmaceutical companies that sponsor the antibodies, Merck, Inc. and Tolerx, Inc.

GITR, a membrane-bound protein on Tregs, transmits a signal to the Treg that blocks the

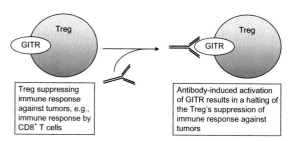

FIGURE 27.2 T-regulatory cell. Tregs have the useful effect of preventing indiscriminate inflammatory diseases in healthy people. However, Tregs can have the undesirable effect of preventing effective immune response in cancer, and in chronic infections such as hepatitis C virus infections. Drugs such as anti-GITR antibody may block the immune-suppressing effects of Tregs.

immunosuppressive activity of the Treg. Therefore, when anti-GITR antibody is used as an anticancer drug, the antibody must be one that provokes GITR-mediated cell signaling. In other words, the antibody must be an activating antibody, and not an inhibitory antibody (Fig. 27.2).

[49]Heier I, Hofgaard PO, Brandtzaeg P, Jahnsen FL, Karlsson M. Depletion of CD4 + CD25 + regulatory T cells inhibits local tumour growth in a mouse model of B cell lymphoma. Clin. Exp. Immunol. 2008;152:381−7.

[50]Kobayashi N, Hiraoka N, Yamagami W, et al. FOXP3 + regulatory T cells affect the development and progression of hepatocarcinogenesis. Clin. Cancer Res. 2007;13:902−11.

[51]Yakirevich E, Resnick MB. Regulatory T lymphocytes: pivotal components of the host antitumor response. J. Clin. Oncol. 2007;25:2506−8.

[52]Leao IC, Ganesan P, Armstrong TD, Jaffee EM. Effective depletion of regulatory T cells allows the recruitment of mesothelin-specific CD8 T cells to the antitumor immune response against a mesothelin-expressing mouse pancreatic adenocarcinoma. Clin. Transl. Sci. 2008;1:228−39.

[53]Vincent J, Mignot G, Chalmin F, et al. 5-Fluorouracil selectively kills tumor-associated myeloid-derived suppressor cells resulting in enhanced T cell-dependent antitumor immunity. Cancer Res. 2010;70:3052−61.

[54]Placke T, Kopp HG, Salih HR. Glucocorticoid-induced TNFR-related (GITR) protein and its ligand in antitumor immunity: functional role and therapeutic modulation. Clin. Dev. Immunol. 2010;2010:239083.

[55]Cohen AD, Schaer DA, Liu C, Li Y, et al. Agonist anti-GITR monoclonal antibody induces melanoma tumor immunity in mice by altering regulatory T cell stability and intra-tumor accumulation. PLoS One 2010;5:e10436.

[56]Berman D, et al. The development of immunomodulatory monoclonal antibodies as a new therapeutic modality for cancer: the Bristol-Myers Squibb experience. Pharmacol. Therap. 2015;148:132−53.

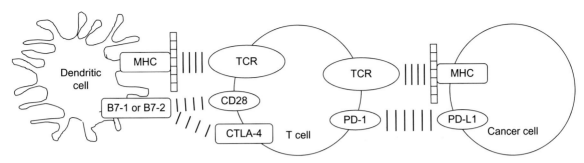

FIGURE 27.3 Signaling via PD-1, PD-L1, and CTLA-4 during communication between a DC, T cell, and cancer cell. The goal of the DC is to stimulate the T cell to mount immune response against the cancer cell. The goal of the cancer cell is to inhibit the T cell.

d. Immune Response Against Cancer Summarized by a Picture of Three Different Cells

Figure 27.3 summarizes the immune response against cancer. The figure shows a DC, a T cell, and a cancer cell. DCs and T cells collaborate and orchestrate the immune response against cancer cells. The T cell recognizes the cancer cell, by way of tumor antigens that are expressed by MHC of the cancer cell. On the other hand, the cancer cell engages in immune evasion, and dampens this immune response, by expressing PD-L1, which directly dampens the activity of T cells. Figure 27.3 illustrates CTLA-4, PD-1, and PD-L1, which are membrane-bound proteins, and which are each a target of a recombinant antibody that has proven success in treating cancer.

In the figure, the rows of vertical lines indicate noncovalent binding interactions between ligands and receptors. A row of vertical lines is conventionally used to represent hydrogen bonds (57). The long segmented rectangles represent oligopeptides that are held and positioned on the outside surface of DCs.

The term, "immune synapse," refers to the point of contact between the T cell and DC, and to the signals that are transmitted when peptides are bound to MHC are presented to the T cell. Membrane-bound proteins of the DC, such as B7-1 and B7-2, are involved in the immune synapse. At a later point in the timeframe of the immune synapse's existence, B7-1 or B7-2 transmits an inhibiting signal to CTLA-4 of the T cell, which limits and dampens the activation of the T cell, thereby preventing pathological consequences, such as autoimmune disease.

After the DC and T cell have parted ways, the T cell infiltrates tumors, where it attempts to kill cancer cells. The T cell recognizes tumor cells by way of tumor antigens that are presented by the cancer cell on the tumor cell's own MHC. However, the cancer cell fights back, and transmits inhibiting signals to the T cell, by way of the cancer cell's PD-L1.

Figure 27.3 discloses targets of antibodies that are used to treat various cancers. Anti-CTLA-4 antibodies reverse the inhibition that results from immune tolerance, and antibodies that target PD-1 or PD-L1 prevent cancer cells from engaging in their tactic of immune evasion.

[57]Nelson DL, Cox MM. Lehninger principles of biochemistry. 5th ed. New York: W.H. Freeman and Co.; 2008. pp. 44–6, 49–50.

According to Hamid et al. (58), "[a]ntibodies that block the inhibitory receptor cytotoxic T-lymphocyte-associated antigen 4 (CTLA-4), such as ipilimumab, have been shown to release one of these negative immune regulatory pathways, leading to durable responses" in cancer patients. CTLA-4 is the target of *ipilimumab*. PD-1 is targeted by the anti-PD-1 antibody *nivolumab*, and also by the anti-PD-1 antibodies, *lambrolizumab* (59) and pembrolizumab. Pembrolizumab is distinguished in that, in December 2015, it was announced that pembrolizumab treatment successfully eliminated President Jimmy Carter's melanoma. The anti-PD-L1 antibody, **BMS-936559**, is being tested for efficacy against NSCLC (60). The term "BMS" refers to the sponsor of the drug, Bristol-Meyers Squibb.

In one clinical trial, both ipilimumab and nivolumab were co-administered to melanoma patients (61). The design of this particular clinical trial serves as a good teaching device, because it ties together the signaling pathways mediated by B7/CTLA-4 and PD-1/PD-L1.

e. Nomenclature and Definitions

- PD-1 is programmed death-1. PD-1 is a receptor. PD-1 is not expressed in resting naive T cells or in resting memory T cells, and it is expressed after engagement of T-cell receptor (TCR) (62).
- PD-L1 is the ligand for PD-1. PD-L1, which is expressed by solid tumor cells and by some hematological cancer cells, is used by these cells to avoid being killed by $CD8^+$ T cells (63).
- CTLA-4 is cytotoxic T-lymphocyte-associated antigen-4. CTLA-4 is not expressed in resting naive T cells or in resting memory T cells, and it is expressed after engagement of TCR (64).
- B7-1 and B7-2 are ligands for the receptor, CD28.
- B7-1 and B7-2 are also ligands for the receptor, CTLA-4.
- B7-1 is also called CD80.
- B7-2 is also called CD86.
- CD means cluster of differentiation.
- TCR means T-cell receptor.
- "Priming" refers to the act where a DC presents an antigen to a T cell.
- Generally, it is the case that when a ligand binds to a receptor, the ligand transmits a signal to the receptor. However, signal transmission can occur in both directions (65).

[58]Hamid O, Robert C, Daud A, et al. Safety and tumor responses with lambrolizumab (anti-PD-L1) in melanoma. New Engl. J. Med. 2013;369:134−44.

[59]Hamid O, Robert C, Daud A, et al. Safety and tumor responses with lambrolizumab (anti-PD-L1) in melanoma. New Engl. J. Med. 2013;369:134−44.

[60]Hall RD, et al. Beyond the standard of care: a review of novel immunotherapy trials for the treatment of lung cancer. Cancer Control. 2013;20:22−31.

[61]Wolchok JD, Kluger H, Callahan MK, et al. Nivolumab plus ipilimumab in advanced melanoma. New Engl. J. Med. 2913;369:122−33.

[62]Topalian SL, et al. Immune checkpoint blockade: a common denominator approach to cancer therapy. Cancer Cell 2015;27:451−61.

[63]Topalian SL, et al. Immune checkpoint blockade: a common denominator approach to cancer therapy. Cancer Cell 2015;27:451−61.

[64]Topalian SL, et al. Immune checkpoint blockade: a common denominator approach to cancer therapy. Cancer Cell 2015;27:451−61.

[65]Kaufmann DE, Walker BD. PD-1 and CTLA-4 inhibitory cosignaling pathways in HIV infection and the potential for therapeutic intervention. J. Immunol. 2009;182:5891−7.

- An antibody that binds to a ligand or to a receptor can be blocking. Alternatively, the antibody can be activating and can result in transmission of a signal into the cell. Whether an antibody is blocking or inhibiting may depend on the exact conformation and contact points between the antibody binds to the ligand (or binds to the receptor).
- *Nivolumab* is an anti-PD-1 antibody. Nivolumab has been tested for treating various cancers (66,67). Novilumab was FDA-approved in March 2015 for the indication of NSCLC, and in Dec. 2015 for melanoma.
- *Pembrolizumab* is an anti-PD-1 antibody that was FDA-approved in September 2014, for melanoma.
- *Ipilimumab* is an anti-CTLA-4 antibody that was FDA-approved in March 2011 for melanoma.
- *BMS-9365559* is an anti-PD-L1 antibody that has been used in clinical trials on subjects with NSCLC, melanoma, colorectal cancer, renal-cell cancer, ovarian cancer, pancreatic cancer, gastric cancer, and breast cancer (68).

f. Priming

CTLA-4 is not expressed on the surface of T cells that are resting. CTLA-4 appears on the surface of T cells only with T-cell activation (69). DCs activate T cells by way of two signals:

- *First signal*. The first signal is delivered by the DC's MHC/antigen complex to TCR. TCR resides on the surface of the T cell.
- *Second signal*. The second signal is delivered by the DC's B7-1 and B7-2 to the T cell's CD28.

Dendritic cells present antigens to T cells in a step called priming. However, priming without more is not enough to result in an effective immune response. What is also needed is a co-stimulatory signal, originating from B7-1 or B7-2, where these signals are transmitted to CD28 of the T cell. In other words, what is needed is priming and also a co-stimulatory signal.

g. B7/CD28 Signaling and B7/CTLA-4 Signaling

B7 proteins have a much higher affinity for CTLA-4 than for CD28, and thus materialization of CTLA-4 on the surface of the T cells persuades B7 to leave CD28 and instead to bind to CTLA-4. This dissipates the B7/CD28 signaling (70).

The time element in T-cell activation is revealed by a scenario that involves CD28, B7-1, and B7-2. When a DC contacts a T cell, initially it is the case that the DC's B7-1 and B7-2 engage CD28 on naive T cells. Subsequently, CTLA-4 is expressed on the activated T cell, with the consequence that B7-1 and B7-2 are distracted from their binding to CD28, and instead bind to CTLA-4, thus dampening and attenuating the activity of the activated T cell (71).

[66]Brahmer J, Drake CG, Wollner I, et al. Phase I study of single-agent anti-programmed death-1 (MDX-11065) in refractory solid tumors. J. Clin. Oncol. 2010;28:3167−75.

[67]Ansell SM, Lesokhin AM, Borrello I, et al. PD-1 blockade with nivolumab in relapsed or refractory Hodgkin's lymphoma. New Engl. J. Med. 2015;372:311-91.

[68]Brahmer JR, Tykodi SS, Chow LQ, et al. Safety and activity of anti-PD-L1 antibody in patients with advanced cancer. New Engl. J. Med. 2012;366:2455−65.

[69]Auchincloss H, Turka LA. CTLA-4: not all costimulation is stimulatory. J. Immunol. 2011;187:3457−8.

[70]Salama AK, Hodi FS. Cytotoxic T-lymphocyte-associated antigen-4. Clin. Cancer Res. 2011;17:4622−8.

[71]Leung J, Shu WK. The CD28-B7 family in anti-tumor immunity: emerging concepts in cancer immunotherapy. Immune Netw. 2014;14:265−76.

CD28 is constitutively expressed by T cells, where it serves as a receptor for ligands that are expressed by DCs, namely, B7-1 and B7-2 (72,73). B7-1 and B7-2 on DCs each can bind to the CD28 of the T cell. The B7-1 and B7-2 on DCs transmit signals to the T cells, that is, to naive T cells, resulting in the activation of the naive T cells. Once activated, the T cells transiently express CTLA-4. This CTLA-4 functions by dampening any immune response of the T cells.

CTLA-4's behavior in inhibiting immune response is by a process where "CTLA-4 rips B7 molecules from the surface of [dendritic cells] ... thereby preventing interactions of B7 with CD28" (74). The researchers who discovered this named the process "trans-endocytosis" (75).

This summarizes one part of the sequence of events involving CTLA-4. After a DC activates a T cell, by way of the T cell's TCR, what happens is that CTLA-4 becomes detectable on the T cell's surface. CTLA-4 is not detectable on the surface of naive T cells. Activation of CTLA-4 in this way occurs on both $CD4^+$ T cells and $CD8^+$ T cells (76). The fact that antibodies that target CTLA-4 or PD-1

can successfully treat cancer, and the fact that features of the mechanisms of CTLA-4 signaling and PD-1 signaling overlap with each other, is summarized by Topalian et al. (77), who state that, "[t]he rapid-fire clinical successes from blocking CTLA-4 and PD-1 ... have opened prospects for extending the potential of cancer immunotherapy ... [i]t is clear that, despite some commonalities, CTLA-4 and PD-1 have distinct patterns of expression, signaling pathways, and mechanisms of action."

h. PD-1/PD-L1 Signaling

PD-1 is expressed by T cells, B cells, monocytes, and NK cells (78). PD-1 is also expressed by macrophages (79).

PD-L1 is expressed by hematopoietic cells and paranchymal cells, and PD-L2 is expressed only on DCs and macrophages (80). Interactions between PD-L1 (ligand) and PD-1 (receptor) frequently occur within tumors, where the interactions are between cancer cells and associated infiltrating lymphocytes. PD-L1 is not expressed by most normal tissues, though it is expressed by

[72]Kaufmann DE, Walker BD. PD-1 and CTLA-4 inhibitory cosignaling pathways in HIV infection and the potential for therapeutic intervention. J. Immunol. 2009;182:5891−7.

[73]Pardoll DM. The blockade of immune checkpoints in cancer immunotherapy. Nat. Revs. Cancer 2012;12:252−64.

[74]Chen L, Flies DB. Molecular mechanisms of T cell co-stimulation and co-inhibition. Nat. Rev. Immunol. 2013;13:227−42.

[75]Qureshi OS, Zheng Y, Nakamura K, et al. Trans-endocytosis of CD80 and CD86: a molecular basis for the cell-extrinsic function of CTLA-4. Science 2011;332:600−3.

[76]Grosso JF, Jure-Kunkel MN. CTLA-4 blockade in tumor models: an overview of preclinical and translational research. Cancer Immunity 2013;13 (14 pp.).

[77]Topalian SL, et al. Immune checkpoint blockade: a common denominator approach to cancer therapy. Cancer Cell 2015;27:451−61.

[78]McDermott DG, Atkins MB. PD-1 is a potential target in cancer therapy. Cancer Med. 2013;2:662−73.

[79]Huang X, Venet F, Wang YL, et al. PD-1 expression by macrophages plays a pathologic role in altering microbial clearance and the innate inflammatory response to sepsis. Proc. Natl Acad. Sci. USA 2009;106:6303−8.

[80]Leung J, Shu WK. The CD28-B7 family in anti-tumor immunity: emerging concepts in cancer immunotherapy. Immune Netw. 2014;14:265−76.

many tumors. In detail, PD-L1 is not expressed in normal epithelial tissues, but it is expressed by cancer cells, including in breast cancer, renal-cell cancer, pancreatic cancer, ovarian cancer, gastric cancer, and hepatocellular cancer (81).

Mechanisms by which cancer cells evade the immune system, where the cancer cells take advantage of PD-1−PD-L1 interactions, are provided by Brahmer et al. (82). In a study of one type of *breast cancer*, researchers found that the breast cancer cells increased their expression of PL-L1, where the result was decreased proliferation of the T cells and increased death of the T cells (83). Histological studies of *melanoma* tumors revealed that PD-L1 can be either nondetectable on the melanoma cells, or expressed diffusely on the surface of melanoma cells, or alternatively, highly localized in "discrete geographic foci" with "highly co-localized" T cells that have infiltrated the melanoma tumor (84). PD-L1 is expressed in 40−50% of melanomas and has limited expression otherwise in most visceral organs with the exception of respiratory epithelium and placental tissue (85).

II. IMMUNE EVASION

Immune evasion by cancer cells involves a number of mechanisms, including T-cell exhaustion, immunosuppressive cytokines that "cool down" the immune system, such as the cytokine interleukin-10 (IL-10). Accounts of IL-10 in immune evasion have been reviewed (86,87). Immune evasion also can involve Tregs (88). The term, "tumor microenvironment" is used in studies of tumors, of the immune cells that infiltrate tumors, and of the immunosuppressive cytokines that are released by the cancer cells.

PD-L1/PD-1-mediated T cell exhaustion is shown in Figure 27.3. Both CD8$^+$ T cells and CD4$^+$ T cells are susceptible to immune exhaustion (89). When CTLA-4 is activated, CTLA-4 can enhance the immunosuppressive functions of Tregs (90).

[81]Mittendorf EA, Philips AV, Meric-Bernstam F, et al. PD-L1 expression in triple-negative breast cancer. Cancer Immunol. Res. 2014;2:361−70.

[82]Brahmer JR, et al. Nivolumab: targeting PD-1 to bolster antitumor immunity. Fut. Oncol. 2015;23 [Epub ahead of print].

[83]Mittendorf EA, Philips AV, Meric-Bernstam F, et al. PD-L1 expression in triple-negative breast cancer. Cancer Immunol. Res. 2014;2:361−70.

[84]Taube JM, Anders RA, Young GD, et al. Colocalization of inflammatory responses with B7-H1. Expression in human melanocyte lesions supports an adaptive resistance mechanism of immune escape. Sci. Trans. Med. 2012;4:127ra37 (22 pp.).

[85]Johnson DB, et al. Nivolumab in melanoma: latest evidence and clinical potential. Therapeutic Adv. Med. Oncol. 2015;7:97−106.

[86]Urosevic M, Dummer R. HLA-G and IL-10 expression in human cancer—different stories with the same message. Semin. Cancer Biol. 2003;13:337−42.

[87]Domagala-Kulawik J, et al. Mechanisms of immune response regulation in lung cancer. Transl. Lung Cancer Res. 2014;3:15−22.

[88]Teague RM, Kline J. Immune evasion in acute myeloid leukemia: current concepts and future directions. J. Immunother. Cancer 2013;1:13 (11 pp.).

[89]Yi JS, et al. T-cell exhaustion: characteristics, causes and conversion. Immunology 2010;129:474−81.

[90]Pardoll DM. The blockade of immune checkpoints in cancer immunotherapy. Nat. Revs. Cancer 2012;12:252−64.

T-cell exhaustion is described. With momentary exposure of a foreign antigens to T cells, as occurs in the immune synapse between a DC and a T cell, CTLA-4 signaling occurs, but it is transient. In contrast, when an antigen is chronically exposed to T cells, as is the case when DC's present tumor antigens to T cells (or when DC's present viral antigens to T cells, during chronic viral infections), the result can be sustained signaling of CTLA-4 in the T cells, and sustained inhibition of T-cell activity (91,92,93). The sustained inhibition of T-cell activity in cancer and in chronic infections is often called T-cell exhaustion (94,95).

Chronic antigen exposure, as is common in certain viral infections, provokes sustained expression of CTLA-4 and PD-1 in T cells, thus dampening the ability of these T cells to kill cancer cells (or to kill virus-infected host cells). The result of this dampening is immune evasion, which can result in prolonged morbidity and eventually death in patients with cancer or viral infections such as hepatitis C virus (96).

Immune tolerance is a mechanism by which all normal tissues in the body avoid attack by the immune system, thus avoiding massive autoimmune diseases and death. Immune tolerance, as it applies during health and during chronic diseases, has been reviewed (97).

Cancer cells can avoid attack from the immune system by way of immune tolerance. Immune tolerance is not the same thing as immune evasion (98). Immune tolerance refers to mechanisms that normally protect healthy tissues from autoimmune damage. Because tumor antigens are often identical in structure to normal antigens, except that the tumor antigens are overexpressed, or because tumor antigens have a minimal change in structure, such as a mutation in one amino acid, researchers are faced with the problem of overcoming immune tolerance to tumor antigens.

Immune tolerance occurring in *melanoma* is described. Trager et al. (99) provide an account of melanoma antigens and immune tolerance to melanoma antigens. Melanoma antigens are normally expressed during the differentiation of melanocytes. However, in transformed melanocytes (melanoma cells), these antigens are often overexpressed. The main melanoma antigens are tyrosinase, an enzyme that catalyzes the production of melanin from tyrosine by

[91]Leung J, Shu WK. The CD28-B7 family in anti-tumor immunity: emerging concepts in cancer immunotherapy. Immune Netw. 2014;14:265–76.

[92]Ha SJ, et al. Manipulating both the inhibitory and stimulatory immune system towards the success of therapeutic vaccination against chronic viral infections. Immunol. Revs. 2008;233:317–33.

[93]Kaufmann DE, Walker BD. PD-1 and CTLA-4 inhibitory cosignaling pathways in HIV infection and the potential for therapeutic intervention. J. Immunol. 2009;182:5891–7.

[94]Pentcheva-Hoang T, et al. Cytotoxic T lymphocyte antigen-4 blockade enhances antitumor immunity by stimulating melanoma-specific T-cell motility. Cancer Immunol. Res. 2014;2:970–80.

[95]Ye B, et al. T-cell exhaustion in chronic hepatitis B infection: current knowledge and clinical significance. Cell Death Dis. 2015;6:e1694.

[96]Grosso JF, Jure-Kunkel MN. CTLA-4 blockade in tumor models: an overview of preclinical and translational research. Cancer Immun. 2013;13 (14 pp.).

[97]Xing Y, Hogquist K. T-cell tolerance: central and peripheral. Cold Spring Harb. Perspect. Biol. 2012;4:9006957.

[98]Teague RM, Kline J. Immune evasion in acute myeloid leukemia: current concepts and future directions. J. Immunother. Cancer 2013;1:13 (11 pp.).

[99]Trager U, et al. The immune response to melanoma is limited by thymic selection to self-antigens. PLoS One 2012;7(4):e35005.

oxidation, the tyrosinase-related proteins TRP-1 and TRP-2, as well as MelanA/MART. Trager et al. disclose the issue of immune tolerance, in their writing that, "[h]owever, as [melanoma antigens] . . . are self-antigens, it is known that the immune system establishes immunological tolerance to them either in the thymus or in the periphery." To summarize, immune tolerance is a problem to be overcome in immunotherapy against various cancers.

III. CONCLUDING REMARKS

The mechanism of action of the study drug is included in the Sponsor's submissions to the FDA and is included in the package insert of the marketed drug. As a word of caution, there does not exist any "generic immune mechanism" that is applicable to all drugs that influence the immune system. For any given drug, and for any given disease that is treated with that drug, the mechanism of action of the drug will be different. For any given anticancer drug, that drug will influence the immune system with a different mechanism, depending on the type of cancer. In initiating the task of drafting the mechanism of action of a given drug, the medical writer should separately consider the influence of the drug on the following cells:

1. the cancer cells,
2. $CD8^+$ T cells,
3. $CD4^+$ T cells,
4. myeloid DCs,
5. plasmacytoid DCs,
6. macrophages,
7. NK cells, and
8. Tregs.

Mechanism of Action—Part III (Immune Disorders)

I. INTRODUCTION

Immune disorders include conditions where a self-antigen is the target of a pathological immune response, where a self-antigen is the target of immune response but where the response is not a major part of the pathology, and disorders such as allergies where self-antigens are not involved. Autoimmune diseases are diseases where a self-antigen is involved in a pathological response. Autoimmune diseases tend to inflict women more than men (1). Inflammatory disorders, as distinguished from autoimmune diseases, include allergies, asthma, and chronic obstructive pulmonary disease (COPD), and these may be initiated by external stimulants, such as pollen or cigarette smoke.

This outlines the mechanisms of action (MOAs) of a number of immune diseases followed by a more detailed account of multiple sclerosis. The example of multiple sclerosis provides a leaping-off point for understanding the MOAs for other immune diseases, and for understanding the MOAs of the relevant drugs.

For immune cells that are T cells or dendritic cells (DC), the following questions can be asked for all types of immune diseases:

- What is the activation state of the T cell?
- What is the antigen-specificity of the T cell?
- For T cells, are the relevant T cells mainly $CD4^+$ T cells, $CD8^+$ T cells, or $CD4^+$ T regulatory cells?
- If the T cell is a memory T cell, is it a central memory T cell or an effector memory T cell? (2,3)
- What is the maturation state of the relevant DC?
- What is the activation state of the relevant DC?

[1]Oliver JE, Silman AJ. Why are women predisposed to autoimmune rheumatic diseases? Arthritis Res. Ther. 2009;11:252.

[2]Ahlers JD, Belyakov IM. Memories that last forever: strategies for optimizing vaccine T-cell memory. Blood 2010;115:1678−89.

[3]Brinkmann V. FTY720 (fingolimod) in multiple sclerosis: therapeutic effects in the immune and the central nervous system. Br. J. Pharmacol. 2009;158:1173−82.

Clinical Trials.
DOI: http://dx.doi.org/10.1016/B978-0-12-804217-5.00028-X

For cytokines, these questions can be asked for each of the immune diseases:

- Does the pathology of the disorder result from activity of Th1-type cytokines, Th2-type cytokines, or Th17 cytokines?
- What is the identity of the cytokines and of the cytokine receptors?
- Does the receptor occur in a form that is intracellular, membrane-bound, or that is a free-floating soluble protein residing in the bloodstream?
- How do the relevant cytokines differ between early stages and late stages of the immune disorder? For example, tumor necrosis factor (TNF) is a cytokine that is protective to the intestines in early stages of ulcerative colitis (UC), but is pathological in later stages of UC (4).
- What is the involvement of chemokines (cytokines that control cell trafficking)?

a. Outlines of Mechanisms of Action for Various Immune Disorders

The immune diseases include disorders that affect the brain (multiple sclerosis), joints (rheumatoid arthritis), skin (psoriasis, atopic dermatitis), kidneys (lupus), gut (Crohn's disease (CD), ulcerative colitis (UC)), and lungs (asthma, COPD). A variety of immune cells and cytokines contribute to the pathology of each of these diseases. Although the players in all of these diseases include white blood cells, cytokines, cytokine receptors, and self-antigens, the contributions of these players to the mechanisms of each of these diseases are strikingly different from each other.

1. Rheumatoid Arthritis

Rheumatoid arthritis is an autoimmune disease of the joints, involving inflammation of the synovium and loss of bone from the joint (5,6). The relevant self-antigens include perinuclear factor, keratin, and citrullinated peptides of various matrix proteins. The cytokines most responsible for the pathology of arthritis include TNF-alpha and interleukin-6 (IL-6). The immune cells most responsible are macrophages, neutrophils, and T cells. Immune cells express toxic oxygen, thereby causing pain to the joints. Certain cytokines expressed by immune cells activate osteoclasts to digest bone in the joints. Bone undergoes continual turnover that is mediated by osteoblasts and osteoclasts (7). FDA's Guidance for Industry on rheumatoid arthritis provides information on trial design and endpoints (8).

---

[4]Corridoni D, et al. Probiotic bacteria regulate intestinal epithelial permeability in experimental Ileitis by a TNF-dependent mechanism. PLoS One 2012;7:e42067.

[5]Goronzy JJ, Weyand CM. Developments in the scientific understanding of rheumatoid arthritis. Arthritis Res. Ther. 2009;11:249.

[6]Dayer JM, Choy E. Therapeutic targets in rheumatoid arthritis: the interleukin-6 receptor. Rheumatology (Oxford) 2010;49:15—24.

[7]Brody T. Nutritional biochemistry. San Diego, CA: Academic Press; 1999. pp. 565—88, 761—85.

[8]U.S. Department of Health and Human Services. Food and Drug Administration. Guidance for industry. Rheumatoid arthritis: developing drug products for treatment; May 2013 (11 pp.).

2. Psoriasis

Psoriasis is a disease of the skin, involving itchy, red scaly plaques covering large areas of the skin (9,10). The stimulus or antigen of psoriasis is not well established, but data suggest that the antimicrobial peptide LL37 may convert the host's DNA into an autoimmune trigger that activates various immune cells. Psoriasis involves the cytokines TNF-alpha, IL-23, and IL-17. This disease involves Th17-type T cells. Keratinocytes (skin cells) respond to the IL-17 by increasing their proliferation rate, causing epidermal thickening. Autoantigens identified in psoriasis include keratin 13, heterologous nuclear ribonuclear protein A1, and FJ00294 (11).

3. Systemic Lupus Erythematosus

Systemic lupus erythematosus (SLE) involves the production of antibodies that recognize various components of the cell nucleus, such as certain chromatin proteins (12,13). These antibodies deposit in the kidneys, causing glomerulonephritis and kidney failure. As with all antibodies, the antibodies responsible for the pathology of SLE are expressed by B cells. The cytokines most responsible for the pathology of SLE are TNF and IL-6. Autoantigens in SLE include Smith proteins, double-stranded DNA, phospholipid, Ro/SS-A (Ro52), Ro/SS-B (La), and U1A (14). The Smith proteins are used in the splicesome. U1A is a component of a ribonucleoprotein. The antibodies against double-stranded DNA have been reviewed (15). The autoantibodies deposit in the kidneys, skin, and joints, causing inflammation. Regarding the kidneys, the most serious complication of SLE is lupus nephritis, which results from deposit of antibodies in the mesangium, subendothelial, and subepithelial spaces, and consequent damage to kidney cells (16,17).

The mechanism of autoantibody formation is outlined. A defect in SLE is reduced clearance of dead cells that are normally produced in healthy individuals. With prolonged residence of the dead cells in the body, the chromatin component of the dead cells is recognized by the immune system, where the immune system reacts as though the chromatin was from a virus. As a consequence, the human

[9]Mak RK, Hundhausen C, Nestle FO. Progress in understanding the immunopathogenesis of psoriasis. Actas Dermosifiliogr. 2009;100(Suppl. 2):2−13.

[10]Krulig E, Gordon KB. Ustekinumab: an evidence-based review of its effectiveness in the treatment of psoriasis. Core Evid. 2010;5:11−22.

[11]Jones DA, et al. Identification of autoantigens in psoriatic plaques using expression cloning. J. Invest. Dermatol. 2004;123:93−100.

[12]Bagavant H, Fu SM. Pathogenesis of kidney disease in systemic lupus erythematosus. Curr. Opin. Rheumatol. 2009;21:489−94.

[13]Lee HM, Sugino H, Nishimoto N. Cytokine networks in systemic lupus erythematosus. J. Biomed. Biotechnol. 2010;2010:676284.

[14]Han S, et al. Mechanisms of autoantibody production in systemic lupus erythrematosus. Front. Immunol. 2015;6: Article 228.

[15]Rekvig OP. Anti-dsDNA antibodies as a classification criterion and a diagnostic marker for systemic lupus erythematosus: critical remarks. Clin. Exp. Immunol. 2014;179:5−10.

[16]Lech M, Anders HJ. The pathogenesis of lupus nephritis. J. Am. Soc. Nephrol. 2013;24:1357−66.

[17]Corapi KM, et al. Comparison and evaluation of lupus nephritic response criteria in lupus activity indices and clinical trials. Arthritis Res. Therapy 2015;17:110−22.

body mounts an immune response against the body's own chromatin. In this response, the chromosomal proteins serve as the autoantigen, while the DNA component of the chromatin serves as an immune adjuvant that stimulates toll-like receptors, for example, TLR7 [18,19]. Regarding T cells, in SLE it is the case that $CD8^+$ T cells lose their ability to kill target cells, because these T cells lack perforin. Because of the lack of perforin, SLE results in an increase in bacterial, viral, and fungal infections [20]. The viral infections include those from Epstein—Barr virus and cytomegalovirus. Moreover, the $CD8^+$ T cells are less effective because they receive suboptimal activation from $CD4^+$ T cells [21]. Regarding this point, in SLE $CD4^+$ T cells have reduced expression of IL-2. IL-2 is a cytokine that supports the differentiation and survival of $CD8^+$ T cells. FDA has provided guidance for trial design and endpoints for clinical trials on SLE [22].

4. Asthma

Asthma has an allergic component called "extrinsic asthma" and a nonallergic component called "intrinsic asthma" [23]. The disease is characterized by a process called airway remodeling. Airway remodeling has the histological features of epithelial shedding, basement membrane thickening, smooth muscle hypertrophy, mucosal hyperplasia, and neovascularization. A number of autoantigens have been identified in asthma, but it is unclear how immune response against these autoantigens contributes to the pathology of the disease. These autoantigens include collagen V, bronchial epithelial cytokeratin, epithelial group factor receptor, activin A type 1 receptor, and alpha-catenin [24]. The pathology of asthma is mediated by Th2-type cytokines, IL-4, IL-5, IL-9, and IL-13. The immune cells most responsible for the pathology of asthma are eosinophils. The following demonstrates that IL-5, IL-13, and IL-4, each contribute to the pathology of asthma. The contribution of IL-5 to asthma pathology is demonstrated by the fact that administering an anti-IL-5 antibody (mepolizumab) to patients with severe asthma results in reductions in eosinophil counts, as well as improvements in lung function, as measured by the forced expiratory volume (FEV_1) test [25]. The role of IL-13 in the pathology of asthma is demonstrated by the fact that administering an

[18]Celhar T, et al. TLR7 and TLR9 in SLE: when sensing self goes wrong. Immunol. Res. 2012;53:58—77.

[19]Soni C, et al. B cell-intrinsic TLR7 signaling is essential for the development of spontaneous germinal centers. J. Immunol. 2014;193:4400—14.

[20]Esposito S, et al. Infections and systemic lupus erythematosus. Eur. J. Clin. Microbiol. Infect. Dis. 2014;33:1467—75.

[21]Grammatikos AP, Tsokos GC. Immunodeficiency and autoimmunity: lessons from systemic lupus erythematosus. Trends Mol. Med. 2012;18:101—8.

[22]U.S. Department of Health and Human Services. Food and Drug Administration. Guidance for industry. Systemic lupus erythematosus-developing medical products for treatment; June 2010. 15 pp.

[23]Liu M, et al. Immune responses to self-antigens in asthma patients: clinical and immunopathological implications. Hum. Immunol. 2012;73:511—6.

[24]Liu M, et al. Immune responses to self-antigens in asthma patients: clinical and immunopathological implications. Hum. Immunol. 2012;73:511—6.

[25]Orgega HG, Liu MC, Pavord ID, et al. Mepolizumab treatment in patients with severe eosinophilic asthma. New Engl. J. Med. 2014;371:1198—207.

anti-IL-13 antibody (lebrikizumab) results in improvement of FEV_1, and a reduction in nitric oxide (NO) in the exhaled breath (26). NO and superoxide are metabolites that are constitutively present in healthy cells and tissues. NO can react with superoxide to generate a form of toxic oxygen, peroxynitrite. Increased NO in exhaled air is a hallmark feature of asthma, and evidence suggests that the NO contributes to the pathology of asthma by directly destroying tissues (27). The fact that IL-4 contributes to the pathology of asthma is demonstrated by the fact that administering an anti-IL-4 antibody (dupilumab) to asthma patients results in improved FEV_1 and decreased exhaled NO (28).

5. Chronic Obstructive Pulmonary Disease

COPD is mainly caused by long-term cigarette smoking (29,30). The disease involves a decreased ability to breath, as measured by FEV_1 per second, with consequent disability and death. Cytokines that mediate COPD include IL-6, TNF-alpha, IL-1beta, while the immune cells most responsible for this disease are macrophages, neutrophils, and T cells. While COPD and asthma both involve the airways (bronchial tree) and alveoli, COPD is distinguished in that its pathology is mostly caused by *neutrophils*, while that of asthma is caused mostly by *eosinophils*. FDA provides guidance for trial design and endpoints for clinical trials on COPD (31).

6. Crohn's Disease and Ulcerative Colitis

CD and UC are two autoimmune diseases of the large intestines. The term *inflammatory bowel disease* (IBD) is used to refer to both of these diseases (32,33). Both diseases result in abscesses in the colon. CD also involves abscesses in the distal ileum. Both diseases result in weakening of the tight junctions between intestinal epithelial cells, distortion of the crypts, disappearance of the mucus layer that coats the lumen side of the epithelial cells, pathological infiltration of white blood cells in the lamina propria (the tissue immediately beneath the layer of epithelial cells), intestinal bleeding, and diarrhea.

CD is characterized as a Th1-mediated disease, while UC is a Th2-mediated disease (34). UC patients express increased IL-5, and have NKT cells that express increased IL-13. IL-5 and IL-13 are Th2-type cytokines. Biopsies from both CD and UC patients show increased levels of

[26]Corren J, Lemanske RF, Hanania NA, et al. Lebrikizumab treatment in adults with asthma. New Engl. J. Med. 2011;365:1088−98.

[27]Eriksson U, et al. Human bronchial epithelium controls TH2 responses by TH1-induced, nitric oxide-mediated STAT5 dephosphorylation: implications for the pathogenesis of asthma. J. Immunol. 2005;175:2715−20.

[28]Wenzel S, Ford L, Pearlman D, et al. Dupilumab in persistent asthma with elevated eosinophil levels. New Engl. J. Med. 2013;368:2455−66.

[29]Halpin DM, Tashkin DP. Defining disease modification in chronic obstructive pulmonary disease. COPD 2009;6:211−25.

[30]van der Molen T. Co-morbidities of COPD in primary care: frequency, relation to COPD, and treatment consequences. Prim. Care Respir. J. 2010;19:326−34.

[31]U.S. Department of Health and Human Services. Food and Drug Administration. Guidance for industry. Chronic obstructive pulmonary disease: developing drugs for treatment; November 2007. 17 pp.

[32]Casanova JL, Abel L. Revisiting Crohn's disease as a primary immunodeficiency of macrophages. J. Exp. Med. 2009;206:1839−43.

[33]Shih DQ, Targan SR. Insights into IBD pathogenesis. Curr. Gastroenterol. Rep. 2009;11:473−80.

[34]Wallace KL, et al. Immunopathology of inflammatory bowel disease. World J. Gastroenterol. 2014;20:6−21.

IFN-gamma. The above distinction regarding Th1 response and Th2 response is not an absolute one, as CD and UC also include Th17-type immune responses. Gut biopsies from both CD and UC patients show increased expression of IL-17A, increased Th17 cells, and increases in the subset of Th17 cells that is "Th1/Th17 cells," which express both interferon-gamma (IFN-gamma) and IL-17. In CD, gut cells express high levels of IL-12, and high levels of IL-18, a cytokine that enhances Th1-type immune response. The gut in CD is infiltrated with Th17 cells, which express IL-17A, IL-17F, IL-21, IL-22, and IL-26 (35).

In lesions of CD, CD4$^+$ T cells express large amounts of the Th1-type cytokine, IFN-gamma. In contrast, in UC, the lesions result from the Th2-type cytokines. Both diseases involve IL-17-producing T cells. These diseases result in gastrointestinal pain, and require diet therapy and the services of a dietician.

A number of self-antigens have been identified as targets in IBD, but the extent to which immune response against these antigens is responsible for the pathology of IBD is not clear. The self-antigens in UC include lyso-sulfatide glycoprotein (36), colonic tropomysin (hTm5) (37), goblet cell glycoproteins (38), and the antigen of "perinuclear antineutrophil cytoplasmic antibodies" (39). The self-antigens in CD include goblet cell glycoproteins (40), prohibitin, calreticulin, apolipoprotein A—I, and protein disulfide isomerase (41). The primary defect in IBD seems not to be related to these self-antigens, but instead is a result of an abnormal gut epithelial barrier, which allows for invasion of gut bacteria past the layer of epithelial cells of the large intestines, and overactive immune response and chronic inflammation (42).

II. DETAILED MECHANISM OF ACTION OF MULTIPLE SCLEROSIS

a. Introduction

Multiple sclerosis is a disorder of the central nervous system (CNS) characterized by chronic inflammation, myelin loss, and progressive neurological dysfunction (43). Symptoms that occur most commonly in multiple sclerosis include tremor, optic neuritis or double vision,

[35]Zorzi F, et al. Distinct profiles of effector cytokines mark the different phases of Crohn's disease. PLoS One 2013;8:e54562.

[36]Fuss IH, et al. NKT cells reactive to sulfatide self-antigen populate the mucosa of ulcerative colitis. Gut 2014;63:1728—36.

[37]Das KM, Bajpai M. Tropomysins in human disease: ulcerative colitis. Adv. Exp. Med. Biol. 2008;644:158—67.

[38]Wen Z, Fiocchi C. Inflammatory bowel disease: autoimmune or immune-mediated pathogensis. Clin. Dev. Immunol. 2004;11:195—204.

[39]Wen Z, Fiocchi C. Inflammatory bowel disease: autoimmune or immune-mediated pathogensis. Clin. Dev. Immunol. 2004;11:195—204.

[40]Wen Z, Fiocchi C. Inflammatory bowel disease: autoimmune or immune-mediated pathogensis. Clin. Dev. Immunol. 2004;11:195—204.

[41]Zhou Z, et al. Immunoproteomic to identify antigens in the intestinal mucosa of Crohn's disease patients. PLoS One 2013;8:81662.

[42]Corridoni D, et al. Probiotic bacteria regulate intestinal epithelial permeability in experimental Ileitis by a TNF-dependent mechanism. PLoS One 2012;7:e42067.

[43]Nicot AB. Gender and sex hormones in multiple sclerosis pathology and therapy. Front. Biosci. 2009;14:4477—515.

dysarthria (speech disorders), and dizziness (44). The term *inflammation* has classically been used to refer to four signs:

- Rubor (redness),
- Tumor (swelling),
- Calor (heat),
- Dolor (pain).

Inflammation also refers to accumulations of white blood cells in the body, for example, accumulations of white blood cells at infected areas of the body, or in parts of the body suffering from an autoimmune disease.

This outlines two of the drugs used against multiple sclerosis. Natalizumab is an antibody that prevents movement of white blood cells into the CNS. But because this drug impairs immunity in the CNS, a rare adverse event is a viral infection of the brain. Glatiramer takes the form of a collection of synthetic polypeptides. Since glatiramer imposes a specific response against antigens that are the targets of the pathological inflammatory response, glatiramer is not associated with any generalized weakened immune response against infections. Additional features of these two drugs and of other drugs are detailed below.

b. Natalizumab

Part of the MOA of multiple sclerosis can be illustrated by the MOA of natalizumab (45).

Natalizumab is an antibody that binds to a membrane-bound protein of T cells, namely, an integrin. The integrin is a dimer of two polypeptides, alpha-4 integrin and beta-1 integrin. The antibody binds to the alpha-4 subunit, thereby inhibiting the biological activity of the integrin. Normally, this integrin binds to a protein located on the blood vessels at the blood−brain barrier, namely, the vascular cell adhesion molecule-1 (VCAM-1) (46). But the antibody prevents the integrin from binding to VCAM-1, where the consequence is that T cells are prevented from binding to the blood vessel, and prevented from moving through the blood vessel's wall to the CNS. Figure 28.1 shows the location in the body of natalizumab's action.

c. Fingolimod

Fingolimod is a small molecule. This molecule is derived from a natural product made by the fungus, *Isaria sinclairii*. The natural product is myriocin (47). Fingolimod acts on T cells that reside in lymph nodes, and prevents these T cells from exiting the lymph nodes, where the end-effect is preventing them from migrating to the CNS. In detail, fingolimod acts on a membrane-bound protein of the T cell, namely, the sphingosine-1-phosphate receptor (48,49). The drug induces internalization of the receptor, that is, transfer from the cell surface to the

[44]Wehman-Tubbs K, Yale SH, Rolak LA. Insight into multiple sclerosis. Clin. Med. Res. 2005;1:41−4.

[45]Brody T. Multistep denaturation and hierarchy of disulfide bond cleavage of a monoclonal antibody. Analyt. Biochem. 1997;247:247−56.

[46]Bauer M, Brakebusch C, Coisne C, et al. Beta1 integrins differentially control extravasation of inflammatory cell subsets into the CNS during autoimmunity. Proc. Natl Acad. Sci. USA 2009;106(6):1920−5.

[47]Adachi K, Chiba K. FTY720 story. Its discovery and the following accelerated development of sphingosine 1-phosphate receptor agonists as immunomodulators based on reverse pharmacology. Perspect. Medicin. Chem. 2007;1:11−23.

[48]Kappos L, Radue EW, O'Connor P, et al. A placebo-controlled trial of oral fingolimod in relapsing multiple sclerosis. New Engl. J. Med. 2010;362:387−401.

[49]Cohen JA, Barkhof F, Comi G, et al. Oral fingolimod or intramuscular interferon for relapsing multiple sclerosis. New Engl. J. Med. 2010;362:402−15.

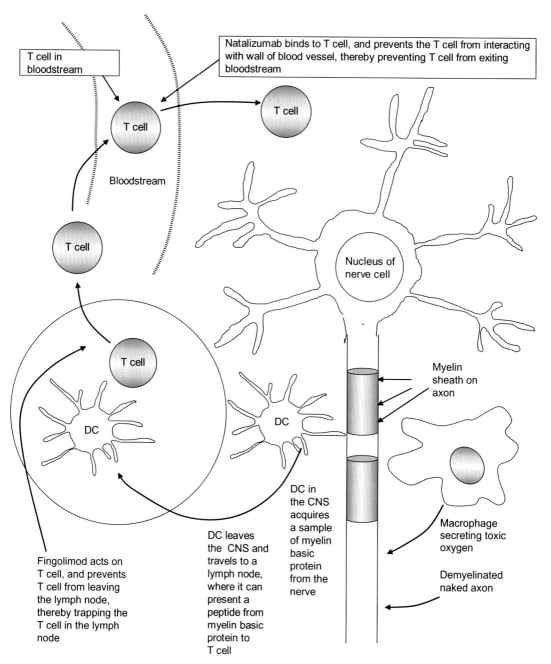

FIGURE 28.1 Mechanism of action of multiple sclerosis. The diagram illustrates physiological mechanisms of multiple sclerosis, as well as the points of action of two drugs, natalizumab and fingolimod.

cell's interior, thereby depriving the T cell of a necessary tool for exiting from the lymph node. Only a small subset of T cells, not all T cells, becomes trapped in the lymph nodes. Figure 28.1 shows the location in the body of fingolimod's action.

d. Interferon-Beta-1

Interferon-beta-1 (IFN-beta-1) is a cytokine. When used for treating multiple sclerosis, IFN-beta-1 has a number of MOAs. IFN-beta-1 acts at a number of points in the immune system (50) and at the blood–brain barrier. The MOAs of interferon in multiple sclerosis treatment are many, and have not been conclusively established (51). The effects of IFN-beta-1 in mitigating the disease include action on:

• Cytokine expression. The effects of IFN-beta-1 on cytokine expression include increases of antiinflammatory cytokines, and reductions of proinflammatory cytokines (52). IFN-beta-1 increases expression of cytokines that are antiinflammatory, namely IL-10 and IL-4. IL-10 and IL-4 are Th2-type cytokines (53).

• Reduces various activities of T cells. INF-beta-1 reduces the migration of T cells (54), the activation of T cells, and the expression by $CD4^+$ T cells of MHC class II. T cells, which occur as two classes, the $CD4^+$ T cells and the $CD8^+$ T cells, play a major role in the pathology of multiple sclerosis (55).

• Decreases expression of proteases by T cells.

• Inhibition of maturation of DCs (56,57).

• Reduces activities of neutrophils. IFN-beta-1 blocks production of toxic oxygen by neutrophils (58). Neutrophils are cells of the immune system that produce toxic oxygen, and have been found to contribute to the pathology of multiple sclerosis (59).

[50]Marckmann S, Wiesemann E, Hilse R, Trebst C, Stangel M, Windhagen A. Interferon-beta up-regulates the expression of co-stimulatory molecules CD80, CD86 and CD40 on monocytes: significance for treatment of multiple sclerosis. Clin. Exp. Immunol. 2004;138:499–506.

[51]Axtell RC, Steinman L. Type 1 interferons cool the inflamed brain. Immunity 2008;28:600–2.

[52]Manfredonia F, Pasquali L, Dardano A, Iudice A, Murri L, Monzani F. Review of the clinical evidence for interferon B 1a (Rebif) in the treatment of multiple sclerosis. Neuropsychiatr. Dis. Treat. 2008;4:321–36.

[53]Manfredonia F, Pasquali L, Dardano A, Iudice A, Murri L, Monzani F. Review of the clinical evidence for interferon beta 1a (Rebif) in the treatment of multiple sclerosis. Neuropsychiatr. Dis. Treat. 2008;4:321–36.

[54]Dressel A, Mirowska-Guzel D, Gerlach C, Weber F. Migration of T-cell subsets in multiple sclerosis and the effect of interferon-beta1a. Acta Neurol. Scand. 2007;116:164–8.

[55]Huseby ES, Liggitt D, Brabb T, Schnabel B, Ohlén C, Goverman J. A pathogenic role for myelin-specific CD8(+) T cells in a model for multiple sclerosis. J. Exp. Med. 2001;194:669–76.

[56]Duddy ME, Dickson G, Hawkins SA, Armstrong MA. Monocyte-derived denddritic cells:a potential target for therapy in multiple sclerosis (MS). Clin. Exp. Immunol. 2001;123:280–7.

[57]Zhang X, Jin J, Speer D, Sujkowska D, Markovic-Plese S. IFN-b1a inhibits the secretion of Th17-polarizing cytokines in human dendritic cells via TLR7 up-regulation. J. Immunol. 2009;182:3928–36.

[58]Huseby ES, Liggitt D, Brabb T, Schnabel B, Ohlén C, Goverman J. A pathogenic role for myelin-specific CD8(+) T cells in a model for multiple sclerosis. J. Exp. Med. 2001;194:669–76.

[59]Sayed BA, Christy AL, Walker ME, Brown MA. Meningeal mast cells affect early T cell central nervous system infiltration and blood–brain barrier integrity through TNF: a role for neutrophil recruitment? J. Immunol. 2010;184:6891–900.

- Maintenance of the integrity of the blood–brain barrier (60). "Integrity of the blood–brain barrier" refers, in part, to the ability of the blood–brain barrier to serve as a wall against migrating immune cells.

e. Cladribine

Cladribine (2-chlorodeoxyadenosine) is a small molecule that is an analog of deoxyadenosine. When administered, cladribine is taken up by cells, including lymphocytes, and is phosphorylated to produce cladribine-triphosphate. Cladribine-triphosphate is then incorporated into the chromosome of lymphocytes during the normal activities of cell division and DNA repair. But when cladribine is incorporated into the cell's DNA, the result is DNA stand breaks, and cell death by apoptosis (61,62), as indicated in the following diagram.

Cladribine's selective action in killing lymphocytes results from the fact that lymphocytes have high levels of deoxycytidine kinase (63,64). This enzyme catalyzes the phosphorylation of cladribine, producing cladribine-triphosphate. Please note that conversion of cladribine to cladribine-triphosphate is required for incorporation of the drug into the chromosome. The killing action of cladribine is increased in cells that contain greater amounts of deoxycytidine kinase (65). Experimentally increased amounts of this enzyme in cells resulted in enhanced killing action by cladribine. One might expect cladribine to be broken down by adenosine deaminase, an enzyme present at strikingly high levels in lymphocytes (66). However, cladribine is distinguished in that it resists breakdown by this enzyme (67). Cladribine does not inhibit

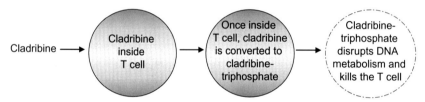

[60]Sheremata WA, Jy W, Delgado S, Minagar A, McLarty J, Ahn Y. Interferon-b1a reduces plasma CD31 + endothelial microparticles (CD31+ EMP) in multiple sclerosis. J. Neuroinflamm. 2006;3:23—7.

[61]Szondy Z. The 2-chlorodeoxyadenosine-induced cell death signalling pathway in human thymocytes is different from that induced by 2-chloroadenosine. Biochem. J. 1995;311:585—8.

[62]Van Den Neste E, Cardoen S, Husson B, et al. 2-Chloro-2′-deoxyadenosine inhibits DNA repair synthesis and potentiates UVC cytotoxicity in chronic lymphocytic leukemia B lymphocytes. Leukemia 2002;16:36—43.

[63]Petzer AL, Bilgeri R, Zilian U, et al. Inhibitory effect of 2-chlorodeoxyadenosine on granulocytic, erythroid, and T-lymphocytic colony growth. Blood 1991;78:2583—7.

[64]Sabini E, Hazra S, Konrad M, Lavie A. Elucidation of different binding modes of purine nucleosides to human deoxycytidine kinase. J. Med. Chem. 2008;51:4219—25.

[65]Hapke DM, Stegmann AP, Mitchell BS. Retroviral transfer of deoxycytidine kinase into tumor cell lines enhances nucleoside toxicity. Cancer Res. 1996;56:2343—7.

[66]Ungerer JP, Oosthuizen HM, Bissbort SH, Vermaak WJ. Serum adenosine deaminase: isoenzymes and diagnostic application. Clin. Chem. 1992;38:1322—6.

[67]Piro LD, Carrera CJ, Beutler E, Carson DA. 2-Chlorodeoxyadenosine: an effective new agent for the treatment of chronic lymphocytic leukemia. Blood 1988;72:1069—73.

adenosine deaminase (68). The MOA by which cladribine induces apoptosis is not settled, and it is likely to have more than one component. The drug may become incorporated into DNA and inhibit the ongoing "housekeeping" activity of DNA repair, or it may directly inhibit DNA polymerases (69). Cladribine kills lymphocytes, and is thus an effective drug for multiple sclerosis (70,71). Because cladribine kills lymphocytes, it is also an effective drug against cancers involving neoplastic T cells, such as the leukemias (72) and lymphomas (73,74,75).

f. Glatiramer Acetate

Glatiramer acetate ("glatiramer") takes the form of a heterogeneous mixture of polypeptides, ranging in length from 20 to 200 amino acid residues, with an average length of 60 amino acids (76). The polypeptides are random polymers of four amino acids, glutamate, lysine, alanine, and tyrosine. Glatiramer was designed so that it would include amino acid residues that promote anchoring to MHC class II, and so that it would also include contact residues that promote binding to T-cell receptor during formation of the immune synapse (77).

The mechanism of action of glatiramer, or more accurately, of certain polypeptides in the glatiramer mixture, is described (78). First, the polypeptide binds to MHC class II, and reduces presentation by the MHC class II of peptides derived from myelin-antigens. When glatiramer binds to MHC class II, it is not processed inside DCs. In other words, when

[68]Piro LD, Carrera CJ, Beutler E, Carson DA. 2-Chlorodeoxyadenosine: an effective new agent for the treatment of chronic lymphocytic leukemia. Blood 1988;72:1069–73.

[69]Van Den Neste E, Cardoen S, Husson B, et al. 2-Chloro-2′-deoxyadenosine inhibits DNA repair synthesis and potentiates UVC cytotoxicity in chronic lymphocytic leukemia B lymphocytes. Leukemia 2002;16:36–43.

[70]Giovannoni G, Comi G, Cook S, et al. A placebo-controlled trial of oral cladribine for relapsing multiple sclerosis. New Engl. J. Med. 2010;362:416–26.

[71]Barten LJ, Allington DR, Procacci KA, Rivey MP. New approaches in the management of multiple sclerosis. Drug Des. Devel. Ther. 2010;4:343–66.

[72]Sigal DS, Miller HJ, Schram ED, Saven A. Beyond hairy cell: the activity of cladribine in other hematologic malignancies. Blood 2010;116:2884–96.

[73]Blum KA, Johnson JL, Niedzwiecki D, et al. Prolonged follow-up after initial therapy with 2-chlorodeoxyadenosine in patients with indolent non-Hodgkin lymphoma: results of Cancer and Leukemia Group B Study 9153. Cancer 2006;107:2817–25.

[74]Inwards DJ, Fishkin PA, Hillman DW, et al. Long-term results of the treatment of patients with mantle cell lymphoma with cladribine (2-CDA) alone (95-80-53) or 2-CDA and rituximab (N0189) in the North Central Cancer Treatment Group. Cancer 2008;113:108–16.

[75]Jaeger G, Bauer F, Brezinschek R, Beham-Schmid C, Mannhalter C, Neumeister P. Hepatosplenic gammadelta T-cell lymphoma successfully treated with a combination of alemtuzumab and cladribine. Ann. Oncol. 2008;19:1025–6.

[76]Conner J. Glatiramer acetate and therapeutic peptide vaccines for multiple sclerosis. J. Autoimmun. Cell Responses 2014;1:3(2054-989X-1-3) (11 pp.).

[77]Duda PW, et al. Glatiramer acetate (Copaxone) induces degenerate, Th2-polarized immune responses in patients with multiple sclerosis. J. Clin. Inv. 2000;105:967–6.

[78]Firdkis-Hareli M. Design of peptide immunotherapies for MHC class-II-associated autoimmune disorders. Clin. Devel. Immunol. 2013;2013:Article ID 826191 (9 p.).

glatiramer binds to MHC class II, it is not processed inside DCs with the subsequent formation of an intracellular complex with MCH class II, prior to insertion of MCH class II into the plasma membrane, as is the case with other antigens. According to Dr Masha Hareli, glatiramer "binds to MHC class II with no processing and displaces the bound autoantigens, e.g., MBP, from the binding site" (79,80).

Second, according to Arnon and Aharoni (81), glatiramer treatment of experimental autoimmune encephalomyelitis (EAE) mice provokes the generation of glatiramer-specific CD4$^+$ T cells. Consequentially, these T cells migrate across the blood−brain barrier and into the CNS, where they accumulate and express antiinflammatory cytokines, that is, Th2-type cytokines. Once in the brain, the glatiramer-specific CD4$^+$ T cells also may stimulate microglia and astrocytes to express Th2-type cytokines, thus further dampening the inflammatory environment in the brain.

MHC class II includes two polypeptide chains, the alpha chain and beta chain, which form a dimer (82). MHC class II resides in a subcellular structure, that is, an endosome, located inside DCs. Peptides derived from extracellular antigens are loaded on to MHC class II, and then the endosome fuses with the plasma membrane, resulting in the peptide-located MHC class II being located in the plasma membrane, where the MHC class II positions the peptide so that it can be presented in the immune synapse. The endosome is called "MHC class II-containing compartment (MIIC)" (83,84,85). Polypeptides, can bind directly to MHC class II that resides on the surface of the DC. This capability results from the fact that the ends of the binding groove on MHC class II are open and allow the polypeptide to extend well beyond the binding groove while, in contrast, with MHC class I, the ends of the binding groove are closed (86,87).

[79]Kind response from Dr Masha Hareli, in e-mail of May 1, 2015.

[80]Fridkis-Hareli M, et al. Synthetic copolymer 1 and myelin basic protein do not require processing prior to binding to class II major histocompatibility complex molecules on living antigen-presenting cells. Cell. Immunol. 1995;163:229−36.

[81]Arnon R, Aharoni R. Mechanism of action of glatiramer acetate in multiple sclerosis and its potential for the development of new applications. Proc. Natl Acad. Sci. 2004;101:14593−8.

[82]Tong JC, et al. Modeling the structure of bound peptide ligands to major histocompatibility complex. Protein Sci. 2004;13:2523−32.

[83]Thery C, et al. MHC class II transport from lysosomal compartments to the cell surface is determined by stable peptide binding, but not by the cytosolic domains of the alpha- and beta-chains. J. Immunol. 1998;161:2106−13.

[84]van Nispen tot Pannerden ME, et al. Spatial organization of the transforming MHC class II compartment. Biol. Cell. 2010;102:581−91.

[85]Burster T, Beck A, Tolosa E, et al. Differential processing of autoantigens in lysosomes from human monocyte-derived and peripheral blood dendritic cells. J. Immunol. 2005;175:5940−9.

[86]Fridkis-Hareli M. Direct binding of myelin basic protein and synthetic copolymer 1 to class II major histocompatibility complex molecules on living antigen-presenting cells—specificity and promiscuity. Proc. Natl Acad. Sci. 1994;91:4872−6.

[87]Greenbaum J, et al. Functional classification of class II human leukocyte antigen (HLA) molecules reveals seven different supertypes and a surprising degree of repertoire sharing across supertypes. Immunogenetics 2011;63:325−35.

MHC class II functions to hold a peptide antigen on the outer surface of the DC, for use in transmitting a signal to a T cell. DCs, as well as other antigen-presenting cells (APCs), such as macrophages, express MHC class I as well as MHC class II on their plasma membrane. *MHC class I* holds antigenic peptides for use in presenting to cytotoxic T cells (CD8$^+$ T cells), while *MHC class II* holds antigenic peptides for presenting to helper T cells (CD4$^+$ T cells). Presentation occurs in a structure called "the immune synapse," and the result is activation of the T cell.

When administered glatiramer arrives, by way of diffusion, near the outside surface of a DC, it binds to MHC class II. After glatiramer's binding to MHC class II, the glatiramer is presented by the DC to T cells. It is likely that glatiramer binds to all types of APCs, that is, to DCs, monocytes, macrophages, and B cells. B cells are particularly relevant, because glatiramer induces antibody (IgG4) responses (88). When the bound glatiramer is presented, by way of the immune synapse, to a T cell, the result is the generation of T cells that express antiinflammatory cytokines, such as one or more of the Th2-type cytokines, IL-4, IL-5, and

IL-10. Glatiramer presumably gets presented to T cells in the draining lymph nodes of the inoculation site first, and later at other secondary lymphoid organs, including the spleen (89).

Regarding animals, glatiramer is equally effective in treating the various models of EAE, that is, EAE that is induced in the animal by administering one of the antigens of nerves: myelin basic protein (MBP), proteolipid protein (PLP), or myelin oligodendrocyte glycoprotein (MOG) (90). Regarding humans, in multiple sclerosis patients, glatiramer treatment results in increased expression of Th2-type cytokines (91). Efficacy of administered glatiramer in humans was shown, for example, by the fact that glatiramer prevents the formation of new lesions in the brain, as determined by magnetic resonance imaging (92). Glatiramer (Copaxone®; Glatopa®) is FDA-approved for treating relapsing-remitting multiple sclerosis (RRMS) (93). Glatiramer is effective only for RRMS, and has little or no efficacy for primary progressive multiple sclerosis (94).

Skihar et al. (95) demonstrated that after administering glatiramer to mice with EAE, the T cells express Th2-type cytokines, such as IL-4, IL-10, and also express the antiinflammatory

[88]The author thanks Prof. Amit Bar-Or, MD, of McGill University for his reply in e-mail of April 21, 2015.

[89]Kind response from Prof. Olaf Stuve, MD, PhD, University of Texas Southwestern Medical Center, e-mail of April 20, 2015.

[90]Duda PW, et al. Human and murine CD4$^+$ T cell reactivity to be a complex antigen:recognition of the synthetic random polypeptide glatiramer acetate. J. Immunol. 2000;165:7300−7.

[91]Arnon R, Aharoni R. Mechanism of action of glatiramer acetate in multiple sclerosis and its potential for the development of new applications. Proc. Natl Acad. Sci. 2004;101:14593−8.

[92]Duda PW, et al. Glatiramer acetate (Copaxone) induces degenerate, Th2-polarized immune responses in patients with multiple sclerosis. J. Clin. Invest. 2000;105:967−76.

[93]The Approval Letter, Medical Review, and other documents drafted by FDA reviewers for Copaxone® are available for NDA 020622 at December 1996, while these documents for Glatopa® for ANDA 090218 are available on FDA website at April 2015.

[94]Wolinsky JS, et al. Glatiramer acetate in primary progressive multiple sclerosis: results of a multinational, multicenter, double-blind, placebo-controlled trial. Ann. Neurol. 2007;61:14−24.

[95]Skihar V, et al. Promoting oligodendrogenesis and myelin repair using the multiple sclerosis medication glatiramer acetate. Proc. Natl Acad. Sci. 2009;106:17992−7.

cytokine, transforming growth factor-beta. Glatiramer treatment also induces T cells to express growth factors (brain-derived neurotrophic factor (BDNF); IGF-1) that promote the CNS to recover from demyelination. In other studies of glatiramer-induced BDNF, it was found that BDNF expression increased by about fourfold in the brain cortex of EAE mice, as compared to untreated EAE mice. This BDNF was expressed by infiltrating T cells, as well as by cells that are dedicated residents of the brain, such as astrocytes (96).

When glatiramer is administered, it has the potential to contact hundreds of different kinds of cells in the body, including dozens of different kinds of immune cells. To establish that glatiramer's influence in treating EAE arises, at least in part, from its effects on T cells, and that *glatiramer-specific T cells alone* can ameliorate EAE, researchers have turned to the technique of adoptive transfer. The adoptive transfer technique is detailed later in this chapter. In short, researchers established that glatiramer-specific T cells alone can ameliorate EAE, by demonstrating that the transfer of glatiramer-specific T cells into the bloodstream

of an animal is followed by their migration into the CNS, with consequent protection against the EAE (97,98).

III. ANIMAL MODELS OF MULTIPLE SCLEROSIS

Most of the available information on the mechanism of multiple sclerosis comes from the animal model, EAE. In this animal model, an animal, such as a mouse, is injected with a protein of myelin, for example, MOG, where neurological disease develops within a few days (99). This animal model had an origin in observations in 1885 by Louis Pasteur, that vaccines contaminated with brain proteins sometimes produced paralysis. These particular vaccines were against rabies, and were prepared from rabbit spinal cord.

Protocols for inducing multiple sclerosis in animals are described (100). Primate models for multiple sclerosis are believed to be more useful than mouse models for predicting efficacy in humans (101,102). The technique of adoptive transfer can be used to create

[96]Chen M, et al. Glatiramer acetate-reactive T cells produce brain-derived neurotrophic factor. J. Neurol. Sci. 2003;215:37—44.

[97]Firdkis-Hareli M. Design of peptide immunotherapies for MHC class-II-associated autoimmune disorders. Clin. Devel. Immunol. 2013;2013:Article ID 826191 (9 p.).

[98]Arnon R, Aharoni R. Mechanism of action of glatiramer acetate in multiple sclerosis and its potential for the development of new applications. Proc. Natl Acad. Sci. USA 2004;101:14593—8.

[99]Friese MA, Montalban X, Willcox N, Bell JI, Martin R, Fugger L. The value of animal models for drug development in multiple sclerosis. Brain 2006;129:1940—52.

[100]Furlan R, et al. Animal models of multiple sclerosis. Methods Mol. Biol. 2009;549:157—73.

[101]Hart BA, et al. The primate autoimmune encephalomyelitis model; a bridge between mouse and man. Ann. Clin. Transl. Neurol. 2015;2:581—93.

[102]Kap YS, et al. Experimental autoimmune encephalomyelitis in the common marmoset, a bridge between rodent EAE and multiple sclerosis for immunotherapy development. J. Neuroimmune Pharmacol. 2010;5:220—30.

[103]Ben-Nun A, et al. The rapid isolation of clonable antigen-specific T lymphocyte lines capable of mediating autoimmune encephalomyelitis. Eur. J. Immunol. 1981;11:195—9.

an animal model of multiple sclerosis (103). Transgenic animal models for multiple sclerosis are available (104,105).

IV. ETIOLOGY AND MECHANISMS OF MULTIPLE SCLEROSIS

a. Introduction

The pathways and networks of inflammatory activities, as they occur in multiple sclerosis, are quite different from those during the immune response against cancer and against infections. First of all, the origin of multiple sclerosis is not clear. Second, the antigens responsible for the pathology of multiple sclerosis are not certain. Third, immune response in multiple sclerosis seems to have a prominent nonspecific immune component, where immune cells, such as macrophages, indiscriminately produce toxic oxygen in the vicinity of nerve cells. The unknown qualities of the mechanisms of multiple sclerosis (MS) were articulated by Lolli et al. (106) in the writing, "[i]n the case of MS, the primary activated T cells may be specific for (but as of yet unknown) CNS-derived self-antigens ... that start the immunological cascade leading to MS."

The unknown quality of the autoantigens in multiple sclerosis (the disease in humans) was articulated by Niland et al. (107) as, "T cell responses to MBP (myelin basic protein) and proteolipid protein, or another oligodendrocyte-specific protein (OSP), MOG, did not differ considerably between MS patients and control donors."

In contrast to the situation with multiple sclerosis, in immune response against cancer and infections, $CD8^+$ T cells mount highly specific and concerted attacks against highly characterized antigens and their target cells, where the killing mechanisms involve granzyme/perforin and Fas-ligand/Fas-receptor.

Ortiz et al. (108) provides a concise account of the role of the immune system in initiating and perpetuating lesions of multiple sclerosis in humans, writing that the disease includes, "breakdown of the blood—brain barrier, the recruitment of lymphocytes, microglia, and macrophages to lesion sites ... multiple lesions ... being more pronounced in the brain stem and spinal cord ... the temporal maturation of lesions from inflammation through demyelination, to gliosis and partial remyelination ... [l]ymphocytes activated in the periphery infiltrate the central nervous system to trigger a local immune response that ultimately damages myelin and axons ... [t]he inflammatory environment in demyelinating lesions leads to the generation of oxygen- and nitrogen-free radicals as well as proinflammatory cytokines which contribute to the development and progression of the disease."

b. Initiating Events in Multiple Sclerosis

It is not certain whether multiple sclerosis originates from a defect in the immune system or from a defect in the CNS. Data from sequencing the genome of patients with multiple sclerosis suggest that the defect lies in the

[104]Mix E, et al. Animal models of multiple sclerosis—potentials and limitations. Prog. Neurobiol. 2010;92:386–404.

[105]Hohlfeld R. Multiple sclerosis: human model for EAE? Eur. J. Immunol. 2009;39:2036–9.

[106]Lolli F, Martini H, Citro A, et al. Increased CD8 + T cell responses to apoptotic T cell-associated antigens in multiple sclerosis. J. Neuroinflamm. 2013;10:94 (12 pp.).

[107]Niland B, Miklossy G, Banki K, et al. Cleavage of transaldolase by granzyme B causes the loss of enzymatic activity with retention of antigenicity for multiple sclerosis patients. J. Immunol. 2010;184:4025–32.

[108]Ortiz GG, Pacheco-Moieses FP, Bitzer-Quintero OK, et al. Immunology and oxidative stress in multiple sclerosis: clinical and basic approach. Clin. Dev. Immunol. 2013;2013:708659. doi:10.1155.

immune system (109). Various stages can be identified in multiple sclerosis. According to Marik et al. (110), an early stage involves microglia in the CNS, where the microglia express an enzyme called *myeloperoxidase*, and another enzyme, *NO synthase*. Myeloperoxidase produces hypochlorite, a form of toxic oxygen that is the active component of bleach (the cleaning product). Nitric oxide synthase produces NO, a form of oxygen that can be converted to peroxynitrite. Peroxynitrite nitrates proteins forming nitrotyrosine residues, leading to loss of protein function and cell death (111). Peroxynitrite is a form of toxic oxygen, which forms from the reaction of NO and superoxide.

In remarks about EAE in experimental animals, Kang et al. (112) referred to "the explosive inflammatory cascade associated with the onset of EAE." This inflammatory cascade provokes damage to the blood—brain barrier, to cells in the spinal cord, and in the brain. The molecules that are the most immediate cause of damage include peroxynitrite and proteolytic enzymes, such as matrix metalloproteinases and elastase (113,114,115,116).

c. CD4$^+$ T Cells and CD8$^+$ T Cells

Areas of inflammation in the lesions of multiple sclerosis contain CD4$^+$ T cells and CD8$^+$ T cells, B cells, macrophages, and DCs (117,118). According to Jain et al. (119), CD4$^+$ T cells circulate in the bloodstream and then gain access to the CNS. DCs within the CNS may present nervous system antigens to these T cells. These CD4$^+$ T cells are presented with nervous system antigen within the CNS, where they develop into activated CD4$^+$ T cells (120).

[109]Friese MA, Fugger LM. T cells and microglia as drivers of multiple sclerosis. Brain 2007;130:2755-7.

[110]Marik C, Felts PA, Bauer J, Lassmann H, Smith KJ. Lesion genesis in a subset of patients with multiple sclerosis: a role for innate immunity? Brain 2007;130:2800-15.

[111]Bishop A, et al. Differential sensitivity of oligodendrocytes and motor neurons to reactive nitrogen species: implications for multiple sclerosis. J. Neurochem. 2009;109:93-104.

[112]Kang Z, Altuntas C, Gulen M, et al. Astrocyte-restricted ablation of interleukin-17-induced Ac1-mediated signaling ameliorates autoimmune encephalomyelitis. Immunity 2010;32:414-25.

[113]Columbo E, et al. Stimulation of the neurotrophin receptor TrkB on astrocytes drives nitric oxide production and degeneration. J. Exp. Med. 2012;209:521-35.

[114]Columbo E, et al. Fingolimod may support neuroprotection via blockage of astrocyte nitric oxide. Ann. Neurol. 2014;76:325-7.

[115]Fabis MJ, et al. Blood brain barrier changes and cell invasion differ between therapeutic clearance of neurotrophic virus and CNS autoimmunity. Proc. Natl Acad. Sci. USA 2008;105:15511-6.

[116]Rumble JM, et al. Neutrophil-related factors as biomarkers in EAE and MS. J. Exp. Med. 2015;212:23-35.

[117]del Pilar Martin M, Cravens PD, Winger R, et al. Decrease in the numbers of dendritic cells and CD4$^+$ T cells in cerebral perivascular spaces due to natalizumab. Arch. Neurol. 2008;65:1596-603.

[118]Batoulis H, Addicks K, Kuerten S. Emerging concepts in autoimmune encephalomyelitis beyond the CD4/T(H)1 paradigm. Ann. Anat. 2010; Jul 15 [Epub ahead of print].

[119]Jain P, Coisne C, Enzmann G, Rottapel R, Engelhardt B. Alpha4beta1 integrin mediates the recruitment of immature dendritic cells across the blood—brain barrier during experimental autoimmune encephalomyelitis. J. Immunol. 2010;184:7196-206.

[120]Jain P, Coisne C, Enzmann G, Rottapel R, Engelhardt B. Alpha4beta1 integrin mediates the recruitment of immature dendritic cells across the blood—brain barrier during experimental autoimmune encephalomyelitis. J. Immunol. 2010;184:7196-206.

Evidence suggests that CD8$^+$ T cells can contribute to the pathology of multiple sclerosis (121,122,123). If CD8$^+$ T cells contribute to the pathology of multiple sclerosis, it is likely that the mechanisms include damage to nerve tissue in the CNS by way of secretion by CD8$^+$ T cells of perforin and granzyme (124,125).

d. DCs Present Antigen to T Cells and Activate the T Cells

Prior to attack of CD4$^+$ T cells or CD8$^+$ T cells on components of the CNS, these T cells must be activated to recognize antigens of the CNS. DCs are required for the full activation of CD8$^+$ T cells and CD4$^+$ T cells. DCs are present within the healthy CNS (126). Therefore, the sampling of CNS antigens by DCs likely plays an integral role in CNS immunity. The term "sampling" generally refers to the DC's uptake of antigens from the physiological environment, followed by processing them to forms that can bind to the DC's MHC, followed by binding of the processed antigens to the MHC. Sampling may be followed by the DC's formation of an immune synapse with a T cell, where the processed antigen (held in place by the DC's MHC) is presented to the T cell. DCs are also found within lesions of multiple sclerosis.

e. Breakdown of the Blood–Brain Barrier

At later stages of multiple sclerosis, there is a massive influx of immune cells at the lesion in the CNS, including T cells, B cells, and macrophages. In human lesions of multiple sclerosis, macrophages and CD8$^+$ T cells also inflict damage on blood vessels, where the result is a breakdown of the *blood–brain barrier*, and where this breakdown permits an ever greater influx of immune cells from the circulatory system into the CNS (127).

f. Toxic Oxygen From Microglia

Microglia, which are macrophage-like cells that reside only in the CNS, also contribute to the lesions of multiple sclerosis (128). Normally, microglia function to protect the CNS against infections, but in multiple sclerosis, microglia

[121]Benkhoucha M, et al. The neurotrophic hepatocyte growth factor attenuates CD8$^+$ cytotoxic T-lymphocyte activity. J. Neuroinflamm. 2013;10:154. doi: 10.1186.

[122]Haile Y, et al. Granule-derived granzyme B mediates the vulnerability of human neurons to T cell-induced neurotoxicity. J. Immunol. 2011;187:4861–72.

[123]Niland B, Miklossy G, Banki K, et al. Cleavage of transaldolase by granzyme B causes the loss of enzymatic activity with retention of antigenicity for multiple sclerosis patients. J. Immunol. 2010;184:4025–32.

[124]Lassmann H, Brück W, Lucchinetti CF. The immunopathology of multiple sclerosis: an overview. Brain Pathol. 2007;17:210–8.

[125]Deb C, Lafrance-Corey RG, Zoecklein L, Papke L, Rodriguez M, Howe CL. Demyelinated axons and motor function are protected by genetic deletion of perforin in a mouse model of multiple sclerosis. J. Neuropathol. Exp. Neurol. 2009;68:1037–48.

[126]Wu GF, Laufer TM. The role of dendritic cells in multiple sclerosis. Curr. Neurol. Neurosci. Rep. 2007;7:245–52.

[127]Lassmann H. Hypoxia-like tissue injury as a component of multiple sclerosis lesions. J. Neurol. Sci. 2003;206:187–91.

[128]Li J, Baud O, Vartanian T, Volpe JJ, Rosenberg PA. Peroxynitrite generated by inducible nitric oxide synthase and NADPH oxidase mediates microglial toxicity to oligodendrocytes. Proc. Natl Acad. Sci. USA 2005;102:9936–41.

contribute to multiple sclerosis lesions by producing NO, which then reacts with superoxide to produce peroxynitrite (129). Microglia are a type of resident macrophage, just as Kupffer cells are resident macrophages of the liver, and alveolar macrophages are resident macrophages of the lung (130).

V. DIAGRAM OF MULTIPLE SCLEROSIS MECHANISM

Figure 28.1 demonstrates the relationships between the CNS, lymph nodes, the circulatory system, and walls of the blood vessels, as well as macrophages, DCs, and T cells. DCs bear dendrites, and hence are typically represented in drawings by a shape resembling that of a starfish.

In multiple sclerosis, DCs may acquire antigens from nerves, and then travel to lymph nodes. As a general feature of immunology, immune presentation by DCs to T cells occurs in lymph nodes. Once in the lymph nodes, the DCs can present nerve antigen to T cells. Fingolimod prevents T cells from exiting the lymph nodes, thereby preventing the T cells from eventually inflicting antigen-specific damage on nerves. The antibody, natalizumab, prevents T cells from exiting the bloodstream, thereby preventing these T cells from entering the CNS and thereby preventing these T cells from inflicting antigen-specific damage on the nerves. Macrophages inflict damage on nerves, where this damage is not specific for any particular antigen, and where this damage results from toxic oxygen produced by the macrophages.

MBP is one of the specific targets of T cells, in the pathology of multiple sclerosis (131). One of the relevant oligopeptides found in the polypeptide sequence of MBP has been identified as (132):

85-Proline-Valine-Valine-Histidine-Phenylalanine-Phenylalanine-Lysine-Asparagine-Isoleucine-Valine-Threonine-Phenylalanine-96.

Using the one-letter abbreviations, this oligopeptide is: 85-PVVHFFKNIVTP-96. The entire polypeptide of human MBP is shown below (133,134). The sequence of MBP, as well as of every human protein, can be found by way of the BLAST searching device, available from the US government, on the world wide web at: www.ncbi.nlm.nih.gov. One of the epitopes implicated in contributing to the pathology of multiple sclerosis is underlined and in bold.

[129]Wu M, Tsirka SE. Endothelial NOS-deficient mice reveal dual roles for nitric oxide during experimental autoimmune encephalomyelitis. Glia 2009;57:1204—15.

[130]Hogg N, Selvendran Y, Dougherty G, Allen C. Macrophage antigens and the effect of a macrophage activating factor, interferon-gamma. Ciba Found. Symp. 1986;118:68—80.

[131]Belogurov Jr AA, Kurkova IN, Friboulet A, et al. Recognition and degradation of myelin basic protein peptides by serum autoantibodies: novel biomarker for multiple sclerosis. J. Immunol. 2008;180:1258—67.

[132]Bates IR, Feix JB, Boggs JM, Harauz G. An immunodominant epitope of myelin basic protein is an amphipathic alpha-helix. J. Biol. Chem. 2004;279:5757—64.

[133]Roth HJ, Kronquist K, Pretorius PJ, Crandall BF, Campagnoni AT. Isolation and characterization of a cDNA coding for a novel human 17.3K myelin basic protein (MBP) variant. J. Neurosci. Res. 1986;16, 227—38.

[134]GenBank Accession No. M30047.1. Human 17.3K myelin basic protein (MBP) mRNA, complete cds.

```
MASQKRPSQRHGSKYLATASTMDHARHGFLPRHRDTG
ILDSIGRFFGGDRGAPKRGSGKDSHHPARTAHYGSLPQK
SHGRTQDENPVVHFFKNIVTPRTPPPSQGKGAEGQRPGF
GYGGRASDYKSAHKGFKGVDAQGTLSKIFKLGGRDSRSG
SPMARR.
```

VI. ADDITIONAL MECHANISMS OF ACTION IN MULTIPLE SCLEROSIS

a. Introduction

This continues to focus on multiple sclerosis and the corresponding animal model, EAE. The duality of Th1-type immune response and Th2-type immune response was initially observed in the mid-1980s by researchers at Schering-Plough, Corp. (135). Although this duality continues to be a mainstream context for understanding all disorders with an immune component, other paradigms have materialized, such as the concept of Th17-type immune response. Immune cells engaged in this response express cytokines in the IL-17 family, including IL-17, and these cells are conventionally called "Th17 cells." CD4$^+$ T cells, and not CD8$^+$ T cells, are the main drivers behind the pathology of multiple sclerosis (136,137,138).

The mechanisms of multiple sclerosis and EAE include, but are not limited to, these elements:

- CD4$^+$ T cells that are Th1-type T cells and express Th1-type cytokines,
- CD4$^+$ T cells that are Th17 cells and express IL-17,
- macrophages,
- astrocytes,
- microglia,
- various myelin antigens.

As a form of shorthand, applicable to all narratives in immunology, it is conventional to identify T cells as Th1 cells, Th2 cells, Tc1 cells, and Tc2 cells. The letter "h" means helper, while the letter "c" means cytotoxic. Th1 cells are CD4$^+$ T cells that express Th1-type cytokines, for example, IFN-gamma. Th2 cells are CD4$^+$ T cells that express Th2-type cytokines, for example, IL-4, IL-5, IL-6, and IL-10. Tc1 cells are CD8$^+$ T cells that express Th1-type cytokines, as listed above, while Tc2 cells are CD8$^+$ T cells that express Th2-type cytokines, as listed above (139,140). This shorthand is used throughout all immunology, including studies on the immunology of cancer, autoimmune diseases, and infections.

[135]Mosmann TR, et al. Two types of murine helper T cell clone. I. Definition according to profiles of lymphokine activities and secreted proteins. J. Immunol. 1986;136:2348−57.

[136]Yadav SK, et al. Advances in the immunopathogenesis of multiple sclerosis. Curr. Opin. Neurol. 2015;28:206−19.

[137]Legroux L, Arbour N. Multiple sclerosis and T lymphocytes: an entangled story. J. Neuroimmune Pharmacol. 2015; May 7 [Epub ahead of print].

[138]Mars LT, et al. Contribution of CD8 T lymphocytes to the immuno-pathogenesis of multiple sclerosis and its animal models. Biochim. Biophys. Acta 2011;1812:151−61.

[139]Kemp RA, Ronchese F. Tumor-specific Tc1, but not Tc2, cells deliver protective antitumor immunity. J. Immunol. 2001;167:6497−502.

[140]Yu Y, Cho H, Wang D, et al. Adoptive transfer of Tc1 or Tc17 cells elicits antitumor immunity against established melanoma through distinct mechanisms. J. Immunol. 2013;190:1873−81.

b. Heterogeneity in Multiple Sclerosis and EAE

In multiple sclerosis, histological presentation can differ between patients, where differing pathological patterns can be distinguished by the distributions of myelin loss, plaque geography, pattern of oligodendrocyte injury, and complement deposits (141). Various animal EAE models take into account the fact that multiple sclerosis occurs in different forms, that is, a progressive disease and as a relapsing-remitting disease. EAE can be induced in animals by injecting myelin antigens, such as peptides derived from MBP, PLP, or MOG (142). As the disease progresses in the animal, lesions develop in the CNS, and these lesions contain activated T cells (in contrast to naive T cells), that specifically recognize the injected myelin antigen. The three antigens used to generate EAE are relevant to multiple sclerosis in human patients, as demonstrated by the fact that multiple sclerosis patients have T cells that are specific for MBP, PLP, and MOG (143,144,145). Although the peripheral blood of healthy persons also has T cells that are specific for MBP, PLP, and MOG, these T cells from multiple sclerosis patients are distinguished by their greater expression of inflammatory cytokines, that is, Th1-type cytokines (146,147,148). Additional autoantigens in multiple sclerosis include myelin-associated oligodendrocyte basic protein and OSP (149,150).

Macrophages in the CNS originate from monocytes, that is, from monocytes entering from the bloodstream and crossing the blood–brain barrier. Yamasaki et al. (151) provide photographs showing nerve cells in the spinal

[141]Simmons SB, et al. Modeling the heterogeneity of multiple sclerosis in animals. Trends Immunol. 2013;34:410–22.

[142]Aharoni R, et al. Copolymer 1 induces T cells of T helper type 2 that crossreact with myelin basic protein and suppress experimental autoimmune encephalomyelitis. Proc. Natl Acad. Sci. 1997;94:10821–6.

[143]Minohara M, et al. Differences between T-cell reactivities to major myelin protein-derived peptides in opticospinal and conventional forms of multiple sclerosis and healthy controls. Tissue Antigens 2001;57:447–56.

[144]Hellings N, et al. T-cell reactivity to multiple myelin antigens in multiple sclerosis patients and healthy controls. J. Neurosci. Res. 2001;60:290–302.

[145]Bornsen L, Christensen JR, Ratzer R, et al. Endogenous interferon-β-inducible gene expression and interferon-β-treatment are associated with reduced T cell responses to myelin basic protein in multiple sclerosis. PLoS One 2015;10:e0118830 (20 pp.).

[146]Zafranskaya M, et al. Interferon-beta therapy reduces CD4 + and CD8 + T-cell reactivity in multiple sclerosis. Immunology 2007;121:29–39.

[147]Tejada-Simon MV, et al. Reactivity pattern and cytokine profile of T cells primed by myelin peptides in multiple sclerosis and healthy individuals. Eur. J. Immunol. 2001;31:907–17.

[148]Hedegaard CJ, et al. T helper cell type 1 (Th1), Th2 and Th17 responses to myelin basic protein and disease activity in multiple sclerosis. Immunology 2008;125:161–9.

[149]Kaushansky N, et al. The myelin-associated oligodendrocytic basic protein (MOBP) as a relevant primary target autoantigen in multiple sclerosis. Autoimmun. Rev. 2010;9:233–6.

[150]de Rosbo NK, Kaye, JF, Eisenstein M, et al. The myelin-associated oligodendrocyte basis protein region MOBP15-36 encompasses the immunodominant major encephalitogenic epitope(s) for SJL/J mice and predicted epitope(s) for multiple sclerosis-associated HLA-DRB1*1501. J. Immunol. 2004;173:1426–35.

[151]Yamasaki R, Lu H, Butovsky O, et al. Differential role of microglia and monocytes in the inflamed central nervous system. J. Exp. Med. 2014;211:1533–49.

cord from animals with EAE, where the nerve cells are encircled by macrophages. The macrophages initiate demyelination, whereas the microglia clear debris that is produced during demyelination.

Administering MOG peptide or MBP antigen to animals induces a progressive form of EAE, while administering PLP peptide induces a relapsing-remitting form of EAE (152).

In addition to inducing EAE by injecting antigens from MBP, PLP, or MOG, EAE can also be induced by the technique of adoptive transfer. Adoptive transfer is used for probing the mechanisms of any disorder having an immune component, including autoimmune diseases, infections, and cancer. Adoptive transfer is also used for therapy against cancer in humans (153). Adoptive transfer can involve inducing a T cell of interest, for example, in an experimental animal, withdrawing blood and purifying the population of T cells of interest, and then injecting the purified T cells into a second experimental animal. In this way, the researcher can distinctly address the influence (therapeutic or pathologic) of a single species of T cells on the disease of interest. Other immune cells, such as NK cells, can also be used for adoptive transfer (154). A technique related to adoptive transfer is the method where immune cells are withdrawn from an animal or human subject, treated with a cytokine or with an antigen, allowed to differentiate or adapt during in vitro culture, and then injected back into the same subject or into a different subject (155).

c. Th1-Type Immune Response and Th17-Type Immune Response Both Contribute to EAE

Lees et al. (156) treated mice with myelin antigen to stimulate the formation of myelin-specific CD4$^+$ T cells. The researchers then purified these cells, cultured them in vitro to generate populations of T cells that were skewed to become either Th1-type T cells (Th1 cells) or Th17-type T cells (Th17 cells). In order to more clearly distinguish Th1 cells from Th17 cells, terms such as "Th1-type T cells" and "Th1-type immune response" are used in this narrative.

For both populations of cells, the cells were specific for myelin antigen. Then, the researchers adoptively transferred either the Th1-type T cells or the Th17 cells into different mice. In both cases, the mice developed EAE. Mice receiving the Th1-type T cells developed signs of classical EAE, which involves paralysis with inflammation of the spinal cord. Mice receiving the Th17 cells developed similar symptoms. To this point, the researchers wrote that, "T cells polarized to produce IL-17 induced

[152]Gold R, et al. Understanding pathogenesis and therapy of multiple sclerosis via animal models: 70 years of merits and culprits in experimental autoimmune encephalomyelitis research. Brain 2006;129:1953—71.

[153]Kalos M, June CH. Adoptive T cell transfer for cancer immunotherapy in the era of synthetic biology. Immunity 2013;39:49—60.

[154]Palucka K, Banchereau J. Dendritic-cell-based therapeutic cancer vaccines. Immunity 2013;39:38—48.

[155]Lees JR, et al. Regional CNS responses to IFN-gamma determine lesion location patterns during EAE pathogenesis. J. Exp. Med. 2008;205:2633—42.

[156]Lees JR, et al. Regional CNS responses to IFN-gamma determine lesion location patterns during EAE pathogenesis. J. Exp. Med. 2008;205:2633—42.

clinical symptoms identical to those produced by ... cells cultured under Th1 polarizing conditions" (157).

Adoptive transfer of either myelin-specific Th1-type T cells, or myelin-specific Th17 cells, can produce EAE. The following studies reveal that Th17 cells, adoptively transferred into mice, spontaneously change inside the mice to become like Th1-type T cells. Each of these types of T cell can produce EAE. With adoptive transfer of Th17 cells, the materialization of EAE is delayed and occurs only after the Th17 cells have acquired the ability to express IFN-gamma in the host mouse (IFN-gamma is a Th1-type cytokine). In the words of O'Connor et al. (158), an analysis of the adoptively transferred Th17 cells, taken out of the recipient mouse and analyzed, revealed that they "had a propensity of IFN-gamma production, suggesting a degree of instability upon encounter with Ag [myelin antigen in the recipient mouse]." The researchers characterized this phenomenon as "organ-specific enrichment ... of IFN-gamma + IL-17 + cells in the CNS." Similarly, Lalor and Segal (159) stated that, "[t]he majority of CNS-infiltrating IFN-gamma-producing T cells could represent transformed Th17 cells that acquire Th1-like characteristics within the CNS environment." Consistently, Simmons et al. (160) acknowledged the fact that in studies of EAE induced by Th17 cells, the Th17 cells in the CNS "converted to IFN-gamma producers."

d. Numbers of Th1-Type T Cells and Th17 Cells, in Response to Induction of EAE With Myelin Antigen, and Subsequently, in Response to Treatment With Glatiramer

Aharoni et al. (161) demonstrated that Th1-type T cells and Th17 cells each account for roughly equal proportions of the accumulation of T cells in the brain, following induction of EAE with myelin antigen. With EAE induction, histological examination of the brain revealed that Th17 cells accounted for about 40% of the T cells in the brain.

An elegant time course study followed clinical score on a daily basis after administration of myelin-antigen, over the course of 5 weeks, and also followed the accumulation of total T cells over the course of 5 weeks. Clinical score was calculated from the parameters of limp tail, hind limb paralysis, all four limbs paralyzed, and death.

On day 0, the total number of T cells was under five T cells per square millimeter, as determined by histology, where, over the course of 5 weeks, this number increased to about 50–150 T cells per square millimeter. As mentioned above, following EAE induction, about 40% of the accumulated T cells were Th17 cells. Total T cells was assessed by the conventionally used biomarker, CD3.

All experiments were conducted in parallel using induction with PLP peptide, which is a

---

[157]Lees JR, et al. Regional CNS responses to IFN-gamma determine lesion location patterns during EAE pathogenesis. J. Exp. Med. 2008;205:2633–42.

[158]O'Connor RA, et al. Cutting edge: Th1 cells facilitate the entry of Th17 cells to the central nervous system during experimental autoimmune encephalomyelitis. J. Immunol. 2008;181:3750–4.

[159]Lalor SJ, Segal BM. Th1-medicated experimental autoimmune encephalomyelitis is CXCR3 independent. Eur. J. Immunol. 2013;43:2866–74.

[160]Simmons SB, et al. Modeling the heterogeneity of multiple sclerosis in animals. Trends Immunol. 2013;34:410–22.

[161]Aharoni R, Eilam R, Stock A, et al. Glatiramer acetate reduces Th-17 inflammation and induces regulatory T-cells in the CNS of mice with relapsing-remitting or chronic EAE. J. Neuroimmunol. 2010;225:110–1.

model for RRMS, and with MOG peptide, which is a model for chronic multiple sclerosis. Some of the histological data were from brain sections and other data are from spinal cord sections.

Both models of EAE (PLP, MOG) resulted in massive inflammation, where Th1-type T cells and Th17 cells each comprised roughly half of the infiltrating T cells. The researchers further probed possible differences between Th1-type T-cell response and Th17 response, in response to glatiramer therapy. Regarding the overall effect of glatiramer on the number of T cells, it was the case that glatiramer reduced the total number of T cells to a level that was from 30% to 50% the number, as compared to without glatiramer therapy. In exploring details of the therapeutic effect of glatiramer, the researchers discovered that glatiramer's influence on reducing T-cell number was disproportionately greater on the population of T cells that was Th17 cells. To view the numbers after glatiramer therapy, Th17 cells accounted for only 5–10% of the total T cells.

e. Modifying the Th1/Th2 Paradigm

In the study of Aharoni et al. (162), the researchers referred to the "Th1/Th2 paradigm," and concluded that, in the context of multiple sclerosis and EAE, this paradigm must be modified to account for the fact that inflammation includes Th17 cells, and for the fact that glatiramer treatment provokes dramatic decreases in the numbers and proportions of Th17 cells. Referring to the effect of glatiramer, the researchers stated that, "GA administered … reduced the amounts of Th-17

cells in both models" (PLP; MOG). Referring to other cells in the CNS, the researchers added that microglia, monocytes, and macrophages also contributed to IL-17 expression, during EAE, and that "[t]he significance of IL-17 … was revealed by the … IL17 expressing cells in lesion sites with myelin loss."

VII. CONCLUDING REMARKS

The commentary on Th1-type T cells and Th17 cells establishes the basic landscape of the mechanism of action of multiple sclerosis and EAE. This landscape provides a context for understanding further details in the mechanism of action of the disease and the mechanisms of action of various drugs, as they unfold during the coming decades. In contemplating data on multiple sclerosis or on EAE, the researcher should consider these variables when assessing the mechanism of action of the disease or of the drug:

- Whether the data were acquired from assays of cells from the lymph node, bloodstream, spinal cord, or brain;
- Whether the data are from early or late stage of EAE;
- Whether EAE was induced by peptides from MBP, PLP, or MOG;
- The genetic background of the experimental animal;
- Whether the mechanism of action of the drug is on T cells in the lymph nodes, on T cells in the bloodstream prior to crossing the blood–brain barrier, or on T cells located in the central nervous system.

---

[162]Aharoni R, Eilam R, Stock A, et al. Glatiramer acetate reduces Th-17 inflammation and induces regulatory T-cells in the CNS of mice with relapsing-remitting or chronic EAE. J. Neuroimmunol. 2010;225:110–1.

29

Mechanisms of Action—Part IV (Infections)

I. INTRODUCTION

Infectious diseases include those caused by bacteria, viruses, and protozoa. These diseases are distinguished from many other diseases in that their cause, namely a specific microbe, is usually unambiguous. This is in contrast to the causes of various cancers, which typically take the form of the cumulative effect of several genetic mutations. This is also in contrast to the causes of all of the autoimmune diseases which, as of this writing, are only partially established.

Microbes responsible for infectious diseases are to be distinguished from the gut microflora, as well as from the microflora that reside on the skin. In healthy individuals, the gut microflora and skin bacteria are not pathological and are not considered to be infections. Please note that except for the case of newborn infants, the human body contains more bacterial cells than human cells (1).

This chapter provides the mechanisms of action of an exemplary infectious disease, namely, hepatitis C virus (HCV), and introduces the mechanisms of immune response against HCV. The term "immune network" is used to refer to the various interactions between immune cells and cytokines in health and disease.

II. HCV INFECTIONS

Hepatitis C is caused by HCV. A related infection is hepatitis B, which is caused by hepatitis B virus (HBV). While both viruses infect the liver, they are members of different viral families. HCV is a *flavivirus*, while HBV is a *hepadnavirus*. HCV and HBV are also distinguished, in that HCV does not have a naturally occurring small-animal model, while the established small-animal model for HBV is the woodchuck (2).

---

[1]Yang X, Xie L, Li Y, Wei C. More than 9,000,000 unique genes in human gut bacterial community: estimating gene numbers inside a human body. PLoS One 2009;4:e6074 (8 p).

[2]Menne S, Cote PJ. The woodchuck as an animal model for pathogenesis and therapy of chronic hepatitis B virus infection. World J. Gastroenterol. 2007;13:104−24.

Each of these viruses causes acute and chronic inflammatory liver disease and eventual hepatocellular carcinoma (HCC) (3). On a worldwide basis, over 500 million people are persistently infected by these viruses and are at risk of dying from HCC. A contrasting feature of HCV and HBV infections is that more than 70% of adult-onset HCV infections *persist*, while more than 95% of adult-onset HBV infections are *self-limited*.

This chapter details the HCV polyprotein. The genome of hepatitis C is a 9.6-kb single-stranded RNA molecule that serves as a template for both translation and replication. Translation of the plus-strand RNA results in production of a single polyprotein that is processed, by various proteases, into structural proteins (C, E1, E2, p7) and nonstructural proteins (NS2, NS3, NS4A, NS4B, NS5A, and NS5B). "NS" means nonstructural. These proteases are encoded by the viral genome. A protease is an enzyme having the catalytic activity of cleaving other proteins.

As mentioned above, the genome of HCV encodes a large protein called a polyprotein. The amino acid sequence of this protein is shown in its entirety at a later point in this chapter. The sequence is from GenBank Accession Number: ADD13463, on the world wide web at www.ncbi.nlm.gov.

Knowledge of the mechanism of action is required for drafting the package insert. For example, the package insert for an anti-HCV drug refers to the drug's ability to inhibit NS5A protein and NS5B polymerase (4). The package insert states that:

> Ledipasvir is an inhibitor of the HCV NS5A protein, which is required for viral replication. Resistance selection in cell culture and cross-

resistance studies indicate ledipasvir targets NS5A as its mode of action. Sofosbuvir is an inhibitor of the HCV NS5B RNA-dependent RNA polymerase, which is required for viral replication. Sofosbuvir is a nucleotide prodrug that undergoes intracellular metabolism to form the pharmacologically active uridine analog triphosphate (GS-461203), which can be incorporated into HCV RNA by the NS5B polymerase and acts as a chain terminator.

Mechanisms of action in the lifecycle of HCV, and mechanisms of anti-HCV drugs, include these compositions and processes:

- Proteins encoded by HCV genome and their functions;
- Immune evasion by HCV;
- Consequences of chronic HCV infection (fibrosis, cirrhosis, HCC);
- Immune response to HCV infection (innate immunity, adaptive immunity).

In developing drugs against HCV, researchers have explored the ability of each of the proteins expressed by HCV's genome to serve as a drug target. Also, researchers have addressed the possibility of stimulating the immune response against HCV and ways to overcome HCV's evasion of the immune system.

Goals in anti-HCV drug development include the need to avoid the safety issues of ribavirin and pegylated interferon-alfa (peg-IFN) (traditional drugs for HCV), the need for broader efficacy against the various HCV genotypes, and the need to overcome drug-resistant mutants (5). The goal of broad efficacy is especially important for HCV patients infected with more than one genotype of the virus.

---

[3]Wieland SF, Chisari FV. Stealth and cunning: hepatitis B and hepatitis C viruses. J. Virol. 2005;79:9369–80.

[4]Package insert for HARVONI® (ledipasvir and sofosbuvir) tablets, for oral use; March 2015 (32 p).

[5]Kayali Z, Schmidt WN. Finally sofosbuvir: an oral anti-HCV drug with wide performance capability. Pharmgenomics Pers. Med. 2014;7:387–98.

III. LIFE CYCLE OF HCV

Kayali et al. (6) and Popescu et al. (7) provide diagrams of the lifecycle of HCV, starting from entry into the host hepatocyte by way of endocytosis, through viral replication, and finally secretion of the completed virus particles into the extracellular fluid. The final steps of HCV's lifecycle include steps when capsid proteins and genomic RNA assemble to form a nucleocapsid, which then buds through intracellular membranes where the result is residence in cytoplasmic vesicles. Mature virus particles leave the cell by way of a secretory pathway (8).

HCV particles enter the hepatocyte by way of clathrin-mediated endocytosis (9). After entry of HCV into the host cell, the viral genome is uncoated, and then translated by ribosomes on the host cell's endoplasmic reticulum, resulting in creating of the polyprotein. The HCV genome is a 9.6-kb single-stranded RNA genome, which encodes a polyprotein that consists of about 3000 amino acids (10,11). Proteases encoded by HCV as well as by the host cell then process the polyprotein, liberating the proteins listed below. Cleavage occurs during translation as well as after translation has been completed results in the liberation of these proteins (12):

- Core protein;
- E1;
- E2;
- P7;
- NS2;
- NS3;
- NS4A;
- NS4B;
- NS5A;
- NS5B.

HCV's nonstructural proteins are NS2, NS3, NS4A, NS5A, NS5A, and NS5B. **NS2** is needed for HCV particles to be secreted from the host cell (13). Also, **NS2** appears to function as an adaptor that mediates interactions between, for example, E2 and NS3 or between E2 and NS5A. **NS3** and **NS4A** form the NS3/4A protease. **NS4B** and **NS5A** bind to RNA, and appear to play a structural role during viral replication. NS4B and NS5A are both integral membrane proteins (14). According to Eyre

---

[6]Kayali Z, Schmidt WN. Finally sofosbuvir: an oral anti-HCVdrug with wide performance capability. Pharmgenomics Pers. Med. 2014;7:387—98.

[7]Popescu CI, et al. Hepatitis C virus life cycle and lipid metabolism. Biology 2014;3:892—921.

[8]Rehermann B. Hepatitis C virus versus innate and adaptive immune responses: a tale of coevolution and coexistence. J. Clin. Invest. 2009;119:1745—54.

[9]Cordek DG, et al. Targeting the NS5A protein of HCV: an emerging option. Drugs Future 2011;36:691—711.

[10]Lohmann V. Hepatitis C virus RNA replication. Curr. Top. Microbiol. Immunol. 2013;369:167—98.

[11]Hundt J. Post-translational modifications of hepatitis C viral proteins and their biological significance. World J. Gastroenterol. 2013;19:8929—39.

[12]Ross-Thriepland D, et al. Serine phosphorylation of the hepatitis C virus NS5A protein controls the establishment of replication complexes. J. Virol. 2015;89:3123—35.

[13]Bentham MJ, et al. NS2 is dispensable for efficient assembly of hepatitis C virus-like particles in a bipartite trans-encapsidation system. J. Gen. Virol. 2014;95:2427—41.

[14]Herod MR, et al. Genetic complementation of hepatitis C virus nonstructural protein functions associated with replication exhibits requirements that differ from those for virion assembly. J. Virol. 2014;88:2748—62.

et al. (15), **NS5A**, which binds to the RNA genome, transfers HCV's RNA between the replication complex to the "lipid droplet," for the purpose of encapsidating the viral genome. **NS5B** is the RNA polymerase that is used for the replication of HCV's genome. **P7** is an ion channel that is a membrane-bound protein of lipid vesicles, and that controls the pH inside the vesicles (16). The changes in pH that are induced by P7 are linked to the production of infectious intracellular viral particles.

IV. INITIATING BIOSYNTHESIS OF THE HCV POLYPEPTIDE

Part of HCV's RNA genome does not encode any proteins, and this is the internal ribosome entry sequence (IRES) sequence. The 5'-end of the RNA genome has an IRES that is required for translation of the viral RNA by the host cell's ribosomes (17). The IRES is responsible for assembling functional ribosomes at the viral start codon in a mechanism that bypasses the host cell's translation initiation, which depends on the 5'-cap modified terminus of eukaryotic mRNA (18).

V. MEMBRANOUS WEB AND LIPID DROPLET

The membranous web is derived from the host cell's endoplasmic reticulum. HCV-encoded proteins function to recruit some of the host cell's proteins, to generate the membranous web. The membranous web consists of lipid membranes in the form of vesicles, where the vesicles contain the HCV-encoded proteins (NS3, NS5A, NS5B) and host cell proteins, such as VAP-A. The membranous web is the site of HCV replication (19). The vesicles that make up the membranous web are dispersed throughout the cytoplasm of the host cell.

In contrast to the membranous web, which is used for replication, packaging of newly bio-synthesized viral proteins to create new HCV particles occurs on the lipid droplets. The lipid droplets are coated with HCV's core proteins, and are recruited to the membranous web (site of HCV replication) to allow encapsidation of viral RNA. NS5A associates with core protein at the surface of the lipid droplet, where it appears to coordinate assembly of the virus particle (20). Lipid droplets are distinguished by the presence of specific proteins that coat the lipid droplets. These proteins, which are

[15]Eyre NS, Fiches GN, Aloia A, et al. Dynamic imaging of the hepatitis C virus NS5A protein during a productive infection. J. Virol. 2014;88:3636–52.

[16]Wozniak AL, et al. Intracellular proton conductance of the hepatitis C virus p7 protein and its contribution to infectious virus production. PLoS Pathogens 2010;6:e1001087 (17 p).

[17]Ross-Thriepland D, et al. Serine phosphorylation of the hepatitis C virus NS5A protein controls the establishment of replication complexes. J. Virol. 2015;89:3123–35.

[18]Dibrov SM, Parsons J, Carnevali M, et al. Hepatitis C virus translation inhibitors targeting the internal ribosomal entry Site. J. Med. Chem. 2014;57:1694–707.

[19]Ross-Thriepland D, et al. Serine phosphorylation of the hepatitis C virus NS5A protein controls the establishment of replication complexes. J. Virol. 2015;89:3123–35.

[20]Clement S, et al. Role of seipin in lipid droplet morphology and hepatitis C virus life cycle. J. Gen. Virol. 2013;94:2208–14.

encoded by the host cell, include TIP47 and ADRP. TIP47 binds to one of HCV's proteins, namely, NS5A. TIP47 is required for HCV replication, as demonstrated by experimentally created mutations in TIP47 that prevent binding and that also prevent HCV replication (21).

VI. NS3/4A PROTEASE

NS3/4A protease is described first, because it is the target of the anti-HCV drugs, boceprevir, telaprevir, and simeprevir. The structure of boceprevir is shown below. The molecule is a mimetic of an oligopeptide:

NS3/4A protease is a heterodimer of two subunits, a catalytic subunit (NS3) and an activating cofactor (NS4A). NS3/4A is responsible for cleaving four sites of HCV's polyprotein. NS3 is a 631-amino-acid polypeptide. In the absence of NS4A, the NS3 protease is able to make one of the cleavages, but it is not able to cleave at the three other sites (22).

As is common with many other proteases, NS3 contains a zinc atom. NS3 holds this zinc atom by way of cysteine-97, cysteine-99, cysteine-145, and histidine-149. This information about amino acid residues is useful, since it provides a context for better understanding the naturally occurring mutations in NS3 that cause HCV to become resistant to drugs that inhibit NS3. Naturally occurring mutations in NS3 have been found that provide resistance to telaprevir, boceprevir, and simeprevir. These include mutations resulting in amino acid substitutions at arginine-155 or at alanine-156 (23,24). Footnote (25) provides a list of NS3/4A protease inhibitors (26).

VII. NS5A—HCV'S RECRUITING AND ASSEMBLY PROTEIN

NS5A is the target of the drugs, ledipasvir, daclatasvir, and samatasvir. The structure of ledipasvir is shown below. As is evident from the backbone of benzene rings, ledipasvir is not a peptide mimetic (oligopeptides do not contain a backbone of benzene rings):

[21]Vogt DA, et al. Lipid droplet-binding protein TIP47 regulates hepatitis C virus RNA replication through interaction with the viral NS5A protein. PLoS Pathogens. 2013;9:e1003302 (14 pp).

[22]Lin C. HCV NS3-4A Serine protease. Chapter 6 (Tan SL, editor) Hepatitis C viruses: genome and molecular biology. Norfolk (UK): Horizon Bioscience; 2006. (64 pp).

[23]Paolucci S, Fiorina L, Piralla A, et al. Naturally occurring mutations to HCV protease inhibitors in treatment-naive patients. Virology J. 2012;9:245 (8 p).

[24]Lenz O, Verbinnen T, Lin TI, et al. In vitro resistance profile of the hepatitis C virus NS3/4A protease inhibitor TMC435. Antimicrob. Agents Chemother. 2010;54:1878–87.

[25]ABT-450/r, faldaprevir, asunaprevir, GS-9256, vedroprevir (GS-9451), danoprevir, MK-5172, vaniprevir, sovaprevir, ACH-2684, narlaprevir simeprevir, telaprevir, and boceprevir.

[26]De Clercq E. Current race in the development of DAAs (direct-acting antivirals) against HCV. Biochem. Pharmacol. 2014;89:441–52.

Eyre et al. (27) provides an account of NS5A that discloses its role in virus assembly at the location of the membranous web, and at the location of the lipid droplet. **NS5A** appears not to possess any enzymatic activity (28). A knowledge of certain amino acids of NS5A's polypeptide chain is needed to understand naturally occurring mutations in NS5A that result in drug resistance, or that are part of the binding site of various anti-HCV drugs.

NS5A has the ability to recruit and activate the lipid kinase phosphatidylinositol-kinase III alpha, to stimulate the local production of phosphatidylinositol 4-phosphate, and to induce morphologically normal *membranous webs*. Also, NS5A is essential for viral genome replication within cytoplasmic replication complexes and virus assembly at the surface of the *lipid droplet* (29). **NS5A** is used for movement

of subcellular particles in the infected hepatocyte, that is, for "vesicular traffic." This vesicular traffic includes movement of endosomes along microtubules, where movement depends on motor proteins, such as dynein and kinesin.

NS5A has several serine residues, which can be phosphorylated during HCV's lifecycle. Serine-225, in particular, is essential for the replication of the HCV genome (30). It has been proposed that serine-225 is used in the regulation of HCV's lifecycle, that is, to switch from intervals in the viral lifecycle that are used for replication, and intervals that are used for viral assembly (31).

This is about mutations. Mutations in **NS5A** that confer resistance to drugs, include the mutation Tyr-93-His, and the mutation Leu-31-Val (32,33). "Tyr-93-His" means that the wild type tyrosine residue has, by the mutation, been replaced by a histidine residue. Footnote (34)

---

[27]Eyre NS, Fiches GN, Aloia A, et al. Dynamic imaging of the hepatitis C virus NS5A protein during a productive infection. J. Virol. 2014;88:3636−52.

[28]Kwon HJ, et al. Direct binding of ledipasvir to HCV NS5A: mechanism of resistance to an HCV antiviral agent. PLoS One. 2015;1:e0122844 (14 pp).

[29]Eyre NS, Fiches GN, Aloia A, et al. Dynamic imaging of the hepatitis C virus NS5A protein during a productive infection. J. Virol. 2014;88:3636−52.

[30]Ross-Thriepland D, et al. Serine phosphorylation of the hepatitis C virus NS5A protein controls the establishment of replication complexes. J. Virol. 2015;89:3123−35.

[31]Kohler JJ, et al. Approaches to hepatitis C treatment and cure using NS5A inhibitors. Inf. Drug Resistance 2014;7:41−56.

[32]Kwon HJ, et al. Direct binding of ledipasvir to HCV NS5A: mechanism of resistance to an HCV antiviral agent. PLoS One. 2015;1:e0122844 (14 p).

[33]Ascher DB, et al. Potent hepatitis C inhibitors bind directly to NS5A and reduce its affinity for RNA. Sci. Rep. 2014;4:4765. doi: 10.1038.

[34]ABT-267, daclatasvir, ledipasvir, ACH-2928, ACH-3102, PPI-668, AZD-7295, MK-8742, and GSK 2336805.

provides a list of drugs that inhibit NS5A (35). HCV acquires mutations in NS5A that cause drug resistance, where these mutations occur at methionine-28, glutamine-30, leucine-31, glutamine-54, histidine-58, and tyrosine-93 (36,37). The exact list of mutations can differ between different genotypes of HCV.

VIII. NS5B—HCV'S RNA POLYMERASE

NS5B is an RNA-dependent RNA polymerase, that is, it uses ssRNA (single-stranded RNA) as a template for the generation of dsRNA (double-stranded RNA). NS5B is a membrane-bound protein that contains a tail that anchors the protein to the membrane. Also, NS5B has domains called finger domains, palm domain, and thumb domain. The thumb and finger domains encircle the active site of the enzyme (38).

A knowledge of these domains is essential when designing drugs that inhibit NS5B, and when classifying mutations that confer resistance to these drugs (39). The drugs filibuvir and lomibuvir bind to the "thumb domain," while the drugs, dasabuvir, HCV-796, and GSK5852 bind to the "palm domain" (40).

This is about mutations in NS5B's polypeptide chain. HCV has a high sequence diversity, resulting in what is called, "viral quasispecies." The presence of several viral quasispecies in any given patient suffering from HCV infection enhances the virus' ability to evade anti-HCV drugs. For example, the mutation Ser-282-Thr encoded by the *NS5B* gene confers resistance to various anti-HCV drugs (41,42). Footnote (43) provides a list of inhibitors of NS5B (44). This list of NS5B inhibitors includes sofosbuvir.

[35]De Clercq E. Current race in the development of DAAs (direct-acting antivirals) against HCV. Biochem. Pharmacol. 2014;89:441−52.

[36]Kohler JJ, et al. Approaches to hepatitis C treatment and cure using NS5A inhibitors. Inf. Drug Resist. 2014;7:41−56.

[37]Fridell RA, Wang C, Sun JH, et al. Genotypic and phenotypic analysis of variants resistant to hepatitis C virus nonstructural protein 5A replication complex inhibitor BMS-790052 in humans: in vitro and in vivo correlations. Hepatology 2011;54:1924−35.

[38]Chevaliez S, Pawlotsky JM. HCV genome and life cycle. In: Chapter 1. Tan SL, editor. Hepatitis C viruses: genomes and molecular biology. Norfolk (UK): Horizon Biosciences; 2006.

[39]Devlogelaere B, Berke JM, Vijgen L, et al. TMC647055, a potent nonnucleoside hepatitis C virus NS5B polymerase inhibitor with cross-genotypic coverage. Antimicrob. Agents Chemother. 2012;56:4676−84.

[40]Kati W, et al. In vitro activity and resistance profile of dasabuvir, a nonnucleoside hepatitis C virus polymerase inhibitor. Antimicrob. Agents Chemother. 2015;59:1505−11.

[41]Bartels DJ, et al. Natural prevalence of hepatitis C virus variants with decreased sensitivity to NS3/4A protease Inhibitors in treatment-Naive Subjects. J. Infect. Dis. 2008;198:800−7.

[42]Gotte M. Resistance to nucleotide analogue inhibitors of hepatitis C virus NS5B: mechanisms and clinical relevance. Curr. Opin. Virol. 2014;8:104−8.

[43]NS5B (nucleoside-type) polymerase inhibitors: sofosbuvir, GS-0938, mericitabine, VX-135, ALS 2158 and TMC 649128; NS5B (non-nucleoside-type) polymerase inhibitors: VX-222, ABT-072, ABT-333, deleobuvir, tegobuvir, setrobuvir, VCH-916, VCH-759, BMS-791325 and TMC-647055.

[44]De Clercq E. Current race in the development of DAAs (direct-acting antivirals) against HCV. Biochem. Pharmacol. 2014;89:441−52.

IX. E1 AND E2—HCV'S ENVELOPE PROTEINS

E1 and E2 are released from the HCV polyprotein by cleavage of specific peptide bonds. Once released, E1 and E2 associate with each other to form a heterodimer. In the intact HCV virus, the E1/E2 heterodimer functions to bind to and enter human hepatocytes. When HCV binds to the host cell, it fuses its own lipid envelope with the host cell's plasmid membrane, resulting in the materialization of a "nucleocapsid" in the host cell's cytoplasm. When HCV infects the hepatocyte, it binds to a protein called tetraspanin (CD81) or to scavenger receptor class B type I (SR-BI), where this binding has a direct role in HCV's entry into the host cell. Also, at a later point in HCV's lifecycle when new HCV virus particles are being assembled, E1 and E2 anchor the HCV to the endoplasmic reticulum of the host cell (45).

X. CORE PROTEIN OF HCV

HCV's core protein is soluble in water, in contrast to the envelope proteins (E1, E2), which are anchored to the phospholipid membranes of the host cell, or anchored to the phospholipid membrane of individual virus particles. Core protein forms an oligomer that surrounds the RNA genome, thus forming a nucleocapsid that protects the viral genome (46). HCV replication occurs in the host cell, in a structure called, "membranous web." The membranous web is derived from the host cell's endoplasmic reticulum, and it appears to be a rearrangement of part of the host cell's endoplasmic reticulum. Membranous web consists of double-membrane vesicles and single-membrane vesicles. Paul et al. (47) provide a cartoon diagram of the double-membrane vesicles.

After HCV replication is completed, viral proteins and RNA occur on a structure called the "lipid droplet." The lipid droplet is surrounded by a phospholipid monolayer, and it likely originates by budding from the endoplasmic reticulum into the cytosol (48).

A transition point occurs when HCV particles are being assembled. The transition is from being associated with membranous web, to being associated with the "lipid droplets." Core protein is retained at the endoplasmic reticulum membrane until cleavage of the signal peptide of the core protein, thus releasing the mature core protein, which then traffics to the surface of cellular lipid droplets (49).

[45]Lavie M, et al. HCV glycoproteins: assembly of a functional E1-E2 Heterodimer. In: Chapter 4. Tan SL, editor. Hepatitis C viruses: genomes and molecular biology. Norfolk (UK): Horizon Biosciences; 2006.

[46]Jones DM, et al. A genetic interaction between the core and NS3 proteins of hepatitis C virus is essential for production of infectious virus. J. Virol. 2011;85:12351−61.

[47]Paul D, et al. Morphological and biochemical characterization of the membranous hepatitis C virus replication compartment. J. Virol. 2013;87:10612−27.

[48]Popescu CI, et al. Hepatitis C virus life cycle and lipid metabolism. Biology 2014;3:892−921.

[49]Jones DM, et al. A genetic interaction between the core and NS3 proteins of hepatitis C virus is essential for production of infectious virus. J. Virol. 2011;85:12351−61.

XI. INNATE IMMUNE RESPONSE AGAINST HCV

a. Introduction

The RNA molecules of HCV stimulate pathways involving:

- Toll-like receptors (TLRs);
- RIG-like receptors;
- NOD-like receptors (50,51).

Of the TLRs, the main sensors of HCV RNA are TLR3 and TLR7. TLR3 recognizes dsRNA. TLR7 recognizes ssRNA. TLR3 and TLR7 reside in the endosomes of the hepatocyte (52). Location inside endosomes provides an environment in which host DNA should not be present, thus avoiding deleterious effects of self-recognition (53). As is the case with all TLRs, when a foreign molecule such as a viral nucleic acid binds to the TLR, the result is that the TLR activates another component of the immune system, with the consequent activation of innate immune response.

RIG-like receptors are especially sensitive to the poly(U/UC) tract that is part of the HCV genome (54,55). The RIG-like receptors include three proteins, RIG-I, MDA5, and LGP2. RIG-I stands for *retinoic acid inducible gene-1*. MDA5 stands for *melanoma differentiation associated gene 5*, and LGP2 stands for, *laboratory of genetics and physiology 2*. RIG-I is an intracellular molecule that responds to viral nucleic acids and activates downstream signaling, resulting in the induction of interferon. The consequence of the activation of RIG-I and TLR3, is that the host cell expresses interferon-beta (56).

b. Innate Immune Response Includes Interferon-Beta

The first cytokine that is involved in innate response against HCV is interferon-beta, which is expressed by infected hepatocytes. Interferon-beta expression is stimulated by HCV's interactions with TLR3 and RIG-I. Secreted interferon-beta induces an antiviral state that extends to not-yet-infected neighboring cells, where the neighboring cells respond by expressing OAS proteins and RNAse L. The OAS proteins are activated when they bind to dsRNA, where in this activated form, the OAS proteins alter RNase L to produce activated RNase L. This activated RNase L degrades viral RNA. When RNase L cleaves viral RNA, thereby generating small pieces of RNA, these small pieces are

[50]Heim MH, Thimme R. Innate and adaptive immune response in HCV infections. J. Hepatol. 2014;61:S14–S25.

[51]Horner SM. Activation and evasion of antiviral innate immunity by hepatitis C virus. J. Mol. Biol. 2013;426:1198–209.

[52]Metz P, et al. Interferon-stimulated genes and their role in controlling hepatitis C virus. J. Hepatol. 2013;59:1331–41.

[53]Funk E, et al. Tickling the TLR7 to cure viral hepatitis. J. Trans. Med. 2014;12:125 (8 p).

[54]Metz P, et al. Interferon-stimulated genes and their role in controlling hepatitis C virus. J. Hepatol. 2013;59:1331–41.

[55]Horner SM. Activation and evasion of antiviral innate immunity by hepatitis C virus. J. Mol. Biol. 2013;426:1198–209.

[56]Kalkeri G, et al. Restoration of the activated rig-I pathway in hepatitis C virus (HCV) replicon cells by HCV protease, polymerase, and NS5A inhibitors in vitro at clinically relevant concentrations. Antimicrob. Agents Chemother. 2013;57:4417–26.

recognized by RIG-I and MDA5, further increasing the innate immune response against HCV. OAS1 means, 2′−5′ oligoadenylate synthase (57,58).

c. HCV Inhibits Immune Responses

HCV impairs immune response by inhibiting innate immune response, and by inhibiting adaptive immune response. HCV evades innate immune response by damaging TLRs. HCV evades adaptive immune response by provoking exhaustion of T cells.

This is about *innate immunity*. HCV's N3/4A protease catalyzes the cleavage and inactivation of host cell proteins that sense the presence of HCV's RNA (59). HCV's proteins and HCV's nucleic acid are sensed by TLRs, where the proteins are sensed by TLR2 and TLR4, and the RNA is sensed by TLR3, TLR7, and TLR9. TLR3 detects double-stranded RNA intermediates that exist during replication of the HCV genome. However, as stated above, N3/4A protease inactivates host cell proteins that mediate innate immune response against HCV. In detail, the N3/4A protease inactivates host cell proteins called MAVS and TRIF.

This concerns *T-cell exhaustion*. Yamada et al. (60) characterized T-cell exhaustion as a mechanism where viruses "subvert host immunity." The mechanisms of T-cell exhaustion concern adaptive immune response. HCV-infected patients have higher PD-1 expression on $CD4^+$ T cells and $CD8^+$ T cells, compared with healthy human subjects. Also, in patients with chronic HCV, NK cells expressed higher levels of PD-1, consistent with their greater functional incompetence and less mature differentiation state (61). Treatment with HCV-drugs consequently results in lower PD-1 expression, that is, expression back to normal low levels.

Exhaustion of $CD8^+$ T cells that follows a pattern of progressive loss of function, that is, decreased IL-2 and TNF-alpha secretion, followed by loss of IFN-gamma production. Exhaustion culminates in loss of cytolytic activity of $CD8^+$ T cells (62). Chronic exposure of viral antigens to T cells provokes increased expression of PD-1 by the T cell (63).

In chronic infection, HCV-specific T cells are focused on only a few HCV antigens, and these T cells decline to such low numbers that they are often undetectable in the blood. The few HCV-specific T cells that are detectable display an

[57]Kristiansen H, Scherer CA, McVean M, et al. Extracellular 2′-5′ oligoadenylate synthetase stimulates RNase L-independent antiviral activity: a novel mechanism of virus-induced innate immunity. J. Virol. 2010;84:1898−11904.

[58]Rehermann B. Hepatitis C virus versus innate and adaptive immune responses: a tale of coevolution and coexistence. J. Clin. Invest. 2009;119:1745−54.

[59]Heim MH, Thimme R. Innate and adaptive immune responses in HCV infections. J. Hepatol. 2014;61:S14−S25.

[60]Yamada DH, et al. Suppression of Fcγ-receptor-mediated antibody effector function during persistent viral infection. Immunity 2015;42:379−90.

[61]Golden-Mason L, et al. Race-dependent differences failure of response to antiviral therapy: chronic hepatitis C virus and predicts expression is increased on immunocytes in cutting edge: programmed death-1. J. Immunol. 2008;180:3637−41.

[62]McMahan RH, et al. Tim-3 expression on PD-1 + HCV-specific human CTLs is associated with viral persistence, and its blockade restores hepatocyte-directed in vitro cytotoxicity. J. Clin. Inv. 2010;120:4546−57.

[63]Kroy DC, Ciuffreda D, Cooperider JH, et al. Liver environment and HCV replication affect human T-cell phenotype and expression of inhibitory receptors. Gastroenterology 2014;146:550−61.

exhausted phenotype with decreased ability to proliferate, to kill infected target cells, or to produce cytokines (64). This T-cell dysfunction is attributed to high levels of persisting viral antigen that drive the expression of PD-1 on virus-specific T cells. The ligand, PD-L1, is expressed on hepatocytes, Kupffer cells, and stellate cells. Interaction of PD-L1 with PD-1 expressed by the T cells that infiltrate the liver, results in inhibition of antiviral functions of the T cells (65). To summarize, when HCV infects the host's T cell, the HCV provokes an increase in the T cell's expression of PD-1, where the result of the increased PD-1 expression is that other host cells transmit a signal via PD-L1 to PD-1, thus inhibiting the T cell.

d. Innate Immune Response by NK Cells

NK cells recognize and lyse virus-infected cells, and inhibit viral replication. NK cells constitute about 30% of resident lymphocytes in a normal liver, and may account for as many as 60% of lymphocytes in HCV infections (66). The NK cell's ability to lyse virus-infected cells is mediated by two proteins of the NK cell, granzyme and perforin. The NK cell's noncytolytic response against HCV is mediated by interferon-gamma that is secreted by the NK cell, which inhibits HCV replication in nearby hepatocytes.

During acute infections, the interferon-gamma that is secreted by NK cells does not kill host cells, but instead it blocks HCV replication (67). Studies with hepatocyte cell lines determined that interferon-gamma inhibits HCV replication, as determined by adding pure interferon-gamma to the cells, and measuring synthesis of NS5A (68). Delving into more detail, the interferon-gamma suppression of HCV replication is mediated by interferon-gamma's stimulation of host cell genes, such as *IFIT3*, *TRIM14*, *IFITM1*, and *IFITM3* (69,70). In the body, interferon-gamma is produced only by NK cells, T cells, and macrophages (71).

XII. CHRONIC INFLAMMATION

a. Introduction

Chronic activation of innate immune response, as it occurs in chronic HCV

[64]Raghuraman S, et al. Spontaneous clearance of chronic hepatitis C virus infection is associated with appearance of neutralizing antibodies and reversal of T-cell exhaustion. J. Inf. Dis. 2012;205:763−71.

[65]Raghuraman S, et al. Spontaneous clearance of chronic hepatitis C virus infection is associated with appearance of neutralizing antibodies and reversal of T-cell exhaustion. J. Inf. Dis. 2012;205:763−71.

[66]Spengler U, et al. Between Scylla and Charybdis: the role of the human immune system in the pathogenesis of hepatitis C. World J. Gastroenterol. 2013;19:7852−66.

[67]Kokordelis P, Kramer B, Korner C, et al. An effective interferon-gamma-mediated Inhibition of hepatitis C virus replication by natural killer cells is associated with spontaneous clearance of acute hepatitis C in human immunodeficiency virus-positive patients. Hepatology 2014;59:814−27.

[68]Frese M, Schwarzle V, Barth K, et al. Interferon-gamma inhibits replication of subgenomic and genomic hepatitis C virus RNAs. Hepatology 2002;35:694−703.

[69]Metz P, Dazert E, Ruggieri A, et al. Identification of type I and type II interferon-induced effectors controlling hepatitis C virus. Hepatology 2012;56:2082−93.

[70]Metz P, et al. Interferon-stimulated genes and their Role in controlling hepatitis C virus. J. Hepatol. 2013;59:1331−41.

[71]Frese M, Schwarzle V, Barth K, et al. Interferon-gamma inhibits replication of subgenomic and genomic hepatitis C virus RNAs. Hepatology 2002;35:694−703.

infections, contributes to various pathologies such as liver fibrosis, cirrhosis, and the development of HCC (72). Cirrhosis is sometimes a component of the study design of clinical trials for anti-HCV drugs. In one trial, cirrhosis was one of the exclusion criteria (73). In another clinical trial, subjects with cirrhosis were permitted to enroll in the trial, but they were required to be stratified according to the presence or absence of cirrhosis (74). Chronic inflammation can result in cirrhosis of the liver as well as liver cancer, that is, HCC. The damage that is caused by the immune system to the liver is separate from, and in addition to, that caused by the virus alone (75,76,77,78).

b. Stellate Cells, Fibrosis, and Cirrhosis

In patients with chronic HCV infections about 20% develop cirrhosis. Progression to cirrhosis takes about 20—50 years. Cirrhosis of the liver is staged according to the Metavir system, with F1 indicating portal fibrosis without septa, F2 portal fibrosis with few septa, F3 septal fibrosis without cirrhosis, and F4 cirrhosis. The Metavir score evaluates data from a liver biopsy (79,80). Dienstag (81) and Ramadori and Bernhard (82) provide accounts of the distinction between portal fibrosis and septal fibrosis.

Hepatic stellate cells are involved in HCV-induced liver fibrosis. The stellate cells reside in the liver in areas called the space of Disse. Stellate cells, which represent about 5—8% of the cells of the liver, are distinguished in that they are rich in vitamin A and store nearly 80% of retinoids of the human body in their lipid droplets in the cytoplasm (83). HCV-infected hepatocytes release transforming growth factor-beta1 (TGF-beta-1) and other profibrogenic factors which, in turn, activate stellate cells.

[72]Spengler U, et al. Between Scylla and Charybdis: the role of the human immune system in the pathogenesis of hepatitis C. World J. Gastroenterol. 2013;19:7852—66.

[73]Gane EJ, et al. Nucleotide polymerase inhibitor sofosbuvir plus ribavirin for hepatitis C. N. Engl. J. Med. 2013;368:34—44.

[74]Afdhal N, Zeuzem S, Kwo P, et al. Ledipasvir and sofosbuvir for untreated HCV genotype 1 infection. N. Engl. J. Med. 2014;370:1889—98.

[75]Cruise MW, Lukens JR, Nguyen AP, Lassen MG, Waggoner SN, Hahn YS. Fas ligand is responsible for CXCR3 chemokine induction in CD4 + T cell-dependent liver damage. J. Immunol. 2006;176:6235—44.

[76]Cruise MW, Melief HM, Lukens J, Soguero C, Hahn YS. Increased Fas ligand expression of CD4 + T cells by HCV core induces T cell-dependent hepatic inflammation. J. Leukoc. Biol. 2005;78:412—25.

[77]Urbani S, Amadei B, Fisicaro P, et al. Heterologous T cell immunity in severe hepatitis C virus infection. J. Exp. Med. 2005;201:675—80.

[78]Bertoletti A, Maini MK. Protection or damage: a dual role for the virus-specific cytotoxic T lymphocyte response in hepatitis B and C infection? Curr. Opin. Immunol. 2000;12:403—8.

[79]Muir AH. Cirrhosis in hepatitis C virus-infected patients: a review for practitioners new to hepatitis C care. Top. Antiviral Med. 2014;22:685—89.

[80]Boursier J, et al. Comparison of fibrosis degree classifications by liver biopsy and non-Invasive tests in chronic hepatitis C. BMC Gastroenterol. 2011;11:132 (13 p).

[81]Dienstag JL. The role of liver biopsy in chronic Hepatitis C. Hepatology 2002;36:S151—S160.

[82]Ramadori G, Bernhard S. Portal tract fibrogenesis in the liver. Lab. Inv. 2004;84:153—9.

[83]Brody T. Nutritional biochemistry. 2nd ed. San Diego, CA: Academic Press; 1999. p. 555—7.

But chronic injury to the liver can activate the stellate cells, resulting in the conversion of *stellate cells* into proliferative, *myofibroblast-like cells*, which produce molecules that result in fibrogenesis (84).

With this conversion, the molecules expressed by stellate cells include proteins of the extracellular matrix, such as collagen types I and III, fibronectin, and laminin (85,86).

During chronic liver injury, as in chronic HCV infections, normal collagen type IV is lost and replaced with collagen types I and III, as well as with other extracellular matrix proteins, such as elastin, hyaluronan, proteoglycans, and fibronectin (87). These changes impair the transport of nutrients and other solutes to the hepatocytes. Another change that impairs transport of nutrients to the hepatocyte is that the hepatocytes lose their microvilli (88). The term "scar deposition" may be used to refer to fibrosis of the liver, where the scar contains high levels of fibrillar collagen type I and type III. Cirrhosis is defined as an abnormal liver architecture, with "fibrotic septa" and altered vascularization (89).

The liver stands out from all other tissues by its ability to regenerate from and reverse fibrotic lesions. Thus, it is the case that fibrosis may be reversed. In other words, with treatment of HCV, it is the case that liver fibrosis may be reversed (90).

XIII. ONCOGENES AND GROWTH FACTORS

a. Introduction to Oncogenes and Growth Factors Relevant to HCC

HCC is a risk with chronic HCV infection. The risk for this type of cancer increases as liver fibrosis progresses, and once cirrhosis is established, the risk for this cancer is about 1−7% per year (91).

Hoshida et al. (92) and Whittaker et al. (93) provide lists of genes, mutations, enzymes, and signaling pathways that connect *chronic HCV* infections to eventual *HCC*. It is not yet known which components in these lists of genes, mutations, and such, are necessary or sufficient for the generation of HCC. But to

---

[84]Nishitsuji H, et al. Hepatitis C virus infection induces inflammatory cytokines and chemokines mediated by the cross talk between hepatocytes and stellate cells. J. Virol. 2013;87:8169−78.

[85]Bandyopadhyay S, et al. Hepatitis C virus infection and hepatic stellate cell activation downregulate miR-29: miR-29 overexpression reduces hepatitis C viral abundance in culture. J. Inf. Dis. 2011;203:1753−52.

[86]Elpek GO. Cellular and molecular mechanisms in the pathogenesis of liver fibrosis: an update. World J. Gastroenterol. 2014;20:7260−76.

[87]Albanis E, Friedman SL. Antifibrotic agents for liver disease. Am J. Transplant. 2006;6:12−9.

[88]Albanis E, Friedman SL. Antifibrotic agents for liver disease. Am J. Transplant. 2006;6:12−9.

[89]Mallat A, Lotersztajn S. Cellular mechanisms of tissue fibrosis. 5. novel Insights into liver fibrosis. Am. J. Physiol. Cell Physiol. 2013;305:C789−C799.

[90]Zeisberg M, Kalluri R. Cellular mechanisms of tissue fibrosis. 1. common and organ-specific mechanisms associated with tissue fibrosis. Am. J. Physiol. Cell Physiol. 2013;304:C216−C225.

[91]Hoshida Y, et al. Pathogenesis and prevention of hepatitis C virus-induced hepatocellular carcinoma. J. Hepatol. 2014;61:S79−S90.

[92]Hoshida Y, et al. Pathogenesis and prevention of hepatitis C virus-induced hepatocellular carcinoma. J. Hepatol. 2014;61:S79−S90.

[93]Whittaker S, et al. The role of signaling pathways in the development and treatment of hepatocellular carcinoma. Oncogene 2010;29:4989−5005.

provide a starting point, this outlines pathways involving the proteins:

- RAS;
- IGF-2;
- PTEN.

For convenience, this glossary is provided:

1. IGF-2 is insulin-like growth factor-2;
2. EGF is epidermal growth factor;
3. ERK is extracellular signal-regulated kinase;
4. HGF is hepatocyte growth factor;
5. MEK means MAPK/Erk kinase;
6. PTEN is phosphatase and tensin homolog deleted on chromosome 10;
7. PI3K is phosphoinositide 3-kinase.

b. Ras

Ras expression has been correlated with HCC in HCV-infected patients. Newell et al. (94) analyzed samples of human HCC in HCV-infected patients, where the results showed increased expression of Ras. More specifically, the samples were analyzed for changes in expression of three kinds of Ras, that is, H-ras, K-ras, and N-ras. Upregulation was found only for H-ras. In some of the samples, H-ras expression was increased by over threefold. Expression levels of K-ras and N-ras was unchanged. Liver samples from normal samples were used a controls, as described elsewhere (95).

This provides a large picture of the view that connects Ras, as well as mutations in Ras, to signals that control expression of various genes. Ras is a membrane-bound protein of the plasma membrane that transduces various signals from the cell membrane to the nucleus. About 30% of all cancers have constitutive activation of the Ras-mediated signaling. With activation, the activated Ras binds to and activates Raf, a serine kinase, which subsequently activates MEK1 and MEK2. Next, the activated MEK1 and MEK2 phosphorylate and activate ERK1 and ERK2. Once activated, ERK1 and ERK2 enter the nucleus, where they influence the expression of various genes (96).

Activation of the *RAS* gene can arise from mutations in the *RAS* gene, as well as from increased levels of growth factors that stimulate various signaling pathways (97). IGF-2 is part of the mechanism of HCC. In HCC, overexpression of IGF-2 is driven by alterations in promoters that are part of the gene encoding IGF-2. The *IGF-2* gene has four promoters, namely, P1, P2, P3, and P4. In HCC, the methylation status of one of these promoters (P4) changes, where the change is that the promoter has fewer methyl groups. The consequence of this reduced methylation is increased expression of IGF-2 (98,99).

Increased expression of both IGF (the ligand) and IGF receptor (the receptor) occurs in HCC, resulting in stimulation of the listed signaling pathways, where the consequence

[94]Newell P, Toffanin S, Villanueva A, et al. Ras pathway activation in hepatocellular carcinoma and anti-tumoral effect of combined sorafenib and rapamycin in vivo. J. Hepatol. 2009;51:725−33.

[95]Villanueva A, Chiang DY, Newell P, et al. Pivotal role of mTOR signaling in hepatocellular carcinoma. Gastroenterology 2008;135:1972−83.

[96]Zhang Q, et al. Activation of the Ras/Raf/MEK pathway facilitates hepatitis C virus replication via attenuation of the interferon-JAK-STAT pathway. J. Virol. 2012;86:1544−54.

[97]Gollob JA, et al. Role of Raf kinase in cancer: therapeutic potential of targeting the Raf/MEK/ERK signal transduction pathway. Semin. Oncol. 2006;33: 392−406.

[98]Tang SH, et al. Hypomethylated P4 promoter induces expression of the insulin-like growth factor-II gene in hepatocellular carcinoma in a Chinese population. Clin. Cancer Res. 2006;12:4171−77.

[99]Nardone G, et al. Activation of fetal promoters of insulin-like growth factors II, in hepatitis C virus-related chronic hepatitis, cirrhosis, and hepatocellular carcinoma. Hepatology 1996;23:1304−12.

is the transformation of hepatocytes to HCC cells:

- RAF/MEK/ERK signaling pathway;
- PI3/Act/mTOR signaling pathway;
- WNT/beta-catenin signaling pathway.

c. HCV Core Protein Stimulates Cell-Signaling Pathways

As stated above, mutations in *Ras* can increase the activity of *Ras*, resulting in increased signaling by various cell-signaling pathways, and where this increased signaling can promote the development of HCC. In addition, HCV core protein may activate one or more cell-signaling pathways. In a study by Giambartolomei et al. (100), researchers modified human cells by adding a plasmid that expressed HCV core protein. With expression of core protein in the cells, the result was phosphorylation of ERK proteins that were endogenous to the cell.

In addition to increased ERK phosphorylation, the core protein induced a prolonged ERK response to the growth factor, EGF. In other words, it was the case that core protein potentiated the effect of EGF. To summarize, the two influences of core protein are to *increase ERK phosphorylation* and to *potentiate EGF's effect in stimulating ERK phosphorylation*.

Core protein's effect on stimulating ERK phosphorylation was also shown by Erhardt

et al. (101) and Hayashi et al. (102), further implicating core protein's possible role in promoting the formation of HCC.

d. PTEN

PTEN antagonizes the PI3K/AKT/mTOR signaling pathway. PTEN is a tumor suppressor, mainly involved in maintaining the phosphatidylinositol 3-kinase (PI3K)/AKT signaling pathway. PTEN reverses the action of PI3K, thereby hampering all downstream functions controlled by AKT/mTOR signaling, such as cycle progression, apoptosis, transcription, translation, and stimulation of angiogenesis (103). PTEN function is commonly lost in many human cancers by way of, for example, genetic mutations or epigenetic mechanisms.

Bao et al. (104) introduced HCV's RNA genome into human hepatocytes, and detected inhibition of transport of PTEN from the cell's cytoplasm to the cell's nucleus. In detail, these researchers discovered that a small RNA (vmr11) encoded by HCV's genome has the influence of downregulating transportin-2, where the reduced levels of transportin-2 are associated with impaired transport of PTEN to the nucleus. These data fit into earlier work, establishing PTEN's role as a tumor suppressor, and characterizing the relative amounts of cytosolic versus nuclear PTEN. As part of the scenario of PTEN's proposed role in the etiology of HCC, Shan et al. (105) provided data

[100]Giambartolomei S, et al. Sustained activation of Raf/MEK/Erk pathway in response to EGF in stable cell lines expressing hepatitis C virus (HCV) core protein. Oncogene 2001;20:2606—10.

[101]Erhardt A, et al. Hepatitis C virus core protein induces cell proliferation and activates ERK, JNK, and p38 MAP kinases together with the MAP kinase phosphatase MKP-1 in a hepG2 tet-off cell line. Virology 2002;292:272—84.

[102]Hayashi J, Aoki H, Kajino K, et al. Hepatitis C virus core protein activates the MAPK/ERK cascade synergistically with tumor promoter TPA, but not with epidermal growth factor or transforming growth factor alpha. Hepatology 2000;32:958—61.

[103]Milella M, et al. PTEN: multiple functions in human malignant tumors. Front. Oncol. 2015;doi:10.3389 (14 p).

[104]Bao W, et al. Loss of nuclear PTEN in HCV-infected human hepatocytes. Infect. Agents Cancer 2014;9:23 (11 p).

[105]Shan SW, Fang L, Shatseva T, et al. Mature miR-17-5p and passenger miR-17-3p induce hepatocellular carcinoma by targeting PTEN, GalNT7 and vimentin in different signal pathways. J. Cell Sci. 2013;126:1517—30.

establishing that inhibiting PTEN had the result of stimulating formation of HCC.

XIV. ACQUIRED IMMUNE RESPONSE AGAINST HCV

a. Introduction

Acquired immune response against HCV is outlined here. Antigens of the infecting agent that may be targeted by human immune response are relevant to the mechanisms of action of any infection. Antigenic peptides are generated by the immune system's processing of the HCV polyprotein. During the life cycle of HCV, the polyprotein is processed to form a number of small proteins. The ability of these proteins, and of portions of these proteins, to stimulate the immune system has been exhaustively studied. One such study was that of Chang et al. (106). This study found that nine short stretches, or *epitopes*, from this protein are unusually immunogenic. In brief, the authors studied CD8$^+$ T cells from patients infected with HCV, and CD8$^+$ T cells from normal human subjects, and found that only the T cells from infected patients displayed an immune response against these nine epitopes. The goal of the study was to identify the most immunogenic regions of the hepatitis C protein, for use as a vaccine against the virus. The nine epitopes are as follows:

1. RLGVRATRK;
2. KTSERSQPR;
3. QLFTFSPRR;
4. RMYVGGVEHR;
5. LGFGAYMSK;
6. LIFCHSKKK;
7. GVAGALVAFK;
8. VAGALVAFK;
9. LPGCSFSIF.

In a separate study, Schultz Zur Wiesch et al. (107) also studied the HCV polyprotein, and identified peptide epitopes that are presented by MHC class II, and are recognized by CD4$^+$ T cells. Two of these peptide epitopes from the Wiesch study are shown below:

1. PAAYAAQGKVLVLNPSVAA;
2. GIQYLAGLSTLPGNP.

For any virus infection, it is important that the viral proteins contain epitopes that are recognized by MHC class I of the human host and also by MHC class II of the human host. The reason for this is that effective immune response against most, or perhaps all, infections requires a concerted effort involving CD8$^+$ T cells and CD4$^+$ T cells. Shown below is the sequence of the entire HCV polyprotein, where the most antigenic epitopes are **bolded**. The two peptides of Schultz Zur Wiesch et al. (108), can easily be found in the polyprotein. The nine peptides of Chang et al. (109), can also be found in the polyprotein:

[106]Chang KM, Gruener NH, Southwood S, Sidney J, Pape GR, Chisari FV, Sette A. Identification of HLA-A3 and -B7-restricted CTL response to hepatitis C virus in patients with acute and chronic hepatitis C. J. Immunol. 1999;162:1156—64.

[107]Schulze Zur Wiesch J, Lauer GM, Day CL, et al. Broad repertoire of the CD4 + Th cell response in spontaneously controlled hepatitis C virus infection includes dominant and highly promiscuous epitopes. J. Immunol. 2005;175:3603—13.

[108]Schulze Zur Wiesch J, Lauer GM, Day CL, et al. Broad repertoire of the CD4 + Th cell response in spontaneously controlled hepatitis C virus infection includes dominant and highly promiscuous epitopes. J. Immunol. 2005;175:3603—13.

[109]Chang KM, Gruener NH, Southwood S, Sidney J, Pape GR, Chisari FV, Sette A. Identification of HLA-A3 and -B7-restricted CTL response to hepatitis C virus in patients with acute and chronic hepatitis C. J. Immunol. 1999;162:1156—64.

```
   1 mstnpkpqrk tkrntnrrpq dvkfpgggqi vggvyllprr gprlgvratr ktsersqprg
  61 rrqpipkarp pegrtwaqpg ypwplygneg mgwagwllsp rgsrpswgps dprrrsrnlg
 121 kvidtltcgf adlmgyiplv gaplggaara lahgvrvled gvnyatgnlp gcsfsiflla
 181 llscltipas ayevrnvsgv yhvtndcsns sivyeaadmi mhspgcvpcv rennisrcwv
 241 altptlaarn vsvpiktirr hvdllvgaaa fcsamyvgdl cgsvflvsql ftfsprrhet
 301 vqdcncslyp ghvsghrmaw dmmmnwspta alvvsqllri pqavvdmvag ahwgvlagla
 361 yysmvgnwak vlivmllfag vdggtyvtgg aqshtvrgla sfftpgpaqk iqlvntngsw
 421 hinrtalncn dslqtgflaa lfyankfnss gcperlascr pidkfaqgwg pityaepdss
 481 dqrpycwhya prpcgivpas evcgpvycft pspvvvgttd rfgvptyawg gnetdvllln
 541 ntrppqgnwf gctwmngtgf tktcggppcn iggvgnntlt cptdcfrkhp eatyakcgsg
 601 pwltprcmvd ypyrlwhypc tvnftifkvr myvggvehrl naacnwtrge rcdledrdrs
 661 elsplllstt ewqilpcsft tlpalstgli hlhqnivdvq ylygvgsaiv sfaikweyvl
 721 llfllladar vcacfwmmll iaqaeaalen lvvlnaasva rehgmlsflv ffcaawyikg
 781 rlvpgaayal ygvwplllll lalppprayam dremaascgg avfvglillt lsphykvila
 841 rliwwlqyfi traeahlhvw ipplnvrggr daiilltcav hpelifditk lllailgplm
 901 vlqagivrip yfvraqglir acmlvrkaag ghyvqmalmk laaltgtyvy dhltplrdwa
 961 haglrdlava vepvifsdme ikiitwgadt aacgdiisgl pvsarrgeei llgpadsfeg
1021 qgwrllapit aysqqtrgll gciitsltgr dknqvegevq vvstatqsfl atcvngvcwt
1081 vyhgagsktl agpkgpvtqm ytnvdqdlvg wpappgarsl tpctcsssdl ylvtrhadvi
1141 pvrrrgdgrg sllsprpvsy lkgssggpll cpsghavgif raavctrgva kavdfvpves
1201 mettmrspvf tdnssppavp qtfqvahlha ptgsgkstkv paayaaqgyk vlvlnpsvaa
1261 tlgfgaymsk ahgtdpnirt gvrtittgap itystygkfl adggcsggay diiicdechs
1321 tdsttilgig tvldqaetag arlvvlatat ppgsvtvphs nieevalsnt geipfygkai
1381 pietikggrh lifchskkkc delaaklsgl glnavayyrg ldvsviptsg dvvvvatdal
1441 mtgftgdfds vidcntcvtq tvdfsldptf tietttvpqd avsrsqrrgr tgrgrrgiyr
1501 fvtpgerpsg mfdssvlcec ydagcawyel tpaetsvrlr aylntpglpv cqdhlefwes
1561 vftglthida hflsqtkqag dnfpylvayq atvctralap ppswdqmwkc lirlkptlhg
1621 ptpllyrlga vqneiilthp itkyimacms pdlevvtstw vlvggvlaal aayclttgsv
1681 vivgrinlsg kpavipdrev lyrefdemee cashlpyieq gmhlaeqfkq kalgllqtat
1741 kqaeaaapvv eskwqaleaf wakhmwnfis giqylaglst lpgnpaiasl maftasitsp
1801 lttqstllfn ilggwvaaql appsaasafv gagiagaavg siglgkvlvd ilagygagva
1861 galvafkvms gempstedlv nllpailspg alvvgvvcaa vlrrhvgpge gavqwmnrli
1921 afasrgnhvs pthyvpesda aarvtqilss ltitqllkrl hqwinedcst pcsgswlrdi
1981 wewictvltd fktwlqskll prlpgvpfls cqrgykgvwr gdgimqttcp cgaqitghvk
2041 ngsmrivgpk tcsnmwcgtf pinayttgpc tpspapnysr alwrvaaeey vevtrvgdfh
2101 yvtgmttdnv kcpcqvpape fftevdgvrl hryapacrpl lrdevafqvg lhqypvgsql
2161 pcepepdvav ltsmltdpsh itaetakrrl argsppslas ssasqlsaps lkatctthhd
2221 spdadliean llwrqemggn itrvesenkv vildsfdplr aeeddrevsv aaeilrktkk
2281 yppampvwar pdynpplles wkdpdyvppv vhgcplpptk appippprrk rtvvltestv
2341 ssalaelatk tfgssessai dsgtatapld casddgdkgs dvesyssmpp legepgdpdl
2401 sdgswstvse easedvvccs msytwtgali tpcaaeeskl pinplsnsll rhhnmvyatt
2461 srsasqrqkk vtfdrlqvld dhyrdvlkem kakastvkak llsveeackl tpphsakskf
2521 gygakdvrnl sskamnhirs vwkdlledte tpidttimak nevfcvqpek ggrkparliv
2581 fpdlgvrvce kmalydvvst lpqavmgssy gfqyspgqrv eflvntwksk knpmgfsydt
2641 rcfdstvten dirveesiyq ccdlapearq airslterly iggpltnskg qncgyrrcra
2701 sgvlttscgn tltcylkasa acraaklqdc tmlvcgddlv vicesagtqe daaslrvfte
2761 amtrysappg dppqpeydle litscssnvs vahdasgkrv yyltrdpttp laraawetar
2821 htpvnswlgn iimyaptlwa rmilmthffs illaqeqlek aldcqiygat ysiepldlpq
2881 iiqrlhglsa fslhsyspge inrvasclrk lgvpplrvwr hrarsvrakl lsqggraatc
2941 grylfnwavr tklkltpipa asqldlsgwf iagysggdiy hslsrarprw fmwclllllsv
3001 gvgiyllpnr
```

As reviewed by Saito et al. (110), recovery from hepatitis C (HCV) infection requires responses by both CD8$^+$ T cells and CD4$^+$ T cells. Moreover, what is required is response by T cells that are specific for, and recognize, a *variety* of epitopes from HCV (not just one epitope). In other words, if the T-cell response involved only T cells specific for one particular epitope, for example, the epitope of RLGVRATRK, the infected person would not be able to effectively combat the infection. Semmo and Klenerman (111) provide a detailed account of the most stimulatory epitopes of the HCV polyprotein.

b. Methodology Tip—GenBank

The following information is relevant to acquiring the primary sequence of nucleic acids and polypeptides from any organisms, including mammals, plants, yeasts, bacteria, archaea, and viruses, including hepatitis C virus. GenBank is a database, provided by the US Government, which can be accessed on the internet at: www.ncbi.nlm.nih.gov.

Where a person has a sequence of a nucleic acid in hand, and where the goal is to find other nucleic acids having a similar sequence, or related sequence, this goal can be accomplished by inputting that sequence at this website. Where a person has the sequence of an oligopeptide or polypeptide in hand, the same goal can be accomplished using search tools at this website.

Where a researcher is interested in comparing the primary sequences of two polypeptides, this comparison can be accomplished using computer software programs available from the *Expasy Proteomics Server* of the Swiss Institute of Bioinformatics, or by using the *Accelrys* program, available from Biovia, San Diego, CA. Side-by-side comparisons of primary sequences can be used, for example, for determining whether the same oncogene from two different tumors contains the same collection of antigenic epitopes, for determining whether two different viral isolates have acquired the same mutations, or for determining the function of a newly discovered cytokine.

c. Dendritic Cells and Antigens of HCV

At the start of HCV infection, dendritic cells (DCs) take up the virus. The DCs process the HCV polyprotein, and present peptides by way of MHC class I and MHC class II. The peptides bound to MHC class I are presented to CD8$^+$ T cells, resulting in the activation and propagation of these T cells. These T cells eventually kill liver cells that are infected with HCV. The peptides bound to MHC class II are presented to CD4$^+$ T cells, resulting in the activation and propagation of these T cells, where the result is that these helper T cells stimulate the CD8$^+$ T cells. The following accounts for the ability of CD8$^+$ T cells to specifically kill infected hepatocytes. Normal liver cells do not contain HCV proteins on the cell membrane, because normal liver cells do not contain the HCV. But when HCV infects a liver cell, epitopes from the virus are processed and presented on the MHC class I of the liver cell. Thus, the complex of MHC class I/HCV

[110]Saito K, Ait-Goughoulte M, Truscott SM, et al. Hepatitis C virus inhibits cell surface expression of HLA-DR, prevents dendritic cell maturation, and induces interleukin-10 production. J. Virol. 2008;82:3320–28.

[111]Semmo N, Klenerman P. CD4 + T cell responses in hepatitis C virus infection. World J. Gastroenterol. 2007;13:4831–38.

peptide, which resides on the outer surface of liver cells, enables the CD8$^+$ T cells to recognize which liver cells need to be killed (112,113).

To view the big picture relating to MHC class I, this molecular complex is likely utilized at two distinct steps during any kind of infection. The first step is when MHC class I expressed by a DC presents antigens to CD8$^+$ T cells. The second step is when MHC class I expressed by a hepatocyte (or other infected host cell) presents antigens, and allows CD8$^+$ T cells to recognize which host cells need to be killed. In the case of HCV, the host cell that needs to be killed is infected hepatocytes.

As reviewed by Kanto and Hayashi (114), dendritic cells residing in the liver take up HCV antigens. As with many viruses, HCV contains certain molecules that bind to TLRs in the dendritic cell, where this binding stimulates the activation of the dendritic cell. Uptake of antigen by dendritic cells is not enough for the dendritic cells to stimulate T cells. More is needed for effective activation by dendritic cells of T cells. What is also needed is activation of dendritic cells by one or more mechanisms. Takahashi et al. (115) found that ribonucleic acid expressed by HCV can stimulate TLR7 of dendritic cells, resulting in the activation of these dendritic cells. Moreover, Ebihara et al. (116) disclosed that HCV ribonucleic acid can stimulate TLR3. In addition, HCV core protein stimulates TLR2, thereby stimulating immune response against HCV (117,118,119). Chang et al. (120) found that HCV NS3 protein and HCV core protein can transmit signals to the host, by way of TLR1, TLR2, and TLR6. RIG-I is another host protein that mediates innate immune response against HCV. RIG-I, which functions in a manner similar to that of the TLRs, is activated by ribonucleic acid of HCV (121,122).

[112]Gleimer M, Wahl AR, Hickman HD, et al. Although divergent in residues of the peptide binding site, conserved chimpanzee Patr-AL and polymorphic human HLA-A*02 have overlapping peptide-binding repertoires. J. Immunol. 2011;186:1575−88.

[113]Herzer K, Falk CS, Encke J, et al. Upregulation of major histocompatibility complex class I on liver cells by hepatitis C virus core protein via p53 and TAP1 impairs natural killer cell cytotoxicity. J. Virol. 2003;77:8299−309.

[114]Kanto T, Hayashi N. Immunopathogenesis of hepatitis C virus infection: multifaceted strategies subverting innate and adaptive immunity. Intern. Med. 2006;45:183−91.

[115]Takahashi K, Asabe S, Wieland S, et al. Plasmacytoid dendritic cells sense hepatitis C virus-infected cells, produce interferon, and inhibit infection. Proc. Natl. Acad. Sci. USA 2010;107:7431−36.

[116]Ebihara T, Shingai M, Matsumoto M, Wakita T, Seya T. Hepatitis C virus-infected hepatocytes extrinsically modulate dendritic cell maturation to activate T cells and natural killer cells. Hepatology 2008;48:48−58.

[117]Chang S, Dolganiuc A, Szabo G. Toll-like receptors 1 and 6 are involved in TLR2-mediated macrophage activation by hepatitis C virus core and NS3 proteins. J. Leukoc. Biol. 2007;82:479−87.

[118]Brown RA, Gralewski JH, Eid AJ, Knoll BM, Finberg RW, Razonable RR. R753Q single-nucleotide polymorphism impairs toll-like receptor 2 recognition of hepatitis C virus core and nonstructural 3 proteins. Transplantation 2010;89:811−15.

[119]Hoffmann M, Zeisel MB, Jilg N, et al. Toll-like receptor 2 senses hepatitis C virus core protein but not infectious viral particles. J. Innate Immun. 2009;1:446−54.

[120]Chang S, Dolganiuc A, Szabo G. Toll-like receptors 1 and 6 are involved in TLR2-mediated macrophage activation by hepatitis C virus core and NS3 proteins. J. Leukoc. Biol. 2007;82:479−87.

[121]Saito T, Owen DM, Jiang F, Marcotrigiano J, Gale M Jr. Innate immunity induced by composition-dependent RIG-I recognition of hepatitis C virus RNA. Nature. 2008;454:523−27.

[122]Tasaka M, Sakamoto N, Itakura Y, et al. Hepatitis C virus non-structural proteins responsible for suppression of the RIG-I/Cardif-induced interferon response. J. Gen. Virol. 2007;88:3323−33.

HCV also has the ability to suppress innate immune response, for example, by subverting the activity of TLRs. This ability has been extensively documented by many investigators (123,124,125,126). This subversion accounts, in part, for the ability of HCV to mount infections that are chronic and that cannot be resolved.

Once the dendritic cell has acquired HCV antigens, the dendritic cell migrates to the lymph nodes, where it presents HCV antigens to CD4[+] T cells and to CD8[+] T cells. This activates the T cells, and the T cells circulate in the bloodstream and eventually encounter the liver. The CD8[+] T cells kill hepatocytes that are infected with HCV, where the CD8[+] T cells use two methods of killing. The first method, which involves Fas ligand, results in apoptosis of the hepatocyte. The second method, which involves granzyme and perforin, also results in apoptosis of the hepatocyte.

d. Dendritic Cells

Dendritic cells (DCs) are antigen-presenting cells that process antigens, and present them to T cells. DCs also secrete various cytokines, including interleukin-12 (IL-12) and IFN-alpha. DCs occur in two lineages, the *myeloid DCs* and the *plasmacytoid DCs*. The myeloid DCs secrete IL-12, which provokes a Th1-type immune response against hepatocytes infected by HCV. The plasmacytoid DCs secrete interferon-gamma (IFN-gamma), a cytokine having a direct inhibitory effect on HCVs. The immune response against HCV involves both types of DCs (127).

e. Sources of Interferons During HCV Infections

Interferon-alpha (IFN-alpha) and interferon-gamma (IFN-gamma), both naturally expressed and administered as a drug, are issues in HCV infections. Therapeutic IFN-gamma, which is not part of the standard of care for HCV, has been tested for potential therapeutic effects, as shown by Balan et al. (128), and Shin et al. (129).

[123]Miyazaki M, Kanto T, Inoue M, et al. Impaired cytokine response in myeloid dendritic cells in chronic hepatitis C virus infection regardless of enhanced expression of Toll-like receptors and retinoic acid inducible gene-I. J. Med. Virol. 2008;80:980–88.

[124]Chang S, Dolganiuc A, Szabo G. Toll-like receptors 1 and 6 are involved in TLR2-mediated macrophage activation by hepatitis C virus core and NS3 proteins. J. Leukoc. Biol. 2007;82:479–87.

[125]Kaukinen P, Sillanpää M, Kotenko S, et al. Hepatitis C virus NS2 and NS3/4A proteins are potent inhibitors of host cell cytokine/chemokine gene expression. Virol. J. 2006;3:66 (13 p).

[126]Atencia R, Bustamante FJ, Valdivieso A, et al. Differential expression of viral PAMP receptors mRNA in peripheral blood of patients with chronic hepatitis C infection. BMC Infect. Dis. 2007;7:136 (6 p).

[127]Kanto T, Hayashi N. Immunopathogenesis of hepatitis C virus infection: multifaceted strategies subverting innate and adaptive immunity. Intern. Med. 2006;45:183–91.

[128]Balan V, Rosati MJ, Anderson MH, Rakela J. Successful treatment with novel triple drug combination consisting of interferon-gamma, interferon alfacon-1, and ribavirin in a nonresponder HCV patient to pegylated interferon therapy. Dig. Dis. Sci. 2006;51:956–59.

[129]Shin EC, Protzer U, Untergasser A, et al. Liver-directed gamma interferon gene delivery in chronic hepatitis C. J. Virol. 2005 Nov;79:13412–20.

IFN-alpha, which is classed as a type I interferon, is secreted by almost all virus-infected cells (130), and in higher amounts by plasmacytoid DCs (131,132).

Expression of IFN-gamma (the only type II interferon) is restricted to T cells, NK cells, and macrophages (133).

f. What IFN-Gamma does During HCV Infections

Interferon-gamma contributes to HCV clearance in several ways. First, IFN-gamma enhances NK cell activity. Second, IFN-gamma promotes the processing and presentation of antigens, that is, processing by DCs and presentation by DCs to T cells. DCs use MHC class I to present antigens to CD8$^+$ T cells, and MHC class II to present antigens to CD4$^+$ T cells. IFN-gamma stimulates expression of various components of the MHC complex of proteins. Thus, according to Meissner et al. (134), both MHC class I and class II genes are inducible by IFN-gamma stimulation.

Third, IFN-gamma facilitates T cell homing from lymph nodes and peripheral blood to the site of infection by way of inducing chemokines (135). To repeat, IFN-gamma stimulates various cells to express chemokines, and the chemokines (a class of cytokines that causes migration of immune cells) causes T cells to migrate to sites of infections. Finally, IFN-gamma directly inhibits replication of HCV.

g. What T Cells Do During HCV Infections Where the Patient Spontaneously Recovers

In acute self-limited hepatitis C, the HCV-specific responses by CD4$^+$ T cells and CD8$^+$ T cells can be vigorous with more than 10% of all the peripheral blood lymphocytes recognizing HCV antigens (136). In patients spontaneously recovering from an acute HCV infection, T cells express IFN-gamma, where this IFN-gamma is thought to be critical for clearing the HCV infection (137).

[130]Frese M, Schwärzle V, Barth K, et al. Interferon-gamma inhibits replication of subgenomic and genomic hepatitis C virus RNAs. Hepatology 2002;35:694−703.

[131]Cella M, Jarrossay D, Facchetti F, et al. Plasmacytoid monocytes migrate to inflamed lymph nodes and produce large amounts of type I interferon. Nat. Med. 1999;5:919−23.

[132]Dolganiuc A, Chang S, Kodys K, et al. Hepatitis C virus (HCV) core protein-induced, monocyte-mediated mechanisms of reduced IFN-alpha and plasmacytoid dendritic cell loss in chronic HCV infection. J. Immunol. 2006;177:6758−68.

[133]Frese M, Schwärzle V, Barth K, et al. Interferon-gamma inhibits replication of subgenomic and genomic hepatitis C virus RNAs. Hepatology 2002;35:694−703.

[134]Meissner TB, Li A, Biswas A, et al. NLR family member NLRC5 is a transcriptional regulator of MHC class I genes. Proc. Natl. Acad. Sci. USA 2010;107:13794−99.

[135]Shin EC, Protzer U, Untergasser A, et al. Liver-directed gamma interferon gene delivery in chronic hepatitis C. J. Virol. 2005;79:13412−20.

[136]Ahlenstiel G, Titerence RH, Koh C, et al. Natural killer cells are polarized toward cytotoxicity in chronic hepatitis C in an interferon-alfa-dependent manner. Gastroenterology 2010;138:325−35.

[137]Ahlenstiel G, Titerence RH, Koh C, et al. Natural killer cells are polarized toward cytotoxicity in chronic hepatitis C in an interferon-alfa-dependent manner. Gastroenterology 2010;138:325−35.

h. What Immune Cells Do During HCV Infections Where the Patient Develops a Chronic HCV Infection

In chronic hepatitis C, T cells that specifically recognize antigens of HCV are ineffective and functionally impaired. They are terminally differentiated and do not proliferate well. Moreover, they are impaired in their effector functions due to upregulation of inhibitory molecules, such as programmed death-1 (PD-1) and cytotoxic T-lymphocyte antigen 4 (CTLA-4).

HCV-specific T cells are present at very low frequency in both blood and liver of chronically HCV-infected patients, typically comprising less than 0.05% of all the peripheral blood lymphocytes (138).

Once chronic HCV infection is established, NK cells are activated, but the activated NK cells are ineffective against the infection. Activation of NK cells is determined by the expression of CD69, a membrane-bound protein of NK cells.

i. In HCV Infections, IL-12 Stimulates NK Cells to Express IFN-Gamma

In HCV infection, plasmacytoid DCs are the main sources of IFN-alpha. This expression of IFN-alpha can influence the behavior of NK cells. The continual expression of IFN-alpha by plasmacytoid DCs, may contribute to the observed polarization of the NK cell phenotype towards cytotoxicity (139). The NK cells' cytotoxicity kills hepatocytes that are infected by HCV, accounting for the elevated levels of serum liver enzymes that occur during HCV infections. NK cells kill HCV-infected

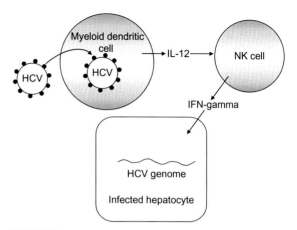

FIGURE 29.1   IFN-gamma-mediated inhibition of HCV replication via IL-12. Hepatitis C virus infects a dendritic cell (DC) where the DC responds by expressing IL-12. The IL-12 induces NK cells to express IFN-gamma.

hepatocytes by the mechanism of antibody-dependent cell cytotoxicity (ADCC). ADCC was explained in this textbook in the earlier chapters on mechanism of action.

The following concerns a mechanism of action that is more subtle than ADCC, namely IL-12's effect of stimulating NK cells to express IFN-gamma (Fig. 29.1). Nellore and Fishman provide a drawing showing one of the sequences of events taking place during HCV infection (140). In this sequence, HCV infects DCs, the DCs express IL-12, the expressed IL-12 contacts NK cells and stimulates the NK cells to express IFN-gamma, and the IFN-gamma travels to nearby HCV-infected hepatocytes and inhibits the replication of the HCV virus inside these hepatocytes (Fig. 29.1).

[138]Ahlenstiel G, Titerence RH, Koh C, et al. Natural killer cells are polarized toward cytotoxicity in chronic hepatitis C in an interferon-alfa-dependent manner. Gastroenterology. 2010;138:325–35.

[139]Ahlenstiel G, Titerence RH, Koh C, et al. Natural killer cells are polarized toward cytotoxicity in chronic hepatitis C in an interferon-alfa-dependent manner. Gastroenterology 2010;138:325–35.

[140]Nellore A, Fishman JA. NK cells, innate immunity and hepatitis C infection after liver transplantation. Clin. Infect. Dis. 2011;52:369–77.

IL-12 in the bloodstream or other extracellular fluids binds to the IL-12 receptor. With binding, the receptor transmits a signal into the cell, resulting in the formation of the Stat4/Stat4 dimer and the Stat3/Stat4 dimer (141). These dimers than travel to the nucleus, where they bind to promoters of IL-12-responsive genes. Stat4 binds to promoters operably linked to a number of genes. The promoter that is used to regulate expression of the IFN-gamma gene has the DNA sequence shown here (142):

TTAAGTGAATTTTTTGAGTTTCTTTTA

j. In HCV Infections, IFN-Alpha Stimulates NK Cells (or CD8⁺ T Cells) to Express IFN-Gamma

The following concerns yet another mechanism of action that involves NK cells, or CD8⁺ T cells, but that is more subtle than ADCC. During HCV infection, plasmacytoid DCs infiltrate the liver, where they are in the proximity of HCV-infected hepatocytes (143). Once inside the liver, contact of HCV-infected hepatocytes with plasmacytoid DCs stimulates these DCs to express IFN-alpha. In turn, the IFN-alpha stimulates NK cells, or CD8⁺ T cells, or both, to express IFN-gamma, where IFN-gamma in turn inhibits replication of HCV (Fig. 29.2) (144).

Evidence for the scenario includes the following (Fig. 29.2). In HCV infections, plasmacytoid DCs are the dominant IFN-alpha-expressing cells (145). IFN-alpha expression is critical for immune response against HCV (146). In turn, the IFN-alpha stimulates CD8⁺ T cells, CD4⁺ T cells, and NK cells to express IFN-gamma (147,148). A number of studies have shown that

[141]Kusaba H, Ghosh P, Derin R, et al. Interleukin-12-induced interferon-gamma production by human peripheral blood T cells is regulated by mammalian target of rapamycin (mTOR). J. Biol. Chem. 2005;280:1037—43.

[142]Xu X, Sun YL, Hoey T. Cooperative DNA binding and sequence-selective recognition conferred by the STAT amino-terminal domain. Science 1996;273:794—97.

[143]Sagan SM, Sarnow P. Plasmacytoid dendritic cells as guardians in hepatitis C virus-infected liver. Proc. Natl. Acad. Sci. USA 2010;107:7625—26.

[144]Huang Y, Yang H, Borg BB, et al. A functional SNP of interferon-gamma gene is important for interferon-alpha-induced and spontaneous recovery from hepatitis C virus infection. Proc. Natl. Acad. Sci. USA 2007;104:985—90.

[145]Anthony DD, Yonkers NL, Post AB, et al. Selective impairments in dendritic cell-associated function distinguish hepatitis C virus and HIV infection. J. Immunol. 2004;172:4907—16.

[146]Dolganiuc A, Chang S, Kodys K, et al. Hepatitis C virus (HCV) core protein-induced, monocyte-mediated mechanisms of reduced IFN-alpha and plasmacytoid dendritic cell loss in chronic HCV infection. J. Immunol. 2006;177:6758—68.

[147]Anthony DD, Yonkers NL, Post AB, et al. Selective impairments in dendritic cell-associated function distinguish hepatitis C virus and HIV infection. J. Immunol. 2004;172:4907—16.

[148]Barnes E, Gelderblom HC, Humphreys I, et al. Cellular immune responses during high-dose interferon-alpha induction therapy for hepatitis C virus infection. J. Infect. Dis. 2009;199:819—28.

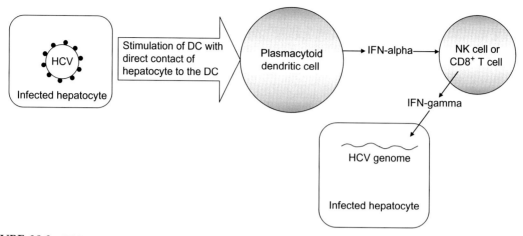

FIGURE 29.2   IFN-gamma-mediated inhibition of HCV replication via IFN-alpha. During HCV infections, plasmacytoid DCs respond by expressing IFN-alpha. The IFN-alpha then induces NK cells or CD8[+] T cells to express IFN-gamma. Evidence suggests that direct contact of infected hepatocytes to the DCs induces the DCs to express IFN-alpha.

IFN-alpha can stimulate NK cells to secrete IFN-gamma (149,150,151).

Moreover, Huang et al. (152) discovered variants in the regulatory region of the IFN-gamma gene (variant nucleotides in the gene's promoter), where one variant is associated with spontaneous recovery from HCV, and where the other variant is associated with chronic HCV infection. The variation of interest is named the "-764C/G polymorphism region." The researchers took leukocytes from 284 patients with chronic HCV, and from 251 patients who had spontaneously cleared HCV infections, determined DNA sequences at the IFN-gamma gene, and discovered this difference.

Regarding the molecular biology of IFN-alpha's ability to stimulate gene expression, Decker et al. (153) identified an element, interferon stimulation response element (ISRE), which is targeted by IFN-alpha, and which mediates IFN-alpha's ability to regulate various target genes. In order to stimulate the ISRE, IFN-alpha promotes formation of a complex of three proteins (STAT 1, STAT2, and p48), to form the IFN-stimulated gene

[149]Miyagi T, Takehara T, Nishio K, et al. Altered interferon-alpha-signaling in natural killer cells from patients with chronic hepatitis C virus infection. J. Hepatol. 2010;53:424−430.

[150]Jewett A, Bonavida B. Interferon-alpha activates cytotoxic function but inhibits interleukin-2-mediated proliferation and tumor necrosis factor-alpha secretion by immature human natural killer cells. J. Clin. Immunol. 1995;15:35−44.

[151]Jewett A, Gan XH, Lebow LT, Bonavida B. Differential secretion of TNF-alpha and IFN-gamma by human peripheral blood-derived NK subsets and association with functional maturation. J. Clin. Immunol. 1996;16:46−54.

[152]Huang Y, Yang H, Borg BB, et al. A functional SNP of interferon-gamma gene is important for interferon-alpha-induced and spontaneous recovery from hepatitis C virus infection. Proc. Natl. Acad. Sci. USA 2007;104:985−90.

[153]Decker T, Lew DJ, Darnell JE Jr. Two distinct alpha-interferon-dependent signal transduction pathways may contribute to activation of transcription of the guanylate-binding protein gene. Mol. Cell Biol. 1991;11:5147−53.

factor 3 (ISGF3) complex, which travels to the cell nucleus, where it binds to the ISRE sequence in IFN-alpha-stimulated gene promoters (154,155,156,157). To repeat, ISGF3 is a complex of three proteins. ISREs are found near the promoters of most genes that are responsive to IFN-alpha (158). Levy et al. (159) identified the target sequence, present in the human genome, as follows. This sequence is a consensus sequence. The "Y" means pyrimidine:

YAGTTTC(A/T)YTTTYCC.

k. Influence of IFN-Alpha on Gene Expression as Measured by Microarrays

The following addresses attempts to measure IFN-alpha's induction of IFN-gamma, by measurements of mRNA in peripheral blood mononuclear cells (PBMCs), using the technique of microarrays. Waddell et al. (160), Lanford et al. (161), Zhu et al. (162), and Ji et al. (163), identified a large number of genes that can be induced by IFN-alpha. The influence of IFN-alpha on expression of IFN-gamma seems not to have been detected by the methods reported in these publications, even though in vivo data do show that IFN-alpha stimulates expression of IFN-gamma. Dr Jake Liang has acknowledged that IFN-alpha is a weak inducer of IFN-gamma in PBMCs in vitro (164).

According to Dr Robert Lanford, the effect of IFN-alpha, as it pertains to IFN-gamma, may not be to stimulate expression of IFN-gamma. Instead, the effect of IFN-alpha, as it pertains to IFN-gamma, may be to potentiate the antiviral effect of IFN-gamma (165). This means that the combination of IFN-alpha and

[154]de Lucas S, Bartolome J, Carreno V. Hepatitis C virus core protein down-regulates transcription of interferon-induced antiviral genes. J. Infect. Dis. 2005;191:93–9.

[155]Kimura T, Kadokawa Y, Harada H, et al. Essential and non-redundant roles of p48 (ISGF3 gamma) and IRF-1 in both type I and type II interferon responses, as revealed by gene targeting studies. Genes Cells 1996;1:115–24.

[156]Morrow AN, Schmeisser H, Tsuno T, Zoon KC. A novel role for IFN-stimulated gene factor 3II in IFN-γ signaling and induction of antiviral activity in human cells. J. Immunol. 2011;186:1685–93.

[157]Ghislain JJ, Wong T, Nguyen M, Fish EN. The interferon-inducible Stat2:Stat1 heterodimer preferentially binds in vitro to a consensus element found in the promoters of a subset of interferon-stimulated genes. J. Interferon Cytokine Res. 2001;21:379–88.

[158]Leung S, Qureshi SA, Kerr IM, Darnell JE Jr, Stark GR. Role of STAT2 in the alpha interferon signaling pathway. Mol. Cell Biol. 1995;15:1312–17.

[159]Levy DE, Kessler DS, Pine R, Reich N, Darnell JE Jr. Interferon-induced nuclear factors that bind a shared promoter element correlate with positive and negative transcriptional control. Genes Dev. 1988;2:383–93.

[160]Waddell SJ, Popper SJ, Rubins KH, et al. Dissecting interferon-induced transcriptional programs in human peripheral blood cells. PLoS One. 2010;5:e9753.

[161]Lanford RE, Guerra B, Lee H, Chavez D, Brasky KM, Bigger CB. Genomic response to interferon-alpha in chimpanzees: implications of rapid downregulation for hepatitis C kinetics. Hepatology 2006;43:961–72.

[162]Zhu H, Zhao H, Collins CD, et al. Gene expression associated with interferon alfa antiviral activity in an HCV replicon cell line. Hepatology 2003;37:1180–88.

[163]Ji X, Cheung R, Cooper S, Li Q, Greenberg HB, He XS. Interferon alfa regulated gene expression in patients initiating interferon treatment for chronic hepatitis C. Hepatology 2003;37:610–21.

[164]Liang J. E-mail of April 6, 2011.

[165]Lanford RE. E-mail of April 7, 2011.

IFN-gamma has stronger anti-HCV activity than either cytokine alone.

l. Diagrams of the Immune Network in Immune Response Against HCV

Figure 29.1 shows a sequence of events that involves IL-12 and IFN-gamma. HCV expresses various viral proteins when it infects a DC, and some of these proteins are processed to antigens, and then presented via MHC to T cells. The event of processing and presentation is not shown in the figure. What is shown, however, is that when the virus infects the DC, the DC responds by expressing IL-12 which, in turn, causes NK cells to express IFN-gamma, where the IFN-gamma then inhibits viral replication.

Figure 29.2 shows a sequence of events involving IFN-alpha and IFN-gamma. A hepatocyte is shown infected with a HCV virus. Evidence suggests that the infected hepatocyte contacts (touches) a plasmacytoid DC, causing the DC to secrete IFN-alpha. Takahashi et al. (166), provide evidence that the infected hepatocyte causes the plasmacytoid DC to secrete IFN-alpha, by direct contact. Once IFN-alpha contacts an NK cell (or a CD8$^+$ T cell), the IFN-alpha may stimulate an NK cell (or CD8$^+$ T cell) to secrete IFN-gamma, where the IFN-gamma has a direct effect on inhibiting HCV replication (167). In characterizing the influence of IFN-alpha on expression of IFN-gamma, Huang et al. (168), found that the G allele at −764 confers a stronger induction of the IFN-gamma gene and favors viral clearance and response to exogenous IFN-alpha-based therapy. The authors also concluded that their discovery took the form of a polymorphism variant in the IFN-gamma promoter (−764C/G), where this variant regulates IFN-gamma gene expression.

m. Methodology Tip—Populations of Leukocytes in the Bloodstream

In assays of gene expression from leukocytes, expression results will depend on the method used for purifying the cells, and the homogeneity of the cell type. The most typical preparation of partially purified white blood cells is peripheral blood mononuclear cells (PBMCs). PBMCs, which include T cells, B cells, NK cells, and monocytes, are typically prepared by isolating leukocytes using density gradient centrifugation (169). This method excludes denser cells, such as red blood cells and polymorphonuclear leukocytes (neutrophils). According to Huang et al. (170),

[166]Takahashi K, Asabe S, Wieland S, et al. Plasmacytoid dendritic cells sense hepatitis C virus-infected cells, produce interferon, and inhibit infection. Proc. Natl. Acad. Sci. USA 2010;107:7431−36.

[167]Huang Y, Yang H, Borg BB, et al. A functional SNP of interferon-gamma gene is important for interferon-alpha-induced and spontaneous recovery from hepatitis C virus infection. Proc. Natl. Acad. Sci. USA 2007;104:985−90.

[168]Huang Y, Yang H, Borg BB, et al. A functional SNP of interferon-gamma gene is important for interferon-alpha-induced and spontaneous recovery from hepatitis C virus infection. Proc. Natl. Acad. Sci. USA 2007;104:985−90.

[169]Delves P, Martin S, Burton D, Roitt I. Roitt's essential immunology. 11th ed. Hoboken (NJ): Wiley-Blackwell; 2006. p. 138.

[170]Huang YH, Rönnelid J, Frostegård J. Oxidized LDL induces enhanced antibody formation and MHC class II-dependent IFN-gamma production in lymphocytes from healthy individuals. Arterioscler. Thromb. Vasc. Biol. 1995;15:1577−83.

human PBMCs contain about 55% CD4$^+$ T cells, 20% CD8$^+$ T cells, and 10% B cells. Somewhat consistent data are available from Porrata et al. (171), who determined that human PBMCs contain about 46% CD4$^+$ T cells, 27% CD8$^+$ T cells, and 8% (5–15%) NK cells. Other researchers found that NK cells account for 5–20% of human peripheral blood lymphocytes (172,173). McLaren et al. (174), found that CD4$^+$ T cells plus CD8$^+$ T cells account for 70% of PBMCs, with B cells (15%), NK cells (10%), monocytes (5%), and DCs under 1.0%.

Dendritic cells can be directly isolated from blood. Circulating DCs are rare in the bloodstream and comprise less than 1% of PBMCs (175). DCs can also be prepared by differentiation of DCs from PBMCs obtained from whole blood. These DCs are called monocyte-derived DCs (moDCs). The monocytes are induced to differentiate into immature DCs by culturing for several days in the presence of IL-4 and GM-CSF. The immature DCs are stimulated to become mature DCs by culturing for an additional 1–2 days in the presence of a maturation stimulus. A recurring issue is that experiments that use moDCs are subject to criticism, because these DCs have a physiology that is not exactly the same as naturally occurring DCs.

Gao et al. (176) reviewed the populations of various lymphocytes residing in the liver.

When evaluating the influence of cytokines on immune cell physiology or on gene expression, or when evaluating the influence of one type of immune cell on another, the results will likely depend on the purity of the cell, the subpopulation of the cell, and status of maturation, differentiation, and activation of the cell.

XV. CONCLUDING REMARKS

The mechanisms of infectious diseases, such as HCV, are used as a starting point in the development of drugs and biomarkers. The Food and Drug Administration (FDA) has approved various small-molecule drugs that inhibit HCV-encoded proteins, such as various structural proteins or HCV's RNA polymerase. In addition, the above material reveals various antigens that are specific to HCV, and describes various tactics by which the immune system mounts an attack against hepatocytes that express these HCV-derived antigens.

Mechanisms of disease, and the natural course of events for a given disease, can guide the design of clinical trials. Relevant aspects of clinical trial design are the inclusion/exclusion

[171]Porrata LF, Inwards DJ, Lacy MQ, Markovic SN. Immunomodulation of early engrafted natural killer cells with interleukin-2 and interferon-alpha in autologous stem cell transplantation. Bone Marrow Transplant. 2001;28:673–80.

[172]Cho D, Campana D. Expansion and activation of natural killer cells for cancer immunotherapy. Korean J. Lab. Med. 2009;29:89–96.

[173]Berrington JE, Barge D, Fenton AC, Cant AJ, Spickett GP. Lymphocyte subsets in term and significantly preterm UK infants in the first year of life analysed by single platform flow cytometry. Clin. Exp. Immunol. 2005;140:289–92.

[174]McLaren PJ, Mayne M, Rosser S, et al. Antigen-specific gene expression profiles of peripheral blood mononuclear cells do not reflect those of T-lymphocyte subsets. Clin. Diagn. Lab. Immunol. 2004;11:977–82.

[175]Sabado RL, Bhardwaj N. Directing dendritic cell immunotherapy towards successful cancer treatment. Immunotherapy 2010;2:37–56.

[176]Gao B, Radaeva S, Park O. Liver natural killer and natural killer T cells: immunobiology and emerging roles in liver diseases. J. Leukoc. Biol. 2009;86:513–28.

criteria, and stratification of study subjects. Also, a knowledge of the mechanisms of action of any given drug can be used to persuade the FDA to grant approval to a proposed clinical trial (177). Furthermore, the mechanism of action is included in the Clinical Pharmacology section of the package insert (178).

[177]Roberts TG, Lynch TJ, Chabner BA. The phase III trial in the era of targeted therapy: unraveling the "go or no go" decision. J. Clin. Oncol. 2003;21:3683–95.

[178]U.S. Dept. of Health and Human Services. Food and Drug Administration Guidance for Industry. Clinical Pharmacology Labeling for Human Prescription Drug and Biological Products—Considerations, Content, and Format; August 2014, (12 p).

30

Consent Forms

I. INTRODUCTION

The main goal of consent forms, in the context of clinical trials, is to protect human subjects enrolled in the clinical trial. Another goal of consent forms is to protect the investigator from liability. In a study of readability of consent forms used in clinical trials, Paasche-Orlow et al. (1) states the general proposition that, "[w]hen documents are incomprehensible, health care providers may risk liability."

Consent forms are required for regulated clinical studies, for example, those that are regulated by the US Food and Drug Administration (FDA) (2) and other regulatory agencies (3), as well as for clinical studies funded by the US Federal Government. Federal funding for studies on human subjects includes grants from the National Institutes of Health (NIH).

The administrative law relating to consent forms reads, in part (4):

[N]o investigator may involve a human being as a subject in research covered by these regulations unless the investigator has obtained the legally effective informed consent of the subject or the subject's legally authorized representative. An investigator shall seek such consent only under circumstances that provide the prospective subject or the representative sufficient opportunity to consider whether or not to participate and that minimize the possibility of coercion or undue influence. The information that is given to the subject or the representative shall be in language understandable to the subject or the representative.

The above quotation is from Title 21 of the Code of Federal Regulations (CFR). Title 21 of the CFR is a body of administrative law that applies to the FDA.

a. The First Clinical Study to Use a Consent Form—Yellow Fever Study

Carlos Finlay originated the theory that mosquitoes are the source of yellow fever.

---

[1] Paasche-Orlow MK, Taylor HA, Brancati FL. Readability standards for informed-consent forms as compared with actual readability. New Engl. J. Med. 2003;348:721–6.

[2] U.S. Department of Health and Human Services. Food and Drug Administration. Guidance for industry. E6 good clinical practice: consolidated guidance; April 1996.

[3] Macrae DJ. The Council for International Organizations and Medical Sciences (CIOMS) guidelines on ethics of clinical trials. Proc. Am. Thorac Soc. 2007;4:176–8.

[4] 21 Code of Federal Regulations (CFR) 50.20 (April 1, 2010 version).

Clinical Trials.
DOI: http://dx.doi.org/10.1016/B978-0-12-804217-5.00030-8

This theory was based on his observation that epidemics occurred coincidently with the peak in the population of the female mosquito, *Aedes aegypti*, during the hot, wet summer months. In 1881, Finlay presented his results in *The Annals of the Academy of Medical, Physical, and Natural Sciences of Havana* (5). Finlay conducted experiments with 102 human volunteers in an attempt to prove that mosquitoes were responsible for the disease. Yellow fever is actually caused by a virus (yellow fever virus) with a small genome encoding 10 proteins (6,7). The mosquito is the vector, that is, the transmitting agent.

The prevailing notion, before 1900, was that yellow fever was caused by bacteria. For example, Giuseppe Sanarelli of the Pasteur Institute in Paris argued that *Bacillus icteroides* was responsible for yellow fever. But George M. Sternberg, later Surgeon General of the United States, doubted Sanarelli's experiment, writing, "I would say it appears to me at the present time that ... the bacillus of Sanarelli is ... present occasionally and accidentally in the blood and tissue of yellow-fever patients, and that its etiological relation to this disease has not been established" (8).

In 1900, Sternberg asked Walter Reed, of the US army, to assemble the *Yellow Fever Commission* to look into the large number of American troops that died in Cuba during the

Spanish—American War (9,10). Over 2000 American soldiers had died of yellow fever compared to the 400 killed in combat. Sternberg had criticized Finlay's experiments on the basis that during the inoculation stage, volunteer subjects were not isolated from the general population, and so one could not completely exclude direct transmission between humans.

Walter Reed arrived in Cuba in Jun. 1900, with three other researchers, Jesse Lazear, Aristides Agramonte, and James Carroll. Reed's tests for the bacteria proved negative. Reed's group established that the vector was filterable through a Berkefeld filter, excluding a bacterial agent (11). A number of problems prevented Walter Reed's experiments with mosquitoes from working right away. First, Reed did not know that, for a mosquito to transmit yellow fever, the virus needed to be sitting in the mosquito's body for 12 days (incubation period). Also, he did not know that during cold weather, you needed to adjust this incubation period. Reed conducted a negative control experiment, where human volunteers wore clothing and bed sheets stained by sweat, vomit, and feces, from yellow fever patients. The goal of this experiment was to prove that contact with fluids from disease victims could not cause yellow fever, and that what was required was exposure to the

[5]Tan SY, Sung H. Carlos Juan Finlay (1833—1915): of mosquitoes and yellow fever. Singapore Med. J. 2008;49:370—1.

[6]McElroy KL, Tsetsarkin KA, Vanlandingham DL, Higgs S. Role of the yellow fever virus structural protein genes in viral dissemination from the *Aedes aegypti* mosquito midgut. J. Gen. Virol. 2006;87:2993—3001.

[7]Yellow fever virus strain Ivory Coast 1999, complete genome. GenBank: AY603338.1.

[8]Editorial. The yellow-fever question. Boston Med. Surg. J. 1899;141:223—4.

[9]Pierce JR, Writer JV. Yellow jack: how yellow fever ravaged America and Walter Reed discovered its deadly secrets. New York: Wiley; 2005.

[10]Malkin HM. The trials and tribulations of George Miller Sternberg (1838—1915) America's first bacteriologist. Perspect Biol. Med. 1993;36:666—78.

[11]Frierson JG. The yellow fever vaccine: a history. Yale J. Biol. Med. 2010;83:77—85.

mosquito. This type of control is exactly like that used by Joseph Goldberger, when he proved that pellagra is not an infectious disease (12).

Jesse Lazear decided to test Finlay's theory on himself, and he allowed himself to be bitten by mosquitoes (13). Lazear died 13 days later of yellow fever. After Lazear's death, Reed created the first written informed consent form, which outlined the risks of the experiments and their possible benefits. Those who agreed to be subjects in the experiments had to sign the forms. Spanish immigrants who volunteered received $100 in gold to participate and $100 more if they got sick. In all, 29 people contracted yellow fever while participating in the *Commission*'s experiments and five died.

b. The Consent Form of the *Yellow Fever Commission*

The consent form, as signed by one of the volunteers in Walter Reed's study, is shown in its English translation:

> Antonio Benino
>
> The undersigned, Antonio Benino being more than twenty-five years of age, native of Cerceda, in the province of Corima, the son of Manuel Benino and Josefa Castro here states by these presents, being in the enjoyment and exercise of his own very free will, that he consents to submit himself to experiments for the purpose of determining the methods of transmission of yellow fever, made upon his person by the *Commission* appointed for this purpose by the Secretary of War of the United States, and that he gives his consent to undergo the said experiments for the reasons and under the conditions below stated.
>
> The undersigned understands perfectly well that in case of the development of yellow fever in him, that he endangers his life to a certain extent but it being entirely impossible for him to avoid the infection during his stay in this island, he prefers to take

the chance of contracting it intentionally in the belief that he will receive from the said *Commission* the greatest care and the most skillful medical service.

> It is understood that at the completion of these experiments, within two months from this date, the undersigned will receive the sum of $100 in American gold and that in case of his contracting yellow fever at any time during his residence in this camp, he will receive in addition to that sum a further sum of $100 in American gold, upon his recovery and that in case of his death because of this disease, the *Commission* will transmit the said sum (two hundred American dollars) to the person whom the undersigned shall designate at his convenience.
>
> The undersigned binds himself not to leave the bounds of this camp during the period of the experiments and will forfeit all right to the benefits named in this contract if he breaks this agreement.
>
> And to bind himself he signs this paper in duplicate, in the Experimental Camp, near Quemados, Cuba, on the 26th day of November nineteen hundred.
>
> The contracting party,
> *Antonio Benigno*
> On the part of the *Commission*:
> Walter Reed
> Maj. & Surg., U.S.A.

c. Summary

The consent form of the *Yellow Fever Commission* contains several vital features that are found in present-day consent forms. First, it is evident that it is a legal document, since it contains the term "contracting party." Second, it states that consent is a matter of the subject's "own very free will" and that the subject is free to leave the study (breaks this agreement). Third, it states the purpose of the clinical study. Fourth, it states that the clinical study is an experiment, not a treatment. Fifth, it discloses some of the risks (endangers his life). Sixth, it provides that the study subject will receive supportive care (greatest care and the

[12]Carpenter KP. Pellagra. New York: Van Nostrand Reinhold; 1981.

[13]Editorial. Jesse William Lazear. Science 1900;12:932–33.

most skillful medical service). The consent form used by the *Yellow Fever Commission* is an exquisite learning device for those involved in present-day clinical trials.

II. SOURCES OF THE LAW IN THE UNITED STATES

Before describing the basis of consent forms in the law, it is first necessary to outline what the law is. In short, the law includes statutes, rules, and published opinions from courtroom cases.

The sources of the law, as it applies to a great variety of human activities, include acts, the legislative history of various acts, federal and state statutes, federal administrative law, federal and state case law, and specialized sources of the law, such as the Restatement of Contracts (14), the Uniform Commercial Code (15), and various ethical doctrines. Federal statutes take the form of the United States Code (USC). Federal administrative law takes the form of the CFR.

The CFR consists of 50 volumes, each volume corresponding to a different arena of federal governance. For example, Title 21 is used by the FDA. Title 37 is used by the United States Patent and Trademark Office. The laws in the CFR constitute "administrative law," because they apply to various administrative agencies of the US Government. Administrative laws are generally not called "laws," but instead are called "rules." Administrative laws generally govern procedures, for example, times for submitting paperwork, while, in contrast, statutes govern activities that are substantive in nature (16).

When new laws and administrative rules are proposed, they are published in the Federal Register. And when they are finalized, they are also published in the Federal Register. The Federal Register is a source of guidance for consent forms. Investigators and medical writers involved in drafting consent forms and re-consent forms need to be aware of 21 CFR 50, which is entitled Informed Consent Elements, which was published in the Federal Register in Jan. 2011 (17).

III. GUIDANCE FOR INDUSTRY

For regulated clinical trials, FDA provides guidance in the form of a collection of about 50 short essays, called Guidance for Industry. These Guidance for Industry documents are clearly written, but they are not detailed, they are rarely revised, and they cover only selected topics relating to FDA-sponsored trials. FDA's Guidance for Industry documents do not have the force of the law.

Guidance for Industry E6 Good Clinical Practice: Consolidated Guidance (18) concerns consent forms. Informed consent is defined as:

> A process by which a subject voluntarily confirms his or her willingness to participate in a particular trial, after having been informed of all aspects of the trial that are relevant to the subject's decision to participate. Informed consent is documented by means of a written, signed, and dated informed consent form.

[14]Byrne JE. Restatement 2nd of contracts and US UCC article 2. 3rd ed. Montgomery Village, MD: Institute of International Banking Law & Practice; 2007. 752 pp.

[15]Uniform Commercial Code, 2009–2010 edition. New York: Thomson West.

[16]Tafas v. Doll. 559 F.3d 1345; 2009 U.S. App. LEXIS 5806; 90 U.S.P.Q.2D (BNA) 1129.

[17]Federal Register. January 4, 2011, Vol. 76, No. 2, p. 256.

[18]U.S. Department of Health and Human Services. Food and Drug Administration. Guidance for industry. E6 good clinical practice: consolidated guidance; April 1996.

Guidance for Industry E6 (19) states that the consent form and relevant instructions to the study subject should include explanations regarding:

a. The trial involves research.
b. The purpose of the trial.
c. The trial treatment and the probability for random assignment to each treatment.
d. The trial procedures to be followed, including all invasive procedures.
e. The subject's responsibilities.
f. Those aspects of the trial that are experimental.
g. The reasonably foreseeable risks or inconveniences to the subject and, when applicable, to an embryo, fetus, or nursing infant.
h. The reasonably expected benefits. When there is no intended clinical benefit to the subject, the subject should be made aware of this.
i. The alternative procedure or course of treatment that may be available to the subject, and their important potential benefits and risks.
j. The compensation and/or treatment available to the subject in the event of trial-related injury.
k. The anticipated prorated payment, if any, to the subject for participating in the trial.
l. The anticipated expenses, if any, to the subject for participating in the trial.
m. That the subject's participation in the trial is voluntary and that the subject may refuse to participate or withdraw from the trial, at any time, without penalty or loss of benefits to which the subject is otherwise entitled.

n. That the monitor, the auditor, the Institutional Review Boards (IRB)/ Independent Ethics Committees (IEC), and the regulatory authority will be granted direct access to the subject's original medical records for verification of clinical trial procedures and/or data, without violating the confidentiality of the subject, to the extent permitted by the applicable laws and regulations and that, by signing a written informed consent form, the subject or the subject's legally acceptable representative is authorizing such access.
o. That records identifying the subject will be kept confidential and, to the extent permitted by the applicable laws and/or regulations, will not be made publicly available. If the results of the trial are published, the subject's identity will remain confidential.
p. That the subject or the subject's legally acceptable representative will be informed in a timely manner if information becomes available that may be relevant to the subject's willingness to continue participation in the trial.
q. The person to contact for further information regarding the trial and the rights of trial subjects, and whom to contact in the event of trial-related injury.
r. The foreseeable circumstances and/or reasons under which the subject's participation in the trial may be terminated.
s. The expected duration of the subject's participation in the trial.
t. The approximate number of subjects involved in the trial.

[19]U.S. Department of Health and Human Services. Food and Drug Administration. Guidance for industry. E6 good clinical practice: consolidated guidance; April 1996.

IV. DISTINCTION BETWEEN STOPPING TREATMENT AND WITHDRAWING FROM THE STUDY

FDA's Guidance for Industry E6 (20) mentions the option of withdrawing from a study.

Fleming (21) provides a fine point regarding dropping out from a study and withdrawal of consent. There are only two valid reasons a subjects can leave a clinical trial, first, withdrawal of consent and second, achieving of all required efficacy and safety end points. According to Fleming (22), it is an unfortunate common practice for Clinical Study Protocols to provide a list of reasons that the subject will be "off study," such as inability to tolerate the intervention, toxicity, physician choice, or need for other therapies. These may be valid reasons for nonadherence (for being off study treatment), but not for being dropped from the study.

Thus, the Clinical Study Protocol should separately list the two reasons a patient could go "off study" and the many reasons the patient could discontinue the treatment, with an indication that efforts should be made to ensure patients who stop the study treatment be consistently followed for outcomes unless they have withdrawn consent.

V. ETHICAL DOCTRINES

Ethical doctrines relevant to consent forms include the Belmont Report (1979), the Declaration of Helsinki (1964), and the Nuremberg Code (1947). The Belmont Report arose from an Act of the US Government, namely, the National Research Act of 1974. This Act created the *National Commission for Protection of Human Subjects of Biomedical and Behavioral Research*, which issued the *Belmont Report*. These ethical doctrines arose, in part, as reactions to notoriously unethical experiments on human subjects. As reviewed by Rice (23), these notorious studies include experiments by Nazis on prisoners, the Willowbrook Hepatitis Studies, and the Tuskegee Syphilis Study.

While the *Belmont Report* was not codified as any law or rule of the US Government, it did serve as a basis for parts of the CFR that concern consent forms used for clinical trials (24). These parts are Title 21 CFR Sections 50 and 56, and Title 45 CFR Section 46. The combination of 21 CFR 50 and 45 CFR 46 is called *The Common Rule* (25,26,27).

---

[20]U.S. Department of Health and Human Services. Food and Drug Administration. Guidance for industry. E6 good clinical practice: consolidated guidance; April 1996.

[21]Fleming TR. Addressing missing data in clinical trials. Ann. Intern. Med. 2011;154:113−7.

[22]Fleming TR. Addressing missing data in clinical trials. Ann. Intern. Med. 2011;154:113−7.

[23]Rice TW. The historical, ethical, and legal background of human-subjects research. Respir. Care 2008;53:1325−9.

[24]Zimmerman JF. The Belmont Report: an ethical framework for protecting research subjects. The Monitor; Summer 1997.

[25]Mehlman MJ, Berg JW. Human subjects protections in biomedical enhancement research: assessing risk and benefit and obtaining informed consent. J. Law Med. Ethics 2008;36:546.

[26]Grimm DA. Informed consent for all! No exceptions. New Mexico Law Rev. 2007;39:39−83.

[27]Luce JM. Informed consent for clinical research involving patients with chest disease in the United States. Chest 2009;135:1061−8.

VI. THE CASE LAW

The great bulk of what is called *law* takes the form of the published case law, also called, *opinions*. Opinions are written by the judge presiding over the case. The published case law results from courtroom cases held before a judge, or a panel of judges. It is rare that a judge will create a law that is entirely new. What almost always occurs, is that the judge incorporates elements from the existing case law into his or her own published opinion. This practice is called *stare decisis*, pronounced, "stah-ray dee-SIGH-siss."

Published courtroom opinions cover various issues relevant to consent forms. One interesting issue, is whether a subject needs to be informed of a potentially toxic side effect that represents only a small risk (under 1% risk). This particular issue can be found in a variety of opinions, notably, Scott v. Wilson (28), Cobbs v. Grant (29), Canterbury v. Spence (30,31), Truman v. Thomas (32), Cruzan v. Director (33), Halushka v. University of Saskatchewan (34,35), and Salgo v. Leland Stanford Jr. University Board of Trustees (36).

Investigators, medical writers, and attorneys can easily find additional guidance by reading subsequent case law that cites these opinions.

The best source of guidance for drafting consent forms is a seasoned attorney, familiar with the case law and having experience in drafting consent forms.

VII. BASIS FOR CONSENT FORMS IN THE CFR

Rules relating to consent forms are found in Title 21, which applies to the FDA. Rules relating to consent forms, also appear in Title 45, which applies to the Department of Health and Human Services (DHHS). The FDA and DHHS are different agencies in the US Government. But the two sets of rules are quite similar to each other.

This concerns Title 45 of the CFR. The DHHS oversees the registration of IRB. An IRB is a small group of volunteers, independent from any given clinical study, consisting of medical experts and laypersons. The IRB reviews and approves consent forms for any given clinical study. Title 45, Part 46, Sections 107–117, provide a legal basis for the IRB and for consent forms.

The following concerns Title 21 of the CFR. Title 21, Part 50, Section 20 (21 CFR §50.20) is reproduced in its entirety below. This part of

---

[28]Scott v. Wilson. 396 S.W.2d 532; 1965 Tex. App. LEXIS 2153.

[29]Cobbs v. Grant. 8 Cal. 3d 229; 502 P.2d 1; 104 Cal. Rptr. 505; 1972 Cal. LEXIS 278.

[30]Canterbury v. Spence. 464 F.2d 772; 150 U.S. App. D.C. 263; 1972 U.S. App. LEXIS 9467.

[31]Couture JJ. The changes in informed consent in experimental procedures: the evolution of a concept. J. Health Biomed. L. 2004;1:125–61.

[32]Truman v. Thomas. 27 Cal. 3d 285; 611 P.2d 902; 165 Cal. Rptr. 308; 1980 Cal. LEXIS 175.

[33]Cruzan v. Director, Missouri DMH, 497 U.S 261, 110 S.Ct. 2841; 1990.

[34]Halushka v. University of Saskatchewan et al. 53 D.L.R. (2d) 436 (Sask. C.A.); 1965.

[35]Tremayne-Lloyd T, Srebrolow G. Research ethics approval for human and animal experimentation: consequences of failing to obtain approval—including legal and professional liability. J. Can. Chiropract. Assoc. 2007;51:56–60.

[36]Salgo v. Leland Stanford Jr. University Board of Trustees. 154 Cal. App. 2d 560; 317 P.2d 170; 1957 Cal. App. LEXIS 1667.

the CFR sets forth the requirement for consent forms for FDA-sponsored clinical trials:

> Except as provided in 50.23 and 50.24, no investigator may involve a human being as a subject in research covered by these regulations unless the investigator has obtained the legally effective informed consent of the subject or the subject's legally authorized representative. An investigator shall seek such consent only under circumstances that provide the prospective subject or the representative sufficient opportunity to consider whether or not to participate and that minimize the possibility of coercion or undue influence. The information that is given to the subject or the representative shall be in language understandable to the subject or the representative. No informed consent, whether oral or written, may include any exculpatory language through which the subject or the representative is made to waive or appear to waive any of the subject's legal rights, or releases or appears to release the investigator, the sponsor, the institution, or its agents from liability for negligence.

Title 21, Part 50, Section 23, as reproduced in part below, provides certain exceptions to the requirement for informed consent:

(a) The obtaining of informed consent shall be deemed feasible unless, before use of the test article (except as provided in paragraph (b) of this section), both the investigator and a physician who is not otherwise participating in the clinical investigation certify in writing all of the following:
  (1) The human subject is confronted by a life-threatening situation necessitating the use of the test article.
  (2) Informed consent cannot be obtained from the subject because of an inability to communicate with, or obtain legally effective consent from, the subject.
  (3) Time is not sufficient to obtain consent from the subject's legal representative.
  (4) There is available no alternative method of approved or generally recognized therapy that provides an equal or greater likelihood of saving the life of the subject.
(b) If immediate use of the test article is, in the investigator's opinion, required to preserve the life of the subject, and time is not sufficient to obtain the independent determination required

in paragraph (a) of this section in advance of using the test article, the determinations of the clinical investigator shall be made and, within 5 working days after the use of the article, be reviewed and evaluated in writing by a physician who is not participating in the clinical investigation.

The elements of the consent form are defined in Title 21, Part 50, Section 25, as reproduced in part below:

(1) A statement that the study involves research, an explanation of the purposes of the research and the expected duration of the subject's participation, a description of the procedures to be followed, and identification of any procedures which are experimental.
(2) A description of any reasonably foreseeable risks or discomforts to the subject.
(3) A description of any benefits to the subject or to others which may reasonably be expected from the research.
(4) A disclosure of appropriate alternative procedures or courses of treatment, if any, that might be advantageous to the subject.
(5) A statement describing the extent, if any, to which confidentiality of records identifying the subject will be maintained and that notes the possibility that the Food and Drug Administration may inspect the records.
(6) For research involving more than minimal risk, an explanation as to whether any compensation and an explanation as to whether any medical treatments are available if injury occurs and, if so, what they consist of, or where further information may be obtained.
(7) An explanation of whom to contact for answers to pertinent questions about the research and research subjects' rights, and whom to contact in the event of a research-related injury to the subject.
(8) A statement that participation is voluntary, that refusal to participate will involve no penalty or loss of benefits to which the subject is otherwise entitled, and that the subject may discontinue participation at any time without penalty or loss of benefits to which the subject is otherwise entitled.

Many academic medical centers have voluntarily complied with the federal rules, regardless of the source of funding. Only five states in the United States of America, which has 50 states in all, have state laws requiring application of the federal rules to all research conducted with human subjects regardless of the source of funding (37).

VIII. SUMMARY

Consent forms used in clinical trials need to conform with the administrative law set forth in the CFR. The conditions imposed by the consent form of the *Yellow Fever Commission* have parallels with the conditions set forth in the CFR. What was, and is, required is that the study subject understands that the clinical study is an experiment (and is not a treatment), that risks be explained to the study subject, that medical treatment will be available if the clinical study results in injury to the study subject, and that participation in the clinical trial is voluntary.

IX. EXAMPLES OF CONTEMPORARY CONSENT FORMS

The following provides, in its entirety, a consent form used for a study of lung cancer (38,39,40). The consent form uses a standard format. In reviewing this particular consent

TABLE 30.1 Comparison of Terms Used in the Consent Form, With Corresponding Medical Terms Used by Physicians

Layperson's Term in the Consent Form	Corresponding Medical Term
Change in sense of taste	Hypogeusia or hypergeusia
Loss of appetite	Anorexia
Side effects	Adverse drug reactions
Hair loss	Alopecia
High blood pressure	Hypertension
Numbness in the hands and feet	Paresthesia

form, the reader might want to keep an eye on Table 30.1. This table contains terms familiar to the layperson (should be in consent forms) and the corresponding medical terms (should be avoided in consent forms) (41).

a. Example of a Contemporary Consent Form (Reproduced in Full) (42,43)

Patient Consent From (E1594).
Research Study.
   I, _____, willingly agree to participate in this study which has been explained to me by Dr. _____. This research study is being conducted by the Eastern Cooperative Oncology Group and by _____ (Institution).

---

[37]Shamoo AE, Katzel LI. How should adverse events be reported in US clinical trials?: ethical considerations. Clin. Pharmacol. Ther. 2008;84:275–8.

[38]Cella D. Consent form was developed by Peter Raich for an ECOG study. E-mail of November 9, 2009.

[39]Coyne CA, Xu R, Raich P, et al. Randomized, controlled trial of an easy-to-read informed consent statement for clinical trial participation: a study of the Eastern Cooperative Oncology Group. J. Clin. Oncol. 2003;21:836–42.

[40]Permission to reproduce provided by Dr P.C. Raich. E-mail of April 6, 2011.

[41]Coyne CA, Xu R, Raich P, et al. Randomized, controlled trial of an easy-to-read informed consent statement for clinical trial participation: a study of the Eastern Cooperative Oncology Group. J. Clin. Oncol. 2003;21:836–42.

[42]Cella D. Consent form was developed by Peter Raich for an ECOG study. E-mail of November 9, 2009.

[43]Coyne CA, Xu R, Raich P, et al. Randomized, controlled trial of an easy-to-read informed consent statement for clinical trial participation: a study of the Eastern Cooperative Oncology Group. J. Clin. Oncol. 2003;21:836–42.

Purpose of the Study.

It has been explained to you that you have advanced non-small cell lung cancer. Your physician has decided that chemotherapy is the best option available. You have been invited to participate in this research study. This study involves treatment with four drug regimens, Arm A (taxol + cisplatin), Arm B (gemcitabine + cisplatin), Arm C (taxotere + cisplatin), and Arm D (carboplatinol + taxol). The drugs gemcitabine and taxotere are considered experimental. Each of these regimens has been used and demonstrated activity (responses) in non-small cell lung cancer. The purpose of this study is to slow or stop the growth of your disease, define the side effects of each treatment arm, and to see if one regime is better at controlling lung cancer than the others.

Description of Procedures.

This study involves treatment with four drug regimens, Arm A (taxol + cisplatin), Arm B (gemcitabine + cisplatin), Arm C (taxotere + cisplatin), and Arm D (carboplatinol + taxol). It is not clear at the present time which of the therapies is better. For this reason, the therapy which is to be offered to you will be based upon chance, using a method of selection called randomizaton. Randomizaton means that your physician will call a statistical office which will assign one of the treatments to you, and the chances of your receiving any one of the therapies are approximately equal.

If you are assigned to Arm A, you will receive taxol and cisplatin. Taxol is given by vein over 24 hours on day one. On day 2 after the taxol is given, you will receive cisplatin by vein over one hour. This treatment is given every 3 weeks. You will continue to receive treatment with taxol and cisplatin until your disease becomes worse, or toxicities become unacceptable, at which time you will be removed from the study and offered other therapy.

If you are assigned to Arm B, you will receive gemcitabine and cisplatin. Gemcitabine is given by vein over 30 minutes on days 1, 8, and 15. Cisplatin is given by vein over one hour on day 1 following gemcitabine. Treatment in Arm B is given every 4 weeks. You will continue to receive treatment with gemcitabine and cisplatin until your disease becomes worse, or toxicities become unacceptable, at which time you will be removed from the study and offered other therapy.

If you are assigned to Arm C, you will receive taxotere and cisplatin. Taxotere is given by vein over 60 minutes on day one. Cisplatin is also given by vein on day 1 over an additional hour.

Treatment in Arm C is given every 3 weeks. You will continue to receive treatment with taxotere and cisplatin until your disease becomes worse, or toxicities become unacceptable, at which time you will be removed from the study, and offered other therapy.

If you are assigned to Arm D, you will receive carboplatin and taxol. Taxol is given by vein over 3 hours on day 1. Carboplatin is also given by vein on day 1 over an additional 30 minutes. Treatment in arm D is given every three weeks. You will continue to receive treatment with carboplatin and taxol until your disease becomes worse, or toxicities become unacceptable, at which time you will be removed from the study and offered other therapy.

At the start of this treatment study, a small amount of urine will be collected and analyzed. We are trying to see if there is a factor in your urine to identify cachexia. Cachexia is a syndrome of severe weight loss and muscle mass that is seen in many cancer patients. We are going to compare the presence or absence of this marker with your treatment outcome. This is for research purposes only, and the results will not influence your treatment. These results will also not be routinely provided to you or to your physician.

Risks and Discomforts.

The drugs used in this program may cause all, some, or none of the side effects listed. In addition, there is always a risk of very uncommon or previously unknown side effects occurring.

Arm A.

Arm A: Taxol and cisplatin may cause lowering of the blood counts (specifically white blood cells that can increase your risk of bleeding), lowering of red blood cells that can lead to anemia, and lowering of platelets, that can result in bleeding. An allergic reaction may also occur. Symptoms of an allergic reaction can be mild-flushing, skin rash, fever or severe-shortness of breath, narrowing of your airway resulting in difficulty breathing and a drop or increase in your blood pressure. Before treatment begins, you will be given medication to try to prevent this type of reaction, and you will be closely watched for such a reaction. Other common side effects are: nausea, vomiting, change in your sense of taste, diarrhea, sores in the mouth or throat, sore throat, loss of appetite, fatigue, muscle weakness, muscle and joint aches, hair loss, lightheadedness, headaches, high blood pressure, blurred vision or a sensation of flashing lights, irritation to the blood vessels at the place where you are given the drugs, damage to nerves causing numbness in the hands and feet, confusion, mood changes, changes in liver and kidney function tests, damage to the kidneys and hearing loss.

Abnormalities of the blood may also occur, that is, low magnesium, low calcium, low sodium or an increase in triglyceride (blood lipid) levels. Rare side effects include fainting, an irregular heart beat (arrhythmia), other rhythm changes (rapid heart rate, heart block, etc.), or heart attack. These can be life-threatening side effects, however, you will be given medication to prevent these and watched closely for such reactions. Other rare side effects include crampy stomach pain, or loss of blood supply to the intestines, which may require surgery; and inflammation of the pancreas, dizziness, and shooting pain down our back when bending your neck forward, liver damage, liver failure, and seizures. In rare cases, acute leukemia or other cancers may develop after treatment with cisplatin, especially when it is given along with other anticancer drugs.

Arm B.

Arm B: Gemcitabine and cisplatin may cause a decrease in the number of white blood cells, which may cause increased possibility of infection, and a decrease in the number of platelets and red blood cells which may cause bleeding, bruising, or tiredness. These effects could possibly result in the need for blood transfusion(s) and/or platelet transfusion (s) which has other risks. Other common side effects include loss of appetite, hair loss, nausea, vomiting, hearing loss, pressure or ringing in the ears, and damage to the kidneys. Other less common, but serious side effects include neurologic symptoms (numbness and tingling of fingers and toes), problems with dexterity (buttoning, handwriting, unsteady walking), allergic reactions, chemical abnormalities of the blood (high uric acid and low magnesium), facial swelling, involuntary shaking, decreased vision, liver damage (which could be fatal), metallic or altered taste, heart damage, and spasms and muscle cramps. Some patients have worsening of the neurologic symptoms for up to 2 months after treatment is stopped. The nerve damage may improve over a year after the cisplatin is stopped, however, the damage may be permanent. Other possible risks include fever, chills, diarrhea, constipation, itchy skin rash, loss of strength and energy, headaches, muscle aches, cough, runny nose, insomnia, sweating, low blood pressure, drowsiness, swelling of arms and legs, shortness of breath, difficulty in breathing, mouth sores, flu-like symptoms and small amounts of protein and blood

may appear in the urine. In rare cases, acute leukemia or other cancers may develop after treatment with cisplatin, especially when it is given along with other anticancer drugs.

Arm C.

Arm C: Taxotere and cisplatin may cause lowering of the blood counts (specifically white blood cells that can increase your risk of infection), lowering of red blood cells that can lead to anemia, and lowering of platelets, that can result in bleeding. Other side effects are: nausea, vomiting, sores in the mouth or throat, sore throat, loss of appetite, fatigue, irritation to the blood vessels at the place where the drugs are given, damage to nerves causing numbness in the hands and feet, changes in liver and kidney function tests, damage to the kidneys, hearing loss, and possible changes in vision. Abnormalities of the blood may also occur, that is, low magnesium, increase in liver function tests, calcium, or sodium levels. An allergic reaction may also occur. Symptoms of an allergic reaction can be mild flushing, skin rash, fever or severe shortness of breath, narrowing of your airway resulting in difficulty breathing, and drop or increase in your blood pressure. Before treatment begins, you will be given medication to try to prevent this type of reaction, and you will be closely watched for such a reaction. Rare side effects include: shooting pain down the back when bending your neck forward, weakness, fluid retention in arms and legs, fluid in the lungs, hair loss, dizziness, and seizures. In rare cases, acute leukemia or other cancers may develop after treatment with cisplatin, especially when it is given along with other anticancer drugs. If your liver function tests are higher than normal, you are at an increased of having ore toxicity from the taxotere. Patients who have higher than normal liver function tests will receive a lower dose of taxotere, but we do not know for sure this is safe. We will take extra precautions and monitor these patients closely.

Arm D.

Arm D: Taxol and carboplatin may lower your blood counts increasing your risk of infection, anemia, tiredness, bruising and bleeding. An allergic reaction (mild flushing, skin rash, fever, severe shortness of breath, difficulty breathing, and a change in blood pressure) may also occur. Before treatment begins you will be given drugs to prevent this type of reaction and we will watch you closely for such a reaction. Other side effects are: nausea, vomiting, change in sense of taste, diarrhea, pain, sores in the mouth or throat, sore throat, loss of appetite, fatigue, muscle weakness, muscle and joint aches, and hair loss. Lightheadedness, headaches, high blood pressure, blurred vision or sensation of flashing light, irritation at the drug injection site, numbness in the hands and feet, confusion, mood changes, reduced liver and kidney function, and kidney damage are also common side effects. Abnormal blood chemistry levels such as low calcium, sodium, or magnesium levels or increased lipid levels may occur. Rare side effects include: fainting, irregular heart beat (arrhythmia), other rhythm changes (rapid heart rate, heart block, etc.), or heart attack. You will be given drugs to help prevent these life-threatening side effects. You will be watched closely for such reactions. Other rare side effects include stomach cramps, loss of blood supply to the intestines that may require surgery, inflamed pancreas, dizziness and shooting back pain when bending your neck forward, liver damage, liver failure, and seizures. Rarely, acute leukemia or other cancers may develop after treatment with carboplatin, especially when given with other anticancer drugs.

Your physician will be checking you closely to see if any of these side effects are occurring. Routine blood and urine tests will be done to monitor the effects of treatment. Many side effects disappear after the treatment is stopped. In the meantime, your doctor may prescribe medication to keep these side effects under control. Schedules and dosages may be altered to reduce the side effects. The use of medications to control side effects could result in added costs. This institution is not financially responsible for the treatment of side effects caused by the study drugs.

The National Cancer Institute will provide you with the taxol and the investigational drugs gemcitabine and taxotere free of charge for this study. Should either of these drugs become commercially available, either you or your insurance company will be responsible for payment of subsequent doses of these drugs.

In the event that physical injury occurs as a result of this research, facilities for treatment of injury will be available; however, you will not automatically be provided with reimbursement for medical care or other compensation. For more information concerning the research and research-related risks or injuries, you can notify Dr. _____, the investigator in charge at _____ (telephone). In addition, you may contact _____ at _____ for information regarding patients' rights in research studies.

Benefits.

It is not possible to predict whether or not any personal benefit will result. Possible benefits are remission of tumors and prolonged survival. It is possible that the investigational drug may prove to be less effective than the standard regimen. If you receive treatment with the experimental drug and do not show any benefit from the treatment, you will receive treatment that has previously been shown to be effective. You have been told that, should your disease become worse, should side effects become very severe, should new scientific developments occur that indicate the treatment is not in your best interest, or should your physician feel that this treatment is no longer in your best interest, the treatment would be stopped. Further treatment would be discussed.

Alternatives.

Alternative treatments which could be considered in your case include treatment with other similar drug combinations. An additional alternative is no further therapy. Your doctor can provide detailed information about your disease and the benefits of the various treatments available. You have been told that you should feel free to discuss your disease and your prognosis with the doctor.

The physician involved in your care would be available to answer any questions you have concerning this program. In addition, you are free to ask your physician any questions concerning this program that you wish in the future. You will be advised of the procedures related solely to research which would not otherwise be necessary. These will be explained to you by your physician. Some of the procedures may result in added costs and some of these costs may not be covered by insurance. Your doctor will discuss these with you.

Voluntary participation.

Participation in this study is voluntary. No compensation for participation will be given. You are free to withdraw your consent to participate in this treatment program at any time without prejudice to your subsequent care. Refusing to participate will involve no penalty or loss of benefits. You are free to seek care from a physician of your choice at any time. If you do not take part in or withdraw from the study, you will continue to receive care. In the event that you withdraw from the study, you will continue to be followed and clinical data will continue to be collected from your medical records.

Confidentiality.

A record of your progress while on the study will be kept in a confidential form at

_____ (Institution) and also in a computer file at the statistical headquarters of the Eastern Cooperative Oncology Group (ECOG). The confidentiality of the central computer record is carefully guarded. During their required reviews, representatives of the Food and Drug Administration (FDA) and the National Cancer Institute (NCI) may have access to medical records which contain your identity. A qualified representative of the drug manufacturer(s) may also have access to your study records. However, no information by which you can be identified will be released or published. Histopathologic material, including slides, may be sent to a central office for review.

I have read all the above, asked questions, received answers concerning areas I did not understand and I willingly give my consent to participate in this program. Upon signing this form, I will receive a copy.

_____ (Patient signature)
_____ (Date)
_____ (Witness signature)
_____ (Date)

I, _____, willingly agree that any unused urine collected for this protocol may be stored at the Central Laboratory. This remaining urine may be used for future research that could include genetic research (about diseases that are passed on in families). This research will not have an effect on my care, therefore, neither I nor my doctor will receive results of this testing. No medical report will be added to my records. My medical records may be reviewed in the future for purposes of obtaining more information about my health, buy my name and address will remain confidential and will not be released. The urine will be used for research purposes only, it will not be sold and may not have a direct benefit to me or my cancer.

If I decide now that my urine can be kept for research, I can change my mind at any time. I just need to contact my doctor and withdraw my consent for the use of my urine for research.

I have read all of the above, asked questions and received answers concerning areas that I did not understand. I willingly consent to allow my urine to be stored for future research.

_____ (Patient signature)
_____ (Date)
_____ (Witness signature)
_____ (Date)

b. Another Example of a Contemporary Consent Form (Reproduced in Part)

The following reproduces, in part, a second consent form. This is the second of two consent forms that were the subject of the study of Coyne et al. (44,45,46). This second consent form contains all of the information as found in the above-reproduced consent form, plus some additional information. But the second consent form takes a more step-by-step approach suitable for understanding by the layperson.

Informed Consent For a Research Study
Chemotherapy Treatments for Non-Small Cell Lung Cancer

Please use the space on the right to write down any questions you might have. You also can put a check in the box if you have questions on that section.

About the Study   **Notes/Questions**
What am I being asked to do?   ☐

You are being asked to make a choice about taking part in a research study. This research study compares four different drug treatments (chemotherapy) for advanced non-small cell lung cancer. You are being asked to be part of this study because you have this type of cancer.

Why are we doing this study?   ☐

Advanced non-small cell lung cancer is very hard to treat. There is no known cure. Better treatments are needed. We are doing the study to see which, if any, of four treatments works best at slowing the growth of this type of cancer. We also want to look at the risks and side effects for each of the

---

[44]Cella D. Consent form was developed by Peter Raich for an ECOG study. E-mail of November 9, 2009.

[45]Coyne CA, Xu R, Raich P, et al. Randomized, controlled trial of an easy-to-read informed consent statement for clinical trial participation: a study of the Eastern Cooperative Oncology Group. J. Clin. Oncol. 2003;21:836–42.

[46]Permission to reproduce provided by Dr P.C. Raich. E-mail of April 6, 2011.

treatments. This study uses two "investigational" drugs, gemcitabine and taxotere. These drugs are "investigational" because they have not been fully tested against other drugs.

Who will be part of this study? ☐

About 1200 patients from many cancer treatment centers will join the study over a period of three years. All patients will have advanced non-small cell lung cancer.

Who is sponsoring the study? ☐

This study is sponsored by the National Cancer Institute (NCI), the Eastern Cooperative Oncology Group (ECOG), and the North Central Cancer Treatment Group (NCCTG). ECOG and NCCTG are groups of cancer specialists from across the country who do studies to find better ways to treat cancer. This study is supported partly by funds from NCI.

Description of Procedures.

What will happen in the study? ☐

If you join the study, you will be treated with two cancer-fighting drugs. Four different combinations of two (2) drugs each will be used in this study. Each of these drug combinations have been used before and have shown some anti-cancer activity. Which two drugs you will get depends on which of four treatment groups you are in. We do not know which, if any, of these treatments is best.

What are the differences between the four treatment groups? ☐

The differences between the four treatment groups are the drugs used in each group and how often they are given. Each patient will get two cancer-fighting drugs. The drugs used in each treatment group are listed in the table below.

Which treatment group will I be in? ☐

If you decide to be part of the study, you will be put into one of the four treatment groups. A computer will pick which group you will be in. This is done by chance, like flipping a coin. You have the same chance of being placed in any of the four treatment groups. Your doctor will tell you which group the computer puts you in. Neither you nor your doctor can pick which treatment group you will be in.

Do these drugs have any side effects or other risks? ☐

Yes. Drugs that are strong enough to kill cancer cells often cause problems in other parts of the body. These added problems are called side effects. We have listed side effects and risks that can be seen in all treatment groups in the study. We have also listed risks and possible side effects for the drugs that are specific to each of the treatment groups. You may have a few or all of the side effects listed and they may be mild or severe. You also could have other unexpected side effects that are not listed. Side effects differ from patient to patient. Be sure to talk with your doctor about any side effects you have while you are in the study.

. . . . . .

What does signing the consent form mean? ☐

Signing the consent form means that you choose to be part of this cancer treatment study. It means that you have read the consent form, your questions have been answered and that you understand what will happen in the study. A copy of this informed consent form will be given to you after you sign it. If you decide not to take part in the study, just give the unsigned form back to the doctor or nurse.

_____ (Patient's signature)
_____ (Date)
_____ (Witness signature)
_____(Date)
_____ (Physician's signature)
_____(Date)

c. Comparison of Standard Consent Form With the More Elementary Consent Form

The two consent forms reproduced above were used as part of a clinical trial of lung cancer patients, as reported by Coyne et al. (47). This trial is distinguished from most other clinical trials, in that the investigators administered two different consent forms to different enrollees.

One of the consent forms was standard. The other consent form contained the same information, but it disclosed the information in a step-by-step manner, similar to instructions that come with toys or gadgets to be assembled by children.

The reader might want to compare the content of the two consent forms with the content that is suggested by FDA's Guidance for Industry E6. For example, it can be seen that

---

[47]Coyne CA, Xu R, Raich P, et al. Randomized, controlled trial of an easy-to-read informed consent statement for clinical trial participation: a study of the Eastern Cooperative Oncology Group. J. Clin. Oncol. 2003;21:836–42.

both consent forms state that enrollment in the clinical trial is voluntary. Both consent forms state that enrollees are randomly assigned to the different treatments. Guidance for Industry E6 suggests that the consent form reveal the number of subjects enrolled in the trial. Only the second of the above two consent forms of Coyne et al. (48) contains this particular number.

Coyne et al. (49) did not find any significant differences in comprehension of the two consent forms. But this lack of difference may have been due to the relatively high education level of the subjects. Higher education has been correlated with better understanding of consent forms (50).

Coyne et al. (51) did observe a general issue with both of their consent forms. In obtaining feedback from the patients, about half of the patients did not understand the fact that the clinical trial was not likely to result in a cure for their cancer. About one-third of the patients did not understand that the goal of the trial was to find a cure for lung cancer.

d. Analysis of Consent Forms—Most Consent Forms Adequately Disclose the Purpose of Trial, and Refrain From Creating Expectations of Benefit

In an analysis of a large number of consent forms (272 forms) used in oncology clinical trials, Horng et al. (52) found that most consent forms adequately reveal that the purpose of the trial was to test for safety, that subjects had the right to withdraw from the trial, and that the trial involved risk of severe or permanent harm.

These authors found that most forms were adequate or appropriate, in acknowledging uncertainty of benefit, in refraining from promising a cure, and in refraining from downplaying risks. Another good point is that only one out of the 272 forms mentioned that the subject should "expect" any benefit. Horng et al. (53) also found certain deficiencies to be common in consent forms. The deficiencies were that the forms tended to use the term "treatment." Treatment is not a good term since it implies hope for recovery. Better terms are "investigational treatment," "experimental treatment," and "research drug."

e. Analysis of Consent Forms—Most Consent Forms Are Written at a Level That Is Too Advanced

Delgado and Leskovac (54) provide an overall guiding light regarding the comprehensibility of consent forms. These authors find that the burden of understanding the experimental treatment, and understanding the consent

[48]Coyne CA, Xu R, Raich P, et al. Randomized, controlled trial of an easy-to-read informed consent statement for clinical trial participation: a study of the Eastern Cooperative Oncology Group. J. Clin. Oncol. 2003;21:836–42.

[49]Coyne CA, Xu R, Raich P, et al. Randomized, controlled trial of an easy-to-read informed consent statement for clinical trial participation: a study of the Eastern Cooperative Oncology Group. J. Clin. Oncol. 2003;21:836–42.

[50]Ryan RE, Prictor MJ, McLaughlin KJ, Hill SJ. Audio-visual presentation of information for informed consent for participation in clinical trials. Cochrane Database Syst. Rev. 2008;(1):CD003717.

[51]Coyne CA, Xu R, Raich P, et al. Randomized, controlled trial of an easy-to-read informed consent statement for clinical trial participation: a study of the Eastern Cooperative Oncology Group. J. Clin. Oncol. 2003;21:836–42.

[52]Horng S, Emanuel EJ, Wilfond B, et al. Descriptions of benefits and risks in consent forms for phase 1 oncology trials. New Engl. J. Med. 2002;347:2134–40.

[53]Horng S, Emanuel EJ, Wilfond B, et al. Descriptions of benefits and risks in consent forms for phase 1 oncology trials. New Engl. J. Med. 2002;347:2134–40.

[54]Delgado R, Leskovac H. Informed consent in human experimentation: bridging the gap between ethical thought and current practice. UCLA Law Rev. 1986;34:67.

TABLE 30.2 Fourth Grade Level Language Versus College-Level Language

	4th Grade Level Language	College-Level Language
Statement of voluntary nature of the clinical trial	"You don't have to be in this research study. You can agree to be in the study now and change your mind later. Your decision will not affect your regular care. Your doctor's attitude toward you will not change."	"You voluntarily consent to participate in this research investigation. You may refuse to participate in this investigation or withdraw your consent and discontinue participation in this study without penalty and without affecting your future care or your ability to receive alternative medical treatment at the University."
Statement of goal of the clinical study	"We may learn about new things that might make you want to stop being in the study. If this happens, you will be informed. You can then decide if you want to continue to be in the study."	"During the course of the study, you will be informed of any significant new findings (either good or bad), such as changes in the risks or benefits resulting from participation in the research or new alternatives to participation, that might cause you to change your mind about continuing in the study. If new information is provided to you, your consent to continue participating in this study will be re-obtained."
Statement that the study does not provide a cure	"There is no benefit to you from being in the study. Your taking part may help patients in the future."	"The research physician treats all subjects under a specific protocol to obtain generalizable knowledge and on the premise that you may or may not benefit from your participation in the study."

form, shifts to the study subject, in the context of a clinical trial. The reason the burden shifts is that only the potential subject can decide whether or not to enroll.

Paasche-Orlow et al. (55) also find that the burden shifts to the study subject. These authors wrote, "[e]ven though consent forms are never used in isolation, text written at a 4th-grade level would promote the autonomy of most candidates for participation in medical research."

Paasche-Orlow et al. (56) obtained 114 consent forms that had been used in clinical studies, and analyzed them using a standard reading level test, the Flesch-Kincaid score. The authors found the average readability to be at the 10th to 11th grade level. In view of evidence that half of American adults read at the 8th grade level (or lower), these authors recommended that the reading level of consent forms be at the 4th grade level. Table 30.2, which is from Paasche-Orlow et al. (57), provides concrete examples of 4th grade language versus college-level language.

Table 30.3, which is from Jefford and Moore (58), also provides a list of language to avoid, along with reasonable alternatives.

[55]Paasche-Orlow MK, Taylor HA, Brancati FL. Readability standards for informed-consent forms as compared with actual readability. New Engl. J. Med. 2003;348:721–6.

[56]Paasche-Orlow MK, Taylor HA, Brancati FL. Readability standards for informed-consent forms as compared with actual readability. New Engl. J. Med. 2003;348:721–6.

[57]Paasche-Orlow MK, Taylor HA, Brancati FL. Readability standards for informed-consent forms as compared with actual readability. New Engl. J. Med. 2003;348:721–6.

[58]Jefford M, Moore R. Improvement of informed consent and the quality of consent documents. Lancet Oncol. 2008;9:485–93.

TABLE 30.3 Comparison of Poor Language Versus Good Language for Consent Forms

	Poor	Good
People are not tumors	You have progressed.	The cancer has grown.
	You have failed the earlier chemotherapy.	The chemotherapy you had received is no longer helping you.
Avoid language that is like an enticing advertisement	You have been invited ...	This trial might be suitable for you.
	If you are eligible ...	If the trial is suitable for you ...
Address the reader as "you"	Study participants will ...	If you choose ...
	Giving study medication intravenously and collecting blood samples might involve temporary discomfort or bruising.	If you choose to join this trial, you will have the drugs through a needle in your arm. The doctor will also use a needle to take blood for testing. You might have a bit of pain or bruising from the needle.

Davis et al. (59) conducted a study with a complex consent form, written at the 16th grade level (college level) and a simple consent form, written at the 7th grade level. The study was conducted on 153 adults. The simple consent form was distinguished in that it contained a drawing, showing a woman receiving an injection (Treatment A) and a woman receiving an injection and a bottle of pills (Treatment B).

The subjects preferred the simpler consent form, and they felt that the complex consent form might discourage them from enrolling in a clinical trial for cancer. However, this survey also determined that there was little or no difference in the comprehension of the two forms.

Coyne et al. (60) conducted a study with a complex consent form (14th grade level) and a simple consent form (12th grade level). The study was conducted with 226 adults. The subjects preferred the simpler consent form, in that

it produced slightly less anxiety. However, this survey also determined that there was little or no difference in comprehension between the two forms. Moreover, this survey found that the two different consent forms, which were configured for an oncology clinical trial, did not influence enrollment into this trial.

Comprehension of any consent form can be reduced for certain populations. Comprehensibility is less where the potential study subject is a child or infant, is the victim of a mental illness, or is in intractable pain.

Tait (61) finds that intractable pain can impair the ability of a patient to make rational decisions, including decisions to sign a consent form. Patients with severe pain, when confronted with complex information, may be impaired in the ability to make rational decisions. Researchers may fail to recognize such deficits, where this failure may expose the

[59]Davis TC, Holcombe RF, Berkel HJ, Pramanik S, Divers SG. Informed consent for clinical trials: a comparative study of standard versus simplified forms. J. Natl Cancer Inst. 1998;90:668–74.

[60]Coyne CA, Xu R, Raich P, et al. Randomized, controlled trial of an easy-to-read informed consent statement for clinical trial participation: a study of the Eastern Cooperative Oncology Group. J. Clin. Oncol. 2003;21:836–42.

[61]Tait RC. Vulnerability in biomedical research: vulnerability in clinical research with patients in pain: a risk analysis. J. Law Med. Ethics 2009;37:59.

patient to a greater risk. Similarly, Hoffman (62) reports that people who are gravely ill are impaired in their ability to make decisions.

X. ETHICAL ISSUES SPECIFIC TO PHASE I CLINICAL TRIALS IN ONCOLOGY

In an excellent review, Daugherty (63) highlighted an ethical conundrum that is somewhat specific to phase I clinical trials, in particular, to phase I clinical trials in oncology. In this type of trial, the chance of therapeutic benefit is usually very low, that is, under 5%. The low therapeutic benefit arises from the fact that the most optimal dose is yet unknown, and from the fact that the goal of phase I trials is to assess safety (not to assess efficacy or to cure the cancer). Another problem is that phase I trials may have a study design of the "dose-escalating" or "dose-finding" format, that is, where dosing is increased to, or beyond, an intolerable level. The ethical conflict arises from the following. Evidence demonstrates that motivation of subjects enrolling in phase I oncology trials takes the form of, "hope for improvement of their condition, by pressure exerted by relatives and friends, or simply because they felt they had no choice" (64).

XI. FDA'S WARNING LETTERS

FDA's Warning Letters, available on FDA's website, provide concrete and reliable guidance to all Sponsors involved in designing and conducting clinical trials. FDA's Warning Letters provide concrete guidance on various topics relating to the conduct of clinical trials, including consent forms.

FDA's Warning Letters sometimes refer to an earlier inspection by FDA employees, where the FDA had issued a Form 483 notice. Form 483 notices are issued spontaneously during a site visit, and FDA's Warning Letters, which are written at an FDA office, are then sent to the investigator (65).

a. Warning Letter Teaching the Investigator the Elements of Informed Consent

This concerns a clinical trial on a topical drug (a lotion). Referring to 21 CFR §50.24, the letter complained about deficiencies in the Sponsor's consent form, and set forth to teach the Sponsor the elements of informed consent. The letter stated that (66):

> The informed consent document is required to contain eight basic elements ... [o]ur investigation found that the informed consent document used in

---

[62]Hoffman S. Regulating clinical research: informed consent. Capital Univ. Law Rev. 2002;31:71−91.

[63]Daugherty CK. Impact of therapeutic research on informed consent and the ethics of clinical trials: a medical oncology perspective. J. Clin. Oncol. 1999;17:1601−17.

[64]Daugherty CK. Impact of therapeutic research on informed consent and the ethics of clinical trials: a medical oncology perspective. J. Clin. Oncol. 1999;17:1601−17.

[65]Cooper RM, Fleder JR. Responding to a form 483 warning letter: a practical guide. Food Drug Law J. 2005;60:479−93.

[66]Warning Letter No. 07-HFD-45-0102 (January 19, 2007) from Gary Zana, Division of Scientific Investigations, Office of Compliance, CDER, U.S. Food and Drug Administration.

your [redacted] study ... did not contain the following required elements.

a. The consent form failed to disclose any reasonably foreseeable risks or discomforts to the subject and appropriate alternative procedures or courses of treatment, if any, that might be advantageous to the subject.

b. The consent form failed to disclose the extent, if any, to which confidentiality of records identifying the subject will be maintained and the possibility of Food and Drug Administration inspection.

c. The consent form failed to describe available medical treatments and further information in case of an injury.

d. The consent form failed to describe the purposes of the research, the procedures to be followed, and the expected duration of the subject's participation.

e. The consent form failed to include a statement that refusal to participate will involve no penalty or loss of benefits to which the subject is otherwise entitled, and that the subject may discontinue participation at any time without penalty or loss of benefits to which the subject is otherwise entitled.

In an unrelated Warning Letter, the FDA provided a similar useful list of consent form elements to the investigator, referring to the list as (67), "[t]hese most basic components of informed consent."

b. Warning Letter About Consent Forms Administered After Performance of Medical Procedures; Consent Forms in the Wrong Language

This discloses the situation where the investigator performed medical procedures without first obtaining a consent form, and the problem consent forms were not in the appropriate language, that is, other than English.

The Warning Letter named the FDA inspectors, and reminded the investigator of the inspection, writing that, "We are aware that at the conclusion of the inspection, Ms. Bellamy and Ms. Kononen presented and discussed with you Form FDA 483, Inspectional Observations." The Warning Letter went a step beyond this reminder, reiterated the procedures that did not conform with the CFR, and warned the investigator that, "Within fifteen (15) working days of your receipt of this letter, you should notify this office in writing of the actions you have taken or will be taking to prevent similar violations in the future (68)."

The Warning Letter read (69):

> You failed to obtain informed consent of subjects involved in research ... 21 CFR §50.20 requires that ... no investigator may involve a human being as a subject in research unless the investigator has obtained the legally effective informed consent of the subject ... [t]he information that is given to the subject ... shall be in **language understandable to the subject** or the representative ... [r]egarding study [redacted], study procedures were conducted prior to obtaining informed consent from subjects [redacted] and [redacted]. Specifically, for subject [redacted], an MRI of the brain was conducted on 10/4/88, but informed consent was not signed by the subject until 10/06/88. For subject [redacted], a liver biopsy was performed on 10/4/94, but informed consent was not signed by the subject until 10/5/94 ... [t]he information that was given to the subject or the subject's legally authorized representative was not in a language understandable to the subject or the subject's legally authorized representative. Specifically, non-English speaking subjects were given informed consent documents written in English.

[67]Warning Letter No. 13-HFD-45-03-01 (March 25, 2013) from Thomas N. Moreno, Office of Scientific Investigations, Office of Compliance, CDER. U.S. Food and Drug Administration.

[68]Warning Letter to George J. Brewer (January 14, 2009) from Dr Leslie K. Ball, MD, Office of Compliance, CDER, U.S. Food and Drug Administration.

[69]Warning Letter to George J. Brewer (January 14, 2009) from Dr Leslie K. Ball, MD, Office of Compliance, CDER, U.S. Food and Drug Administration.

c. Warning Letters About Expired Consent Forms

This concerns an intersection between the investigator, IRB, and study subjects. This type of intersection occurs, for example, when the IRB approves a revised consent form, and where the result is that study subjects are required to sign the revised consent form. The Warning Letter complained that the investigator required that the study subjects sign the expired consent form (70):

> [y]ou failed to obtain the legally effective informed consent before involving a subject in research ... [w]hen you signed the Form FDA 1572 on July 1, 2003, you agreed to ensure that the requirements relating to informed consent were met. The IRB approved a revised Informed Consent Document (ICD) on July 9, 2003 (to incorporate a protocol amendment). The previous version ... specified that the form expired on July 22, 2003. Subjects #2190 and 2192 signed the outdated version of the ICD on August 7, 2003, subject #2223 signed the outdated version on August 4, 2003, and subject #2224 signed the outdated version on August 5, 2003.

A variation of this issue is revealed in another Warning Letter, where FDA complained that one of the study subjects, "was consented with a consent form with hand-written information/language added to the form, which denied payment to subjects for inpatient visits. This additional information/language was not approved by the IRB" (71). The letter added that this additional, handwritten language had not even been approved by the Sponsor.

d. Warning Letter About Consent Form Failing to Disclose Right to Withdraw From Study

Gross inadequacies in the consent form are also revealed from a Warning Letter issued for a clinical trial on cystic fibrosis. As one can see, some of the features of the yellow fever study consent form were absent from the cystic fibrosis consent form. The Warning Letter complained that (72):

> You failed to include the expected **duration** of study participation ... the informed consent document did not disclose that the plan was to treat subjects for approximately 5 months 2 months and 2 weeks treatment ... informed consent document also failed to specify the evaluations that study subjects would be required to undergo, including a physical exam and medical history, pulmonary **function testing**, oximetry, bacterial culture, and a 6-minute walk test ... [y]ou failed to include an explanation in the consent document as to whether any **compensation** or medical treatments would be available if injury occurs ... [y]ou failed to include a statement in the consent form that **refusal to participate or discontinuation** would involve no penalty or loss of benefits to which the subject is otherwise entitled.

e. Warning Letter About Re-Consent Forms

Issues relating to revised consent forms (re-consent forms) are disclosed in a Warning Letter that complained about re-consent forms. This letter provides an exemplary account of

---

[70]Warning Letter No. 06-HFD-45-0803 (September 14, 2006) from Joseph P. Salewski, Division of Scientific Investigations, Office of Compliance, CDER, U.S. Food and Drug Administration.

[71]Warning Letter No. 10-HFD-45-04-01 (April 9, 2010) from Dr Leslie K. Ball, MD, Office of Compliance, CDER, U. S. Food and Drug Administration.

[72]Warning Letter No. 05-HFD-45-0601 (June 7, 2005) from Dr Leslie K. Ball, MD, Office of Compliance, CDER, U.S. Food and Drug Administration.

the rationale for administering re-consent forms. The letter complained that (73):

> [y]ou failed to re-consent 11 subjects (#001, 007, 013, 024, 036, 041, 043, 048, 049, 053, and 056) in a timely manner at their next scheduled visit per the IRB's requirement . . . [i]n FDA's review of the documents, we note that several months had elapsed prior to your site re-consenting these subjects with the revised consent form. The revised informed consent document, version 5/23/06, provided information that may have affected the subjects' willingness to stay in the study, because it warned them of additional risks of participating in the study and also provided new information about the study. Thus, your delay in re-consenting these subjects with the revised consent document leads to significant concerns about the adequacy of your oversight over the study to ensure the protection of the rights, safety and welfare of the subjects enrolled in this study.

f. Warning Letter About Using a Consent Form That Had Not Been Approved by the IRB

This concerns a consent form that had been modified by hand-writing, and where the modification was not approved by the IRB. The Warning Letter complained that (74):

> You violated this requirement [21 CFR §312.66] by administering the investigational new drug . . . to Subject 1010 without obtaining IRB approval of the modified informed consent document. Specifically, the IRB-approved version of the informed consent . . . was altered by hand to state that the subject

would not receive payment for participation . . . and this altered form was signed by the parent of Subject 1010.

XII. DECISION AIDS

Decision aids can be used in conjunction with a consent form, in the course of a clinical trial, as well as in conventional medical care. Brehaut et al. (75) advocate the use of decision aids for subjects contemplating enrolling in a clinical trial, in view of the fact that consent forms can be confusing. Where confusion occurs with consent forms, it usually takes the form of not understanding "randomization," (76). Confusion also occurs because the subject incorrectly expects the study drug to be effective, even though it might only be an experimental drug.

This example is from an account from a published courtroom opinion. In one particular clinical trial for breast cancer, patients were randomized to receive a biopsy either of the axillary lymph node or of the sentinal lymph node. One patient from this clinical trial was confused about the meaning of randomization. The confusion arose from being "explained that the clinical trial would let the computer decide whether plaintiff [the patient] would have an axillary lymph node or sentinal lymph node biopsy, plaintiff [the patient] thought that the computer would decide the choice that was right for her" (77).

---

[73]Warning Letter No. 09-HFD-45-06-01 (June 12, 2009) from Dr Leslie K. Ball, MD, Office of Compliance, CDER, U.S. Food and Drug Administration.

[74]Warning Letter No. 10-HFD-45-01-02 (February 24, 2010) from Dr Leslie K. Ball, MD, Office of Compliance, CDER, U.S. Food and Drug Administration.

[75]Brehaut JC, Lott A, Fergusson DA, Shojania KG, Kimmelman J, Saginur R. Can patient decision aids help people make good decisions about participating in clinical trials? A study protocol. Implement Sci. 2008;3:38.

[76]Stead M, Eadie D, Gordon D, Angus K. "Hello, hello—it's English I speak!": a qualitative exploration of patients' understanding of the science of clinical trials. J. Med. Ethics 2005;31:664–9.

[77]Compton v. Pass. 2010 Mich. App. LEXIS 556.

Featherstone and Donovan (78) character-ized the patient's confusion about randomiza-tion as, "[m]any of these men were struggling to come to terms with different (sometimes competing) views about randomisation."

Flory and Emanuel (79) found that compre-hension may or may not be improved by video presentations and that, in contrast, comprehen-sion can be reliably increased by having a study team member or a neutral educator spend more time talking one-on-one to study participants.

Decision aids are not standard within the pharmaceutical industry. Using a decision aid is a matter of the investigator's discretion and of the available budget (80). The decision aid, as well as the consent form, need to be approved by the IRB, or other ethics committee. Decision aids provide balanced, neutral infor-mation about treatment options, and can lead to more realistic expectations, reduce negative emotions, and promote better adherence (81,82). Decision aids take the form of literature, audiotapes, and videotapes. Also, a decision aid can take the form of verbal counseling (83).

A decision aid can take the form of a card to help understand specific parts of the clinical trial. For instance, a decision aid may outline the "Schedule of Events" and help the subject to understand the number of visits to the clinic, and what each visit entails (84). One goal is to enable the potential subject to deter-mine whether he or she can afford the time or want to undergo all the necessary procedures. Shillington et al. (85) provide a decision aid for use with diabetes patients, which includes a colored chart showing six different medicines (eg, insulin, dipeptidyl peptidase-4 inhibitor, or thiazolidione), with six corresponding columns, each column showing little icons that indicate whether the medicine requires a pill or injection, whether the medicine results in weight loss or weight gain, whether the medicine poses a risk for low blood sugar (hypoglycemia risk), the cost (icons showing $, $$, or $$$), and number of years on the market.

A decision aid for cystic fibrosis patients considering a lung transplant provides information on prognosis (in absence of any lung transplant), advantages of refusing the lung transplant, and advantages of accepting the lung transplant (86,87). Although the medical treatment was surgery, and not a drug or medical device, the decision aid is

[78]Featherstone K, Donovan JL. Random allocation or allocation at random? Patients' perspectives of participation in a randomised controlled trial. Br. Med. J. 1998;317:1177–80.

[79]Flory J, Emanuel E. Interventions to improve research participants' understanding in informed consent for research: a systematic review. J. Am. Med. Assoc. 2004;292:1593–601.

[80]Mosher KA. E-mail of October 21, 2010.

[81]Shillington AC, et al. Development of a patient decision aid for type 2 diabetes mellitus for patients not achieving glycemic control on metformin alone. Patient Prefer. Adherence 2015;9:609–17.

[82]Sawka AM, Straus S, Brierley JD, et al. Decision aid on radioactive iodine treatment for early stage papillary thyroid cancer—a randomized controlled trial. Trials 2010;11:81.

[83]Brehaut JC. E-mail of October 22, 2010.

[84]Mosher K. E-mail of October 21, 2010.

[85]Shillington AC, et al. Development of a patient decision aid for type 2 diabetes mellitus for patients not achieving glycemic control on metformin alone. Patient Prefer. Adherence 2015;9:609–17.

[86]Stacey D, Vandemheen KL, Hennessey R, et al. Implementation of a cystic fibrosis lung transplant referral patient decision aid in routine clinical practice: an observational study. Implement. Sci. 2015;10:17.

[87]The decision aid is available on the world wide web at: <http://decisionaid.ohri.ca/decaids.html>.

interesting because of its thorough disclosure of risks and benefits, and because of its request for input from the patient.

The decision aid has about 50 check boxes, where the patient provides feedback regarding his or her understanding of the options, and degree of interest in having the lung transplant. The decision aid recites, "As time goes by, you may have more frequent chest infections and more trouble breathing. The infections cause a decline in lung function. Generally when your lung function is less than 30% of normal, your doctor would consider referring you for lung transplantation." The decision aid lists advantages of refusing lung transplant, such as the 3% risk of death due to having the transplant, the 50% risk of transplant rejections, and the discomfort of surgery. The decision aid also lists advantages of moving forward and having a lung transplant, such as 78% chance of survival for at least 3 years (vs only 50% chance of survival for at least 3 years with no transplant).

Elwyn et al. (88) warn that decision aids should be unbiased, and that the motivation to draft and use a decision aid should arise from the need to rectify variations in practice due to poor comprehension. In particular, these authors warn that use of "patient stories" can have undue influence on the patient. Patient stories can introduce bias since decisions by the patient are strongly influenced by identification with patients featured, for example, in video presentations.

Waljee et al. (89) find that when a decision aid is used, improved "health literacy is correlated with improved patient outcomes, and patients with inadequate knowledge of their disease states are more likely to be hospitalized and have poorer disease management."

Juraskova et al. (90,91) believe that a decision aid can increase enrollment, improve subject adherence to the Clinical Study Protocol, and reduce drop-out rates. Mathibe (92) has also commented on methods to reduce drop-out rates in study subjects, for example, the technique of providing a small payment.

In a study of decision aids used for breast cancer surgery, it was found that women found that photographs were useful aspects in the decision aid, and that few women found them inappropriate or frightening (93). Palladino (94) provides another example of a decision aid, namely, a videotape showing a patient discussing methods for making decisions, along with interviews of medical

[88]Elwyn G, O'Connor A, Stacey D, et al. Developing a quality criteria framework for patient decision aids: online international Delphi consensus process. Br. Med. J. 2006;333:417.

[89]Waljee JF, Rogers MA, Alderman AK. Decision aids and breast cancer: do they influence choice for surgery and knowledge of treatment options? J. Clin. Oncol. 2007;25:1067–73.

[90]Juraskova I, Butow P, Lopez AL, et al. Improving informed consent in clinical trials: successful piloting of a decision aid. J. Clin. Oncol. 2007;25:1443–4.

[91]Juraskova I, Butow P, Lopez A, et al. Improving informed consent: pilot of a decision aid for women invited to participate in a breast cancer prevention trial (IBIS-II DCIS). Health Expect. 2008;11:252–62.

[92]Mathibe LJ. Drop-out rates of cancer patients participating in longitudinal RCTs. Contemp. Clin. Trials 2007;28:340–2.

[93]Waljee JF, Rogers MA, Alderman AK. Decision aids and breast cancer: do they influence choice for surgery and knowledge of treatment options? J. Clin. Oncol. 2007;25:1067–73.

[94]Palladino ML. Challenges in the informed consent process: identifying design strategies that enhance communication in adult clinical trials. Res. Practitioner 2002;3:164–71.

experts. The goal of the videotape was to encourage patient involvement by showing other patients as role models.

XIII. CONCLUDING REMARKS

Consent forms are required for clinical trials. The administrative law provides guidelines for writing consent forms. Consent forms may be written by an investigator, medical writer, or attorney, and they must be approved by an IRB or by an ethics committee.

The primary goal of consent forms, in the context of clinical trials, is to ensure that the potential subject makes an autonomous decision regarding whether to enroll in the trial. Other goals are to promote communication between the study subject and healthcare providers, promote patient enrollment, reduce drop-out rate, and reduce liability.

When new information on safety and efficacy becomes available, as the clinical trial progresses, a revised consent form may be needed (95,96). The IRB needs to review the revised consent form (97). According to Dal-Ré et al. (98), the information in a re-consent form should be new and relevant to the subject's consent. The information in the re-consent form should be relevant to the subject's willingness to continue participation in the trial. Administering re-consent forms can be appropriate when subjects are in the run-in phase, treatment phase, and even in the follow-up phase.

Regarding some fine points, consent forms also include the issues of informed consent to allow research in medical emergencies (99), informed consent for Alzheimer's disease patients (100), the problem that patients with advanced cancer have decreased comprehension, memory change, and concentration difficulty (101), allowing a surrogate to sign an informed consent for medical emergencies such as stroke (102,103), using cartoon drawings to enable children to understand their informed

[95]Dal-Ré R, Avendaño C, Gil-Aguado A, Gracia D, Caplan AL. When should re-consent of subjects participating in a clinical trial be requested? A case-oriented algorithm to assist in the decision-making process. Clin. Pharmacol. Ther. 2008;83:788—93.

[96]Resnik DB. Re-consenting human subjects: ethical, legal and practical issues. J. Med. Ethics 2009;35:656—7.

[97]Bankert EA, Amdur RJ. Institutional Review Board: management and function. 2nd ed. Sudbury, MA: Jones and Bartlett; 2005. p. 259.

[98]Dal-Ré R, Avendaño C, Gil-Aguado A, Gracia D, Caplan AL. When should re-consent of subjects participating in a clinical trial be requested? A case-oriented algorithm to assist in the decision-making process. Clin. Pharmacol. Ther. 2008;83:788—93.

[99]Yamal J-M, et al. Enrollment of racially/ethnically diverse participants in traumatic brain injury trials: effect of availability of exception from informed consent. Clin. Trials 2014;11:187—94.

[100]Rose D, et al. Taking part in a pharmacogenetic clinical trial: assessment of trial participants understanding of information disclosed during the informed consent process. BMC Med. Ethics 2013;14:34 (9 p.).

[101]Malik L, Mejia A. Informed consent for phase I oncology trials: form, substance and signature. J. Clin. Med. Res. 2014;6:205—8.

[102]Bryant J, et al. The accuracy of surrogate decision makers: informed consent in hypothetical acute stroke scenarios. BMC Emerg. Med. 2013;13:18 (6 p.).

[103]U.S. Department of Health and Human Services. Food and Drug Administration. Guidance for Institutional Review Boards, Clinical Investigators, and Sponsors. Exception from informed consent requirements for emergency research; April 2013 (55 pp.).

consent form (104), and low literacy rates, for example, in parts of Australia or Texas (105) and the opinion that one-third of all Americans have a low "health literacy" (106). Malik et al. (107) recommend that consent forms include the study schema and treatment calendar.

[104]Grootens-Wiegens, P, et al. Comic strips help children understand medical research: tailoring the informed consent procedure to children's needs. Design4Health 2013 Conference Guidebook. Sheffield: Sheffield Hallam University; 2013. pp. 42–3.

[105]Malik L, et al. How well informed is the informed consent for cancer clinical trials? Clin. Trials 2014. doi:10.1177/1740774514548734 (3 p.).

[106]U.S. Department of Health and Human Services. Food and Drug Administration. Guidance for IRBs, Clinical Investigators, and Sponsors. Informed consent information sheet; July 2014 (42 pp.).

[107]Malik L, et al. How well informed is the informed consent for cancer clinical trials? Clin. Trials 2014. doi:10.1177/1740774514548734 (3 p.).

31

Package Inserts

I. INTRODUCTION

The package insert can take the form of folded paper tucked inside the drug enclosure, or a paper separately provided by pharmacies to patients. The terms package insert and label are often discussed together, as indicated in the cited references (1,2,3,4), though package inserts may contain much more information than a label. The primary purpose of the package insert is to give healthcare professionals information needed to prescribe drugs. The primary purpose is not to give information to patients, though it should be noted that the patient counseling information section of the package insert is written for the lay audience (5).

Information that is in package inserts can be acquired from Drugdex®, one of several databases for use in acquiring information about medicines, including information on drug safety. According to Rehman (6), Drugdex is more detailed than other databases, for example, Lexi-Comp® (Lexi-Comp, Inc., Hudson, OH). Drugdex and Lexi-Comp databases can be consulted for blackbox warnings for any drug. Cheng et al. (7) determined that Drugdex provides more complete information on the blackbox warnings that are printed on package labels and package inserts, while Lexi-Comp tends to provide this type of information in the form of a summary. Similarly, Kupferberg et al. (8) determined that Drugdex

[1]Lal R, Kremzner M. Introduction to the new prescription drug labeling by the Food and Drug Administration. Am. J. Health Syst. Pharm. 2007;64:2488−94.

[2]United States of America v. Evers. 643 F.2d 1043; 1981 U.S. App. LEXIS 13844.

[3]Ramirez v. Plough, Inc. 6 Cal. 4th 539; 863 P.2d 167; 25 Cal. Rptr. 2d 97; 1993 Cal. LEXIS 6012.

[4]Papike v. Tambrands, Inc. 107 F.3d 737; 1997 U.S. App. LEXIS 2870.

[5]Kremzner ME, Osborne SF. An introduction to the improved FDA prescription drug labeling (68 pp.) (undated document obtained from www.fda.gov in February 2011).

[6]Rehman B. Micromedix and lexicomp: considerations to aid choice between products. Northwick Park and St. Mark's Hospital, NHS Trust, Harrow, Middlesex, UK: UK Medicines Information; September. 2011 (2 pp.).

[7]Cheng CM, et al. Boxed warning inconsistencies between drug information sources and the prescribing Information. Am. J. Health Syst. Pharm. 2011;68:1626−31.

[8]Kupferberg N, et al. Evaluation of five full-text drug databases by pharmacy students, faculty, and librarians: do the groups agree? J. Med. Libr. Assoc. 2004;92:66−71.

Clinical Trials.
DOI: http://dx.doi.org/10.1016/B978-0-12-804217-5.00031-X

is more informative than Lexi-Comp. In 2012, ownership of the Drugdex database was transferred from Thomson Reuters to a new corporation, Truven Health Analytics (9).

The package insert must provide a statement of the ingredients, the indication (disorder to be treated), and directions for use. Directions for use include quantity, frequency of administration, and duration of administration. Duration refers to the number of days, weeks, or years. The directions also provide the time of administration, that is, relation to time of meals, or relation to time of onset of symptoms. The package insert also provides warnings regarding adverse drug reactions (ADRs). These and other requirements are summarized by the following bullet points:

- Indications;
- Warnings and precautions;
- List of adverse reactions;
- Dosage and administration;
- Dosage forms and strengths;
- Black box warning, if applicable;
- Interactions of the drug with other drugs;
- The name and place of the manufacturer;
- Use in specific populations, such as pregnant women, nursing mothers, children, and the elderly;
- Contraindications, for example, regarding special populations, such as pregnant women, nursing mothers, children, and the elderly;
- The order in which contraindications are listed is based on the likelihood of occurrence and the size of the population affected (10).

Effective June 30, 2006, the FDA's rule, "Requirements on Content and Format of Labeling for Human Prescription Drug and Biological Products," mandated that package inserts be organized as shown in Table 31.1. Lal and Kremzer (11) provide side-by-side comparisons of the new labeling format and the old labeling format, where the new labeling format is disclosed in Table 31.1. These authors also provide an example of a label filled out in the new format.

a. FDA's Guidance for Industry Documents Relating to Package Inserts

Several of FDA's Guidance for Industry documents relate to the package insert, and these pertain to the dosage and administration section (12), warnings and precautions section (13), adverse reactions section (14), mechanism

---

[9]Press release (June 6, 2012) Veritas completes purchase of Thomson Health unit (1 p.).

[10]Kremzner ME, Osborne SF. An introduction to the improved FDA prescription drug labeling (68 pp.) (undated document obtained from www.fda.gov in February 2011).

[11]Lal R, Kremzner M. Introduction to the new prescription drug labeling by the Food and Drug Administration. Am. J. Health Syst. Pharm. 2007;64:2488–94.

[12]Department of Health and Human Services. Food and Drug Administration. Guidance for industry. Dosage and administration section of labeling for human prescription drug and biological products—Content and Format; March 2010.

[13]Department of Health and Human Services. Food and Drug Administration. Guidance for industry. Warnings and precautions, contraindications, and boxed warning sections of labeling for human prescription drug and biological products—Content and Format; January 2006 (11 pp).

[14]Department of Health and Human Services. Food and Drug Administration. Guidance for industry. Adverse reactions section of labeling for human prescription drug and biological products—Content and Format; January 2006 (13 pp.).

TABLE 31.1 Format of Label Mandated by Requirements on Content and Format of Labeling for Human Prescription Drug and Biological Products

Highlights of prescribing information (1/2 page)

Brand name	Contraindications
Initial approval date	Warnings and precautions
Indications and usage	Adverse reactions
Dosage and administration	Drug interactions
Dosage forms and strengths	Revision date

Full prescribing information: Contents (1/2 page)

1 Indications and usage	**9** (information not given)
2 Dosage and administration	**10** Overdosage
2.1 Dosing information	**11** Description
2.2 Dose modifications	**12** Clinical pharmacology
2.3 Dosing in special populations	**12.1** Mechanism of action
3 Dosage forms and strengths	**12.2** (information not given)
4 Contraindications	**12.3** Pharmacokinetics
5 Warnings and precautions	**13** Nonclinical toxicology
6 Adverse reactions	**14** Clinical studies
6.1 Clinical trials experience	**15** References
7 Drug interactions	**16** How supplied/storage and handling
8 Use in specific populations	**17** Patient counseling information
8.1 Pregnancy	**17.1** Instructions
8.2 Nursing mothers	**17.2** FDA-approved patient labeling
8.3 Pediatric use	
8.4 Geriatric use	
8.5 Use in patients with hepatic impairment	
8.6 Use in patients with renal impairment	

of action section (15), clinical studies section (16), drugs for hypertension (17), geriatric drugs (18), and estrogen drugs (19).

In detail, the guidance on dosage and administration recommends including these subparts (20):

A. Basic dosing information;
B. Monitoring to assess effectiveness;
C. Monitoring to assess safety;
D. Monitoring for therapeutic blood levels;
E. Dosage modifications because of drug interactions;
F. Dosage modifications in specific patient populations;
G. Important considerations concerning compliance with dosage regimen;
H. Premedication and concomitant medication information; and
I. Important administration instructions.

Regarding the first of these subparts, the Guidelines further recommend that the basic dosing information encompasses the recommended starting dose (if different from the usual recommended dose), the usual dose, the duration of use, and the route of administration.

In detail, the Guidance document on warnings and precautions, provides the following criteria for inclusion in the package insert (21). Adverse drug reactions to include in the warnings and precautions include those associated with use of the drug where there is evidence (but not necessarily proof) for a causal association. The ADR should only be included in the package insert: (1) if it is serious; (2) if it is clinically significant, for example, if it requires dose modification; or (3) if the drug interferes with a laboratory test. What should also be included is ADRs that are expected to occur (but have not yet been observed in humans), based on what is known about the pharmacology, chemistry, or class of drug, or if animal data (toxicological data) show potential for a corresponding ADR in humans.

At the time FDA grants approval to a drug, FDA publishes the package insert on FDA's website. The administrative law relating to

---

[15]Department of Health and Human Services. Food and Drug Administration. Guidance for industry. Clinical pharmacology section of labeling for human prescription drug and biological products—Content and Format; February. 2009.

[16]Department of Health and Human Services. Food and Drug Administration. Guidance for industry. Clinical studies section of labeling for human prescription drug and biological products—Content and Format; January 2006 (22 pp.).

[17]Department of Health and Human Services. Food and Drug Administration. Guidance for industry. Hypertension indication: drug labeling for cardiovascular outcome claims; March 2008.

[18]Department of Health and Human Services. Food and Drug Administration. Guidance for industry. Content and format for geriatric labeling; October 2001 (10 pp.).

[19]Department of Health and Human Services. Food and Drug Administration. Guidance for industry. Noncontraceptive estrogen drug products for the treatment of vasomotor symptoms and vulvar and vaginal atrophy symptoms—recommended prescribing information for health care providers and patient labeling; November 2005.

[20]Department of Health and Human Services. Food and Drug Administration. Guidance for industry. Dosage and administration section of labeling for human prescription drug and biological products—Content and Format; March 2010.

[21]Department of Health and Human Services. Food and Drug Administration. Guidance for industry. Warnings and precautions, contraindications, and boxed warning sections of labeling for human prescription drug and biological products—Content and Format; January 2006 (11 pp.).

labeling is set forth in Title 21, Part 201, of the Code of Federal Regulations (CFR) (21 CFR §201.10). An excerpt from 21 CFR §201.10 discloses that (22):

> If the drug is in tablet or capsule form or other unit dosage form, any statement of the quantity of an ingredient contained therein shall express the quantity of such ingredient in each such unit … [s]uch statements shall be in terms that are informative to licensed practitioners, in the case of a prescription drug, and to the layman, in the case of a nonprescription drug.

Other requirements from 21 CFR §201.56, include (23):

(1) The labeling must contain a summary of the essential scientific information needed for the safe and effective use of the drug.

(2) The labeling must be informative and accurate and neither promotional in tone nor false or misleading in any particular. The labeling must be updated when new information becomes available that causes the labeling to become inaccurate, false, or misleading.

(3) The labeling must be based whenever possible on data derived from human experience. No implied claims or suggestions of drug use may be made if there is inadequate evidence of safety or a lack of substantial evidence of effectiveness. Conclusions based on animal data but necessary for safe and effective use of the drug in humans must be identified as such and included with human data in the appropriate section of the labeling.

b. Classes of Drugs

Drugs can be classed by the *Anatomical Therapeutic Chemical* (ATC) system (24,25,26,27,28). This system is based on the assumption that compounds with similar physical and chemical properties exhibit similar biological activities (29). Lin et al. (30) describe the utility of the ATC system, and also identify a number of databases that list drugs, their associated adverse events, and drug targets. One such database is Drugbank, available from the University of Alberta. Drugdex, provided by Thomson Reuters, is another database on dosage, pharmacokinetics, indications, and ADRs. The ATC system, as well as the listed databases, can aid in drafting package inserts.

[22]21 Code of Federal Regulations 201.10 (April 1, 2010 version).

[23]21 Code of Federal Regulations 201.56 (April 1, 2010 version).

[24]Takarabe M, Shigemizu D, Kotera M, Goto S, Kanehisa M. Characterization and classification of adverse drug interactions. Genome Inform. 2010;22:167−75.

[25]Imming P, Sinning C, Meyer A. Drugs, their targets and the nature and number of drug targets. Nat. Rev. Drug Discov. 2006;5:821−84.

[26]Bender A, Scheiber J, Glick M, et al. Analysis of pharmacology data and the prediction of adverse drug reactions and off-target effects from chemical structure. ChemMedChem. 2007;2:861−73.

[27]Imming P, Buss T, Dailey LA, et al. A classification of drug substances according to their mechanism of action. Pharmazie. 2004;59:579−89.

[28]Gurulingappa H, Kolárik C, Hofmann-Apitius M, Fluck J. Concept-based semi-automatic classification of drugs. J. Chem. Inf. Model 2009;49:1986−92.

[29]Dunkel M, Günther S, Ahmed J, Wittig B, Preissner R. SuperPred: drug classification and target prediction. Nucleic Acids Res. 2008;36:W55−W59.

[30]Lin SF, Xiao KT, Huang YT, Chiu CC, Soo VW. Analysis of adverse drug reactions using drug and drug target interactions and graph-based methods. Artif. Intell. Med. 2010;48:161−6.

c. Black Box Warning

Where a drug presents a serious risk that can lead to death or serious injury, FDA may require that the package insert include a black box warning. This warning informs the physician that patients taking the drug need to be closely monitored (31). Black box warnings include those that require laboratory testing, avoiding other drugs (warning regarding drug–drug interactions), avoiding prescribing in the presence of another specified health condition, or knowing the risks associated with a specific population, such as pregnant women.

Black box warnings take the form of a writing that resides inside a black box. Examples appear below. These examples, which are from drugs discussed earlier in this book, include an anticancer drug (cisplatin), an antiviral drug (ribavirin), and an antidepressant (Zoloft®).

The black box warning for cisplatin (32) is reproduced here:

> **WARNINGS.** Cisplatin injection should be administered under the supervision of a qualified physician experienced in the use of cancer chemotherapeutic agents. Appropriate management of therapy and complications is possible only when adequate diagnostic and treatment facilities are readily available. Cumulative renal toxicity associated with cisplatin is severe. Other major dose-related toxicities are myelosuppression, nausea, and vomiting. Ototoxicity, which may be more pronounced in children, and is manifested by tinnitus, and/or loss of high frequency hearing and occasionally deafness, is significant. Anaphylactic-like reactions to cisplatin have been reported. Facial edema,

> bronchoconstriction, tachycardia, and hypotension may occur within minutes of cisplatin administration. Epinephrine, corticosteriods, and antihistamines have been effectively employed to alleviate symptoms.
>
> **Exercise caution to prevent inadvertent cisplatin overdose.** Doses greater than $100 \, mg/m^2/$ cycle once every 3–4 weeks are rarely used. Care must be taken to avoid inadvertent cisplatin overdose due to confusion with carboplatin or prescribing practices that fail to differentiate daily doses from total dose per cycle.

The black box warning for ribavirin (33) reads:

> **WARNING.** COPEGUS (ribavirin) monotherapy is not effective for the treatment of chronic hepatitis C virus infection and should not be used alone for this indication. The primary clinical toxicity of ribavirin is hemolytic anemia. The anemia associated with ribavirin therapy may result in worsening of cardiac disease that has led to fatal and nonfatal myocardial infarctions. Patients with a history of significant or unstable cardiac disease should not be treated with ribavirin.
>
> Significant teratogenic and/or embryocidal effects have been demonstrated in all animal species exposed to ribavirin. In addition, ribavirin has a multiple dose half-life of 12 days, and it may persist in non-plasma compartments for as long as 6 months. Ribavirin therapy is contraindicated in women who are pregnant and in the male partners of women who are pregnant. Extreme care must be taken to avoid pregnancy during therapy and for 6 months

[31]Ricci JR, Coulen C, Berger JE, Moore MC, McQueen A, Jan SA. Prescriber compliance with black box warnings in older adult patients. Am. J. Manag. Care 2009;15:e103–8.

[32]Package insert. Bedford Laboratories, Cisplatin injection, (June 2004).

[33]Package insert. Copegus Roche Laboratories, Inc. (May 2004).

after completion of therapy in both female patients and in female partners of male patients who are taking ribavirin therapy. At least two reliable forms of effective contraception must be utilized during treatment and during the 6-month posttreatment follow-up period.

The black box warning for sertraline (34) reads, in part:

> **WARNING**. Antidepressants increased the risk compared to placebo of suicidal thinking and behavior (suicidality) in children, adolescents, and young adults in short-term studies of major depressive disorder (MDD) and other psychiatric disorders. Anyone considering the use of Zoloft or any other antidepressant in a child, adolescent, or young adult must balance this risk with the clinical need. Short-term studies did not show an increase in the risk of suicidality with antidepressants compared to placebo in adults beyond age 24; there was a reduction in risk with antidepressants compared to placebo in adults aged 65 and older. Depression and certain other psychiatric disorders are themselves associated with increases in the risk of suicide. Patients of all ages who are started on antidepressant therapy should be monitored appropriately and observed closely for clinical worsening, suicidality, or unusual changes in behavior. Families and caregivers should be advised of the need for close observation and communication with the prescriber.

II. DRUG−DRUG INTERACTIONS

a. Introduction

The term "drug−drug interactions" concerns a first drug's influence on the metabolism of a

second drug. For example, the first drug can influence parameters of the second drug, such as its plasma concentration, rate of transport into cells, rate of efflux out of cells, rate of catabolism, and rate of conjugation. Where drug−drug interactions have been found for a study drug, issues that can arise include unexpected changes in the safety and efficacy of the drug. For these reasons, package inserts for drugs include a section entitled, "Drug−drug interactions." Drug−drug interactions find a basis in 21 CFR §201.57, which requires the following. The emphasis is added:

> (8) *Drug interactions*. (i) This section must contain a description of clinically significant interactions, either observed or predicted, with other prescription or over-the-counter drugs, classes of drugs, or **foods** (e.g., dietary supplements, grapefruit juice), and specific practical instructions for preventing or managing them. The mechanism(s) of the **interaction**, if known, must be briefly described. Interactions that are described in the "Contraindications" or "Warnings and Precautions" sections must be discussed in more detail under this section.

Please note that the influences of *foods* on the study drug should be included in the *Drug−Drug Interactions* section of the package insert. A concrete example of food−drug interactions is provided below, in the account of *everolimus*. Further regarding drug−drug interactions, the *Dose and Administration* part of the package label requires a disclosure of (21 CFR §201.57):

> (H) Modification of dosage needed because of **drug interactions** or in special patient populations (e.g., in children, in geriatric age groups, in groups defined by genetic characteristics, or in patients with renal or hepatic disease).

A concept related to drug−drug interactions is the interference of the study drug with a laboratory test. Section 201.57 also requires that

---

[34]Package insert. Pfizer, Zoloft (October 2008).

the *Warnings and Precautions* part of the package insert disclose the drug's interference with laboratory tests:

> (iv) *Interference with laboratory tests.* This section must briefly note information on any known interference by the product with laboratory tests and reference the section where the detailed information is presented (e.g., "Drug Interactions" section).

Characterizing drug–drug interactions includes in vitro studies to see whether a drug is a substrate, inhibitor, or inducer of enzymes that metabolize drugs. Enzymes that metabolize drugs include those that catalyze drug oxidation, as well as those catalyzing conjugation with sugars, sulfate groups, and so on. Various isozymes of cytochrome P450 are the most commonly studied of these enzymes, and these isozymes include cytochrome P450 enzymes known by the abbreviations:

- CYP1A2;
- CYP2B6;
- CYP3A.

Other enzymes and proteins that are the subject of drug–drug interaction studies include uridine diphosphate (UDP)-glucuronosyltransferase, as well as transport proteins such as:

- BCRP;
- OATP1B1;
- OTP1B3.

FDA's Guidance for Industry describes the isozymes of cytochrome P450, drug conjugating enzymes, and transport systems, as well as some of the more notorious examples of drug–drug interactions (35).

b. Instructions in a Clinical Study Protocol That Prohibit Concomitant Drugs

The issue of drug–drug interactions is so prevalent that the Clinical Study Protocol may include instructions that prohibit study subjects from taking certain medications that are expected to modify in vivo metabolism of the study drug.

The following provides a set of instructions that are somewhat generic, in view of the fact that the pharmacokinetics of the drug was only partly characterized. The excerpt is from a Protocol on prostate cancer. The warning refers to a list in an appendix in the Protocol (36,37):

> APPENDIX G provides a list of potent CYP enzyme inhibitors and inducers that may have a theoretical concern of potential drug–drug interactions with [the study drug]. In vitro drug metabolism studies suggest that [the study drug] may have the potential to induce CYP3A4 and to inhibit CYP1A2, CYP2B6, CYP2C8, CYP2C9, CYP2C19, CYP2D6, and CYP3A4/5; therefore, concomitant medications that are substrates of any of these enzymes should be used with caution, and relevant monitoring should be considered, especially for substrates known to cause seizure, because the possibility of drug–drug interactions cannot be fully excluded. Since the metabolism of [the study drug] is not known, caution should be taken for the

[35]U.S. Department of Health and Human Services. Food and Drug Administration. Guidance for industry. Drug interaction studies—study design, data analysis, implications for dosing, and labeling recommendations; February 2012 (75 pp.).

[36]Clinical Research Protocol. Study Title: PREVAIL: A multinational phase 3, randomized, double-blind, placebo-controlled efficacy and safety study of oral MDV3100 in chemotherapy-naïve patients with progressive metastatic prostate cancer who have failed androgen deprivation therapy protocol no: MDV3100-03.

[37]Clinical Study Protocol available as supplement to: Beer TM, Armstrong AJ, Rathkopf DE, et al. Enzalutamide in metastatic prostate cancer before chemotherapy. New Engl. J. Med. 2014;371:424–33.

concomitant use of strong inhibitors and inducers of CYP enzymes and alternative products used when available.

The following second example provides instructions that are relatively specific and distinct. The excerpt is from a Protocol from a cancer clinical trial, where the study drug was LDK378, also known as ceritinib (38). The Protocol contained the following instructions (39). The Protocol includes tables that list the prohibited concomitant drugs. The instructions stated that:

> **Permitted concomitant therapy requiring caution and/or action**. LDK378 [study drug] may result in a 2- to 5-fold increase in the AUC of sensitive CYP3A4/5 substrates. In addition, LDK378 is a potent inhibitor of CYP2C9. Prior to starting study treatment, investigators should carefully review the study subject's current medications for drugs metabolized by these isoenzymes. Caution is required when prescribing drugs that are known to be metabolized by CYP3A4/5 and 2C9 to patients taking LDK378. The investigator and patients should be aware of potential signs of overdose of these drugs, and in the event of suspected toxicity should stop either the substrate or LDK378 according to the clinical judgment of the investigator.

The instructions in the Protocol continued with:

> **CYP3A4/5 substrates with narrow therapeutic index**. Based on *in vitro* data, LDK378 is a potent inhibitor of CYP3A4/5 substrates. Drugs of this class which have a narrow therapeutic index are prohibited … CYP3A4/5 strong inhibitors and

inducers. CYP3A4/5 strong inhibitors and inducers are also prohibited … CYP2C9 substrates with narrow therapeutic index. Based on in vitro data, LDK378 is a potent inhibitor of CYP2C9 substrates. The only CYP2C9 substrate with narrow therapeutic index is warfarin and phenytoin which are not permitted for the duration of the study.

c. Example of Drug–Drug Interactions Involving Mibefradil

The following narrative takes its inspiration from the FDA's examples, and solidifies these examples with more recently published information. The FDA's Guidance for Industry provides the example of *mibefradil* (Posicor®) which when used in combination with *statins*, such as simvastatin, causes an increase in plasma statin and consequent rhabdomyolysis (skeletal muscle injury). The mechanism in this drug–drug interaction is that mibefradil inhibits CYP3A, where this inhibition provokes increased levels of the statin. *Mibefradil* is used for the indication of heart failure (40). A study of some 871 cases of statin-associated rhabdomyolysis revealed that 99 of these were associated with *mibefradil*. The statins in these reports were simvastatin, atorvastatin, and cerivastatin (41).

One year after its introduction into the market, the Sponsor of the drug voluntarily withdrew the drug, after receiving reports of dangerous interactions with various other drugs. Regarding the mechanism of action,

---

[38]Khozin S, Blumenthal GM, Zhang L, et al. FDA approval: ceritinib for the treatment of metastatic anaplastic lymphoma kinase-positive non-small cell lung cancer. Clin. Cancer Res. 2015;21:2439–39.

[39]Oncology Clinical Trial Protocol CLDK378X2101. A phase I, multicenter, open-label dose escalation study of LDK378, administered orally in adult patients with tumors characterized by genetic abnormalities in anaplastic lymphoma kinase (ALK) (August 19, 2010).

[40]van der Vring, JA, et al. Evaluating the safety of mibefradil, a selective T-type calcium antagonist in patients with chronic congestive heart failure. Clin. Ther. 1996;18:1191–206.

[41]Omar MA, Wilson JP. FDA adverse event reports on statin-associated rhabdomyolysis. Ann. Pharmacother. 2002;36:288–95.

mibefradil was found to inhibit CYP3A4, and CYP2D6, resulting in increases of the concomittantly used other drugs to dangerous levels. When first marketed, the package label warned against concurrent use with astemizole, cisapride, and terfenadine. After a few months, statins (lovastatin, simvastatin) were added to this list of drugs that must not be co-administered with mibefradil (42).

d. Naturally Occurring Genetic Variations That Influence Drug–Drug Interactions

Genetic variations that influence drug–drug interactions exist naturally in the human population. The most frequent source of concern is variation in the expression and activity of isozymes of cytochrome P450 and, in particular, the isozymes that are:

- CYP2D6;
- CYP2C19;
- CYP2C9.

CYP2D6 is responsible for catabolizing about 25% of drugs that are antidepressants, antiarrhythmias, and tamoxifen (43). To provide an example of people with CYP2D6 variants that are expressed at abnormally low levels, Schultz discloses that, "Caucasians are more likely than people of Asian and African ancestry to have abnormally low levels of … CYP2D6" (44). A danger arising from the variability of expression in one or more of the cytochrome P450 isozymes is that some patients will exhibit, as a consequence, unexpected drug–drug interactions that have an adverse influence on efficacy or safety of either drug.

e. Drug–Drug Interactions Involving Fluoxetine and Atomoxetine

The following illustrates the situation where a patient is given *fluoxetine* and *atomoxetine*. Each of these drugs may be used alone, or in combination with each other, for treating depression (45). Fluoxetine (Prozac®) inhibits CYP2D6. When administered, fluoxetine's inhibition of CYP2D6 provokes increases in concentrations of various drugs that would otherwise have been oxidized by CYP2D6. These oxidized drugs include atomoxetine (Strattera®). But for people who naturally fail to express CYP2D6, administered fluoxetine cannot inhibit CYP2D6 (because there does not exist any CYP2D6), and as a consequence any administered fluoxetine will not influence the levels of atomexetine (46).

f. Atomoxetine's Package Insert Warns That Fluoxetine Increases Levels of Atomexetine in the Body

The package insert for atomoxetine warns that fluoxetine will increase amoxetine levels

[42]SoRelle R. Withdrawal of Posicor from market. Circulation. 1998;98:831–2.

[43]Samer CF, et al. Applications of CYP450 testing in the clinical setting. Mol. Diagn. Ther. 2013;17:165–84.

[44]Schultz J. FDA Guidelines on race and ethnicity: obstacle or remedy? J. Natl. Cancer Inst. 2003;95:425–6.

[45]Kratochvil CD, et al. Atomoxetine alone or combined with fluoxetine for treating ADHD with comorbid depressive or anxiety syndromes. J. Am. Acad. Child Adolesc. Psychiatry. 2005;44:915–24.

[46]U.S. Department of Health and Human Services. Food and Drug Administration. Guidance for industry. Drug interaction studies—study design, data analysis, implications for dosing, and labeling recommendations; February 2012 (75 pp.).

in most people, but does not have this effect in a fraction of the population (47). This warning is:

> [a] fraction of the population (about 7% of Caucasians and 2% of African Americans) ... have reduced activity in [CYP2D6] resulting in ... higher ... plasma concentrations ... of atomoxetine compared with people with normal activity. Drugs that inhibit CYP2D6, such as fluoxetine, paroxetine, and quinidine, cause similar increases in exposure.

The package insert warns that, where fluoxetine is co-administered with atomoxetine, the result is atomoxetine-specific adverse reactions, such as liver injury and jaundice.

g. Transporters

Konig et al. (48) provide an excellent account of drug−drug interaction studies that involve transporters. These include transporters that are dedicated to mediating either entry into cells, or mediating efflux of drugs out of cells. In drug−drug interaction studies, the transporters of greatest interest include the hepatic transporters, OATPB1 and OATP1B3, and the transporters mediating efflux, such as P-glycoprotein (Pgp), Breast Cancer Resistance Protein (BCRP), and Multi-Drug Resistance Protein 2 (MRP2). Despite being named BCRP, this efflux transporter is expressed by intestines, liver, kidney, and brain. OATP means "Organic Anion-Transporting Protein."

h. Drug−Drug interactions Between Statins and Cyclosporin A

Statins, such as atorvastatin (Lipitor®), reach their target enzyme in liver cells by way of the transporter, OATP1B1. This transporter is a membrane-bound protein on hepatocytes (49). Impaired transport of atorvastatin into liver cells occurs with naturally occurring variants of OATP1B1 in the human population. A knowledge of the genotype of the gene encoding this transporter, for any given patient, can predict whether statin therapy in that patient will be reduced because of that impairment. In other words, if the statin cannot enter the hepatocyte, the statin will not work.

Naturally occurring variants in OATP1B1 can impair the transport activity of OATP1B1 and, as a consequence, result in unexpectedly high levels of any statin drugs that are administered. This scenario is illustrated by the following excerpts from Nies et al. (50):

"The common variant c.521T > C (rs4149056; Val174Ala) is highlighted by a genome-wide association study (GWAS) suggesting an increased risk for simvastatin-induced myopathy in variant carriers."

"The increased atorvastatin [plasma concentration] ... in carriers of the *15 haplotype in our pharmacokinetic study revealed impaired atorvastatin uptake, indicating that the variant OATP1B1*15 protein is associated with decreased intrinsic transport activity."

The quotations refer to the variants in OATP1B1 that are the Val174Ala variant and

---

[47]STRATTERA® (atomoxetine) CAPSULES for Oral Use; April 2015 (18 pp.).

[48]Konig J, et al. Transporters and drug-drug Interactions: important determinants of drug disposition and effects. Pharmacol. Rev. 2013;65:944−96.

[49]Kunze A, et al. Prediction of OATP1B1 and OATP1B3 mediated hepatic uptake of statins based on transporter protein expression and activity data. Drug Metab. Dispos. 2015;43:424−32.

[50]Nies AT, Niemi M, Burk O, et al. Genetics is a major determinant of expression of the human hepatic uptake transporter OATP1B1, but not of OATP1B3 and OATP2B1. Genome Med. 2013;5:1 (11 pp.).

the OATP1B1*15 haplotype. Separate studies have demonstrated that the OATP1B*15 haplotype has reduced transporting activity for atorvastatin (51).

Van de Steeg et al. (52) provides an excellent "big picture" summary of the consequences of the Val174Ala variant:

> In particular, the OATP1B1*15 variant (Asn130Asp and Val174Ala), with an average ... frequency of 16–24% in Europe and America ... is generally known to have a ... **reduced transport activity** and has been associated with ... increased plasma levels of certain OATP1B1 substrates ... **decreased hepatic uptake** by OATP1B1*15 might result in decreased pharmacological response and give rise to unforeseen toxic side effects. Indeed, it has been demonstrated that patients carrying the OATP1B1*15 variant show ... increased plasma levels, decreased pharmacological response, and even increased extra-hepatic toxicity, for instance, after pravastatin, pitavastatin, or rosuvastatin treatment.

A number of drugs, such as cyclosporin A, can inhibit the transporting activity of OATP1B1. As a consequence, when patients are treated with statin and cyclosporin A, the plasma levels of the statin drug can increase to unexpectedly high levels (53). Increased levels of statins in the bloodstream, for example, as caused by impaired transport into hepatocytes, can result in statin-induced adverse events such as myopathy and rhabodomyolysis (skeletal muscle damage) (54,55).

i. Drug—Drug Interactions Distinguished From Adverse Events From Other Drugs That Do Not Involve Drug—Drug Interactions

Adverse events resulting from drug—drug interactions should be distinguished from adverse events from concurrent medications that result from mechanisms that do not involve drug—drug interactions. For example, the package label for televancin (56), which is an antibiotic that kills some types of bacteria, warns against diarrhea resulting from overgrowth of another type of gut bacterium, *Clostridium difficile*. It can readily be understood that this mechanism of action for producing diarrhea is independent from (and does not involve any drug—drug interaction) the mechanism of action for diarrhea, when taking drugs that prevent digestion of fats or carbohydrates (57). The following is another example of the same adverse events from two different drugs, but where there is no drug—drug interaction. According to the package label for the antibiotic, televancin, this drug may result in renal toxicity. The package label warns against taking concurrent medications that act on the kidneys,

[51]Tamraz B, Fukushima H, Wolfe AR, et al. OATP1B1-related drug—drug and drug—gene interactions as potential risk factors for cerivastatin-induced rhabdomyolysis. Pharmacogenet. Genomics 2013;23:355–64.

[52]van de Steeg E, Greupink R, Schreurs M, et al. Drug—drug interactions between rosuvastatin and oral antidiabetic drugs occurring at the level of OATP1B1. Drug Metab. Dispos. 2013;41:592–601.

[53]Karlgren M, et al. In vitro and In silico strategies to identify OAT1B1 inhibitors and predict clincal drug-drug interactions. Pharm. Res. 2012;29:411–26.

[54]Amundsen R, et al. Cyclosporin A, but not tacrolimus, shows relevant inhibition of organic anion-transporting protein 1B1-mediated transport of atorvastatin. Drug Metab. Dispos. 2010;38:1499–504.

[55]Ballantyne CM, et al. Risk for myopathy with statin therapy in high-risk patients. Arch. Intern. Med. 2003;163:553–64.

[56]Package insert for VIBATIV (telavancin) for injection, for intravenous use; December 2014 (37 pp.).

[57]Chassany O. Drug-induced diarrhoea. Drug Safety. 2000;22:53–72.

that is, diuretics. The package label warns that, "renal adverse event rates were also higher in patients who received concomitant medications known to affect kidney function (e.g., non-steroidal antiinflammatory drugs, ACE inhibitors, and loop diuretics)" (58). The company marketing televancin provided the kind guidance, that this type of interaction, that is, televancin's action on the kidney versus loop diuretic's action on the kidney, is not categorized as a drug–drug interaction, writing that, "[t]he medication guide provides information to the patient—specifically to warn their health care provider (HCP) about any other medications they are taking. *This is not due to any drug–drug interactions with Telavancin*, but due to the potential for increasing adverse event rates with the medications listed in the Med Guide (i.e. NSAIDs, loop diuretics, ACEIs, ARBs, and antiarrhythmics)" (59).

j. Summary

Recurring themes in drug–drug interaction studies include:

- *Variants that change activities of catabolic enzymes or of transporters.* Naturally occurring variants of a given enzyme or a transporter, can result in *increased plasma levels* of that drug, and consequent adverse events. This statement refers to variants in catabolic enzymes that destroy the drug, and to transporter variants with reduced transporter activity.
- *Drugs that change activities of catabolic enzymes or of transporters.* The following relates to a totally different scenario. A drug (a first drug) administered to a patient, that inhibits

an enzyme or inhibits transporter, can result in *increased plasma levels* of a second drug, and consequent adverse events. This statement refers to enzymes that catabolize the second drug. In other words, if the first drug inhibits the catabolic enzyme, the levels of the second drug will increase.

- *Protein variants.* Naturally occurring variants in catabolic enzymes, conjugating enzymes, and transporter proteins, can influence what is written in the package insert. If the variant results in a change in efficacy or safety of a drug, in absence of any second administered drug, these changes may be disclosed in the *Warnings and Precautions* section of the package insert. In the case that two drugs are administered to a patient, and if the variant results in a change in a protein that metabolizes the *first drug*, or if the variant results in a change in a protein that metabolizes the *second drug*, and if the end result is any change in efficacy or safety of either drug, then the results may be disclosed in the *Drug–Drug Interactions* section of the package label.

III. FDA'S DECISION-MAKING PROCESS IN EVALUATING DRUG–DRUG INTERACTIONS

Medical Reviews, as well as other reviews, are published along with the FDA's *Approval Letter*, at the time a drug is approved. All of these documents can be acquired from FDA's website by the footnoted procedure (60). The *Medical Reviews* take the form of data provided by the Sponsor, together with FDA's analysis

---

[58]Package insert for VIBATIV (telavancin) for injection, for intravenous use; December 2014 (37 pp.).

[59]Kind guidance from Dr Christina Slover, PharmD, in e-mail of April 7, 2015.

[60]On the FDA website, click on DRUG tab, click on Search Drug Approvals by Month Using Drugs @FDA, then choose the month and year, then choose the drug, and finally click on Approval History, Letters, Reviews, and related documents.

and conclusions from the data. It is the case that FDA reviews the data and draws its own conclusions, even though the Sponsor has already arrived at its conclusions. Some of the material in FDA's reviews takes the form of text that is copied from documents provided by the Sponsor (61). The *Medical Reviews* provide a candid insider's account of how FDA addresses gray areas, on topics such as drug–drug interactions, drug safety, and subgroup analysis.

a. Imatinib, for the Indication of Chronic Myeloid Leukemia

This concerns *imatinib* for treating chronic myeloid leukemia (CML), from the *Medical Review* of NDA 21588 at Jan. 2013 on the FDA website. In the following three studies with human subjects, the results demonstrated an increase, an increase, and a decrease in concentration of imatinib in the bloodstream. The three studies involved administering ketoconazole, simvastatin, or rifampin, as indicated below. The commentary reveals the experimental results and the reviewer's conclusions:

Study 1. *Ketoconazole*, a drug that inhibits CYP3A4. With administration of both ketoconazole and imatinib, it was the case that imatinib concentrations increased in the plasma of healthy subjects. These results suggest that imatinib is normally catabolized by CYP3A4.

Study 2. *Simvastatin*, a drug that is a substrate of CYP3A4. With administration of both simvastatin and imatinib, it was the case that simvastatin concentrations increased. The reviewer concluded that imatinib inhibited CYP3A4.

Study 3. *Rifampin*, a drug that induces CYP3A4. With administration of both rifampin and ibrutinib, it was the case that there was a decrease in plasma concentration of ibrutinib. This result also suggests that imatinib is normally catabolized by CYP3A4.

Another review, the *Clinical Pharmacology and Biopharmacology Review*, commented on the catabolism of imatinib, stating that "[c]learance is primarily hepatic, by the cytochrome P450 . . . enzyme system. CYP3A4 is the specific enzyme that metabolized imatinib."

The package insert reiterated the biochemical information from the *Medical Review* (62). The *Drug–Drug Interactions* section of the package insert read:

- CYP3A4 inducers may decrease Gleevec Cmax and AUC;
- CYP3A4 inhibitors may increase Gleevec Cmax and AUC;
- Gleevec is an inhibitor of CYP3A4 and CYP2D6 which may increase the Cmax and AUC of other drugs;

b. Everolimus for Astrocytoma

The following *Medical Review* provides an excellent take-home lesson regarding various dramatic topics:

- *Drugs that are non-study drugs.* The fact that study subjects were permitted to be medicated with drugs (antiepileptic drugs) that were not study drugs, and that were known to modulate cytochrome P450.
- *Stratification.* Use of stratification of the population, enabling separate analysis of the efficacy and safety results on subjects who were taking, and not taking, concurrent drugs, such as antiepileptics.
- *Food–drug interactions.* The need to take into account food–drug interactions, such as those involving grapefruit juice.

---

[61]Kind advice from Dr. Patrick Archdeacon, MD, FDA, CDER, in e-mail dated March 5, 2015.

[62]GLEEVEC® (imatinib mesylate) tablets for oral use; January 2015 (44 pp.).

The *Medical Review* for *everolimus* (Afinitor®) included comments about drugs and foods that modulated cytochrome P450, in particular CYP3A4, and Pgp. This information is from January 2015 on the FDA's website.

The reviewer provided comments on drug–drug interactions and food–drug interactions, writing, "[a]void the use of concomitant strong CYP3A4 inhibitors … e.g., ketoconazole, itraconazole, clarithromycin … in patients receiving AFINITOR … [d]o not ingest foods … grapefruit, grapefruit juice … that are known to inhibit cytochrome P450 or PgP activity."

The FDA reviewer also made comments regarding the Clinical Study Protocol. The reviewer noted that the Clinical Study Protocol stated that drugs that inhibit, induce, or are substrates for CYP3A4 or Pgp should not be used by study subjects. One exception was made in the Clinical Study Protocol. Antiepileptic drugs, which are known to induce CYP3A4, were permitted to be taken by the subjects enrolled in the clinical trial.

The following discloses the intersection between the concept of *patient stratification* and the concept of drug–drug interactions. In order to acquire higher-quality data and higher-quality interpretations on efficacy and safety of the study drug, the clinical trial was designed so that subjects were stratified into whether they were taking antiepileptics along with the study drug. The reviewer wrote, "[i]n addition, relationships between the use of enzyme-inducing antiepileptic drugs and response and pharmacokinetic endpoints should be explored."

Regarding *foods*, the FDA reviewer commented on foods that influence the activity of CYP3A4 or Pgp, writing that, "[i]nvestigators were instructed to avoid … consumption [by subjects] of the following … foods … Seville orange, starfruit, grapefruit, and other juices known to affect CYP450 and PgP activity."

As published, the *Drug–Drug Interactions* section of the package label read (63):

- Strong CYP3A4/PgP inhibitors: Avoid concomitant use.
- Moderate CYP3A4/PgP inhibitors: If combination is required, use caution and reduce dose of AFINITOR.
- Strong CYP3A4/PgP inducers: Avoid concomitant use. If combination cannot be avoided, increase dose of AFINITOR.

The *Patient Medication Guide*, which was published as part of the package label, contained a warning about foods:

"What should I avoid while taking AFINITOR or AFINITOR DISPERZ? You should not drink *grapefruit juice* or eat grapefruit during your treatment with AFINITOR or AFINITOR DISPERZ. It may make the amount of AFINITOR in your blood increase to a harmful level."

To conclude, the *Medical Review* for everolimus (Afinitor) provides a clear-cut account of the FDA's decision-making process regarding drug–drug interactions and food–drug interactions, and how these decisions resulted in instructions residing in the Clinical Study Protocol, and in warnings appearing in the package insert and *Patient Medication Guide*.

c. Lapatinib (In Vitro Drug–Drug Interaction Data Inspired the FDA to Require In Vivo Studies)

This illustrates the situation where FDA imposed requirements to conduct in vivo experiments on drug–drug interactions, in order to supplement existing data from in vitro studies. This is from NDA 22059 from

---

[63]AfinitorDISPERZ (everolimus tablets for oral suspension) (January 2015) (44 pp.).

March 2015 of the FDA's website. The study drug is *lapatinib*.

The *Medical Review, Clinical Pharmacology and Biopharmaceutics Review,* and the *Approval Letter* all referred to the fact that the study drug inhibited CYP3A4, CYP2C8, and Pgp. The *Clinical Pharmacology and Biopharmaceutics Review* referred to the Sponsor's in vitro studies, stating that "[i]n vitro studies in human hepatocytes ... indicate that lapatinib is primarily metabolized by CYP3A4 and CYP3A5 with smaller contributions from CYP2C8, and CYP2C19."

The *Approval Letter* referred to the fact that the Sponsor had agreed to perform in vivo experiments on the ability of the study drug (lapatinib) to influence the pharmacokinetics of a second drug. This information is from NDA22059 at March 2015 of the FDA's website. In short, FDA required that the Sponsor test the influence of *lapatinib* on the pharmacokinetics of *midazolam, paclitaxel, rosiglitazone,* and *digoxin.* The *Approval Letter* imposed the requirement:

> Description of Commitment: Based upon the ability of lapatinib to act as a **CYP3A4** inhibitor in vitro, [Sponsor] ... agrees to perform an in vivo drug interaction study of the ability of steady-state lapatinib dosing to alter the pharmacokinetics of a single dose of midazolam ... [b]ased upon the ability of lapatinib to act as a **CYP2C8** inhibitor in vitro, [Sponsor] ... agrees to perform an in vivo drug interaction study of the ability of steady-state lapatinib dosing to alter the pharmacokinetics of a single dose of paclitaxel or rosiglitazone ... [b]ased upon the ability of lapatinib to act as a **Pgp inhibitor** in vitro, [Sponsor] ... agrees to perform an in vivo drug interaction study of the ability of steady-state lapatinib dosing to alter the pharmacokinetics of a single dose of digoxin.

The take-home lesson is as follows. If a Sponsor has data from in vitro experiments that demonstrate drug–drug interactions, it is possible that the FDA will still grant approval to the drug, even if there are no in vivo studies

with animals or human subjects. However, it is also possible that the FDA will impose the requirement, in the postmarketing time frame, that the Sponsor conduct additional studies to assess in vivo drug–drug interactions.

d. Lapatinib (Drug–Drug Interaction Data Compelled Changes in Study Design)

This is about *lapatinib*, described immediately above, and is also from NDA 22059 from March 2015 of the FDA's website. The observed drug–drug interactions compelled the following features of the study design, as set forth in the Clinical Study Protocol:

- Inclusion/exclusion criteria;
- Wash-out period.

The reviewer referred to the fact that the study design included the following exclusionary criteria. These criteria included the fact that, "the patients excluded from the study, such as ... people on medications that are known CYP3A4 and CYP3A5 inhibitors or inducers."

In general, a wash-out period can be part of the study design of any clinical trial, and it may be incorporated into the study schema. The FDA reviewer commented on the fact that the clinical trial on lapatinib included a "wash-out period that required for prohibited CYP3A4 inhibitors and inducers." With this comment, the *Medical Review* included a table of a dozen drugs, as well as a dietary supplement (St. John's wort) that were prohibited during the clinical trial. The table included the requirement for the wash-out period in its writing, "for a period of time specified prior to administration of the first dose of lapatinib."

The take-home lesson is that data from drug–drug interactions can provide valuable guidance for the study design of any clinical trial, including the inclusion/exclusion criteria and the wash-out period.

e. Tocilizumab, for the Indication of Rheumatoid Arthritis

This concerns *tocilizumab*, an antibody that binds to interleukin-6 (IL-6), from the *Medical Review* of BLA 125276 (Jan. 2011 of FDA website). The reviewer acknowledged that the antibody is not metabolized by cytochrome P450 enzymes, and that direct interactions between the antibody and cytochrome P450 do not occur. However, the FDA reviewer further stated that, "there is the possibility of indirect effects of tocilizumab on P450 enzymes … [because] IL-6 decreases P450 activity, suggesting that [binding of] … IL-6 by tocilizumab could increase P450 activity."

The reviewer then pointed out that, "[i]n vitro studies with human hepatocytes demonstrated that tocilizumab could indeed prevent the IL-6 mediated reduction in P450 activity."

The drug–drug interaction scenario was completed by the reviewer's account of the drug–drug interaction between tocilizumab (a biological) and omeprazole (a small-molecule drug). The scenario was completed by the observation that, "an in vivo study showed that co-administration of tocilizumab … resulted in a decrease" in concentrations of omeprazole, as a result of the antibody-induced up-regulation of P450.

A view of the *package insert*, reveals the same scenario (64). The package insert referred to the influence of the antibody on the small-molecule drugs, omeprazole and simvastatin:

> Cytochrome P450s in the liver are down-regulated by infection and inflammation stimuli including cytokines such as IL-6. Inhibition of IL-6 signaling in RA patients treated with **tocilizumab** may restore CYP450 activities to higher levels than

those in the absence of tocilizumab leading to increased metabolism of drugs that are CYP450 substrates. In vitro studies showed that tocilizumab has the potential to affect expression of multiple CYP enzymes including CYP1A2, CYP2B6, CYP2C9, CYP2C19, CYP2D6 and CYP3A4 … [i]n vivo studies with **omeprazole**, metabolized by CYP2C19 and CYP3A4, and **simvastatin**, metabolized by CYP3A4, showed up to a 28% and 57% decrease in exposure one week following a single dose of ACTEMRA, respectively.

f. Ledipasvir in Combination with Vedroprevir for Hepatitis C Virus, and the Issue of Combination Treatment, Where a First Drug Interferes With Pharmacokinetics of Second Drug

This concerns a clinical trial on *ledipasvir* in combination with *vedroprevir*, for hepatitis C virus. The information is from NDA 205834, from October 2014 on the FDA's website. In assessing drug–drug interactions, the adverse event in question was elevated levels of bilirubin. In the *Medical Review*, the FDA reviewer wrote:

> [t]his case of … bilirubin elevation, with resolution following [discontinuing] study medication … is supportive of a drug-related event; however, the concomitant use of VDV [vedroprevir] … confounds causality assessment … VDV is known to increase bilirubin due to inhibition of OATP1B1 hepatic transporters … [w]hile the contribution of LDV [ledipasvir] cannot be fully excluded, the presence of … coadministered drugs are significant confounders.

The take-home lesson is that, in a clinical trial where a study drug is administered in combination with another drug that is already on the market, the Sponsor needs to be vigilant in assessing any adverse event, including adverse events that take the form of abnormal laboratory values, and assess the contribution of both drugs that are in the drug contribution.

---

[64]ACTEMRA (tocilizumab) injection for intravenous use, injection, for subcutaneous use.

The following provides the scientific background on how drugs can provoke increases in serum bilirubin. Bilirubin in the bloodstream may be taken up by way of the organic anion transporter proteins OATP1B1 and OATP1B3. It is recognized that genetic diseases that impair activity of OATP1B1 transporters can provide increases in serum bilirubin, as well as exacerbate the toxicity of drugs (methotrexate, statin drugs) that are cleared from the bloodstream by way of these transporters (65). Thus, the FDA's reviewer's comments about vedroprevir can be seen as a reasonable explanation for the observed adverse event of increased bilirubin.

IV. SUMMARY OF DRUG–DRUG INTERACTIONS

Information on drug–drug interactions is required on the package insert of FDA-approved drugs. Sponsors conduct drug–drug interaction studies using purified enzymes, subcellular particles such as microsomes, in vitro cultured cells, animal studies, and studies on human subjects. Information on drug–drug interactions, as well as on drug–food interactions, may be included in the *Medication Guide*. Most typically, the enzyme of interest is one or more of the cytochrome P450 enzymes.

Because of the heterogeneity of genes encoding the drug-metabolizing enzymes and transport systems, in the human population, biomarkers have been devised to identify variants in these genes. Where a variant has been identified in an enzyme that metabolizes the study drug, or in a transport system, and if this variant changes the rate of metabolism or transport, corresponding information may be placed in the *Warnings and Precautions* section of the package insert.

V. ANIMAL TOXICITY DATA AND THE PACKAGE INSERT

a. Animal Toxicity Data and FDA's Guidance for Industry

Safety data from animal studies can be included in the package insert, even in the absence of corresponding safety data from human subjects. This concerns the *Warnings and Precautions* section and the *Contraindications* section of the package insert.

Regarding package inserts, FDA's Guidance for Industry provides advice for adverse reactions that have not been observed in humans. For these adverse reactions, FDA recommends that, "[t]he Warnings and Precautions section should include serious or otherwise clinical significant adverse reactions ... that are anticipated to occur with the drug if ... animal data raise substantial concern about the potential for occurrence of the adverse reaction in humans ... e.g., animal data demonstrating that a drug has teratogenic effects" (66). Consistent with this, is the fact that researchers have commented on the fact that, "serious animal toxicity may also be the basis of a boxed warning in the absence of clinical data" (67).

FDA's Guidance for Industry provides a similar recommendation for the

[65]Sticova E, Jirsa M. New insights in bilirubin metabolism and their clinical implications. World J. Gastroenterol. 2013;19:6398–407.

[66]U.S. Department of Health and Human Services. Food and Drug Administration. Guidance for industry. Warnings and precautions, contraindications, and boxed warning section of labeling for human prescription drug and biological products—Content and Format; October 2011 (13 pp.).

[67]Halloran K, Barash PG. Inside the black box: current policies and concerns with the United States Food and Drug Administration's highest drug safety warning system. Curr. Opin. Anaesthesiol. 2010;23:423–27.

Contraindications section of the package insert, "[o]rdinarily, a drug should be contraindicated on the basis of an anticipated adverse reaction if the risk of the adverse reaction in the clinical situation … based on both likelihood and severity of the adverse reaction, outweighs any potential benefit to any patents … and … animal data raise substantial concern about the potential for occurrence of the adverse reaction in humans" (68). In other words, the information on *Contraindications* should be disclosed only where risk outweighs the benefit of the drug.

b. FDA's Decision-Making Process in Evaluating Animal Toxicity Data and Information on the Package Insert

This concerns the drug approval process for dimethyl fumarate (DMF), for treating multiple sclerosis. The information is from the Medical Review for NDA 204063, on Mar. 2013 of the FDA's website. The FDA reviewer observed that, "DMF is toxic to the kidney in multiple species. Renal pathology, including tubular basophilia, tubular dilation, nephropathy … were seen in the rat … similar findings were seen in the dog … [i]n a one year monkey study, tubular necrosis and regeneration were also seen."

Regarding the labeling recommendations, the FDA reviewer wrote, "Please refer to approved label." A view of the package insert reveals information regarding renal toxicity (69). This information does not occur in the *Warnings and Precautions* section of the package insert. The information does not occur in the *Contraindications* section. Instead, it occurs in the *Animal Toxicology and/or Pharmacology* section of the package insert, where it reads:

> Kidney toxicity was observed after repeated oral administration of dimethyl fumarate (DMF) in mice, rats, dogs, and monkeys. Renal tubule epithelia regeneration, suggestive of tubule epithelial injury, was observed in all species.

The take-home lesson is that, where safety data from animals are available, the Sponsor should ensure that the relevant information is properly included in the package insert in one or more of the *Warnings and Precautions* section, the *Contraindications* section, and the *Animal Toxicology and/or Pharmacology* section.

FDA refrained from requiring that the package label disclose renal toxicity issues in the *Warnings and Precautions* section, and in fact, the FDA reviewer stated that, "the clinical trials did not suggest that [study drug] … exposed patients were at increased risk for renal toxicity."

However, FDA went a step further by disclosing the Sponsor's agreement to conduct additional studies on renal toxicity in patients taking the marketed drug. Referring to this agreement, the reviewer wrote that, "the Sponsor states that they intend to conduct a large, global, observational study with the … objective of determining the nature and incidence of … serious renal … events." The take-home lesson is as follows. Where a gray area occurs as to toxicity issues, the Sponsor may choose to include information in the *Animal Toxicology and/or Pharmacology* section, and also to conduct additional studies after the drug goes on the market.

---

[68]U.S. Department of Health and Human Services. Food and Drug Administration. Guidance for industry. Warnings and precautions, contraindications, and boxed warning section of labeling for human prescription drug and biological products—Content and Format; October 2011 (13 pp.).

[69]Package insert for TECFIDERA (dimethyl fumarate) delayed-response capsules for oral use; March 27, 2013 (12 pp.).

VI. SUMMARY

Black box warnings include statements that the drug should be administered by a physician experienced with that particular drug. Black box warnings can identify specific populations especially susceptible to toxicity, such as children or patients with cardiac disease. The warnings may refer to animal studies, such as animal toxicity studies showing that the drug results in death to embryo. Moreover, black box warnings can mandate that the patient be closely monitored or observed. Drug–drug interactions and food–drug interactions take into account adverse reactions that can interfere with the safety or efficacy of the drug that is marketed with the package insert. The package insert can also include animal toxicity data, thereby improving vigilance for adverse effects that may present in the patient.

VII. BRAND NAMES, CHEMICAL NAMES, PACKAGING

a. Introduction to Brand Names

This concerns the proprietary name (brand name) and accompanying chemical name (non-proprietary name, established name) of drugs.

The CFR establishes that the brand name or proprietary name be unique. Title 21 of the CFR warns that labeling of a drug is misleading where, "[d]esignation of a drug or ingredient by a proprietary name that, because of similarity in spelling or pronunciation, may be confused with the proprietary name or the established name of a different drug or ingredient" (21 CFR §201.10).

FDA's Guidance for Industry requires using a brand name that prevents confusion with other drugs. The Sponsor must submit, and FDA reviews, proposed proprietary names as part of its NDA or BLA. Many drug manufacturers prefer to have the FDA evaluate a proposed brand name even earlier in the drug development process. FDA permits the Sponsor to seek FDA's evaluation of the name when the product is in the IND stage, that is, in a timeframe before the Sponsor is able to submit an NDA or BLA (70). Brand names find a basis in the CFR. For example, 21 CFR §201.10 requires that the brand name should be written next to the established name, "the established name shall be placed in direct conjunction with the proprietary name ... and the established name shall be made clear by use of ... brackets surrounding the established name."

FDA requires "pharmaceutical companies to test proposed drug names to identify and remedy potential sound-alike and look-alike confusion with existing drug names" (71). To further prevent medication errors, FDA recommends using different packaging, capsule color, and so on, where the same product is marketed in different strengths. FDA's Guidance for Industry states that (72):

> [i]f multiple strengths are being developed, they should look different from each other, especially to reduce the chances of use errors that can result in harm if an overdose occurs due to administration of an incorrect strength ... error has been attributed to inadequate differentiation among dosage strengths with respect to tablet/capsule color, size, and shape.

[70]U.S. Department of Health and Human Services. Food and Drug Administration. Guidance for industry. Contents of a complete submission for the evaluation of proprietary names; February 2010 (19 pp.).

[71]U.S. Department of Health and Human Services. Food and Drug Administration. Guidance for industry. Safety considerations for product design to minimize medication errors; December 2012 (15 pp.).

[72]U.S. Department of Health and Human Services. Food and Drug Administration. Guidance for industry. Safety considerations for product design to minimize medication errors; December 2012 (15 pp.).

A question that might arise is, "Why not just print the name of the active ingredient on the package label?" Anton et al. (73) provides the answer that, "[t]he use of brand names serves to distinguish products with the same active ingredient but different formulation or indication."

Medication errors can arise because of confusion caused by the brand name, or from the packaging. FDA recognizes that, "medication errors are a significant public health concern that accounts for an estimated 7000 deaths annually in the United States" (74). Confusion can arise during prescribing, administration, and monitoring recovery of a patient. According to FDA's Guidance for Industry, "FDA considers the potential for confusion throughout the entire U.S. medication-use system, including product procurement, prescribing and ordering, dispensing, administration, and monitoring the effects of the medication" (75).

Gershman and Fass (76) point out that consumers and healthcare professionals can report medication errors through a program administered by the Institute for Safe Medication Practices (ISMP), that individuals can describe the medication error, and the drug, and this is followed by ISMP distributing alerts.

The documents medication errors resulting from inconsistent units. The inconsistent units were milligrams and teaspoonfuls, in a container of oseltamivir (Tamiflu®) for children. Parker et al. (77) revealed that the problem was that, "[t]he medication bottle was accompanied by a prepackaged syringe with markings of 30, 45, and 60 mg ... [t]he label attached by the pharmacy specified the dose in volume units (3/4 teaspoonful) but the syringe provided only markings in mass units (milligrams). Despite these disparate directions, the parents were eventually able to determine the correct dose."

b. Division of Medication Error Prevention and Analysis

An office in the FDA, *Division of Medication Error Prevention and Analysis* (DMEPA), reviews the proposed names of drugs, and evaluates the brand name as well as the chemical name. Comments in the *Medical Review* for BLA 125418, on Aug. 2012 of FDA's website, provides a general account of the tasks performed by DMEPA. The reviewer wrote:

> The DMEPA considers the spelling of the name, pronunciation of the name when spoken, and appearance of the name when scripted. DMEPA compares the proposed proprietary name with the proprietary and established name of existing and proposed drug products and names currently under review at the FDA. DMEPA compares the pronunciation of the proposed proprietary name with the pronunciation of other drug names because verbal communication of medication names is common in clinical settings. DMEPA examines the phonetic similarity using patterns of speech. If provided, DMEPA will consider the Sponsor's intended pronunciation of the proprietary name. However, DMEPA also considers a variety of pronunciations that could occur in the English language because

[73]Anton C, et al. Using trade names: sometimes it helps. Arch. Intern. Med. 2002;162:2630.

[74]U.S. Department of Health and Human Services. Food and Drug Administration. Best practices in developing proprietary names for drugs; May 2014 (33 pp.).

[75]U.S. Department of Health and Human Services. Food and Drug Administration. Guidance for industry. Contents of a complete submission for the evaluation of proprietary names; February 2010 (19 pp.).

[76]Gershman JA, Fass AD. Medication safety and pharmacovigilance resources for the ambulatory care setting: enhancing patient safety. Hosp. Pharm. 2014;49:363–8.

[77]Parker RM, et al. Risk of confusion in dosing tamiflu oral suspension in children. New Engl. J. Med. 2009;361:1912–3.

the Sponsor has little control over how the name will be spoken in clinical practice. The orthographic appearance of the proposed name is evaluated using a number of different handwriting samples.

c. FDA Recommends Changing the Brand Name

A practical application of DMEPAs's tasks is shown as part of FDA's evaluation of NDA 050810, available on Apr. 2007 on the FDA's website. DMEPA had made a recommendation for a name change, but the FDA reviewer refused to accept this recommendation. The brand name of the study drug was AzaSite® and the brand name of the other drug was AquaSite®. The FDA reviewer stated that, "DMETS does not recommend the use of the name AzaSite ... the primary concerns were relating to look-alike confusion with ... AquaSite." However, the FDA reviewer disagreed with DMETS, stating that, "AquaSite is not ... a concern because the product ... was removed from the market and has not been marketed in several years."

Please note that DMPEA was formerly named, Division of Medication Errors and Technical Support (DMETS).

d. FDA Recommended Changing the Chemical Name

Another practical application of DMEPA's tasks is shown as part of FDA's evaluation of NDA 022250, located on Jan. 2010 of FDA's website. The *Summary Review* stated that:

> [l]ate in the review process, it became clear that the established chemical name "fampridine" was very similar (especially in appearance when hand written) to the established name for "famotidine", and that therefore there was a risk for medication errors involving these two drugs. Although famotidine is an over-the-counter (OTC) drug at low doses, higher doses that overlap with the

fampridine dose are available by prescription. For this reason, we asked the sponsor to propose another established name. They have done so, proposing "dalfampridine", which we find acceptable.

e. FDA's Decision-Making Process in Recommending a Prefix Be Added to a Name

This is from FDA's *Proprietary Name Review*, for *trastuzumab emtansine*. The information is for BLA 125418, on Aug. 2012 of the FDA's website.

This review concerned confusion of the chemical name (trastuzumab emtansine) with the chemical name of another drug, *trastuzumab*. The issue was that, even though the brand names for the two drugs were extremely different from each other (Kadcyla® vs Herceptin®), the chemical names were very similar.

In a nutshell, FDA recommended that the Sponsor modify the chemical name of the drug to include a prefix. As is evident from the package label, the Sponsor complied with the FDA's request, and changed the chemical name to include a prefix. The new name was, "*ado-trastuzumab emtansine*."

The similarities were not just in the chemical names, but also in the type of clinic and patient population. The FDA reviewer outlined a general problem, occurring when physicians fill out prescriptions, writing that:

> Due to the fact that healthcare providers may use nonproprietary names instead of proprietary names when prescribing and ordering products, and confusion has already occurred in clinical trials, FDA has determined the use of **distinct proprietary names is insufficient** to adequately address the Agency's safety concerns with use of "trastuzumab emtansine" as the proper name for Kadcyla.

The FDA reviewer complained that the chemical name, "trastuzumab emtansine," is similar to that of the chemical name, "trastuzu-mab," writing that:

> This ... name is extremely similar to the currently marketed Herceptin (Trastuzumab). In addition to similar established names, the products have the following overlaps: both are oncology products, both are prepared and diluted in 250 mL bags, and both are administered over the same rates (30 minutes, 60 minutes, or 90 minutes) and with the same frequency of administration (every 3 weeks). Additionally, both products would be prescribed by oncologists and utilized in similar settings (infusion or cancer centers) for similar patients (women with breast cancer). However, the Trastuzumab Emtansine dose of 3.6 mg/kg for single-agent treatment is almost one half the 6 mg/kg dose of the currently marketed Trastuzumab.

The reviewer referred to a very similar situation for another drug. See, review of BLA 125418, on Aug. 2012 of the FDA's website. In the review of BLA 125418, the FDA rationalized its proposal to use a chemical name that contained a hyphen, writing that, "there is precedent for using a hyphen in biological product nonproprietary names, e.g., interferon alpha-2b."

As is evident from the FDA's Approval Letter for BLA 125427, the chemical name of Kadcyla was changed to include a prefix, "ado-trastuzumab emtansin."

f. Conclusions Regarding the Trade Name and Chemical Name

During the timeline of the drug approval process, FDA evaluates the brand name and the chemical name of the study drug for potential confusion between the study drug and other drugs. Even if the brand name is distinct from other brand names, FDA separately evaluates the potential for confusion of the chemical name. The brand name is separately evaluated by the United States Patent and Trademark Office (USPTO). Protection of brand names is acquired by filing a trademark application with the USPTO. The most common reason for the USPTO refusing to register a brand name is confusion with existing brand names (78).

VIII. AMBIGUOUS WRITING ON PACKAGE INSERTS

The issue of ambiguity of writing on package inserts has found its way into popular culture, as demonstrated by the dialog in an episode of *Leave It To Beaver* (79), involving an 8th grade boy (Wally) and his mother (June):

> Wally: Mom, it says here, "TAKE ONE PILL TWICE A DAY."
> June: That's right!
> Wally: Well gee, how do you take the same pill twice?

Of particular interest to medical writers, is guidance from FDA on potential sources of ambiguity, for example, ambiguity relating to timing. FDA informs us that, "[i]f it is particularly important that doses be given 8 hours apart, as opposed to three times a day at convenient intervals, the section should explain the importance of 8-hour spacing of doses" (80). Also regarding the need to reduce ambiguity, is FDA's recommendation that some

[78]United States Patent and Trademark Office Protecting Your Trademark. Enhancing your rights through federal registration; 2015 (29 pp.).

[79]Connelly J, Mosher R. New Doctor. In: Leave it to beaver. Gomalco Productions; 1958.

[80]Department of Health and Human Services. Food and Drug Administration. Guidance for industry. Dosage and administration section of labeling for human prescription drug and biological products—Content and Format; March 2010.

information be reiterated in more than one section of the package insert (81).

Moreover, in an analysis of about 70 package inserts, Fuchs and Hippius (82), found that package inserts can confuse patients where a page break occurs in the package insert in the middle of a dosing paragraph, or where doses are expressed in terms of milligrams, rather than in pill number. In general, package inserts in the United States tend to address the reading level of physicians, while package inserts in Europe tend to address the reading level of the patient (83).

The Canadian Public Health Association provides an account of readability of package inserts as it relates to patients, and recommends that parts of the insert that are especially relevant to the patient, for example, information on safety and dosing instructions, be written at the level of a 6th grader (84).

IX. PACKAGE INSERT MAY PROTECT MANUFACTURER FROM LIABILITY

The content of the package insert can protect the manufacturer from liability in the event of a drug-induced injury to the patient. The following published opinions illustrate situations where there was a drug-induced injury, where the patient filed a lawsuit, and where the manufacturer argued that the warning on the package insert satisfied its duty to warn the physician.

In some of these cases, the argument of the manufacturer succeeded. In other cases, the argument seemed to mitigate the manufacturer's liability. But in other cases, the argument failed.

Writing on package inserts plays a central role in liability cases. These cases serve as learning tools for medical writers needing to draft package inserts. The best sources of the case law from the state and federal courts are in databases from two vendors, LexisNexis®, Albany, NY, and Westlaw®, Eagen, MN. Courtroom opinions can also be found on Google Scholar®. The present commentary does not in any way constitute a comprehensive review of the applicable law. Where there is a desire to use published opinions as a source of guidance, guidance should be provided with the help of an attorney with experience in package inserts.

The drug-induced injuries from a small sampling of the available cases include brain damage, blindness, deafness, massive damage to the intestinal tract, and the case of a patient giving birth to a brain-damaged, paralyzed infant.

These courtroom cases do not involve obscure drugs that had never been widely marketed. These cases involve widely used drugs such as kanamycin (antibiotic), dilantin (antiepileptic), dicoumarol (anticoagulant), oxytocin (a naturally occurring hormone), and norethindrone (for treating endometriosis and a contraceptive).

a. Opinion Concerning Dicumarol

Baker v. St. Agnes Hospital (85), an opinion from a court in New York, involved dicumarol, an anticoagulant. Anticoagulants

---

[81]Kremzner ME, Osborne SF. An introduction to the improved FDA prescription drug labeling (68 pp.) (undated document obtained from www.fda.gov in February 2011).

[82]Fuchs J, Hippius M. Inappropriate dosing instructions in package inserts. Patient Educ. Couns. 2007;67:157−68.

[83]Fuchs J, Hippius M. Inappropriate dosing instructions in package inserts. Patient Educ. Couns. 2007;67:157−68.

[84]Canadian Public Health Assoc. National Literacy and Health Program. Ottowa, Ontario. Good medicine for seniors: guidelines for plain language and good design in prescription medication; 2002.

[85]Baker v. St. Agnes Hospital. 70 A.D.2d 400; 421 N.Y.S.2d 81; 1979 N.Y. App. Div. LEXIS 12729.

prevent pathological blood clots. Dicumarol has the same mechanism of action as warfarin. Dicumarol inhibits vitamin K epoxide reductase.

The package insert contained a warning, "Dicumarol passes the placental barrier. When pregnant women are treated with the drug, fetal bleeding ... may occur and cause fetal death *in utero* ... [t]herefore, the drug is contraindicated for pregnant patients ... [i]f anticoagulant therapy is required for such patients, heparin is considered the drug of choice, because it does not pass through the placenta."

The problem was that the physician supplied dicumarol to the patient for the treatment of phlebitis, even though he knew that the patient was pregnant. The patient gave birth to a child with brain damage and paralysis. A related problem is that the doctor had failed to read the package insert. In the words of the opinion, "[h]e did not consult the package insert or any other source of information on dicumarol before ordering it for Ms. Baker."

In the courtroom, the drug company argued that it should not be held liable, first, because its warning on the package insert was adequate, and second, because the doctor had ignored the package insert. Surprisingly, the court rejected the argument of the drug manufacturer. The court's basis for refusing the manufacturer's argument, was that the manufacturer should have gone a step further to warn the medical community, by transmitting "Dear Doctor" letters to the medical community, warning of the hazards of dicumarol to the fetus. This case has at least two take-home lessons. First, package inserts should provide warnings regarding ADRs. Second, even where the package insert does provide an adequate warning, this does not provide iron-clad defense against liability.

b. Opinion Regarding Kanamycin

Bristol-Myers Co. v. Gonzales (86), taking place in Texas, involved kanamycin. Kanamycin is a common antibiotic. This drug kills bacteria. The package insert contained a warning, but the warnings were not adequate. The warning on the package insert failed to recommend that less toxic antibiotic drugs be used where appropriate. Moreover, the package insert failed to warn that the patient's hearing should be tested. The case turned on evidence showing that the manufacturer knew of the potential toxic effects to hearing (ototoxicity). In writing the opinion, the judge wrote, "[i]f a manufacturer knows or should know of potential harm to a user because of the nature of its product, the manufacturer is required to give an adequate warning of such dangers." The take-home lesson is relatively simple. If a company is aware of an ADR, for example, toxicity to hearing, it should include it in the package insert.

c. Opinion Regarding Dilantin

Peterson v. Parke Davis (87), which took place in Colorado, concerns dilantin, a drug for treating epilepsy. The patient was a 17-year-old boy with epilepsy. The package insert contained a warning, where the warning stated that, "if toxic effects occurred, the drug dosage should be reduced or discontinued."

But there were three problems. First, the doctor had failed to read the package insert. Second, the doctor switched from administering dilantin in capsule form (absorbed slowly) to dilantin in liquid form (absorbed quickly). This was a problem, because the liquid form results in greater serum levels of dilantin. And third, the doctor did not have blood serum tests done on the boy, even when the boy

---

[86]Bristol-Myers Co. v. Gonzales. 561 S.W.2d 801; 1978 Tex. LEXIS 302; 21 Tex. Sup. J. 179.

[87]Peterson v. Parke Davis & Co. 705 P.2d 1001; 1985 Colo. App. LEXIS 1062; 58 A.L.R.4th 1.

showed signs of dilantin toxicity. The result was that the boy suffered brain damage.

The drug manufacturer was held not liable. The take-home lesson is that medical writers need to disclose ADRs, and to provide instructions on dose reduction or on discontinuing the drug. The package insert was, in these respects, sufficient and adequate.

d. Opinion Concerning Oxytocin

Fornoff v. Parke Davis (88), which took place in Illinois, involved oxytocin, a drug for inducing labor in pregnant mothers. Oxytocin stimulates the uterus to contract. The package insert warned that administration of the drug, "must be adapted to the patient's response." The package insert warned that, "administration of oxytocin … in untrained hands is dangerous … [m]aternal deaths … and fetal deaths due to various causes have resulted from the injudicious use of parenteral oxytocic drugs."

The injury to the patient (the mother), which occurred some time after the child's healthy birth, took the form of severe damage to the mother's intestinal track and rectum. The damage to the mother could not be reversed by surgery.

The issue in the courtroom was whether the warnings given were adequate. The court found that the warnings were, in fact, adequate, and the manufacturer was found not liable. The take-home lesson is that the package insert should warn of possible ADRs. This case also implies that package inserts should also state, where relevant, that specially trained personnel should be consulted before administering the drug.

e. Opinion Regarding Oral Polio Vaccine

Tenuto v. Lederle (89), which took place in New York, involved Orimune®, an oral polio vaccine. The patient was an infant receiving the vaccine, but the person who suffered the ADR was the infant's father. The infant received the vaccine in May 1979. At this time, the infant was 5 months old.

Morbidity and Mortality Weekly Report is a publication of the Centers for Disease Control and Prevention (CDC) (90). The Oct. 7, 1977 issue of this publication disclosed a danger of Orimune called contact polio. Contact polio refers to situations where a patient receives the Orimune vaccine, and where another person touches the patient, or touches the patient's feces, and where the other person contracts polio.

Contact polio is what happened to the infant's father. After the infant received the vaccine, the father touched the infant's feces, possibly while changing her diapers, and he contracted polio and became permanently paralyzed. According to the published opinion, "[f]rom October of 1977, when Lederle knew of the federal government's recommendations regarding vaccination of adults who may be in close contact of children receiving Orimune, until the 1979 Orimune package insert, there is no indication that [the drug company] took any steps to bring that knowledge to the attention of the medical profession."

[88]Fornoff v. Parke Davis & Co. 105 Ill. App. 3d 681; 434 N.E.2d 793; 1982 Ill. App. LEXIS 1712; 61 Ill. Dec. 438.

[89]Tenuto v. Lederle Laboratories. 2010 NY Slip Op 50255U; 26 Misc. 3d 1225A; 907 N.Y.S.2d 441; 2010 N.Y. Misc. LEXIS 309.

[90]The CDC is a United States federal agency encompassed by the Department of Health and Human Services. The applicable rules (regulatory laws) are found in Title 45 of the Code of Federal Regulations (CFR).

It was not until May 1979 that the drug company updated its package insert to include a warning on contact polio. The warning on the package insert read:

> The risk of vaccine-associated paralysis is extremely small for vaccinees, susceptible family members and other close personal contacts. However, the responsible physician should convey or specifically direct personnel acting his authority to convey the warnings to the vaccinee [or] parent ... of the possibility of vaccine-associated paralysis propr to administration of the vaccine. When the attenuated vaccine strains are to be introduced into a household with adults who have never been vaccinated, some physicians may choose to give these adults at least two doses of IPV a month apart before the children receive Orimune.

The court found the drug company liable for its failure to timely update its package insert. The take-home lesson to medical writers is to be vigilant in searching for and acquiring information on drug toxicity, and to be expedient in up-dating package inserts.

f. Opinion Regarding Norethindrone

McEwen v. Ortho (91), which took place in Oregon, involved norethindrone, a contraceptive. The patient began taking norethindrone in Dec. 1966, and by Nov. 1967, experienced difficulty with vision. In Dec. 1967, the patient's physician switched the patient to a different brand of norethindrone, that is, from Norinyl® to Ortho-Novum®. A year later, in Dec. 1968, the patient noticed black lines, dots, and streaks, in her vision. And it was not until this time, Dec. 1968, that the patient stopped taking the contraceptive. But the patient became permanently blind in one eye.

The package insert available in Sep. 1966 contained the warning, "Discontinue medication ... if there is sudden partial or complete loss of vision ... [i]f examination reveals ...

retinal vascular lesions, medication should be withdrawn."

In May 1967, more definitive evidence of a cause-and-effect relationship, between the drug and vision problems, was published in a British journal. But the manufacturer did not mention this in its package insert until 1 year later (May 1968), and this warning took the form, "available evidence is suggestive on an association ... [between the drug] and neuroocular lesions, e.g., retinal thrombosis."

Three problems contributed to the manufacturer's liability. The first problem was that, in effect, the package insert told doctors that they could still prescribe the drug, even if there was loss of vision—just as long as there no vascular lesions. The second problem was the manufacturer's failure to issue a "Dear Doctor" letter. The third problem was the manufacturer's 1-year delay in updating the package insert.

The package insert warned that the drug was to be withdrawn only if an examination revealed retinal vascular lesions (damage to blood vessels in the eye), even if the patient has suffered vision loss. The Jan. 1968 exam of the patient's eyes failed to reveal any retinal vascular lesions, and for this reason, the doctor continued to prescribe the drug. The court found the manufacturer liable, based mainly on the failure to include a more timely reference to the British study in the package insert. The take-home lesson for the investigator is to ensure timely incorporation of data on adverse events into the package insert and, where appropriate, to issue a *Dear Healthcare Professional* letter.

g. Summary of Legal Opinions

Lawsuits are published in the form of an opinion of the court. Typically, the judge presiding over the case writes the opinion, but often an attorney assisting the court writes the

---

[91]McEwen v. Ortho Pharmaceutical Corp. 270 Ore. 375; 528 P.2d 522; 1974 Ore. LEXIS 311.

opinion. Opinions are published for several reasons. One goal is to memorialize the decision of the court, enabling that particular decision to be enforced. Another goal is to establish stare decisis, that is, the custom in all aspects of law where the court bases its decision on earlier decisions that concern similar issues. Still another goal is to provide society with guidelines as to how it should behave and carry out its business. For example, quality control units in pharmaceutical companies are required to comply with the Barr decision (92). The Barr decision held that lots or batches of drugs must not be tested and re-tested, until the data somehow, that is, by chance, comply with the specifications. The opinion from the Barr decision is read by directors of regulatory affairs and directors of quality control in pharmaceutical companies. Where a pharmaceutical company wants to ensure that a package insert is consistent with the case law the company should consult an attorney with experience in the case law, as it applies to package inserts.

X. PACKAGE INSERT COMPARED WITH CONSENT FORM

A context for understanding package inserts can be provided by comparing package inserts with consent forms. Consent forms are read by study subjects before the study drug is administered to humans for the first time. In contrast, package inserts are read by physicians and patients, after FDA-approval of the drug, and long after the clinical trials have been completed. Consent forms and package inserts are both regulated by the CFR.

Another similarity is that, during the course of a clinical trial, the consent form may need to be changed in view of newly observed ADRs, and study subjects may be required to sign a re-consent form, while package inserts are sometimes changed, in view of adverse event reporting through the MedWatch device, and requirements mandated by the FDA regarding the package insert.

XI. RELATION BETWEEN PACKAGE INSERTS TO THE STANDARD OF CARE, AND TO OFF-LABEL USES

A further understanding of package inserts can be acquired by a knowledge of what a package insert is not. The dosing instructions and indications on a package insert are not the "standard of care." Also, the dosing instructions and indications on the package insert are not an off-label use. Herrmann and Bownas (93) describe the relations between the package insert, the standard of care, and off-label uses.

The standard of care has been characterized as, "treatment that experts agree is appropriate, accepted, and widely used. HCPs are obligated to provide patients with the standard of care" (94). The standard of care, for any given treatment, may be a topic of continual debate. For example, certain treatments, while acceptable and common at one time, may later be found no longer to be the standard of care

---

[92] United States of America v. Barr Laboratories, Inc. 812 F. Supp. 458; 1993 U.S. Dist. LEXIS 1932.

[93] Herrmann M, Bownas P. Keeping the label out of the case. Northwestern Univ. Law Rev. Colloquy. 2009;103:477−89.

[94] National Cancer Institute, U.S. National Institutes of Health. Dictionary of cancer terms; 2010.

(95,96). Moss and Lee (97) describe how the publication of results from clinical trials can influence the adoption of a new standard of care.

Second, the package insert does not describe off-label uses of the drug. An off-label use is any use that deviates substantially from what is on the package insert, that is, from the indication, patient population, dosage, and route of administration. For example, off-label uses are common for some pediatric cancers. Where an anticancer drug has been approved for use with adult cancer patients, and where no clinical trials with children have been conducted, the physician will have little or no choice but to prescribe the drug for an off-label use.

FDA prohibits drug manufacturers from promoting off-label use. Physicians, however, are not prohibited from prescribing drugs for an off-label use or from independently publishing information, or communicating information to the medical community, on off-label uses. On the other hand, it may be illegal for a physician to promote an off-label use, where the physician is paid by the manufacturer (98).

Other legal implications of off-label uses are as follows. Where a physician uses an FDA-approved drug, but uses it for an off-label use, an adverse party may make the following argument. The adverse party may argue that

the physician, by ignoring the package insert, had also ignored the standard of care, and that the physician is therefore liable for injuries to the patient. Herrmann and Bownas (99) have shown that, while this type of argument has been made, it is an erroneous argument. It is erroneous because it is incorrect to identify what is on a package insert with the standard of care. But the argument that a package insert establishes the standard of care has been found to be persuasive in some parts of the United States, for example, in Minnesota (100).

What is on the package insert may differ from the standard of care, or may differ from the approach taken by an individual physician, for various reasons. FDA's Guidance for Industry states that, "[o]nce a drug or medical device has been approved ... by FDA ... healthcare professionals may lawfully use or prescribe that product for uses or treatment regimens that are not included in the product's approved labeling ... [t]hese off-label uses or treatment regimens may be important and may even constitute a medically recognized standard of care" (101).

Additionally, once a drug is approved and is on the market, and where the medical public arrives at and embraces a new off-label treatment, a pharmaceutical company might not

[95]Bolanos-Meade J. To the Editor. New Engl. J. Med. 2004;351:98–9.

[96]Verma S, Lavasani S, Mackey J, et al. Optimizing the management of her2-positive early breast cancer: the clinical reality. Curr. Oncol. 2010;17:20–33.

[97]Moss RA, Lee C. Current and emerging therapies for the treatment of pancreatic cancer. Onco. Targets Ther. 2010;3:111–27.

[98]Watson KT, Barash PG. The new Food and Drug Administration drug package insert: implications for patient safety and clinical care. Anesth. Analg. 2009;108:211–8.

[99]Herrmann M, Bownas P. Keeping the label out of the case. Northwestern Univ. Law Rev. Colloquy. 2009;103:477–89.

[100]Moyer CA. Off-label use and the medical negligence standard under Minnesota law. Wm. Mitchell L. Rev. 2005;31:927–38.

[101]Department of Health and Human Services. Food and Drug Administration. Guidance for Industry. Good reprint practices for the distribution of medical journal articles and medical or scientific reference publications on unapproved new uses of approved drugs and approved or cleared medical devices; January 2009.

have any particular motivation (or resources) to conduct clinical trials to test the new off-label treatment (102). Moreover, once a drug is on the market, and the ensuing years result in the acceptance of new forms of off-label treatment, the patent on the drug may have expired (103,104). In other words, once a patent on a drug expires, it would not make much sense for a pharmaceutical company to conduct clinical trials on the off-label uses. Once a patent expires, the pharmaceutical company would no longer be able to control the manufacture, sale, or use of a particular drug.

To summarize, what is on the package insert is not the same as the standard of care. And it is not the same as the off-label use.

XII. CONCLUDING REMARKS

Package inserts are written by the drug manufacturer, reviewed and approved by a regulatory agency, and read by physicians and patients. In reading the package insert, the physician sometimes serves as a "learned intermediary" (105), and teaches the patient the safety issues and dosing schedule. The package insert is a living document, as it is periodically updated in view of new safety data acquired from various sources. These sources include MedWatch forms. Failure to update package inserts on a timely basis can raise grave legal issues.

It might also be noted that drug manufacturers may provide information, other than the package insert, to consumers. These include the Patient Package Insert (PPI), and Consumer Medication Information (CMI) (106). PPIs are developed by the manufacturer and approved by the FDA. Some PPIs are mandatory, and are required to be dispensed with specific products, such as oral contraceptives, while other PPIs are submitted to the FDA voluntarily by the manufacturer and approved by FDA, but their distribution is not mandated.

[102]Herrmann M, Bownas P. Keeping the label out of the case. Northwestern Univ. Law Rev. Colloquy. 2009;103:477−89.

[103]Herrmann M, Bownas P. Keeping the label out of the case. Northwestern Univ. Law Rev. Colloquy. 2009;103:477−89.

[104]United States Patent and Trademark Office. Manual of patent examining procedure (Rev. 6, September 2007).

[105]Hall TS. Reimaging the learned intermediary rule for the new pharmaceutical marketplace. Seton Hall Law Rev. 2004;35:193−261.

[106]Development and distribution of patient medication information for prescription drugs. Federal Register. August 27, 2010;75:52765−8.

32

Warning Letters

I. INTRODUCTION

FDA's Warning Letters provide reliable and consistent guidance on substantive and procedural aspects of clinical trials (1). Warning Letters are available on FDA's website. Please note that FDA inspects pharmaceutical companies, medical device companies, and companies that manufacture foods and dietary supplements, and issues Warning Letters to all of these entities. Where a Warning Letter is sent to a food or dietary supplement company, the complaint usually concerns sanitation, inconsistencies between the package label and regulations in the CFR, and exaggerated health claims on the package label.

Although it is not often that a company fails to comply with the demands in the FDA's Warning Letters, failure can result in product seizure, debarment, or injunctions (FDA shuts down operations) (2). The consistent nature of FDA's Warning Letters is ensured by the fact that the draft letters are reviewed, before issue, by the FDA's Office of Chief Counsel (3,4). The bold font in the Warning Letters was added to emphasize certain phrases, and was not in the original Warning Letters.

---

[1]This author acquired 3 years of experience with FDA's Warning Letters during employment at Baker Hostetler, a law firm in Costa Mesa, CA. As part of his work on drafting package labels, he published: Brody T (2015) Food and Dietary Supplement Package Labeling—Guidance from FDA's Warning Letters and Title 21 of the Code of Federal Regulations. Comprehensive Reviews In Food Science and Food Safety. DIO: 10.1111/1541-4337. 12172 (38 pages).

[2]Fleder JR. Who decides your fate in FDA enforcement matters? Update Magazine. Food and Drug Law Institute; May/June 2007. p. 38—41.

[3]Advice from Reynaldo, R. Rodriguez, District Director, U.S. Food and Drug Administration (e-mail of April 7, 2014).

[4]Fleder JR. Who decides your fate in FDA enforcement matters? Update Magazine. Food and Drug Law Institute; May/June 2007. p. 38-41.

II. LIST OF TOPICS

This chapter mainly concerns the FDA's Warning Letters that are issued to a Sponsor during clinical trials on human subjects. As such, this chapter does not much concern letters that are issued relating to issues that arise during the marketing or manufacture of drugs that have already received FDA-approval. The topics in this chapter include:

- Authority of FDA inspectors to monitor clinical trials;
- Relation between FDA's Form 483 notices and FDA's Warning Letters;
- How a Sponsor should respond to a Warning Letter;
- Institutional Review Board (IRB);
- Data Monitoring Committee (DMC);
- Consent Forms;
- Protocol violations;
- Drug accountability and record keeping.

These particular topics are related to each other. For example, the most frequent issues of complaint include the IRB's failure to approve consent forms, and the IRB's failure to comply with the FDA's requirements for record keeping.

III. WARNING LETTER DESCRIBING AUTHORITY OF FDA INSPECTORS

As a starting point, the following Warning Letter establishes part of the FDA's regulatory authority, namely, the authority to acquire the investigator's records. Warning Letters are issued as a result of records obtained during the FDA's inspection of the Sponsor's workplace. Thus, it should be taken for granted that the Sponsor actually allows FDA inspectors to enter the workplace and see the records. But on rare occasions, inspection is denied by the Sponsor.

The cited Warning Letter stated that (5), "[b]etween May 24 and June 8, 2005, Ms Barbara Breithaupt, representing the Food and Drug Administration (FDA), met with you to review your conduct of the following clinical study of the investigational drug ... for which you served as the sponsor and clinical investigator." The letter went on to state that the investigator had refused to allow the inspector to see the records and, as a result, the inspector issued a Form 483 notice to the investigator.

The Warning Letter complained that, "[y]ou failed to permit an authorized officer of FDA to have access to, copy, or verify records or reports related to the conduct of the study noted above ... Ms Breithaupt made multiple attempts over a two week period from May 24, 2005 to June 7, 2005, to obtain access to your study records for the above-referenced study, for purposes of copying and verifying those records. Despite Ms Breithaupt's repeated and persistent efforts to obtain access to your study records, you failed to provide access to any of the records that would have been responsive to the inspection request" (6).

The letter listed reasons for the FDA's routine procedure for acquiring records from companies throughout the United States. The FDA's list of reasons was that, "[a]bsent access to source records, FDA is unable to verify any aspect of your study, including, but not limited to, whether adequate informed consent

---

[5] Warning Letter No. 07-HFD-45-0601 (June 22, 2007) from Gary Della'Zanna of Division of Scientific Investigations, Office of Compliance, CDER, U.S. Food and Drug Administration.

[6] Warning Letter No. 07-HFD-45-0601 (June 22, 2007) from Gary Della'Zanna of Division of Scientific Investigations, Office of Compliance, CDER, U.S. Food and Drug Administration.

was obtained, whether protocol-required pregnancy testing was performed prior to administration of study drug to female subjects with child-bearing potential, protocol-required assessments of the extent of periodontal disease, the number of subjects enroled, the formulation of the study drug, the amount of study drug administered to subjects, and the occurrence and reporting of adverse events" (7). Thus, it is evident that all of these reasons correlate with instructions set forth in a typical Clinical Study Protocol.

The Warning Letter concluded with a statement found at the end of all of the FDA's many thousands of Warning Letters:

> Within fifteen (15) working days of your receipt of this letter, you must notify this office in writing of the actions you have taken or will be taking to prevent similar violations in the future. Failure to adequately and promptly explain the violations noted above may result in regulatory action without further notice.

The same issue is revealed by another Warning Letter, where the investigator refused the FDA access to records, and where the FDA issued a Form 483 notice. The investigator (Synergy Health) stubbornly responded to the Form 483 by writing that, "FDA has no jurisdiction to inspect or review Synergy Health's studies" (8). Yet another Warning Letter documents the investigator's refusal to allow the FDA inspectors to see records (9).

IV. ANECDOTAL DESCRIPTION OF AN FDA INSPECTION, FDA'S REQUIREMENTS FOR RECORD KEEPING DURING DRUG MANUFACTURE, AND GUIDANCE FOR RESPONDING TO FDA'S COMPLAINTS

The following letter, which concerns a drug manufacturing facility, provides an anecdotal description of an FDA inspection. The letter provides an anecdotal description that refers to company employees as being "panicked" by the FDA inspection, but what is more important is the letter's account of corrective action that is needed. The anecdotal account in the Warning Letter referred to panic by company employees, and revealed that (10):

> In your response, you refer to an investigation and indicate that two analysts momentarily panicked upon (1) learning that FDA Investigators were approaching the microbiology Lab and (2) seeing used petri plates from the weekend scattered throughout the laboratory ... and directed the lab technician to immediately remove the petri plates from the microbiology lab ... in an utterly misguided and ill-conceived attempt to clean up the microbiology lab prior to the start of the FDA inspection.

Following the account of this anecdote, FDA's Warning Letter complained about failures in quality control during manufacturing, and poor record keeping. Please note that

---

[7]Warning Letter No. 07-HFD-45-0601 (June 22, 2007) from Gary Della'Zanna of Division of Scientific Investigations, Office of Compliance, CDER, U.S. Food and Drug Administration.

[8]Warning Letter to Synergy Health Concepts (there is no Warning Letter number) (September 5, 2012) from Steven D. Silverman, Office of Compliance, Center for Devices and Radiological Health, U.S. Food and Drug Administration.

[9]Warning Letter 10-HFD-45-10-02 (October 19, 2009) from Dr Leslie K. Ball, MD, Office of Compliance, CDER, U.S. Food and Drug Administration.

[10]Warning Letter No. WL: 320-15-06 (January 13, 2015) from Thomas Cosgrove, JD, Office of Manufacturing Quality, Office of Compliance, CDER, U.S. Food and Drug Administration.

quality control during manufacturing is an issue in FDA-regulated clinical trials on small molecules and biologicals. FDA's Guidance for Industry for manufacturing drugs for use in clinical trials, states that (11):

> As indicated in previous sections, **manufacturers should keep complete records** relating to the quality and operation of the manufacturing processes, including but not limited to:
> - Equipment maintenance and calibration;
> - Manufacturing records and related analytical test records;
> - Distribution records QC functions;
> - Component records;
> - Deviations and investigations;
> - Complaints.

Regarding record keeping, FDA's Warning Letter complained that (12):

> Your response lacks a comprehensive risk assessment of your failure to follow procedures, your **inadequate documentation** system and your inadequate practices related to microbiological control. Your response failed to evaluate the effect of these violations on product quality, and did not include an assessment as to whether any other batches have been compromised.
>
> [Sponsor's] inability to prevent and detect **poor record keeping** practices raises serious concerns regarding the quality system in place at the time of the inspection. Appropriate controls are essential to assure that the information used for making decisions is trustworthy, accurate, and reliable.

The corrective action requested by FDA's Warning Letter took the following form. The letter requested an evaluation of inaccuracies in data, and a risk assessment analysis (13):

> In response to this letter and including the specific requests noted above, provide the following to the Agency:

- A comprehensive evaluation of the extent of the inaccuracy of recorded and reported data. As part of your comprehensive evaluation, provide a detailed action plan to investigate the extent of the deficient documentation practices noted above;
- A risk assessment of the potential effect of the observed failures on the quality of drug products. As part of your risk assessment, determine the effects of your deficient documentation practices on the quality of the drug product released for distribution; and
- A management strategy for your firm that includes the details of your global corrective action and preventive action plan.

V. FDA'S WARNING LETTER DISTINGUISHED FROM FDA'S FORM 483 NOTICE

Where Warning Letters are issued to a Sponsor conducting a clinical trial, the letters tend to complain about failure to comply with the instructions set forth in the Clinical Study Protocol, failures of an investigator to engage with an Institutional Review Board (IRB), and discrepancies in record-keeping.

FDA's Warning Letters are to be distinguished from another format used by the FDA

---

[11]U.S. Department Health and Human Services. Food and Drug Administration. Guidance for industry. CGMP for phase 1 investigational drugs; July 2008 (17 pp.).

[12]Warning Letter No. WL: 320-15-06 (January 13, 2015) from Thomas Cosgrove, JD, Office of Manufacturing Quality, Office of Compliance, CDER, U.S. Food and Drug Administration.

[13]Warning Letter No. WL: 320-15-06 (January 13, 2015) from Thomas Cosgrove, JD, Office of Manufacturing Quality, Office of Compliance, CDER, U.S. Food and Drug Administration.

for complaining about violations. This format is Form 483. FDA's Form 483, "is issued by one or more FDA investigators at the conclusion of a site inspection, and usually is not reviewed by a compliance officer, district director, or an official in FDA's headquarters before it is issued. An FDA Warning Letter, on the other hand, is issued by a district director or headquarters official of similar seniority, and only after review by FDA's Office of Chief Counsel" (14).

FDA provides the following outline regarding the timeline of FDA inspections and duties of FDA inspectors (15). Typically, the FDA inspector makes a comparison, and compares what is set forth in the Sponsor's submissions to the FDA with documents that are possessed by the investigator, such as case report forms:

> When the inspection occurs as a result of FDA's receipt of a marketing application/submission, it will include a comparison of the data submitted by the sponsor to FDA with source documents at the clinical investigator's site ... and case report forms (CRFs) in the clinical investigator's files ... [i]f it is a ... surveillance inspection of an on-going study, data comparison will generally involve only source documents and case report forms ... [s]ource documents may include office records, hospital records, laboratory reports, records of consultations, etc.

One of FDA's Warning Letters provides guidance for responding to a Form FDA 483. The guidance states that the Sponsor should not merely assert that corrective actions will be taken, but should detail the corrective steps that will be taken. In the FDA's words, "Your firm's response stated that procedures will be put into place to ensure compliance with the FDA regulations in the future. We acknowledge your firm's assurance that corrective actions will be taken. However, we note that the response did not contain a detailed outline of procedures or processes that would be implemented to prevent the future occurrence of these observations" (16). This Warning Letter includes an exemplary account of correcting a procedural issue. The example is from a chronic problem of dosing errors of a pediatric drug. The remedial steps taken by the Sponsor were to suspend enrolment at various study sites pending retraining of personnel, reassessing the ability of personnel to follow the Clinical Study Protocol, and increasing monitoring of drug accountability to 100% for all study sites (17).

Most Warning Letters are preceded by a Form 483 notice (18). Copies of issued Form 483 notices can be acquired by the public, but requests must be made via the Freedom of Information Act Office. This Office will cooperate and provide these documents, but only

---

[14]Cooper, RM and Fleder, JR. Responding to a form 483 warning letter: a practical guide. Food Drug Law J. 2005;60:479–93.

[15]Inspections, Compliance, Enforcement, and Criminal Investigations (April 15, 2015) U.S. Food and Drug Administration. Accessed by author from FDA website on July 3, 2015.

[16]Warning Letter No. 10-HFD-45-04-01 (April 9, 2010) from Dr Leslie K. Ball, MD, Office of Compliance, CDER, U.S. Food and Drug Administration.

[17]Warning Letter No. 10-HFD-45-04-01 (April 9, 2010) from Dr Leslie K. Ball, MD, Office of Compliance, CDER, U.S. Food and Drug Administration.

[18]On July 9, 2015, this author conducted searches, demonstrating that most Warning Letters are preceded by a Form 483. These searches were: "institutional review board" (167 hits), "institutional review board" + 483 (163 hits); "consent form" (128 hits), "consent form" + 483 (125 hits); "adverse events" (277 hits), "adverse events" + 483 (204 hits); and "protocol deviations" (50 hits), "protocol deviations" + 483 (50 hits).

DEPARTMENT OF HEALTH AND HUMAN SERVICES		
FOOD AND DRUG ADMINISTRATION		

DISTRICT ADDRESS AND PHONE NUMBER

1431 Harbor Bay Parkway
Alameda, CA 94502-7070
(510) 337-6700 Fax: (510) 337-6702
Industry Information: www.fda.gov/oc/industry

DATE(S) OF INSPECTION

04/27/2011-05/06/2011

FEI NUMBER

3005615655

NAME AND TITLE OF INDIVIDUAL TO WHOM REPORT IS ISSUED

TO: - - -

FIRM NAME
- - -

STREET ADDRESS
- - -

CITY, STATE, ZIP CODE, COUNTRY

Palo Alto, CA 94304-1212

TYPE ESTABLISHMENT INSPECTED

Sponsor

DURING AN INSPECTION OF YOUR FIRM I OBSERVED:

OBSERVATION 1

Not all adverse drug experiences that are both serious and unexpected have been reported to FDA within 15 calendar days of initial receipt of the information. Specifically, on 4/21/2001, your firm was made aware of seventy four (74) confirmed death reports for drug product Xyrem retained by your specialty pharmacy during the time period of November 2002-April 2001 that were not expeditiously reported within 15calendar days to the agency. These seventy four (74) confirmed death reports were previously undetected through the monitoring of your specialty pharmacy. A representative sample of these seventy four (74) confirmed death reports exceeding the 15-day reporting time-frame andthat are more than 2000 days late are summarized as follows:

Date Information Received at Specialty Pharmacy	15-Day Report Submission Due Date	15-Day Report Submission Date	Days Late	
7/1/2003	7/16/2003	5/6/2011	2851	
7/29/2003	8/13/2003	5/6/2011	2823	
11/3/2003	11/18/2003	5/6/2011	2726	
12/3/2003	12/18/2003	5/6/2011	2696	
3/17/2004	4/1/2004	5/6/2011	2591	

SEE REVERSE OF THIS PAGE	**EMPLOYEE(S) SIGNATURE** Daniel J. Roberts, Investigator	**DATE ISSUED** 05/06/2011
FORM FDA 483 (09/08)	**PREVIOUS EDITION OBSOLETE**	**INSPECTIONAL OBSERVATIONS**

FIGURE 32.1 Example of an FDA Form 483, as filled out by an FDA investigator. The issue of this Form 483 was adverse event reporting.

after a delay of many months (19,20). A small number of issued Form 483s are posted on the FDA's website and are available without delay, but the number is too small to provide any real guidance. Fig. 32.1 provides an example of an issued Form 483 (the names of the company and company employees are redacted) (Fig. 32.1).

[19]In this author's own experience, acquired at Cerus Corporation in Concord, CA, it took about 8 months to acquire a document from the Freedom of Information Act Office. The document was a grant application that had been submitted to National Institutes of Health (NIH).

[20]Chen T. Who can see Form FDA 483s, and where do I get them? FDAzilla.com. Yorkville, IL; 2011 (accessed from internet on July 10, 2015).

VI. WARNING LETTER ON CORRECTIVE RESPONSES, BY SPONSOR, FOR A TUMOR CLINICAL TRIAL

a. Overview of FDA's Complaint

A Warning Letter against a Sponsor engaged in a clinical trial on tumors complained about inaccurate measurements of tumor size and volumes, and about the consequent inaccurate measurements of the endpoint of objective response (21). The Warning Letter focused on procedures in conducting the clinical trial, such as managing data and reporting adverse events, and the Sponsor's assertion that newly drafted SOPs will prevent future problems from arising.

b. Details of FDA's Complaint About Incorrect Classification of Tumor Size and Number

The Warning Letter referred to the Sponsor's failures in monitoring the clinical trial, and failures to comply with the instructions in the Clinical Study Protocol. To this end, the Warning Letter complained that (22):

> Our investigation found that [Sponsor] failed to ensure proper monitoring of the studies referenced above and did not ensure that a clinical investigator conducted the investigations in accordance with the **protocols contained in the IND**. As a result of inadequate monitoring, [Sponsor] did not identify, and correct in a timely manner, a clinical investigator's incorrect classification of therapeutic responses and failure to obtain informed consent from subjects in accordance with FDA regulations. Specifically

> ... Protocols BT-09, BT-10, and BT-21 define each possible therapeutic response (Complete Response, Partial Response, Stable Disease, and Progressive Disease), and include specific criteria the clinical investigator must use to classify a subject as having one of those responses. [Sponsor's] monitoring failed to identify and correct the clinical investigator's incorrect classification of therapeutic responses for 9 of the 27 subjects whose therapeutic response classifications were reviewed during the inspection ...

> Subjects 006389 and 013660 did not have complete disappearance of all contrast-enhancing tumors for at least four weeks and, therefore, were incorrectly classified by the clinical investigator as having a Complete Response ... [h]owever, the Tumor Measurements CRF shows that none of the neuroimaging studies showed complete disappearance of contrast-enhancing tumor for at least four weeks. Therefore, the subject did not meet the criteria for Complete Response.

c. Warning Letter on Corrective Responses, Taken by Sponsor, for a Brain Tumor Clinical Trial

This concerns a Warning Letter that reveals a Sponsor's appropriate corrective action. In other words, FDA's Warning Letter was favorable towards the Sponsor. The letter stated that (23):

> [Sponsor's] April 5, 2013 written response identified several corrective actions related to [Sponsor's] general monitoring practices. The response acknowledged that as of 2005, [the Sponsor] ceased using the Study Monitoring Plan dated 23 April 2004, and that "[e]rroneously our revised monitoring practices were not formally acknowledged in the form of revised monitoring guidelines."

---

[21]Warning Letter No. 13-HFD-45-11-05 (December 3, 2013) from Thomas N. Moreno, Office of Scientific Investigations, Office of Compliance, CDER, U.S. Food and Drug Administration.

[22]Warning Letter No. 13-HFD-45-11-05 (December 3, 2013) from Thomas N. Moreno, Office of Scientific Investigations, Office of Compliance, CDER, U.S. Food and Drug Administration.

[23]Warning Letter No. 13-HFD-45-11-05 (December 3, 2013) from Thomas N. Moreno, Office of Scientific Investigations, Office of Compliance, CDER, U.S. Food and Drug Administration.

The response contained several attachments, including, for example, the following new SOPs:

- Study Monitoring Guidelines (SOP 420) . . .
- Clinical Trial Material Management (SOP 430)
- Reporting and Processing Adverse and Serious Adverse Events (SOP 702)

In addition to the implementation of these new SOPs, [Sponsor] has committed to immediately reinstituting the use of a dedicated monitor to review data and Good Clinical Practice (GCP) documentation according to the new SOPs. These corrective actions related to [Sponsor's] general monitoring practices, if properly carried out, **appear adequate to prevent the recurrence of similar violations in the future**.

d. Warning Letter Concerning Corrective Action, Taken by Sponsor, for a Clinical Trial on a Drug With Cardiovascular Risks

FDA's Warning Letter referred to failures of the Institutional Review Board (IRB) to take into account risks of the study drug, and complained about the IRB's ineffective response to correct this failure. The letter stated that (24):

The IRB's written response indicates that the IRB agrees that it incorrectly identified these studies as presenting no more than minimal risk to subjects, and outlines proposed corrective actions that include revision of an SOP to include the regulatory definition of minimal risk, and training on the new SOP for IRB members and administrator . . . [t]his response is incomplete because it does not describe the criteria the IRB intends to establish and follow to ensure adequate interpretation and application of this regulatory definition in the future (i.e., the procedure describing how the IRB will determine whether a study involves no more than minimal risk).

VII. DEFINITIONS

The Code of Federal Regulations (CFR) provides the following definitions of "investigator" and "Sponsor." Although not reproduced here, the CFR also defines "Sponsor—investigator." These definitions are important in determinations of the chain of responsibility for conducting a clinical trial.

According to 21 CFR §50.3, *investigator* is defined as, "*Investigator* means an individual who actually conducts a clinical investigation, i.e., under whose immediate direction the test article is administered or dispensed to, or used involving, a subject, or, in the event of an investigation conducted by a team of individuals, is the responsible leader of that team."

According to 21 CFR §50.3, *Sponsor* is defined as, "*Sponsor* means a person who initiates a clinical investigation, but who does not actually conduct the investigation, i.e., the test article is administered or dispensed to or used involving, a subject under the immediate direction of another individual. A person other than an individual (e.g., corporation or agency) that uses one or more of its own employees to conduct a clinical investigation it has initiated is considered to be a sponsor (not a sponsor-investigator), and the employees are considered to be investigators."

According to 21 CFR §312.3, the *responsibilities of the Sponsor* are defined as, "*Sponsor* means a person who takes responsibility for and initiates a clinical investigation. The sponsor may be an individual or pharmaceutical company, governmental agency, academic institution, private organization, or other organization."

According to 21 CFR §56.102, Institutional Review Board (IRB), is defined as, "*Institutional Review Board (IRB)* means any board, committee, or other group formally designated by an institution to review, to approve the initiation

---

[24]Warning Letter No. 10-HFD-45-04-03 (April 26, 2010) from Dr Leslie K. Ball, MD, Office of Compliance, CDER, U.S. Food and Drug Administration.

of, and to conduct periodic review of, biomedical research involving human subjects. The primary purpose of such review is to assure the protection of the rights and welfare of the human subjects."

Regulations that apply to IRBs are found in 21 CFR §§50, 56, and in 45 CFR §46. According to Emanuel and Menikoff (25), these two sets of regulations that apply to the IRB are, "[s]imilar but not identical regulations." This author also points out that a rule found in Title 21 that applies to clinical trials on drugs many not have a corresponding rule that applies to clinical trials on medical devices, and vice versa. In this chapter, where an excerpt from a Warning Letter concerns a rule applying to medical devices, this suggests but does not necessarily mean that the FDA may have a corresponding rule that applies to drugs.

FDA's Guidance for Industry provides a definition for the Data Monitoring Committee (DMC), also known as Data Safety Monitoring Committee (DSMC). The definition is (26), "A clinical trial DMC is a group of individuals with pertinent expertise that reviews on a regular basis accumulating data from one or more ongoing clinical trials. The DMC advises the sponsor regarding the continuing safety of trial subjects and those yet to be recruited to the trial, as well as the continuing validity and scientific merit of the trial."

VIII. FAILURE OF SPONSOR TO HAVE AN FDA-APPROVED IND

Failure to submit an IND prior to administering drug to subjects, or refusal of the FDA to approve a submitted IND, was an issue in a number of Warning Letters, as cited (27,28,29,30,31,32,33,34). The layperson can readily understand that this represents a gross and blatant failure to comply with FDA-regulations.

[25]Emanuel EG, Menikoff J. Reforming the regulations governing research with human subjects. New Engl. J. Med. 2011;365:1145–50.

[26]U.S. Department of Health and Human Services. Food and Drug Administration Guidance for industry. Establishment and operation of clinical trial data monitoring committees; March 2006 (34 pp.).

[27]Warning Letter No.CBER-06-006 (June 14, 2006) from Mary A. Malarkey, Office of Compliance and Biologics Quality, CBER, U. S. Food and Drug Administration.

[28]Warning Letter No. 07-HFD-45-01-02 (January 19, 2007) from Gary Della 'Zanna, Division of Scientific Investigations, Office of Compliance, CDER, U.S. Food and Drug Administration.

[29]Warning Letter No. 14-HFD-45-04-01 (April 10, 2014) from Sean Y. Kassim, PhD, Office of Scientific Investigations, Office of Compliance, CDER, U.S. Food and Drug Administration.

[30]Warning Letter No. 15-HFD-45-04-01 (April 1, 2015) from Sean Y. Kassim, PhD, Office of Scientific Investigations, Office of Compliance, CDER, U.S. Food and Drug Administration.

[31]Warning Letter No. 07-HFD-45-01-02 (January 19, 2007) from Gary Della 'Zanna, Division of Scientific Investigations, Office of Compliance, CDER, U.S. Food and Drug Administration.

[32]Warning Letter No. 05-HFD-45-06-01 (June 5, 2005) from Dr Leslie K. Ball, MD, Office of Compliance, CDER, U.S. Food and Drug Administration.

[33]Warning Letter No. 06-HFD-45-06-03 (June 15, 2006) from Joseph Salewski, Division of Scientific Investigation, Office of Compliance, CDER, U.S. Food and Drug Administration.

[34]Warning Letter No. 15-HFD-45-04-01 (April 1, 2015) from Sean Y. Kassim, PhD, Office of Scientific Investigations, Office of Compliance, CDER, U.S. Food and Drug Administration.

a. Failure to Have an Approved IND

The following discloses a consequence of conducting a clinical trial on human subjects, without first submitting an IND to the FDA. The letter referred to 21 CFR §312.20(a) and complained that (35):

> You failed to submit an Investigational New Drug Application to FDA for your clinical investigation ... [i]n Study 1 you administered an unapproved attenuated strain of Listeria vaccine ...to at least 20 subjects between October 14, 1999 and December 2001 and continued this study until August 2, 2004, **without submitting an Investigational New Drug Application (IND) to the FDA**. During the inspection you explained that in 2001, after you had dosed the last subject with the Study 1 investigational vaccine, you sought FDA guidance for the need for an IND. An FDA representative told that you needed an IND to conduct the study. Nevertheless, **you failed to submit an IND to FDA**, and continued to follow the subjects from this study through August 2004 when you informed the IRB that the study was closed. In your letter you acknowledge and accept responsibility for this violation.

In another clinical trial, also on cystic fibrosis, the Warning Letter issued a similar complaint. The letter read (36), "[o]n that same day, notwithstanding the safety concerns communicated to you by DPADP, and without an IND in effect, you initiated the clinical investigation in which you administered [study drug]to children and adolescents with cystic fibrosis." In this situation, the Sponsor had submitted an IND, but FDA officials complained about safety issues, and as a consequence, the Sponsor withdrew the IND.

The abbreviation DPADP means, *Division of Pulmonary and Allergy Drug Products.*

b. Refusal of FDA to Approve a Submitted IND

FDA's Warning Letter complained that an IND had been submitted, but that the IND had never been approved. FDA refused to approve the IND because of safety issues. The letter complained that (37):

> Our investigation indicates that you initiated and were responsible for the conduct of a clinical investigation designed to determine whether [redacted] or inhalation, an investigational drug, is an effective treatment for cystic fibrosis. Accordingly, you were the sponsor and should have had an IND in effect before proceeding with the above-referenced study. Our records indicate that, on May 20, 2002, you submitted an IND ... to the FDA ... and ... [d]uring a June 17, 2002 teleconference, you were advised ...that, for safety reasons, your proposed study could not be allowed to proceed ... [o]n that same day, notwithstanding the safety concerns communicated to you ... and without an IND in effect, you initiated the clinical investigation in which you administered [redacted] to children and adolescents with cystic fibrosis.

c. Situation Where FDA Does not Require an IND Prior to Administering Study Drug to Subjects

This illustrates the situation where a Sponsor believed that the clinical trial fit into one of the FDA's regulations that permitted drug administration without an IND. The FDA pointed out that the procedures in the Clinical

---

[35]Warning Letter CBER-06-007 (July 10, 2006) from Mary A. Malarkey, Office of Compliance and Biologics Quality, CBER, U.S. Food and Drug Administration.

[36]Warning Letter No. 05-HFD-45-06-01 (June 5, 2005) from Dr Leslie K. Ball, MD, Office of Compliance, CDER, U.S. Food and Drug Administration.

[37]Warning Letter 05-HFD-45-06-01 (June 7, 2005) from Dr Leslie K. Ball, MD, Office of Compliance, CDER, U.S. Food and Drug Administration.

Study Protocol were such that a submitted IND was, in fact, required. This issue narrowly applies only to drugs that are radioactive, and narrowly applies to radioactive drugs that are used for basic research in humans. The Warning Letter stated that (38):

> FDA regulations require that a sponsor submit an IND to FDA if the sponsor intends to conduct a clinical investigation with an investigational new drug …and have IND in effect before the investigational drug is used in a clinical investigation … [o]ur investigation indicates that you initiated and were responsible for the conduct of a clinical investigation intended to evaluate the use of [redacted] an investigational new drug, as a diagnostic agent, and that you did not have an IND in effect when the study drug was administered to study subjects.

FDA's Warning Letter stated that the Sponsor, "originally believed that the study could be conducted under 21 CFR §361 … and, therefore, did not require an IND." This section of the Code of Federal Regulations, which concerns drugs that are recognized as safe, states that:

> Radioactive drugs … are generally recognized as safe and effective when administered … to human research subjects during the course of a research project intended to obtain basic information regarding the metabolism (including kinetics, distribution, and localization) of a radioactively labeled drug or regarding human physiology, pathophysiology, or biochemistry, **but not intended for immediate therapeutic**, diagnostic, or similar purposes **or to determine the safety and effectiveness** of the drug in humans.

Unfortunately for the Sponsor, FDA's Warning Letter pointed out that the Sponsor's *radioactive drug could have a pharmacological influence* on the human subjects. The letter complained that, "[t]here was no documentation to indicate that the proposed dose of … 75 µg … would not induce an immunological response in humans."

Further referring to Section 361, the Warning Letter referred to additional potential pharmacological effects of the study drug (pyrogenicity), and complained that, "the radioactive drug used in the research must meet … standards of identity, strength, quality, and purity as needed for safety and be prepared in sterile and pyrogen-free form … [y]ou failed to ensure that the **[study drug]** which was derived from human biological material, was appropriately processed or tested to ensure at it was free of transmissible human pathogens and that it was in a sterile and pyrogen-free form."

IX. INSTITUTIONAL REVIEW BOARD

a. Introduction

FDA's Guidance for Industry provides some of the responsibilities of the Institutional Review Board (IRB). These responsibilities include (39):

- IRB must determine that risks to subjects are minimized;
- IRB must determine that risks to subjects are reasonable in relation to anticipated benefits, if any, to subjects;
- IRB must determine that informed consent will be sought from each prospective subject or the subject's legally authorized representative;
- IRB must determine that safeguards are included to protect vulnerable subjects;

---

[38]Warning Letter No. 06-HFD-45-06-03 (June 15, 2006) from Joseph Salewski, Division of Scientific Investigation, Office of Compliance, CDER, U.S. Food and Drug Administration.

[39]U.S. Department of Health and Human Services. Food and Drug Administration Guidance for industry. IRB continuing review after clinical investigation approval; February 2012 (25 pp.).

- IRB must determine that where the study involves children, the research complies with 21 CFR part 50, Subpart D.

The initial steps in working with an IRB have been outlined. The outline refers to *expedited review* and to *review that is not expedited, that is, full IRB review* (40):

> Once you have completed your written protocol and supporting documents, such as the informed-consent form, you will submit them to your IRB for initial administrative review ... [t]he IRB must ensure that clinical investigators have completed any required training before the study can be approved ... [i]n many situations your research protocol may involve no more than minimal risk to the research subjects ... and **can be approved in an accelerated manner** by the chair of the IRB, without going to the **full IRB**. This is called **expedited review** and approval ... where the investigational procedures involve interventions that have greater than minimal risk, your protocol must be reviewed and approved by the **full IRB**.

Institutional Review Boards conform to sets of ethical standards that have been set forth, for example, by the Nuremberg Code, the Belmont Report: Ethical Principles and Guidelines for the Protection of Human Subjects of Research, and Protection of Human Subjects (45 CFR §46.101) (41).

b. Requirements to Keep Written Procedures

The following Warning Letters complain about the IRB's failures to keep written records. These records include a list of the procedures carried out by the IRB, minutes from meetings, and lists of professional qualifications of IRB members. One Warning Letter complained that the IRB did not draft and maintain a *list of these procedures* for its own use. Failure to possess this list resulted in the FDA issuing the Warning Letter. These procedures are listed in this excerpt of the letter (42):

- Conducting its initial and continuing review of research and for reporting its findings and actions to the investigator and the institution;
- Determining which projects require review more often than annually and which projects need verification from sources other than the investigator that no material changes have occurred since previous IRB review;
- Ensuring that changes in approved research, during the period for which IRB approval has already been given, may not be initiated without IRB review and approval except where necessary to eliminate apparent immediate hazards to the human subjects.

FDA's Warning Letter had simply reiterated parts of the Code of Federal Regulations (21 CFR §56.108; 21 CFR §56.115). The CFR states that, "each IRB shall ... [f]ollow written procedures ... [f]or conducting its initial and continuing review of research and for reporting its findings and actions to the investigator and the institution."

Please note that in addition to maintaining the above written procedures, Section 56.115 also requires that the IRB keep "[c]opies of all research proposals reviewed, scientific evaluations ... approved consent documents, progress reports submitted by investigators, and reports of injuries to subjects ... [m]inutes of IRB meetings ... actions taken by the IRB;

---

[40]Schwenzer KJ. Practical tips for working effectively with your institutional review board. Respiratory Care. 2008;53:1354–61.

[41]Enfield KB, Truwit JD. The purpose, composition, and function of an institutional review board: balancing priorities. Respiratory Care. 2008;53:1330–6.

[42]Warning Letter No. 13-HFD-45-03-01 (March 25, 2013) from Thomas N. Moreno, Office of Scientific Investigations, Office of Compliance, CDER. U.S. Food and Drug Administration.

the vote on these actions including the numbers voting for, against, and abstaining"(43).

An unrelated Warning Letter also issued the same complaint regarding the IRB's failure to possess a document disclosing the IRB's written procedures (44). In addition to its document that sets forth these written procedures, IRBs are required to possess other documents. In another Warning Letter, FDA complained about failure of the IRB to maintain records of other IRB procedures, such as meeting minutes, and records of professional qualifications of IRB members.

The letter also provides a concrete "you-are-there" account of the frequency of IRB meetings and of the number of and nature of documents that are reviewed by IRB members at each IRB meeting. The letter complained that (45):

> minutes of the IRB meetings do not document all actions taken by the IRB, and the vote on those actions, including the number of members voting for, against, and abstaining. The minutes from meetings on 3/21/02, 5/9/03, 7/18/03, 10/14/03, and 7/12/04 all **failed to show the actions taken** and the members voting for, against, and abstaining ... [m]eeting minutes do not always record the basis for requiring changes in or disapproving research, and a summary discussion of controverted issues and their resolution. For example, the meeting minutes for the 07/18/03 meeting showed that eight new proposals, three annual renewals, and two amendments were approved **without documenting the discussions** and the basis for approval ... [t]he **IRB failed to maintain records** of the current

members' earned degrees ... indications of experience ... and any employment or other relationship between each member and the institution.

Note that the complaint in the above Warning Letter that the, "IRB failed to maintain records of the current members' earned degrees ... indications of experience." An unrelated Warning Letter also complained about lack of competence of IRB members, in it writing that (46), "[r]eview of the IRB's records indicates that the IRB **lacked the professional competence** necessary to review this study ... IRB meeting minutes from April 20, 2011, and May 25, 2011, show that an attendee [redacted] ... participated in voting. According to the IRB membership rosters, [redacted] **was not a member** of the IRB."

IRB membership needs to include one person who is a "nonscientific member." This requirement was the subject of one Warning Letter, which complained that (47), "[t]he meeting minutes for February 7 and 14, 2003, document that the IRB did not have a nonscientific member present when the IRB approved new research proposals and approved continuation of studies." Professional qualifications of IRB members was also an issue in many other letters, one of which also complained about failure of the IRB to keep records, failure to have the required number of voting members, and failure to notify the investigator of its decisions (48).

[43]21 CFR §56.115.

[44]Warning Letter to Florida Atlantic University (no Warning Letter No.) (December 17, 2009) from Timothy A. Ulatowski, Office of Compliance, Center for Devices and Radiologic Health, U.S. Food and Drug Administration.

[45]Warning Letter No.CBER-06-003 (December 15, 2005) from Mary A. Malarkey, Office of Compliance and Biologics Quality, CBER, U.S. Food and Drug Administration.

[46]Warning Letter No.CBER-12-03 (March 19, 2012) from Mary A. Malarkey, Office of Compliance and Biologics Quality, CBER, U.S. Food and Drug Administration.

[47]Warning Letter No.CBER-06-005 (May 25, 2006) from Mary A. Malarkey, Office of Compliance and Biologics Quality, CDER, U.S. Food and Drug Administration.

[48]Warning Letter No. 12-HFD-45-050502 (June 1, 2012) from Dr Leslie K. Ball, MD, Office of Compliance, CDER, U.S. Food and Drug Administration.

Regarding the requirement for one "nonscientific member" of the IRB, it is the case that FDA scrutinizes the membership list to ensure that it includes a nonscientific letter. One Warning Letter complained that (49), "[t]he membership roster ... lists [redacted] as a nonscientific member. [Redacted] obtained a Bachelor's Degree in Biology ... as well as a Masters in Public Health ... and appears to be involved in scientific areas. She should be listed as a scientific member."

FDA will issue a Warning Letter for failure of an IRB to have a written procedure, even if the IRB had never violated any requirement of the procedure, and even though the same procedure is set forth by the Code of Federal Regulations. In a Warning Letter issued as a follow-up to a Form 486 notice, FDA complained that (50), "there were no written procedures for ... ensuring prompt reporting to the Food and Drug Administration of any unanticipated problems ... for reporting all IRB findings and actions to the investigator and the institution." Regarding the IRB's procedure for expedited review, FDA complained that this procedure, "does not state who is authorized to conduct the review."

c. Requirement to Train IRB Members on the Written Procedures

In addition to possessing written procedures, the IRB is required to train its members on these procedures and, when asked, to

provided evidence to the FDA that its members had been trained. The following Warning Letter complained about failure to train its members, and about the IRB's inadequate response to the FDA's earlier complaint about this failure. The letter stated (51):

> The IRB's written response to the Form FDA 483 ... states that the IRB has drafted new policies and procedures, and that it will **educate IRB members on these processes**. However, the new policies and procedures submitted with this response have not received final approval from the IRB. In addition, the IRB's statement that it will **educate IRB members on the processes** is inadequate because it does not describe the process that the IRB will use to train and educate IRB members and staff on these regulatory requirements, nor does it provide projected completion dates for the training of the IRB members and staff.

d. Requirement of IRB to Follow its Own Written Procedures

Although it might be self-evident that an IRB should comply with its own written procedures, an IRB's failure to act was the subject of the following Warning Letter. The letter provides a concise example of an IRB's failure to follow its own procedures. Citing 21 CFR §56.108(a), the letter referred to the IRB's procedure (Standard Operating Procedure 221) and complained that (52):

> The IRB failed to follow SOP 221 "Conducting Continuing Review" which states that "Particular

[49]Warning Letter to Staten Island University Hospital (the letter had no Warning Letter No.) (June 29, 2009) from Timothy A. Ulatowski, Office of Compliance, Center for Devices and Radiological Health, U.S. Food and Drug Administration.

[50]Warning Letter (to Freeport Health Network, there is no Warning Letter No.) (March 14, 2007) from Timothy A. Ulatowski, Center for Devices and Radiological Health, Office of Compliance, U.S. Food and Drug Administration.

[51]Warning Letter No. 12-HFD-45-050502 (June 1, 2012) from Dr Leslie K. Ball, MD, Office of Compliance, CDER, U.S. Food and Drug Administration.

[52]Warning Letter No.CBER-07-06 (February 1, 2007) from Mary A. Malarkey, Office of Compliance and Biologics Quality, CDER, U.S. Food and Drug Administration.

attention is paid to new information, changes to the protocol, or if unanticipated risks were discovered during the research." In reference to one of the...-studies, the IRB received reports of serious and unanticipated events, and reports of a total of 131 protocol deviations. Nevertheless, the IRB allowed the studies to continue without paying "particular attention" to this new information. In fact, the IRB meeting minutes simply state, *The Board reviewed and noted the deviations. No further action was required.*

The serious nature of the adverse events was of especial interest to the FDA, in view of the fact that the subjects were economically disadvantaged. According to the letter (53), "[m]any of the protocol deviations were directly related to the economically and educationally disadvantaged subjects that the IRB had allowed to be enrolled."

e. Failure of Investigator to Inform IRB of Protocol Deviations

The following Warning Letter, which was mentioned in an earlier chapter in this textbook, describes the bizarre situation where an investigator had mistakenly performed randomization after, rather than before, performing a medical procedure on the study subjects. This Warning Letter is further described here, because of its disclosure of the issue of failure to notify the IRB. The letter emphasizes the importance of protocol deviations. What is emphasized by the letter is that any protocol deviations must be promptly reported to the IRB. The letter complained that (54):

[a]ddditionally, in your written response, you indicated that you notified the IRB of this protocol deviation. We note that **under section 5.2 of the protocol, any protocol deviations were to be submitted to the IRB as soon as possible.** However, you did not notify the IRB until April 8, 2009, almost a year following notification of your site's closure of the study on April 24, 2008, and almost two years after you were notified by the monitor that randomization was to occur prior to surgery.

f. Failure of Investigator to Inform IRB of Unanticipated Problems or Risks, and Investigator's Behavior in Undermining the IRB

FDA requires that the investigator be prompt in reporting unanticipated problems to the IRB. For example, one Warning Letter complained that the investigator's failures in prompt reporting "undermined" the IRB. The letter complained that (55):

Subject 6002 was admitted to the hospital for bilateral deep venous thrombosis (DVT) and pulmonary embolism ... [y]ou did not report this hospitalization to the IRB until 11/2/09 ... [f]ailure to report to the IRB unanticipated problems involving risks to subjects raises concerns about subject safety by **undermining the IRB's role** in continuing review and evaluating risks to subjects.

The following Warning Letter, which concerned a clinical trial on cystic fibrosis, reveals the requirement to inform the IRB about certain adverse events. These adverse events fall into the category of, "unanticipated problems

---

[53]Warning Letter No.CBER-07-06 (February 1, 2007) from Mary A. Malarkey, Office of Compliance and Biologics Quality, CDER, U.S. Food and Drug Administration.

[54]Warning Letter No. 10-HFD-45-11-03 (November 24, 2009) from Dr Leslie K. Ball, MD, Office of Compliance, CDER, U.S. Food and Drug Administration.

[55]Warning Letter No. 11-HFD-45-08-02 (August 26, 2011) from Dr Leslie K. Ball, MD, Office of Compliance, CDER, U.S. Food and Drug Administration.

or risks." The letter referred to the requirement set forth in 21 CFR §312.66, that the *Sponsor report unanticipated problems* to the IRB (56). The letter reiterated the fact that the Sponsor's Clinical Study Protocol did not include any discussion of anticipated risks. The letter then went on to complain that, because of this failure, the Sponsor should have reported "all problems" to the IRB. The letter provided teachings to the Sponsor, and also complaints to the Sponsor, in its writing that (57):

> Protocols typically include discussion of anticipated problems involving risks to human subjects or others; however, your protocol did not adequately describe any anticipated problems or risks to subjects. Since you provided the IRB no information to assess the likelihood that subjects would experience an anticipated problem or category of problems, you should have reported all problems experienced by subjects to the IRB as potential adverse events.

The letter concluded that the Sponsor had failed to report adverse events to the IRB, in its writing that, "[o]ur investigation found, however, that you failed to promptly report multiple adverse events experienced by subjects ... examples of adverse events that were reported by the subjects but not reported by you to the

IRB ... headache ...brochospasm [sic] ... sore throat, headache ... emergency room visit and CT scan for severe headache."

Yet another Warning Letter referred to the fact that the Clinical Study Protocol required reporting medical emergencies within 5 days, and to the failure of the Sponsor to submit the report on a timely basis (58). What was required was that the investigator report the emergencies to the IRB and to the Sponsor. The letter read cited 21 CFR 812.150(a)(4) and complained that (59), "[i]t is also your responsibility, as a clinical investigator, to notify the sponsor and the reviewing IRB, within five working days, of any deviation from the investigational plan to protect the life ... of a subject in an emergency." Another letter complained that (60), "the IRB required serious adverse events to be reported within three business days of your site becoming aware of the event."

In addition to the requirement that the Sponsor report unanticipated problems to the IRB, it is the case that the *IRB must require the Sponsor* to submit unanticipated problems to the IRB. Thus, in a Warning Letter, the FDA complained that (61), "[a]ldditionally, the IRB has not been requiring **clinical investigators to submit unanticipated problems** or progress reports to the IRB."

[56]Warning Letter No. 05-HFD-45-06-01 (June 7, 2005) from Dr Leslie K. Ball, MD, Office of Compliance, CDER, U.S. Food and Drug Administration.

[57]Warning Letter No. 05-HFD-45-06-01 (June 7, 2005) from Dr Leslie K. Ball, MD, Office of Compliance, CDER, U.S. Food and Drug Administration.

[58]Warning Letter to Providence Spokane Heart Institute (there was no Warning Letter No.) (January 14, 2013) from Steven D. Silverman, Office of Compliance, Center for Devices and Radiological Health, U.S. Food and Drug Administration.

[59]Warning Letter to Providence Spokane Heart Institute (there was no Warning Letter No.) (January 14, 2013) from Steven D. Silverman, Office of Compliance, Center for Devices and Radiological Health, U.S. Food and Drug Administration.

[60]Warning Letter No. 09-HFD-45-04-02 (April 20, 2009) from Dr Leslie K. Ball, MD, Office of Compliance, CDER, U.S. Food and Drug Administration.

[61]Warning Letter No. 13-HFD-45-03-01 (March 25, 2013) from Thomas N. Moreno, Office of Scientific Investigations, Office of Compliance, CDER.U.S. Food and Drug Administration.

g. Failure of IRB to Notify Investigator of its Own Decisions

It might appear a matter of common sense that an IRB should notify the Sponsor of its analysis and decisions. However, the FDA has complained about failures of an IRB to report its analysis and decisions to the Sponsor. The Warning Letter refers to an excuse referring to the lack of secretarial support. The Warning Letter cited 21 CFR §56.109(e) and complained that (62):

> [t]he IRB did not notify the investigator in writing that the IRB approved the study protocol, the associated consent forms ... the IRB failed to notify the investigator of the IRB's approval of several revisions to the informed consent forms ... [i]n your letter, you propose corrective actions, including adding more details to correspondence and recruitment of additional support personnel.

It is interesting to point out that, in another Warning Letter, another investigator also blamed its shortcomings on lack of support personnel. The Warning Letter stated that (63), "in Dr. Bice's response, he stated that *the clerical errors will be alleviated when a full time IRB support person has been hired.*" The Warning Letter concluded that, "[t]his is not an acceptable response."

h. Failure of Investigator to Provide IRB With Enough Information to Evaluate the Risks and Benefits of the Clinical Trial

The issue in the next Warning Letter was a poorly written Clinical Study Protocol and the inability of this Protocol to enable the IRB to evaluate the efficacy and safety of the clinical trial under review. The letter complained that:

> Based on ...our review ... [the] IRB did not have sufficient information to identify potential risks to subjects and to determine that risks to subjects are minimized ...For example, the protocol provided to [the] IRB mentioned use of the ADHESIABLOC® Gel in "preclinical animal models"... without providing any further information. Without a complete device description or results from preclinical testing, a determination that risks to subjects are minimized could not be made.

The letter went on to complain that:

> [a]s noted above, [the] **IRB did not have sufficient information to identify risks to subjects**; nor was sufficient information available to assess anticipated benefits. For example, while the background information in the protocol states, "In clinical evaluations ...Propylene Glycol ...is found to be safe and marginally effective" ...the results of these evaluations were not provided ... [b]ased on this limited information, [the] IRB could not determine that the risks to subjects were reasonable in relation to the anticipated benefits, as required under 21 CFR §56.111(a)(2).

i. IRB Suspends or Withdraws Approval of a Clinical Study Protocol

The IRB has the ability to suspend or withdraw its approval of a Clinical Study Protocol. The Code of Federal Regulations provides for the ability of the IRB to suspend a study, or to withdraw approval of a study.21 CFR §56.113 states that:

> An IRB shall have authority to **suspend or terminate approval of research** that is not being conducted in accordance with IRB's requirements or

[62]Warning Letter to Oklahoma Blood Institute Institutional Review Board (no Warning Letter No.) (July 10, 2006) from Mary A. Malarkey, Office of Compliance and Biologics Quality, CBER, U.S. Food and Drug Administration.

[63]Warning Letter to Wellmont Holston Valley Medical Center (the letter did not have a Warning Letter No.) (August 30, 2008) from Timothy A. Ulatowski, Office of Compliance, Center for Devices and Radiological Health, U.S. Food and Drug Administration.

that has been associated with unexpected serious harm to subjects. Any suspension or termination of approval shall include a statement of the reasons for the IRB's action and shall be reported promptly to the investigator, appropriate institutional officials, and the Food and Drug Administration.

Additional requirements apply, where the study concerns a medical device (21 CFR §812.150(a)(2)).21 CFR §812.150(a)(2) states, "Withdrawal of IRB approval. An investigator shall report to the sponsor, within 5 working days, a withdrawal of approval by the reviewing IRB of the investigator's part of the investigation."

One letter complained that the IRB had failed to report its decision to the Sponsor. The letter, which cited part of the CFR that applies to medical devices (21 CFR §812.150(a)(2), complained that (64):

> [a]n investigator shall report to the sponsor within 5 working days, a withdrawal of approval by the reviewing Institutional Review Board (IRB) of the investigator's part of an investigation. An example of your failure is ...[t]he IRB terminated approval of the LeMaitre Vascular study, Protocol LMV-AUI-P2-001, on December 11, 2009. However, this termination was not reported to the sponsor until January 12, 2010.

In another Warning Letter, FDA referred to Sections 312.66 and 56.103(a), and complained that (65):

> [y]ou continued to conduct clinical investigation related activities despite the fact that IRB approval had been withdrawn ... [y]ou violated these

requirements by continuing to see and treat study subjects after ...Human Research Review Board [the IRB] withdrew approval of your clinical investigation site on May 12, 2005. Despite your awareness of the withdrawal of IRB approval ... you continued to obtain informed consent ... from 27 of the 33 subjects previously entered into the study after May 12, 2005 ... [i]n your written response, you stated that you did not know you were not permitted to conduct follow up visits after approval had been withdrawn. Your response is inadequate. **The IRB correspondence to you clearly documents that approval for the study had been withdrawn.**

The following letter concerns the requirement for reporting approval suspensions to the FDA. The letter, which cited 21 CFR §56.113 and 21 CFR §56.115(a)(6), and complained that the IRB failed to report its decision to the FDA. The letter stated that (66), "[y]our IRB failed to report to the FDA the February 22, 2010, suspension of approval."

j. FDA Terminates Patient Enrollment in a Clinical Trial Because of Chronic Failures of the IRB

This concerns the situation where the FDA stopped patient enrollment because of deficiencies of the IRB. Citing 21 CFR §56.120 (b). In a Warning Letter, FDA complained that (67):

> Based on the repeated deficiencies found during the last three inspections ... FDA will withhold approval of all new studies... [n]o new subjects are to be enrolled in any ongoing studies subject to

---

[64]Warning letter to Coastal Vascular and Interventional (the letter has no Warning Letter No.) from Timothy A. Ulatowski, Office of Compliance, Center for Devices and Radiological Health, U.S. Food and Drug Administration.

[65]Warning Letter No. 08-HFD-45-02-02 (June 6, 2008) from Dr Leslie K. Ball, MD, Office of Compliance, CDER, U.S. Food and Drug Administration.

[66]Warning Letter to St. Joseph Mercy Oakland Health System (the letter has no Warning Letter No.) (August 1, 2013) from Steven Silverman, Office of Compliance, Center for Devices and Radiological Health, U.S. Food and Drug Administration.

[67]Warning Letter No.CBER-12-09 (September 24, 2012) from Mary A. Malarkey, Office of Compliance and Biologics Quality, CBER, U.S. Food and Drug Administration.

21 CFR Part 56 and approved by the IRB. These restrictions will remain in effect until such time as FDA has evidence of adequate corrective actions and notifies you in writing that the IRB's corrective actions are satisfactory.

Another Warning Letter reveals FDA's termination of patient enrollment is set forth by the letter's statement that (68), "[a]s a result of the IRB's continuous non-compliance with FDA regulations, FDA hereby directs that no new subjects be enrolled into ongoing studies … that are reviewed by your IRB … [t]his restriction will remain in effect until FDA has evidence of adequate corrective actions." Other examples where repeated IRB failures provoked the FDA to suspend enrollment of subjects in a clinical trial are cited (69,70,71).

k. FDA's Warning Letters About Relation Between the IRB and the Investigator's Amendments to the Clinical Study Protocol

1. Failure of Investigator to Notify IRB of an Amendment

FDA's Warning Letter complained that the investigator failed to promptly report to the IRB a change in the research activity, that is, a change that took the form of an amendment to the Protocol. The letter complained that (72):

> [t]he following **Protocol Amendments** were not submitted to the IRB for review and approval … Amendment A4 dated April 14, 2008, which increased the frequency of physical examination, review of systems, review of laboratory results, and review of radiologic findings from only at screening and baseline to every 6 months.

2. Failure of the IRB to Vote on and Approve an Amendment

Another Warning Letter also concerned the relationship between the IRB and amendments, namely, the requirement for the IRB to vote on amendments. The letter complained about failure of the IRB to vote on and approve an amendment to the Clinical Study Protocol. The letter cited 21 CFR §56.108 and complained that (73):

> The IRB failed to follow its written procedures … that … state: "The IRB must approve any protocol changes before they are instituted." Our review of the IRB meeting minutes, dated May 22, 2008, determined that the following protocol changes were noted by the IRB without being voted on and approved by a majority of the members present.

[68]Warning Letter to Wellmont Holston Valley Medical Center (the letter did not have a Warning Letter No.) (August 30, 2008) from Timothy A. Ulatowski, Office of Compliance, Center for Devices and Radiological Health, U.S. Food and Drug Administration.

[69]Warning Letter No.CBER-12-09 (September 24, 2012) from Mary A. Malarkey, Office of Compliance and Biologics Quality, CBER, U.S. Food and Drug Administration.

[70]Warning Letter to Genetics & IVF Institute (the letter had no Warning Letter No.) (December 23, 2009) from Timothy A. Ulatowski, Office of Compliance, Center for Devices and Radiological Health, U.S. Food and Drug Administration.

[71]Warning Letter to St. Elizabeth Medical Center (the letter had no Warning Letter No.) (May 8, 2007) from Timothy A. Ulatowski, Office of Compliance, Center for Devices and Radiological Health, U.S. Food and Drug Administration.

[72]Warning Letter No. 10-HFD-45-03-03 (April 1, 2010) from Dr Leslie K. Ball, MD, Office of Compliance, CDER, U.S. Food and Drug Administration.

[73]Warning Letter 10-HFD-45-04-02 (April 22, 2010) from Dr Leslie K. Ball, MD, Office of Compliance, CDER, U.S. Food and Drug Administration.

The letter identified these amendments as:

> **Amendment 1 for Protocol** [redacted] included the addition of concomitant medications such as intravenous opioids, inhaled steroids, and Demerol. Amendment 2 for Protocol [redacted] included substantial changes to the inclusion criteria, such as extending the upper age limit from 75 years to 80 years of age and allowing the inclusion of subjects with types of [redacted] different from those indicated in the initial protocol.

l. Chain of Responsibility for Making Amendments (Sponsor, Investigator, IRB)

This concerns an amendment to the Protocol's instruction for screening study subjects. FDA's Warning Letter provides the generally applicable lesson that only a Sponsor of a study may amend a study protocol, and that the Sponsor is responsible for submitting such amended protocols to FDA and the IRB for review. As revealed by the letter, the investigator's mistakes included failing to perform laboratory screening procedures and incorrectly assuming that the Clinical Study Protocol no longer required these screening procedures. This false assumption was based on the notion that the investigator had the authority to amend the Protocol to not require the laboratory tests. The letter complained that (74):

> You failed to follow the protocols for Studies 1 and 2. The required screening, treatment, and follow-up procedures are described in Study 1 protocol sections 5.1 to 5.4, and in Study 2 protocol sections 4.1, 4.2, and 4.3, and 6.0. You failed to perform the protocol-required procedures as illustrated in the following table.

The table revealed that the overlooked screening procedures involved assays for phosphorous, magnesium, glucose, calcium, and platelets. The letter further complained that (75):

> In your letter of May 1, 2009, **you state that the protocols have been amended** because you determined that some tests were not … appropriate for the screening or ongoing assessment of the eligibility of subjects. You also described that you have developed new protocol-specific forms to ensure that the appropriate tests are performed. However, **only a sponsor of a study may amend a study protocol** requiring omission of tests and that the sponsor is responsible for submitting such amended protocols to the FDA and the Institutional Review Board (IRB) for review … [y]ou are not the sponsor of Study 1 and therefore are not authorized to amend a study protocol requiring omission of tests … [w]e further remind you that any such revisions made to the protocol regarding study procedures be reflected on the consent form and approved by the IRB.

m. Arbitrary Decision-Making by IRB Regarding Risks to Study Subjects

As might be self-evident to the layperson, an ethics board has the responsibility to evaluate a proposed clinical study, and to evaluate the risks and benefits to the subjects enroled in the study. The following Warning Letter reveals an instance where the IRB's evaluation of risks was, in the words of the FDA reviewer, "arbitrary." The IRB's arbitrary evaluation took the form of failure to recognize the well-known risks associated with a specific class of drugs. The letter complained that (76):

> [t]he …protocol and the Investigator's Brochure submitted to [the] IRB by the … sponsor clearly indicate that the test article is a [redacted]. With this

---

[74]Warning Letter CBER-09-08 (September 15, 2009) from Mary A. Malarkey, Office of Compliance and Biologics Quality, CBER, U.S. Food and Drug Administration.

[75]Warning Letter CBER-09-08 (September 15, 2009) from Mary A. Malarkey, Office of Compliance and Biologics Quality, CBER, U.S. Food and Drug Administration.

[76]Warning Letter No. 10-HFD-45-04-03 (April 26, 2010) from Dr Leslie K. Ball, MD, Office of Compliance, CDER, U.S. Food and Drug Administration.

drug class, there is a **well established association with the potential for increased risk of serious cardiovascular events**. However, there is no evidence in the IRB meeting minutes …to indicate that the IRB considered this risk in determining whether risks to subject were minimized. The potential for associated cardiovascular risks was also not included in the IRB-approved informed consent form … it is incumbent upon the IRB to conduct a thorough, independent, systematic, **non-arbitrary analysis** of risks and benefits.

Although decisions that are arbitrary or incorrect are rarely the topic of FDA's Warning Letters, the following provides one more example. This concerned the IRB's mistaken approval of a study drug that contained a pyrogen and immunogenic substances. The Warning Letter referred to the IRB's mistake, and documented the fact that the IRB had corrected the problem (77):

> [o]ur investigation found that the … protein used to prepare the investigational drug … was derived from human placenta and … should have been prepared under conditions that would assure that it was sterile and pyrogen-free … it has the potential to cause untoward immunogenic reactions. Written IRB records … of the IRB meetings … contain no discussion of … the risk of non-sterility and pyrogenicity… or the immunogenic potential of the component … [i]n its December 7, 2004 written response, the IRB acknowledged that the study was "incorrectly" approved and maintained that new procedures have been implemented to ensure that a protocol will not be approved until all relevant issues are considered.

n. Enrollment of Disadvantaged Subjects

Enrollment of disadvantaged subjects may prompt the FDA to question the procedures used by the IRB. The FDA issued a Warning Letter regarding the issue of disadvantaged subjects, and stated that the IRB should have considered whether the "economically and educationally disadvantaged subjects were appropriate candidates for these studies." The letter stated that the IRB should have requested further "information about the source of the vulnerable population." The letter complained that (78):

> In a letter to the IRB dated 2/24/04, investigator … requested approval to enroll economically and educationally disadvantaged subjects into those … studies, and to amend the informed consent document by adding a signature line for an impartial witness. The IRB's meeting minutes of 3/2/04, show that the IRB approved the changes to the informed consent form. The IRB's "Amended Certificate of Approval" for the … studies indicates only that the IRB approved the revised consent form; it does not include documentation that the IRB specifically discussed, voted on, and approved the use of economically and educationally disadvantaged subjects for the … studies.

The letter also complained that:

> There is no indication that the IRB considered, among other issues, whether … economically and educationally disadvantaged subjects were appropriate candidates for these studies … the economically disadvantaged subjects would be vulnerable to coercion or undue influence by the $150 monetary compensation for study participation …the educationally disadvantaged subjects would be able to fully understand the requirements of the study and the potential risks to others … the 19-page consent form containing complex medical and technical terminology was appropriate for educationally disadvantaged subjects.

o. Protocol Deviations. Sponsor must Submit Requests to IRB Prior to Deviating from the Clinical Study Protocol

The FDA categorizes protocol deviations as those that are "initiated by the clinical investigator" and those that are "unplanned."

[77]Warning Letter No. 06-HFD-45-06-03 (June 6, 2015) from Dr Leslie K. Ball, MD, Office of Compliance, CDER, U.S. Food and Drug Administration.

[78]Warning Letter No.CBER-07-06 (February 1, 2007) from Mary A. Malarkey, Office of Compliance and Biologics Quality, CBER, U.S. Food and Drug Administration.

FDA states that the protocol deviations that are "initiated by the clinical investigator" must be reviewed and approved by the IND. As set forth by a document on FDA's website (79):

> A protocol deviation/violation is generally an unplanned excursion from the protocol that is not implemented or intended as a systematic change ...**[l]ike protocol amendments, deviations initiated by the clinical investigator must be reviewed and approved by the IRB** and the sponsor prior to implementation, unless the change is necessary to eliminate apparent immediate hazards to the human subjects ... or to protect the life or physical well-being of the subject ... and generally communicated to FDA. "Protocol deviation" is also used to refer to any other, unplanned ... protocol noncompliance. For example, situations in which the investigator failed to perform tests or examinations as required by the protocol.

FDA issued a Warning Letter to a Sponsor because of failure to request permission from the IRB, before engaging in activities that were protocol deviations. The letter illustrates various recurring themes in FDA Warning Letters. The recurring themes are complaints about deviations from the Clinical Study Protocol, and problems with drug accountability, drug storage, and drug shipping. The letter cited 21 CFR §812.150(a)(4), and complained that (80):

> [y]ou failed to submit required reports to the Institutional Review Board (IRB) ... **[y]ou did not request IRB review or receive IRB approval for the following two protocol deviations**... [c]hange in

finger-stick procedure: Although you received a letter dated November 21, 2003, from the sponsor's representative ... that permitted you to conduct the testing using three ... devices per single fingerstick and to test whole blood in the lab, you never sought or received IRB approval to deviate from the protocol in that manner; and ... [c]hange in sample shipping requirement: You also received an email ... stating it is "OK to ship samples on the next day following collection." You did not, however, seek or obtain approval from the IRB for that protocol deviation.

p. Conflict of Interest of an IRB Member

FDA's guidelines state that an IRB member should abstain from voting when there is a *conflict of interest*. The guidelines state that (81):

> IRB regulations ... prohibit any member from participating in the IRB's ... review of any study in which the member has a conflicting interest ... [w]hen members frequently have **conflicts** and must absent themselves from deliberation and **abstain from voting**, their contributions to the group review process may be diminished and could hinder the review procedure. Even greater disruptions may result if this person is chairperson of the IRB.

A Warning Letter cited 21 CFR §56.107(e) and complained that (82):

> This is a recurrence of a violation cited in the last IRB inspection and in the last Warning Letter issued to you in 2006. You failed to ensure that IRB members with **conflicting interests** in the projects

[79]Inspections, Compliance, Enforcement, and Criminal Investigations (April 15, 2015) U.S. Food and Drug Administration. Accessed by the author from the FDA website on July 3, 2015.

[80]Warning Letter No.CBER-05-016 (May 26, 2005) from Mary A. Malarkey, Office of Compliance and Biologics Quality, CBER, U.S. Food and Drug Administration.

[81]Institutional Review Boards Frequently Asked Questions—Information Sheet Information Sheet—Guidance for Institutional Review Boards and Clinical Investigators (June 25, 2014) (accessed from the FDA's website on July 9, 2015).

[82]Warning Letter to Wellmont Holston Valley Medical Center (the letter did not have a Warning Letter No.) (August 30, 2008) from Timothy A. Ulatowski, Office of Compliance, Center for Devices and Radiological Health, U.S. Food and Drug Administration.

being reviewed did not participate ... [t]he minutes of nearly every IRB meeting ... contain statements noting that IRB members [redacted] ... both abstained from voting on oncology protocol actions ... [h]owever, documentation in the minutes regarding the votes ... indicates that **these two people voted for approvals**.

The following Warning Letter provides another account of the conflict of interest requirements for IRB members. The issue was that one of the IRB members was also an investigator on the clinical trial. The Warning Letter cited 21 CFR §56.107, which states that, "No IRB may have a member ... in which the member has a conflicting interest." The letter complained that (83):

> The IRB failed to ensure that no member participated in the initial or continuing review of a project in which the member had a conflicting interest ... [f]or the ... study, you (IRB Chairman [redacted], Ph.D.) are listed as a clinical investigator ... [m]inutes of the August 8, 2008 IRB meeting indicate that you attended this meeting and participated in the discussion of the ... study. At this meeting, the IRB voted to draft a letter... to inquire about the status of the animal toxicity studies ... therefore, according to the minutes of these ... IRB meetings, you participated in the review of this study and voted on it even though you had a conflict of interest.

If there is a conflict of interest, one approach is for the conflicting IRB member to refrain from voting. This approach was suggested in the following Warning Letter. The letter referred to 21 CFR §56.107(e) and stated that (84):

[n]o IRB may have a member participate in the IRB's initial or continuing review of any project, in which the member has a conflicting interest, except to provide information requested by the IRB. You failed to adhere to the above stated regulation. Examples of this failure include, but are not limited to, the following: At the ... September 26, 2002 IRB meetings ... a principal investigator and then Chairman of the IRB, was present during the review of three studies in which he had a conflicting interest. There is no documentation in the minutes that Dr. Opsahl **refrained from voting** on the approval of these three studies.

q. IRB needs to Resolve Controversies before IRB Proceeds to Approve the Research that is Set Forth by the Clinical Study Protocol

FDA's Warning Letter complained that the IRB had observed a "controverted issue," but has approved of the Clinical Study Protocol without resolving the issue (85). The letter referred to 21 CFR §56.115(a)(2), which requires that: "Minutes of IRB meetings ... shall be in sufficient detail to show ... actions taken by the IRB; the vote on these actions ...; the basis for requiring changes in or disapproving research; and a written summary of the discussion of **controverted issues** and their resolution."

FDA complained that (86), "[t]he IRB failed to prepare and maintain adequate documentation of IRB activities including a written summary of the discussion of controverted issues and their resolution ... making it appear that

---

[83]Warning Letter 10-HFD-45-09-01 (October 5, 2009) from Dr Leslie K. Ball, MD, Office of Compliance, CDER, U.S. Food and Drug Administration.

[84]Warning Letter to Genetics and IVF Institute (there was no Warning Letter No.) (December 23, 2009) from Timothy A. Ulatowski, Office of Compliance, Center for Device and Radiologic Health, U.S. Food and Drug Administration.

[85]Warning Letter No. 11-HFD-45-09-01 (October 7, 2011) from Dr Leslie K. Ball, MD, Office of Compliance, CDER, U.S. Food and Drug Administration.

[86]Warning Letter No. 11-HFD-45-09-01 (October 7, 2011) from Dr Leslie K. Ball, MD, Office of Compliance, CDER, U.S. Food and Drug Administration.

the IRB failed to determine that risks to subjects were minimized." Specifically, the problem was that an IRB member had "questioned if the placebo group of the study would be receiving less than the standard of care in this study since the national professional association was recommending the use of [redacted] currently."

A further problem occurring at the IRB meeting was that, "[h]owever, after the standard of care for prevention of preterm birth issue was raised, there is no evidence in the correspondence between the IRB and the clinical investigator that the IRB queried the clinical investigator with respect to this issue."

The letter further complained about this shortcoming, adding that (87), "[f]inally, the meeting minutes do not document any discussion or its resolution prior to approval at the December 2009 meeting. The IRB identified a potential risk and did not document discussion of the **controverted issue**, and its resolution, before approving the research. Thus, it appears that the IRB approved research without making a determination that risks to subjects were minimized and reasonable in relation to the anticipated benefit."

r. Quorum

An issue in IRB procedures is the requirement for a specific number of IRB members to be present where a vote was taken, but where a quorum was not present. In the words of the Warning Letter (88), "[a] review of IRB meeting minutes ... revealed that the IRB consistently reviewed and approved new studies and conducted continuing review **without a majority of the IRB membership present**. Individuals not on the IRB membership rosters, including the IRB Chair, attended meetings and voted. Many meetings also failed to include at least one non-scientific member."

Further concerning lack of a quorum, another Warning Letter complained that (89), "[t]his is a recurrence of a violation cited in the last IRB inspection and in the last Warning Letter issued to you in 2006. Examples of this failure include: The minutes for the March 14, 2006, IRB meeting lists eleven members, including [member A] and [member B]. However, the March 2006 **IRB roster lists only nine voting members**, and does not include [member A] or [member B]."

s. Expedited Review by the Institutional Review Board

Expedited review is a periodic and continuing issue in the FDA's Warning Letters. For an expedited review to be permissible, there is not a requirement for a quorum. FDA's Guidance for Industry provides for expedited review of proposed changes in the Clinical Study Protocol. FDA's Guidance for Industry states that a proposed change (90):

> may be eligible for expedited review: (a) Where (i) the research is permanently closed to the enrollment of new subjects; (ii) all subjects have

---

[87]Warning Letter No. 11-HFD-45-09-01 (October 7, 2011) from Dr Leslie K. Ball, MD, Office of Compliance, CDER, U.S. Food and Drug Administration.

[88]Warning Letter No.CBER-09-06 (March 12, 2009) from Mary A. Malarkey, Office of Compliance and Biologics Quality, CBER, U.S. Food and Drug Administration.

[89]Warning Letter to Wellmont Holston Valley Medical Center (the letter did not have a Warning Letter No.) (August 30, 2008) from Timothy A. Ulatowski, Office of Compliance, Center for Devices and Radiological Health, U.S. Food and Drug Administration.

[90]U.S. Department of Health and Human Services. Food and Drug Administration. Guidance for industry. IRB continuing review after clinical investigation approval; February 2012 (25 pp.).

completed all research-related interventions; and (iii) the research remains active only for long-term follow-up of subjects; or (b) Where no subjects have been enrolled and no additional risks have been identified; or (c) Where the remaining research activities are limited to data analysis.

The Federal Register also states these same requirements for eligibility for an expedited review (91).

Expedited review is used to review requests by a Sponsor to alter the Clinical Study Protocol to include a *low-risk procedure*. Green et al. (92) provide a context and background information on the timeframe for IRB reviews. Green et al. determined the time taken by various IRBs for conducting ordinary (nonexpedited) reviews, and for conducting expedited reviews. According to these authors:

> The median time to IRB approval at the 43 sites was 286 days, with a minimum of 52 days and a maximum of 798 days. (The median time to approval for the 10 sites that granted **expedited review** was 289 days, ranging from 127 to 546; the median time from submission to first review was 1 week shorter for the 10 expedited review sites.

In continuing to comment on delays and on the IRB's request for multiple revisions, Green et al. (93) stated that:

> Most IRBs returned applications for revision, requiring changes to consent procedures, study

protocols, and forms. Especially in the beginning of the study, this feedback was often helpful in refining the protocol and clarifying the consent form. However, revisions continued to be requested at an undiminished rate even late in the recruitment phase of the study.

One characteristic of an expedited review is that it does not require participation by all IRB members. As stated by a number of FDA letters (94,95,96), "[e]xcept when an expedited review procedure is used, the IRB may only review proposed research at convened meetings at which **a majority of the IRB members** (i.e., a **quorum**) is present, including at least one member whose primary concerns are in nonscientific areas."

Continuing on the topic of the required "**quorum**," another Warning Letter concerned the possibility that IRB voting can be made by mail. In a nutshell, regular review must not be conducted by mail while, in contrast, it might be permitted to conduct an expedited review by mail. The Warning Letter complained that (97):

> [m]ail ballot voting was used for … the … approval to a study involving an exception from informed consent requirements for emergency research … [e]xcept for **expedited review** of certain kinds of research involving no more than minimal risk, or minor changes in research; review of proposed research must be conducted at a **convened meeting** at which a majority of the membership of

[91]Federal Register: November 9, 1998 (Volume 63, Number 216).

[92]Green LA, et al. IRB and methodological issues. Health Res. Educ. Trust. 2006;214–30.

[93]Green LA, et al. IRB and methodological issues. Health Res. Educ. Trust. 2006;214–30.

[94]Warning Letter No. 10-HFD-45-04-03 (April 26, 2010) from Dr Leslie K. Ball, MD, Office of Compliance, CDER, U.S. Food and Drug Administration.

[95]Warning Letter No. 09-HFD-45-02-02 (February 11, 2009) from Dr Leslie K. Ball, MD, Office of Compliance, CDER, U.S. Food and Drug Administration.

[96]Warning Letter No. 13-HFD-45-01-01 (February 1, 2013) from Thomas N. Moreno, Office of Scientific Investigations, Office of Compliance, CDER, U.S. Food and Drug Administration.

[97]Warning Letter No.CBER-09-03 (February 5, 2009) from Mary A. Malarkey, Office of Compliance and Biologics Quality, CDER, U.S. Food and Drug Administration.

the IRB is present, including one member whose primary concerns are non-scientific. The use of a mail ballot to vote ... is not permitted because this method does not constitute a **convened meeting**.

The Federal Register states that conditions for IRB use of the expedited review procedure include the fact that (98), "[r]esearch activities that ... present no more than minimal risk to human subjects." Federal Register provides a list of *low-risk procedures*, where this list includes (99):

> [c]ollection of blood samples by finger stick, heel stick, ear stick, or venipuncture... [c]ollection of data through noninvasive procedures (not involving general anesthesia or sedation) routinely employed in clinical practice, excluding procedures involving x-rays or microwaves.

To provide an excerpt from a Warning Letter, one letter complained that (100), "Dr. Bice approved the renewal of at least four significant risk studies. None of these approvals meet the **criteria for expedited review** since the research involves more than minimal risk and the approval was for renewal of the studies, not for minor changes to them."

Another and more expansive letter reiterated the applicable rules, in its writing that (101): "under an **expedited review** procedure, the review may be carried out by the IRB chairperson ... [a]n IRB may use the expedited review process to review ... [procedures] found by the reviewer(s) to involve no more than minimal risk; or ...minor changes in previously approved research during the period for which approval is authorized."

The same letter further reiterated the applicable rules, which included the fact that (102), "the expedited review procedure may be used for continuing review as follows:

[w]here ... the research is permanently closed to the enrollment of new subjects." Finally, the letter arrived at its complaint, namely, that (103):

> On May 18, 2011, the IRB Chairman used the **expedited review** procedure for the continuing review and approval of study ...[h]owever, on March 21, 2011, the IRB was notified that one subject had been enrolled ...and the study was still open for subject accrual. Therefore, the ...study was not eligible for expedited continuing review.

To repeat, because "the study was still open for subject accrual," the FDA determined that expedited review by the IRB could not be used and, as a consequence, issued this Warning Letter.

As stated above, for an expedited review to take place, the procedure under review must be a low-risk procedure. A Warning Letter addressed this requirement. According to this

---

[98]Federal Register: November 9, 1998 (Volume 63, Number 216).

[99]Federal Register: November 9, 1998 (Volume 63, Number 216).

[100]Warning Letter to Wellmont Holston Valley Medical Center (the letter did not have a Warning Letter No.) (August 30, 2008) from Timothy A. Ulatowski, Office of Compliance, Center for Devices and Radiological Health, U.S. Food and Drug Administration.

[101]Warning Letter No. 12-HFD-45-12-01 (December 2, 2011) from Dr Leslie K. Ball, MD, Office of Compliance, CDER, U.S. Food and Drug Administration.

[102]Warning Letter No. 12-HFD-45-12-01 (December 2, 2011) from Dr Leslie K. Ball, MD, Office of Compliance, CDER, U.S. Food and Drug Administration.

[103]Warning Letter No. 12-HFD-45-12-01 (December 2, 2011) from Dr Leslie K. Ball, MD, Office of Compliance, CDER, U.S. Food and Drug Administration.

letter, the issue was that (104), "The IRB used the **expedited review** procedure to review and approve the use of . . . in the treatment of **pregnant women with recent. . . infection** under two expanded access protocols." The FDA reviewer pointed out that the procedure in question was *not a low-risk procedure*, writing that (105): "[t]he use of expedited review for the approval of these studies violates FDA regulations because they involve more than minimal risk and are not a minor change in previously approved research."

X. CONSENT FORMS

The topic of Chapter 30, Consent Forms, is further developed here. This concerns the issue of using an obsolete consent form. The warning letter referred to 21 CFR §312.60 and complained that (106):

> You failed to ensure that informed consent was obtained according to the provisions of . . . 21 CFR §312.60 . . . [y]ou obtained informed consent from some subjects using consent form versions for Study 1 that were not approved by the Institutional Review Board (IRB). Informed consent from the subject is not legally effective if the form that is signed has not been approved by the IRB or if the consent form describes the wrong procedures. The following table illustrates the deficiencies noted in the informed consent process for 8 of the 20 enrolled subjects . . . [s]igned a revised informed consent form before it was approved by the IRB . . . [s]igned an **obsolete . . . version of the informed consent form**.

Consent forms can require that the Sponsor provide compensation to the study subject. As stated earlier in this book, the consent form in the Yellow Fever Study recited, "within two months from this date, the undersigned will receive the sum of $100 in American gold." The following Warning Letter concerns a discrepancy in the stated compensation. The letter complained (107):

> Based on our review of Study 1, we request further explanations for the discrepancies between the amount of **monetary compensation** to subjects provided on the consent form approved by the lRB and the amount of monetary compensation calculated in the protocol. For example, the consent forms approved by the IRB . . . advised that the subject would receive compensation of [redacted] and [redacted] respectively, whereas the corresponding compensation calculations in the protocol for the required hospital stay and outpatient study visits included amounts of [redacted] and [redacted] respectively.

Failure to include conventional information in consent forms was a topic in the following Warning Letter. This omitted information was disclosure of risk, and disclosure that the clinical trial was merely an experiment. As written in the consent form from the Yellow Fever Study, "[t]he undersigned understands perfectly well that in case of the development of yellow fever in him, that he **endangers his life** to a certain extent but it being entirely impossible for him to avoid the infection during his stay in this island." Also, the Yellow Fever Study consent form stated that, "he consents to

---

[104]Warning Letter No. 11-HFD-45-09-01 (October 7, 2011) from Dr Leslie K. Ball, MD, Office of Compliance, CDER, U.S. Food and Drug Administration.

[105]Warning Letter No. 11-HFD-45-09-01 (October 7, 2011) from Dr Leslie K. Ball, MD, Office of Compliance, CDER, U.S. Food and Drug Administration.

[106]Warning Letter CBER-06-007 (July 10, 2006) from Mary A. Malarkey, Office of Compliance and Biologics Quality, CBER, U.S. Food and Drug Administration.

[107]Warning Letter CBER-06-007 (July 10, 2006) from Mary A. Malarkey, Office of Compliance and Biologics Quality, CBER, U.S. Food and Drug Administration.

submit himself to experiments." The Warning Letter complained about failure to describe risks, and failure to state that the study drug is "investigational," in its writing that (108):

> The IRB-approved consent forms used for the study **lack a complete description of reasonably foreseeable risks** and discomforts to the subjects. For example, the consent forms do not include the risk of [redacted], which may require a [redacted] to correct, as described in the study protocol ... [n]one of the versions of the IRB-approved consent forms used for the study informed subjects that the [redacted] used in the [redacted]...is investigational.

A similar deficiency was documented in another Warning Letter, where the issue was that the consent form had failed to mention the type of therapy. This Warning Letter complained that the (109) "Study Procedures section of the informed consent document does not describe the study procedures outlined in the protocol ... **there is no description of the therapy.**"

XI. DATA MONITORING COMMITTEE (DMC)

a. Introduction

DMC is alternatively called Data Monitoring Committee (DMC), Data Safety Monitoring Committee (DSMC), and Data and Safety Monitoring Board (DSMB). The following Warning Letter addresses the basis of the DMC, namely 21 CFR §312.50, which requires "monitoring." Section 312.50 reads, "Sponsors are responsibile [sic, responsible]

for ... ensuring proper monitoring of the investigation(s), ensuring that the investigation(s) is conducted in accordance with the general investigational plan and protocols contained in the IND."

The Warning Letter complained that the Sponsor had only instructed the DMC of its responsibilities, but that there was no evidence that the Sponsor had actually done any active monitoring of the clinical trial.

The letter complained that (110), "[o]ur inspection found that you did not monitor any aspect of the study. As the sponsor of Protocol [redacted] conducted under Investigational New Drug Application (IND) [redacted], you were responsible for ensuring that this study was adequately monitored for compliance with regulatory requirements, thereby ensuring the data quality, and that the rights, safety, and welfare of study subjects were adequately protected."

The letter further complained that, "you informed the FDA investigator that the study was monitored by the Data Safety Monitoring Board (DSMB) ... you informed the FDA Investigator that **the DSMB was to oversee the study** and issue reports every four months ... [w]e find your explanations to be insufficient."

Complaining about lack of any documentation that the DMC had actually done any monitoring, the letter concluded that, "[y]ou provided no additional documentation with your response, relying only on the DSMB research monitoring plan dated February 6, 2007, and DSMB Review dated September 9, 2009, collected during the 2009 inspection, to support the assertion that the DSMB provided

[108]Warning Letter to Christopher D. Saudek (no Warning Letter No.) (November 13, 2008) from Timothy A. Ulatowski. Office of Compliance. Center for Devices and Radiologic Health. U.S. Food and Drug Administration.

[109]Warning Letter 10-HFD-45-09-01 (October 5, 2009) from Dr Leslie K. Ball, MD, Office of Compliance, CDER, U.S. Food and Drug Administration.

[110]10-HFD-45-03-01 (March 8, 2010) from Dr Leslie K. Ball, MD, Office of Compliance, CDER, U.S. Food and Drug Administration.

adequate monitoring … **[t]hose two documents indicate only that the DSMB was to monitor adverse events.**"

b. FDA's Warning Letters Concerning Data Safety Monitoring Committee; Corrective Action Taken by Investigator

This illustrates the well-known fact that Sponsors *need to report SAEs to the DMC* on a timely basis. The letter provides a dramatic example of what constitutes an SAE. The SAEs in question included an infected melanoma lesion that required amputation, pain requiring surgery, and a cellulitis infection. The Warning Letter also provides an exemplary account of how a Sponsor should respond to a Warning Letter, that is, the nature of the corrective action. The corrective actions taken, in response to the letter, included *regular meetings between the investigators and nursing staff*. The letter complained that (111):

> **You failed to report serious adverse events (SAEs)** experienced by three subjects enrolled in Study 1 in a timely manner to the … DSMC … as required by the protocol. Protocol … requires the investigator and study staff to meet weekly to review the study data and subject safety issues, and to submit a cumulative summary of all adverse events occurring during the study to the IRB according to the established IRB guidelines on an annual basis. **You failed to report the following SAEs** until this inspection:

1. On 11/6/06, subject # [redacted] experienced *infected melanoma lesions which resulted in amputation* on 11/27/06. These SAEs were not reported to the DSMC until 4/14109, more than 2 years later.

2. Subject # [redacted] experienced the SAEs of pleural effusion, *left sided chest pain, and subsequent surgery* in March 2008. These SAEs were not reported to the DSMC until 4/1/09.

3. Subject # [redacted] experienced the SAE of a *lower leg cellulitis infection which resulted in hospitalization* on 12/19/08. This SAE was not reported to the DSMC until 4/1/09.

> In your May 1 letter you acknowledged the lapses in your reporting of the SAEs to the DSMC as required by the protocol and describe corrective action plans to be implemented, including **regular meetings between the investigators, nursing staff, clinical research coordinators, and associates**.

This particular Warning Letter has a happy ending. As available on the FDA's website, the Warning Letter has an associated Closeout Letter, dated several months after the Warning Letter. The Closeout Letter read, "[t]he Food and Drug Administration has completed an evaluation of your corrective actions in response to our Warning Letter CBER-09-08 dated September 15, 2009. Based on our evaluation, it appears that you have addressed the violations contained in this Warning Letter."

c. Interactions between the DMC and the Institutional Review Board (IRB)

This concerns interactions between the DMC and the IRB. The Warning Letter illustrates the fact that FDA officials review records from IRB meetings. Also, the Warning Letter reveals the fact that the DMC and IRB communicate with each other. The letter complained that (112):

> In our review of the IRB meeting minutes dated April 28, 2008, FDA determined that the **IRB**

[111]Warning Letter CBER-09-08 (September 15, 2009) from Mary A. Malarkey, Office of Compliance and Biologics Quality, CBER, U.S. Food and Drug Administration.

[112]Warning Letter 10-HFD-45-04-02 (April 22, 2010) from Dr Leslie K. Ball, MD, Office of Compliance, CDER, U.S. Food and Drug Administration.

requested a copy of the preceding two quarterly **Data Safety Monitoring Board reviews**... because they had concerns about reports of bleeding, embolus formation, and death occurring in the [redacted] protocol. Despite this concern, **there is no evidence that the IRB ever received the requested reports**, and the study was permitted to continue until it closed on April 23, 2009.

d. Instructions in the Clinical Study Protocol Regarding the DMC

The Clinical Study Protocol can provide instructions to the Data Monitoring Committee (DMC), regarding its participation during the course of the clinical trial. An excerpt from a Clinical Study Protocol for a trial on leukemia, establishes some of the responsibilities of the DMC (113). Although the excerpt consists only of generic background information, the following might be observed: (1) DMC is autonomous from Sponsor; (2) DMC must be a neutral party; (3) DMC operates under the DMC charter; (4) A goal of DMC is to protect safety of study subjects; (5) DMC reviews, for example, protocol violations; and (6) DMC can only recommend changes, and not mandate changes. The term "SSC" refers to a committee of physicians, such as the medical monitor, directly engaged in running the clinical trial. The excerpt from the Protocol reads:

> **Data Monitoring Committee**. A DMC, operating autonomously from [the Sponsor], the clinical investigators, and the SSC, will be responsible for providing independent recommendations to [the Sponsor] about evolving risk-benefit observed in the course of the study and any modifications required during the course of the study. The DMC will consist of a biostatistician and ≥ 2 physicians experienced in treating patients with lymphoid malignancies ...

DMC members must not be actively involved in study design, conduct, or subject accrual and must not have financial, proprietary, professional, or other interests that may affect impartial, independent decision-making ...

The DMC will formally interact with the external SSC members through the sharing of meeting minutes. Informal interactions between the DMC and external SSC members will be limited. The DMC will operate under a **charter** developed as a collaborative document between [the Sponsor] and the DMC. The primary responsibility of the DMC is **to protect the safety and welfare of subjects** participating in this clinical trial ... [i]n general, the DMC will be responsible for:

- Examining accumulated safety, efficacy, and other relevant data during the course of the study in order to make recommendations concerning continuation, termination, or modification of the study
- Reviewing the general progress of the study as regards subject accrual, study conduct, and **protocol violations** ...

> Based on the results of its deliberations during the course of the study, **the DMC can recommend** continuation of the study unchanged, study interruption, study termination, modification of the trial, or alteration in the DMC monitoring plan.

The Protocol for another clinical trial, and from a different Sponsor, included the following instructions regarding the DMC (114). These instructions provided information regarding timing that was unique to this clinical trial:

> An independent Data Monitoring Committee (DMC) will be formed and constituted according to regulatory agency guidelines. Detailed information regarding the composition of the DMC and detailed

---

[113]A Phase 3, Randomized, Double-Blind, Placebo-Controlled Study Evaluating the Efficacy and Safety of GS-1101 (CAL-101) in Combination with Rituximab for Previously Treated Chronic Lymphocytic Leukemia. Protocol GS-US-312-0116. November 18, 2011.

[114]A Randomized, Multicenter, Open-label, Phase 3 Study of the Bruton's Tyrosine Kinase (BTK) Inhibitor Ibrutinib versus Ofatumumab in Patients with Relapsed or Refractory Chronic Lymphocytic Leukemia/Small Lymphocytic Lymphoma. NCT01578707; Phase 3.ORIGINAL PROTOCOL PCYC-1112-CA.

DMC procedures will be provided in a separate charter. The DMC will review the safety data periodically and the interim analysis results, and provide recommendations according to the charter. One interim analysis using classical O'Brien & Fleming boundary for superiority and Gamma family boundary for futility is planned for the study.

As is evident from the following excerpt, the information in the Protocol is similar to information provided in a typical DMC Charter, such as the parameters for determining when the DMC should perform its analyses. The excerpt is:

> The safety of this study will be monitored by an independent DMC. An early safety analysis will be performed after at least 50 patients have been treated for a minimum of 8 weeks. This analysis will focus on deaths, treatment discontinuations, SAEs, and grade 3/4 AEs as well as special events of interest ... [t]he chair of the DMC ... will issue a recommendation as to whether the study should be interrupted during this period. If the DMC recommends the trial be continued, the DMC will review safety data every 6 months. Otherwise, the DMC may request further safety analyses. Results from a pre-specified interim analysis will also be reviewed by the DMC ... [t]he DMC will review data and provide recommendations regarding stopping or continuing the trial in accordance with the DMC charter. The Sponsor may attend only the blinded portion of the DMC meetings to answer questions as necessary. The DMC charter will provide provisions for restricted communications between the DMC and the Sponsor in the event the DMC recommends stopping the study for safety, futility, or superiority.

Referring to the interim analysis performed by the DMC, the Clinical Study Protocol further stated that:

> A pre-specified interim analysis for both superiority and futility will be performed after approximately 117 PFS [progression-free survival] events are reported. One-hundred and seventeen (117) PFS events correspond to 50% of the required number of 234 PFS events for the final analysis.

XII. PROTOCOL DEVIATIONS

a. FDA's Position on Protocol Deviations

FDA's Information Sheet Guidance provides information on protocol deviations (115). This Information Sheet Guidance states that FDA inspectors frequently find deficiencies that are protocol deviations and that inspectors also find, "failure to appropriately document and report any medically necessary protocol deviations ... [s]ee 21 CFR §312.66 and §812.150(a)(4)." This Information Sheet Guidance further refers to, "[a] Warning Letter that identifies serious deviations from applicable statutes and regulations. A Warning Letter is issued for violations of regulatory significance. Significant violations are those violations that may lead to enforcement action if not promptly and adequately corrected. Warning Letters are issued to achieve voluntary compliance, and include a request for correction and a written response to the agency."

Use of the terms "protocol deviations" and "protocol violations" can result in confusion (116,117). To avoid this confusion, the FDA recommends that (118), "[t]o avoid confusion over terminology, sponsors are encouraged to replace the phrase 'protocol violation' ... with protocol deviation."

[115]U.S. Department of Health and Human Services. Food and Drug Administration. Information sheet guidance for irbs, clinical investigators, and sponsors. FDA inspections of clinical investigators; June 2010 (9 p.).

[116]Sweetman EA, Doig GS. Failure to report protocol deviations in clinical trials: a threat to internal validity? Trials. 2001;12:214–22.

[117]Mehra M et al. The life cycle and management of protocol deviations. Therapeutic Innovation Regulatory Science. 2014;http://dx.doi.org/10.1177/2168479014530119 (16 pp.).

[118]U.S. Department of Health and Human Services. Food and Drug Administration Guidance for Industry. E3 Structure and Content of Clinical Study Reports. Questions and Answers (R1); January 2013 (8 p.).

b. Significant and Insignificant Protocol Deviations

FDA has recognized the gray area where a given protocol deviation can be significant versus insignificant. This concerns a clinical trial on economically disadvantaged subjects. The applicable Warning Letter is cited (119), while a letter attached to this particular Warning Letter, discloses this type of gray area. The attached letter refers to protocol deviations that can be considered to be "routine or nonsignificant" or that can be considered to be "significant" (120):

> Further, we believe that protocol deviations that might initially appear to be **routine or nonsignificant may be significant** in vulnerable populations. Although it is not uncommon for subjects to miss scheduled study visits, the clinical investigator and IRB bear additional responsibility to ensure that educationally and economically disadvantaged subjects be seen for study visits. Educationally disadvantaged subjects simply might not have understood the importance of each visit to make sure that they were appropriately followed for recognized complications associated with the studies.

c. Selected Issues Regarding Protocol Deviations

Mehra et al. (121) acknowledged the sources mentioned above (FDA's Information Sheet Guidance; 21 CFR §312.66 and §812.150(a)(4)) but *observed that*, "[t]here is currently no clear guidance from regulators or consistency in terminology across pharmaceutical companies to detect, assess, classify, or report protocol deviations."

A number of sources have categorized protocol deviations as those that are minor, major, and critical. Critical deviations are those that have direct negative effect on the rights, safety, or well-being of subjects or integrity of data for conclusions on efficacy or safety (122). Critical deviations also include fraud, as well as enrolling patients that do not meet eligibility criteria and incorrect administration of study drug.

Major deviations are those that reasonably have a negative effect on the rights, safety, or well-being of subjects or integrity of data. Examples of major deviations include a pattern of deviations classified as minor or poor quality of the data, as well as inaccurate recording, failure in recording, or incorrectly recording nonserious adverse events or secondary efficacy assessments. Critical protocol deviations and also major protocol deviations should be reported to regulatory authorities and IRBs (123).

Referring to the causes of protocol deviations, Mehra et al. (124) suggested that these include, "[t]oo specific detail (i.e., very strict

---

[119]Warning Letter No. CBER-07-06 (February 1, 2007) from Mary A. Malarkey, Office of Compliance and Biologics Quality, CDER, U.S. Food and Drug Administration.

[120]Warning Letter to Emord and Associates, P.C. (the letter has no Warning Letter No.) (March 16, 2007) from Mary Malarkey, Office of Compliance and Biologics Quality, CBER, U.S. Food and Drug Administration.

[121]Mehra M, et al. The life cycle and management of protocol deviations. Therapeutic Innovation Regulatory Science. 2014; http://dx.doi.org/10.1177/2168479014530119 (16 pp.).

[122]Mehra M, et al. The life cycle and management of protocol deviations. Therapeutic Innovation Regulatory Science. 2014; http://dx.doi.org/10.1177/2168479014530119 (16 pp.).

[123]Mehra M, et al. The life cycle and management of protocol deviations. Therapeutic Innovation Regulatory Science. 2014; http://dx.doi.org/10.1177/2168479014530119 (16 pp.).

[124]Mehra M, et al. The life cycle and management of protocol deviations. Therapeutic Innovation Regulatory Science. 2014; http://dx.doi.org/10.1177/2168479014530119 (16 pp.).

precise requirements regarding who needs to do what and when) can result in the trial not reflecting 'real world' clinical practice, as well as causing too many protocol deviations." Moreover, "[t]oo many complex assessments can tire subjects and site personnel, resulting in missed or inaccurate evaluations as well as subjects discontinuing from the study."

A variety of protocol deviations are described in the Warning Letters cited below. These deviations include:

• Failure to report deviations to the FDA;
• Failure to comply with the protocol's inclusion/exclusion criteria;
• Failures in randomization;
• Failure to comply with dosing schedule;
• Failure to comply with instructions to carry out laboratory procedures;
• Failure to comply with dose modification requirements;
• Failure to report illnesses during the study;
• Failure to report concomitant treatments on the case report form.

d. Failure to Report Deviations to FDA

Referring to the "investigational plan," the letter referred to various protocol deviations. The letter complained that (125):

> An investigator is responsible for ensuring that an investigation is conducted according to the signed agreement, the investigational plan, and all applicable regulations for protecting the rights, safety, and welfare of subjects under the investigator's care, and for the control of devices under clinical investigation.

Our investigation reveals that you failed to fulfill your responsibilities as a clinical investigator under 21 CFR 812.100 and 21 CFR 812.110(b) in that **you failed** to maintain an adequate internal quality control program and **to immediately document and report all protocol deviations**, as required by the protocol. More specifically, on several occasions, your staff falsified study subject consent forms, which falsifications you have admitted the existence of in a letter dated January 20, 2004.

Examples of some of the falsifications are as follows: The consent forms for subjects ... were apparently filled out by a clinic staff member who signed as both the study subject and as the staff member administering the consent, as you explained in your letter ... [t]he consent forms for study subject [redacted] and [redacted] were apparently filled out by a staff member who signed as a study subject using false names, as you explained in your letter ... [o]ne study subject was apparently enrolled three times under the same name but under different study subject numbers (... on 6/10/03, ... on 8/28/03, and ... on 11/04/03); as you explained in your letter.

e. Failure to Comply With the Protocol's Inclusion/Exclusion Criteria

The letter complained that (126), "the protocol and the HIV-1 Sample Collection Case Report Form Instructions require that enrolled subjects be 18 years of age or older. However, on at least three occasions detailed in the table below, you enrolled subjects ... in the study despite the fact that **they were under the age of 18** at the time of study enrollment, all this in violation of 21 CFR 812.100."

In another Warning Letter concerning failure to comply with inclusion/exclusion criteria, FDA complained that (127), "[t]he study protocol excluded subjects with severe

[125]Warning Letter No.CBER-07-001 (October 12, 2006) from Mary A. Malarkey, Office of Compliance and Biologics Quality, CBER, U.S. Food and Drug Administration.

[126]Warning Letter No.CBER-07-001 (October 12, 2006) from Mary A. Malarkey, Office of Compliance and Biologics Quality, CBER, U.S. Food and Drug Administration.

[127]Warning Letter to Allegheny General Hospital (no Warning Letter No.) (May 23, 2007) from Timothy A. Ulatowski, Office of Compliance, Center for Devices and Radiological Health, U.S. Food and Drug Administration.

hypertension as defined by blood pressure greater than 180 systolic and/or 110 diastolic. There was **no documentation in any of these study subjects' records to indicate that you evaluated their eligibility** for enrollment in the study."

Yet another letter complained about failure to use a microbiology test at screening. The letter referred to the participation of a contract research organization (CRO). According to the letter (128), "[f]urthermore, in ... [f]orms submitted by your site to the CRO, in a protocol deviation list submitted to the IRB, and/or in memos to files, you reported that additional ...Subjects 389129, 389137, and 389142, were enrolled into the study **without documentation of a current negative H. pylori test** performed at the screening visit."

And in another letter, FDA observed that the Protocol excluded subjects that had received insulin, in its writing that (129), "[o]f fifteen subjects randomized ... twelve subjects were enrolled in violation of protocol inclusion and exclusion criteria ... [t]he excluded subjects that had received insulin within the prior year. The following subjects reportedly received insulin at their first visit to the clinical site, but were enrolled in the study **in violation of protocol exclusion criteria** ... Subject # 3511-001 was consented and screened on August 7, 2006, even though he received 6 units of Humalog® subcutaneously on June 5, 2006."

The letter also observed that the Protocol required subjects to be on a dose of an "oral agent" before entering the screening phase of the study, writing that, "[t]he required subjects to be on a stable dose of two or three of the following oral agents for at least three months before the screening visit: Sulfonylureas, Biguanides, or Thiazolidinediones. The following subjects were enrolled in the study in violation of this criterion ... Subject # 3511-007 was not on a stable dose of the protocol-required classes of oral agents."

f. Failures in Randomization

The letter complained that (130), "[w]hile assigning subjects to study treatment, our investigation found that **you skipped the randomization number 1533 twice**, thereby violating the protocol specified randomization plan of not missing or substituting any numbers. This protocol deviation involved the randomization of subjects #47045, 47046 and 47047."

g. Failure to Comply with Dosing Schedule

Regarding the dose schedule the letter complained (131):

> With respect to Subject [redacted] source documents showed that the baseline study procedures including but not limited to the physical exam, neurological assessment, and [redacted] performance status evaluation were performed on March 23, 2006. The **subject did not receive the first dose of investigational drugs until either April 15 or April 17, 2006, which was greater than the 14 days allotted by the protocol.**

[128]Warning Letter No. 11-HFD-45-02-03 (February 17, 2011) from Leslie K. Ball, M.D., Office of Compliance, CDER, U.S. Food and Drug Administration.

[129]Warning Letter No. 09-HFD-45-04-02 (April 20, 2009) from Dr Leslie K. Ball, MD, Office of Compliance, CDER, U.S. Food and Drug Administration.

[130]Warning Letter No. 06-HFD-45-1201 (February 28, 2007) from Gary Della'Zanna, Office of Compliance, CDER, U.S. Food and Drug Administration.

[131]Warning Letter No. 09-HFD-45-12-01 (January 3, 2009) from Leslie K. Ball, MD, Office of Compliance, CDER, U.S. Food and Drug Administration.

In our comparison of the case histories found at your site with the protocol in effect during the time of each visit, protocol deviations were identified ... [a]lthough laboratory samples were taken for certain tests, including the hematology, biochemistry, coagulation ... these laboratory samples were not performed within the protocol specified time periods prior to study drug administration for the Day 1 visits of Cycles 1, 2, 3, 4, 5 and/or 6.

h. Failure to Comply With Instructions to Carry Out Laboratory Procedures

The letter complained that (132):

Protocol 08-110 stated that ...**a chest X-ray must be performed at Visit 1** ... [s]ubject 385-101 was enrolled into the study on September 10, 2008, and received study drug on **September 17, 2008 at Visit 2**... [s]ource documents confirm that the **chest X-ray for this subject was taken on September 17, 2008**, approximately an hour after the subject had received the first dose of investigational drug.

The letter further observed that the investigator had a standard operating procedure (SOP) for "Protocol Deviations and Study Amendments." Regarding this SOP, the letter commented that the SOP would serve as corrective actions to prevent the recurrence of this finding, but the investigator had failed to take the measures required by the SOP.

i. Failure to Comply With Dose Modification Requirements

The letter complained that (133):

Protocol ... requires that you stop dosing ... subjects with an increase of 0.5 mg/dL from a normal baseline creatinine that is greater than the institutional upper limit of normal (IULN), or any increase of at least 1 mg/dL from an abnormal baseline creatinine that is greater than the IULN, until serum creatinine returns to within 10% of baseline.

Subject 222626, who was randomized to Treatment Arm 2 (clodronate), met this protocol criterion for stopping the dosing of clodronate, and yet the subject continued to receive clodronate for more than one year after meeting the criterion ... the subject's serum creatinine increased to 1.7 mg/dL on January 11, 2011, and remained more than 0.5 mg/dL above the institutional upper limit of normal (1.0 mg/dL) for over 10 months... [f]or Subject 222626, **you failed to stop dosing of clodronate** until January 24, 2012, more than one year after you should have done so.

j. Failure to Report Illnesses During the Study

According to the Warning Letter, the Clinical Study Protocol required that (134), "[i]llnesses detected during the study, **concomitant illnesses that worsened** during the study, and concomitant medications **were not reported** as required by the protocol."

The letter complained about violations of this requirement, adding that, "Subject # 3511-008 was hospitalized in December 2006 due to complications of a viral infection (pneumonia), but this serious adverse event was not reported to the sponsor until July 13, 2007."

The Warning Letter reiterated the Protocol's instruction of reporting SAEs, stating that the protocol required that, "the protocol required this SAE to be recorded on the 'Serious Adverse Event/Expedited Report from a Clinical Trial' form, and faxed to the sponsor's Pharmacovigilance department within 24 hours, with a copy faxed to the study monitor."

---

[132]Warning Letter No. 10-HFD-45-01-03 (January 28, 2010) from Leslie K. Ball, MD, Office of Compliance, CDER, U.S. Food and Drug Administration.

[133]Warning Letter No. 14-HFD-45-04-04 (April 28, 2014) from Sean Y. Kassim, PhD, Office of Compliance, CDER, U.S. Food and Drug Administration.

[134]Warning Letter No. 09-HFD-45-04-02 (April 20, 2009) from Dr Leslie K. Ball, MD, Office of Compliance, CDER, U.S. Food and Drug Administration.

k. Failure to Report Concomitant Treatments on the Case Report Form

The Warning Letter complained about failure of the Sponsor to record the use of a concomitant treatment, as was required by the Protocol. The treatment was a drug for neuropathic pain. The letter complained that (135):

> Subject # 3511-019's case report form (CRF) lacks information on the reported use of Cymbalta® and the clinical condition corresponding to the use of this medication ... all treatments taken by subjects ... at any time during the study, in addition to the investigational product, are regarded as **concomitant treatments** and must be documented on the appropriate pages of the CRF.

XIII. CLINICAL HOLD

This concerns the decision tree facing a Sponsor when the FDA issues a *Clinical Hold*. As documented in Chapter 33, excessive protocol violations can result in the FDA issuing a *Clinical Hold*. One of the requirements facing the Sponsor is that the Sponsor must inform the Institutional Review Board (IRB) of the fact of the *Clinical Hold*. This requirement is made evident from the following Warning Letter. The letter referred to 21 CFR §312.66 and complained that (136):

> You failed to promptly report to the IRB all changes to the research activity and failed to promptly report all unanticipated problems involving risk to human subjects ... [y]ou failed to promptly notify the IRB that Study 2 was placed on clinical hold. In your absence, FDA notified

[redacted]... that the study was placed on clinical hold, and FDA sent you a letter dated 10/17/03 listing the clinical hold issues. You did not inform the IRB about the clinical hold until 1/2/04, when you submitted a protocol amendment and revised consent form.

Another Warning Letter, which also concerned a *Clinical Hold*, revealed that the reason for the *Clinical Hold* was the issue of animal toxicity data. This particular Warning Letter is a "poster-boy" for major violations of the Code of Federal Regulations (CFR). The letter documents the following violations:

- The IRB warned the Sponsor that additional toxicity studies on animals were needed.
- Despite warning the Sponsor that more toxicity studies were needed, the IRB recommended that the Sponsor move forward with dosing in humans.
- The Sponsor began dosing human subjects, even though the Sponsor did not have an approved IND.
- The IRB failed to inform the FDA that the Sponsor was dosing human subjects, without any approved IND in place.

These violations are documented in the letter, which complained that (137):

> Minutes of the February 1, 2008 IRB meeting indicate that the IRB was aware that the clinical investigator had already dosed human subjects with the investigational drug ... [d]espite knowledge that Dr. [redacted] was dosing human subjects without IRB approval, as required by 21 CFR 312.66, the IRB failed to report Dr. [redacted] noncompliance to the FDA pursuant to 21 CFR 56.108(b)(2) ... [h]owever, in a letter dated February 15, 2008, the IRB

---

[135]Warning Letter No. 09-HFD-45-04-02 (April 20, 2009) from Dr Leslie K. Ball, MD, Office of Compliance, CDER, U.S. Food and Drug Administration.

[136]Warning Letter CBER-06-007 (July 10, 2006) from Mary A. Malarkey, Office of Compliance and Biologics Quality, CBER, U.S. Food and Drug Administration.

[137]Warning Letter No. 10-HFD-45-09-01 (October 5, 2009) from Leslie K. Ball, MD, Office of Compliance, CDER, U.S. Food and Drug Administration.

wrote the following to the clinical investigator, [redacted] M.D. "... additional toxicity studies on animals will need to be completed ... [o]n behalf of the Committee, you may go forward with the study and we look forward to your continued success in this area".

The Warning Letter then went on to complain that, "It is unclear why the IRB allowed the study to go forward in humans when additional toxicity studies in animals were requested. In addition, it is unclear why the IRB allowed Dr. [redacted] to continue ... the study when it appears that he initiated this research study, i.e., began dosing subjects, prior to obtaining IRB approval."

[T]he IRB sent a letter to ... the study sponsor ... regarding the status of the animal toxicity studies. The August 18, 2008 letter ... stated "At this time, I must remind you that human studies, according to the protocol, cannot proceed until your Investigative [Investigational, sic] New Drug (IND) Application is approved by the FDA." This letter to the sponsor appears to contradict the February 15, 2008 IRB letter sent to Dr. [redacted] in which the IRB permitted the study to go forward.

During the inspection in December 2008, you told the FDA investigator that you were unaware that this IND was on **clinical hold**. However, [redacted] responded to the IRB in a letter dated September 4, 2008, and referenced the **clinical hold** placed on the IND by FDA.

XIV. CONCOMITANT MEDICATIONS

a. Warning Letters About Concomitant Medications

A number of Warning Letters issued regarding concomitant medications concern failure to enter the medications on the case report form (138,139,140,141,142). These medications include acetaminophen and rosiglitazone.

Another Warning Letter complained about failure to comply with the exclusion criteria in the Clinical Study Protocol forbidding certain concomitant medications (143), "[p]rotocol ... specifically stated that subjects with current use of postmenopausal oral hormone replacement therapy were to be excluded from the clinical investigation ... [s]ubject #0011 was ... allowed to continue in the clinical investigation despite clinic records dated 8/8/06 and 1/24/07 documenting the use of the disallowed concomitant medication." The same type of violation was a complaint in other letters (144,145).

[138]Warning Letter No. 08-HFD-45-05-02 (May 28, 2008) from Dr Leslie K. Ball, MD, Office of Compliance, CDER, U.S. Food and Drug Administration.

[139]Warning Letter No. 10-HFD-45-03-02 (March 17, 2010) from Dr Leslie K. Ball, MD, Office of Compliance, CDER, U.S. Food and Drug Administration.

[140]Warning Letter No. 09-HFD-45-04-02 (June 18, 2009) from Dr Leslie K. Ball, MD, Office of Compliance, CDER, U.S. Food and Drug Administration.

[141]Warning Letter No. CBER-10-05 (March 11, 2010) from Mary A. Malarkey, Office of Compliance and Biologics Quality, CBER, U.S. Food and Drug Administration.

[142]Warning Letter No. CBER-07-008 (March 29, 2007) from Mary A. Malarkey, Office of Compliance and Biologics Quality, CBER, U.S. Food and Drug Administration.

[143]Warning Letter No. 10-HFD-45-11-01 (November 9, 2009) from Dr Leslie K. Ball, MD, Office of Compliance, CDER, U.S. Food and Drug Administration.

[144]Warning Letter No. 08-HFD-45-01-11 (March 19, 2008) from Dr Leslie K. Ball, MD, Office of Compliance, CDER, U.S. Food and Drug Administration.

[145]Warning Letter No. 05-HFD-45-102 (December 19, 2005) from Dr Leslie K. Ball, MD, Office of Compliance, CDER, U.S. Food and Drug Administration.

Where the Clinical Study Protocol prohibits certain medications in the timeframe prior to initiating the study, these may optionally also be referred to as concomitant medications, as is evident from the writing that (146), "[t]he protocol excluded subjects that had taken ... treatment for pulmonary arterial hypertension within 30 days **before study entry**. The concomitant medication ... document ... shows that subject 095 was taking both Lasix and Aldactone for pulmonary arterial hypertension within several days **prior to study entry**."

b. Clinical Study Protocol's Instructions for Concomitant Medications

This provides an example of a list, from a Clinical Study Protocol, of prohibited concomitant medications. The clinical trial compared the efficacy of **tofacitinib** with methotrexate, for rheumatoid arthritis. This reveals the statements about concomitant medications, at various parts of the Protocol (147).

One of the *inclusion criteria* requires: "Patient has discontinued all disallowed **concomitant medications** for the required time prior to the first dose of study drug and is taking only those concomitant medications in doses and frequency allowed by the protocol."

Instructions for administration of one of the study drugs (methotrexate; MTX) also provide guidance for using a permitted concomitant medication (antiemetic): "[s]imple medical management of adverse events typical of lack of tolerance to MTX may include allowed **concomitant medications** (e.g., anti-emetic medication)."

The text of the Protocol includes further brief instructions, regarding a concomitant medication, "[i]ntravenous or intramuscular corticosteroids are not allowed during this study either as a stable *concomitant medication* or as rescue medication."

Throughout the Protocol, in narratives corresponding to each patient visit, is the same repeated instruction regarding concomitant medications, "[m]onitoring of adverse events and **concomitant medications**: Record any modifications, deletions or additions."

Finally, an appendix at the end of the Protocol contains a long list of prohibited concomitant medications, along with comments on whether the concomitant medications inhibit cytochromes (CYP3A) or induce cytochromes (CYP3A).

This list of prohibited medications was included in the Protocol, apparently because of a publication demonstrating the fact that CYP3A is capable of metabolizing the study drug (tofacitinib) (148). The publication states that (149), "[a]n understanding of the pharmacokinetics (PK) ... of **tofacitinib** is important to ... inform the potential for drug–drug interactions."

The connection between the Clinical Study Protocol and the published pharmacokinetic study is obvious—both were authored by the same company. A goal of the list of prohibited concomitant medications was to prevent

---

[146]Warning Letter No. 06-HFD-45-08-04 (November 6, 2003) from Dr Leslie K. Ball, MD, Office of Compliance, CDER, U.S. Food and Drug Administration.

[147]Phase 3 randomized, double-blind study of the efficacy and safety of 2 doses of CP690,550 compared to methotrexate in methotrexate-naive patients with rheumatoid arthritis. Compound Name: tofacitinib. US IND No: 70,903. Protocol No: A3921069 (November 2012).

[148]Dowty ME, et al. The pharmacokinetics, metabolism, and clearance mechanisms of tofacitinib, a Janus kinase inhibitor, in humans. Drug Metab. Dispos. 2014;42:759–73.

[149]Dowty ME, et al. The pharmacokinetics, metabolism, and clearance mechanisms of tofacitinib, a Janus kinase inhibitor, in humans. Drug Metab. Dispos. 2014;42:759–73.

unexpected increases or decreases in the concentration of *tofacitinib* in the patient's bloodstream and tissues.

The list of CYP3A inhibitors includes cimetidine, erythromycin, and verapamil. The list of CYP3A inducers includes phenytoin, rifampin, and St John's Wort.

This appendix that concerns concomitant medications reads, in part (150):

> **Appendix 4. Prohibited Concomitant Medications**. All prohibited drugs require discontinuation at least 7 days or 5 half lives prior to first dose of study drug, whichever is longer. In the table version below those drugs requiring washout longer than 7 days are in bold and italicized. Please note that efavirenz, nevirapine, barbiturates, carbamazepine, phenobarbital, St. John's Wort, rifabutin and rifapentene should be discontinued at least 30 days prior to first dose of study based on the half life of these drugs, and that amiodarone should be discontinued at least 290 days prior to the first dose of study drug based on a half life of 58 days.

XV. INCLUSION/EXCLUSION CRITERIA

This further develops issues relating to the inclusion and exclusion criteria. One Warning Letter concerned the exclusion criterion that subjects must not have seizures in the timeframe before enrollment. The letter referred to 21 CFR §312.60, and complained that (151), "[y]ou failed to conduct the studies according to the investigational plan ... [t]he research plan for study [redacted] specified that **subjects with concurrent seizure activities should**

be excluded. Subject [redacted] had tonic-clonic seizures on 5/8/99, but was enrolled in the study in violation of the study."

Another Warning Letter concerned inclusion criteria that were results from laboratory tests. The first problem was that the investigator did not perform the laboratory test before administering the study drug to the subject in question. The second problem was that the investigator stated that the subjects had met the inclusion criteria, even though the investigator's statement was not supported by any paperwork.

The Warning Letter referred to 21 CFR §812.100 and 21 CFR §812.110(b), and complained that (152):

> you failed to conduct the investigation in accordance with the investigational plan for ...**[s]ubjects who did not meet the eligibility criteria were enrolled** in the study. Examples of your failure include ... the following ... [t]he protocol states that all subjects will receive routine laboratory work including...test results were not obtained prior to study treatment to determine if the subject met the exclusion criteria ...test results were never obtained.

XVI. DRUG ACCOUNTABILITY, DRUG STORAGE, DRUG DISPENSING, AND RECORD KEEPING

a. Introduction to the Variety of Topics

The Clinical Study Protocol can optionally include information on handling, storing, and

---

[150]Phase 3 randomized, double-blind study of the efficacy and safety of 2 doses of CP690,550 compared to methotrexate in methotrexate-naive patients with rheumatoid arthritis. Compound Name: tofacitinib. US IND No: 70,903. Protocol No: A3921069 (November 2012).

[151]Warning Letter to George J. Brewer (January 14, 2009) from Dr Leslie K. Ball, MD, Office of Compliance, CDER, U.S. Food and Drug Administration.

[152]Warning Letter to Sarah H. Lisanby (no Warning Letter No.) (October 6, 2008) from Timothy A. Ulatowski, Office of Compliance, Center for Devices and Radiological Health, U.S. Food and Drug Administration.

dispensing the study drug. A Clinical Study Protocol for a cystic fibrosis drug provided information on tablets. The instructions referred to a Pharmacy Manual, which provided instructions for storing study drug before, as well as after, dispensation to subjects. The Protocol's information on tablets included (153):

- Color of the tablets;
- Coating for the tables;
- Packaging (blister cards);
- Storage.

> **Study Drug Supply, Storage, and Handling**. Lumacaftor/ivacaftor (200/125) and matching placebo will be supplied as pink film-coated tablets of similar size and appearance containing 200 mg lumacaftor/125 mg ivacaftor and 0 mg lumacaftor/ 0 mg ivacaftor, respectively. Lumacaftor/ivacaftor (200/83) and matching placebo will be supplied as pink film-coated tablets ...Ivacaftor and matching placebo will be supplied as blue film-coated tablets ... Blister cards must be stored at room temperature according to ... instructions provided in the Pharmacy Manual. While at the clinical site, the study drug must be stored in a secure, temperature-monitored area of limited access and only at the location(s) listed on the Form FDA 1572.

The Pharmacy Manual also detailed how to dispose of unused study drug (154):

> **Disposal, Return, or Retention of Unused Drug**. Subjects must be instructed to return all used, partially used, and full study drug blister cards. The site staff or pharmacy personnel (as appropriate) will retain all materials returned by the subjects until the site monitor has performed drug accountability. The site monitor will instruct the site when it is appropriate to return or destroy study drug ...**[d]estruction** must be adequately documented. Procedures for destruction or return of the study drug will be detailed in the Pharmacy Manual.

A Clinical Study Protocol from a different trial established the generality of the following categories of information (155):

> **Supply, receipt, and storage**. Study drugs must be received by a designated person at the study site, handled and stored safely and properly, and kept in a secured location to which only the investigator and designated assistants have access. Upon receipt, the [study drug] should be stored according to the instructions specified on the drug labels.
>
> **Dispensing and preparation**. The site pharmacy will receive open label bottles containing [study drug] capsules. Patients will receive one or multiple bottles according to the appropriate dose with instructions from the investigator on how to take the medication.
>
> **Drug accountability**. The investigator or designee must maintain an accurate record of the shipment and dispensing of study drug per local institutional guidelines. Drug accountability will be noted by the field monitor during site visits and at the completion of the study. Patients will be asked to return all unused study drug and packaging on a regular basis, at the end of the study or at the time of study drug discontinuation. At study close-out, and, as appropriate during the course of the study, the investigator will destroy all used and unused study drug, packaging, drug labels per institutional

---

[153]Clinical Study Protocol A Phase 3, Randomized, Double-Blind, Placebo-Controlled, Parallel-Group Study to Evaluate the Efficacy and Safety of Lumacaftor in Combination With Ivacaftor in Subjects Aged 12 Years and Older With Cystic Fibrosis, Homozygous for the F508del-CFTR Mutation Vertex Study Number: VX12-809-103 Lumacaftor IND No: 79,521 Ivacaftor IND No: 74,633 EUDRACT No: 2012-003989-40.

[154]Clinical Study Protocol A Phase 3, Randomized, Double-Blind, Placebo-Controlled, Parallel-Group Study to Evaluate the Efficacy and Safety of Lumacaftor in Combination With Ivacaftor in Subjects Aged 12 Years and Older With Cystic Fibrosis, Homozygous for the F508del-CFTR Mutation Vertex Study Number: VX12-809-103 Lumacaftor IND No: 79,521 Ivacaftor IND No: 74,633 EUDRACT No: 2012-003989-40.

[155]Oncology Clinical Trial Protocol CLDK378X2101. A phase I, multicenter, open-label dose escalation study of LDK378, administered orally in adult patients with tumors characterized by genetic abnormalities in anaplastic lymphoma kinase (ALK) (August 19, 2010).

guidelines. A copy of completed drug accountability will be sent ... to the [Sponsor's] address provided in the investigator folder at each site. **Disposal and destruction**. The drug supply can be destroyed at the local [Sponsor's] facility.

Further information on the composition of the ivacaftor tablets for cystic fibrosis can be found in FDA's Medical Review. The Medical Review was for NDA No. 203,188, which is on March 2015 of the FDA's website. The formulation, which included the excipient and the tablet's coating, is revealed in the footnote (156).

One more example of instructions on drug accountability, from another Clinical Study Protocol, is as follows (157). Highlights of these instructions, include the need to count tablets, and the need to record which patients in the clinical trial received the study drug,

> **Drug Accountability**. Drug inventory and accountability records will be kept by the Investigator and the Pharmacy of the hospital. In general, the following rules are to be followed:

> a) The Investigator will keep the IMP [investigational medicinal product] refrigerated between 2°C and 8°C in a pharmacy or in a locked and secure area or storage facility, accessible only to those individuals authorized by the Investigator to dispense the IMP.
> b) The inventory will be maintained by the Investigator or pharmacist ...[t]he inventory will be done by means of a "Drug Accountability Log" and will include details of IMP received and a clear record of when they were dispensed and to which patient. The inventory record shall

indicate the quantity and description of all IMP on hand at any time during the course of the clinical trial.

> c) At the conclusion ... of the clinical trial, the Investigator agrees to conduct a final IMP inventory and to record the results of the inventory on an appropriate form provided by the CRO (Drug Supply Return Form). The Investigator will perform the drug accountability to calculate the number of tablets left. According to instructions, the Investigator will return all original drug containers, whether empty or containing IMP, for disposition.
> d) The Investigator agrees not to supply IMP to any person except those named as Investigators/Co-Investigators in the Study Personnel Form and patients in this study.
> e) No investigational product stock or returned inventory from this trial may be removed from the investigational site where originally shipped without prior knowledge and consent by CRO or sponsor, as appropriate.

The need for including drug accountability instructions in the Clinical Study Protocol is apparent from the fact that accountability failures often result in Warning Letters from the FDA (158). FDA's Warning Letters that complain about drug accountability include the following.

One Warning Letter complained that, "[f]ailure to retain study records as required by FDA regulations compromises the validity and integrity of data significantly. Because **you failed to retain drug accountability records** and case histories for both studies, we consider the data generated at your site for Protocols [redacted] and [redacted] unreliable in support

---

[156]The study drug was "formulated as a waxed, light blue film-coated tablet containing 150 mg of drug substance. Each tablet contains the following excipients: colloidal silicon dioxide, croscarmellose sodium, hypromellose acetate succinate, lactose monohydrate, magnesium stearate, microcrystalline cellulose, and sodium lauryl sulfate. The tablet film coat contains carnauba wax, FD&C Blue #2, PEG 3350, polyvinyl alcohol, talc, and titanium dioxide. The printing ink contains ammonium hydroxide, iron oxide black, propylene glycol, and shellac."

[157]A phase II multicenter, randomized, double-blind, controlled versus placebo, dosefinding study on the efficacy and safety of GED-0301, in patients with active Crohn's disease (Ileo-Colitis). Protocol: GED-301-01-11. EUDRACT NUMBER 2011-002640-27.

[158]Marwah R, et al. Good clinical practice regulatory inspections: lessons for Indian investigator sites. Perspect. Clin. Res. 2010;1:151−5.

of a research or marketing application" (159). As is evident, the deficiency in drug accountability contributed to the FDA's refusal to grant marketing approval to the study drug.

To provide an additional example, another Warning Letter issued the following complaint. Please note the Letter's mention of records of the disposition of the drug, product accountability documents, and a case report form (160):

> You failed to maintain adequate records of the disposition of the drug, including dates, quantity, and use by subjects [21 CFR 312.62(a)]. As a clinical investigator, you are required to maintain adequate **records of the disposition of the drug**, including dates, quantity, and use by subjects. According to Protocol GLP112757, the disposition of the investigational drug should be recorded in **product accountability documents** stating the amounts of albiglutide/matching placebo ... administered to study subjects; the amounts returned by study subjects; and the amounts received from and returned to the sponsor, when applicable. You did not adequately maintain records of these documents. Examples of this failure include ... [f]or Subject 1398757002 ... [t]he Investigational Supplies Inventory Log notes that Container #2592361 was administered on November 21, 2010, but the **case report form** notes that this container was administered on January 21, 2011.

b. Record Keeping

FDA frequently issues letters about failures to maintain records. The following letter referred to the requirement in the Code of Federal Regulations (CFR) to keep records for at least 2 years, and complained (161):

> You failed to retain records required to be maintained ... until 2 years after the investigation was discontinued and FDA was notified [21 CFR 312.62(c)].

> On October 1, 2009, the sponsor discontinued your participation in Protocol [redacted]. FDA was notified in a letter dated October 5, 2009, that your participation in Protocol [redacted] was discontinued ... Mr. Watson and Mr. Thomas, representing FDA, conducted an inspection and met with you ... [a]t the time of the inspection, which was less than two years after your investigation was discontinued and FDA was notified, the inspection revealed that you failed to retain the following records:

> Electronic case report forms (eCRFs). During FDA's inspection, you stated that your study coordinator used a sponsor-provided laptop to enter data into the eCRF for each subject .... [h]owever, it was your responsibility as the investigator to retain copies of the eCRFs for two years after the investigation was discontinued and FDA was notified [21 CFR 312.62(c)].

The Clinical Study Protocol can optionally include instructions for record keeping. An excerpt from the Protocol used in a clinical trial on an autoimmune disease is as follows (162). These instructions refer to case report forms (CRFs), signed informed consents, and records of efficacy and safety:

> **STUDY DOCUMENTATION, CRFS AND RECORD KEEPING. Investigator Files/Retention of Documents.**
> The investigator must maintain adequate and accurate records to enable the conduct of the study to be fully documented and the study data to be subsequently verified. These documents should be classified into two different separate categories (1) investigator's study file, and (2) subject clinical source documents. The investigator's study file will contain the protocol/amendments, CRF and query

---

[159]Warning Letter No. 14-HFD-45-08-01 (August 12, 2014) from Dr Sean Y. Kassim, PhD, Office of Compliance, CDER, U.S. Food and Drug Administration.

[160]Warning Letter No. 14-HFD-45-04-03 (April 30, 2014) from Dr Sean Y. Kassim, PhD, Office of Compliance, CDER, U.S. Food and Drug Administration.

[161]Warning Letter No. 11-HFD-45-03-02 (March 21, 2011) from Dr Leslie K. Ball, MD, Office of Compliance, CDER, U.S. Food and Drug Administration.

[162]Clinical Study Protocol. Protocol Number WX17801. Aspreva Lupus Management Study (ALMS). April 12, 2007.

forms, IEC/IRB and governmental approval with correspondence, sample informed consent, drug records, staff curriculum vitae and authorization forms, and other appropriate documents/correspondence etc. Subject clinical source documents (usually defined in advance to record key efficacy/safety parameters independent of the CRFs) would include subject hospital/clinic records, physician's and nurse's notes, appointment book, original laboratory reports, ECG, pathology and special assessment reports, signed informed consent forms, consultant letters, and subject screening and enrollment logs.

The next letter referred to the person dispensing the drug, and to keeping records of unused study drugs. The drugs took the form of tablets and injectables.

The letter referred to a patient's failure to return unused tablets, discrepancies in tablet counting, and failures in entering tablet numbers. Citing 21 CFR §312.62(a), the letter complained that (163), "[y]ou failed to maintain adequate drug disposition records" and added that the Clinical Study Protocol requires that, "[d]rug administration will be documented (date, time, dose and signature of dispensing person). Drug account of the unused study medication will be performed."

The letter further complained that, "[f]or Subject **[redacted]** the Drug Dispensing log documents that the **amount of drug used was**

'unknown' with no explanation provided for the lack of drug accountability ... [f]or Subject [redacted] the Drug Dispensing log documents the number of tablets and injections administered as unknown and that the patient **never returned study medication**... [f]or Subject [redacted] the drug Dispensing log documents that 21 tablets and 16 injections were administered to the subject and that the subject returned 19 tablets, with **no explanation provided in the 'discrepancy'** column."

Another Warning Letter complained that the number of tablets used by one patient was recorded on two different case report forms, and that the numbers on these case report forms disagreed with each other (164), "[t]he case history for Subject #002 had two different copies of CRF page 77 from Visit 7. One copy indicated that 168 tablets were dispensed on 8/22/07, while the other copy had 168 crossed out and 140 written instead on 10/10/07, with no documentation to support this change." Similar Warning Letters are cited (165,166,167,168).

In one clinical trial, instructions in the Clinical Study Protocol coupled low compliance with dropping the subject from the trial. The Warning Letter disclosed that (169), "[t]he protocol specified that a secondary measure of

[163]Warning Letter No. 08-HFD-45-05-02 (May 28, 2008) from Dr Leslie K. Ball, MD, Office of Compliance, CDER, U.S. Food and Drug Administration.

[164]Warning Letter No. 09-HFD-45-07-03 (July 27, 2009) from Dr Leslie K. Ball, MD, Office of Compliance, CDER, U.S. Food and Drug Administration.

[165]Warning Letter No. 10-HFD-45-11-01 (November 9, 2009) from Dr Leslie K. Ball, MD, Office of Compliance, CDER, U.S. Food and Drug Administration.

[166]Warning Letter No. 07-HFD-45-03-01 (July 7, 2003) from Gary Della'Zanna, Office of Compliance, CDER, U.S. Food and Drug Administration.

[167]Warning Letter No. 06-HFD-45-08-01 (August 18, 2006) from Dr Leslie K. Ball, MD, Office of Compliance, CDER, U.S. Food and Drug Administration.

[168]Warning Letter No. 10-HFD-45-09-05 (September 30, 2010) from Dr Leslie K. Ball, MD, Office of Compliance, CDER, U.S. Food and Drug Administration.

[169]Warning Letter No. 06-HFD-45-09-05 (February 8, 2007) from Gary Della'Zanna, Office of Compliance, CDER, U.S. Food and Drug Administration.

patient compliance would be determined by weighing the ciclesonide spray bottles to determine the amount of study drug used by each patient … [t]he protocol required that if patients were found to be less than 80% compliant at repeat visits, they should be withdrawn from study."

The next Warning Letter complained about failures in keeping track of shipments of the study drug. As is apparent from this, and other warning letters, the Sponsor believed that it could persuade the FDA that it had complied with FDA regulations by submitting a bare, conclusory statement, without any corroborative evidence. The letter referred to 21 CFR §312.57 and complained that (170):

> You failed to maintain adequate records showing the receipt, shipment, or other disposition of the investigational drug … [a]s a sponsor, you are required to maintain drug disposition records to include … the name of the investigator to whom the drug is shipped, and the date, quantity, and batch or code mark of each such shipment. Our investigation found that you did not maintain these records.
>
> You stated in your written response dated July 27, 2009, that it was your understanding at the time of the FDA inspection that you were to provide a letter from the …Pharmacy verifying proper shipment to the FDA investigator. You further stated that you obtained records showing receipt and shipment of the study drug. Your response, however, provided no documentation to corroborate your statements that you had obtained these documents.

c. Clinical Study Protocol's Instructions for Drug Accountability

The following Clinical Study Protocol provides information on medication accountability, as well as other techniques for monitoring compliance of drug administration. The Protocol was published as a supplement to a

medical journal article (171). The Protocol included general guidance on drug accountability methods, referring to self-assessment by study subjects, pill-counting by study personnel, and checking drug levels in urine or blood, as revealed by this excerpt:

> Compliance with a medical regimen can be quantified by patient self assessment, pill counting, inspection of pharmacy databases, checking blood or urine samples for the presence of a medication or a marker substance, and/or by electronic monitoring of dispenser use … Patient self-assessment of compliance is easy to record, but the accuracy of the information is questionable. Patients who admit to not following prescribed regimens tend to describe their compliance accurately … while those who claim good compliance may be consciously falsifying their response or have inaccurate recall … Pill counting is also easy to accomplish, but also generally overestimates compliance. Finding excessive numbers of pills clearly indicates poor compliance, but finding the appropriate number of pills does not confirm that the medication was actually taken … Electronic monitoring systems utilize microprocessors to record the time and date that a medication container was opened or when a blister pack was accessed … Systems that assess pill bottle or blister pack opening have limited utility if patients use daily pill containers that are filled once weekly … Finally, all monitoring methods are susceptible to the Hawthorne effect, i.e., compliance being improved because the patients know that their drug use is being monitored.

XVII. WITHDRAWAL OF SUBJECTS FROM THE CLINICAL TRIAL

a. Warning Letter About Failure of Clinical Study Protocol to Include Instructions for Withdrawing Subjects because of Adverse Events

This concerns a clinical trial for cystic fibrosis, a disease of the lungs, and the lack of

---

[170]10-HFD-45-03-01 (March 8, 2010) from Dr Leslie K. Ball, MD, Office of Compliance, CDER, U.S. Food and Drug Administration.

[171]Albert RK, Connett J, Bailey WC, et al. Azithromycin for prevention of exacerbations of COPD. New Engl. J. Med. 2011;365:689−98.

instructions for safety monitoring. In addition to failing to provide instructions for withdrawing subjects because of adverse events, the Clinical Study Protocol also failed to configure the inclusion/exclusion criteria to minimize risks, and failed to include instructions for monitoring adverse events of the subjects. The Warning Letter complained that (172):

> The protocol lacked sufficient detail concerning inclusion/exclusion criteria and in-study safety assessments to ensure that risks to subjects were minimized. The protocol did not sufficiently describe the clinical procedures, laboratory tests, or other measures to be taken to monitor the effects of [redacted] in human subjects and to minimize risk ... [y]our protocol did not provide for adequate safety **monitoring**. Specifically, your protocol lacked adequate provisions for **monitoring adverse events, serious adverse events, withdrawals due to adverse events**, exacerbations, hospitalizations, vital signs, physical examinations, laboratory studies, and electrocardiograms, and **did not include specific rules for discontinuation of patients from the study**.

Where a study subject withdraws or drops out of a study, the Sponsor is required to keep records of the withdrawal. Regarding failure to keep records of patient withdrawal, one Warning Letter complained (173):

> [a]s the clinical investigator, you were required to ... maintain ... case histories that record all observations ... on each individual administered the investigational drug or employed as a control in the investigation ... [c]ase histories include

information related to ... participation in ... the study. However, during the inspection, you indicated ... that you did not keep records of ... how many subjects withdrew from the study ... [a]s a result, it appears that you failed to maintain adequate and accurate case histories as required by 21 CFR 312.62(b).

b. Clinical Study Protocol's Requirement for Withdrawing Subjects Due to Adverse Events

This concerns a Protocol's requirements for safety monitoring. The Protocol concerned cystic fibrosis. The study drug was *ivacaftor* (Kalydeco®). Ivacaftor received FDA-approval on March 18, 2015. The Protocol does not indicate whether it was associated with the same clinical trial which was the subject of the above-cited Warning Letters (174).

The Clinical Study Protocol (175) for ivacaftor included instructions to withdraw subjects from the clinical trial because of adverse events. The Protocol's instructions for withdrawal included:

• Withdrawal because of an adverse event that requires treatment with a medication that is not allowed by the Clinical Study Protocol;
• Withdrawal because of an SAE;
• Withdrawal because of an adverse event taking the form of abnormal laboratory values (transaminases);
• Withdrawal because of electrocardiogram data (increase in QTc).

[172]Warning Letter 05-HFD-45-06-01 (June 7, 2005) from Dr Leslie K. Ball, MD, Office of Compliance, CDER, U.S. Food and Drug Administration.

[173]Warning Letter No. 12-HFD-45-11-01 (November 21, 2011) from Dr Leslie K. Ball, MD, Office of Compliance, CDER, U.S. Food and Drug Administration.

[174]Warning Letter 05-HFD-45-06-01 (June 7, 2005) from Dr Leslie K. Ball, MD, Office of Compliance, CDER, U.S. Food and Drug Administration.

[175]Clinical Study Protocol A Phase 3, Randomized, Double-Blind, Placebo-Controlled, Parallel-Group Study to Evaluate the Efficacy and Safety of Lumacaftor in Combination With Ivacaftor in Subjects Aged 12 Years and Older With Cystic Fibrosis, Homozygous for the F508del-CFTR Mutation Vertex Study Number: VX12-809-103 Lumacaftor IND No: 79,521 Ivacaftor IND No: 74,633. EUDRACT No: 2012-003989-40.

The relevant excerpt from the Protocol reads, "a subject will be withdrawn from study drug treatment for any of the following reasons ... [a] subject develops a medical condition that requires prolonged concomitant therapy with a prohibited medication or prolonged interruption of the study drug. A subject develops a life-threatening AE or a serious AE (SAE) that places him/her at immediate risk, and discontinuation of study drug treatment and withdrawal from the study are deemed necessary ... a subject has an increase in transaminases (ALT or AST) ... a subject has an increase in QTc... [a] subject develops a cataract or lens opacity."

c. Clinical Study Protocol Concerning Withdrawal of Study Subjects and Missing Data

Missing data can result from simple oversight by clinical trial personnel, as well as by withdrawals of study subjects from the clinical trial. An excerpt from a Clinical Study Protocol for an antihepatitis C drug proves instructions for the analysis of data, where the data are characterized by missing values (laboratory values, clinical values). The excerpt refers to the option of imputing missing data (making a reasonable guess as to the missing value) and to missing data due to withdrawal (premature discontinuation).

The excerpt reads (176):

> Data Handling Conventions. Missing data can have an impact upon the interpretation of the trial data. In general, values for missing data **will not be imputed**. For the analysis of post-baseline ... efficacy endpoints, if a data point is missing and is

immediately preceded and followed in time by values that are deem successes, then the missing data point will be termed a success; otherwise the data point will be termed a failure. Any subject with missing data due to **premature discontinuation** of the study will be considered a failure at the time points on, or following, the date of discontinuation. If no HCV RNA [hepatitis C virus RNA] values are obtained after the last dose of study medication, the subject will be considered a treatment failure for the [efficacy] endpoints. Where appropriate, safety data for subjects that did not complete the study will be included in summary statistics.

d. Clinical Study Protocol Concerning Subject Retention

A Clinical Study Protocol on a drug for treating COPD included a general account of methods for enhancing patient retention (177). The Protocol provided various types of advice, all of which can be translated to diseases other than COPD.

The Protocol provided advice regarding finance, "[a] variety of factors contribute to patients failing to complete trials or comply with prescribed regimens ... [i]n addition to the cost of buying medications patients frequently need sufficient financial resources to cover the cost of traveling to the health care provider, arranging childcare, taking time off from work. Unstable living conditions, low levels of education and poor social support systems contribute to these problems. Patients agreeing to participate in this study will bear no additional expense for medications or testing, and will be reimbursed for their travel-related time and effort."

The Protocol provided guidance regarding continuity of care, "continuity of care, and the communication style of the provider may

---

[176]The Clinical Study Protocol was included as a supplement to Jacobson IM, Gordon SC, Kowdley KV, et al. Sofosbuvir for hepatitis C genotype 2 or 3 in patients without treatment options. New Engl. J. Med. 2013;368:1867–77.

[177]The Clinical Study Protocol was published as a supplement to Albert RK, Connett J, Bailey WC, et al. Azithromycin for prevention of exacerbations of COPD. New Engl. J. Med. 2011;365:689–98.

improve retention and adherence to a pre-scribed regimen ... [w]e will structure the ini-tial evaluation and all follow-up phone contacts and clinic visits such that the patients interact with the **same study coordinator** on each occasion."

Also, the Protocol provided advice regard-ing a need for simple dosing, "[t]he most important therapy-related factors affecting compliance are the complexity of the medical regimen, the duration of treatment, frequent changes in treatment, the immediacy of benefi-cial effects, the frequency of side effects ... [i]n an attempt to facilitate compliance with the prescribed regimen **we have chosen a daily dosing regimen (250 mg once daily)** despite the fact that it will provide a slightly higher total weekly dose, and run the risk of causing a slightly higher rate of side effects than the 500 mg three times weekly dose that was alter-nately considered."

Moreover, the Protocol taught the impor-tance of educating subjects and conferring the ability of self-management, "all patients will receive education about their disease as described above and information pertaining to COPD Support Groups in their respective areas, and they will be queried on a monthly basis about their disease management, their understanding of their treatment instructions and the success or lack thereof they are seeing in response to the intervention. We will also attempt to increase the patient's motivation by discussing the perceived importance of

adherence, and by teaching self-management skills (e.g., correct bronchodilator inhalation techniques, the importance of exercise, purse-lipped breathing)."

e. Publications Commenting on Study Subject Withdrawal and Subject Retention

Where subjects withdraw during the course of a clinical trial, the result could be lack of enough subjects to arrive at statistically signifi-cant conclusions on efficacy and safety. Also, where subjects withdraw, the result could be disruption of the study's stratification scheme, that is, it could result in imbalances in one of the subgroups (number of subjects in the study drug arm and in the control arm, of that subgroup).

Methods for enhancing patient retention most obviously include the fact that the clinical trial may reduce risk for the disease under study, especially where the control arm is an active control (and not a placebo) (178). Other methods include providing 24-hour availabil-ity of a nurse to the study subjects (179), engaging study subjects in periodic clinic visits (once every 4 weeks) with intervening tele-phone calls (180), and using psychological screening prior to enrollment to exclude non-motivated subjects (181). Another commenta-tor suggests the methods of using educational tools for patients, and reimbursement of

[178]Mor M, et al. Patient retention in a clinical trial: a lesson from the rofecoxib (VIOXX) study. Dig. Dis. Sci. 2006;51:1175–8.

[179]Proietto J, et al. A clinical trial assessing the safety and efficacy of the CB1R inverse agonist taranabant in obese and overweight patients: low-dose study. Int. J. Obesity. 2010;34:1243–54.

[180]Proietto J, et al. A clinical trial assessing the safety and efficacy of the CB1R inverse agonist taranabant in obese and overweight patients: low-dose study. Int. J. Obesity. 2010;34:1243–54.

[181]Bemder BG, et al. Retention of asthmatic patients in a longitudinal clinical trial. J. Allergy. Clin. Immunol. 1997;99:197–203.

expenses (travel, telephone usage, missed work, babysitter, lunch) (182).

XVIII. CONTRACT RESEARCH ORGANIZATIONS

a. Chain of Responsibilities of Sponsor, Investigator, and CRO

FDA's Warning Letters reveal some of the responsibilities of contract research organizations (CRO) that conduct clinical trials for a Sponsor (183). The same responsibilities also apply to the Sponsor, irrespective of whether the Sponsor performs the investigation on its own or uses a CRO. The following provides a granular account of some of the routine paperwork that needs to be done, in the course of a clinical trial.

FDA's Warning Letter stated that the Sponsor had (184), "specifically transferred the following tasks associated with site monitoring to [the CRO]." The tasks that were transferred to the CRO were:

- Develop and write monitoring plan;
- Schedule and conduct on-site monitoring visits;
- Schedule and conduct telephone follow-up visits;
- Write follow-up letters;
- Notify sponsor of any critical site issues (ie, good clinical practice violations,

non-compliance trends noticed at site) and for providing a proposed resolution plan;
- Conduct weekly teleconferences to review site-monitoring schedule;
- Provide tracking of monitoring visits, telephone follow-up visits, monitoring-visit reports, and protocol violations.

The Warning Letter provides an excellent view of the responsibilities of the Sponsor and CRO, in its writing that (185):

> The regulations permit the transfer of obligations to a CRO by a sponsor (21 CFR 312.52(a)), and describe the responsibilities that the CRO incurs when obligations are transferred (21 CFR 312.52(b)). Specifically, a CRO that assumes any obligation of a sponsor shall be subject to the same regulatory action as a sponsor for failure to comply with any obligation assumed under part 312. From our review … we conclude that you did not adhere to the applicable statutory requirements and FDA regulations governing the conduct of clinical investigations.

An unrelated Warning Letter provides an exemplary account of the supervisory role of the clinical investigator. (This letter did not concern any Contract Research Organization.) The letter focuses on the meaning of delegating responsibilities, as is evident from its writing that (186), "[w]hile **you may delegate certain study tasks** to individuals qualified to perform them, as clinical investigator, **you may not delegate your general responsibilities**." The Warning Letter listed violations that

---

[182]Vondraskova A. Customizing patient retention in clinical trials. Pharmanet Development Group. Obere Wiltisgasse 52, CH-8700, Switzerland.

[183]Warning Letter No. 10-HFD-45-11-04 (November 27, 2009) from Dr Leslie K. Ball, MD, Office of Compliance, CDER, U.S. Food and Drug Administration.

[184]Warning Letter No. 10-HFD-45-11-07 (November 27, 2009) from Dr Leslie K. Ball, MD, Office of Compliance, CDER, U.S. Food and Drug Administration.

[185]Warning Letter No. 10-HFD-45-11-04 (November 27, 2009) from Dr Leslie K. Ball, MD, Office of Compliance, CDER, U.S. Food and Drug Administration.

[186]Warning Letter No. 06-HFD-45-11-01 (January 16, 2007) from Gary Zana, Division of Scientific Investigations, Office of Compliance, CDER, U.S. Food and Drug Administration.

had earlier been documented on several Form FDA483 notices, cited 21 CFR §312.60, and complained that (187):

> You failed to personally conduct or supervise the clinical investigation ...
>
> When you signed ... **Form FDA 1572**... you agreed to take on the responsibilities of a clinical investigator at your site. Your ... responsibilities ... include ensuring that the investigation is conducted according to the signed investigator statement, the investigational plan, and applicable regulations; protecting the ... safety ... subjects under your care; and ensuring control of drugs under investigation ... [w]hile **you may delegate certain study tasks** to individuals qualified to perform them ... **you may not delegate your general responsibilities**. Our investigation indicates that your supervision of personnel to whom you delegated study tasks was not adequate to ensure that clinical trials were conducted according to the signed investigator statement, the investigational plan, and applicable regulations, and in a manner that protected the ... safety ... of human subjects.

An unrelated Warning Letter also complained about failures in the chain of responsibilities. The letter referred to Form FDA 1572 and to the agreement to supervise and failure to supervise individuals to whom tasks were delegated, stating that (188), "[y]ou did not adequately supervise individuals to whom you delegated study tasks ... [y]our lack of oversight resulted in protocol violations, inadequate drug accountability, inadequate informed consent." Failure to supervise was also the issue in yet another Warning Letter,

where the problem was failure to supervise "new study coordinators" (189). Yet another Warning Letter provides guidance of the relative responsibilities of the investigator and the monitor. The issue was the responsibility to report amendments of the Clinical Study Protocol to the Institutional Review Board (IRB). The investigator tried to blame the monitor for failing to notify the IRB of the amendment. However, the Warning Letter corrected the investigator's false notion, by writing (190):

> In your December 24, 2012, written response to the violation ... you said, "The **monitor** failed to inform and educate the site about the amendment to the Protocol ..." [h]owever, it is **your responsibility as the investigator (not the monitor's responsibility)** to ensure that the IRB has approved any changes in the research prior to implementing those changes. In addition, your response is inadequate because you failed to provide evidence of IRB approval.

b. Record Keeping Failure of CRO

This concerns a problem in record keeping. The problem was that the written record stated that one of the study personnel did something that was impossible, namely, giving study drug to two subjects at exactly the same time. The letter complained that it is impossible for one person, the "study coordinator," to administer study drug to two people at exactly the same time.

---

[187]Warning Letter No. 06-HFD-45-1101 (January 16, 2007) from Gary Zana, Division of Scientific Investigations, Office of Compliance, CDER, U.S. Food and Drug Administration.

[188]Warning Letter No. 08-HFD-45-09-01 (October 1, 2008) from Dr Leslie K. Ball, MD, Office of Compliance, CDER, U.S. Food and Drug Administration.

[189]Warning Letter No. 09-HFD-45-06-01 (June 12, 2009) from Dr Leslie K. Ball, MD, Office of Compliance, CDER, U.S. Food and Drug Administration.

[190]Warning Letter No. 13-HFD-45-08-04 (September 3, 2013) from Thomas N. Moreno, Office of Compliance, CDER, U.S. Food and Drug Administration.

The letter complained that (191), "[s]tudy monitors failed to identify that on multiple occasions, site personnel documented administration of study drug to different subjects at precisely the same time ... at Site #520, study monitors failed to identify that on multiple occasions, study coordinators documented administration of study drug to two different subjects at the same time ... study coordinators documented administration of study drug to two different subjects at the same time, and study monitors should have sought an explanation for these observations ... Subject #1266 at 09:00–10:00 and Subject #1267 at 09:00–10:00 on 7/2/05 ... study monitors should have noted that on multiple occasions, study site personnel documented administration of study drug to different subjects at precisely the same time, and further investigated the reason for this irregularity ... it would not be possible for the same study coordinator to begin study infusions on more than one subject at precisely the same time, even if the two subjects had been treated at the same location."

According to FDA's letter, the persons responsible for this oversight in record keeping included the study coordinator, the study monitor, and site personnel.

c. Drug Accountability Failure of CRO

The letter complaining about the record-keeping oversight, where one person administered study drug to two subjects at the same time, also complained about a drug accountability failure. The issue was the Clinical Study Protocol's requirement that (192), "receiving site storage conditions must be confirmed upon delivery of the study medication. Clinic, investigator office and/or patient refrigerator temperatures must be recorded and the plan must specify where and by whom." FDA's Warning Letter complained that, "at Site #509, study monitors failed to ensure that reconstituted study drug infusion solutions were stored appropriately. Protocol [redacted] stated that reconstituted study drug infusion solutions should ... be stored at room temperature (25°C) and used within 6 hours ... [a]lthough they were asked by [CRO] monitors, the personnel at the site never addressed how they would document the temperature storage conditions of the product in subjects' homes ... storage temperatures for these medications could not be confirmed as complying with storage conditions specified by the protocol."

The above complaint concerned deviations at Site#509. The same Warning Letter also complained about an out-of-range temperature reading, which occurred at another site (Site #520). The letter complained that (193), "at Site #520, study monitors failed to document the out-of-range temperature readings noted at this site, and failed to provide appropriate follow-up instructions to the site regarding the usage of the kits in a particular shipment." The layperson can easily understand the seriousness of this out-of-range temperature, by the Warning Letter's further complaint that,

---

[191]Warning Letter No. 10-HFD-45-11-04 (November 27, 2009) from Dr Leslie K. Ball, MD, Office of Compliance, CDER, U.S. Food and Drug Administration.

[192]Warning Letter No. 10-HFD-45-11-04 (November 27, 2009) from Dr Leslie K. Ball, MD, Office of Compliance, CDER, U.S. Food and Drug Administration.

[193]Warning Letter No. 10-HFD-45-11-04 (November 27, 2009) from Dr Leslie K. Ball, MD, Office of Compliance, CDER, U.S. Food and Drug Administration.

"[b]ased on documentation available at the time, study monitors … should have recognized that drug kits … should not have been administered to subjects."

d. Close-Out Letter

The issues regarding the CRO, as described above, had a happy ending. The above Warning Letter, which complained about study drug to two subjects at exactly the same time, and about the out-of-range temperature, was followed by a favorable Close-Out Letter. As stated by FDA (194), "[a] close-out letter will not be issued based on representations that some action will or has been taken. The corrective actions must actually have been made and verified by FDA. Usually, the standard for verifying that corrections have been implemented will be a follow-up inspection. If the Warning Letter contains violations that by their nature are not correctable, then no close-out letter will issue." On occasion, the FDA's website provides, along with its Warning Letter, a second letter that is a Close-Out Letter. The Close-Out Letter discloses if or how the problem was eventually resolved.

Regarding the deficiencies of the CRO described above, the Close-Out Letter stated that (195), "[t]he Food and Drug Administration has completed an evaluation of your firm's corrective actions in response to our Warning Letter … [b]ased on our evaluation, it appears that you have addressed the violations contained in this Warning Letter." The Close-Out Letter was dated about 5 years after the initial Warning Letter.

XIX. CASE REPORT FORMS

a. Case Report Form was Generic and was not Relevant to the Clinical Trial

Case report forms are drafted to be aligned with details of the clinical trial. Bellary et al. (196) state that the "CRF should be designed for optimal collection of data in accordance with the study protocol compliance, regulatory requirements and shall enable the researcher test the hypothesis or answer the trial related questions. A well-designed CRF should represent the essential contents of the study protocol and in an ideal situation, CRF is designed once the study protocol is finalized."

Real-world guidance on the content and filling-out of case report forms comes from Warning Letters that are issued by the FDA against personnel involved in regulated clinical trials. A failure of a case report form to be aligned with goals of a clinical trial resulted in a Warning Letter complaining that (197):

> We do not find it acceptable for you to assign these responsibilities to study coordinators without first considering the **specifics and requirements of each study** that you undertake and determining the extent, if any, to which the study coordinator is qualified to be the primary author of all source documents and **Case Report Forms**… [w]ith respect to the sample **Case Report Form** that you provided, we are unable to determine the purpose of this sample Case Report Form and when you plan to use it. We are concerned that you may introduce error into future studies by using Case Report Forms that are **not study-specific**.

---

[194]U.S. Food and Drug Administration. About Warning and Close-Out Letters. December 8, 2011. Accessed from the FDA website on July 30, 2015.

[195]Warning Letter No. 10-HFD-45-11-04 (November 27, 2009) from Dr Leslie K. Ball, MD, Office of Compliance, CDER, U.S. Food and Drug Administration.

[196]Bellary S, et al. Basics of case report form designing in clinical research. Perspect. Clin. Res. 2014;5:159–66.

[197]Warning Letter No. 14-HFD-45-12-01 (April 30, 2014) from Dr Sean Y. Kassim, PhD, Office of Compliance, CDER, U.S. Food and Drug Administration.

As is the case with all Warning Letters issued by the FDA, the letter concluded with the warning that, "[w]ithin fifteen (15) working days of your receipt of this letter, you should notify this office in writing of the actions you have taken to prevent similar violations in the future. Failure to address the violations noted above adequately and promptly may result in regulatory action without further notice."

b. Garbled Filling Out of Case Report Forms by Study Personnel

Another Warning Letter complained about inconsistencies in start and stop dates, and inconsistencies in the number of pills (tablets) (198):

> Multiple concomitant therapy case report forms documenting medications used by subject #0003 contain conflicting information with respect to start and stop dates. There is no written documentation to explain these inconsistencies ... Visit 7: The study medication case report form for visit 7 documents 200 tablets returned on 2/20/07, yet the study medication compliance check for visit 7 documents 38 tablets returned on 2/20/07.

c. Failure to Fill Out the Study Subject Number on the Case Report Form

Yet another Warning Letter from the FDA complained about failure to fill out all of the required information. The letter complained that (199):

[a] clinical investigator is responsible for maintaining accurate, complete, and current records of each subject's case history and exposure to the device, which includes the case report forms (CRFs) and supporting data. You failed to adhere to the above-stated regulation in that several CRFs were not complete. Examples of your failure include ... [s]creening and **subject number identification were left blank on the CRFs** for most subjects in the study. The investigator and observer names and signatures noting when an intervention was performed were not completed on most CRFs.

d. Failure to Record Concomitant Therapy on the Case Report Form

FDA's Warning Letter complained that (200): "Concomitant therapy was not always reported in the CRFs as required by the protocol. For example ... [p]rescriptions dated November 9, 2005, and November 30, 2005 indicate Dilaudid was prescribed for the subject. Neither medication was reported on the Other Medications and Supplements CRF."

e. Failure of Physician to Conduct Physical Examination, Even Though Physician's Signature was on Case Report Form

The letter concerned the fact that the Clinical Study Protocol required that subjects have a weekly physical examination, and the fact that the case report form be signed, but that one case report form had a signature where there had not been a corresponding physical examination. The letter complained that (201):

---

[198]Warning Letter No.10-HFD-45-11-01 (November 9, 2009) from Dr Leslie K. Ball, MD, Office of Compliance, CDER, U.S. Food and Drug Administration.

[199]Warning Letter to Mark Pinsky (no Warning Letter number) (January 14, 2013) from Steven Silverman, Office of Compliance, Center for Devices and Radiological Health. U.S. Food and Drug Administration.

[200]Warning Letter No. 06-HFD-45-11-01 (January 16, 2007) from Gary Zana, Division of Scientific Investigations, Office of Compliance, CDER, U.S. Food and Drug Administration.

[201]Warning Letter No. 06-HFD-45-11-01 (January 16, 2007) from Gary Zana, Division of Scientific Investigations, Office of Compliance, CDER, U.S. Food and Drug Administration.

The protocol required that subjects have physical examinations at each study visit. The Physical Exam **Case Report Form** (CRF) ... had missing or discrepant documentation of one or more physical exams, and several had physical exam **CRFs** without physician signatures. For example ... Subject 41806: there is no documentation in the record of a physical exam at the baseline visit of December 6, 2005 ... [f] or the ... visit on October 25, 2005, **the physical exam form** is not filled out **but is signed by a physician** ... the study coordinator states that **the physician can't recall the physical exam** and therefore can't comment on whether it was performed.

f. ICH Guidelines Provide Guidance for Case Report Forms

The ICH Guidelines define a case report form (CRF) as "[a] printed, optical, or electronic document designed to record all of the protocol-required information to be reported to the sponsor on each trial subject" (202). FDA's Guidance for Industry defines the electronic case report form as, "[a]n auditable electronic record of information that generally is reported to the sponsor on each trial subject, according to a clinical investigation protocol. The eCRF enables clinical investigation data to be systematically captured, reviewed, managed, stored, analyzed, and reported" (203).

According to one commentator,"[c]ase report forms (CRF) are tools used by the sponsor of a clinical trial to collect data ... [a]ll data on participating subjects ... (including adverse events) should be documented in the CRF. A copy of the CRF should be included with the IND application."

During this planning stage of any clinical trial, various documents that need to be generated and be on file before the trial formally starts, include the case report form, Clinical Study Protocol, Investigator's Brochure, consent form, and curriculum vitae of the investigators. Further regarding the case report form, what is also required is documentation that the Institutional Review Board (IRB) has approved the case report form, consent form, and Clinical Study Protocol (204).

Case report forms are used to capture adverse events of individual study subjects, during the course of a clinical trial. Various features of the case report form include data such as protocol ID, site code, subject ID, and patient initials. The case report form may also specify units of measurement to be used, the number of decimal places that need to be recorded, and use of pre-coded answer sets such as yes/no, male/female, method of administration of medicine, and severity of adverse event (AE) (mild/moderate/severe) (205). Bellary et al. (206) provide excellent examples of a well-designed case report form and of a poorly designed case report form. Kelly et al. (207) also provide an example of a well-written case report form.

g. Instructions in Clinical Study Protocol Regarding Case Report Forms

A Clinical Study Protocol for a trial on systemic lupus erythromatosus (SLE) provides concrete, general guidance for filling out case

[202]ICH guidance E6: good clinical practice: consolidated guideline. US HHS, US FDA, CDER, CBER; 1996.

[203]U.S. Department of Health and Human Services. Food and Drug Administration. Guidance for industry. Electronic source data in clinical investigations; September 2013 (11 pages).

[204]ICH guidance E6: good clinical practice: consolidated guideline. US HHS, US FDA, CDER, CBER; 1996.

[205]Bellary S, et al. Basics of case report form designing in clinical research. Perspect. Clin. Res. 2014;5:159−66.

[206]Bellary S, et al. Basics of case report form designing in clinical research. Perspect. Clin. Res. 2014;5:159−66.

[207]Kelly CR, et al. A how to guide: investigational new drug application for fecal microbiota transplantation. Clin. Gastroenterol. Hepatol. 2014;12:283−8.

report forms. The instructions refer to the need for completion and signature, and for the **need to note patient withdrawals** on the case report form (208):

> **Case Report Forms (CRFs)**. For each subject enrolled, a CRF must be completed and signed by the principal investigator or authorized delegate from the study staff. This also applies to records for those subjects who fail to complete the study (even during a pre-randomization screening period if a CRF was initiated). **If a subject withdraws from the study, the reason must be noted on the CRF**. If a subject is withdrawn from the study because of a treatment limiting adverse event, thorough efforts should be made to clearly document the outcome. All forms should be typed or filled out using indelible ink, and must be legible. Errors should be crossed out but not obliterated, the correction inserted, and the change initialed and dated by the investigator or his/her authorized delegate.

A Clinical Study Protocol on another disease, Crohn's disease, instructs study personnel to use the case report form to record deviations in study drug administration. The Protocol provides instructions for assessing treatment compliance, and for recording deviations on the case report form (209):

> **Drug dispensing and administration**. This will be a randomized, Phase II dose-finding study in 160 patients with active Crohn's disease ... [p]atients will be instructed to take the Study Medication in the morning, 30 minutes before breakfast, with a glass of water, and patients will also be instructed to store the Clinical Drug Supply in a refrigerator between 2°C and 8°C. The **treatment compliance** will be calculated on basis of the ratio between the number of tablets actually taken (verified by the

Investigator) and the number of theoretical tablets expected by the protocol. Full details and **the deviation will be recorded on the corresponding pages of the CRF** as well as in the source documents.

XX. INVESTIGATOR'S BROCHURE

A Warning Letter concerned one aspect of the Investigator's Brochure, namely, the requirement that the Sponsor provide copies of the Investigator's Brochure to medical personnel involved in conducting the clinical trial. The letter referred to 21 CFR§312.23 and 21 CFR §312.55 and complained that (210):

> You failed to give each participating investigator an investigator brochure ... [o]ur inspection found that you failed to provide the clinical investigator with an investigator brochure ... [e]nrollment began on February 20, 2007 ... [i]n your written response dated July 27, 2009, you state that no further action is needed. You attached to your written response a copy of a fax from Dr. [redacted], stating that she had submitted the investigator brochure to the Institutional Review Board (IRB) along with her IRB application on 12/6/06. We find your response inadequate. There was no investigator brochure attached to your written response, nor was it attached to the fax from Dr. [redacted], to document that the investigator brochure was given to Dr. [redacted] prior to the start of the study.

XXI. OFF-LABEL USES

a. Warning Letters Concerning Off-Label Use

Although off-label uses of drugs are widespread in the United States, it must first be the

---

[208]Clinical Study Protocol. Protocol Number WX17801. Aspreva Lupus Management Study (ALMS). April 12, 2007.

[209]A phase II multicenter, randomized, double-blind, controlled versus placebo, dosefinding study on the efficacy and safety of GED-0301, in patients with active Crohn's disease (ileo-colitis). Protocol: GED-301-01-11. EUDRACT NUMBER 2011-002640-27.

[210]Warning Letter 10-HFD-45-03-01 (March 8, 2010) from Leslie K. Ball, MD, Office of Compliance, CDER, U.S. Food and Drug Administration.

case that the drug be FDA-approved for a first use, before it is permissible to use the drug for a second, off-label use. FDA issued a Warning Letter complaining that a company had advertised a drug as suitable for a particular off-label use, where the problem for the company was that the drug had never been FDA-approved for any use. The Warning Letter complained that (211):

> FDA ... has reviewed your website, www.spa35.com ... your website contains false or misleading claims related to your LipoDissolve products ... [y] our LipoDissolve products are intended to cure, treat, mitigate, or prevent disease in humans or to affect the structure or function of the body. Statements on your websites that document these intended uses include ... "LipoDissolve uses a pharmaceutical compound called phosphatidylcholine deoxycholate, or PCDC, which is administered through a series of microinjections to permanently dissolve fat."

The letter referred to the fact that the drug (phosphatidylcholine) had been approved in some countries, but not in the United States, writing that (212), "[a]lthough intravenous phosphatidylcholine has been approved in some countries for the treatment of a variety of conditions, it has not been approved in the U.S. Currently there is no FDA-approved injectable PCDC; therefore, **any claim that PCDC is being used 'off-label' is false or misleading.**"

b. FDA's Guidance for Industry on Off-Label Uses

FDA's Guidance for Industry defines off-label uses as, "The terms *unapproved new use*, *unapproved use*, and *off-label use* are used interchangeably in this guidance to refer to a use of an approved or cleared medical product that is not included in the product's approved labeling or cleared indications for use statement" (213).

Because any "off-label" uses have not been approved by the FDA, because off-label uses are sometimes published in medical journals, and because pharmaceutical companies sometimes distribute these publications (in order to promote their drug), it is the case that FDA reacted by issuing the warning described below. The FDA observed that these publications "have also been commonly distributed by manufacturers to health care professionals and health care entities" (214).

In its Guidance for Industry, FDA issued the ethical imperative that the distributed publication, "should ... [b]e disseminated with the approved labeling." Also, FDA issued the ethical imperative that the publication "should ... [b]e disseminated with a representative publication, when such information exists, that reaches contrary or different conclusions regarding the unapproved use"

---

[211]Warning Letter to www.spa35.com (the letter had no Warning Letter No.) from Michael M. Levy, Esq., Office of Compliance, CDER. U.S. Food and Drug Administration.

[212]Warning Letter to www.spa35.com (the letter had no Warning Letter No.) from Michael M. Levy, Esq., Office of Compliance, CDER. U.S. Food and Drug Administration.

[213]U.S. Depertment of Health and Human Services. Food and Drug Administration. Guidance for industry. Distributing scientific and medical publications on unapproved new uses—recommended practices; February 2014 (17 pp.).

[214]U.S. Department of Health and Human Services. Food and Drug Administration. Guidance for industry. Distributing scientific and medical publications on unapproved new uses—recommended practices; February 2014 (17 pp.).

(215). Moreover, FDA's Guidance states that the publication should, "[b]e distributed separately from the delivery of information that is promotional in nature. For example, if a sales representative delivers a reprint to a physician in his or her office, the reprint should not be attached to any promotional material the sales representative uses or delivers during the office visit."

"Off-label" refers to use of a drug, where the use is not included in the package label or package insert. For a drug to be used "off-label," it is the case that the physician uses his or her own judgment to determine whether the contemplated off-label use is appropriate. Frequent off-label uses include use for diseases and age groups that are not included on the package label.

The term "off-label" does not imply a use that is contraindicated by any package label or merely experimental (216). Also, lack of labeling does not mean that therapy is unsupported by clinical experience, for example, that it is unsupported by any published case reports or by any clinical trials detailed in a medical journal.

The physician's judgment for off-label use can be based on medical journal publications of clinical trials, medical journal publications of case studies, as well as anecdotal information from colleagues (217). Physicians can also acquire guidance for off-label use from review articles that provide an account of published off-label treatments for a given disease. For example, Brezinski and Armstrong (218) reviewed the available information on off-label drugs for psoriasis, where the drugs were antibodies and fusion proteins.

But FDA's review process for a new drug (the process that results in an FDA-approved package label) may be compared with a medical journal's review of a manuscript. According to one FDA official, "peer review is not a replacement for a strong FDA. FDA uses multidisciplinary teams—physicians, pharmacologists, toxicologists, chemists, and statisticians, as well as experts in the conduct of clinical trials ...to independently analyze the rawdata from the studies ... [p]eer review, on the other hand, is generally conducted by a more limited set of experts and involves only the articleunder consideration for publication" (219).

Lack of labeling refers to the specifics of the physician's off-label use, such as for a disease that does not have any corresponding FDA-approved drug, a population age group that has never been subjected to a clinical trial leading to FDA-approval, a route of administration that is not on the label (220), a stage of a disease where that particular stage is not on the

[215]U.S. Department of Health and Human Services. Food and Drug Administration. Guidance for industry. Distributing scientific and medical publications on unapproved new uses—recommended practices; February 2014 (17 pp.).

[216]American Academy or Pediatrics. Policy statement. Off-label use of drugs in children. Pediatrics. 2014;133:563–7.

[217]Mullins CD, et al. Recommendations for clinical trials of off-label drugs used to treat advanced-stage cancer. J. Clin. Oncol. 2012;30:661–6.

[218]Brezinski EA, Armstrong AW. Off-label biologic regimens in psoriasis: a systematic review of efficacy and safety of dose escalation, reduction, and interrupted biologic therapy. PLoS One. 2012;7:e33486 (10 pp.).

[219]Hamburg MA. Innovation, regulation, and the FDA. New Engl. J. Med. 2010;363:2228–32.

[220]Danes I, et al. Outcomes of off-label drug uses in hospitals: a multicentric prospective study. Eur. J. Clin. Pharmacol. 2014;70:1385–95.

label (221), or a combination of drugs that is not on the label (222).

Populations that are commonly underserved by FDA-approved medicines include cancer patients, children, and pregnant women (223). For many cancers, such as rare tumors, there may never be enough evidence to support a labeling indication because of the inability to conduct the appropriate trial as a result of inadequate patient numbers (224). Another factor that impairs the ability to recruit subjects for off-label uses is as follows. Patients are reluctant to participate in a randomization process that only provides investigational treatment to some patients, especially when the drug is already widely available (225).

Cost is another factor that encourages off-label use. This example is for antibody drugs (ranibizumab; bevacizumab) that are effective for treating a disease of the eye, age-related macular degeneration. Both drugs bind to a growth factor, VEGF. Ranibizumab has been FDA-approved for macular degeneration (226).

Bevacizumab has been FDA-approved for cancer treatment (227,228), but not for macular degeneration. According to Schmucker et al. (229), "[t]he costs of ranibizumab, however, are immense." The cost of bevacizumab is 40 times lower. Both drugs have similar efficacy against macular degeneration (230). Unfortunately, bevacizumab has increased safety risks. Schmucker concluded that if the, "higher rates of adverse effects [for bevacizumab] are subsequently confirmed to be higher in bevacizumab than in ranibizumab, some of the cost savings with bevacizumab may be negated" (231).

Yet another factor that enhances the prevalence of off-label use, and impairs utilization of the FDA-approval process where the result is an FDA-approved package label, is the following. This factor is expiration of the patent for the drug (232). In other words, if a patent that covers a specific drug has already expired, a pharmaceutical company would have little incentive to spend a million dollars on a

---

[221]Conti RM, et al. Prevalence of off-label use and spending in 2010 among patent-protected chemotherapies in a population-based cohort of medical oncologists. 2013;31:1134–9.

[222]Perrone F, et al. Tackling off-label use of anticancer drugs. J. Clin. Oncol. 2012;30:2800–2.

[223]Radley DC, et al. Off-label prescribing among office-based physicians. Arch. Intern. Med. 2006;166:1021–6.

[224]Krzyzanowska MK. Off-label use of cancer drugs: a benchmark is established. J. Clin. Oncol. 2913;31:1125–7.

[225]Mullins CD, et al. Recommendations for clinical trials of off-label drugs used to treat advanced-stage cancer. J. Clin. Oncol. 2012;30:661–6.

[226]Package insert. Lucentis® (ranibizumab injection) intravitreal injection; February 2015. 20 pp.

[227]Suh DH, et al. Major clinical research advances in gynecologic cancer in 2014. J. Gynecol. Oncol. 2015;26:156–67.

[228]Conti RM, et al. The impact of emerging safety and effectiveness evidence on the use of physician-administered drugs: the case of bevacizumab for breast cancer. Med. Care. 2013;51:622–7.

[229]Schmucker C, et al. A safety review and meta-analyses of bevacizumab and ranibizumab: off-Label versus gold standard. PLoS One. 2012;7:e42701 (15 pp.).

[230]CATT Research Group. Ranibizumab and bevacizumab for neovascular age-related macular degeneration. New Engl. J. Med. 2011;364:1897–908.

[231]Schmucker C, et al. A safety review and meta-analyses of bevacizumab and ranibizumab: off-Label versus gold standard. PLoS One. 2012;7:e42701 (15 pp.).

[232]Pfister DG. Off-label use of oncology drugs: the need for more data and then some. J. Clin. Oncol. 2012;30:584–6.

clinical trial for testing an off-label use, when it is the case that generic drug manufacturers are already making and selling the drug.

If the off-label use is based on sound medical evidence, no additional informed consent beyond that routinely used in therapeutic decision-making is needed. But, if the off-label use is experimental, then the patient (or the patient's mother or father in the case of pediatric patients) should be informed that the treatment is experimental (233).

In a study of 232 off-label medicines requested and administered in the hospital setting it was determined that the most frequent pharmacological groups were the monoclonal antibodies and muscle relaxants. The most frequent monoclonal antibodies used off-label were rituximab and obalizumab, and the most frequent off-label muscle relaxant was botulinum toxin (234). Another study revealed that off-label use was most common among cardiac medications and anticonvulsants. This study found that most (about 61−84%) off-label drug uses had little scientific support (235).

Another example of an off-label use is that for a recombinant blood-clotting factor, factor VIIa. Recombinant factor VIIa was FDA-approved in 1999 for treatment of spontaneous or surgical bleeding episodes in patients with hemophilia A or B who have inhibitors to factor VIII or factor IX. When first introduced, rFVIIa was mostly used for these FDA-approved indications. But later on, it was increasingly used for preventing or treating bleeding in other conditions. After 2002, the off-label use for traumatic bleeding became popular, and in 2008, off-label use in cardiac surgery became popular. According to Logan et al. (236), use for off-label indications eventually greatly exceeded the FDA-approved use.

In a study of anticancer drugs, it was determined that for the year 2010, doxetaxel (Taxotere®) had total sales of $1198 million and $271 million in off-label sales, ritixumab (Rituxan®) had total sales of $2320 million and $530 million in off-label sales, bevacizumab (Avastin®) had $3,100 million in total sales and $1942 million in off-label sales, and cetuximab (Erbitux®) had $709 million in total sales and $192 million in off-label sales (237). These numbers demonstrate that off-label uses are a critical part of the physicians' set of therapeutic tools, but the numbers also suggest the temptation of pharmaceutical companies to engage in aggressive promotion for off-label uses for their drugs. FDA's Guidance for Industry directly addresses this type of aggressive behavior of pharmaceutical companies (238).

Ethical questions are raised when considering medications where it is not readily possible to assess risk for benefit and risk for toxicity.

[233]American Academy or Pediatrics.Policy statement. Off-label use of drugs in children. Pediatrics. 2014;133:563−7.

[234]Danes I, et al. Outcomes of off-label drug uses in hospitals: a multicentric prospective study. Eur. J. Clin. Pharmacol. 2014;70:1385−95.

[235]Radley DC, et al. Off-label prescribing among office-based physicians. Arch. Intern. Med. 2006;166:1021−6.

[236]Logan AC, et al. Off-label use of recombinant factor VIIa in United States hospitals: 2000−2008. Ann. Intern. Med. 2011;154:516−22.

[237]Conti RM, et al. Prevalence of off-label use and spending in 2010 among patent-protected chemotherapies in a population-based cohort of medical oncologists. 2013;31:1134−9.

[238]U.S. Department of Health and Human Services. Food and Drug Administration. Guidance for industry. Distributing scientific and medical publications on unapproved new uses—recommended practices; February 2014 (17 pp.).

According to one commentator (239), case reports suggest that anticoagulants might play a role in migraine prophylaxis. The question that arises is, should a physician consider prescribing warfarin for migraine prophylaxis? There are no randomized controlled trials and there is little published literature on this indication, and the mechanism of warfarin's effect on migraines is not well understood. As further opined by this commentator, most physicians would not prescribe warfarin for migraine prophylaxis. However, for an individual patient, this treatment would be reasonable, if a patient has already tolerated warfarin that had earlier been used for a different indication (for reducing risk for stroke), or has reported a decreased incidence of migraines while taking it, or cannot tolerate other prophylaxis medications.

c. Off-Label Uses and Genetic Biomarkers

Biomarkers that identify genetic mutations or chromosomal rearrangement are sometimes used as part of the inclusion criteria or exclusion criteria. For some drugs, evidence demonstrates that the drug is effective only for patients who possess the genetic biomarker in question, and that the drug does not work in other patients. Because of the natural urge of patients with a certain disease, such as breast cancer or cystic fibrosis, to seek and receive treatment, patients are likely to overlook the fact that the drug works only in the subset that is carved out by the biomarker. This illustrates the situation where the genetic biomarker found its way into the package insert. The take-home lesson is applicable to all drugs, where efficacy is found only in a subset that possesses the biomarker and where the drug has been shown not to work in other patients having a disease with the same name (but not with the same biomarker expression).

Cystic fibrosis is caused by mutations in *Cystic Fibrosis Transmembrane Conductance Regulator* (CFTR) protein activity. The most common mutation in CFTR is a deletion of phenylalanine-508 (240). This mutation can be abbreviated as "delta508." FDA's *Medical Review* pointed out that the study drug (ivacaftor (Kalydeco)) is *not effective* in cystic fibrosis patients where the delta508 mutation occurs in both copies of the CFTR gene, writing that the study (241), "demonstrates the **lack of efficacy** in the CF population who are **homozygous** for the deltaF508 deletion in CFTR."

In the *Medical Review* for a cystic fibrosis drug (ivacaftor), the FDA reviewer commented about off-label uses of this drug (242). The FDA reviewer pointed out that the study drug (ivacaftor alone) was not effective for patients homozygous for the deltaF508 mutation, writing that:

> [l]ack of efficacy in this deltaF508/deltaF508 CF population is important to note, because [ivacaftor] represents the first entity that appears to treat one underlying defect of CFTR function that causes the disease. **It is therefore important to state that [ivacaftor] demonstrated no clinical benefit in patients homogeneous for the deltaF508-CFTR mutation.**

[239]Fitzgerald AS, O'Malley PG. Staying on track when prescribing off-label. Family Physician. 2014;89:4−5.

[240]Wainwright CE, Elborn JS, Ramsey BW, et al. Lumacaftor-ivacaftor in patients with cysticfibrosis homozygous for Phe508del CFTR. New Engl. J. Med. 2015;May 17 [Epub ahead of print].

[241]Medical Review for NDA 203,188.Ivacaftor (Kalydeco®) FDA's website at March 2015.

[242]Medical Review for NDA 203,188.Ivacaftor (Kalydeco®) FDA's website at March 2015.

The reviewer went on to warn about the possibility of widespread off-label uses by patients homozygous for this mutation, writing that (243).:

> [i]f not clearly stated in labeling, this reviewer could imagine a large proportion of deltaF508/deltaF508 patients, providers, and families willing to use [ivacaftor] in an **off-label usage** for individual patients to see if any perceived benefit could be achieved. Strong evidence from the double-blind, placebo controlled trial should be able to prevent much **off-label usage**, which would not presumably provide benefit, but **could lead to financial burden** to these patients and families.

The package label for ivacaftor (Kalydeco) warns against administering the drug to patients with the homozygous mutation, in its writing that, *"Limitations of Use.* KALYDECO is not effective in patients with CF who are homozygous for the *F508del* mutation in the *CFTR* gene."

Please note that the study that was evaluated by the above *Medical Review* was not the same clinical trial, as another clinical trial where a combination of two drugs was administered. This combination was ivacaftor plus lumacaftor, both of which influence the behavior of the CGTR protein. This combination enabled effectiveness even in homozygous deltaF508 mutation patients (244,245). The reader might take note of a distinction in the study design in these two clinical trials.

The package insert for another drug, the antibody known as *trastuzumab*, includes a statement warning that the drug must only be used for breast cancer patients where the tumor expresses a certain biomarker. The biomarker takes the form of overexpressed HER2. Overexpression of HER2 (human epidermal growth factor type-2) occurs in 15−20% of invasive breast cancers (246). The package insert reads (247):

> **HER2 Testing**. Detection of HER2 protein overexpression is necessary for selection of patients appropriate for Herceptin therapy because these are the only patients studied and for whom benefit has been shown. Due to differences in tumor histopathology, use FDA-approved tests for the specific tumor type … to assess HER2 protein overexpression and HER2 gene amplification. Tests should be performed by laboratories with demonstrated proficiency in the specific technology being utilized.

XXII. CONCLUSION

FDA's Warning Letters provide consistent and reliable guidance on procedural aspects of clinical trials. Most of these letters are issued in the timeframe between a Sponsor's submission of an IND, and on through the phase I, phase II, and phase III clinical trials. Some Warning Letters are issued in the postmarketing situation, and these usually concern issues in drug manufacturing. The consistent nature

---

[243]Medical Review for NDA 203,188.Ivacaftor (Kalydeco®) FDA's website at March 2015.

[244]Clinical Study Protocol. A Phase 3, Randomized, Double-Blind, Placebo-Controlled, Parallel-Group Study to Evaluate the Efficacy and Safety of Lumacaftor in Combination With Ivacaftor in Subjects Aged 12 Years and Older With Cystic Fibrosis, Homozygous for the F508del-CFTR Mutation Vertex Study Number: VX12-809-103 Lumacaftor IND No: 79,521 Ivacaftor IND No: 74,633 EUDRACT No: 2012-003989-40.

[245]Wainwright CE, Elborn JS, Ramsey BW, et al. Lumacaftor-ivacaftor in patients with cystic fibrosis homozygous for Phe508del CFTR. New Engl. J. Med. 2015;May 17 [Epub ahead of print].

[246]Tolaney SM, Barry WT, Dang CT, et al. Adjuvant paclitaxel and trastuzumab for node-negative, HER2-positive breast cancer. New Engl. J. Med. 2015;372:134−41.

[247]Package insert for HERCEPTIN® (trastuzumab) intravenous infusion. 2015 (36 pp.).

of the FDA's Warning Factors stems from the fact that each complaint in any given letter closely tracks a section in Title 21 of the Code of Federal Regulations, and from the fact that the draft letters are viewed by FDA's Office of Chief Counsel. The most frequent issues in these letters include those relating to the Institutional Review Board and the closely related topic of Consent Forms. Other frequent issues are protocol violations, drug accountability, and record keeping.

In contrast to the procedural focus of the FDA's Warning Letters, the FDA's *Medical Reviews*, *Clinical Reviews*, *Pharmaceutical Reviews*, and *Statistical Reviews*, which are published at the same time as the FDA's *Approval Letter*, provide guidance on substantive aspects of clinical trials.

33

Regulatory Approval

I. ORIGINS OF THE FEDERAL FOOD, DRUG AND COSMETIC ACT AND ITS AMENDMENTS

This outlines the history of the U.S. Food and Drug Administration (FDA), the European Medicines Agency (EMA), and the International Conference on Harmonisation (ICH). Also described is the organization and content of various regulatory submissions, as well as various milestones in the process of obtaining regulatory approval.

Federal regulation of drugs began with the Pure Food and Drug Act of 1906. That law made the manufacture of an adulterated or misbranded drug a misdemeanor, carrying a punishment not to exceed a $200 fine and/or one year in prison for the first conviction.

Harvey W. Wiley is known as the "Father of the Pure Food and Drugs Act of 1906." Dr Wiley received his medical degree at Indiana Medical College in 1871, then did laboratory work on sugar chemistry, with the aid of a polariscope, in the Imperial Food Laboratory in Germany (1). Then he returned to the mid-west in the United States, where he studied sorghum and sugars at Purdue University, and in 1883 became a chemist at the US Department of Agriculture. Dr Wiley created the "Poison Squad" in 1902, which was a group of 20 healthy men who were chosen to eat foods containing suspected poisons that were dyes or preservatives. He determined that borax, a food preservative at the time, was poisonous to man. Dr Wiley became a crusader for national food and drug regulation, and was FDA Commissioner from 1907 to 1912.

The Pure Food and Drug Act of 1906 did not require government clearance for new drugs, and companies were still permitted to market new drugs without first proving their safety or effectiveness (2).

By the mid-1930s, dissatisfaction with the 1906 law led to efforts to strengthen this law.

[1]Wong V, Tan SY. Harvey Washington Wiley (1844–1930): champion of the Pure Food and Drugs Act. Singapore Med. 2009;50:235–6.

[2]Nelson RJ. Regulation of investigational new drugs: "giant step for the sick and dying?" 77 Georgetown Law J. 1988;77:463.

Clinical Trials.
DOI: http://dx.doi.org/10.1016/B978-0-12-804217-5.00033-3

Senator Royal S. Copeland, a physician and former New York City health commissioner, worked to reform the old statute, and argued (3):

> A law which permits the continued manufacture and sale of utterly worthless remedies for cancer, tuberculosis, diabetes, and other maladies considered incurable by such means, is certainly defective. Because their manufacturers cannot be shown to know that their products are worthless creates a legal situation which is unbearable. That actually poisonous cosmetics and injurious slenderizing compounds can be distributed without interference from the Federal Government is positively indecent.

TABLE 33.1   Manufacture of Elixir Sulfanilamide by S.E. Massengill Co

Component	Quantity
Sulfanilamide	58.5 pounds
Elixir flavor	1 gallon
Raspberry extract	1 pint
Saccharin soluble	1 pound
Amaranth solution	1.5 pints
Caramel	2 fluid ounces
Diethylene glycol	60 gallons
Water q.s.	80 gallons

II. FEDERAL FOOD, DRUG AND COSMETIC ACT OF 1938

Efforts to reform the 1906 law produced the Federal Food, Drug and Cosmetic Act of 1938 (4). Passage of this new law was motivated, in part, by the fact that in 1937, 105 people died after ingesting a drug marketed as "Elixir Sulfanilamide," where the deaths resulted from the excipient, ethylene glycol. The Elixir Sulfanilamide disaster of 1937 occurred shortly after the introduction of sulfanilamide, the first sulfa antimicrobial drug. Under the existing drug regulations, premarketing toxicity testing was not required. Elixir Sulfanilamide was manufactured and sold by the S.E. Massengill Company of Bristol, Tennessee. About 240 gallons were manufactured. Since the Federal Food

and Drugs Act contains no provision against dangerous drugs, seizures had to be based on a charge that the word "elixir" implies an alcoholic solution, whereas this product was a diethylene glycol solution. Had the product been called a "solution," rather than an "elixir," no charge of violating the law could have been brought (5).

The elixir was manufactured as shown in Table 33.1 (6). No tests had been made to determine the toxicity of the separate ingredients or of the finished product.

The Federal Food, Drug and Cosmetic Act of 1938 created a new drug approval process under which the FDA had 60 days to reject a new drug application. After 60 days, if the FDA had not acted, the drug was automatically approved. Under this law, the FDA had

---

[3]78 Congressional Record 4,572 (March 15, 1934), *reprinted in* Dunn C. FEDERAL FOOD, DRUG, AND COSMETIC ACT 88 (1938).

[4]Merrill RA. Regulation of drugs and devices: an evolution. Health Aff. (Millwood). 1994;13:47−69.

[5]Report of the United States Secretary of Agriculture. Elixir sulfanilamide-Massengill. California and Western Medicine 48:68−70.

[6]Report of the United States Secretary of Agriculture. Elixir sulfanilamide-Massengill. California and Western Medicine 48:68−70.

the option of requiring drug sponsors to provide evidence of safety before marketing the drug. But the 1938 law did not require evidence of efficacy (7).

In 1937, George P. Larrick led a team of FDA inspectors in tracking down Elixir Sulfanilamide and, in effect, served as the "point man" for gathering evidence that argued for the passage of the Federal Food, Drug and Cosmetic Act of 1938. Mr Larrick received an undergraduate degree in Ohio, and in 1923 became a food inspector in Cincinnati, Ohio. At a later time, Mr Larrick served as the Commissioner of the FDA, that is, in the years 1954–1965 (8).

But at the time of the Federal Food, Drug and Cosmetic Act of 1938, the FDA Commissioner was Walter G. Campbell. Mr Campbell received a law degree from the University of Louisville in 1905, where he helped enforce Kentucky's food and drug laws. Campbell was selected by Harvey Wiley to be chief inspector at the FDA, where he enforced inspections of whiskey, milk, eggs, vinegar, oysters, and medicines marketed by charlatans, that is, "patent medicines" (9). Campbell, FDA Commissioner from 1921 to

1924 and from 1927 to 1944, was to the Federal Food, Drug and Cosmetic Act of 1938 what Harvey Wiley was to the 1906 Act.

In 1960, thalidomide was characterized as a new sedative that "produces no toxic effects when administered orally to animals in massive doses," and that was found to have "no deleterious side effects and does not affect the heart, respiration or autonomic nervous system" (10). However, in 1961, the drug was implicated in an epidemic of congenital malformations (11). Pregnant women who took thalidomide to relieve morning sickness delivered babies without arms or legs, some blind, and some mentally retarded. There were about 8000 such deformed births (12).

The requirement for efficacy for regulatory approval was motivated, in part, by the thalidomide tragedy. In 1962, partially as a result of the thalidomide disaster, Congress amended the 1938 Act to strengthen FDA control over new drugs. The amendments required the FDA to obtain evidence of the drug's efficacy as well as its safety, and granted the FDA powers to determine clinical testing of proposed drugs for safety and efficacy (13,14).

[7]Nelson RJ. Regulation of investigational new drugs: "giant step for the sick and dying?" 77 Georgetown Law J. 1988;77:463.

[8]Editorial. Personal profile: George P. Larrick. J. Agric. Food Chem. 1956;6:572 (one page only).

[9]Hickmann MA. The food and drug administration. Hauppauge (NY): Nova Science Publishers; 2003.

[10]Somers GF. Pharmacological properties of thalidomide (alpha-phthalimido glutarimide), a new sedative hypnotic drug. Br. J. Pharmacol. Chemother. 1960;15:111–6.

[11]Diggle GE. Thalidomide: 40 years on. Int. J. Clin. Pract. 2001;55:627–31.

[12]Nelson RJ. Regulation of investigational new drugs: "giant step for the sick and dying?" 77 Georgetown Law J. 1988;77:463.

[13]Nelson RJ. Regulation of investigational new drugs: "giant step for the sick and dying?" 77 Georgetown Law J. 1988;77:463.

[14]Stepp DL. The history of FDA regulation of biotechnology in the twentieth century. Food and Drug Law 1999;46:1–116.

III. DRUG AMENDMENTS ACT OF 1962

The Drug Amendments Act of 1962, also known as Public Law 87-781, and also known as the Kefauver-Harris Amendments, became effective on Oct. 10, 1962. The text of Public Law 87-781 (15) can be found on the HeinOnline database (16).

This law changed the pre-existing definition of a new drug by adding the words, "effectiveness" and "effective" to the existing definition. A view of the law reveals that it reads, *Public Law 87-781-Oct. 10, 1962*. An Act to protect the public health by amending the Federal Food, Drug, and Cosmetic Act to assure the safety, effectiveness, and reliability of drugs ... is amended by ... inserting therein, immediately after the words "to evaluate the safety," the words "and effectiveness," and ... inserting therein, immediately after the words "as safe," the words "and effective."

Therefore from 1938 to 1962 an "old drug" was one generally recognized by qualified experts as safe for its intended uses. There was no requirement that an old drug generally be regarded as effective (17). Today, it might seem self-evident that the FDA should review the efficacy of proposed drugs before granting approval. However, this was not at all self-evident prior to passage of the Drug Amendments Act of 1962. After the passage of this law, the FDA reacted as follows, at least in the words of one commentator (18), "[t]he FDA has wavered, procrastinated, and quaked with indecision on rulings which often they are unqualified to make, owing to the multifaceted areas of medical science and medical practice involved. In addition, the volume of work has become so enormous that the staff has become inundated by its size and complexity ... the FDA staff has made a monumental effort to cope with its additional responsibilities."

As revealed by comments in *New England Journal of Medicine* (19), "[t]he amendments granted the FDA the power to demand proof of efficacy – in the form of 'adequate and well-controlled investigations' – before approving a new drug for the US market. They also led to a retrospective review of all drugs approved between 1938 and 1962 (the Drug Efficacy Study Implementation program), which by the early 1970s had categorized approximately 600 medicines as 'ineffective' and forced their removal from the market."

IV. FDA MODERNIZATION ACT OF 1997 AND PHASE IV CLINICAL TRIALS

Later developments in FDA law included the option to impose a requirement for phase IV clinical trials. Phase IV clinical trials involve capturing data on safety and efficacy after FDA approval of a drug. In phase IV trials, data are captured from experiences of ordinary consumers (not from subjects enrolled in clinical

---

[15]HeinOnline 76 Stat. 780–796 (1962) (17 pp.).

[16]William S. Hein and Co., Inc. & HeinOnline, 1285 Main Street, Buffalo, NY 14209. At HeinOnline, statutes can be accessed at the bulletpoint, "U.S. Statutes at Large."

[17]United States v. An Article of Drug "Bentex Ulcerine." 469 F.2d 875; 1972 U.S. App. LEXIS 6476.

[18]Krantz JC. New drugs and the Kefauver-Harris Amendment. J. Clin. Pharmacol. 1966;6:77–9.

[19]Greene JA, Podolsky SH. Reform, regulation, and pharmaceuticals—the Kefauver-Harris amendments at 50. N. Engl. J. Med. 2012;367:1481–3.

trials). As reviewed by Steenburg (20), the first FDA-regulated phase IV clinical trial occurred in 1970. This phase IV trial involved levodopa, used for treating Parkinson's disease. At this time, evidence suggested that levodopa was a therapeutic breakthrough for a previously untreatable disease. The issue was that levodopa required chronic treatment, while long-term safety studies with animals were not available. Nevertheless, FDA granted approval for the drug, but with the requirement that the sponsors, Roche and Shire, conduct a series of formal postapproval tests to assess long-term safety.

FDA's regulatory authority to require phase IV trials finds a basis in the 1997 Food and Drug Administration Modernization Act. This requirement occurs in the context of drugs that are approved by FDA's fast-track approval program. In other words, FDA's authority to require the capture of data by way of phase IV trials applies only to drugs that were approved by the avenue of fast-track approval. The relevant statute is 21 USC 356 (21). Please note the statute's requirement for evidence for a clinical endpoint, evidence on a surrogate endpoint, requirement for a showing of clinical benefit or for a reasonable prediction of clinical benefit, and the requirement for postapproval (phase IV) studies (22):

> (b) APPROVAL OF APPLICATION FOR A FAST TRACK PRODUCT.—
> (1) IN GENERAL.—The Secretary may approve an application for approval of a fast track product under section 505(c) or section 351 of the Public Health Service Act upon a determination that the product has an effect on a clinical endpoint or on a surrogate endpoint that is reasonably likely to predict clinical benefit.
> (2) LIMITATION.—Approval of a fast track product under this subsection may be subject to the requirements—
> (A) that the sponsor conduct appropriate postapproval studies to validate the surrogate endpoint or otherwise confirm the effect on the clinical endpoint.

According to FDA's Guidance for Industry, the fast track program of the FDA is designed to expedite the review of new drugs. Products regulated by CBER are eligible for priority review if they improve the safety or effectiveness of the treatment, diagnosis, or prevention of a serious or life-threatening disease, while products regulated by CDER are eligible for priority review if they improve the treatment, diagnosis, or prevention of a disease (23). In the latter case, eligibility is not limited to drugs for a serious or life-threatening disease. Legislation in the United States can be found on the world wide web at: http://home.heinonline.org.

V. HISTORY OF EUROPEAN MEDICINES AGENCY

European Medicines Agency (EMA) was established by EU Regulation 2309/93, where the goal of the EMA was to coordinate the evaluation of scientific data associated with

---

[20]Steenburg C. The food and drug administration's use of postmarketing (phase IV) study requirements: exception to the rule? Food Drug Law J. 2006;61:295—400.

[21]21 USC 356, in effect as of January 24, 2002.

[22]21 USC 356, in effect as of January 24, 2002.

[23]U.S. Department of Health and Human Services. Food and Drug Administration. Guidance for Industry Fast Track Drug Development Programs-Designation, Development, and Application Review. January 2006. Revision 2 (25 pp.).

the approval, manufacturing, and inspection of medicines in the EU (24). This EU Regulation is dated Jul. 22, 1993.

EU Regulation 2309/93 contains 74 parts, that is, Articles 1 to 74. Article 1 provides that, "[t]he purpose of this Regulation is to lay down Community procedures for the authorization and supervision of medicinal products for human and veterinary use and to establish a European Agency for the Evaluation of Medicinal Products." Article 3 establishes that, "[n]o medicinal product referred to in Part A of the Annex may be placed on the market within the Community unless a marketing authorization has been granted by the Community in accordance with the provisions of this Regulation." Article 4 requires that, "[i]n order to obtain the authorization referred to in Article 3, the person responsible for placing a medicinal product on the market shall submit an application to the European Agency for the Evaluation of Medicinal Products, hereinafter referred to as 'the Agency', set up under Title IV."

From these excerpts of the Articles, it is evident that the EMA is an organization that regulates medicinal products, that marketing requires approval by the EMA, and that an application must be submitted to the EMA in order to acquire approval.

As of 1994, the leadership of the EMA comprised Strachan Heppell, Fernand Sauer, Romano Marabelli, and Fernand Van Hoeck (25). The EMA was designed to be an advisory board, where advice was to be given to national regulatory authorities (26). In the initial years of the EMA, sponsors submitted their drug applications directly to the EMA which, in turn, referred the matter to the Committee for Proprietary Medicinal Products (CPMP) for review. The EMA was formerly known as EMEA, but in Dec. 2009, EMEA was changed to EMA (27).

Some earlier history of European regulatory law is as follows. The process of centralization of regulatory approval for drugs was begun in Europe in 1965 by the publication of Directive 65/65 EEC (28). This Directive required Member States to establish premarket approval requirements (29).

In 1975 the EC established a multistate procedure for mutual recognition of national approval systems, and the EU created the CPMP to coordinate the procedure (30). The CPMP generated an opinion, reached by consensus or by a majority vote, where the opinion recommended approval or disapproval, or approval with special conditions such as postmarketing studies or special labeling. Where

[24]First General Report on the Activities of the European Agency for the Evaluation of Medicinal Products. EMEA/MB/065/95; January 15, 1996 (47 pp.).

[25]First General Report on the Activities of the European Agency for the Evaluation of Medicinal Products. EMEA/MB/065/95; January 15, 1996 (47 pp.).

[26]Kidd D. The international conference on harmonization of pharmaceutical regulations, the European Medicines Evaluation Agency, and the FDA: who's zooming who? Ind. J. Global Legal Stud. 1996–1997;4:183–206.

[27]Pennanen T. European Medicines Agency, 7 Westferry Circus, London, UK. E-mail of February 22, 2011.

[28]Eakin DV. The international conference on harmonization of pharmaceutical regulations: progress or stagnation? Tulsa J. Comp. Int. Law 1999;6:221.

[29]Kingham RF, Bogaert PWL, Eddy PS. The New European medicines agency. Food Drug Law J. 1994;49:301.

[30]Kingham RF, Bogaert PWL, Eddy PS. The New European Medicines Agency. Food Drug Law J. 1994;49:301.

CPMP rendered a favorable opinion, the CPMP transmitted the opinion to the European Commission, to the Member States, and to the applicant (31).

At a later time, the CPMP was replaced by a new agency, namely the Committee for Medicinal Products for Human Use (CHMP). The name of the CPMP was changed to CHMP, together with other changes to European Regulatory committees, upon the expansion of the EU from 15 member states to 25 member states in May 2004 (32). The EMA/CHMP system is superior to and less cumbersome than the previously used multistate system in Europe, but the EMA/CHMP system still does not take the form of a centralized authority, in the way that the US Food and Drug Administration is a centralized authority (33).

VI. INTERNATIONAL CONFERENCE ON HARMONISATION

The ICH has the goals of harmonizing pharmaceutical regulations in Europe, Japan, and the United States, shortening the time from development to marketing of new drugs (34), eliminating redundant and duplicative requirements for registering new medicines, and increasing patient access to new drugs (35). The ICH is not intended to replace the drug approval procedures.

The ICH provides a set of guidelines that are similar, and sometimes identical, to the FDA's Guidance for Industry documents. The ICH Guidelines can be found on the world wide web at: www.ich.org/products/guidelines. There exist 11 quality guidelines, 10 efficacy guidelines, and 11 safety guidelines. There are also eight multidisciplinary guidelines, which cover miscellaneous topics such as MedDRA terminology and the Common Technical Document (CTD).

This concerns the history of the ICH. In the 1980s, the European Community (EC), now called the European Union (EU), began plans for a single market for pharmaceuticals. The WHO Conference of Drug Regulatory Authorities in 1989 in Paris marked a starting point for plans leading to the ICH (36). The idea for the ICH originated in a joint mission between Japan and the EU in 1988, where the mission's goal was to resolve differences in safety and efficacy requirements of the various countries (37).

[31]Kingham RF, Bogaert PWL, Eddy PS. The New European medicines agency. Food Drug Law J. 1994;49:301.

[32]Brown D, Volkers P, Day S. An introductory note to CHMP guidelines: choice of the non-inferiority margin and data monitoring committees. Stat. Med. 2006;25:1623−7.

[33]Kidd D. The international conference on harmonization of pharmaceutical regulations, the European Medicines Evaluation Agency, and the FDA: who's zooming who? Ind. J. Global Legal Stud. 1996−1997;4:183−206.

[34]Kidd D. The international conference on harmonization of pharmaceutical regulations, the European Medicines Evaluation Agency, and the FDA: who's zooming who? Ind. J. Global Legal Stud. 1996−1997;4:183−206.

[35]Booth PM. FDA implementation of standards developed by the international conference of harmonisation. Food Drug Law J. 1997;52:203.

[36]Allport-Settle MJ. International Conference on Harmonisation (ICH) quality guidelines: pharmaceutical, biologics, and medical device guidance documents concise reference. Willow Spring (NC): PharmaLogika; 2010. p. 4−5.

[37]Kidd D. The international conference on harmonization of pharmaceutical regulations, the European Medicines Evaluation Agency, and the FDA: who's zooming who? Ind. J. Global Legal Stud. 1996−1997;4:183−206.

The ICH was born at a meeting in Brussels in April 1990. Representatives of regulatory authorities and industry from Europe, Japan, and the United States, met at this meeting. This meeting established the ICH Steering Committee, a committee that has since met at intervals of at least twice per year, with locations rotating between Europe, Japan, and the United States (38). The Brussels meeting was hosted by the International Federation of Pharmaceutical Manufacturers Associations (39).

After the first ICH Steering Committee meeting in Brussels, subsequent larger ICH Conferences took place in Brussels (Nov. 1991), Orlando, Florida (Oct. 1993), Yokohama, Japan (Nov. 1995), Brussels (Jul. 1997), San Diego, California (Nov. 2000), and Osaka, Japan (Nov. 2003) (40). The conference in Orlando, for example, concerned animal-based toxicity experiments, the establishment of guidelines for drug studies in the elderly, and the establishment of standards for clinical safety data management (41). The conference in San Diego concerned MedDRA, CTD, ethnic factors in designing clinical trials, process control of biotech materials, and packaging (42,43). The conference in Osaka concerned the CTD and MedDRA, as well as risk management, immunotoxicity studies, stability testing guidelines, impurity testing guidelines, and harmonization of pharmacopoeial chapters, QT/QTc interval prolongation safety studies, and ethnic factors in clinical trials (44).

In addition to the EMA and the ICH, another organization based in Europe is the European Clinical Infrastructure Network (ECRIN; www.ecrin.org). ECRIN is not a regulatory agency, but is an association of academic researchers working to help academic investigators in the EU develop their clinical trials (45). ECRIN is not a competitor of the ICH. To provide one example of ECRIN's interests, this group conducted a survey of clinical centers in Europe and identified the various types of software used for capturing data from study subjects, and used for data management (46).

VII. HISTORY OF THE MEDICINES AND HEALTHCARE PRODUCTS REGULATORY AGENCY

The Medicines and Healthcare Products Regulatory Agency (MHRA) was formed in

[38]WHO Drug Information. 200;21 (52 pp.).

[39]Moreira A. Happy Birthday, ICH! PDA J. Pharm. Sci. Technol. May–June 2010;64:189–90.

[40]http://private.ich.org/cache/html/325-272-1.html.

[41]Kidd D. The international conference on harmonization of pharmaceutical regulations, the European Medicines Evaluation Agency, and the FDA: who's zooming who? Ind. J. Global Legal Stud. 1996–1997;4:183–206.

[42]Program. The fifth international conference on harmonisation of technical requirements for registration of pharmaceuticals for human use; November 9–11, 2000, San Diego (CA) (32 pp.).

[43]Background Papers. November 2000. The fifth international conference on harmonisation of technical requirements for registration of pharmaceuticals for human use, San Diego (CA); November 9–11, 2000 (36 pp.).

[44]Sixth international conference on harmonisation. new horizons and future challenges, Osaka (Japan), Summary report; November 13–15, 2003 (40 pp.).

[45]Haubenreisser S. E-mail of March 4, 2011.

[46]Kuchinke W, Ohmann C, Yang Q, et al. Heterogeneity prevails: the state of clinical trial data management in Europe—results of a survey of ECRIN centres. Trials 2010;11:79.

Apr. 2003 with the merger of the Medicines Control Agency (MCA) and the Medical Devices Agency (47). The MHRA is the British equivalent of the US FDA (48).

At a much earlier time, the control of medicines in England was practiced during the reign of King Henry VIII of England (1491–1547) (49). The Royal College of Physicians of London was empowered to appoint inspectors of apothecaries' wares in the London area with power to destroy defective stock. Somewhat later, in the early 17th century these inspecting physicians were joined by representative members of the Society of Apothecaries. During the 19th century the Pharmaceutical Society of Great Britain was established, and legislation was enacted for controlling the retail sale of poisons. The 1925 Therapeutic Substances Act introduced this control. It applied to vaccines, sera, toxins, antitoxins, antigens, arsphenamines, insulin, pituitary hormone, and surgical sutures (50). Thalidomide was used as a drug for morning sickness in the years 1957 to 1961. In response to the thalidomide tragedy, the Medicines Act was drafted, and it became effective in September 1971. The Act covered the development, manufacture, packaging, labeling, distribution, and advertising of medicinal products (51).

As one of the steps in the drafting of this Act, a speech given in Parliament in May 1963 stated that, "The House and the public suddenly woke up to the fact that any drug manufacturer could market any product, however inadequately tested, however dangerous, without having to satisfy any independent body as to its efficacy and safety and the public was almost uniquely unprotected in this respect." The Committee on Safety of Drugs, chaired by Derrick Dunlop, was established in 1963 as an interim measure prior to establishing a formal legal framework for licensing new medicines in the United Kingdom (52). The 1968 Medicines Act set up the Medicines Commission. Somewhat later in 1989, the MCA was created. Keith Jones was the first director of the MCA. Legislation from Great Britain can be found on the world wide web at: http://www.legislation.gov.uk.

VIII. OUTLINE OF REGULATORY APPROVAL IN THE UNITED STATES

Regulatory approval for any given drug involves submitting a series of documents, over the course of months or years, to a regulatory agency such as the US FDA. In the United States, regulatory approval finds a basis in Title 21 of the United States Code (21 USC §355), and Title 21 of the Code of Federal Regulations (21 CFR §314.3; 21 CFR §§314.100-314.153). The following is a comment on the

[47]Jones KH. Towards safer medicines. A guide to the control of safety, quality and efficacy of human medicines in the United Kingdom. 2nd ed. London (UK): Medicines Control Agency; 1997.

[48]Barry DC. E-mail of March 27, 2011.

[49]Goodhall C. Royal college of physicians library. An historic account of the College's Proceedings against empiricks and unlicensed practitioners. 1864.

[50]Jones KH. Towards safer medicines. A guide to the control of safety, quality and efficacy of human medicines in the United Kingdom. 2nd ed. London (UK): Medicines Control Agency; 1997.

[51]Harman RJ. Development and control of medicines and medical devices. Great Britain (UK): Pharmaceutical Press; 2004.

[52]Winship K, Hepburn D, Lawson DH. The review of medicines in the United Kingdom. Br. J. Clin. Pharmacol. 1992;33:583–7.

numbers used to refer to the rules in the CFR. The two section marks together refer to the plural of section, that is, they mean "sections."

The first submission to the FDA is likely to contain only animal data, where this submission is the basis for approval of a phase I clinical trial. A second submission to the FDA contains data from the phase I trial, and may contain additional animal data, and is the basis for approval of a phase II trial. The third submission contains data from the phase II trial, as well as any additional animal data, and is the basis for approval of a phase III trial. These submissions, in the context of the FDA, include INDs, Clinical Study Protocols, Amendments to the Clinical Study Protocols, Investigator's Brochures, Briefing Documents, and real-time reports of unexpected serious adverse events (SAEs). Following completion of the phase I, II, and III clinical trials, the investigator submits a CTD. The CTD is a request for approval of the drug.

IX. INVESTIGATIONAL NEW DRUG

The Investigational New Drug (IND) application is used to initiate clinical trials in the United States. The IND is the first step in initiating clinical trials on a new chemical entity in humans, and the first step in initiating clinical trials in a drug that is already FDA-approved, but where the goal is for a new clinical indication (53). In short, the IND is a request for permission to start phase I, phase II, and phase III clinical trials.

The IND discloses nonclinical data on pharmacology, absorption, distribution, metabolism, excretion, and toxicology. The IND also describes the chemistry, manufacturing, and quality control of the proposed drug. Also, the IND details the proposed use of the drug in human clinical trials.

FDA does not respond to the IND by granting approval. "Approval" is a passive response. Instead, once submitted, a sponsor must wait 30 days to allow FDA to make an assessment of the safety of the proposed trials (54). If FDA raises no objections, the sponsor is allowed to begin the proposed clinical trial.

The United States Code (USC) sets forth statutes, whereas the CFR sets forth rules, also known as administrative law. Material from Title 21 of the USC is quoted below. As far is the investigator and medical writer are concerned, the most critical part of this is the phrase, "will enable him to evaluate the safety and effectiveness of such drug."

(A) the submission to the Secretary, before any clinical testing of a new drug is undertaken, of reports, by the manufacturer or the sponsor of the investigation of such drug, of preclinical tests (including tests on animals) of such drug adequate to justify the proposed clinical testing;

. . .

(C) the establishment and maintenance of such records, and the making of such reports to the Secretary, by the manufacturer or the sponsor of the investigation of such drug, of data (including but not limited to analytical reports by investigators) obtained as the result of such investigational use of such drug, as the Secretary finds will enable him to evaluate the safety and effectiveness of such drug in the event of the filing of an application pursuant to subsection (b) of this section; and

. . .

(2) Subject to paragraph (3), a clinical investigation of a new drug may begin 30 days after the Secretary has received from the manufacturer or sponsor of the investigation a submission containing such information about the drug and the clinical investigation, including—

[53]Ferkany JW, Williams M. The IND application. Curr. Protoc. Pharmacol. 2008;9.10.1−9.10.23.
[54]Ferkany JW, Williams M. The IND application. Curr. Protoc. Pharmacol. 2008;9.10.1−9.10.23.

TABLE 33.2 Location of the Law, as It Applies to the Investigational New Drug (IND), in the United States Code

Number of the Title, Chapter, or Section in the United States Code	Name of the Title, Chapter, or Section in the United States Code
Title 21	Food and Drugs
Chapter 9	Federal Food, Drug, and Cosmetic Act
Subchapter V	Drugs and Devices
Section 355	New Drugs

(A) information on design of the investigation and adequate reports of basic information, certified by the applicant to be accurate reports, necessary to assess the safety of the drug for use in clinical investigation; and

(B) adequate information on the chemistry and manufacturing of the drug, controls available for the drug, and primary data tabulations from animal or human studies.

This particular quotation is from Title 21, Chapter 9, Subchapter V, Section 355, of the USC. The full names of these "addresses" are shown in Table 33.2.

The interested reader can see that material from this part of the USC (shown above) tracks some of the topics found in the CFR (shown below). Where an agency of the US government is regulated by both the USC and the CFR, the USC will contain more general demands, and the CFR will contain more specific demands. To some extent, the demands in the USC and CFR will track each other, and sometimes duplicate each other.

The IND includes the following sections or parts. The pharmacology and toxicology section includes animal data, but no human data.

This format finds a basis in 21 CFR 312.23 (55), as shown after the following bullet-points:

- Cover sheet.
- Table of contents.
- Introductory statement and general investigational plan.
- Investigator's Brochure.
- Clinical Study Protocol.
- Chemistry, manufacturing, and control information.
- Pharmacology and toxicology.
- Prior human experience.

Part 312.23 of Title 21 of the Code of Federal Regulations, which organizes the IND, includes the following writings. As is evident, the investigator must identify whether the trial is to be phase I, II, or III. What is also required is that an IRB review and approve the study.

(1) *Cover sheet (Form FDA-1571)*. A cover sheet for the application containing the following:

(i) The name, address, and telephone number of the sponsor, the date of the application, and the name of the investigational new drug.

(ii) Identification of the phase or phases of the clinical investigation to be conducted.

(iii) A commitment not to begin clinical investigations until an IND covering the investigations is in effect.

(iv) A commitment that an Institutional Review Board (IRB) that complies with the requirements set forth in part 56 will be responsible for the initial and continuing review and approval of each of the studies in the proposed clinical investigation and that the investigator will report to the IRB proposed changes in the research activity in accordance with the requirements of part 56.

. . .

(vi) The name and title of the person responsible for monitoring the conduct and progress of the clinical investigations.

. . .

[55]Ferkany JW, Williams M. The IND application. Curr. Protoc. Pharmacol. 2008;9.10.1–9.10.23.

What is also required is details on the rationale for the proposed study drug, number of study subjects that need to be enrolled, and expected risks based on data from animal studies:

(2) A table of contents.

(3) Introductory statement and general investigational plan. (i) A brief introductory statement giving the name of the drug and all active ingredients, the drug's pharmacological class, the structural formula of the drug (if known), the formulation of the dosage form(s) to be used, the route of administration, and the broad objectives and planned duration of the proposed clinical investigation(s).

(ii) A brief summary of previous human experience with the drug, with reference to other INDs if pertinent, and to investigational or marketing experience in other countries that may be relevant to the safety of the proposed clinical investigation(s) . . .

(iv) A brief description of the overall plan for investigating the drug product for the following year. The plan should include the following: (a) The rationale for the drug or the research study; (b) the indication(s) to be studied; (c) the general approach to be followed in evaluating the drug; (d) the kinds of clinical trials to be conducted in the first year following the submission (if plans are not developed for the entire year, the sponsor should so indicate); (e) the estimated number of patients to be given the drug in those studies; and (f) any risks of particular severity or seriousness anticipated on the basis of the toxicological data in animals or prior studies in humans with the drug or related drugs.

If an Investigator's Brochure is warranted, the CFR provides the organization for this document. The Investigator's Brochure contains:

(i) A brief description of the drug substance and the formulation, including the structural formula, if known.

(ii) A summary of the pharmacological and toxicological effects of the drug in animals and, to the extent known, in humans.

(iii) A summary of the pharmacokinetics and biological disposition of the drug in animals and, if known, in humans.

(iv) A summary of information relating to safety and effectiveness in humans obtained from prior

clinical studies. (Reprints of published articles on such studies may be appended when useful.)

(v) A description of possible risks and side effects to be anticipated on the basis of prior experience with the drug under investigation or with related drugs, and of precautions or special monitoring to be done as part of the investigational use of the drug.

The IND must also include the Clinical Study Protocol. The CFR expressly requires the following components for the Clinical Study Protocol:

(iii) A protocol is required to contain the following, with the specific elements and detail of the protocol reflecting the above distinctions depending on the phase of study:

(a) A statement of the objectives and purpose of the study.

(b) The name and address and a statement of the qualifications (curriculum vitae or other statement of qualifications) of each investigator, and the name of each subinvestigator (eg, research fellow, resident) working under the supervision of the investigator; the name and address of the research facilities to be used; and the name and address of each reviewing Institutional Review Board.

(c) The criteria for patient selection and for exclusion of patients and an estimate of the number of patients to be studied.

(d) A description of the design of the study, including the kind of control group to be used, if any, and a description of methods to be used to minimize bias on the part of subjects, investigators, and analysts.

(e) The method for determining the dose(s) to be administered, the planned maximum dosage, and the duration of individual patient exposure to the drug.

(f) A description of the observations and measurements to be made to fulfill the objectives of the study.

(g) A description of clinical procedures, laboratory tests, or other measures to be taken to monitor the effects of the drug in human subjects and to minimize risk.

The Chemistry, Manufacturing, and Controls sections provide information on the chemical or biological characteristics of the drug substance, information on stability of the drug, and information on the placebo, as indicated:

(a) *Drug substance.* A description of the drug substance, including its physical, chemical, or biological characteristics; the name and address of its manufacturer; the general method of preparation of the drug substance; the acceptable limits and analytical methods used to assure the identity, strength, quality, and purity of the drug substance; and information sufficient to support stability of the drug substance during the toxicological studies and the planned clinical studies. Reference to the current edition of the United States Pharmacopeia – National Formulary may satisfy relevant requirements in this paragraph.

(b) *Drug product.* A list of all components, which may include reasonable alternatives for inactive compounds, used in the manufacture of the investigational drug product, including both those components intended to appear in the drug product and those which may not appear but which are used in the manufacturing process, and, where applicable, the quantitative composition of the investigational drug product, including any reasonable variations that may be expected during the investigational stage; the name and address of the drug product manufacturer; a brief general description of the manufacturing and packaging procedure as appropriate for the product; the acceptable limits and analytical methods used to assure the identity, strength, quality, and purity of the drug product; and information sufficient to assure the product's stability during the planned clinical studies. Reference to the current edition of the United States Pharmacopeia – National Formulary may satisfy certain requirements in this paragraph.

(c) A brief general description of the composition, manufacture, and control of any placebo used in a controlled clinical trial.

(d) *Labeling.* A copy of all labels and labeling to be provided to each investigator.

The pharmacology and toxicity section of the IND includes the following information:

(i) *Pharmacology and drug disposition.* A section describing the pharmacological effects and mechanism(s) of action of the drug in animals, and information on the absorption, distribution, metabolism, and excretion of the drug, if known.

(ii) *Toxicology.* (a) An integrated summary of the toxicological effects of the drug in animals and in vitro. Depending on the nature of the drug and the phase of the investigation, the description is to include the results of acute, subacute, and chronic toxicity tests; tests of the drug's effects on reproduction and the developing fetus; any special toxicity test related to the drug's particular mode of administration or conditions of use (eg, inhalation, dermal, or ocular toxicology); and any in vitro studies intended to evaluate drug toxicity.

The categories of information required for initiating clinical trials, as set forth in the IND, can also be found in documents submitted after completion of clinical trials, when the sponsor or investigator believes that the drug is worthy of regulatory approval. The document submitted for regulatory approval may be an NDA, BLA, or CTD, as reviewed below.

X. IND AND THE COMMON TECHNICAL DOCUMENT

To review the timeline of regulatory approval, the sponsor submits an IND in order to conduct phase I, II, and III clinical trials. The IND is used for both traditional drugs, as well as for drugs that are biologicals. After submitting the IND, the sponsor is required, under 21 CFR §312.33, to submit an annual report. The annual report is a brief report of the progress of the investigation. It is submitted by way of an amendment to the IND (56).

Before submitting the IND to the FDA, the sponsor has the option of scheduling a pre-IND meeting. Pre-IND meetings are often held from 6 months to 1 year before filing the

---

[56]Poole K. The sponsor's guide to regulatory submissions for an investigational new drug. Biological Resources Branch, DCTD, NCI-Frederick, Biopharmaceutical Development Program, SAIC-Frederick, Inc.; 2005.

IND (57). As outlined by Poole (58), the sponsor submits a Pre-IND Information Package prior to the pre-IND meeting. This Package describes the chemical structure of the drug, the proposed dosages, the proposed indications and studies, and other information.

After conducting the phase I, II, and III clinical trials, the sponsor submits an NDA, in the case of traditional drugs, and a BLA, in the case of biologicals.

The entire timeframe for conducting phase I, II, and III clinical trials takes an average of 5 years, while the subsequent timeframe for the FDA's review of the NDA takes an average of 2 years (59).

Instead of filing an NDA or BLA, the sponsor may submit a Common Technical Document (CTD), which can be used for small molecule drugs as well as for biologicals. The format of the CTD was devised by the ICH. The CTD is accepted by regulatory agencies in the United States, Europe, and Japan.

Table 33.3 discloses the organization and titles of the CTD (60,61). The CTD contains five modules. Module 1 is region-specific, while Modules 2, 3, 4, and 5 are common for the United States, Europe, and Japan (62,63). Module 1, which is for administrative information and prescribing information, contains documents specific to each region, for example, the proposed label for use in the region. The content and format of this module can be specified by the relevant regulatory authorities. Module 2 contains overviews and summaries. Module 3 contains information on quality control topics, Module 4 contains the nonclinical study reports, and Module 5 contains clinical study reports. "Quality control" refers to the routine behaviors of personnel who follow the standard operating procedures (SOPs), the keeping of records of the acts of obeying or following the directions in the SOPs, and the collection of quality control data. Generally, SOPs are followed by personnel involved in routine predetermined tasks, such as testing and manufacturing.

Table 33.3 highlights the organization of the CTD. The table shows the classes of information that are submitted, by way of the CTD, to regulatory agencies in United States, Europe, and Japan (64).

[57]Poole K. The sponsor's guide to regulatory submissions for an investigational new drug. Biological Resources Branch, DCTD, NCI-Frederick, Biopharmaceutical Development Program, SAIC-Frederick, Inc.; 2005.

[58]Poole K. The sponsor's guide to regulatory submissions for an investigational new drug. Biological Resources Branch, DCTD, NCI-Frederick, Biopharmaceutical Development Program, SAIC-Frederick, Inc.; 2005.

[59]Poole K. The sponsor's guide to regulatory submissions for an investigational new drug. Biological Resources Branch, DCTD, NCI-Frederick, Biopharmaceutical Development Program, SAIC-Frederick, Inc.; 2005.

[60]U.S. Department of Health and Human Services. U.S. Food and Drug Administration. Electronic Common Technical Document (eCTD) (accessed November 19, 2010).

[61]Guidance for Industry. Providing Regulatory Submissions in Electronic Format—Human Pharmaceutical Product Applications and Related Submissions Using the eCTD Specifications. Rev. 2 (June 2008).

[62]Molzon JA. The international conference on harmonization common technical document—global submission format? Food Drug Law J. 2005;60:447–51.

[63]Juillet Y. Internationalization of regulatory requirements. Fundam. Clin. Pharmacol. 2003;7:21–5.

[64]U.S. Department of Health and Human Services. U.S. Food and Drug Administration. Electronic Common Technical Document (eCTD) (accessed November 19, 2010).

TABLE 33.3 Contents of the Common Technical Document[a]

MODULE 1. ADMINISTRATIVE (DIFFERENT PAPERWORK FOR EACH REGION)

Application forms

Contact information

Fast track designation request (if any); special protocol assessment request (if any)

Draft of package label

MODULE 2. SUMMARIES

Quality summary

Nonclinical summary

Clinical summary

MODULE 3. QUALITY

Drug Substance—name and manufacturer

Description of Manufacturing Process and Process Controls

Impurities

Excipients

Batch Analyses

Container Closure System

Stability Data

MODULE 4. NONCLINICAL STUDY REPORTS

Pharmacology

Pharmacodynamics

Pharmacokinetics (ADME). Absorption, distribution, metabolism, and excretion

Single dose toxicity [Species and route]

Repeat dose toxicity [Species, route, duration]

Genotoxicity

Carcinogenicity

Reproductive and developmental toxicity

MODULE 5. CLINICAL STUDY REPORTS

Clinical Study Protocol

Sample case report form

List and description of investigators and sites

Signatures of principal or coordinating investigator(s) or sponsor's responsible medical officer

Randomization scheme

Statistical methods

(Continued)

TABLE 33.3   (Continued)

Publications based on the study
Discontinued patients
Protocol deviations
Patients excluded from the efficacy analysis
Case report forms
ECG waveform datasets
IND safety reports
Plasma protein binding study reports
Hepatic metabolism and drug interaction studies
Human pharmacokinetic (PK) studies
Healthy subject PK and initial tolerability study reports
Patient PK and initial tolerability study reports
Reports of efficacy and safety studies
Integrated summary of safety report
Integrated summary of efficacy report

[a]*US Department of Health and Human Services. Food and Drug Administration (Aug. 2001) Guidance for Industry. M4Q:The CTD-Quality (29 pages); US Department of Health and Human Services. Food and Drug Administration (Aug. 2001) M4E. The CTD-Efficacy (58 pp.).*

XI. INSTITUTIONAL REVIEW BOARD

a. Introduction to the IRB

An Institutional Review Board (IRB) is not used for routine medical care, but is required for research on human subjects. The possibility of the need for an IRB is raised in the situation where a "project involves gathering or using specimens, tissue, cells, data, documents, or information about or derived from humans for purposes other than medical care" (65). An IRB must have a minimum of five members including a scientist, a nonscientist, and at least one person who is not affiliated with the IRB's supporting institution. Members review the Clinical Study Protocol, informed consent, Investigator's Brochures, and any recruitment material. Following review and discussion, the IRB will vote to approve, disapprove, or require modifications for each study (66,67).

The IRB finds a basis in 21 CFR §56.201, which states that the IRB is, "any board, committee, or other group formally designated by an institution to review, to approve the initiation of, and to conduct periodic review of, biomedical research involving human subjects. The primary purpose of such review is to assure the protection of the rights and welfare of the human subjects."

[65]Byerly WG. Working with the institutional review board. Am. J. Health Syst. Pharm. 2009;66:176–84.

[66]Byerly WG. Working with the institutional review board. Am. J. Health Syst. Pharm. 2009;66:176–84.

[67]21 CFR 56.107 (April 1, 2014)

b. Summary of Responsibilities of the IRB

As summarized by the *American Society of Clinical Oncology*, the responsibilities of the IRB are (68):

- Ensuring that risks to research participants are minimized and that risks are reasonable in relation to anticipated benefits.
- Ensuring that the research plan makes adequate provision for monitoring the data collected to ensure the safety of research participants, and that there are adequate provisions to protect the privacy of research participants and to maintain the confidentiality of data.
- Ensuring that the consent document contains standard elements and that patients give fully informed consent.
- Ensuring that research participant selection is equitable and that appropriate protections are in place for vulnerable research participants.
- Conducting ongoing assessment of risks, potential benefits, and the adequacy of the consent document, by periodic re-review of the research and assessment of adverse events.
- Assessing the competency of investigators to conduct research and the institution's resources for conducting the trial in a safe manner.

c. FDA's Warning Letters Provide a Real-World Account of the Responsibilities of the IRB

Guidance for the conduct of the IRB comes, in part, from Warning Letters issued by the FDA. FDA's Warning Letters issued to an IRB have a basis in 21 CFR §56.120. The most common source of complaint is failure to follow written procedures on how the IRB reviewed the clinical research (69). For example, in one Warning Letter, the FDA complained that the Sponsor had failed to notify the FDA that the IRB at University of Washington had withdrawn its approval of the clinical trial (70). A Warning Letter to another Sponsor complained that the IRB had failed to ensure that Informed Consent was acquired from the study subjects (71). The clinical trial was called "The Effect of Etomidate on Patient Outcomes After Single Bolus Doses." FDA complained that the IRB had failed to ensure that informed consent was sought from all prospective study subjects, and that the IRB had approved of a clinical trial even though the Sponsor had failed to obtain informed consent.

Chapter 32 provides a detailed account of FDA's Warning Letters, as well as further information on IRBs, as provided by Warning Letters issued by FDA to various Sponsors.

---

[68] Am. Soc. Clin. Oncol. American Society of Clinical Oncology policy statement: oversight of clinical research. J. Clin. Oncol. 2003;21:2377–86.

[69] Bramstedt KA, Kassimatis K. A study of warning letters issued to institutional review boards by the United States Food and Drug Administration. Clin. Invest. Med. 27:316–23.

[70] Warning Letter, dated August 28, 2014, from Steven D. Silverman, Director, Office of Compliance Center for Device and Radiological Health, FDA, to Brava, LLC.

[71] Warning Letter, dated June 1, 2012, from Leslie K. Ball, MD, Acting Branch Chief of CDER, FDA to Advocate Health Care.

XII. TIMELINE OF FDA APPROVAL

a. Introduction

The timeline of FDA approval is activated when a Sponsor takes on the responsibility for product development and initiates a clinical investigation. The term "Sponsor" can refer to a person, organization, or pharmaceutical company. Submitting an IND is the first major step in the timeline. FDA assigns an IND number and reviews the application within 30 days. If no deficiencies are found, the IND becomes active and the study may proceed. In this textbook, the terms applicant and sponsor are generally used to mean the same thing. This textbook preferably uses Sponsor because the Sponsor is the party with the greater burden for complying with the rules in Title 21 of the Code of Federal Regulation.

But if deficiencies are found, FDA can impose a Clinical Hold. The Sponsor may request guidance for drafting the IND, prior to submitting the IND. This guidance can take the form of meetings with the FDA, and here, the Sponsor needs to submit information prior to the meeting. The Sponsor may also share new data during the meeting itself. Meetings prior to submitting an IND include informal discussions, mainly for reviewing preclinical data and their relevance to supporting entry of the drug in a clinical trial (72).

Legal aspects of an IND are described. By filing an IND, and by receiving FDA's approval of the IND, the Sponsor acquires an exception to laws that forbid the transport of drugs across state lines (73). In acquiring this exemption, the Sponsor is then free to conduct a typical clinical trial in human subjects, that is, a trial that involves transport of the study drug across state lines.

Prior to approving the initiation and conduct of any clinical trial on human subjects, FDA reviews the IND. The IND is reviewed by the Office of Pharmaceutical Science to provide feedback on drug quality, the Office of Clinical Pharmacology to evaluate data on pharmacokinetics (PK) and pharmacodynamics (PD), and the Office of Biostatistics to evaluate statistical plans (74).

After completing phase I, II, and III clinical trials, the Sponsor submits a NDA or a BLA. FDA has 180 days to review the NDA. If it finds deficiencies, such as missing information, the clock stops until the manufacturer submits the additional information. If and when the manufacturer is able to provide the information, the clock resumes and the FDA continues the review. When the FDA makes a final determination, it sends the Sponsor a "complete response letter" (75).

b. Formal Meetings with FDA

Formal meetings with the FDA include the pre-IND meeting (21 CFR §312.82), end-of-phase I meeting (21 CFR §312.82), end-of-phase 2 and prephase 3 meeting (21 CFR §312.47), and pre-NDA and pre-BLA meeting (21 CFR

[72]Feigal EG, et al. Perspective: communications with the Food and Drug Administration on the development pathway for a cell-based therapy: why, what, when, and how? Stem Cells Transl. Med. 2012;1:825–32.

[73]Feinsod M, Chambers WA. Trials and tribulations a primer on successfully navigating the waters of the Food and Drug Administration. Opthalmology 2004;111:1801–6.

[74]U.S. Department of Health and Human Services. Food and Drug Administration. Center for Drug Evaluation and Research (CDER) Good review practice: good review management principles and practices for effective IND development and review. Manual of Policies and Procedures (MAPP 6030.9); April 29, 2013 (42 pp.).

[75]Thaul S. How FDA approves drugs and regulates their safety and effectiveness. Congressional Research Service; June 25, 2012 (19 pp.).

§312.47) (76). These meetings find a basis in the Code of Federal Regulations, as indicated. Prior to these meetings, the Sponsor is required to submit information relevant to the issues to be discussed. Thus, the information may take the form of nonclinical data, clinical data, or study design. The information needs to be submitted in a document, which has names, such as the briefing package, briefing document, and briefing book (77,78).

The Meeting Package should include a list of questions to be answered, and relevant non-clinical and clinical data. Prior to the meeting, the FDA holds an internal meeting that typically occurs within a week prior to conferring with the Sponsor. The FDA may prepare responses to the questions submitted in the Meeting Package, and then transmit these responses to the Sponsor a day or so before the meeting. Within a month of the meeting, the FDA provides a summary of the meeting to the Sponsor, where the summary includes agreements, disagreements, and recommendations. Feigal et al. (79) warn that Sponsors should take care not to ignore advice from the FDA. FDA does not require pre-IND meetings, but a pre-IND meeting can prevent a Clinical Hold (80).

Phase I clinical trials, which are sometimes called "first in human" trials, are designed to assess the safety of the drug and to acquire data on pharmacokinetics (81). The focus on the end-of-phase I meeting is on safety. In these meetings, FDA provides suggestions that are not binding on the investigator. In these meetings, the FDA and the Sponsor arrive at nonbinding agreements. The focus of the end-of-phase 2 meeting is to determine the safety of proceeding to a phase 3 trial, and to evaluate study design, as it applies to efficacy. At this meeting, it is critical that the Sponsor reaches agreement with FDA on elements of the clinical trial that are intended to persuade FDA to approve of the package label. These elements of the clinical trial include endpoints, statistical power, the acceptability of the control arm, techniques for blinding and unblinding, and validation of the manufacturing processes of the drug entity (82). The end-of-phase 2 meeting signifies the Sponsor's expectation that a drug will proceed to phase 3 development and presumably to a marketing/licensing application (83).

After the phase 3 clinical trial, the Sponsor submits one of two different kinds of marketing applications. These marketing applications are

---

[76]U.S. Department of Health and Human Services. Food and Drug Administration Guidance for Industry. Formal meetings between the FDA and Sponsors or applicants; May 2009 (11 pp.).

[77]Milstein J. FDA Meetings. Center for Drug Evaluation and Research (CDER). U.S. Food and Drug Administration (slide presentation); June 20, 2013 (40 pp.).

[78]Harnett M. The role of statistics in briefing books for FDA meetings. Waltham (MA): NovusLife, LLC (internet posting); September 30, 2014.

[79]Feigal EG, et al. Perspective: communications with the Food and Drug Administration on the development pathway for a cell-based therapy: why, what, when, and how? Stem Cells Transl. Med. 2012;1:825−32.

[80]Shapiro A. Relevant applications for drug development and approval. Retina Today. September 2014;26−44.

[81]Tonkens R. An overview of the drug development process. Physician Exec. May−June 2005;48−52.

[82]Feigal EG, et al. Perspective: communications with the Food and Drug Administration on the development pathway for a cell-based therapy: why, what, when, and how? Stem Cells Transl. Med. 2012;1:825−32.

[83]U.S. Department of Health and Human Services. Food and Drug Administration. Center for Drug Evaluation and Research (CDER) Good review practice: good review management principles and practices for effective IND development and review. Manual of Policies and Procedures (MAPP 6030.9); April 29, 2013 (42 pp.).

the NDA, for small-molecule drugs, and the BLA, for drugs that are biologicals. Before submitting the NDA or BLA, the Sponsor meets with FDA personnel in a pre-NDA meeting or a pre-BLA meeting. The subject matter of these meetings can include, for example, a review of the name for the drug, the planning of pediatric clinical trials, discussions of the risk management plan for use in the marketing phase, and the identification of manufacturing facilities (84).

Pre-NDA and pre-BLA meetings find a basis in 21 CFR §312.47b (2), which states that the main goal of these meetings is to uncover unresolved problems, to identify those studies that the Sponsor is relying on as adequate and well-controlled to establish the drug's effectiveness, to discuss methods for statistical analysis of the data, and to discuss the best approach to the presentation and formatting of data in the marketing application.

The purpose of the pre-NDA or pre-BLA meeting is to discuss filing and format issues. Topics of discussion include the adequacy of the data and information possessed by the Sponsor to warrant submission of the NDA or BLA, the need for an Advisory Committee, and the need for a Risk Evaluation and Mitigation Strategy (85). Also, discussions in these meetings concern the relationship between the manufacturing, formulation, and packaging of the drug product used in the phase 3 studies

and the final drug product (as intended for marketing), and assurance that any comparability or bridging studies agreed upon at the end-of-phase 2 meeting have been completed, assuring that the NDA or BLA submission will contain adequate stability data in accordance with stability protocols agreed upon at the EOP2 meeting, and confirming that all facilities (eg, manufacturing, testing, packaging) will be ready for inspection by the time of the NDA or BLA submission (86).

The most important meetings with the FDA are the pre-IND meetings, end-of-phase II meetings, pre-NDA/BLA meetings, advisory committee meetings, and labeling meetings, as summarized below (87,88):

- *Pre-IND Meetings.* The sponsor presents nonclinical test data on efficacy and safety, data on the characterization and manufacturing of the drug, and the proposed Clinical Study Protocol. The goal is to acquire feedback from the FDA, in an effort to place the clinical trial on "active status," rather than on "hold."
- *End-of-Phase II Meetings.* After completing the phase II trial, the sponsor provides proof of concept for the drug or medical device, through data on efficacy from phase I and phase II trials, and from nonclinical data. Phase III trial designs are discussed,

[84]U.S. Department of Health and Human Services. Food and Drug Administration. Center for Drug Evaluation and Research (CDER) Good review practice: good review management principles and practices for effective IND development and review. Manual of Policies and Procedures (MAPP 6030.9); April 29, 2013 (42 pp.).

[85]Milstein J. FDA Meetings. Center for Drug Evaluation and Research (CDER). U.S. Food and Drug Administration. (slide presentation); June 20, 2013 (40 pp.).

[86]U.S. Department of Health and Human Services. Food and Drug Administration Guidance for Industry. IND meetings for human drugs and biologicals. Chemistry, manufacturing, and controls information; May 2001 (10 p).

[87]U.S. Department of Health and Human Services. Food and Drug Administration. Guidance for Industry. Formal meetings with sponsors and applicants for PDUFA products; February 2000 (13 pp.).

[88]Grignolo A. Meeting with the FDA in FDA regulatory affairs. 2nd ed. In: Pisano DJ, Mantus DS, editors. New York (NY): Informa Healthcare, Inc. p. 109–123.

including information on indications, doses, safety, and manufacturing, suitable for the NDA or BLA.

- *Pre-NDA/BLA Meetings.* The sponsor and the FDA discuss how the application (NDA or BLA) will be organized.
- *Advisory Committee Meetings.* These meetings take place after submitting an NDA or BLA, and are conducted when the FDA needs advice from external experts and thought-leaders about the approvability of an application. Advisory Committee Meetings are open to the public. Advisory Committee members discuss the benefits and risks of the drug, and vote on whether to recommend it for FDA approval. The FDA is not required to follow the recommendations of its Advisory Committees, but it usually does. An Advisory Committee is used for about one third of new drugs (89).
- *Labeling Meetings.* Labeling meetings are held after an NDA or BLA is submitted and prior to the FDA approval of a drug. These meetings occur at the end of the NDA review process, when the FDA and the sponsor meet to agree on writing that informs physicians of the indications the product has been approved for, the dosages, and adverse drug reactions.

At these meetings, FDA expects the discussions to be driven by the data, with an emphasis on science and medicine, and that discussions focus on issues directly related to the product and to FDA regulations.

According to Grignolo (90), the Sponsor should not direct open-ended questions to the FDA, such as, the following: "The phase II trials demonstrated that several different doses were effective. Which dose do you recommend for our phase III trial?" Or, "How many subjects should be included in our phase III trial?" Or, "Our drug is effective against several diseases. Which should we select for further development?" Instead, at meetings with the FDA, the Sponsor's questions should take the form of reasoned proposals, such as the following. "Several different doses were tried, and the 5 mg and 10 mg doses were the most promising for our phase III trial. Do you agree?" Or, "Our statistical calculation shows that a phase III study with 1000 subjects will provide statistically significant results. Do you agree that 1000 subjects will be sufficient?"

c. Submitting the IND

The IND is submitted by way of *FDA Form 1571.* Form 1571 includes check boxes, indicating whether the IND is for a phase 1, phase 2, or phase 3 clinical trial. Form 1571 also has check boxes, indicating whether the IND submission includes, for example, a Clinical Study Protocol, an Investigator's Brochure, or a Pharmacology and Toxicology section.

After receipt of FDA Form 1571 and accompanying documents, the IND is routed to the appropriate division for review. FDA sends a letter of acknowledgment to the Sponsor, where the letter provides an IND number, date received, and name and telephone number of the FDA project manager (91). The Sponsor is permitted to begin the clinical trial at the time point of 30 days after the data are

[89]Lurie P. Financial conflicts of interest are related to voting patterns at FDA Advisory Committee meetings. MedGenMed. 2006;8:22 (1 p).

[90]Grignolo A. Meeting with the FDA in FDA regulatory affairs. 2nd ed. In: Pisano DJ, Mantus DS, editors. New York (NY): Informa Healthcare, Inc. p. 109–123.

[91]Holbein ME. Understanding FDA regulatory requirements for investigational new drug applications for sponsor-investigators. J. Invest. Med. 2009;57:689–93.

received. Following submission of the IND, receipt of the IND number, and initiation of the clinical trial, the Sponsor is required to provide FDA with other submissions, where applicable. These submissions include annual reports and amendments to the Clinical Study Protocol.

Further concerning FDA Form 1571, Holbein (92) reveals that "the serial number is 0000 with the initial application (section 10). Subsequent IND amendments increase the serial number by 1 in the order of submission."

The IND may or may not contain clinical data. According to Huff et al. (93), "[r]esults from a drug's CMC and nonclinical development programme are reported to the FDA in an IND application. This document is reviewed to see if clinical trials should be allowed to start." CMC means chemical manufacturing and controls (94). Title 21 CFR §312.23 also takes into account that a Sponsor may use one or more Contract Research Organizations (CRO) for conducting its laboratory research, clinical research, statistical analysis, drug manufacturing, and so on. Thus, with regard to the IND submission, the CFR states that what is required is a statement about the obligations transferred to the CRO. Referring to this statement, the CFR mandates that:

> [i]f a Sponsor has transferred any obligations for the conduct of any clinical study to a contract research organization, [what is required is] a

statement containing the name and address of the contract research organization, identification of the clinical study, and a listing of the obligations transferred.

d. Submitting the New Drug Application or the Biological License Application

FDA defines the NDA and BLA, as follows (95). The New Drug Application (NDA) is the format for Sponsors to propose that a new drug be approved for sale and marketing in the United States. The Biologics License Application (BLA) is a request for permission to introduce a biologic product into interstate commerce. A BLA is submitted by the manufacturer and must contain data derived from nonclinical laboratory and clinical studies which demonstrate that the manufactured product meets prescribed requirements of safety, purity, and potency.

When *FDA Form 356h* is initially submitted, the space requesting the NDA number or BLA number is left blank (96). After submission of this form, FDA provides the NDA or BLA number, and the number is then used when the Sponsor subsequently submits supplemental information to the NDA or BLA.

The Investigator's Brochure is one of the components of the IND. The Investigator's Brochure finds a basis in 21 CFR §312.23 and 21 CFR §312.55. In short, the IND takes the form of a cover sheet (Form FDA-1571),

---

[92]Holbein ME. Understanding FDA regulatory requirements for investigational new drug applications for sponsor-investigators. J. Investig. Med. 2009;57:689–93.

[93]Huff R, et al. The role of regulatory agencies in new drug development: a global perspective. J. Clin. Stud. 2014;6:20–22.

[94]U.S. Department of Health and Human Services. Food and Drug Administration Guidance for Industry. IND Meetings for Human Drugs and Biologics. Chemistry, Manufacturing, and Controls Information; May 2001 (15 pp.).

[95]U.S. Department of Health and Human Services. Food and Drug Administration SOPP 8401: administrative processing of Biologics License Application (BLA) and New Drug Application (NDA). Ver. no. 7; April 15, 2013 (35 pp.).

[96]Guidance kindly provided by Ms. Patricia Harley of FDA, in teleconference of February 11, 2015.

Table of Contents, Investigator's Brochure, Clinical Study Protocol, and a document called Chemistry, Manufacturing, and Controls (CMC) (97,98).

The Investigator's Brochure must include sections with the information indicated by the following bullet points (21 CFR §312.23 (a)(5)):

- A description of the drug substance and the formulation, including the structural formula.
- A summary of the pharmacological and toxicological effects of the drug in animals and, to the extent known, in humans.
- A summary of the pharmacokinetics and disposition of the drug in animals and, if known, in humans. This author points out that "disposition" can refer to Absorption, Distribution, Metabolism, and Excretion (ADME).
- A summary of information relating to safety and efficacy in humans obtained from prior clinical studies.
- A description of possible risks and side effects to be anticipated on the basis of prior experience with the drug under investigation or with related drugs, and of precautions or special monitoring to be done as part of the investigational use of the drug.

The Investigator's Brochure is like a typical review article, as might be published in an academic journal, in that it provides information that provides summaries on various topics. A goal of these summaries is to establish a context for understanding other documents in the FDA-submission, such as the Clinical Study Protocol.

XIII. SPECIAL PROTOCOL ASSESSMENT

The Special Protocol Assessment (SPA) is a procedure involving meetings with FDA and a binding agreement from the FDA. The SPA takes the form of a submission from the Sponsor, where this submission addresses specific questions about, for example, study design, endpoints, data analysis, and package labeling. According to FDA's Guidance for Industry, the request for an SPA must include "specific questions about the protocol design and scientific or regulatory requirements to which the Agency can respond" (99).

The SPA includes a cover letter that reads, "REQUEST FOR SPECIAL PROTOCOL ASSESSMENT," a protocol, and a document containing questions from the Sponsor. Form FDA 1571 is used to transmit the SPA to the FDA. Usually, the SPA is used to submit questions about a protocol that is the Clinical Study Protocol. However, the SPA can also be used to submit questions about two other types of protocols, namely, Carcinogenicity Protocol and Stability Protocol. Since the SPA is submitted only after an IND is already in place, it should be noted that the SPA must be submitted in the form of an amendment to the

---

[97]U.S. Department of Health and Human Services. Food and Drug Administration Guidance for Industry. INDs for Phase 2 and Phase 3 Studies. Chemistry, Manufacturing, and Controls Information; May 2003 (22 pp.).

[98]Sheinin E, Williams R. Chemistry, manufacturing, and controls information in NDAs and ANDAs, supplements, annual reports, and other regulatory filings. Pharm. Res. 2002;19:217–26.

[99]U.S. Department of Health and Human Services. Food and Drug Administration Guidance for Industry. Special Protocol Assessment; May 2002 (11 pp.).

Sponsor's IND. A unique feature about the SPA is that any agreements are binding on the FDA. Once the Sponsor and the FDA come to an agreement, it is the case that, "the Agency will not later alter its perspective on the issues of design, execution, or analysis" (100). Submission of an SPA is optional, and is not required by the FDA during the regulatory process of any drug. Through the SPA process, the Sponsor and FDA negotiate the design of a clinical trial that will support an efficacy claim for licensure (101).

According to one survey of Special Protocol Assessments submitted to FDA, a minority of these submissions resulted in agreements, and about a quarter of SPA agreements resulted in the submission of an NDA/BLA (102).

XIV. TARGET PRODUCT PROFILE

The Target Product Profile (TPP) is an optional part of the drug development process, and it may be included with the submission of an IND (103). The TPP is a living document that memorializes the goals of the drug development program, as it progresses, where the focus is on what the Sponsor would like to state on the package label. As stated by FDA, the TPP is a "dynamic summary" that gives information about the drug "at a particular time" in its development (104).

In one characterization of the subject matter of the Target Product Profile, the FDA has stated that it "is a concise version of the prototype package label ... used to enhance communication and promote a shared understanding of the drug development program by delineating the Sponsor's goals" (105). In addition, to assist in the maturation of the eventual package label, the TPP enhances the Sponsor's ability to prepare any Briefing Documents (106). The FDA has provided a template for the TPP, where the suggested sections cover indications, dosage and administration, contraindications, warnings and precautions, adverse reactions, drug–drug interactions, and a reference section (107).

[100]U.S. Department of Health and Human Services. Food and Drug Administration Guidance for Industry. Special Protocol Assessment; May 2002 (11 pp.).

[101]Feigal EG, et al. Perspective: communications with the Food and Drug Administration on the development pathway for a cell-based therapy: why, what, when, and how? Stem Cells Transl. Med. 2012;1:825–32.

[102]Maher VE, Kacuba A, Ning YM, et al. Special protocol assessments: 10 years of experience in FDA's Office of Hematology and Oncology Products. 2014 ASCO Annual Meeting. J. Clin. Oncol. 2014;32:2014 (suppl. abstr. e17511).

[103]U.S. Department of Health and Human Services. Food and Drug Administration. Center for Drug Evaluation and Research (CDER) Good review practice: good review management principles and practices for effective IND development and review. Manual of Policies and Procedures (MAPP 6030.9); April 29, 2013 (42 pp.).

[104]U.S. Department of Health and Human Services. Food and Drug Administration Guidance for Industry and Review Staff. Target product profile—a strategic development process tool; March 2007 (22 pp.).

[105]U.S. Department of Health and Human Services. Food and Drug Administration. Center for Drug Evaluation and Research (CDER) Good review practice: good review management principles and practices for effective IND development and review. Manual of Policies and Procedures (MAPP 6030.9); April 29, 2013 (42 pp.).

[106]U.S. Department of Health and Human Services. Food and Drug Administration Guidance for Industry and Review Staff. Target product profile—a strategic development process tool; March 2007 (22 pp.).

[107]U.S. Department of Health and Human Services. Food and Drug Administration Guidance for Industry and Review Staff. Target product profile—a strategic development process tool; March 2007 (22 pp.).

Lambert (108) has cautioned that, without a TPP in place, one group in a company may have certain assumptions about the composition and use of a drug in development, while another group in the same company may harbor different assumptions. Regarding information in the TPP, Lambert has also stated that, while a product is in development, the TPP can be used to keep track of acceptable and unacceptable features of the product, such as the acceptable pH range of the formulation. Moreover, the TPP may be used to keep track of patents (owned by competitors) that have the potential to pose a roadblock to particular variations of the drug and its method of use. As elegantly stated by Wyatt et al. (109), "[t]he TPP has to be periodically reassessed with regard to meeting essential, preferred or minimal acceptable criteria, as the unmet clinical need changes with the development of competing drug candidates and emerging data from clinical trials." To be used effectively, a Sponsor updates the TPP before each discussion with the FDA throughout all phases of the IND (110).

XV. COMPANY CORE DATA SHEET

The Company Core Data Sheet (CCDS) is similar to the Target Product Profile, in that it contains information that tracks the same classes of information that appear on the package label. As defined by the FDA, the Company Core Data Sheet is a document that contains material relating to indications, dosing, pharmacology, safety, and other information concerning the product (111). Companies use a CCDS as a reference for labeling. The content of the Company Core Data Sheet is for in-house use, and it is not negotiated between pharmaceutical companies and regulatory authorities. With respect to the safety information, the CCDS contains a set of data and advice that the company intends to have reflected in national and regional labeling worldwide (112). The CCDS can be prepared at various times, for example, at the time of the final internal approval but before submission of NDA to the regulatory agency, after the first submission, that is, at the time that the labeling information is the company opinion, or after approval, at which time the labeling reflects the opinion of the regulatory agency (113). CCDS are usually prepared by a Sponsor for a drug substance (active ingredient) rather than for the finished drug product.

The CCDS is also used as a reference for safety reporting, in that it can serve as a reference for determining whether a particular adverse event is expected or not. The CCDS includes a section that discloses adverse drug

---

[108]Lambert WJ. Considerations in developing a target product profile for parenteral pharmaceutical products. AAPS PharmaSciTech. 2010;11:1476–81.

[109]Wyatt PG, et al. Target validation: linking target and chemical properties to desired product profile. Curr. Top. Med. Chem. 2011;11:1275–83.

[110]Patrick DL, et al. Patient-reported outcomes to support medical product labeling claims: FDA perspective. Value Health. 2007;10(Suppl. 2): S125–37.

[111]U.S. Department of Health and Human Services. Food and drug administration guidance for industry E2C clinical safety data management: periodic safety update reports for marketed drugs; November 1996 (21 pp.).

[112]International Federation of Pharmaceutical Manufacturers and Associations (IFPMA) MedDRA and Product Labeling: "Best Practices" Recommendations; April 15, 2005 (9 pp.).

[113]Nijveldt G-J. Introduction to core labeling. Drug Information Association. slide show; October 7, 2011 (22 pp.).

reactions. This information can be used to govern labeling in various countries (114). Adverse events should be included in the CCDS where there is a reasonable possibility, or some basis to believe, that the study drug caused the AE. The threshold for including an AE in the CCDS is more than mere temporal association of the drug with the AE (115).

Please note that another document, the Investigator's Brochure, is also used during the course of a clinical trial to determine whether a particular adverse event is *unexpected or expected*. According to the Code of Federal Regulations (21 CFR §312.32), "[a]n adverse event or suspected adverse reaction is considered *unexpected* if it is not listed in the *investigator brochure* or is not listed at the specificity or severity that has been observed; or, if an investigator brochure is not required or available, is not consistent with the risk information described in the general investigational plan or elsewhere in the current application, as amended." [emphasis added] Referring to the above definition (21 CFR §312.32) of "unexpected" and "expected," the FDA's Guidance for Industry states that:

> [t]his definition relies entirely on the adverse events or suspected adverse reactions listed in the **investigator brochure** for the particular drug under investigation (or elsewhere in the general investigational plan if an investigator brochure is not required or available) as the basis for determining whether newly acquired information generated from clinical trials or reported from other sources is **unexpected**. [emphasis added]

This use of the Investigator's Brochure was emphasized by Sherman et al. (116), who stated that an SAE that must be reported to the FDA, by way of expedited reporting, is an SAE that is not listed in the Investigator's Brochure.

To summarize, it is the case that identification of a particular SAE in the Investigator's Brochure, in the CCDS, or elsewhere in the investigational plan, can determine how the investigator reports and routes information on that SAE, during the course of a clinical trial.

XVI. ACCELERATED APPROVAL

a. Introduction

FDA provides a pathway called accelerated approval. This pathway is available where the study drug is intended to treat a serious condition that provides an advantage over other available therapies, and that demonstrates an effect on a surrogate endpoint. The effect on the surrogate endpoint must be one that is, "reasonably likely to predict clinical benefit that can be measured earlier than irreversible morbidity or mortality ... or other clinical benefit ... [such as] an intermediate clinical endpoint" (117).

The Sponsor should discuss the possibility of accelerated approval with the FDA during development. Where a Sponsor receives approval by the FDA for using the accelerated approval pathway, the Sponsor must conduct postmarketing confirmatory clinical trials to

---

[114]Fontaine L, Lachmann B. The adverse reactions and interactions section of a CCDS. Drug Information Association; October 2011 (22 pp.).

[115]Fontaine L, Lachmann B. The adverse reactions and interactions section of a CCDS. Drug Information Association; October 2011 (22 pp.).

[116]Sherman RB, et al. New FDA regulation to improve safety reporting in clinical trials. N. Engl. J. Med. 2011;365:3—5.

[117]U.S. Department of Health and Human Services. Food and Drug Administration Guidance for Industry. Expedited Programs for Serious Conditions—Drugs and Biologics; May 2014 (36 pp.).

confirm that the predictive influence on mortality or other clinical benefit actually occurs.

The confirmatory clinical trials must be developed as early as possible, including the Sponsor's timeline for enrolling subjects and completing the trials. The confirmatory clinical trial must use clinical benefit as a primary endpoint. This means that, for the example of antitumor drugs, prolongation of survival should be a primary endpoint, and it means that objective tumor response cannot be used as the only primary endpoint. If a drug was approved under the accelerated approval pathway, and if the confirmatory trial fails to verify the predicted clinical benefit, then FDA may withdraw the approval of the drug. Also, if the Sponsor fails to conduct the confirmatory trial, FDA may withdraw approval of the drug (118).

According to Dr Richard Pazdur and other FDA officials, the average time for gaining approval by the accelerated approval pathway is about 6 years, while the average time for gaining approval by the regular approval pathway is about 7 years (119). Accelerated approval of an anticancer drug may be based on endpoints, such as objective response rate, complete response, disease-free survival (DFS), and progression-free survival (PFS) (120).

When FDA approves a drug submitted by way of accelerated approval, FDA may publish a paper outlining features of the clinical trial that led to the approval. For example, when *bevacizumab* for glioblastoma was approved, by way of the accelerated approval pathway, FDA published a paper disclosing, for example, that the primary endpoint was objective response rate, and that this endpoint was defined as complete response (CR) or partial response (PR), where the response was required to be confirmed 4 weeks (or later) after the initial measurement (121).

b. Basis in Code of Federal Regulations for Accelerated Approval

Accelerated approval finds a basis in 21 CFR §314, which states that the accelerated approval pathway:

> applies to certain new drug products that have been studied for their safety and effectiveness in treating serious or life-threatening illnesses and that provide meaningful therapeutic benefit to patients over existing treatments (eg, ability to treat patients unresponsive to, or intolerant of, available therapy, or improved patient response over available therapy).

Title 21 CFR §314 also refers to the use of a surrogate endpoint, to the requirement for a confirmatory trial, and to the fact that the confirmatory trial must be conducted promptly and be initiated at the time the Sponsor applies for accelerated approval:

> FDA may grant marketing approval for a new drug product on the basis of adequate and well-controlled clinical trials establishing that the drug product has an effect on a **surrogate endpoint** that is reasonably likely ... to predict clinical benefit ...

---

[118]U.S. Department of Health and Human Services. Food and Drug Administration Guidance for Industry. Expedited Programs for Serious Conditions—Drugs and Biologics; May 2014 (36 pp.).

[119]Lanthier ML, et al. Accelerated approval and oncology drug development timelines. J. Clin. Oncol 2010;28: e226−7.

[120]McKee AE, et al. The role of U.S. Food and drug administration review process: clinical trial endpoints in oncology. Oncologist. 2010;15(Suppl. 1):13−18.

[121]Cohen MH, et al. FDA drug approval summary: bevacizumab (Avastin®) as treatment of recurrent glioblastoma multiforme. Oncologist. 2009;14:1131−8.

[a]pproval under this section will be subject to the requirement that the applicant study the drug further, to verify and describe its clinical benefit ... [p]ostmarketing studies would usually be studies already underway ... [t]he applicant shall carry out any such studies with due diligence.

c. FDA's Decision-Making Process in Approving a Drug, Where the Drug Had Been Subjected to a Clinical Trial That Took Advantage of the Accelerated Approval Pathway

This concerns panitumumab for treating colorectal cancer. The information is from the *Medical Review* for BLA 125147, from March 2015 of the FDA's website. The FDA reviewer disclosed the reason for the FDA's approval, stating that, "[t]he recommendation for accelerated approval is based on demonstration of ... progression-free survival (PFS) ... which is a surrogate endpoint reasonably likely to predict ... survival." The study drug arm received panitumumab, while the control arm received no drug, but instead only received best supportive care. Efficacy was clearly demonstrated by the PFS endpoint, where the mean PFS was 96.4 days for the study drug arm and only 59.7 days for the control arm.

The FDA reviewer commented on the fact that overall survival was measured, but that this endpoint demonstrated lack of efficacy. In the words of the FDA reviewer, "[t]he trial failed to show evidence of an impact on overall survival. This may be a result of a large number of patients from the best supportive care crossing over to the active treatment arm within a short period of time on study ... about 50% crossed over within 8 weeks."

As stated above, where a Sponsor requests the accelerated approval pathway, and where the results of the clinical trial are sufficiently persuasive to convince FDA to grant approval

to the drug, the Sponsor is committed to conduct a subsequent clinical trial where the primary endpoint is overall survival. To this point, the FDA reviewer stated that, the Sponsor "has committed to conduct a randomized trial [where] ... [t]he primary endpoint of this trial is overall survival and the trial is intended to verify the benefit of" the study drug. FDA's Approval Letter, after its review of the trial that used the accelerated approval pathway, reiterated this commitment, stating that:

[a]pproval under these regulations requires ... that you conduct adequate and well-controlled studies to verify and describe ... increased survival ... [i]f postmarketing studies fail to verify the clinical benefit ... we may, following a hearing ... withdraw or modify approval.

XVII. REFUSE TO FILE

a. Purpose of a Refuse to File Notice

The topic of a *Refuse to File* (RTF) notice was introduced earlier in this book in the descriptions of animal models. *Refuse to File*, which has a basis in 21 CFR §314.101(d), can be applied against a New Drug Application (NDA) and against a Biological License Application (BLA). According to FDA's *Manual of Policies and Procedures*, a *Refuse to File* under is a:

tool to help CDER [or CBER] avoid unnecessary review of incomplete applications ... [i]ncomplete applications can lead to multiple-cycle reviews and inefficient use of CDER resources. CDER also believes an RTF action can allow an applicant to begin repair of critical deficiencies in the application far sooner than if these were identified much later ... and may lead to more rapid approval of safe and effective drug products (122)

---

[122]U.S. Department of Health and Human Services. Food and Drug Administration Manual of Policies and Procedures. Good Review Practice: Refuse to File; October 11, 2013. (22 pp.).

In detail, FDA may issue a *Refuse to File* if certain forms have not been filled out, for example if, "[t]he application does not contain a statement for each nonclinical laboratory study that it was conducted in compliance with the requirements set forth in 21 CFR part 58 [Good Laboratory Practice]" (123). FDA has commented on the fact that *Refuse to File* notices are not common (124).

b. FDA's Decision-Making Process in Issuing a Refuse to File Notice

This is an example of FDA's comments, regarding a *Refuse to File* against an application for the drug, cetuximab (Erbitux®), for the indication of colorectal cancer. Although the drug was eventually approved by FDA for marketing, the following provides an example of a glitch in the FDA approval process. What had happened, was that, "FDA refused to file ... [the company's] application not just because of missing documentation and data discrepancies, but also because the ... study was neither adequate nor sufficiently well-controlled to meet Federal requirements" (125).

This provides an excerpt from the *Refuse to File* notice. The *Refuse to File* notice was issued in Dec. 2001, and the excerpt is from the *Medical Review* for BLA 125084, available at Feb. 2004 on the FDA's website. The clinical study involved the combination of two drugs, an antibody (cetuximab) and a small molecule (irinotecan). The *Refuse to File* notice stated:

> The application does not contain data that isolates the contribution of irinotecan to the combination regimen ... the data do not show that the response rate observed with the combination of Cetuximab with irinotecan could not also be observed with the single agent Cetuximab ... [y]ou must provide evidence ... which isolates and establishes the individual contributions of irinotecan and Cetuximab (126).

The presence of this *Refuse to File* letter, with the fact that the study drug eventually met with FDA approval, demonstrates that a hurdle that was encountered in the FDA's timeline was successfully overcome by the Sponsor.

The *Refuse to File* notice provides guidance on study design, where a clinical trial requires administering a combination of two drugs. In other words, as a general proposition, where the study drug is administered as a combination with other drugs, FDA prefers that parameters of each individual drug be separately examined. FDA's *Medical Review* for another drug also addresses the issue where the study drug is administered as a combination with a second drug. See the *Medical Review* for a clinical trial on diabetes, which involved the combination of metformin and sitagliptin for treating diabetes (NDA 022044, at Jan. 2015 on FDA's website).

[123]U.S. Department of Health and Human Services. Food and Drug Administration Manual of Policies and Procedures. Good Review Practice: Refuse to File; October 11, 2013 (22 pp.).

[124]According to Janet Rehnquist, "[a]lthough FDA can refuse to file applications, it rarely does so. The CDER refused to file 4 percent of submitted applications in FY 2000, down from 17 percent in 1993. In part, this decrease may be attributable to the advice FDA provides Sponsors that helps them prepare higher quality applications." See, Rehnquist, J (March 2003) FDA's review process for New Drug Applications. A management review. Department of Health and Human Services (47 pp.).

[125]Hearings Before the Subcommittee on Oversight and Investigations of the Committee on Energy and Commerce. House of Representatives. June 13 and Oct. 10, 2002. Ser. No. 107142. U.S. Government Printing Office, Washington (DC).

[126]U.S. Department of Health and Human Services. Food and Drug Administration. Clinical Review for Biological License Application (BLA) 125084; February 12, 2004 (50 page pdf file).

XVIII. CLINICAL HOLD

a. Introduction

A *Clinical Hold* is a notification issued by FDA to the Sponsor to delay a proposed clinical trial or to suspend an ongoing clinical trial. *Clinical Hold* has a basis in 21 CFR §312.42. Section 312.42 states, for example, that "[w]hen an ongoing study is placed on *Clinical Hold*, no new subjects may be recruited to the study … patients already in the study should be taken off therapy … unless specifically permitted by FDA in the interest of public safety."

Section 312.42 further discloses that the grounds for a Clinical Hold include FDA's assessment that human subjects are exposed to an unreasonable risk of injury, that the clinical investigators named in the IND are not qualified by reason of their training and experience to conduct the clinical trial, and that the Investigator's Brochure is misleading or erroneous. Where FDA imposed the clinical hold because of misconduct by the Sponsor, this misconduct can take various forms. Examples of misconduct include failure to report SAEs, enrollment of study subjects having conditions that put them at increased risk with exposure to the study drug, repeated failure to administer informed consent forms, and failure of the IRB to review and approve significant changes in the Clinical Study Protocol, and falsification of safety data (127).

This concerns the *Partial Clinical Hold*. According to FDA's Guidance for Industry, *Partial Clinical Hold* is "[a] delay or suspension of only part of the clinical work requested under the IND (eg, a specific protocol or part of

a protocol is not allowed to proceed; however, other protocols or parts of the protocol are allowed to proceed under the IND)" (128).

b. Examples of a Clinical Hold

This provides an example of a *Clinical Hold*. A phase 3 clinical trial on an *inhaled drug* was suspended by the FDA, because of data showing that the drug was carcinogenic, as determined in a chronic study with rats. In the *Clinical Hold*, FDA requested additional information from the rat study (129). The press release stated that the company expected to provide all of the information to the FDA within a month.

FDA issued a *Clinical Hold* against a phase 2 clinical trial on fingolimod, a drug for multiple sclerosis, because of insufficient monitoring of adverse events. The clinical trial, which was under IND no. 70,139, was put on hold on June 29, 2005 because of insufficient monitoring of macular edema, pulmonary conditions, and pancreatitis. Shortly after the trial was put on *Clinical Hold*, the Sponsor requested an "End of Phase 2" meeting to discuss why the trial was put on hold. A year later the Sponsor was eventually able to convince FDA of sufficient monitoring, and FDA lifted the hold on May 19, 2006 (Medical Review dated August 26, 2010, NDA 22-527, FDA website).

In a *Clinical Hold* against a drug for *osteoarthritis*, FDA complained about an adverse event that took the form of a single occurrence of an infection in the injected knee joint of a study subject (130). In a *Clinical Hold* against an *anticoagulant drug*, FDA halted an ongoing phase 3 trial because of SAEs that were allergic

---

[127]U.S. Department of Health and Human Services. Food and Drug Administration Guidance for Industry and Clinical Investigators. The use of clinical holds following clinical investigator misconduct; September 2004 (8 pp.).

[128]U.S. Department of Health and Human Services. Food and Drug Administration Guidance for Industry. Submitting and Reviewing Complete Responses to Clinical Holds; April 1998 (3 pp.).

[129]Press release Insmed announces clinical hold on ARIKACE® Phase 3 clinical trials; August 1, 2011.

[130]Press release Flexion Therapeutics announced clinical hold of FX006 Phase 2b clinical trial in osteoarthritis of the knee; September 17, 2014.

reactions (131). The issue of these allergic reactions was detected and raised, while the trial was in-progress, by the Data Safety Monitoring Board (DSMB). Thus, the facts underlying this particular *Clinical Hold* provide an insight regarding one of the subjects of this textbook, namely, the DSMB.

In a *Clinical Hold* against a drug for *hepatitis B virus*, FDA required the company to cut the dose in half, and requested additional information on study subjects that had received elevated doses (132).

Upon receipt of an FDA *Clinical Hold Letter*, the Sponsor can respond by preparing an amendment to the IND that addresses the issues set forth in the Letter. An FDA reviewer then evaluates the amendment, and determines whether the Sponsor's response is satisfactory (133).

c. FDA's Decision-Making Process in Imposing a Clinical Hold

This is from FDA's *Medical Review* of *dinutiximab*, for treating neuroblastoma. The information is from BLA 125516 on Mar. 2015 of the FDA's website. FDA had imposed a *Partial Clinical Hold*, during the course of the clinical trial. The FDA reviewer wrote that the "IND placed on partial hold to prevent treatment of patients ... where two patients received an overdose of IL-2."

About a half year later, the FDA imposed another *Partial Clinical Hold*, and the FDA reviewer wrote that the:

> IND placed on partial hold to prevent enrollment of new patients ... [d]eficiencies included inadequate dose modification rules for IL-2 ... lack of on-site training of

principal investigator, and lack of criteria for screening clinical sites for their ability to administer toxic biologic therapies ... [a]dditionally, pre-printed orders ... appeared to be the cause of the IL-2 overdose.

Several years later, the clinical trial under the same IND was again placed on a *Partial Clinical Hold*, because of allergic reactions to the study drug. The *Medical Review* also documented the fact, that for each partial hold, it was the case that "FDA removed partial hold."

To conclude, in the clinical trial on dinutiximab, the *Partial Clinical Holds* mainly concerned adverse events to one of the drugs administered in the study. However, the available information suggests that essentially any aspect of the clinical trial, such as training of personnel, can result in a *Clinical Hold*.

XIX. EXEMPLARY ACCOUNT OF FDA TIMELINE, AFTER SUBMISSION OF NDA OR BLA

Archdeacon et al. (134) provides an exemplary account of communications and activities occurring following submission of an NDA or BLA. This particular example was with a BLA, and the drug under review was for the indication of preventing organ rejection. The following account demonstrates how various concepts, introduced at earlier points in this textbook, fit into the context of the FDA-approval process. These concepts include:

- Advisory Committee;
- Risk Evaluation and Mitigation Strategy (REMS);

[131]Press release Regado Biosciences announces clinical hold of REGULATE-PCI trial following voluntary halt of trial by Regado; July 9, 2014.

[132]Calia M. FDA informs Arrowhead of partial clinical hold for hepatitis B drug. Wall Street J.; July 12, 2015. Dow Jones & Co., Inc.

[133]Poole K. The Sponsor's guide to regulatory submissions for an investigational new drug. biological resources branch, DCTD, NCI-Frederick. SAIC-Frederick, Inc; March 2005 (104 pp.).

[134]Archdeacon P, et al. Summary of the US FDA approval of Belatacept. Am. J. Transpl. 2012;12:554−62.

- Registry;
- Postmarketing clinical studies.

The following narrative begins with the BLA submission, dated June 30, 2009. FDA agreed to give the standard 10-month review, that is, regarding safety, efficacy, pharmacokinetics, and manufacturing. During this 10-month period, FDA held an Advisory Committee meeting (March 1, 2010) in order to get independent opinions from outside experts. The Advisory Committee voted to approve the drug, but the vote was not unanimous. After the Advisory Committee's meeting and vote, FDA declined to approve the drug, the reasons being mainly because of problems with manufacturing the drug. The Sponsor then submitted additional information, and the FDA determined that all of the issues were adequately addressed, and the drug was approved on June 15, 2011.

At the time of FDA approval, FDA also imposed the requirement that the Sponsor prepare a REMS. The goal of this REMS was to ensure that the benefits of the approved drug outweighed the risks of the disease. FDA determined that a REMS was needed to ensure that physicians and patients were aware of the serious risks of the diseases (posttransplant lymphoproliferative disorder), and how to mitigate those risks. FDA also imposed the requirement for postmarketing clinical studies. The goal of these studies was to provide an estimate of the prevalence of the disease in clinical practice, where the information was deposited in a registry called, "ENLIST." The goal of another of the postmarketing studies was to analyze patterns of use of the approved drug, that is, as used in routine clinical practice.

XX. FDA APPROVAL LETTER

This documents one element of the feedback from the FDA, when it approves an NDA or BLA, namely the approval letter. The example is from the approval letter for *ibrutinib* for the indication of mantle cell lymphoma, a type of hematological cancer. The NDA had been submitted on June 28, 2013, and the date of the approval was Nov. 13, 2013.

The approval letter illustrates these concepts:

- *Accelerated approval.* The study on ibrutinib was conducted under a provision by the FDA for accelerated approval under 21 CFR §314.500. A Sponsor can submit a NDA or BLA under the accelerated approval program, where approval is based on data from a *surrogate endpoint*. In other words, the approval is based on data from an endpoint that is different from actual recovery from the disease. The FDA's *Guidance for Industry Expedited Programs for Serious Conditions* details the requirements, where a Sponsor wishes to submit its NDA or BLA in the accelerated approval program. The requirement for use of a *surrogate endpoint* is reproduced in footnotes (135,136). In commentary on the FDA's accelerated approval program, Dr Richard Pazdur and coworkers outlined the use of *surrogate endpoints* versus the "gold standard" endpoint of survival, and details regarding the successes and failures of postmarketing data

[135]"a product for a serious or life-threatening disease or condition . . . upon a determination that the product has an effect on a surrogate endpoint that is reasonably likely to predict clinical benefit, or on a clinical endpoint that can be measured earlier than irreversible morbidity or mortality, that is reasonably likely to predict an effect on irreversible morbidity or mortality or other clinical benefit, taking into account the severity, rarity, or prevalence of the condition and the availability or lack of alternative treatments."

[136]U.S. Department of Health and Human Services. Food and Drug Administration Guidance for Industry. Guidance for Industry Expedited Programs for Serious Conditions; May 2014 (36 pp.).

intended to confirm the safety and efficacy of the drug (137).

- *Timeline of FDA approval.* The letter documents the date of submission of the NDA, dates of all of the submitted amendments, date of submission of the final printed package label, and dates that are required for postmarketing studies on safety when used in a population of patients.
- *Package label.* The letter documents the fact that approval tracks the elements of the package label, by its writing that the drug "is approved ... for use as recommended in the enclosed agreed-upon labeling text."
- *Requirement for postmarketing safety data.* The letter required that the Sponsor conduct a clinical trial, with a final report due on Dec. 2016. Also, the letter required that the Sponsor collect safety data from all patients (outside of any clinical trial) being treated with the drug, with a final report due on Nov. 2018. The requirement for collecting safety data, in the postmarketing timeframe, is called *pharmacovigilance.* The FDA's *Guidance for Industry Good Pharmacovigilance Practices* (138) discloses that the need to collect safety data, following FDA approval, is:

Risk assessment during product development should be conducted in a thorough and rigorous manner; however, it is impossible to identify all safety concerns during clinical trials. Once a product is marketed, there is generally a large increase in the number of patients exposed, including those with co-morbid conditions and those being treated with concomitant medical products.

FDA's approval letter, which was signed by Dr Richard Pazdur (139), Director of Hematology and Oncology Products, Center for Drug Evaluation and Research (CDER), of the FDA, is reproduced (in part) below:

Dear Ms. [redacted],

Please refer to your New Drug Application (NDA) dated June 28, 2013 ... submitted ... for Imbruvica (ibrutinib) Capsules, 140 mg.

We acknowledge receipt of your amendments dated May 6, 2013; May 13, 2013; June 6, 2013.

We have completed our review of this application, as amended. It is approved under the provisions of accelerated approval regulations (21 CFR 314.500) ... for use as recommended in the enclosed agreed-upon labeling text. Marketing of this drug product and related activities must adhere to the substance and procedures of the referenced ... approval regulations.

Your application ... was not referred to an FDA advisory committee because the application did not raise significant safety or efficacy issues in the intended issues.

Products approved under the accelerated approval regulations ... require further ... studies/clinical trials to verify and describe clinical benefit. You are required to conduct such studies/clinical trials with due diligence. If post marketing studies/clinical trials fail to verify clinical benefit ... we may ... withdraw this approval. Continue follow-up on patients ... and submit a final analysis report of trial PCYC-1104-CA ... [i]n addition, submit ... information regarding all sites of extranodal disease at baseline and follow-up.

We have determined that an analysis of spontaneous postmarketing adverse events ... will not be sufficient to identify an unexpected serious risk of inhibition of platelet function or assess a known serious risk of bleeding. Therefore ... FDA has determined that you are required to ... [d]etermine the effect of a broad range of concentration of

[137]Johnson JR, et al. Accelerated approval of oncology products: the Food and Drug Administration experience. J. Natl. Cancer Inst. 2011;103:636—44.

[138]U.S. Department of Health and Human Services. Food and Drug Administration Guidance for Industry. Good Pharmacovigilance Practices and Pharmcoepidemiologic Assessment; March 2005 (20 pp.).

[139]With the approval any given anticancer drug, it is sometimes the case that Dr Richard Pazdur publishes a paper concerning FDA's decision to approve that drug. For example, with FDA's approval of a drug for mantle cell lymphoma, Dr Pazdur published the following paper Kane RC, et al. Bortezomib for the treatment of mantle cell lymphoma. Clin. Cancer Res. 2007;13:5291—4.

ibrutinib on the potential to inhibit platelet function by conducting in vitro studies … [e]valuation should include samples from subjects with and without concomitant conditions associated with platelet dysfunction, e.g., severe renal dysfunction, use of a concomitant anticoagulant, and use of aspirin.

You will conduct this study according to the following schedule:

Final Protocol Submission: 12/2014
Study Completion: 06/2016
Final Report Submission: 12/2016

Conduct an assessment and an analysis of data from clinical trials and all post-marketing sources in order to characterize the risk of serious bleeding in patients treated with … ibrutinib … [t]he risks of special interest are major hemorrhagic events. This enhanced pharmacovigilance study will include … continue … for a period of four years … [with a] Final Report Submission: 11/2018.

Sincerely, Richard Pazdur, M.D.

XXI. FDA FEEDBACK AT TIME OF ISSUE OF THE FDA APPROVAL LETTER

a. Introduction

At the time FDA issues the Approval Letter, FDA reviewers also provide their reasons for approving the drug, as set forth on the package label, in the format of the following documents. These documents can be found, on FDA's website, by following the footnoted instructions (140). Any given review may contain comments from different FDA employees (141). These reviews include:

- *Medical Review* or *Clinical Review;*
- *Pharmacology Review;*
- *Microbiology Review;*
- *Statistical Review.*

The following compares the writing and analysis that was submitted by the Sponsor, and the writing found in the Reviews that are prepared and published by the FDA. FDA reviewers use both Sponsor's analysis and the FDA's independent analyses in their reviews. In many cases, the FDA checks the data provided by the Sponsor.

In preparing the reviews, FDA officials use primary data acquired from the Sponsor, and then use the data to create tables and graphs. Thus, the majority of tables and graphs are prepared by an FDA reviewer. Some of the material in FDA's reviews may take the form of text that is copied and pasted from documents provided by the Sponsor (142). If the FDA get the same information in the FDA's own analysis, the FDA may simply recreate the tables and writing provided by the Sponsor (143).

The following provides excerpts from the *Medical Reviews* that accompanied FDA's Approval Letter for a selection of drugs. These drugs, which track the content of this textbook, are from *oncology*, autoimmune diseases, as exemplified by *multiple sclerosis*, and infectious diseases, as exemplified by *hepatitis C virus.*

---

[140]On the FDA website, under Drugs, first click, "Search Drug Approvals by Month Using Drugs@FDA." Then, click "Approval History, Letters, Reviews, and Related Documents." Finally, click on "Review."

[141]"Note that there may be differences among reviewers since the FDA review divisions and teams operate slightly differently from one another." Response by RL, Drug Information Specialist, Division of Drug Information, Center for Drug Evaluation and Research, FDA. E-mail response dated March 2, 2015.

[142]Kind advise from Dr Patrick Archdeacon, MD, FDA, CDER, in e-mail dated March 5, 2015.

[143]The author is grateful to Dr Michelle Eby, PharmD, of FDA, CDER for providing this advice, in an e-mail of March 3, 2015.

Excerpts from FDA's *Medical Reviews* are worthy of reiteration in this textbook, because they disclose the nature of the FDA's feedback at the time that approval is granted, and because they demonstrate the practical application of concepts taught in earlier chapters in this textbook.

b. Oncology

This is from the *Medical Review* of *ibrutinib*, used to treat a type of hematological cancer. The information is from NDA 205552, from Nov. 2013 of the FDA's website. The FDA reviewer made the following recommendation:

> This reviewer recommends accelerated approval for this new drug application (NDA). The Applicant has demonstrated the efficacy of patients with mantle cell lymphoma (MCL) who have been previously treated.

1. Need for Pharmacovigilance on Blood Clotting Adverse Events

In comments on risks and benefits, the reviewer made note of the risk for SAEs, writing that, "hemorrhagic adverse reactions occurred in about half (48%) of the trial population," and commented on how the Sponsor proposed to address this safety issue, writing that, "Applicant has pharmacovigilance plans in place to further characterize hemorrhagic events ... confirmatory trials are ongoing to better define the benefit–risk profile."

2. Need for Sponsor to Correlate an Older Test with a Newer Test

The reviewer referred to a revised version of the criteria for assessing efficacy of the drug, writing that the present NDA "represents the first regulatory application" of the revised criteria. The revised version of the criteria is simply called "2007 Response Criteria." The reviewer noted that the new criteria incorporate a new type of test, namely, *fludeoxyglucose positron emission tomography* (FDG-PET) scans. The reviewer suggested that the Sponsor collect information on whether this new test provides data that are consistent with a test (computed tomography) used in the older set of criteria. The reviewer expressly requested that, "A longer duration of follow-up is needed to further characterize the correlation of on-treatment FDG-PET scans with long-term outcome."

3. Requirement for In Vitro Experiments on Drug's Influence on Blood Clotting

In addition to requesting information serving to validate the new test (FDG-PET), the reviewer recommended that the Sponsor conduct in vitro laboratory experiments relating to drug safety. To this end, the reviewer asked for experiments on the influence of the study drug (ibrutinib) on platelets, writing that the Sponsor should, "[d]etermine the effect of a broad range of concentrations of ibrutinib on the potential to inhibit platelet function." This recommendation was made, because of the high rate of bleeding in the study subjects.

4. Requirement for Clinical Trial Designed to Assess Relation of Study Drug to Adverse Event of Renal Failure

Further concerning drug safety, the reviewer referred to the adverse event of renal failure in some of the study subjects, and recommended that the Sponsor conduct an entirely new clinical trial to determine whether the study drug contributes to renal failure. The reviewer commented that the present study (subject of the Approval Letter) was only a single-arm study and thus was not designed to be sensitive to determine whether adverse events were caused by the study drug. At the time of the *Medical Review*, the most plausible reason for the renal failure was the extreme old age of all of the study subjects. Thus the reviewer was interested in the possible influence of the study drug (independent of old age) on renal failure. Further regarding renal failure, the reviewer stated that the Sponsor should consider including a warning, on the package label, that the study drug might increase the risk for renal failure, even though approval was based only on a single-arm clinical trial.

5. Need to Explore Efficacy of Lower Doses for Patients

At the time of the Approval Letter, FDA also issued a *Clinical Pharmacology Review*. The information is from NDA 205552, from Nov. 2013 on the FDA's website.

FDA's review commented on the dosing level, and suggested that the Sponsor explore the efficacy of doses that were lower than that which had been approved by the Approval Letter. To this end, the reviewer stated that:

> [a]lthough the proposed dose ... [is] acceptable based on the limited effectiveness and safety data in the ... study population, the proposed doses are ... higher than the lowest dose that resulted in maximum BTK occupancy and maximum response. Therefore, the applicant should consider exploring lower doses in further development programs.

"BTK" refers to the target of the drug. The drug's target is an enzyme, *Bruton's Tyrosine Kinase* (BTK). In the review's comment, the term "occupancy" refers to the binding of the study drug to the enzyme, thus inhibiting the enzyme.

6. Issue of Toxicity of Excipient in Animal Tests

Further regarding concerns about toxicity of the drug formulation, the reviewer also commented on the excipient in the drug formulation. In comments about a dosing study in dogs, he remarked that "intolerance to the treatment of 100 mg/kg/day of ibrutinib ...

may possibly be due to the intolerance to the vehicle which contained 28% (w/v)."

The following bulletpoints summarize the reviewer's comments:

- *Efficacy*. The FDA reviewer stated that the reviewer recommends approval, because the data showed that the drug was effective in humans.
- *Safety*. Regarding safety, the reviewer requested an entirely new clinical trial designed to examine certain adverse events, that is, relating to blood clotting disorders and renal failure. Also regarding safety, the reviewer commented on the possible toxicity of the excipient, as determined by data from animals, but refrained from making any recommendation.
- *Endpoint*. Regarding criteria for evaluating an efficacy endpoint, the reviewer requested information that correlated an older method (computed tomography) with a newer method (FDG-PET).
- *Dose*. Regarding the dose, which is a vital component of all package labels, the reviewer requested additional clinical studies addressing the efficacy of lower doses.

c. Autoimmune Diseases, As Exemplified by Multiple Sclerosis

This is from the *Medical Review* of *pegylated interferon-beta-1a*, a drug used for treating multiple sclerosis. The information is from BLA 125499, from Jan. 2014, on the FDA's website.

The reviewer recommended approval of the study drug, writing, "[t]his review recommends approval of ... 125 micrograms given subcutaneously every 2 weeks for the treatment of adults with relapsing forms of multiple sclerosis ... [t]he trial data supports that the benefits of peginterferon-beta-1a outweigh the risks."

1. Lack of Any Recommendation to Conduct Postmarketing Safety Studies

The reviewer also commented on the lack of need for "Postmarket Risk Evaluation and Mitigation Strategies," and stated that he did not have any recommendations. The reviewer explained that, "[p]rior experience with the interferon drug products … do not suggest that any additional measures are required to evaluate or mitigate risks after approval."

2. Issue of Whether Subgroups of Study Subjects, Residing in Locations Outside of North America, Were Representative of Patients in the United States

The reviewer commented on the subgroups. As is the case with many clinical trials, one category of subgroup is the study site. The study sites for this BLA included clinics in North America, Europe, Eastern Europe, India, and elsewhere. The reviewer addressed the possibility that the results could not justifiably support approval for use in the United States (FDA grants approval for use in the United States). Then, the reviewer rationalized approval in the United States.

In stating the problem, the reviewer commented on the fact that, "[o]nly 3% of the population was from North America which includes the US and Canada … the Sponsor provided a rationale for the applicability of the data from the overall study to the US population as follows."

The rationalization took the form of a list. The goal of this list was to convey the fact that the populations of overseas subjects had similar characteristics to the subjects in the United States:

- "The US data was [sic] analyzed as part of Region 1 which included Canada, Belgium, Netherlands, Germany, France and Spain which were considered to have similar health care systems.

- The baseline demographic and disease characteristics did not differ significantly in Region 1 from Region 2 (mainly Eastern Europe) or Region 3 (South America, Georgia, India and New Zealand).
- The results in Region 1 do not differ significantly from those in Regions 2 and 3 or from the overall result."

3. Need to Explore a More Frequent Dosing Schedule in Human Subjects

The reviewer also commented about the dose of the study drug, and recommended that the Sponsor address the value of using a more frequent dose. This recommendation compared the more frequent dose of once every 2 weeks (q2w) with once every 4 weeks (q4w). The reviewer referred to the Kaplan–Meier plot, and observed that with the passage of months, improvement in the q2w dose study arm became progressively superior, when compared to the study arm with q4w dosing.

The reviewer suggested that the Sponsor continue to monitor and analyze this trend, in order to support a recommendation for q2w dosing. The reviewer's exact comment was, "[t]here may be a continuing separation of the … q2W group from the q4W group over time based on the above Kaplan–Meier curve. This may further support the superiority of the q2W dosing. This should be reviewed when the dataset for 2-year results is complete."

The bulletpoints summarize the reviewer's comments:

- *Postmarket Risk Evaluation.* Unlike the reviewer's comments for ibrutinib (describe above), which recommended additional studies on drug safety, the reviewer for the *pegylated interferon beta-1a* stated that there was not any need for further studies on drug safety.

- *Subgroups.* The clinical trial design included subgroups taking the form of overseas study subjects. The reviewer rationalized the use of data from the overseas study subjects, that is, why data from these subjects were likely to be applicable to potential patients in the United States.
- *Dosing.* The reviewer noticed a trend in efficacy, as disclosed in one of the Kaplan–Meier plots, perceived that the plot indicated that a more frequent dose would have greater efficacy, and recommended further analysis of data on the more frequent dose.

d. Infectious Diseases, as Exemplified by Hepatitis C Virus

This is from FDA's review of *sofosbuvir*, a drug used for treating hepatitis C virus. The information is from NDA 204671, September 6, 2013 on the FDA's website.

1. Further Studies of HCV Genotype 3

The reviewer reiterated the established fact that hepatitis C virus occurs in various genotypes, and provided comments on two of these genotypes. Regarding genotype 2, the reviewer stated that the 12-week treatment for HCV genotype 2 is satisfactory, and that the Sponsor had no plans to change the package label's current writing about the 12-week treatment for HCV genotype 2. Regarding another genotype (HCV genotype 3), the reviewer stated that the Sponsor had agreed with FDA's recommendation to test longer duration treatment (16 weeks) of patients infected with HCV genotype 3.

2. Further Studies on Subgroup of Subjects With Renal Impairment

Regarding the subgroup of study subjects with renal impairment, the reviewer reiterated the fact that the Sponsor had agreed to design and conduct an additional clinical trial, on HCV-infected subjects with renal impairment.

3. Observations About Baseline Characteristics

The reviewer also provided a table of all of the baseline characteristics of the study subjects, for example, the genotype of the virus, whether the subject had cirrhosis, the baseline titer of the virus, and whether the subject had received prior treatment against the virus. Regarding the baseline characteristics, the reviewer stated that, "[t]here were no notable imbalances between the two treatment groups for the baseline characteristics."

4. Association of Adverse Events With Study Drug

In comments about adverse events, the reviewer stated that the adverse events were not likely related to the study drug. For example, regarding allergies (blotchy rash and difficulty in breathing), the reviewer stated that these adverse events occurred "several weeks after initiation of study drug." Also, the reviewer referred to "the resolution of the event with continuation of study drug." Regarding the adverse event of eczema and swelling of the legs, the reviewer pointed out that these adverse events occurred, "4 weeks after the completion of study treatment." Further criteria for assessing whether an adverse event was caused by a study drug are revealed, in this textbook, on the account of the Naranjo algorithm (144,145).

[144]Kane-Gill SL, et al. Comparison of three pharmacovigilance algorithms in the ICU setting: a retrospective and prospective evaluation of ADRs. Drug Saf. 2012;35:645–53.

[145]Son YM, et al. Causality assessment of cutaneous adverse drug reactions. Ann. Dermatol. 2011;23:432–8.

5. Drug–Drug Interactions Study and Need to Follow FDA's Guidance for Industry

This provides an example from the FDA's published reviews, of application of a conventional test used for gaining FDA approval (146,147). This is from the *Clinical Pharmacology and Biopharmaceutics Reviews*, occurring with the FDA's approval of NDA 204671, available on September 2013 of the FDA's website.

The FDA reviewer commented about the influence of the study drug, *sofosbuvir*, on the induction of cytochrome P450. The data submitted to the FDA were from a test that evaluated in vitro induction, by sofosbuvir, on cytochrome P450 in cultured human hepatocytes.

The goal was to assess whether sofosbuvir induced any of the cytochrome P450 enzymes, with the consequent increase in catabolism of other drugs by these enzymes. FDA's Guidance for Industry describes drug–drug interaction tests by way of cytochrome P450 assays, as cited (148,149,150).

The reviewer complained that, in conducting the cytochrome P450 tests, the Sponsor had failed to use any "predefined threshold," as is required by FDA's Guidance for Industry. The Guidance requires that, "[i]f the in vitro induction results are positive according to predefined thresholds … the investigational drug is considered an enzyme inducer" (151).

6. Pharmacokinetics Test and Blood Sampling Times

The reviewer also complained about the design of the pharmacokinetics tests, in particular, about the fact that the Sponsor had taken only a few blood samples over the course of time. The reviewer complained that:

> [i]t is recognized that due to the rapid half life of [sofosbuvir] … it is difficult to characterize the pharmacokinetics, especially given the sparse sampling schedule used in the … trials.

Because a sparse sampling schedule had been used, the reviewer rejected the Sponsor's conclusion that "HCV-infected subjects have a higher sofosbuvir explosure."

Please note that the goal of the pharmacokinetic studies was to determine bioavailability. Bioavailability, which refers to the extent and rate at which a drug enters the circulatory system, is a measure of the drug's access to its target and site of action. Bioavailability is generally assessed by a parameter known as area under the curve (AUC) (152). The EMA recommends

[146]Murayama N, et al. Human HepaRG cells can be cultured in hanging-drop plates for cytochrome P450 induction and function assays. Drug Metab. Lett. 2015 January 2015 [Epub ahead of print].

[147]Ke AB, et al. Expansion of a PBPK model to predict disposition in pregnant women of drugs cleared via multiple CYP enzymes, including CYP2B6, CYP2C9 and CYP2C19. Br. J. Clin. Pharmacol. 2014;77:554–70.

[148]U.S. Department of Health and Human Services. Food and Drug Administration Guidance for Industry. Drug metabolism/drug interaction studies in the drug development process: studies in vitro; April 1997 (10 pp.).

[149]U.S. Department of Health and Human Services. Food and Drug Administration Guidance for Industry. Drug Interaction Studies—Study Design, Data Analysis, Implication for Dosing, and Labeling Recommendations; February 2012 (75 pp.).

[150]Zhang L, et al. Predicting drug–drug interactions: an FDA perspective. AAPS J. 2009;11:300–6.

[151]U.S. Department of Health and Human Services. Food and Drug Administration Guidance for Industry. Drug Interaction Studies—Study Design, Data Analysis, Implication for Dosing, and Labeling Recommendations; February 2012 (p. 3 of 75 pp.).

[152]Beers MH, et al. The Merck manual of diagnostics and therapy. 18th ed. Rahway (NJ): The Merck Publishing Group; 1999. p. 2559–60.

that sampling be continued for at least 80% of the area under the curve (AUC) (153).

The following bulletpoints summarize FDA's comments for the antihepatitis C virus drug, sofosbuvir:

- *Longer duration tests on some study subjects.* The reviewer referred to the Sponsor's agreement to conduct a longer duration study of patients infected with HCV genotype 3.
- *Subgroup of subjects with renal impairment.* The reviewer referred to the Sponsor's agreement to design and conduct clinical studies on the possible influence of the study drug on subjects with impaired kidney function.
- *Baseline characteristics.* The reviewer agreed that the baseline characteristics in the various subgroups of study subjects were reasonably balanced.
- *Association of adverse events and study drug.* The reviewer provided reasons why the adverse events were not likely caused by the study drug.
- *In vitro drug−drug interaction tests.* The reviewer complained about the analysis of the results from the drug−drug interaction test, namely, that the analysis had failed to comply with the recommendations in the FDA's Guidance for Industry.

XXII. PROCESSES OF ADMINISTRING CLINICAL TRIALS

Dilts, Sandler, and coworkers (154,155,156) published a number of articles on the daunting task of administering a clinical trial. These authors describe the various concurrent timelines that need to be administered, and reveal how communications with regulatory agencies, ethics committees, and so on, fit into these timelines. In particular, these authors warn about a managerial problem called a circular mismatch loop. An example is where the Sponsor cannot collect information from an outside agency, unless the Sponsor first approves of the clinical trial—but where the Sponsor cannot approve of the trial, unless it first gets the information from the agency. Steensma (157) provides examples of circular mismatch in clinical trials, where changes in the Clinical Study Protocol, "can upset trial development homeostasis, creating endless loops or Catch-22s that then require special intervention to resolve. Committee A may need the approval of Committee B to move a protocol forward to Committee C, but Committee B may be silent because it is waiting on something from Committee A ... some protocols have been delayed because study sponsors are reluctant to sign contracts until IRBs approve the protocol, yet some IRBs have been hesitant to approve protocols until contract language is agreed."

---

[153]European Medicines Agency. Guideline on the investigation of bioequivalance; January 2010 (27 pp.).

[154]Dilts DM, Sandler AB. Invisible barriers to clinical trials: the impact of structural, infrastructural, and procedural barriers to opening oncology clinical trials. J. Clin. Oncol. 2006;24:4545−52.

[155]Dilts DM, Sandler AB, Cheng SK, et al. Steps and time to process clinical trials at the Cancer Therapy Evaluation Program. J. Clin. Oncol. 2009;27:1761−6.

[156]Dilts DM, Sandler A, Cheng S, et al. Development of clinical trials in a cooperative group setting: the eastern cooperative oncology group. Clin. Cancer Res. 2008;14:3427−33.

[157]Steensma DP. The ordinary miracle of cancer clinical trials. J. Clin. Oncol. 2009;27:1737−9.

a. Persons That Cooperate With Each Other

This lists most of the persons, offices, and agencies that need to cooperate with each other during a typical clinical trial:

- Principal investigators;
- Sponsor;
- Clinical trials office;
- Regulatory staff;
- Institutional Review Board;
- Scientific review committee;
- Contracts and grants office;
- Division chair;
- Department head;
- Core medical team;
- Secondary clinical research center;
- Compliance office;
- Director, medical affairs/oncology administration;
- Food and Drug Administration;
- Finance department;
- General hospital review board;
- Human subjects radiation committee;
- Institutional biosafety committee;
- Legal department;
- Medical ethics board;
- Office of sponsored research;
- Pharmacy;
- Radioactive drug research committee;
- Site coordinator.

b. Process of Medical Writing

Residing in the above list is the Sponsor, and a key employee of the Sponsor is the medical writer. The most important concept for the medical writer, as it applies to the process of medical writing, is ownership. Ownership refers to one aspect of the management for any given regulatory document. Typically, the medical writer is the owner, but a project manager or drug safety director can also be the owner. The owner maintains a computer file, for example, a document in MicroSoft® Word, which matures through several versions. At the start of the medical writing process, this document can take the form of a blank template, or it can take the form of an earlier version of the document, for example, as used for an earlier regulatory submission. Ownership is used only when people in addition to the medical writer contribute to the writing or editing of the document. For example, when a physician needs to contribute writing, the owner transmits a copy of the computer file to the physician, and the physician adds or deletes writing, where these changes are indicated in red or by a track changes device. When the physician is finished, she transmits the file back to the medical writer, and the medical writer copies all of the changes into the owned document. At the same time, the owner may transmit another copy of the file to a research director, and the research director will input changes, and then transmit the file back to the owner. In turn, the owner copies these changes into the owned document.

Ownership can be maintained manually, or by way of software programs known as Sharepoint® (158), Documentum® (159), FirstDoc® (160), Hummingbird® (161), or Livelink® (162).

It is possible for the principle of ownership to be violated, and when it is violated the result can be chaos. For example, the owner may transmit the document to a physician,

---

[158] MicroSoft Corp., Redmond (WA).

[159] EMC Corporation, Hopkinton (MA).

[160] Computer Sciences Corporation (CSC), Falls Church (VA).

[161] Hummingbird, Ltd, Toronto, Ontario, Canada.

[162] Open Text Corporation, Waterloo, Ontario, Canada.

who then inputs extensive changes to the document, with the presumption that his computer file will be submitted to the regulatory agency. When the physician completes his draft, he transmits it to the sponsor's director of regulatory affairs who, in turn, submits it to the FDA (163). But chaos results because the physician has failed to realize that, all along, the owner has been collecting additional changes and edits from personnel involved in manufacturing, statistics, basic research, and drug safety, and has been inputting these changes in the owner's copy of the document. Failure to observe strict ownership results in failure to input-needed changes and revisions.

c. Grammatical Issues

Where a pharmaceutical company does not have a writing style guide, the medical writer might consider creating one. In drafting a writing style guide, the medical writer should ensure that the content finds a consensus with other employees of the company. Typically, a company's style guide incorporates elements from the *American Medical Association's Manual of Style*, such as citation styles (164). The following provides a handful of examples of what might be included in a company's writing style guide.

1. Abbreviations

A potentially vexing stylistic issue is abbreviations. It has been recommended that the number of abbreviations used in any particular document be kept to a minimum, to prevent the document from resembling an alphabet soup (165). A related issue is whether it is appropriate for sentences to begin with an abbreviation, or if instead what is meant by the abbreviation should be spelled out (as actual words) at the beginning of the sentence.

2. Buried Verbs

A common problem is the use of buried verbs (166). A buried verb occurs where a verb is changed to a noun. An example is, "the drug will be administered at noon" (good writing) and "the drug administration will be at noon" (bad writing with buried verb). Another example is, "three subjects violated the clinical study protocol" (good writing) and "three subjects were in violation of the clinical study protocol" (bad writing with buried verb). Guffey and Loewy (167) provide several examples of buried verbs, and caution that their use, "increases sentence length, drains word strength, slows the reader, and muddies the thought." These authors provide the examples of: (1) "conduct a discussion of" (buried) and "discuss" (unburied); (2) "engage in the preparation of" (buried) and "prepare" (unburied), and (3) "reach a conclusion about" (buried) and "conclude" (unburied).

3. Zeugmas

The zeugma is another recurring problem. A zeugma occurs where a single verb, or a

---

[163] Hypothetical example.

[164] AMA Manual of Style. A guide for authors and editors. 10th ed. New York (NY): Oxford University Press; 2007.

[165] Wood LF, Foote MA. Targeted regulatory writing techniques. Clinical documents for drugs and biologics. Basel (Switzerland): Birkhäuser Verlag, 2009. p. 56.

[166] Garner BA. Advanced legal writing and editing. Dallas (TX): LawProse, Inc., 2002. p. 21–4.

[167] Guffey ME, Loewy D. Essentials of business communication. Mason (OH): South-Western Cengage Learning; 2013. p. 86–7.

single noun, applies to two different phrases (168,169,170). Examples of zeugmas where a single verb applies to two different phrases are as follows. Examples are, "He put out the light and the cat," "They covered themselves with dust and glory" (171), and "You can leave in a taxi. If you can't get a taxi, you can leave in a huff" (172). Another example of speech that is similar to a zeugma, from dialog in *Some Like it Hot* (173), is as follows. Businessman: "Do you play the market?" Woman: "No, the ukelele."

While zeugmas may be desired in literature because of their built-in ambiguity, ambiguity is not a virtue in medical writing or scientific writing. The following provides a concrete example of a zeugma from a scientific journal. The example is from an article on an anticancer drug (174):

> A compound that interferes with the activity of RNR leads to the inhibition of DNA synthesis and cell proliferation.

The sentence is ambiguous, in a manner similar to the drawing of an animal's head that can be either that of a duck or a rabbit (175). The ambiguity is:

1. Does the compound lead to the *inhibition* of DNA synthesis and also to the *inhibition* of cell proliferation?; or
2. Does the compound leads to the *inhibition* of DNA synthesis and also to the *stimulation* of cell proliferation?

A better version of the sentence is, "A compound that interferes with the activity of RNR leads to the inhibition of DNA synthesis and to the inhibition of cell proliferation." An alternative better version is, "A compound that interferes with the activity of RNR leads to the inhibition of both DNA synthesis and cell proliferation."

The same type of ambiguity is found in an article on Crohn's disease (176). The article reads:

> In a mouse model of intestinal fibrosis, blockade of IL-13Rα2 and TGF-β signalling reduced levels of colonic IGF-I and collagen deposition.

The sentence is ambiguous, as in the drawing of an animal's head that can be a duck or a

168Cruse A. Meaning in language: an introduction to semantics and pragmatics. 3rd ed. New York (NY): Oxford Univ. Press; 2011. p. 102−22.

169McGuigan B, Grudzina D, Moliken P. Rhetorical devices: a handbook and activities for student writers. Clayton (DE): Prestwick House, Inc.; 2007. p. 169−72.

170Wimsatt WK. The verbal icon: studies in the meaning of poetry. Lexington (KY): University Press of Kentucky; 1954. p. 178, 208, 288.

171Twain M. The adventures of Tom Sawyer. Knoxville (TN): Wordsworth Classics; 1876. p. 10.

172Sheekman A, Kalmar B, Ruby H, Perrin N. Duck Soup (Marx brothers film), Paramount Pictures; 1933.

173Wilder B, Diamond IAL, Logan M, Thoeren R. Some like it hot. MGM Studios; 1959.

174Hashemy SI, Ungerstedt JS, Zahedi Avval F, Holmgren A. Motexafin gadolinium, a tumor-selective drug targeting thioredoxin reductase and ribonucleotide reductase. J. Biol. Chem. 2006;281:10691−7.

175Wittgenstein L. Philosophical investigations. 4th ed. United Kingdom: John Wiley and Sons; 2009. p. 204.

176Bailey JR, et al. 1L-13 promotes collagen accumulation in Crohn's disease fibrosis by down-regulation of fibroblast MMP synthesis: a role for innate lymphoid cells? PLoS One 2012;7:e52332 (13 pp.).

rabbit (177). The ambiguous sentence can be interpreted in two different ways:

1. Was it the case that blockade of IL-13Rα2 reduced collagen deposition, and also the case that blockade of TGF-β signaling reduced collagen deposition?
2. Or was it the case that blockade of IL-13Rα2 reduced collagen deposition, and also the case that active TGF-β signaling reduced collagen deposition?

In other words, did the author really intend to write about a blockade that was a blockade of IL-13Rα2 and a type of signaling that was TGF-β signaling? Or was it the case that the author had actually intended to write about a blockade that was a blockade of IL-13Rα2 and about another type of blockade that was a blockade of, TGF-β signaling?

The ambiguity can be completely removed by using the same sentence where the word "of" is repeated, as indicated:

> In a mouse model of intestinal fibrosis, blockade of IL-13Rα2 and of TGF-β signalling reduced levels of colonic IGF-I and collagen deposition.

Alternatively, the ambiguity can be completely removed, by adding the word "both":

> In a mouse model of intestinal fibrosis, blockade of both IL-13Rα2 and TGF-β signalling reduced collagen deposition.

In medical writing, the goal of avoiding ambiguity is always more important than the goal of literary elegance.

4. Compound Nouns

Oxford Modern English Grammar (178) and other sources (179,180,181,182,183) recognize the fact that a compound noun can take the form of a *noun + noun* such as "city dweller," "window cleaner," and "city planner," a *noun + verb/noun* such as "fleabite" or "footstep," a *verb + noun* such as "blow torch" or "pay day," or a *noun + gerund* such as "walking stick." *The Chicago Manual of Style* (184) provides examples of compound nouns, such as "small animal hospital" where a noun modifies a noun. *The Chicago Manual of Style* also recognizes the fact that some compound nouns can be ambiguous, and

[177]Wittgenstein L. Philosophical investigations. 4th ed. United Kingdom: John Wiley and Sons; 2009. p. 204.

[178]Aarts B. Oxford modern english grammar. Oxford (UK): Oxford University Press; 2011. p. 34.

[179]Bauer L, Lieber R, Plag I. The oxford reference guide to english morphology. Oxford (UK): Oxford University Press; 2013. p. 625.

[180]Downing P. On the creation and use of English compound nouns. Language 53:810−42.

[181]Balyan R, Chatterjee N. Translating noun compounds using semantic relations. Comput. Speech Lang. 2015;32:91−108.

[182]Fleming IP. Analysis of the English language. London (UK): Longmans, Green, and Co; 1869. Giving example of walking stick. p. 22.

[183]Nakov PI. Using the web as an implicit training set: application to noun compound syntax and semantics. Technical Report No. UCB/ EECS-2007-173. University of California at Berkeley; 2007 (405 pp.).

[184]University of Chicago Press Staff. The Chicago manual of style. 16th ed. Chicago (IL): University of Chicago Press; 2010. p. 227.

recommends that "small animal hospital" be written as "small-animal hospital" (with a hyphen) in order to avoid the unintended meaning that the hospital is a small-sized facility. Regarding compound nouns in general, Plag (185) has stated that "[a] given noun–noun compound is in principle ambiguous and can receive very different interpretations depending on . . . the context."

In an essay on compound nouns, this author provides examples of compound nouns, such as "bee smoker," "primer sequence," and "topical composition" (186). Some compound nouns can be ambiguous. For example, is a "bee smoker" a machine that is used to direct smoke towards bees? Here, the word "smoker" is the object, and the word "bee" confines or dictates the function of the object. Or is a "bee smoker" a person who smokes powdered bees in a pipe? Similarly, Nakov (187) points out that the compound noun "French teacher" can mean either a person who teaches French, or a teacher who is French.

If a term to be used in a technical document is a compound noun that is entirely new, and if the context of the document does not provide examples or definitions, then ambiguity can result.

An example of an ambiguous compound noun from the scientific literature is the term, "sickle cell pain." The word "pain" is the object, and the term "sickle cell" confines and dictates the source of the pain. What is potentially ambiguous is whether this refers to pain that is felt by the red blood cell, or whether it refers to pain that is felt by a patient with sickle cell disease (where the pain arises from abnormalities in the red cells) (188). This author suggests that, where a medical writer needs to devise a new type of compound noun, such as "sickle cell pain," the medical writer should include a definition that removes all potential for ambiguity.

To give another example from the scientific literature, Nakov (189) commented on the compound noun, "tumor suppressor protein," and asked if this term unambiguously means, "protein acting as a tumor suppressor." Remarking on the frequent susceptibility of compound nouns for ambiguity, Nakov observed the "abundance of noun compounds – sequences of nouns acting as a single noun," and added that, "[w]hile eventually mastered by domain experts, their interpretation poses a major challenge for automated analysis." "Tumor suppressor protein" is potentially ambiguous, as

---

[185]Plag I. Word-formation in English. Cambridge textbooks in linguistics. Cambridge University Press; 2003. p. 148.

[186]Brody T. Functional elements in patent claims, as construed by the Board of Patent Appeals and Interferences. J. Marshall Rev. Intell. Prop. Law. 2014;13:251–320.

[187]Nakov PI. Using the web as an implicit training set: application to noun compound syntax and semantics. Technical report No. UCB/ EECS-2007-173. University of California at Berkeley; 2007 (405 pp.).

[188]This ambiguity was observed by the author's 8-year-old daughter, Dawnia, during the course of reading an article on sickle cell disease.

[189]Nakov PI. Using the web as an implicit training set: application to noun compound syntax and semantics. Technical report No. UCB/ EECS-2007-173. University of California at Berkeley; 2007 (405 pp.).

TABLE 33.4 Contrasting Formatting Styles Available for a Given Document

Version A	Alternative Format (version B)
US clinical studies are integrated together with clinical studies from Europe, China, and Russia, and are compared with each other in the same discussion section	US clinical studies are segregated apart from non-US clinical studies, and are discussed separately
A given nonclinical study report contains four different tests: genotoxicity, drug–drug interactions, albumin binding test, and PBMC activation test. The document uses *one heading (one title) to identify the summary* of these four tests	A given nonclinical study report contains four different tests: genotoxicity, drug–drug interactions, albumin binding test, and PBMC activation test. The document breaks up this study report into *four different summaries*, and uses four different headings
The document has only one list of references	The document has four separate lists of references: (1) Publications, (2) US preclinical study reports, and (3) Non-US preclinical study reports, and (4) Patents
The document describes studies with an excessive and inappropriate detail, for example, by identifying buffer concentrations, incubation temperatures, or needle gauges	The document describes studies with an appropriate amount of detail, and does not disclose buffer concentrations and other granular details, unless these details constitute points of novelty in the particular study
The writing style is clumsy and burdensome. For example, the beginning of every nonclinical narrative might begin with the following clumsy and uninformative phrase: "The goal of the following study was to determine the characteristics and physiological properties of the study drug."	The writing style is straightforward and free of mannerisms. Instead of writing, "The goal of the following study was to determine the characteristics and physiological properties of the study drug," what is used as a first sentence in the narrative is: "The pharmacokinetics of cisplatin was determined in dogs."
The document discloses all of the nonclinical studies by way of tables only, with short narratives of 2 or 3 sentences occurring in each cell of the table	The document discloses all of the nonclinical studies by way of 1-page written summaries, with no tables

follows. Although the correct meaning is, "protein acting as a tumor suppressor," it could also mean, "a suppressor protein found in tumors." This alternate meaning is reasonable, in view of the fact that some proteins are named after the type of cell where the protein is found. Example of protein names where the name includes a type of cell, are "muscle actin" and "lymphocyte actin" (190).

This is not to discourage use of compound nouns. Compound nouns are, almost by necessity, a part of medical and scientific writing. Without compound nouns, technical writing would become cumbersome, and would result in "sickle cell pain" being changed to the cumbersome "pain caused by sickle cells," "primer sequence" being changed to the cumbersome "nucleic acid sequence that is used for

[190]Rosenblatt HM, et al. Antibody to human lymphocyte actin regulates immunoglobulin secretion by an EBV-transformed human B-cell line. Biochem. Biophys. Res. Commun. 1986;140:399–405.

priming," and "topical composition" being changed to the cumbersome, "composition for topical application."

d. Formatting Issues

Another aspect of process is formatting. Typically, the source documents for a regulatory submission include earlier FDA-submissions, as well as published research articles. The earlier-filed FDA-submissions are likely to use different types of formatting. Failure of the medical writer to anticipate these types of formatting will lead to delays in the medical writing process.

Table 33.4 documents how formatting can vary, from document to document. The problem of this variability, and the consequent confusion, can be avoided by using a company writing style guide. The table illustrates various formatting issues (191) that can impede the process of regulatory submission. The medical writer should confer with management to choose the preferred styles from the following table, that is, the style shown in Version A versus Version B.

The CONSORT Statement (192) provides guidance on formatting, and ensuring that all of the relevant topics are included in a given document. The medical writer needs to ensure that the subject matter is adequately disclosed. The CONSORT Statement provides guidance on the nature of a complete disclosure. This Statement is the product of a group which describes itself as, "an international and eclectic group, comprising trialists, methodologists and medical journal editors" (193). This statement provides a 25-item checklist which includes: title; abstract; trial design; inclusion criteria; how sample size (number of subjects) was determined; methods for blinding, allocation, and allocation concealment; baseline demographic data; dates of recruitment and follow-up; the registration number of the trial; and sources of funding. The CONSORT Statement also recommends including a flow chart that tracks the number of study subjects, as they move from enrollment, through the treatment phase, and on through follow-up. This type of flow chart is not the same as the study schema. As mentioned earlier in this

---

[191] All of these are real examples from the author's work in preparing regulatory submissions to the FDA.

[192] Schulz KF, Altman DG, Moher D; CONSORT Group. CONSORT 2010 statement: updated guidelines for reporting parallel group randomised trials. PLoS Med. 2010;7:e1000251.

[193] www.consort-statement.org (quotation acquired on February 27, 2011).

textbook, flow charts of the same type, which identify the number of subjects in the ITT group, modified ITT group, and per protocol group, occur in many published clinical trials, as cited (194,195,196,197,198,199,200,201,202, 203,204,205,206,207).

[194]Chiasson JL, Josse RG, Gomis R, Hanefeld M, Karasik A, Laakso M. Acarbose treatment and the risk of cardiovascular disease and hypertension in patients with impaired glucose tolerance: the STOP-NIDDM trial. J. Am. Med. Assoc. 2003;290:486—94.

[195]Emery P, Fleischmann RM, Moreland LW, et al. Golimumab, a human anti-tumor necrosis factor alpha monoclonal antibody, injected subcutaneously every four weeks in methotrexate-naive patients with active rheumatoid arthritis: twenty-four-week results of a phase III, multicenter, randomized, double-blind, placebo-controlled study of golimumab before methotrexate as first-line therapy for early-onset rheumatoid arthritis. Arthritis Rheum. 2009;60:2272—83.

[196]Hesketh PJ, Grunberg SM, Gralla RJ, et al. The oral neurokinin-1 antagonist aprepitant for the prevention of chemotherapy-induced nausea and vomiting: a multinational, randomized, double-blind, placebo-controlled trial in patients receiving high-dose cisplatin—the Aprepitant Protocol 052 Study Group. J. Clin. Oncol. 2003;21:4112—9.

[197]Manegold C, Gravenor D, Woytowitz D, et al. Randomized phase II trial of a toll-like receptor 9 agonist oligodeoxynucleotide, PF-3512676, in combination with first-line taxane plus platinum chemotherapy for advanced-stage non-small-cell lung cancer. J. Clin. Oncol. 2008;26:3979—86.

[198]Rijnders BJ, Van Wijngaerden E, Vandecasteele SJ, Stas M, Peetermans WE. Treatment of long-term intravascular catheter-related bacteraemia with antibiotic lock: randomized, placebo-controlled trial. J. Antimicrob. Chemother. 2005;55:90—4.

[199]Strasser F, Demmer R, Böhme C, et al. Prevention of docetaxel- or paclitaxel-associated taste alterations in cancer patients with oral glutamine: a randomized, placebo-controlled, double-blind study. Oncologist. 2008;13:337—46.

[200]Waltzman R, Croot C, Justice GR, Fesen MR, Charu V, Williams D. Randomized comparison of epoetin alfa (40,000 U weekly) and darbepoetin alfa (200 microg every 2 weeks) in anemic patients with cancer receiving chemotherapy. Oncologist. 2005;10:642—50.

[201]Warr DG, Hesketh PJ, Gralla RJ, et al. Efficacy and tolerability of aprepitant for the prevention of chemotherapy-induced nausea and vomiting in patients with breast cancer after moderately emetogenic chemotherapy. J. Clin. Oncol. 2005;23:2822—30.

[202]Cohen JA, Barkhof F, Comi G, et al. Oral fingolimod or intramuscular interferon for relapsing multiple sclerosis. N. Engl. J. Med. 2010;362:402—15.

[203]Haldar P, Brightling CE, Hargadon B, et al. Mepolizumab and exacerbations of refractory eosinophilic asthma. N. Engl. J. Med. 2009;360:973—84.

[204]Jonas MM, Mizerski J, Badia IB, et al. Clinical trial of lamivudine in children with chronic hepatitis B. N. Engl. J. Med. 2002;346:1706—13.

[205]Shiffman ML, Suter F, Bacon BR, et al. Peginterferon alfa-2a and ribavirin for 16 or 24 weeks in HCV genotype 2 or 3. N. Engl. J. Med. 2007;357:124—34.

[206]Leroy O, Saux P, Bédos JP, Caulin E. Comparison of levofloxacin and cefotaxime combined with ofloxacin for ICU patients with community-acquired pneumonia who do not require vasopressors. Chest. 2005;128:172—83.

[207]Kreijkamp-Kaspers S, Kok L, Grobbee DE, et al. Effect of soy protein containing isoflavones on cognitive function, bone mineral density, and plasma lipids in postmenopausal women: a randomized controlled trial. J. Am. Med. Assoc. 2004;292:65—74.

34

Patents

I. INTRODUCTION

Patents provide a monopoly for a limited period of time, where this monopoly gives the patent owner the right to prevent other parties from making, using, or selling what is claimed. During the time that this monopoly is in effect the patent owner can take legal action to prevent other parties from making, using, or selling the composition, device, or method that is described by the claims. The goals of the patent owner in acquiring a patent include recouping the investment costs needed to research and develop the invention, ensuring eventual profit, and using the patent as a tool for raising investment funds. The main purpose of the patent system is to encourage commercial development, while a secondary purpose is to reward the inventor (1). The main intersection between Food and Drug Administration (FDA) regulations and patent law is as follows. By following FDA regulations, a Sponsor can obtain permission to conduct a clinical trial and, eventually, acquire permission for marketing the tested drugs. By engaging in patenting,

the Sponsor can use its patent applications as a tool for raising funding, and to prevent competitors from copying its drug. In other words, without a patent in place, a Sponsor will not likely be able to recover the expenses needed to develop the drug and to conduct the clinical trial. The same information (nonclinical results; clinical results) that is submitted to FDA can be submitted in patent applications.

II. SERVICES PROVIDED BY THE PATENT ATTORNEY OR AGENT

Management, researchers, and engineers work with their patent attorney or patent agent in performing various tasks. For every patent application, it is customary for the patent attorney or agent to perform each of the following tasks:

- Review the invention disclosure;
- Draft the specification;
- Draft the claims;
- Prior art search;
- Validity analysis;

[1]Walterscheid EC. To promote the progress of useful arts: American patent law and administration 1798–1836. Littleton (CO): Rothman & Co.; 1999. p. 281–282, 321.

829

- Freedom to operate (FTO) analysis;
- Prosecution.

a. The Invention Disclosure

Researchers provide the patent attorney or agent with experimental data, such as from cell culture assays, gene expression assays, animal model studies and, on occasion, from clinical studies. At the time that a reasonable drug candidate is first identified, for example, through screening of a library of candidate drugs, through synthetic organic chemistry, or by way of genetic engineering, laboratory experiments are initiated to establish the efficacy of the drug candidate. Efficacy of the drug through in vitro and in vivo studies is best established where some aspect of the in vitro or in vivo study tracks one or more physiological mechanisms in humans (2). It is typical to file a patent application as soon as enough evidence is available to support an argument that the drug is likely to have a real-world use. The term "file" means to submit or to mail a patent application to the United States Patent and Trademark Office (USPTO). For patents on drugs, what is typically claimed is the drug, formulations of the drug, methods for administering the drug to a mammalian subject, methods for manufacturing the drug, and methods for assessing the efficacy and safety of the drug in the mammalian subject.

b. Specification

Patent applications include a specification and set of claims, as well as formal paperwork, such as the Oath. The content of the specification is similar to that of a typical scientific or medical manuscript, with some exceptions. For example, the specification should refrain from admitting that the ideas for the invention were inspired by publications from other researchers. Also, unlike scientific publications, it is acceptable for the specification to include only prophetic examples of the invention and no working examples of the invention.

It is to the advantage of the inventors for the specification to include working examples with laboratory data, and even more preferable to include a family of related experiments. For example, where the goal is to patent an anticancer drug, it is better to include tests showing efficacy with three different types of cultured cancer cell lines, instead of with just one cancer cell line.

c. Claims

The claims define what the invention is. A useful adage to remember, is that, "the name of the game is the claim" (3,4). It would rarely be the case that an employee would be capable of writing claims, unless that employee was a patent attorney or registered patent agent. Claims include phrases that are referred to by way of specific legal terms, such as "functional elements"

---

[2]Brody T. Enabling claims under 35 USC §112 to methods of medical treatment or diagnosis, based on in vitro cell culture models and animal models. J. Pat. Trademark Off. Soc. 2015;97:328−411.

[3]In re Hiniker Co., 150 F.3d 1362, 1369 (Fed. Cir. 1998).

[4]Hilton Davis Chemical Co. v. Warner-Jenkinson Co., Inc. 62 F.3d 1512 (1995).

(5,6), "negative limitations" (7), and "claim differentiation" (8). Thus, it is not likely that any employee not having a patent bar number could draft a reasonable set of patent claims. However, it is to the company's advantage that management and lab research employees be able to read, understand, and evaluate the scope of a set of claims.

d. Prior Art

The patent attorney, often in collaboration with company personnel, searches for scientific and medical publications, patents, and published patent applications, for possible disclosures of compositions, devices, and methods, that are relevant to the invention. All company personnel have the duty to disclose relevant publications to their patent attorney or agent, who in turn has the duty to disclose these to the Patent Office (9). The term "prior art" refers to documents that disclose compositions, devices, and methods, that appear to be exactly the same as the invention, that are merely similar to the invention, or that provide background information on how to synthesize or build the invention. The term "prior art" refers to documents, as well as other types of disclosures, that were made available to the public up until the date of filing the patent application with the Patent Office. "Prior art" does not encompass documents or other types of disclosures that

were made available to the public in the timeframe after the date of submitting the patent application to the Patent Office. Generally, company employees and their attorneys should refrain from characterizing publications and patent documents as "prior art," and instead should just call them "references."

e. Validity Analysis

Validity analysis compares the prior art with the claims. The patent attorney or agent compares what is disclosed with the prior art with what is encompassed by the claim set, and drafts an analysis that evaluates whether the compositions, devices, and methods that are described in the prior art are identical to or are similar to what is encompassed by the claims. The results of the validity analysis can predict whether the patent examiner will reject the claims. The validity analysis also guides the patent attorney or agent in drafting the claims. This means that the claims are drafted in a way that avoids the invalidating influences of the prior art.

f. Freedom To Operate Analysis

Freedom to operate (FTO) analysis compares the claims of patents that are owned by competitors, with the composition, device, or method, that a company intends to make, use, and sell. In short, FTO analysis determines whether a

---

[5]Brody T. Functional elements in patent claims, as construed by the Board of Patent Appeals and Interferences. John Marshall Rev. Intel. Prop. Law 2014;13:251–320. Please note that, "Spring 2015 meeting of American Intellectual Property Law Association (AIPLA)" (15 p) included the comment,"[a]n excellent review on PTAB treatment of functional claiming is: Tom Brody, Functional Elements in Patent Claims as Construed by the Patent Trial and Appeal Board (PTAB), 13 J. Marshall Rev. Intel. Prop. Law 251(2014).

[6]Brody T. Functional elements can ensure allowance of genus claims. J. Pat. Trademark Off. Soc. 2008;90 (9):621–56. Cited by American Intellectual Property Law Association (AIPLA) in Amicus Brief of March 3, 2014, for U.S. Supreme Court case, Nautilus v. Biosig.

[7]Brody T. Negative claim limitations in patent claims. AIPLA Q. Rev. 2013;41:29–72.

[8]Lemley MA. The limits of claim differentiation. Berkeley Tech. Law J. 2008;22:1389–401.

[9]Brody T. Duty to disclose: Dayco Products v. total containment. John Marshall Law School Rev. Intel. Prop. Law. 2008;7:325–75.

company's proposed product is likely to infringe a competitor's claims. If the FTO analysis reveals that a competitor has claims that encompass the company's composition, device, or method, the company may choose to license the competitor's patent or, alternatively, decide to refrain from making and selling the composition, device, or method. Also, if the FTO analysis reveals that the competitor's patent has already expired, or that it will expire within a few months, then the company may decide to move forward and make and sell its composition, device, or method.

g. Prosecution

After the patent application is submitted to the Patent Office, the patent examiner responds by writing a rejection and mailing it to the company. The patent attorney or agent reviews the rejection, and responds by drafting a rebuttal argument, and by submitting the rebuttal to the Patent Office. Rejections are based on a statute that is called "anticipation" (35 USC §102), which means that there is a one-to-one correspondence between what is in one particular prior art reference and what is in the rejected claim. Rejections are also based on a statute that is called "obviousness" (35 USC §103), which usually means that the combination of two prior art references renders obvious what is in the rejected claim. Guidance on rebutting obviousness rejections is available (10).

It is to the company's advantage that management read the rejections, and provide ideas for rebuttal arguments. The goal of the prosecution phase of all patent applications is to gain allowance of one or more claims. Generally, about 2% of biotechnology claims and about 5% of mechanical device claims are allowed on the first Office Action, that is, allowed by the patent examiner without any rejections (11). The term "prosecution" refers to the sum of the submitted specification and claims, the rejections, the rebuttal arguments, and the eventual Notice of Allowance, that is involved in a particular patent application.

III. HISTORY OF PATENTING

Patents originated in the city-state of Venice in 1474 (12). Modern patent law originated in England in 1623 in an Act of Parliament called *The Statute of Monopolies*. This Statute did away with the earlier practice, where patents were used as a form of patronage to reward the favored subjects of the crown (13). What is notable is that this statute set the patent term at 14 years. In present day US patent law, design patents have a term of 14 years, while patents on devices, machines, compositions of matter (chemicals), and methods, have a term of 20 years. Nicolas (14) details the early case law of patents in England. Walterscheid (15)

---

[10]Brody T. Rebutting obviousness rejections based on impermissible hindsight. J. Pat. Trademark Off. Soc. 2014;96:366−424. For this article, the author won the 2016 *Rossman Memorial Award* ($1,500) from the Patent and Trademark Office Society.

[11]Determined by this author, during a survey of 300 issued patents in biotechnology and in mechanical devices. The survey was conducted during the preparation of Brody T. Obviousness in patents following the U.S. Supreme Court's decision of KSR International Co. v. Teleflex, Inc. J. Pat. Trademark Off. Soc. 2010;92:26−70.

[12]Nard CA, Morriss AP. Constitutionalizing patents. Rev. Law Econ. 2004;2 (70 p).

[13]Glenn MA, Nagle PJ. Article I and the first inventor to file: patent reform or doublespeak? Idea 2010;50:441−62.

[14]Nicolas V. The law and practice relating to letters patent for inventors. London (United Kingdom): Butterworth & Co.; 1904. (307 p).

[15]Walterscheid EC. To promote the progress of useful arts: American patent law and administration 1798−1836. Littleton (CO): Rothman & Co.; 1998. p. 281−282, 321.

describes the early history of patent law in the United States.

Of general interest is the fact that Abraham Lincoln is the inventor for U.S. Pat. No. 6,469, entitled *Manner of Buoying Vessels*. Lincoln's patent issued in May 1849. Also of interest is US Pat. No. 141,072, entitled *Manufacture of Beer and Yeast*, which issued to Louis Pasteur in May 1873 (16). Pasteur's patent is notable by the fact that it claims a form of life, a concept that has recently sparked controversy (17). The most important of the older patents include those of Alexander Graham Bell, such as US Pat. No. 174,465, which issued in March 1876, and US Pat. No. 186,787, which issued on January 1877. The controversy surrounding these patents continues to be relevant today, as is evident from a decision from the US Supreme Court in 2010 (18). In part, the controversy surrounding Mr Bell's patents stemmed from evidence that Mr Bell had misappropriated one of his ideas from another prominent inventor, Elisha Gray (19). Also of general interest is Lawrence Page's US Pat. No. 6,285,999, issued in September, 2001, which helped establish *Google, Inc.* A number of articles on techniques for drafting and interpreting claims is available (20,21,22,23,24,25).

Because it is the case that the *name of the game is the claim*, the claims from Louis Pasteur's patent are reproduced:

Claim 1: The method of obtaining pure yeast by eliminating the organic germs of disease from brewer's yeast, in the manner described.

Claim 2: Yeast, free from organic germs of diseases, as an article of manufacture.

Claim 1 is a methods claim. Where an inventor or a company owns this patent, and where a competitor prepares a pure yeast by the method described in Pasteur's claim, ownership of the patent provides the owner with a legal basis to sue the competitor. Claim 2 is a composition of matter claim. Where a company owns this patent, and where a competitor makes, sells, or uses the yeast that is described in Pasteur's claim, this ownership provides a legal basis for the owner to sue the competitor.

All patents have an expiration date. Once a patent expires, any party is free to make, use, or sell the invention that is described by the

[16]Federico PJ. Louis Pasteur's patents. Science 1937;86:327.

[17]Diamond v. Chakrabarty, 447 U.S. 303 (1980).

[18]Bilski v. Kappos, 130 S. Ct. 3218 (2010).

[19]Evenson AE. The telephone patent controversy of 1876. Jefferson (NC): McFarland & Co., Inc.; 2000 (259 p).

[20]Brody T. Obviousness in patents following the U.S. Supreme Court's decision of KSR International Co. v. Teleflex, Inc. J. Pat. Trademark Off. Soc. 2010;92:26−70.

[21]Brody T. Functional elements can ensure allowance of genus claims. J. Pat. Trademark Off. Soc. 2008;90:621−56.

[22]Brody T. Preferred embodiments in patents. John Marshall Rev. Intel. Prop. Law. 2009;9:398−452.

[23]Brody T. Claim construction using contexts of implication. Virginia J. Law Technol. 2008;13(1):28.

[24]Brody T. Enabling claims under 35 USC §112 to methods of medical treatment or diagnosis, based on in vitro cell culture models and animal models. J. Pat. Trademark Off. Soc. 2015;97:328−411.

[25]Brody T. Negative claim limitations in patent claims. AIPLA Q. Rev. 2013;41:29−72.

claims of the expired patent, without fear of being sued. The following is a word of caution. Any person interested in making, using, or selling, an invention described in an expired patent needs to make certain that no other patent, that is, no other *nonexpired* patent, claims the same or similar activities.

This is a disclaimer. The present writing does not constitute legal advice, and it does not establish any relationship between the reader and the author. A goal of the present writing is to facilitate communication between researchers in pharmaceutical companies and their patent attorneys or patent agents. The opinions set forth herein do not necessarily reflect the opinions of the author's past, present, or future employers.

IV. OUTLINE OF THE PATENTING PROCESS

Patents are organized in the following sections:

- A first page containing names of the inventors, title of the invention, the patent's serial number, and assignee;
- A background section;
- An examples section;
- The claims;
- Drawings and figures.

The combination of the first page, background, examples, and figures, is called the "specification." A patent may or may not have an assignee. Where there is no assignee, the inventors are the default owners of the patent. Where there is an assignee, the assignee owns the patent.

After a patent application is submitted to the Patent Office, the application is reviewed by a patent examiner. Typically, patent applications in mechanical engineering and electrical engineering are reviewed by examiners with only undergraduate degrees, while patent applications in the fields of chemistry or biology are reviewed by examiners with doctorate degrees. The examiner reviews the claims from the standpoint of the ordinary skilled artisan. In doing this, the examiner determines whether the background section of the patent, the examples section of the patent, and the knowledge generally possessed by the skilled artisan, provide enough information to enable the skilled artisan to make and use what is described in each claim.

The routine of the patent examiner is to evaluate the claims, and to determine whether the claims are supported by what is in the working examples. Here, the examiner determines whether the claims satisfy the requirement for enablement (35 USC §112). The examiner also determines whether the invention described by the claims had already been described in earlier publications. Here, the examiner determines whether the claims satisfy the requirement that what is claimed be new. This requirement for being new (or novel) is evaluated from two standpoints, namely, anticipation (35 USC §102) and obviousness (35 USC §103). A rejection for anticipation is called a *102-rejection*, while a rejection for obviousness is called a *103-rejection*.

Where a claim is rejected for anticipation, it means that all of elements in the rejected claim have a one-to-one correspondence with elements that are found in one prior art document. Where a claim is rejected for obviousness, it means that all of the elements in the rejected claim can be found in a combination of two or more prior art documents.

In rebutting the rejection, the attorney typically argues that the examiner had made a mistake. The following example concerns a claim to a chemical having a methyl group. The mistake might be that what the examiner thought was a methyl group in a prior art chemical structure was actually a propyl group. Or it could be a mistake where the examiner had overlooked the fact that none of the prior art documents disclosed any methyl group. Rebuttal arguments that point out mistakes of this type are the most common type of rebuttal argument used against rejections for anticipation or obviousness. Obviousness rejections are distinguished, in that the examiner is required to include a "rationale" for combining the prior art references. The most important courtroom case that sets forth this requirement is, In re Kahn (26). Where an examiner imposes an obviousness rejection, but fails to include a "rationale" in this rejection, it is conventional to refer to the examiner's reasoning as involving "impermissible hindsight" or "hindsight reconstruction." One technique for rebutting obviousness rejections, is to argue that the examiner had failed to articulate the required "rationale." This rebuttal approach has been described in detail (27).

Rebuttals also take the following form. Often the attorney argues that the date the inventor's patent was submitted to the Patent Office was earlier than the date of the prior art publication. Where the date of the inventor's patent is earlier than the date of the so-called prior art publication, the publication cannot be used as a basis for a 102-rejection or a 103-rejection. This rebuttal can take the form "Applicant submits that the patent application has a filing date that is before the publication date of the cited prior art publication, and respectfully requests withdrawal of the rejection."

Once the patent application is submitted, the inventor is not permitted to make corrections or changes to the writing, aside from correcting typographical errors. The inventor is not permitted to add more working examples. This is the prohibition against adding new matter (35 USC §132). If it is essential to provide new laboratory data to an examiner, for example, to make a stronger rebuttal argument, this is routinely and conventionally done by way of a Declaration, where the Declaration is filed with the Patent Office. But new data, as might be submitted via a Declaration, cannot become part of the writing in the specification and cannot become part of the writing in the claim set.

The standard of enablement required for patenting is only that the information be convincing to the skilled artisan, and not that the information be conclusive to the skilled artisan (28). In this way, the standard for all patents is less than the standard that is used for prestigious medical and scientific journals. In fact, the case law establishes that a reasonable amount of experimentation is permitted in order to make up for deficiencies in the guidance that is provided by the patent (29). Typically, these acceptable deficiencies take the form of failure to identify common reagents, failure to identify commercial suppliers of reagents, and failure to identify what is the preferred reagent (30).

[26]In re Kahn.441 F.3d 977 (Fed. Cir. 2006).

[27]Brody T. Rebutting obviousness rejections based on impermissible hindsight. J. Pat. Trademark Off. Soc. 2014;96:366—424.

[28]United States Patent and Trademark Office. Manual of Patent Examining Procedure (Rev. 6, Sept. 2007) Section 2164.05, p. 2100-199.

[29]United States Patent and Trademark Office. Manual of Patent Examining Procedure (Rev. 6, Sept. 2007) Section 2164.06, p. 2100—201.

[30]Brody T. Preferred embodiments in patents. John Marshall Rev. Intel. Prop. Law. 2009;9:398—452.

V. TYPES OF PATENT DOCUMENTS

Patent documents include published patent applications and patents. A published patent application is a patent application that has been filed (submitted; mailed) with the Patent Office, where the application is subsequently published. Publication of patent applications occurs about 18 months after the filing date.

Published patent applications also include those filed under the Patent Cooperation Treaty (PCT) (31). PCT patent applications are administered by the World Intellectual Property Organization (WIPO), which is located in Geneva, Switzerland. Although WIPO is located in Switzerland, WIPO provides a convenient office in the United States, as an address for US inventors to file patent applications. PCT patent applications are published about 18 months after the filing date. PCT patent applications never mature into issued patents. Instead, additional paperwork and fees are required, resulting in the broadcast of the PCT application to patent offices throughout the world, for example, offices in the United States, Japan, India, China, and a European regional office. After broadcast to these offices, the patent applications are examined and eventually issued.

When made available to the public, patents and patent applications can be found at the websites www.uspto.gov and www.epo.org.

After a patent application is submitted to the Patent Office, the only corrections that are permitted in the specification are corrections of typographical errors. Inventors are not permitted to add new data or new examples to their patent application. Actually, new data can be added, but this requires the filing of a patent application called a Continuation-in-Part (CIP) (32,33). The CIP application claims priority on the filing date of the original, earlier patent application, as well as the filing date of the CIP application. Patent examining focuses almost exclusively on the claims, not so much on the quality or integrity of the experimental data. During examination, the claims are almost always re-written to make them narrower in scope. The main reason to amend the claims to make them narrower in scope is to avoid the invalidating influence of prior art publications that were cited by the examiner in the rejections.

When published, a US patent application will have a publication number, for example, US 2006/135786. The inventors of this particular patent application are Saha, Kavarana, Evindar, Satz, and Morgan. The title of the invention is, *Methods and compositions for modulating sphingosine-1-phosphate (S1P) receptor activity*. The publication date of the published patent application is June 22, 2006. The patent concerns a drug used for treating multiple sclerosis.

After a US patent application is reviewed by the patent examiner, and after one or more claims are allowed, the examiner mails a paper called *Notice of Allowance and Fees Due* to the inventor, where this *Notice* provides a list of the allowed claims. Shortly thereafter, the examiner will mail another paper called *Issue Notification*, which bears the number of the actual issued patent (not the number of the published patent application).

The above patent application was examined, allowed by the examiner, and eventually issued by the Patent Office. When it was issued, it was given the patent number, US 7,241,812. As was the case with the published patent application, the inventors listed on the issued patent are

---

[31]United States Patent and Trademark Office. Manual of Patent Examining Procedure (Rev. 7, Sept. 2008) Chapter 1800 Patent Cooperation Treaty, p. 1800-1 to 1800-220.

[32]37 CFR §1.53.

[33]Manual of Patent Examining Procedure (MPEP), 9th ed., March 2014. §201.08.

Saha, Kavarana, Evindar, Satz, and Morgan. The title was the same, namely, *Methods and compositions for modulating S1P receptor activity*. And the issue date is July 10, 2007.

The inventors had filed the same application as a PCT application, and the corresponding published PCT application has the serial number WO2006020951. The inventors are Saha, Kavarana, Evindar, Satz, and Morgan. The title is *Methods and compositions for modulating sphingosine-1-phosphate (S1P) receptor activity*. And the publication date is, February 23, 2006. This date is a few months before the publication date (June 22, 2006) of the corresponding US application.

Thus, any person reading patents should be aware of the following three formats for many patents, that is, the published US patent application, the issued US patent, and the published PCT patent application. It is often the case that the laboratory data in these three documents are identical. But it is rarely the case that the claims in all three documents are identical.

VI. ORGANIZATION OF INFORMATION IN A PATENT

Patents begin with one or more pages of formal information, including the names of the inventors, the title of the invention, the serial number, the filing date, and the date of issue.

The formal information is followed by a lengthy background section, which serves to orient the patent examiner in the field of the invention, as well as to describe special assay methods, manufacturing methods, commercial suppliers, and prophetic examples. Prophetic examples are usually called "prophetic embodiments." The background section is also used to assess the meaning of terms in the claims,

for example, where a word in the claims is ambiguous or unclear.

After the background section, patents contain an examples section. Typically, these examples are working examples, but they may also include examples that are purely prophetic. Prophetic examples can be included for a number of reasons. First, the inventors did not have enough time to complete, or even initiate, any of the relevant experiments before the patent application was filed. Second, the inventors may have included one or more prophetic examples, in order to ensure that the combination of the working examples and the prophetic examples supported, and corresponded to, the genus of compositions that is encompassed by the claims.

The following shows the first page of a patent, namely, US Pat. No. 6,084,100. The inventors are Stampa, Camps, Rodriguez, Bosch, and Onrubia. The assignee is a company called *Medichem*. The issue date is July 4, 2000. The filing date is April 13, 1998. The serial number is US Ser. No. 09/058,837. The Abstract occurs on the right-hand column of the first page. The abstract contains writing, as well as a diagram of a molecule (Fig. 34.1).

a. The Claims

To provide an example of claims, the following shows the claims from two patents. These particular patents were chosen because the patents were the subject of a lawsuit, and because the courtroom opinion provides information useful to pharmaceutical companies. The term "opinion" refers to the write-up of the case that was penned by one of the judges hearing the case. The name of the lawsuit was *Medichem v. Rolabo* (34). The lawsuit concerned

[34]Medichem v. Rolabo 437 F.3d 1157 (Fed. Cir. 2006).

US006084100A

United States Patent [19]

Stampa et al.

[11] **Patent Number:** 6,084,100

[45] **Date of Patent:** Jul. 4, 2000

[54] **PROCESS FOR THE PREPARATION OF LORATADINE**

[75] Inventors: **Alberto Stampa; Pelayo Camps**, both of Barcelona; **Gloria Rodriguez; Jordi Bosch**, both of Girona; **Maria del Carmen Onrubia**, Barcelona, all of Spain

[73] Assignee: **Medichem, S.A.**, Barcelona, Spain

[21] Appl. No.: 09/058,837

[22] Filed: **Apr. 13, 1998**

Related U.S. Application Data

[60] Provisional application No. 60/048,083, May 30, 1997.

[51] **Int. Cl.⁷** **C07D 221/06**
[52] **U.S. Cl.** **546/93**
[58] **Field of Search** 546/93

Primary Examiner—Dwayne C. Jones
Attorney, Agent, or Firm—Scully, Scott, Murphy & Presser

[57] **ABSTRACT**

The process consists of the reductive coupling between the compounds: 8-chloro-5,6-dihydrobenzo[5,6]cyclohepta[1, 2-b]pyridin-11-one (formula VII)

VII

and ethyl 4-oxopiperidine-1-carboxylate (formula IV)

IV

through the action of low-valent titanium species.

13 Claims, No Drawings

FIGURE 34.1 First page of US Pat. No. 6,084,100. The first page of patents contains the serial number of the issued patent, the date of issue, the title of the invention, and the list of inventors. An earlier date is also listed, namely, the date that the patent application was submitted, and the serial number of the patent application. The abstract of this patent is unusual, in that it includes a picture of a molecule.

two patents, namely, US Pat. No. 6,084,100 of Medichem and US Pat. No. 6,093,827 of Rolabo.

Rolabo's claims were broad and covered a "genus" of chemicals. Medichem's claims were relatively narrow, and covered only a chemical "species." The claims of both patents covered *loratidine*. Loratidine is commonly known by the brand name, Claritin®. Regarding the claims, Medichem's claim 1 reads as follows:

> Claim 1. A process for the preparation of loratidine consisting of reacting, in an organic solvent and in the presence of a tertiary amine, 8-chloro-5,6 dihydrobenzo[5,6]cyclohepta[1,2-b]pyridine-11-one...

Medichem's claim 1 is a *species claim*. The claim contains the name of a specific chemical, that is, *loratidine*.

Rolabo's claim1 is as follows:

> Claim 1. A process for preparing 5,6-dihydro-11H-dibenzo[a,d]cyclohept-11-enes comprising reacting a dibenzosuberone or an aza derivative

thereof with an aliphatic ketone in the presence of low valent titanium wherein said low valent titanium is generated by zinc.

Rolabo's claim 1 is a *genus claim*, as it covers a *family of related compounds* called, 5,6-dihydro-11H-dibenzo[a,d]cyclohept-11-enes. Loratidine is a member of this family of related compounds.

Generally, it is to the advantage of the inventor for the claims to be as broad as possible, and to encompass a genus. However, because of its breadth, a genus claim may fall under the invalidating influence of the prior art. Hence, when a patent application is first submitted, it is to the company's advantage to submit a claim set that includes a genus claim and also another claim that is a species claim. In addition, the specification should include a "bank" of written descriptions that correspond to claims of various claim breadths. This bank serves as a reservoir, for use in importing corresponding broader or narrower claims into the claim set, during the prosecution phase of the patent.

VII. TIME-LINE FOR PATENTING

A typical time-line for patenting a new invention is as follows.

1. During a weekly meeting of the company's research director and four lab bench researchers, Jose Vazquez (35) (one of the lab bench researchers) proposes to test a newly synthesized compound (curitol) on a newly available animal model for multiple sclerosis. The novel compound has the properties of low toxicity and a long lifetime in the bloodstream. A second lab bench researcher, Mai Fong (36), suggests administering the curitol by way of a well-known timed-release formulation. At this point, the issue of inventorship may be raised. Dr Vazquez is an inventor and should be listed on the patent application. But Dr Fong is not an inventor, and should not be included in the list of inventors, since she has suggested only something that is well-known in the field of pharmacology.

2. Over the course of 2 months, Dr Vazquez and Dr Fong perform experiments on mice. They work together in the same room. The compound works. The mice partially recover from their neurological disorder. The two researchers are careful to keep all of their records in hardcover laboratory notebooks having sewn bindings, to date and sign all pages with blue ink, and to ask a witness (a trained scientist) to read each page and to co-sign each page. During the course of the 2-month period, Dr Fong suggested use of a new type of excipient that prevents the vexing problem of precipitation of curitol, where precipitation occurs during long-term storage, as well as in the bloodstream. Because of this suggestion, management has decided to identify this excipient in one of the claims in

this patent. Because Dr Fong had suggested the excipient, because the excipient would not likely have been suggested by a typical pharmacology researcher, and because Dr Fong's excipient appears in one of the claims, it is essential that Dr Fong be named as one of the inventors.

3. Dr Vazquez and Dr Fong fill out an Invention Disclosure Form, a standard form used to document in-house inventions. The company's attorney is careful to inform them of the fact that the appearance of their names on the Invention Disclosure Form does not guarantee that they will be named as inventors in the patent application. The attorney is careful to inform them that inventorship is determined by a body of opinions in the published case law from the Federal Circuit. The attorney separately interviews the first researcher, the second researcher, the research director, and possibly other personnel, to determine who should properly be included in the list of inventors. The attorney informs the researchers that, during the prosecution process, some of the claims may be dropped. And the attorney informs the researchers that, as a consequence, the names of inventors who contributed only to the dropped claims need to be removed from the list of inventors. The attorney may or may not want to inform the inventors of the following. If the inventorship is listed incorrectly on the patent as eventually issued, then the entire patent may be rendered invalid during a lawsuit.

4. After a few more months of laboratory testing, the research director puts together a slide presentation, and completes a manuscript for publication, and transmits these to the patent attorney.

[35]Imaginary name.

[36]Another imaginary name.

5. The patent attorney uses the slide presentation and an unpublished manuscript for writing the patent application. The attorney also drafts a sample claim set, and confers with the research director to ensure that they encompass the results of the research project. The research director informs the attorney that the same general method could be used to treat not only multiple sclerosis, but also other diseases having an autoimmune component, such as, rheumatoid arthritis, ulcerative colitis, and Crohn's disease. The attorney drafts the claims to encompass use of the drug to treat all diseases having an autoimmune component, not just the three diseases mentioned by the lab director.

6. The patent attorney completes the patent application and asks the research director to review the claim set once more. The claim set includes a genus claim that covers methods to treat any autoimmune disease, as well as a species claim that covers a method to treat one feature of the mechanism of multiple sclerosis.

   The genus claim reads, "A method for using curitol to prevent or treat an autoimmune disease in a mammal, comprising administering curitol to the mammal."

   The species claim reads, "A method for using curitol to reduce migration of T cells from the circulation to the central nervous system, in a patient diagnosed with multiple sclerosis, wherein the method comprises administering curitol to the patient." The species claim is narrower than the genus claim, because it requires a specific disease (multiple sclerosis), and because it requires a specific mechanism (reducing migration).

7. The patent attorney files the patent application. About 2 weeks later, the attorney receives a Filing Receipt from the Patent Office, where the Filing Receipt bears the names of the inventors, the title of the invention, the filing date, and a serial number. The attorney checks that all of the names and dates on the Filing Receipt are correct.

8. The patent attorney prepares and files various standard documents, namely, the Declaration, Information Disclosure Statement, and Assignment.

9. Several months go by, and the attorney receives a Restriction Requirement from the patent examiner. According to the Restriction Requirement, the attorney must choose or elect between two or three or more groups of claims. The elected group of claims will be prosecuted first, while the other two groups of claims are set aside, for possible use in submitting in a future patent application. The attorney elects one of the groups of claims, responds to the Restriction Requirement, and informs the examiner which of the three groups claims was chosen.

10. Several more months pass by, and the examiner transmits an Office Action to the attorney. The Office Action contains several rejections. These rejections are under 35 USC §102 and 35 USC §103. Rejections under 35 USC §102 are called, rejections for "anticipation." Rejections under 35 USC §103 are called "obviousness rejections." The "Office Action" contains the rejections and other complaints from the patent examiner.

11. The attorney reviews the rejections, drafts a rebuttal, and asks the research director to review the rebuttal. The attorney understands that the research director is an authority in the field, and is interested in feedback on the examiner's way of thinking, as articulated in the examiner's rejection, and feedback on the attorney's proposed rebuttal.

12. The patent application gets published. The published patent application is available to

the public at www.uspto.gov and at www.epo.org. The relevant inventors are told about the published patent application, that the patent application is no longer confidential, and that they may now include the published patent application on their curriculum vitae.

13. Eventually, about 3 years after the filing date, the attorney receives, in the mail, a Notice of Allowance and Fees Due. At this point, the research director and the attorney remember the groups of claims that had been set aside in response to the Restriction Requirement. The company still has an interest in these claims. The research director thus instructs the attorney to file a Divisional patent application, where this application contains all of the claims that had been set aside.

Inventorship must track the claims (37,38). The attorney reviews notes that were kept in the docket folder, and makes sure that each and every one of the named inventors has contributed to at least one of the allowed claims. To be included in the list of inventors, all that is needed is for the person to have contributed to only one claim in the entire claim set. If a person who does not meet the requirements of inventorship, as set forth in the case law, is included in the list of inventors, or if one of the inventors was left off of the list, adverse consequences can occur during a subsequent lawsuit (if there is a lawsuit).

14. After receiving the Notice of Allowance and Fees Due, the attorney pays the fees, and shortly thereafter the patent issues. Most of the communications between the

examiner and the attorney are available to the public at www.uspto.gov, on a device called Public PAIR. As mentioned above, these communications are called the "file history" or the "prosecution history."

VIII. PROVISIONAL PATENT APPLICATIONS

The time-line for patenting usually includes the filing of a provisional patent application. Typically, as soon as the inventors or company management are satisfied that a useful and novel composition, device, or method, has been identified, the provisional application is written and then filed with the Patent Office. The provisional application automatically expires exactly 1 year after the filing date. During the course of that year, if the company continues to show an interest in patenting the invention that is described in the provisional, then the provisional must be converted to a nonprovisional application before the 1-year period is over. The legal term for converting the provisional to a nonprovisional is "conversion" (39). To ensure clarity in communication with the inventor or company management, patent attorneys sometimes use the term, "basic application" or "utility application," instead of the less distinct term, "nonprovisional application."

Two of the most important things in patenting are: (1) to have an invention that is new; and (2) to have the earliest possible priority date. By having a provisional application on file with the Patent Office, the inventor firmly establishes a priority date (this is the date that the provisional

---

[37]University of Colorado Foundation, Inc. v. American Cyanamid Co. 196 F.3d 1366 (Fed. Cir. 1999).

[38]United States Patent and Trademark Office. Manual of Patent Examining Procedure. Rev. 5, Aug. 2006, Section 201.3, p. 200−3 to 200−14.

[39]"Claiming the benefit of the provisional application under 35 USC 119(e) ... will result in a longer patent term. The procedure requires the filing of a request for the *conversion* of the provisional application to a nonprovisional application" (United States Patent and Trademark Office (USPTO). Manual of Patent Examining Procedure (MPEP) §601.01(c)(II). March 2014).

is filed). The advantage of the priority date is that it prevents any publications or other public disclosures, published after the priority date, from having an invalidating influence on the claims (this statement refers only to the claims in the subsequentlyfiled basic patent application).

Although a basic patent application also establishes a priority date, filing a provisional application before filing the basic application has advantages over only filing the basic application. The advantages include allowing time to generate more working examples, allowing time for lab researchers to sort through examples that work well from those that are not particularly reproducible, and providing a patent term that is 1 year longer.

The provisional is often filed as soon as the inventor has established, by experimental data or by prophetic writing, that the new invention is workable. The Patent Office does not allow claims, where the "invention" that is described in the claims merely takes the form of something that is desired and where there is doubt that it is workable (40).

Claims in provisional applications are never examined by the patent examiner. Typically, the goal of a claim is to cover a genus of closely related group of compositions, devices, or methods (not just one species of composition, device, or method). Thus, in the year between filing the provisional and conversion to the basic application, the inventor continues with laboratory work to acquire more types of working examples, where these additional examples are described in the specification of the basic application. The first page of the specification of the basic application must state that the application claims priority from the earlier-filed provisional.

Regarding patent term, it is the case for basic applications that patent term "ends on the date that is 20 years from the date on which the application was filed in the United States" (41). This date can be pushed into the future by 1 year, by first filing a provisional application followed by conversion at the 1-year mark (42). In other words, filing a provisional can establish a priority date for whatever inventive material is in the provisional application, but without starting the 20-year patent term clock. If your basic patent application does not claim priority on a provisional, then competitors will be free to begin making and selling your invention as soon as your basic application has expired. However, if your basic patent application does claim priority on a provisional, then your competitors will have to wait 1 year longer before they can make and sell your invention. To provide a concluding remark about provisional patent applications, the only thing that can exist is the "provisional patent application," that is, there does not exist anything called a "provisional patent."

IX. SOURCES OF THE LAW FOR PATENTING

Patent law has a basis in the US Constitution, in various statutes in Title 35 of the United States Code (USC), in various rules found in Title 37 of the Code of Federal Regulations (CFR), and in the case law from the Federal Circuit. The Federal Circuit is a court of appeals that specializes in hearing cases in intellectual property.

[40]University of Rochester v. G.D. Searle and Co., 358 F.3d 916 (Fed. Cir. 2004).

[41]United States Patent and Trademark Office (USPTO).Manual of Patent Examining Procedure (MPEP) §2701. March 2014.

[42]"Priority ... to one or more U.S. provisional applications is not considered in the calculation of the twenty-year term" (United States Patent and Trademark Office (USPTO). Manual of Patent Examining Procedure (MPEP) §2701. March 2014).

This is about the US Constitution. Article 1, Section 8, of the US Constitution reads, in part, "The Congress shall have Power ... [t]o promote the Progress of Science and useful Arts, by securing for limited Times to Authors and Inventors the exclusive Right to their respective Writings and Discoveries" (43).

The most relevant statutes are 35 USC §101, 35 USC §102, 35 USC §103, and 35 USC §112. These statutes are cited by the patent examiner when making rejections against claims. These same statutes are also cited in the courtroom setting, during litigation of a patent in a federal court. The relevant federal courts are the US District Courts, the Federal Circuit, and the US Supreme Court.

The patent examiner cites 35 USC §101 when rejecting a claim for lack of utility. Utility rejections are often imposed against newly discovered genes, in the situation where the inventor provides the nucleic acid sequence of the gene, but has no convincing evidence that the gene has any particular use or function. Even where an inventor discovers a new gene, and provides conclusive evidence of its function, the claims can still be rejected for lack of utility (35 USC §101). In this particular §101-rejection, the examiner complains that what is claimed is merely a product of nature.

Recently, that is, in the years 2013–2015, the US Supreme Court and the Federal Circuit, have imposed drastic constraints on the patentability of products of nature, such as isolated gene sequences and isolated small molecules. The drastic nature of the relevant courtroom decisions is evident from the fact that, even though a PCR primer never exists in nature, the PCR primer is not patentable under 35 USC §101, merely because the ordering of nucleotides in the PCR primer has a corresponding exact order somewhere in the genome of a human or other organism. Some of the relevant courtroom decisions are cited (44,45,46). Guidance for overcoming 101-rejections that are imposed against genes or other compositions derived from, or that are products of nature, is available from the Patent Office (47).

Patent examiners cite 35 USC §102, when the examiner finds a publication where the publication discloses every aspect of the claim. The examiner can properly cite this publication only where it was published before the filing date of the applicant's patent.

In other words, rejections under 35 USC §102 are imposed where there is a one-to-one correspondence between every element (or phrase) in the claim, and elements that are disclosed in the publication. As mentioned above, rejections under 35 USC §102 are called rejections for "anticipation." They are also called 102-rejections.

Patent examiners cite 35 USC §103, when the examiner finds two or more publications, where the combination of these publications (when taken together) discloses every element of a given claim. In other words, rejections under 35 USC §103 are imposed where there is a one-to-one correspondence between every element in the claim (every phrase in the claim), and elements found in the combination of the two or more publications. Rejections under 35 USC §103 are called rejections for obviousness.

[43]Walterscheid EC. The nature of the intellectual property clause: a study in historical perspective. Buffalo (NY): William S. Hein & Co., Inc.; 2002.

[44]Association for Molecular Pathology v. Myriad Genetics, Inc. 133 S. Ct. 2107 (2013).

[45]In re: BRCA$_1$- and BRCA$_2$- Based Hereditary Cancer Test Patent Litigation. 774 F.3d 755 (Fed. Cir. 2014).

[46]Ariosa Diagnostics, Inc. v. Sequenom, Inc. Fed. Cir. (June 12, 2015).

[47]2014. Interim Guidance on Patent Subject Matter Eligibility. Federal Register. December 16, 2014;79 (241):74618–74633.

Examiners cite 35 USC §112 when the examiner believes the claim to be nonenabled. The examiner imposes a 112-rejection for nonenablement, when the examiner believes that a typical skilled artisan would not be able to make and use the invention as claimed, when provided with the written guidance that is in the specification.

Now, let us turn our attention to sources of law that are found in published courtroom opinions. Patent opinions from the US Supreme Court, the Federal Circuit, and the US district courts can be found on LEXIS NEXIS®, Westlaw®, and Google Scholar®. Patent opinions from the European courts can be found at www.epoline.org.

A few examples of holdings in the case law from the Federal Circuit are as follows. The case law holding that only working examples (and not prophetic examples) can be written in the past tense can be found in Hoffmann-LaRoche, Inc. v. Promega Corp (48). Case law holding that inventors must submit publications to the Patent Office that are relevant to the claims, during the time when a patent application is in the prosecution phase, includes *Bristol-Myers Squibb Co. v. Rhone-Poulenc Rorer, Inc.* (49). If the inventors prefer to keep these publications to themselves, and if the inventors hope that the patent examiner will never find them on her own, the result can have adverse consequences for the company.

Case law holding that people who only supply "common knowledge" must not be named as inventors, includes *Hess v. Advanced Cardiovascular Sys., Inc.* (50). Case law holding that rejections for anticipation must be based on a one-to-one correspondence between what is found in a prior art publication, and all of the elements in one particular claim, include Verdegaal Bros. v. Union Oil Co. of California (51). This courtroom opinion held that, "A claim is anticipated only if each and every element as set forth in the claim is found, either expressly or inherently described, in a single prior art reference." This opinion serves as guidance or as a supplement to 35 USC §102. The case law also provides guidance regarding rejections under 35 USC §103. For example, the opinion of Stratoflex, Inc. v. Aeroquip Corp. (52) held that, "[i]n determining the differences between the prior art and the claims, the question under 35 USC §103 is not whether the differences themselves would have been obvious, but whether the claimed invention as a whole would have been obvious."

Regarding the enablement requirement under 35 USC §112, the inventor can satisfy this requirement in situations where the examples section contains only working examples, where the examples section contains only prophetic examples, and where there are both working examples and prophetic examples (53). Moreover, if the patent contains several examples, and one is believed not to work, or is actually determined not to work, this will not necessarily mean that the claim that covers all of the examples in the patent should be rejected under 35 USC §112 (54).

[48]Hoffmann-LaRoche, Inc. v. Promega Corp., 323 F.3d 1354 (Fed. Cir. 2003).

[49]Bristol-Myers Squibb Co. v. Rhone-Poulenc Rorer, Inc. 326 F.3d 1226 (Fed. Cir. 2003).

[50]Hess v. Advanced Cardiovascular Sys., Inc., 106 F.3d 976, 980-81 (Fed. Cir. 1997).

[51]Verdegaal Bros. v. Union Oil Co. of California, 814 F.2d 628 (Fed. Cir. 1987).

[52]Stratoflex, Inc. v. Aeroquip Corp., 713 F.2d 1530, (Fed. Cir. 1983).

[53]United States Patent and Trademark Office. Manual of Patent Examining Procedure (Rev. 6, Sept. 2007) Section 2164.02, p. 2100−196.

[54]United States Patent and Trademark Office. Manual of Patent Examining Procedure (Rev. 6, Sept. 2007) Section 2164.08(b), p. 2100−212.

The Federal Circuit's practice of adhering to its own past decisions, as memorialized in its own published case law, is set forth by a principle called *stare decisis*. The Federal Circuit has characterized its relationship with the principle of stare decisis as:

> This court respects the principle of *stare decisis* and follows its own precedential decisions unless the decisions are overruled by the court *enbanc*, or by other controlling authority such as an intervening Supreme Court decision (55).

X. INTERSECTIONS BETWEEN THE FDA REVIEW PROCESS AND PATENTS

The FDA and the USPTO are two different administrative agencies in the US government. There is some overlap in the tasks of these two agencies. This provides a glimpse of this type of overlap. As part of the Hatch-Waxman Act, the term of a patent that claims a new drug product or a method of using the drug product can be extended for up to 5 years, if delays occur during the FDA's regulatory review of the drug product. This extension restores a portion of the patent term that was consumed by the FDA review process. The algorithm for calculating the increase in patent term is found in Title 37 of the Code of Federal Regulations (37 CFR §1.775). This section is entitled, "Calculation of patent term extension for a human drug, antibiotic drug or human biological product." Details on extending patent term to compensate for delays due to FDA review can be found in the cited references (56,57). Persons needing to determine patent term extension should consult an attorney or a patent agent with experience in calculating patent term extensions.

FDA regulations and patents interact in another context, as follows. Where an investigator submits to the FDA an application for a new drug, this submission must identify the investigator's patents that cover the active ingredient, the formulation that contains the drug, and methods of use for the drug (21 CFR §314.53) (58). To submit this information to the FDA, the investigator must use FDA Form 3542. If the applicant believes that there are no relevant patents, this must be stated on FDA Form 3542.

To summarize, a knowledge of FDA regulations and patents both become relevant, when it is time to calculate patent term extension. Also, a knowledge of FDA regulations and patents both become relevant, when complying with 21 CFR §314.53.

---

[55]Teva Pharmaceuticals USA, Inc. v. Novartis. Pharmaceuticals Corp., 482 F.3d 1330 (Fed. Cir. 2007).

[56]Eisenberg RS, The Role of FDA in Innovation Policy, 13 Mich. Telecomm. Tech. Law Rev. 2007; 345–399.

[57]Rosen DL. Generic drug approval process: pre-1984 history concerning generic drugs. In: Swarbrick J, editor. The pharmaceutical regulatory process. New York: Marcel Dekker;2005. p. 99–163.

[58]"An applicant . . . shall submit the required information . . . for each patent that claims the drug or a method of using the drug that is the subject of the new drug application . . . and with respect to which a claim of patent infringement could reasonably be asserted . . . such patents consist of drug substance (active ingredient) patents, drug product (formulation and composition) patents, and method-of-use patents. For patents that claim the drug substance, the applicant shall submit information only on those patents that claim the drug substance that is the subject of the pending or approved application . . ." (21 CFR §314.53; version of April 1, 2010).

Index

Printed in the United States
By Bookmasters